Textbook of Basic and Advanced Electrocardiography

‘Simplicity Is Complexity Resolved’

— **Constantin Brancusi** (1876–1957)

Reviewed by

Dr Mokaddas Hossain Sadi
Dr Fahmida Zaman
Dr Rashiduzzaman
Dr Farzana Razzaque Shwarna
Dr Sharmistha Datta Gupta
Dr Md Abul Khayer
Dr Shiblee Sadik Pathan
Dr Ahmed Aldnane Alam
Dr Monasyr Saquiff Amanullah
Dr Shudipan Chakraborty

Textbook of Basic and Advanced Electrocardiography

Baren Chakraborty

MBBS (DMC) MCPS (Med), FCPS (Med) FACA (USA), FCCP (USA), FRCP (Ireland)
FRCP (Edinburgh), FRCP (Glasgow), FACC (USA)

Professor, School of Health Science, State University of Bangladesh and
Chief, Medical Education and Research and Senior Consultant Cardiologist
Labaid Cardiac Hospital, Dhaka, Bangladesh

JAYPEE

JAYPEE BROTHERS MEDICAL PUBLISHERS

The Health Sciences Publisher

New Delhi | London

Jaypee Brothers Medical Publishers (P) Ltd

Headquarters
EMCA House
23/23-B, Ansari Road, Daryaganj
New Delhi 110 002, India
Landline: +91-11-23272143, +91-11-23272703
+91-11-23282021, +91-11-23245672
E-mail: jaypee@jaypeebrothers.com

Corporate Office
4838/24, Ansari Road, Daryaganj
New Delhi 110 002, India
Phone: +91-11-43574357
Fax: +91-11-43574314
E-mail: jaypee@jaypeebrothers.com

Overseas Office
J.P. Medical Ltd
83 Victoria Street, London
SW1H 0HW (UK)
Phone: +44 20 3170 8910
E-mail: info@jpmedpub.com

EU GPSR Authorised Representative
Logos Europe, 9 rue Nicolas Poussin
17000, La Rochelle, France
Phone: +33 (0) 6 67 93 73 78
E-mail: contact@logoseurope.eu

Website: www.jaypeebrothers.com
Website: www.jaypeedigital.com

Textbook of Basic and Advanced Electrocardiography

First Edition: **2020**

Reprint: **2026**

ISBN 978-93-5270-288-6

Printed at: Samrat Offset Pvt. Ltd.

Dedicated to

My Gifted Clinical Teacher

Major General (Prof) Anis Waiz FRCP

Who taught me ECG

Preface

Last two decades saw phenomenal progress and development in the field of Cardiology. Procedures once thought impossible have been made possible, practices once were unsafe are safe now and conditions once considered beyond care are within the grip of the cardiologists. Even during the last decade, Primary Percutaneous Coronary Intervention (PPCI) for ST-segment Elevation Myocardial Infarction (STEMI) and Cardiac Resynchronization Therapy (CRT) devices implantation for heart failure were not very popular around the globe, particularly in the developing countries. Nowadays, PPCI for STEMI and CRT for heart failure are realities and considered as routine procedures all over the world. All clinicians, therefore, need to know the electrocardiographic (ECG) signs of successful reperfusion after STEMI, ECG signs of failed fibrinolytic therapy with a view to rescue angioplasty, difference between the benign and malignant reperfusion arrhythmias, ECG criteria of assessing the suitability of device implantation, ECG evidences of proper device placement, etc. During, last few years, a plethora of articles have been published in different peer-reviewed journals on the diagnostic and prognostic ECG signs of these new techniques/therapies. Most of these newer ECG findings/signs have remained confined to the pages of those well-admired journals; and unfortunately, there is little reflection of these new ECG signs in the standard ECG textbooks. Keeping in view this reality, '*Textbook of Basic and Advanced Electrocardiography*' has been written to keep pace with newer developments in the field of electrocardiogram. As such, this book will be a means of updating one's knowledge on every aspects of electrocardiographic diagnosis both old and new.

All the chapters of this book have been divided into two separate parts: 'Text' and 'summary'. 'Text' part is for better understanding of the particular subject and for broadening the concept in detail. And the 'summary' part is for easy understanding and quick recapitulation, aiding an examinee to revise and re-read the whole book even before night prior to examination.

Throughout the whole book, my utmost endeavor was to keep the simple things simple and to make complicated things concise, easily understandable and of course simple too. This book will prove worthy to the uninitiated undergraduate students, who will find here the fundamentals of electrocardiography based on time honored electrophysiological concepts and facts, and it will be also equally deserving to the cardiologists and internists, who will find it rewarding to review the concepts already acquired and as an update of the latest electrocardiographic disclosures.

To understand the enigmatic smile of 'Monalisa', it is not necessary that one should be an art genius like Leonardo da Vinci and to be a good gardener, it is also not necessary to be a glorious botanist like Carl Linnaeus. In the same way, to become a good interpreter of ECG, it is not necessary that one should be an electrical engineer or intuitive electrophysiologist. Understanding the genesis of the different waves of ECG may be intricate but their clinical interpretation are easy. Keeping this fact in view, I designed this book in such a way that this textbook will be an immense educational resource to both the beginners as well as to the enlightened readers. Throughout the text, I have tried to describe the tricky and knotty subjects in a very simplified way.

This book has been written in a lucid language in my own style and is intended for MBBS students, PG trainees (FCPS, MD, DM, MRCP, DNB students) and of course for the cardiologists and clinicians for updating their existing knowledge. ECG interpretation is an art, and I firmly believe that this textbook will certainly turn the unawareness into awareness, ignorance into knowledge and knowledge into wisdom.

Baren Chakraborty

Acknowledgments

As the author of the book I must testify my gratitude to my late esteemed teachers and astute clinicians Major General (Dr) Anis Waiz, Colonel (Dr) Quazi Shafiuddin Ahmed and Dr A Johan (Singapore). All through my career, I was groomed up as a physician and cardiologist under their able guidance. I also wish to make special mention of my late senior colleague Dr Matiur Rahman, MP for his constant academic inspiration.

I wish to express heartfelt appreciation to my senior and junior colleagues, Maj Gen (Dr) AKM Shafiullah Khan, Maj Gen (Dr) Ziauddin Ahmed, Maj Gen (Dr) M Abdul Moyeed Siddiqui, Maj Gen (Dr) MG Rabbani, Maj Gen (Dr) Rabiul Hossain, Brig Gen (Dr) ABM Syeed Hosain, Brig Gen (Dr) SM Mamunur Rhaman, Brig Gen (Dr) Mamun Mostafi and Col (Dr) Shaila Perveen of Combined Military Hospital, Dhaka and Dr Fazlul Kadir, Dr Lutful Kabir, Dr Md Liaquat Ali, Lt Col (Dr) Md Mofazzel Hossain, Dr Monzur Rahman Galib, Dr Muzibul Haque Mollah, Dr Taimor Nawaz and Dr Ziaul Haque of Bangladesh Medical College, Dr Arthur Tan, Dr Amy Ng, Dr Charles Chan, Dr Chee Tek Siong, Dr Ding Zee Pin, Dr Koh Tian Hai, Dr K Gunasegaran, Dr Lau Kean Wah, Dr Lim Soo Teik, Dr Lee Chung Yin, Dr Mak Koon Hou, Dr Melvin Tan, Dr Philip Koh, Dr Ruth Kam, Dr Susan Quek, Dr Terrance Chua and Dr Teo Wee Siong of Singapore General Hospital, Dr AG Ravi Kishore, Dr Bijay Kumar Mahala, Dr George Cherian, Dr J Kanan, Dr Keshore, Dr Pradeep Kumar Shetty, Dr PV Suresh, Dr Sanjay Mehrotra, Dr Shashi Dhar, Dr Sunitha Abraham, Dr Sunita Maheshwari and Dr R Bagirath of Narayana Hrudayalaya Institute of Cardiac Science, Bengaluru, India for their unforgettable help in shaping up my academic career in various phases.

I am ardently grateful to my teachers and colleagues Dr Abduz Zaher, Dr AK Miah, Dr APM Sohrabuzzaman, Dr Arun Kumar Sharma, Dr Atikuzzaman Sohel, Dr AHM Abul Monsur, Dr ASM Nazmul Islam, Dr Azizur Rahman, Dr Fahmida Zaman, Dr Habibur Rahman, Dr Lutfor Rahman, Dr Md Lokman Hossain, Dr Mahbubor Rahman, Dr Mahbubul Islam, Dr Md Elias Ali, Dr Md Abul Khayer, Dr Mokaddas Hossain Sadi, Dr Nur Mohammad, Dr Reyan Anis, Dr Rabiul Islam, Dr Samiran Kumar Saha, Dr Shaheena Nazneen, Dr Shiblee Sadik Pathan and Dr Ziaul Kabir of Labaid Cardiac Hospital, who, in many ways, have helped and advised me in preparing the manuscript. I particularly express my indebtedness to my present hospital colleagues for furnishing this textbook with rare ECGs.

I wish to thank Dr Abdullah Al Shafi Majumder, Dr Abdul Wadud Chowdhury, Dr Atahar Ali, Dr Fazilatunnesa Malik, Dr Fatema Begum, Dr Kaisar Nasrullah Khan, Dr KMHS Sirajul Haque, Brig Gen (Dr) MA Malik, Dr M Amanullah, Dr M Abdul Kader Akanda, Dr M Afzalur Rahman, Dr MG Azam, Dr Mir Jamal Uddin, Dr M Jalaluddin, Dr M Khaled Mohsin, Dr M Maksumul Haq, Dr Md Mohosin Hossain, Dr Mohosin Ahmed, Maj Gen (Dr) M Shahjahan, Dr NAM Momenuzzaman, Dr Nazrul Islam, Brig Gen (Dr) Nurunnahar Fatema, Dr Razia Sultana Mahmud, Dr Rashiduzzaman, Lt Col (Dr) Rezaul Karim, Dr Sajal Banerjee, Dr Shams Munwar, Dr Shahabuddin Talukder, Dr SM Mustafa Zaman, Dr Sufia Rahman, Dr Syed Ali Ahsan, Dr Syed Azizul Haque and Col (Dr) Zehad Khan of Bangladesh, Dr Atifur Rahman (Australia), Dr Zhang Bin, Dr Zhimin Du, Dr Rong Bai and Dr Wenyi Guo (China), Dr Angela Hoye, Dr Nicholas P Gall (England), Dr Anil Saxena, Dr Ashok Seth, Dr N N Khanna, Dr Praveen Chandra, Dr Rabin Chakraborty, Dr Rakesh Gupta, Dr Satish K Parashar, Dr Shuvo Dutta, Dr Sunip Banerjee, Dr Suvro Banerjee, Dr TS Kler and Dr Upendra Kaul of India, Dr Dicky A. Hanafy, Dr Gunawan, Dr Muhammad Munawar and Dr Yoga Yuniadi (Indonesia), Dr Takashi Akasaka (Japan), Dr Azmee Mohd Ghazi, Dr Kenneth Chin, Dr Razali Bin Omar, Dr Rosli Bin Mohd Ali and Dr Shaiful Azmi Bin Yahaya (Malaysia), Dr Arun Maskey and Dr Yadav Bhatta (Nepal), Dr Alex T Junia, Dr Eugene B Reyes, Dr Jorge Sison (Philippines), Dr Jayaram Lingamanaicker, Dr Lim Yean Teng and Dr Paul TL Chiam (Singapore), Dr Do-Sun Lim, Dr Hyung Joon Joo and Dr Kyung Woo Park (South Korea), Dr Gotabhaya Ranasinghe and Dr WS Santharaj (Sri Lanka), Dr Paul Hsien Li Kao (Taiwan), Dr Rapin Kukreja and Dr Shakti Ranjan Paul (Thailand), Dr Chowdhury Hafiz Ahsan, Dr Chowdhury M Hasan and Dr Rafique Ahmed (USA) and Dr Phong D Phan (Vietnam), with whom I enjoyed a long clinical association.

I am fervently grateful to Brig Gen (Dr) Manzoor A Mollah for taking all the trouble in reviewing the manuscript and editing it. I also express my appreciation to all my intimate friends and well wishers, Dr AM Shamim, Mr Amirul Islam, Mr Alamgir Rahman, Mr Al Emran Chowdhury, Dr Debashish Ganguly, Mr Faridur Reza Sagor, Mr Mazharul Islam, Dr Mehbub Majid Himel, Mr M Mosaddek Hossain, Munni Saha, Mr Suvas Singho Roy, Dr Rita Saha, Mr Tapash Majumder for their constant inspiration in writing a professional book. I am also obligated to Shri Jitendar P Vij (Group Chairman), Mr Ankit Vij (Managing Director) and Mr MS Mani (Group President) of M/s Jaypee Brothers Medical Publishers (P) Ltd, New Delhi, India, for their incentive and effort in the publication of the book. It is needless to say that, it is they, who transformed my dream into reality.

I shall be failing if I do not thank my young scientific designers Mr S Alam, Mr Samiul Haque and Mr Zahidul Islam Sohag for their praiseworthy accomplishments in support of the book.

At last, I earnestly confesses that this book might not have been written, or would have been very different, without the decisive influence of my wife Dr Shikha Ganguly Chandana (Professor of Gynaecology and Obstetrics, Medical College) and Hospital Dhaka, Bangladesh, son, Dr Shudipan Chakraborty (Resident Doctor, Medical College Hospital, Dhaka) and daughter Anindita Chakraborty (5th year, medical student, Armed Forces Medical College, Dhaka). These three lovable and precious family members ceaselessly and consistently pushed me to write at least one academic textbook. Unyielding effort of this trio ultimately turned a novelist to an academic scientific author!

Contents

Chapter 1. Electrocardiogram: The Basics 1

- Parts of the Electrical System 3
- Waves of the Electrocardiogram 3
- Electrocardiogram Representation of Systole and Diastole 3
- Electrocardiogram Tracing 4

Chapter 2. Electrocardiogram Lead Placement and Standardization 5

- Electrode Placement 7
- Limb Leads 7
- Augmented Limb Leads 8
- Precordial (Chest) Leads 8
- Standardization of Voltage and Timing Intervals 9

Chapter 3. Interpretation and Identification of Different Waves in Electrocardiogram and Calculation of Heart Rate 13

- P Wave 14
  - » Characteristics of Normal P Wave 16
- PR Interval 16
  - » Causes of Prolonged PR interval 17
  - » Causes of Short PR interval 17
- PR Segment 17
- QRS Complex 18
- J-Point 19
- ST Segment 19
  - » Common Causes of ST Segment Elevation 19
  - » Less Common Causes of ST Segment Elevation 20
  - » Rare Causes of ST Segment Elevation 20
  - » Common Causes of ST Segment Depression 20
  - » Uncommon Causes of ST Segment Depression 21
- T Wave 22
  - » Patterns of Different "T" Waves 23
  - » Causes of T Wave Inversion 24
- QT interval 27
  - » Causes of Prolonged QT_c 29
  - » Drugs Causing QT Prolongation 30
  - » Causes of Short QT_c 31
- U Wave 32
  - » Causes of Prominent U Waves 32
- TP Segment 32
- Calculation of Heart Rate 32
- Sinus Bradycardia 34
- Sinus Tachycardia 35

Chapter 4. Axis Determination and Rotation of the Heart 39

- Normal and Abnormal Axis on Electrocardiogram 41
- Axis Determination from QRS Configuration in LI, LII, and LIII 41
- Axis Calculation from Lead I and aVF 41
- Rotation of Heart 43
- Interpretation of QRS Axis 45
- Axis Determination by Isoelectric (Equiphasic) Lead Method 45
- Quick and Easy Determination of Electrocardiogram Axis 45

Chapter 5. Normal Variant Electrocardiogram 55

- Sinus Arrhythmia 55
- Inverted P Waves 55
- PR Interval Variation 55
- QRS Duration: Bundle Branch Block Pattern 55
- Axis Deviation 58
- Q-Wave Abnormality 58
- Early Repolarization Pattern 58
- Nonspecific T-Wave Inversion 61
- Persistent Juvenile Pattern 64
- Wandering Pacemaker 64
- Tall R in V1 64

Chapter 6. Chamber Enlargement 68

- Electrocardiographic Criteria for the Diagnosis of Left Ventricular Hypertrophy 68
  - Increased QRS Amplitude (Voltage Criteria) 68
  - Delayed Intrinsicoid Deflection (Increased Ventricular Activation Time) 70
  - Widened QRS/T Angle 70
  - Left Axis Deviation 70
  - Secondary ST-T Abnormalities 70
  - Left Atrial Abnormalities 73
- Diagnostic Criteria of Left Ventricular Hypertrophy Based on QRS Voltage 73
  - Factors Influencing QRS Voltage 74
  - Sokolow–Lyon Criteria 74
  - Cornell Criteria to Detect Left Ventricular Hypertrophy 75
  - Romhilt–Estes Score 75
  - Perugia Score 75
  - Framingham Electrocardiographic Score and Other System 75
  - Left Ventricular Strain Pattern 76
  - Differentiation Between Left Ventricular Hypertrophy with Strain and Ischemia 76
  - Diagnosis of Left Ventricular Hypertrophy in the Presence of Left Bundle Branch Block 77
  - Electrocardiographic Diagnosis of Left Ventricular Hypertrophy in Presence of Right Bundle Branch Block 77
  - Left Ventricular Hypertrophy in Presence of Left Anterior Fascicular Block 77
  - Left Ventricular Hypertrophy Pressure Versus Volume Overload 78

- Right Ventricular Hypertrophy 79
- Biventricular Hypertrophy 82
  - » Katz–Wachtel Sign 83
- Atrial Abnormalities 84
  - » Left Atrial Abnormality/Enlargement 84
  - » Right Atrial Abnormality/Enlargement 85
  - » Pseudo-P Pulmonale 85
  - » Biatrial Abnormality/Enlargement 85

Chapter 7. Myocardial Ischemia **98**

- ECG Features of Stable Angina 98
- ECG Features of Acute Coronary Syndromes 98
- ST-Segment Depression 99
  - » Causes of ST Depression 99
  - » Patterns of ST-Segment Depression 99
  - » Primary and Secondary ST Depression 100
  - » Reciprocal ST-Segment Depression 103
- True Posterior ST-Segment Elevation Myocardial Infarction 104
- Wellens' Syndrome 104
- Nonspecific ST- and T-Wave Changes 104
- Diffuse ST-Segment Depression 108
- Prinzmetal Angina 111
- MINOCA (Myocardial Infarction with Nonobstructive Coronary Arteries) 112

Chapter 8. ECG Diagnosis of ST-Elevation Myocardial Infarction (STEMI) **117**

- Hyperacute T Waves 117
- ST-Segment Elevation 119
  - » Causes of ST Elevation with Convexity Upward 121
  - » Causes of ST Elevation with Concavity Upward 121
  - » Causes of Saddle-Shaped ST Elevation in Leads V1–V3 121
- Appearance of Pathological Q-Waves 121
- T-Waves Inversion 122
- Normalization of the ST-Segment 122
- Significance of Reciprocal ST-Segment Depression in STEMI 125
- Localization of Site of Infarction 125
  - » ECG Criteria of Acute Anterior Myocardial Infarction 126
  - » ECG Criteria of Acute Inferior Myocardial Infarction 127
  - » ECG Criteria of Right Ventricular Infarction 129
  - » ECG Criteria of Posterior Infarction 131
- High Lateral ST-Elevation Myocardial Infarction 131
- Tombstone ST Elevation 134
- Diagnosis of ST-Elevation Myocardial Infarction in Presence of Bundle-Branch Block 134
  - » ECG Diagnosis of ST-Elevation Myocardial Infarction in Presence of Left Bundle-Branch Block 134
  - » Sgarbossa Scoring System for Diagnosis of ST-Elevation Myocardial Infarction in Presence of Left Bundle Branch Block 136
  - » ECG Diagnosis of ST-Elevation Myocardial Infarction in Presence of Right Bundle Branch Block 138
- Differential Diagnosis of ST-Segment Elevation 138

- Causes of ST-Segment Elevation Other Than ST-Elevation Myocardial Infarction 138
- Identification of the Exact Site of the Infarct-Related Artery 140
  - » ECG Criteria of Left Main Coronary Artery Occlusion 140
  - » ECG Criteria of Left Anterior Descending Artery Occlusion 141
  - » ECG Signs of Different Sites of Left Anterior Descending Artery Occlusion in the Context of Anterior ST-Elevation Myocardial Infarction 142
  - » Electrocardiogram Criteria of Left Circumflex Artery Occlusion 143
  - » ECG Criteria of Right Coronary Artery Occlusion 143
  - » de Winter's T Wave 143
  - » ECG Distinction Between Right Coronary Artery Versus Left Circumflex Coronary Artery Related Acute Inferior Myocardial Infarction 145
- Atrial Infarction 149
- Arrhythmias and Conduction Disturbances in the Acute Phase of STEMI 150
- ECG Evidence of Prior Myocardial Infarction 151
- Poor R-Wave Progression 151
- Significance of Persistently Elevated ST Segment After STEMI 151

Chapter 9. Electrocardiogram Documentation of Reperfusion in ST-Elevation Myocardial Infarction 161

- Electrocardiogram Assessment of Resolution of ST Elevation 164
  - » Sum ST-Segment Resolution 164
  - » Single-Lead ST-Segment Resolution 164
  - » Max ST-Segment Elevation 164
- Appearance of Early T-Wave inversion 166
- Arrhythmias Following ST Elevation Myocardial Infarction 168
- Resolution of ST-Segment Depression 169
- ECG Criteria of Successful Reperfusion 170
- Calculation of ST-Segment Change 170

Chapter 10. Ectopic and Escape Beats 172

- Premature Atrial Complex 173
- Premature Junctional Complex 176
- Premature Ventricular Complex 176
  - » Electrocardiogram Criteria for Diagnosis of Premature Ventricular Complex 178
  - » Causes of Premature Ventricular Contraction 181
- R-On-T Phenomenon 182
- Interpolated Beat 182
- Parasystole 183
- Differentiation Between Aberrant Ventricular Conduction and Premature Ventricular Complex 186
- Escape Beats 190
- Differences Between Premature Atrial Complex and Premature Ventricular Complex 193
- Differences Between Ectopic Beat and Escape Beat 193

Chapter 11. Narrow Complex Tachycardia 195

- Sinus Tachycardia 195
- Sinus Node Reentrant Tachycardia 196
- Multifocal Atrial Tachycardia 196

- Atrial Fibrillation 197
  - » Mechanisms of Atrial Fibrillation 197
  - » Causes of Atrial Fibrillation 197
  - » Classification of Atrial Fibrillation Based on the Temporal Pattern of the Arrhythmia 199
  - » Lone Atrial Fibrillation 201
- Atrial Flutter 202
- Paroxysmal Supraventricular Tachycardia 206
- Atrioventricular Nodal Reentrant Tachycardia (AVNRT) 207
  - » Types of Atrioventricular Nodal Reentrant Tachycardia 208
  - » ECG Characteristics of Atrioventricular Nodal Reentrant Tachycardia 208
- Atrioventricular Reentrant Tachycardia (AVRT) 209
  - » ECG Difference Between Atrioventricular Nodal Reentrant Tachycardia and Atrioventricular Reentrant Tachycardia 210
- Atrial Tachycardia 211

Chapter 12. Broad Complex Tachycardia **217**

- Causes of Broad Complex Tachycardia 217
- Ventricular Tachycardia 217
  - » Electrocardiogram Criteria of Ventricular Tachycardia 217
  - » Monomorphic Ventricular Tachycardia 220
  - » Polymorphic Ventricular Tachycardia 222
- Torsades de Pointes 222
- Ventricular Flutter 223
- Ventricular Fibrillation 224
- Fascicular Ventricular Tachycardia 225
- Right Ventricular Outflow Tract Tachycardia 226
- Bidirectional Ventricular Tachycardia 227
- Accelerated Idioventricular Rhythm 227
- Broad Complex Tachycardias of Supraventricular Origin 227
  - » Supraventricular Tachycardia with Aberrant Conduction 229
  - » Supraventricular Tachycardia with Accessory Pathway 229
- Broad Complex Tachycardias: Ventricular Tachycardia Versus Supraventricular Tachycardia with Aberrancy 229
- Fusion Beats 231
- Capture Beats 231
- Josephson's Sign 233
- Tachycardia QRS More Narrow Than Sinus QRS 233
- Newer Criteria to Differentiate Between Ventricular Tachycardia and Supraventricular Tachycardia with Aberrancy 233
  - » The Brugada Algorithm 235
  - » Vereckei "the AVR" Algorithm 236
  - » Griffith Algorithm 236
  - » The Bayesian Approach 236
  - » Ultra Simple Brugada Criterion: R Wave Peak Time 237

Chapter 13. Bundle-Branch Block **242**

- Bundle-Branch Block: Basic Principles 242

- Types of Bundle-Branch Blocks 243
- Right Bundle Branch Block 244
  - » ECG Criteria of Complete Right Bundle Branch Block 244
  - » ECG Criteria of Incomplete Right Bundle Branch Block 245
- Left Bundle Branch Block 247
  - » ECG Criteria of Left Bundle Branch Block 249
- Hemiblock Concept 252
  - » Left Anterior Hemiblock (LAHB) 255
  - » Left Posterior Hemiblock (LPHB) 255
  - » Left Septal Hemiblock 255
- Bifascicular/Trifascicular Block 259
- Peri-infarction Block 265
- Nonspecific Intraventricular Conduction Disturbance 265

Chapter 14. Sick Sinus Syndrome 271

- Sinus Bradycardia 271
- Sinus Arrest 271
- Escape Rhythms 271
- Tachycardia-Bradycardia Syndrome 272
- Sinoatrial Exit Block 279

Chapter 15. Atrioventricular Block 282

- First-Degree Atrioventricular Block 282
  - » Electrocardiogram Criteria of First-Degree Heart Block 285
- Second-Degree Atrioventricular Block 285
  - » Mobitz Type I Second-Degree Atrioventricular Block (Wenckebach Phenomenon) 285
  - » Mobitz Type II Second-Degree Atrioventricular Block (Hay Phenomenon) 286
  - » Site of Block 286
  - » Vagally-Mediated Atrioventricular Block and Atrioventricular Block in Athletes 293
- Third-Degree Atrioventricular Block (Complete Heart Block) 294

Chapter 16. Electrocardiographic Diagnosis of Cardiac Channelopathies 307

- Brugada Syndrome 307
  - » Types of Brugada Pattern Electrocardiograms 308
  - » Electrocardiographic Criteria for the Diagnosis of Brugada Syndrome 308
  - » Electrocardiogram Differentiation: Brugada Syndrome/Pattern Versus Right Bundle Branch Block 310
- Long QT Syndrome 312
  - » Different Varieties of Inherited Long QT Syndrome 313
  - » Acquired Long QT Syndrome 313
  - » QT and QTc Interval 314
  - » T-Wave Morphology in Long QT Syndrome 315
  - » Arrhythmias in Long QT Syndrome 315
  - » Drugs Associated with QTc Prolongation 315
- Short QT Syndrome 317
- Catecholaminergic Polymorphic Ventricular Tachycardia 317

Chapter 17. Preexcitation Syndromes **325**

- Types of Preexcitation Syndromes 326
- Wolff–Parkinson–White Syndrome 326
- Concealed Accessory Pathways 328
- Arrhythmias in Wolff-Parkinson-White Syndrome 328
- Diagnosis of Coronary Artery Disease in Presence of Wolff-Parkinson-White Syndrome 331
- Localization of the Accessory Pathways 332
- Atrial Fibrillation in Wolff–Parkinson–White Syndrome 335
- Sudden Death in Wolff–Parkinson–White Syndrome 338
- Lown–Ganong–Levine Syndrome 338
- Mahaim-Type Preexcitation 338

Chapter 18. Electrocardiographic Diagnosis of Cardiomyopathies **345**

- Hypertrophic Cardiomyopathy 345
  - » Basic Criteria for ECG Diagnosis of Hypertrophic Cardiomyopathy 351
  - » Anis-Baren ECG Triad 351
  - » Apical Cardiomyopathy 351
  - » Sudden Cardiac Death in Hypertrophic Cardiomyopathy 355
- Dilated Cardiomyopathy 361
  - » Goldberger's Triad 361
- Restrictive Cardiomyopathy 365
- Arrhythmogenic Right Ventricular Cardiomyopathy/Dysplasia 365
- Left Ventricular Noncompaction 367
- Takotsubo Cardiomyopathy 368
  - » Differentiation Between Acute Anterior Myocardial Infarction and Takotsubo Cardiomyopathy 368

Chapter 19. Electrocardiogram Diagnosis of Pericarditis and Other Cardiac Inflammatory Conditions **375**

- Pericarditis 375
  - » Spodick's Sign 376
  - » Differentiation of Acute Pericarditis from Acute ST-Elevation Myocardial Infarction 378
  - » Differentiation of Acute Pericarditis from Early Repolarization Pattern 380
  - » Electrocardiogram Changes in Pericardial Effusion 382
  - » Cardiac Tamponade 383
- Electrocardiographic Diagnosis of Myocarditis 384
- Electrocardiographic Diagnosis of Endocarditis 387
- Electrocardiogram Changes in Rheumatic Carditis 387

Chapter 20. Electrocardiographic Manifestations of Electrolyte Abnormalities **392**

- Hyperkalemia 392
  - » Different Stages of Hyperkalemia 393
- Hypokalemia 394
- Hypercalcemia 398
- Hypocalcemia 401
- Hypermagnesemia 401
- Hypomagnesemia 401
- Electrocardiogram Features of Multiple Electrolyte Imbalances 401

Chapter 21. Electrocardiograms in Specific Clinical Conditions **404**

- Chronic Obstructive Pulmonary Disease (COPD) 404
- Pulmonary Embolism 406
  - » McGinn-White Sign 407
- Hypothermia 409
- Thyrotoxicosis 409
- Hypothyroidism 411
- Electrocardiogram Features of Increased Intracranial Pressure 412
- Parkinson's Disease 415
- Electrocardiogram Changes in Neuromuscular Disorders 415
- Friedreich's Ataxia: Cerebellar Ataxia 415
- Electrocardiogram After Heart Transplantation 416
- Electrocardiogram Features of Primary Pulmonary Hypertension (PPH) 417

Chapter 22. Effects of Various Drugs on the Electrocardiogram **425**

- Digitalis 425
  - » Digoxin Effect 425
  - » Reverse Tick Sign 425
  - » ECG Manifestations of Digitalis Toxicity 426
- Tricyclic Antidepressants 430
- Beta-Blockers 430
- Verapamil 431
- Fluoroquinolones 432
- Macrolide Antibiotics 432
- Antiarrhythmic Drugs 432

Chapter 23. Electrocardiogram Features of Congenital Heart Diseases **435**

- Atrial Septal Defect (ASD) 435
  - » ECG Features of Secundum ASD 435
- Crochetage Sign 437
- ECG Features of Primum ASD 440
- ECG Features of Sinus Venosus Type ASD 440
- ECG Findings in Ventricular Septal Defect (VSD) 444
- Tetralogy of Fallot 444
- Ebstein's Anomaly 446
- Dextrocardia 446
- Technical Dextrocardia 450
- Patent Ductus Arteriosus 450
- Coarctation of Aorta 450
- Pulmonary Stenosis 450
- Eisenmenger Syndrome 450
- Transposition of the Great Arteries 453
- Tricuspid Atresia 453
- Mitral Valve Prolapse (MVP) 453

Chapter 24. Pacemaker Electrocardiogram Interpretation **459**

- Indications for Permanent Pacing 459
- Atrial Pacing 460

- Ventricular Pacing 460
- Pacemaker Types 462
- Pacemaker Codes 462
- Pacemaker Terminology 465
  - » Interpretation of Pacemaker ECG 466
- Effects of Pacemaker on ECG 466
- Pacemaker Malfunctions/Complications 466
- Diagnosis of ST-Elevation Myocardial Infarction (STEMI) in Presence of Pacemaker 466
- Diagnosis of Hyperkalemia in Presence of Pacemaker 468
- Electrocardiogram Interpretation After Cardiac Resynchronization Therapy 469

Chapter 25. Pediatric Electrocardiogram Interpretation **473**

- Heart Rate 473
- Age-related Changes in Ventricles and QRS Axis 473
- Variations from Sinus Rhythm 476
  - » High Grade AV Block in Children 478
  - » Extrasystoles 478
- Influence of Sex 480
- Complete Heart Block in Pediatric ECG 480

Chapter 26. Exercise Tolerance Test **484**

- Safety 485
  - » Normal Electrocardiographic Changes During Exercise 485
- Criteria for a Positive Exercise Test 485
  - » ST-Segment Depression 485
  - » ST-Segment Elevation 486
- Significance of ST-Segment Depression Limited to the Recovery Phase of Exercise Stress Test 488
- J-Point Depression During Exercise Tolerance Test 489
- Blood Pressure Response During Exercise Tolerance Test 489
- False-Positive Test 491
- False-Negative Test 491
- Exercise-Induced Arrhythmias 491
- Limitations 491

Chapter 27. Ambulatory Electrocardiogram Monitoring (Holter Monitoring) **496**

- Arrhythmia and Ambulatory Electrocardiogram Monitoring 496
- Continuous Monitors (Holter Technology) 496
- Indications for Holter Monitoring 496
- Diagnostic Value of Holter Monitoring 497

Index *503*

Chapter 1

Electrocardiogram: The Basics

INTRODUCTION

Electrocardiogram (ECG) is nothing but the graphical representation of the electrical activity of the heart during each cardiac cycle. ECG has grown to be one of the most commonly used medical tests in modern medicine. Its utility in the diagnosis of a myriad of cardiac pathologies ranging from myocardial ischemia, arrhythmia, and infarction to syncope has been invaluable to clinicians for decades. The ECG is a tool of extraordinary clinical power, extraordinary both for the ease with which it can be mastered and also for the extraordinary range of situations in which it can provide helpful clinical information. One glance at an ECG can diagnose an evolving myocardial infarction, can predict the possibility of acute coronary syndromes, identify potentially life-threatening arrhythmias, can suggest the possibility of a massive pulmonary embolism or simply provide a measure of reassurance to someone who is worried about his atypical chest symptoms.

While the first electrical current associated with a heartbeat was identified in 1842 by an Italian physicist, it was a British scientist, Augustus Waller, who published the first human ECG in 1887. Adding further, it was not until 1893 that Dutch scientist, Willem Einthoven (21st May 1860 to 29th September 1927) introduced the term "electrocardiogram" and subsequently refined the concept of cardiac electrical conduction, naming the deflections *P, Q, R, S, T, and U-waves* (Fig. 1.1). The same basic waves are used today to identify and interpret the ECG rhythm strip.[1] Willem Einthoven was a doctor and physiologist, he invented the first practical ECG and received the Nobel Prize in Medicine in 1924 for it.[1-7]

Einthoven's concept was a triangle, an imaginary area on the body, formed by the intersection of the standard bipolar limb leads with the heart at the center (Fig. 1.2). The bipolar leads have a negative and positive pole that captures the direction of the electrical activity of the heart in the various lead configurations (Fig. 1.3). Looking at the heart from the various electrical vectors that are produced helps to determine the way in which the impulse is traveling.[3,7]

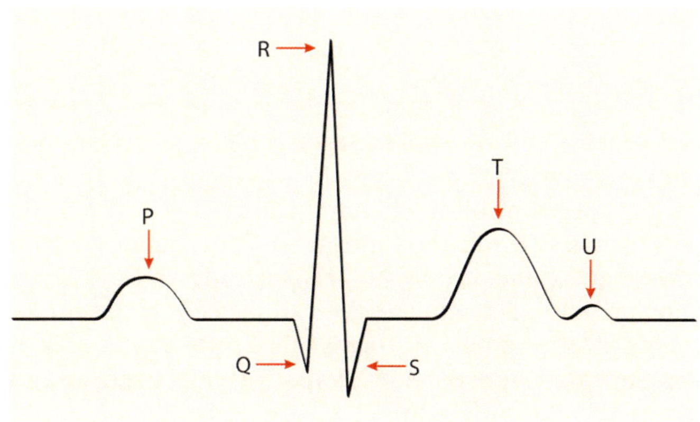

Fig. 1.1: Normal electrocardiogram (ECG).

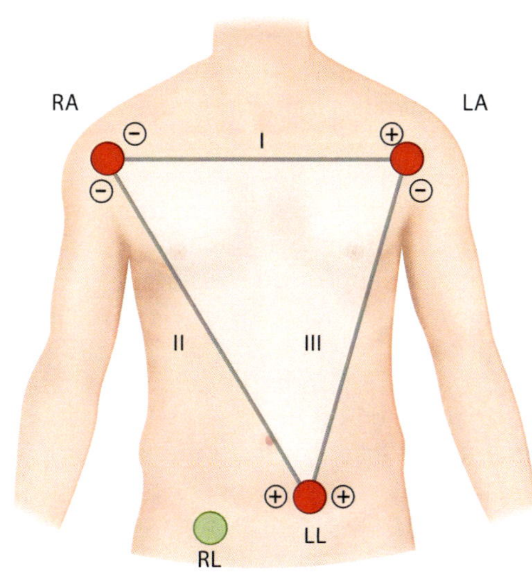

Fig. 1.2: Einthoven's triangle. This triangle is an imaginary formation of three limb leads in a triangle used in electrocardiography. The shape forms an inverted equilateral triangle with the heart at the center that produces zero potential when the voltages are summed.
(RA: right arm, LA: left arm, LL: left leg, RL: right leg).

In resting state, the cardiac cells are electrically polarized; their insides are negatively charged with respect to their outsides. This polarity is maintained by membrane

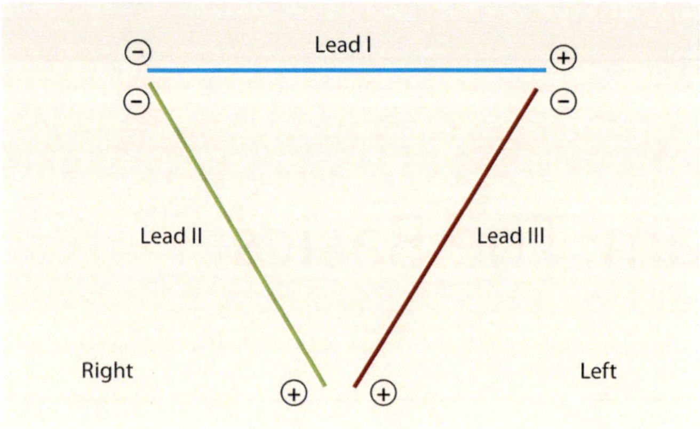

Fig. 1.3: Triangle, formed by the intersection of the standard bipolar limb leads.

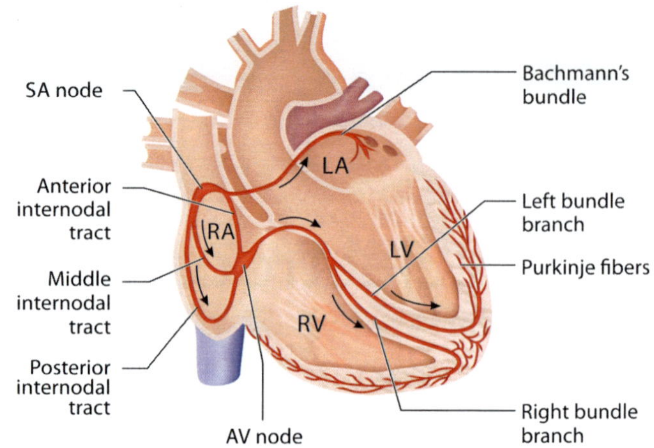

Fig. 1.4: Normal anatomy of the conductive system of heart. SA node (sinoatrial node) and AV node (atrioventricular node).

pump system. Cardiac cells lose their internal negativity in a process called *depolarization*. This depolarization is the key electrical event of the heart. This depolarization propagates from cell-to-cell producing a wave, which can be transmitted across the entire heart. These depolarization waves can be detected by surface electrodes in ECG. Once depolarization is complete, the cardiac cells restore their resting polarity through a process called *repolarization*. Both depolarization and repolarization waves can be sensed and detected in the surface ECG.

An ECG lead consists of two surface electrodes of opposite polarity (one positive and one negative) or one positive surface electrode and a reference point. A lead composed of two electrodes of opposite polarity is called *bipolar lead*. A lead composed of a single positive electrode and a reference point is a *unipolar lead*.

The heart consists of three different types of cells:

1. *Pacemaker cells*: Generates impulse
2. *Electricity conducting cells*: Transmits impulse
3. *Myocardial cells*: Maintains contractile function of heart.

The waves those appear on the surface ECG primarily represent the electrical activities of the myocardial cells, which comprise the vast bulk of the heart. Pacemaker activity and transmission by the conducting cells are generally not reflected on the surface ECG, these events do not generate sufficient voltage to be recorded by the surface electrodes. The waves generated by the myocardial depolarization and repolarization are recorded on the ECG graph and have three primary characteristics:

1. *Duration*: Measured in fractions of a second or a millisecond, in a horizontal direction on the ECG paper
2. *Amplitude*: Measured in millivolts (mv), in a vertical direction
3. *Configuration*: Indicates the shape and appearance of a particular wave.

Pacemaker cells are able to depolarize spontaneously, at a particular rate. Each spontaneous depolarization serves as a source of a wave of depolarization that initiates all the electrical activities of each cardiac cycle, cardiac contraction, and relaxation. The dominant pacemaker of heart is located high up in the right atrium (RA) and is called sinoatrial node (SA node). During normal sinus rhythm the electrical stimulus is always generated by the SA node (Fig. 1.4). This is a small mass of specialized tissue located in the RA (right upper chamber) of the heart. The SA node generates an electrical stimulus regularly (60–100 times per minute under normal conditions). The atrias are then activated. The electrical stimulus travels down through the conduction pathways and stimulates the ventricles. Anatomic evidence suggests the presence of three intra-atrial pathways: (1) anterior internodal pathway, (2) middle internodal tract, and (3) posterior internodal tract. All these internodal fibers convey the impulse from SA node to atrioventricular (AV) node. Apart from these three internodal pathways there is another pathway called the Bachmann bundle which is a large muscle bundle that appears to conduct the cardiac impulse preferentially from the RA to the left atrium (LA). From SA node the impulse travels to AV node. There, impulses are slowed down for a very short period and then continued down the conduction pathway via the His-Purkinje system into the ventricles. The bundle of His divides into right and left pathways to provide electrical stimulation to the right ventricle (RV) and left ventricle (LV). The distal ends of the His-Purkinje system are called Purkinje fibers. The terminal Purkinje fibers connect with the ends of the bundle branches to form interweaving networks on the endocardial surface of both ventricles, which transmit the cardiac impulse almost simultaneously to the entire right and left ventricular endocardium.[7-13] The terminal filaments–Purkinje fibers spread out and terminate beneath the endocardium that lines both left and right ventricular cavities. So, ventricular depolarization begins at the endocardial surface and proceeds toward outer surface, epicardium of the ventricles. In fact, the Purkinje fibers do not penetrate into the myocardium but the terminal ends of the Purkinje fibers subdivide just beneath the endocardium.

PARTS OF THE ELECTRICAL SYSTEM (FIG. 1.5)

Sinoatrial node: It is known as the heart's natural pacemaker, the SA node has special cells that create the electricity that makes heartbeat.

Atrioventricular node: The AV node is the bridge between the atria and ventricles. Electrical signals pass from the atria down to the ventricles through the AV node.

His-Purkinje system: The His-Purkinje system carries the electrical signals throughout the ventricles to make them contract. The parts of the His-Purkinje system include:

- His bundle (the start of the system)
- Right bundle branch (RBB)
- Left bundle branch (LBB)
- Purkinje fibers (the end of the system).

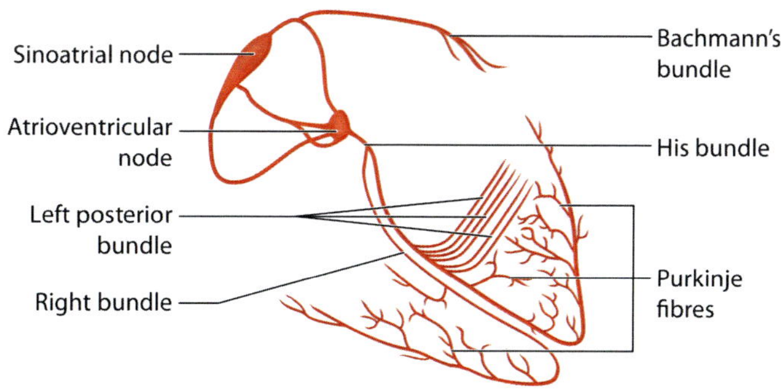

Fig. 1.5: Conductive system of the heart.

WAVES OF THE ELECTROCARDIOGRAM

The ECG tracing shows the electrical conduction of the heart as the cells depolarize and repolarize through each beat. Each individual beat is represented on the ECG as the *PQRST complex* (Fig. 1.6). Each sequential letter represents a sequential discrete part of the complex and each represents a different portion of the cardiac cycle.

The first part of the complex is called the *P-wave*. The P-wave represents the initiation of depolarization in the sinus node and subsequent atrial contraction. It is relatively small in amplitude due to the thin muscle mass of the atrium.

After P-wave the next part of the ECG tracing is called the *QRS complex*. The QRS complex represents the conductance and sequential depolarization of the ventricles. It is a much larger wave form than the P-wave due to the large muscle mass of the ventricles. An initial downward (negative) deflection in the QRS is termed the Q wave. *Q wave* may or may not be present depending on the lead and the presence of any cardiac disease. The *R-wave* is large and upright (positive) after Q-wave. The *S-wave* follows the R-wave and is a downward (negative) deflection. The *ST segment* follows the QRS complex. The ST segment represents the period of time in which the ventricles are isoelectric.

The *T-wave* follows the ST segment of the PQRST complex. The T-wave represents the repolarization of the ventricles. The T-wave is normally upright in all leads except V1 and aVR (isolated T-wave inversion in III can also be normal). The *U-wave* is a wave on the ECG that is not always seen. It is typically small, and, by definition, follows the T-wave. U-waves are thought to represent repolarization of the papillary muscles or Purkinje fibers.

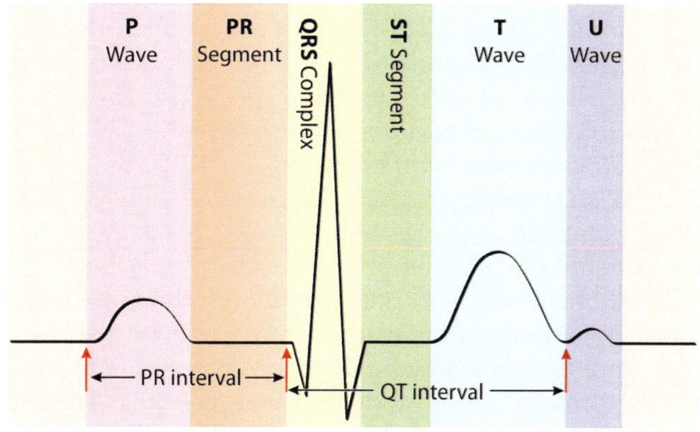

Fig. 1.6: Waves and segments of the normal ECG.

ELECTROCARDIOGRAM REPRESENTATION OF SYSTOLE AND DIASTOLE

The period during which mechanical contraction occurs is termed as *systole* and the remaining periods of time during which the atria or ventricles are relaxing and filling with incoming blood are called *diastole*. Ventricular systole denotes contraction of the ventricles and it is represented on the surface ECG as the interval between the peak of the R-wave and the end of the T-wave. The ventricular diastole is the interval between the end of the T-wave and the peak of the next R-wave (Fig. 1.7).

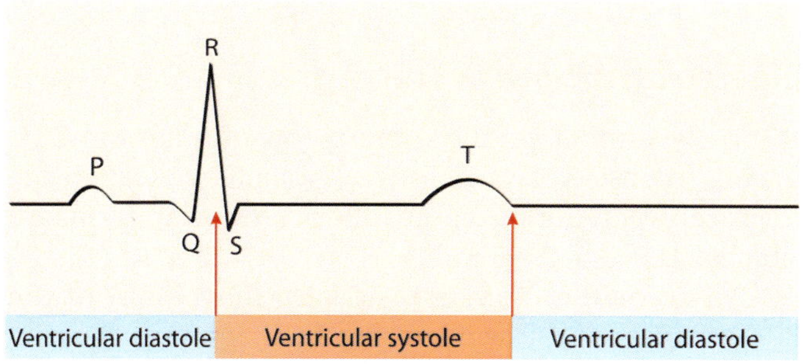

Fig. 1.7: Electrocardiogram representation of systole (*in between two arrows*) and diastole.

SUMMARY

The ECG is a graphic record of the direction and magnitude of the electrical activity generated by the depolarization and repolarization of the atria and ventricles of the heart. This electrical activity is readily detected by electrodes attached to the skin.

The normal electrical conduction in the heart allows the impulse that is generated by the SA node of the heart to be propagated to, and stimulate, the cardiac muscle (myocardium). The myocardium contracts after stimulation. It is the ordered, rhythmic stimulation of the myocardium during the cardiac cycle that allows efficient contraction of the heart, thereby allowing blood to be pumped throughout the body. SA node is the normal pacemaker of the heart and the cardiac impulse is generated here.

- *Sinoatrial node* normally generates the action potential, i.e. the electrical impulse that initiates contraction.
  - The SA node excites the RA, and the impulse travels through Bachmann's bundle to excite LA.
  - The impulse also travels through internodal pathways in RA to the AV node.
- From the AV node, the impulse then travels through the *bundle of His* and down the bundle branches, fibers specialized for rapid transmission of electrical impulses, on either side of the interventricular septum.
  - *Right bundle branch* depolarizes the RV.
  - *Left bundle branch* depolarizes the LV and interventricular septum.
- Both bundle branches terminate in *Purkinje fibers*.

Millions of small Purkinje fibers terminate beneath the endocardium and transmits depolarization wave from endocardium to epicardium. Depolarization wave conducts slowly through the AV node and then conducts rapidly through the His bundle to the right and left bundle branches into the terminal filaments of the Purkinje system, which depolarize the ventricular myocardium (Flowchart 1.1).

Flowchart 1.1: Sequences of cardiac activation.

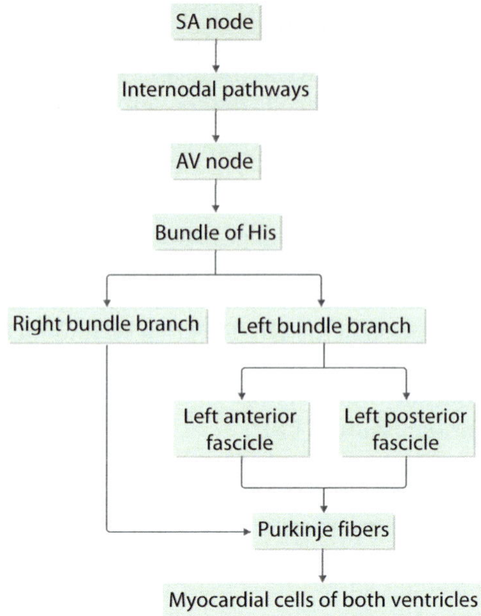

Electrocardiogram Tracing

To briefly summarize the components of a normal ECG tracing, it consists of waveform components which indicate electrical events during one heartbeat. These waveforms are labelled as P, Q, R, S, T, and U.

P-wave is the first short upward movement of the ECG tracing. The P-wave in the ECG represents atrial depolarization, which results in atrial contraction.

The *PR interval* indicates the transit time for the electrical signal to travel from the sinus node to the ventricles.

The *QRS complex* represents ventricular depolarization.

The *ST segment* connects the QRS complex and the T-wave.

T-wave represents ventricular repolarization.

The *U-wave* is a small (0.5 mm) deflection immediately following the T-wave, usually in the same direction as the T-wave.

Ventricular systole: Interval between the peak of the R-wave and the end of the T-wave.

Ventricular diastole: Interval between the end of the T-wave and the peak of the next R-wave.

REFERENCES

1. ECG library. (2011). A Brief History of Electrocardiography. Retrieved from the World Wide Web. [online] Available from http://www.sh.lsuhsc.edu/fammed/OutpatientManual/EKG/ecghist.html. [Accessed Sept., 2017].
2. Waller AD. Introductory address on the electromotive properties of the human heart. Br Med J. 1888;2(1449):751-4.
3. Einthoven W. Le telecardiogramme. Arch Int de Physiol. 1906;4:132-64.
4. Hurst JW. Naming of the waves in the ECG, with a brief account of their genesis. Circulation. 1998;98(18):1937-42.
5. Moukabary T. Willem Einthoven (1860-1927): father of electrocardiography. Cardiol J. 2007;14(3):316-7.
6. Shouldice RB, Bass G. From bench to bedside—developments in electrocardiology. Eng J Inst Eng Ireland. 2002; 56(4):47-9.
7. Einthoven W. Ueber die Form des menschlichen Electrocardiogramms. Arch f d Ges Physiol. 1895;60:101-23.
8. Anderson RH, Yanni J, Boyett MR, et al. The anatomy of the cardiac conduction system. Clin Anat. 2009;22(1):99-113.
9. Sanchez-Quintana D, Yen Ho S. Anatomy of cardiac nodes and atrioventricular specialized conduction system. Rev Esp Cardiol. 2003;56(11):1085-92.
10. Renwick J, Kerr C, McTaggart R, et al. Cardiac electrophysiology and conduction pathway ablation. Can J Anaesth. 1993; 40(11):1053-64.
11. Anderson RH, Ho SY, Smith A, et al. The internodal atrial myocardium. Anat Rec. 1981;201(1):75-82.
12. Nerbonne JM, Kass RS. Molecular physiology of cardiac repolarization. Physiol Rev. 2005;85(4):1205-53.
13. Amin AS, Tan HL, Wilde AA. Cardiac ion channels in health and disease. Heart Rhythm. 2010;7(1):117-26.

Chapter

2

Electrocardiogram Lead Placement and Standardization

INTRODUCTION

The system of positioning of leads for performing a 12-lead electrocardiogram (ECG) is universal. This helps to ensure that, when a person's ECGs are compared, any changes in the ECG are due to a cardiac injury, not due to a difference in the placement of leads. There are universal standards in lead placement throughout the world. Interpretation of the findings can vary from doctor to doctor but methods for obtaining the information are the same all over the world.

The standard 12-lead ECG consists of three limb leads (leads I, II, and III), three augmented limb leads [leads augmented vector right (aVR), augmented vector left (aVL), and augmented vector foot (aVF)], and six precordial leads (Figs. 2.1 to 2.4). All leads are effectively "bipolar", and the term "unipolar" in the description of the augmented limb leads and the precordial leads lack precision.[1-5] Skin preparation by cleaning and gentle abrasion before electrode application can reduce noise and improve the quality of the recorded ECG.[6] Historically, limb lead electrodes have been attached at the wrists and the ankles, with the patient in the supine position, generally with a pillow under the head. For routine 12-lead recording, the American Heart Association (AHA) statement of 1975 recommended placement of the four limb lead electrodes on the arms and legs distal to the shoulders and hips and thus not necessarily on the wrists and ankles.[4,7] Evidence exists that different placement of electrodes on the limbs can alter the ECG, a phenomenon that appears to be more marked with respect to the left arm (LA) electrode.[7] Therefore, reevaluation of the magnitude of changes due to variation in limb electrode placement in clinical practice is required. Six electrodes are placed on the chest in the following locations: V1, 4th intercostal space at the right sternal border; V2, 4th intercostal space at the left sternal border; V3, midway between V2 and V4; V4, 5th intercostal space in the midclavicular line; V5, in the horizontal plane of V4 at the anterior axillary line, or if the anterior axillary line is ambiguous, midway between V4 and V6; and V6, in the horizontal plane of V4 at the midaxillary line (Figs. 2.3 and 2.4).[1]

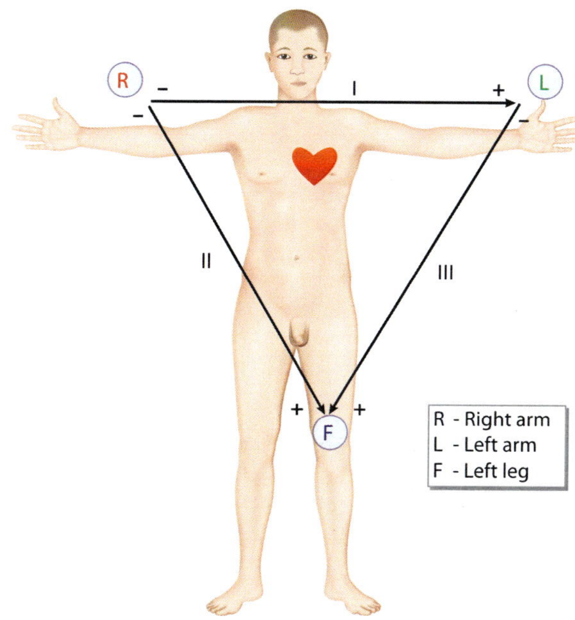

Fig. 2.1: Bipolar limb lead positions.

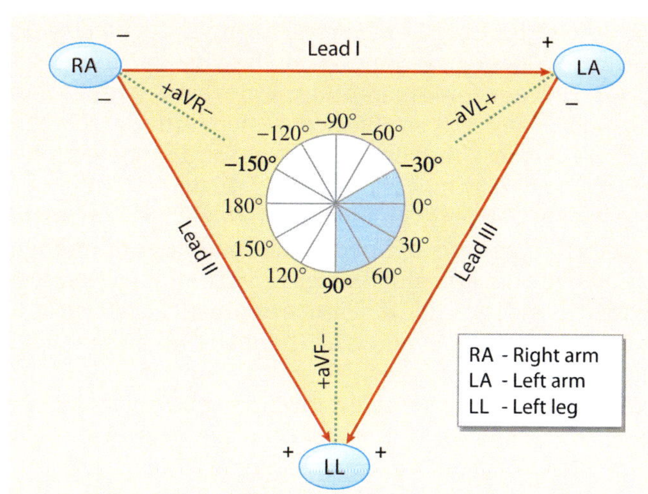

Fig. 2.2: Both unipolar and bipolar lead orientation.

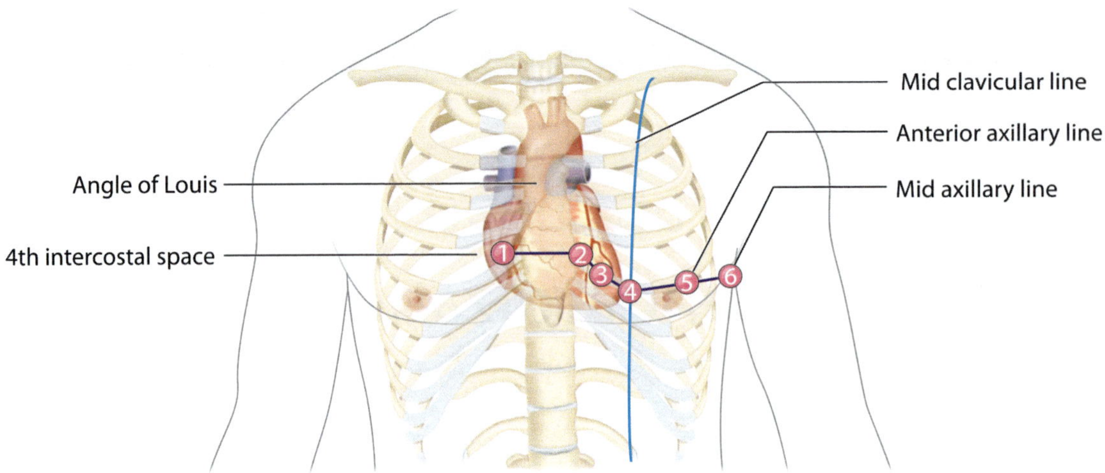

Fig. 2.3: Chest lead placement positions.

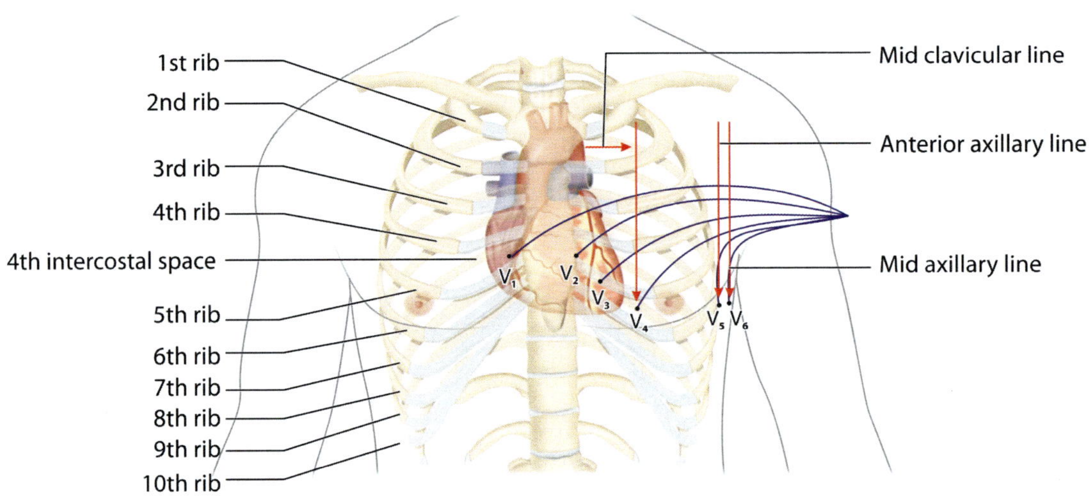

Fig. 2.4: Proper positioning and placement of chest leads.

The four limb electrodes define the standard frontal plane limb leads those were originally defined by Einthoven. With the right leg (RL) electrode acting as an electronic reference that serves to improve common mode (unwanted noise) rejection, three pairs of electrodes exist. Within each pair, one electrode is established as the positive end of the lead in the sense that current flow toward that electrode is inscribed in an upward (positive) direction. The other electrode of the pair would inscribe the exactly opposite waveform. *Lead I* is defined as the potential difference between the left arm and the right arm (LA - RA), *lead II* is defined as the potential difference between the left leg and the right arm (LL - RA), and *lead III* is defined as the potential difference between the left leg and the left arm (LL - LA). In each case, net current flow toward the first electrode of the pair is defined as a positive voltage deflection in the recorded waveform. According to Kirchhoff's law, the sum of the voltage gains and voltage drops in a closed circuit is equal to zero. Therefore, lead II = lead I + lead III at any instant in the cardiac cycle. This relationship is known as Einthoven's law.[1]

Skin preparation and electrode placement have important effects on the ECG, and a patient's positional change, such as elevation and rotation, can change recorded amplitudes and axis. It has been widely accepted for many years that ECG amplitudes, durations, and axis are independent of the distal or more proximal location of the limb electrodes. As a result, routine recording of the ECG from the upper arm rather than from the wrist to "reduce motion artifact" has become popular and is facilitated by the development of disposable tab electrodes. However, one study has shown that electrode placement along the limbs can affect ECG voltages and durations, most importantly in the limb leads.[7] Whether these differences are large enough to alter routine diagnostic criteria, such as voltage for left ventricular hypertrophy (LVH) or Q-wave duration for inferior infarction is unknown.

From the time of their initial standardization by a joint committee of the AHA and the Cardiac Society of Great Britain and Ireland the normal precordial electrode positions have been relatively horizontal in orientation. When precordial electrodes are positioned without reference to the underlying bony landmarks, the placement pattern often is erroneously vertical in orientation.[1,8] A common error is superior misplacement of V1 and V2 in the second or third intercostal space. This can result in reduction of initial R-wave amplitude in these leads, approximating 0.1 mV per interspace, which can cause poor R-wave progression or erroneous signs of anterior infarction.[9] Superior displacements of the V1 and V2 electrodes will often result in rSr′ complexes with T-wave inversion, resembling the complex in lead aVR. It also has been shown that in patients with low diaphragm position, as in obstructive pulmonary disease, V3 and V4 may be located above the ventricular boundaries and record negative deflections that simulate anterior infarction.[1,10] Another common error is inferior placement of V5 and V6, in the sixth intercostal space or even lower, which can alter amplitudes used in the diagnosis of ventricular hypertrophy. Precordial lead misplacement explains a considerable amount of the variability of amplitude measurements that is found between serial tracings.[11] Some residual disagreement persists in current guidelines and texts on the standard for location of V5 and V6, with some sources retaining an early recommendation that these leads follow the course of the 5th intercostal space rather than the horizontal plane of V4. In addition, it is common to refer to the anterior axillary line as an anatomic marker for the placement of V5. These alternatives are discouraged because the course of the intercostal space is variable and the definition of an anterior axillary line is only vague. Placement of precordial electrodes in women with large breasts remains problematic. Electrodes are most commonly placed beneath the breasts, which should reduce amplitude attenuation caused by the higher torso impedance in women and, intuitively, would seem to favor reproducibility of positioning during routine practice. Conversely, one study has suggested that reproducibility of ECG measurements is slightly increased when electrodes are positioned on top of the breasts.[12] Another study using precisely ascertained electrode placement has suggested that precordial potential attenuation by the breasts is very small.[13] Yet another study has found attenuation only in V3 and an increase in voltage in V5 and V6 when electrodes are placed over the breasts; this may result from V5 and V6 being correctly placed at the level of V4 rather than more inferiorly when V4 is positioned under the breasts.[14] Clearly, the magnitude of this effect in ordinary ECGs will depend greatly on the care with which electrodes are ordinarily placed and also on breasts' size, breasts' shape, and small changes in the patients' position. Similar considerations apply in relation to subjects with breast implants and in subjects who are obese. It is recommended that electrodes continue to be placed under the breasts in women until additional studies using electrodes placed on top of the breasts are available.[1]

ELECTRODE PLACEMENT

The electrode placement should adhere to the recommendations and guidelines as per the AHA to ensure consistency between recordings. Any alterations to the positions of the electrode placements should be clearly and accurately documented on the printed ECG recording. This should include how and why the alteration was performed.[15,16]

LIMB LEADS

Evidence confirms that inconsistency with limb lead placement alters the appearance of the ECG.[15,16] To ensure consistency; it is recommended that the limb lead electrodes are placed slightly proximal to the wrists and ankles (Fig. 2.5 and Table 2.1).[16]

But practically, RA and LA leads can also be placed anywhere between the shoulder and the elbow, and LL and RL anywhere above the ankle and below the torso. The limb

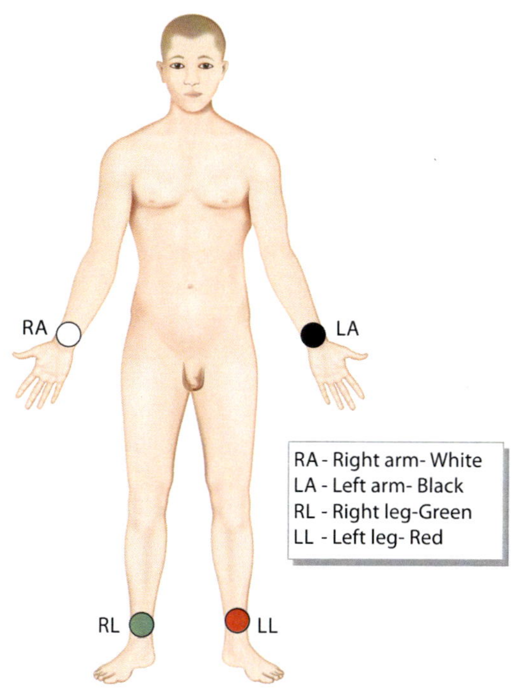

Fig. 2.5: Usually recommended limb lead electrode positions, slightly proximal to the wrists and ankles.

Table 2.1: Placement of limb leads.

Electrode	*Usual position*
RA (Right arm)	Right forearm, proximal to the wrist
LA (Left arm)	Left forearm, proximal to the wrist
LL (Left leg)	Left lower leg, proximal to the ankle
RL (Right leg)	Right lower leg, proximal to the ankle

electrodes can be far down on the limbs or close to the hips/shoulders as long as they are placed symmetrically (Fig. 2.6).

AUGMENTED LIMB LEADS

In a 12-lead ECG, the limb leads (I, II, and III) are bipolar leads. Unipolar leads also have two poles, as a voltage is measured; however, the negative pole is a composite pole. So the term unipolar is somehow misnomer. Leads aVR, aVL, and aVF are augmented limb leads and they are derived from the same three electrodes as leads I, II, and III.

Lead aVR has the positive electrode on the RA, lead aVL has the positive electrode on the LA, and lead aVF has the positive electrode on the LL (Table 2.2).

PRECORDIAL (CHEST) LEADS

Attention should be paid to the correct placement of the precordial leads as variation can produce diagnostically significant differences to the ECG.[15-17]

Correct anatomical positions have been defined and every effort should be made to always ensure correct electrode placement (Table 2.3).[16]

The center of the active surface area of the electrode should be aligned with the relevant anatomical landmark.[15,16]

The standard 12-lead ECG does not directly examine the right ventricle, and is relatively poor at examining the posterior basal and lateral walls of the left ventricle. In particular, acute myocardial infarction in the distribution of the circumflex artery is likely to produce a nondiagnostic ECG. The use of additional ECG leads like right-sided leads V3R and V4R and posterior leads V7, V8, and V9 may improve sensitivity for right ventricular and posterior myocardial infarction (MI). In addition to the standard 12 leads, three posterior chest leads (V7 to V9) may be helpful in diagnosing posterior MI. Leads V7 to V9 are recorded in the same horizontal plane as lead V6 and on the posterior axillary line (lead V7), inferior angle of the scapula (lead V8), and the left border of the spine (lead V9) (Fig. 2.7).[18,19] An easy way to diagnose a posterior MI is flipping the ECG over and looking at leads V1 to V3 in the light. A standard 12-lead ECG is turned over at 180° to look at the back of the upside-down paper. ST elevation in these leads V1 to V3 with Q waves is consistent with posterior ST elevation myocardial infarction (STEMI).

Misconnection or misplacement of the electrodes while performing a 12-lead ECG can lead to a variety of electrocardiographic changes that must be recognized so as not to ascribe pathology where there is none. Similarly, failure to diagnose electrocardiographic artifact may lead to the misattribution of disease to the patient. Fortunately, the presence of electrode misplacement can be discovered through a systematic review of the ECG; patterns suggestive of electrocardiographic artifact can likewise be recognized through an awareness of the characteristics typical of artifact.[20] In both cases, the cardinal rule when reviewing an ECG with unsuspected changes is to repeat this relatively simple, noninvasive, and inexpensive test before acting on electrocardiographic findings that do not make clinical sense.

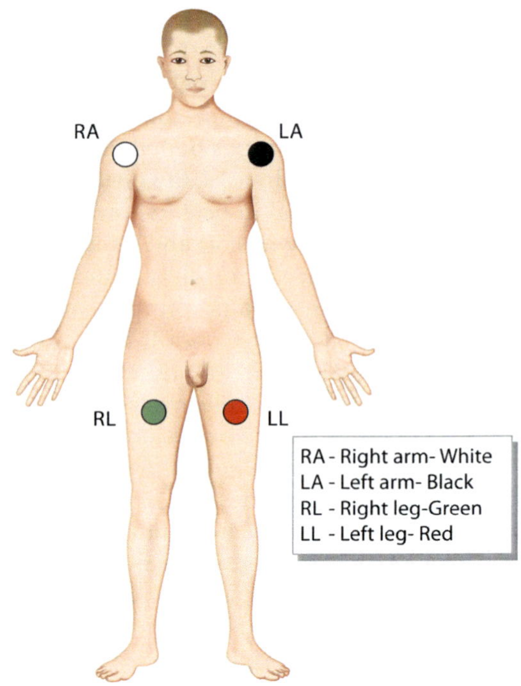

Fig. 2.6: Alternate limb lead positions: for right arm (RA) and left arm (LA) leads can also be placed anywhere between the shoulder and the elbow and for left leg (LL) and right leg (RL) anywhere above the ankle and below the torso. The limb electrodes can be far down on the limbs or close to the hips/shoulders as long as they are placed symmetrically.

Table 2.2: Meaning of the labels and position of augmented limb leads.

Label	*Meaning of label*	*Position of lead on body*
aVR	Augmented vector right	Right wrist
aVL	Augmented vector left	Left wrist
aVF	Augmented vector foot	Left foot

Table 2.3: Electrode position of precordial (chest) leads.

Electrode	*Position*
V1	Fourth intercostal space at the right sternal edge
V2	Fourth intercostal space at the left sternal edge
V3	Midway between V2 and V4
V4	Fifth intercostal space in the mid-clavicular line
V5	Left anterior axillary line at same horizontal level as V4
V6	Left mid-axillary line at same horizontal level as V4 and V5

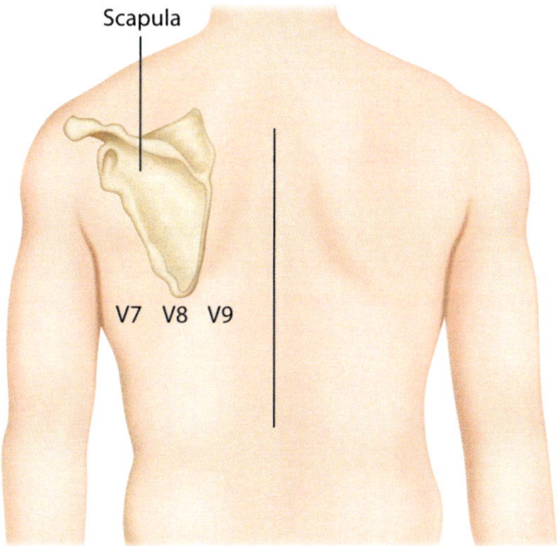

Fig. 2.7: Posterior chest lead positions may be helpful in diagnosing posterior myocardial infarction. Leads V7 to V9 are recorded in the same horizontal plane as lead V6 and on the posterior axillary line (V7), inferior angle of the scapula (V8), and the left border of the spine (V9).

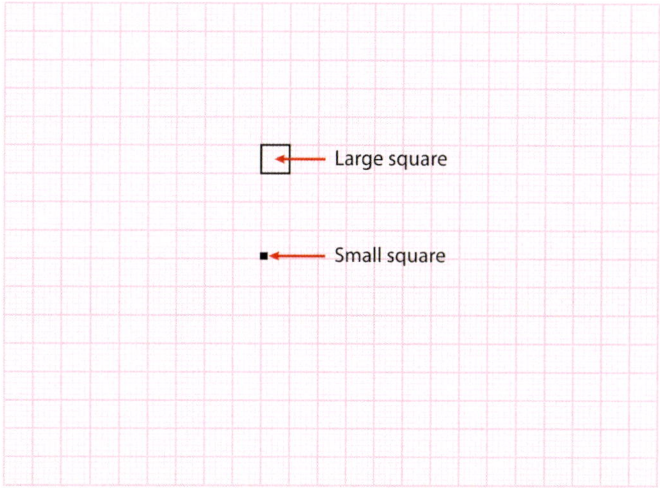

Fig. 2.8: Standard ECG graph paper, showing both large and small square.

STANDARDIZATION OF VOLTAGE AND TIMING INTERVALS

It is conventional to record the ECG using standard measures for amplitude of the electrical signal and for the speed at which the paper moves during the recording. This allows:

- Easy appreciation of heart rates and cardiac intervals and
- Meaningful comparison to be made between ECGs recorded on different occasions or by different ECG machines.

Electrocardiogram is a plot of voltage on the vertical axis against time on the horizontal axis. The electrodes are connected to a galvanometer that records a potential difference. Stylus (needle) of ECG machine moves up and down with changing voltage.

The ECG waves are recorded on special graph paper that is divided into 1 mm^2 grid-like boxes. The ECG paper speed is ordinarily 25 mm/sec. As a result, each 1 mm (small) horizontal box corresponds to 0.04 seconds (40 ms), with heavier lines forming larger boxes that include five small boxes and hence represent 0.20 seconds (200 ms) intervals (Figs. 2.8 to 2.11). On occasion, the paper speed is increased to 50 mm/sec to better define waveforms. In this situation, there are only six leads per sheet of paper. Each large box is therefore only 0.10 seconds (100 ms) and each small box is only 0.02 seconds (20 ms). In addition, the heart rate appears to be one-half of what is recorded at 25 mm/sec paper speed, and all of the ECG intervals are twice as long as normal.

Vertically, the ECG graph measures the height (amplitude) of a given wave or deflection, as 10 mm (10 small boxes) equals 1 mV with *standard calibration* (Fig. 2.12). On occasion, particularly when the waveforms are small, double standard is used (20 mm equals 1 mV). When the wave forms are very large, half standard may be used (5 mm equals 1 mV). Paper speed and voltage are usually printed on the bottom of the ECG.[21]

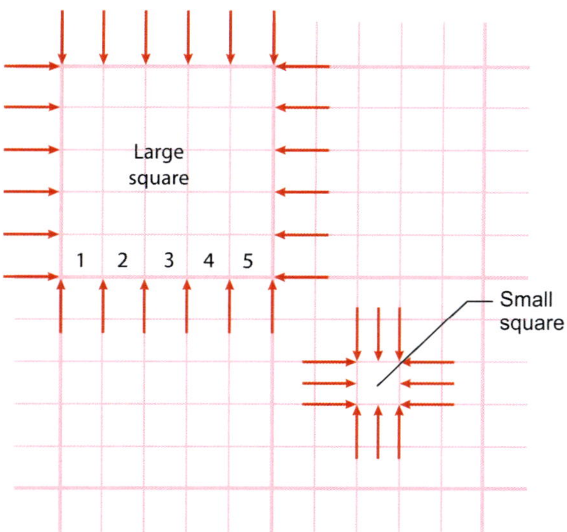

Fig. 2.9: Large square and small square of electrocardiogram (ECG) paper. Each large square contains five small squares inside.

SUMMARY

In a 12-lead ECG, leads I, II, and III are called limb leads (standard leads). The electrodes that form these signals are located on the limbs—one on each arm and one on the LL. The limb leads form the points of what is known

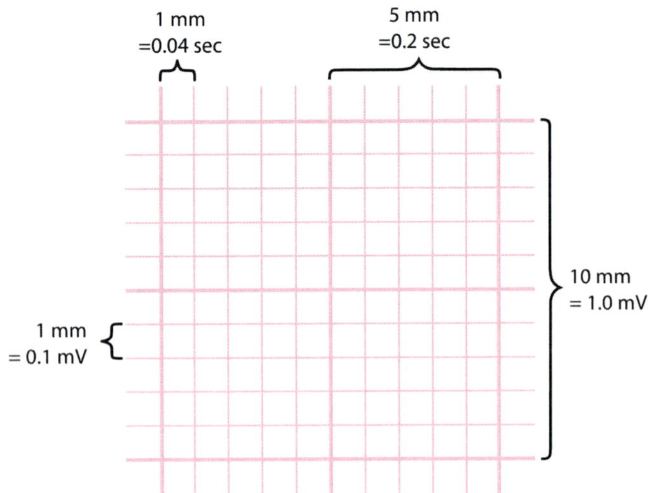

Fig. 2.10: Depiction of time and voltage on ECG paper. Time is recorded in the horizontal direction and amplitude (voltage) in the vertical direction.

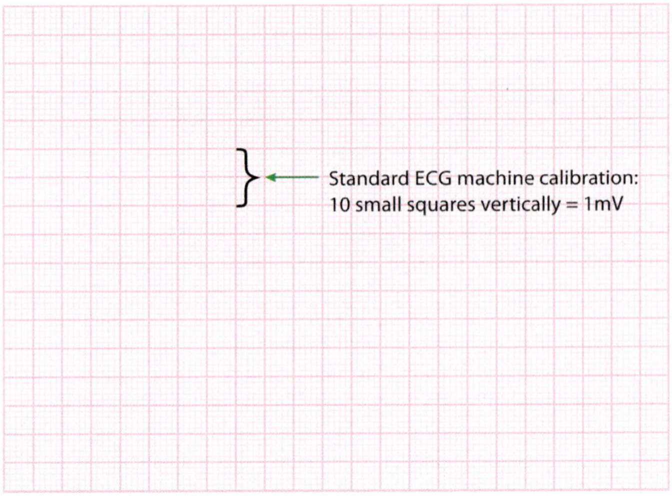

Fig. 2.11: Calculation of voltage on the ECG paper.

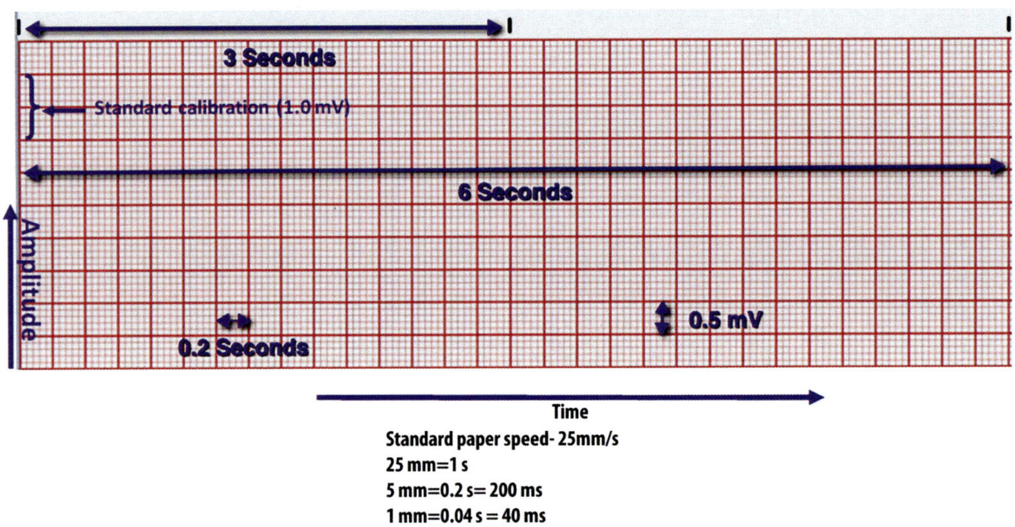

Fig. 2.12: Standard calibration of ECG machine, 10 mm (10 small boxes = 2 large squares) equals 1 mV. Before starting ECG interpretation the clinician must judge, whether the standardization of voltage and timing intervals on the ECG paper is proper or not. If standardization is not proper then ECG interpretation will be wrong.

as Einthoven's triangle. To ensure consistency it is recommended that the limb lead electrodes are placed slightly proximal to the wrists and ankles but the limb electrodes can be far down on the limbs or close to the hips/shoulders as long as they are placed symmetrically.

Arm leads are placed between shoulders and wrists, away from bony prominences and leg leads placed between hips and ankles, away from bony areas. Electrodes are placed on the RA, LA, and LL. The RL electrode is the ground electrode.

- Lead I is the voltage between the (positive) LA electrode and RA electrode:

  LI = LA - RA.
- Lead II is the voltage between the (positive) LL electrode and the RA electrode:

  LII = LL - RA.
- Lead III is the voltage between the (positive) LL electrode and the LA electrode:

  LIII = LL - LA.

Augmented Limb Leads

The same three leads that form the standard leads also form the three unipolar leads known as the augmented leads. These three leads are referred to as aVR (RA), aVL (LA), and aVF (LL) and also record a change in electric potential in the frontal plane. These leads are unipolar in that they measure the electric potential at one point with respect to a null point (one which does not register any significant variation in electric potential during contraction of the heart). This null point is obtained for each lead by adding the potential from the other two leads. For example, in lead aVR, the electric potential of the RA is compared to a null point which is obtained by adding together the potential of lead aVL and lead aVF. Though they are called unipolar leads, but the term unipolar lacks precision.

- *aVR*: Augmented voltage, RA. From heart to RA.
- *aVL*: Augmented voltage, LA. From heart to LA.
- *aVF*: Augmented voltage, left foot. From heart to left foot.

Chest leads, unipolar looks at heart via horizontal plane and they are also called precordial, vector leads. The six chest leads are arranged as follows: V1, 4th intercostal space, right of sternum; V2, 4th intercostal space, left of sternum; V3, halfway between V2 and V4; V4, 5th intercostal space, left midclavicular line; V5, 5th intercostal space, left anterior axillary line; and V6, 5th intercostal space, left midaxillary line.

Correct Placement of Leads V7 to V9

- V7: Posterior axillary line
- V8: Inferior angle of the scapula
- V9: Just to the lateral to the vertebrae.

Flip Test

- Get a standard 12-lead ECG
- Turn it over 180° to look at the back of the upside-down paper.
- Aim the paper at a bright light source to enable seeing the "flipped" tracings.
- ST elevation in these leads V1toV3 with Q waves is consistent with posterior STEMI.

A cheap and easy way to diagnose a posterior MI is flipping the ECG over and looking at the leads V1 to V3 in the light, but using posterior leads (V7 to V9) will more accurately diagnose patients with posterior MI.

Standardization of Voltage and Timing Intervals

The amplitude, or voltage, of the recorded electrical signal is expressed in an ECG in the vertical dimension and is measured in millivolts (mV). On standard ECG paper 1 mV is represented by a vertical deflection of 10 mm. An increase in the amount of muscle mass, such as with LVH, usually results in a larger electrical depolarization signal, and so, a larger amplitude of vertical deflection on the ECG. An essential feature of the ECG is that the electrical activity of the heart is shown as it varies with time. In other words, we can think of the ECG as a graph, plotting electrical activity on the vertical axis against time on the horizontal axis. Standard ECG paper moves at 25 mm per second during real-time recording. This means that when looking at the printed ECG from a distance of 25 mm along the horizontal axis represents 1 second in time. ECG paper is marked with a grid of small and large squares. Each small square represents 0.04 seconds (40 ms) in time along the horizontal axis and each larger square contains five small squares, thus representing 0.2 seconds (200 ms). Standard paper speeds and square markings allow easy measurement of cardiac timing intervals. This enables calculation of heart rates and identification of abnormal electrical conduction within the heart.

REFERENCES

1. Kligfield P, Gettes LS, Bailey JJ, et al. Recommendations for the standardization and interpretation of the electrocardiogram. Part I: The electrocardiogram and its technology: a scientific statement from the American Heart Association, Electrocardiography and Arrhythmias Committee, Council on Clinical Cardiology; the American College of Cardiology Foundation; and the Heart Rhythm Society Endorsed by the International Society for Computerized Electrocardiology. J Am Coll Cardiol. 2007;49(10):1109-27.
2. Kligfield P. The centennial of the Einthoven electrocardiogram. J Electrocardiol. 2002;35(Suppl.):123-9.
3. Fye WB. A history of the origin, evolution, and impact of electrocardiography. Am J Cardiol. 1995;76:641.
4. Pipberger HV, Arzbaecher RC, Berson AS. Recommendations for standardization of leads and of specifications for instruments in electrocardiography and vectorcardiography. Report of the Committee on Electrocardiography. American Heart Association. Circulation. 1975;52:11-31.
5. American National Standards Institute. Diagnostic Electrocardiographic Devices (ANSI/AAMI EC11:1991/(R)2001). Arlington, VA: Association for the Advancement of Medical Instrumentation; 2000.
6. Berson AS, Pipberger HV. Skin-electrode impedance problems in electrocardiography. Am Heart J. 1968;76: 514-25.
7. Pahlm O, Haisty WK Jr, Edenbrandt L. Evaluation of changes in standard electrocardiographic QRS waveforms recorded from activity-compatible proximal limb lead positions. Am J Cardiol. 1992;69(3):253-7.
8. Wenger W, Kligfield P. Variability of precordial electrode placement during routine electrocardiography. J Electrocardiol. 1996;29(3):179-84.
9. Zema MJ, Kligfield P. ECG poor R-wave progression: review and synthesis. Arch Intern Med. 1982;142(6):1145-8.
10. Zema MJ, Kligfield P. Electrocardiographic poor R wave progression. I: correlation with the Frank vectorcardiogram. J Electrocardiol. 1979;12(1):3-10.
11. Farb A, Devereux RB, Kligfield P. Day-to-day variability of voltage measurements used in electrocardiographic criteria for left ventricular hypertrophy. J Am Coll Cardiol. 1990;15(3):618-23.

12. Macfarlane PM, Colaco R, Stevens K, et al. Precordial electrode placement in women. Neth Heart J. 2003;11(3):118-22.
13. Rautaharju PM, Park L, Rautaharju FS, et al. A standardized procedure for locating and documenting ECG chest electrode positions: consideration of the effect of breast tissue on ECG amplitudes in women. J Electrocardiol. 1998;31(1):17-29.
14. Colaco R, Reay P, Beckett C, et al. False positive ECG reports of anterior myocardial infarction in women. J Electrocardiol. 2000;33(Suppl.):239-44.
15. Mason JW, Hancock EW, Gettes LS, et al. Recommendations for the standardization and interpretation of the electrocardiogram: part II: electrocardiography diagnostic statement list: a scientific statement from the American Heart Association Electrocardiography and Arrhythmias Committee, Council on Clinical Cardiology; the American College of Cardiology Foundation; and the Heart Rhythm Society: endorsed by the International Society for Computerized Electrocardiology. Circulation. 2007;115(10):1325-32.
16. The Society for Cardiological Science and Technology. (2010). Clinical Guidelines by Consensus: Recording a Standard 12-Lead Electrocardiogram: An Approved Methodology. [online] Available from: http://www.scst.org.uk/pages/page_box_contents.asp. [Accessed Sept., 2017].
17. Adult and Paediatric Resting Electrocardiography (ECG) Cardiac Sciences Queensland Health. Informed Decision Making in Health Care 2012. [online] Available from http://www.health.qld.gov.au/consent/default.asp. [Accessed Sept., 2017].
18. Matetzky S, Freimark D, Chouraqui P, et al. Significance of ST segment elevations in posterior chest leads (V7 to V9) in patients with acute inferior myocardial infarction: application for thrombolytic therapy. J Am Coll Cardiol. 1998;31(3):506-11.
19. Lindridge J. True posterior myocardial infarction: the importance of leads V7–V9. Emerg Med J. 2009;26(6):456-7.
20. Harrigan RA, Chan TA, Brady WJ. Electrocardiographic Electrode Misplacement, Misconnection, and Artifact. J Emerg Med. 2012;43(6):1038-44.
21. Price D. How to read an Electrocardiogram (ECG). Part One: Basic principles of the ECG. The normal ECG. SSMJ. 2010;3(2):1-4.

Chapter 3

Interpretation and Identification of Different Waves in Electrocardiogram and Calculation of Heart Rate

INTRODUCTION

The standard electrocardiogram (ECG) paper speed is 25 mm/sec or 25 small squares per second. In this way it is possible to calculate the duration of individual waves (Fig. 3.1). Ten small squares (two large squares) vertically are equal to 1 millivolt (mV) (Fig. 3.2). So it is possible to calculate the amount of voltage being released within the heart. If the line is flat at any time in the duration of a series of waves, it indicates no electrical activity at that particular moment. The direction in which the waves point indicates whether electricity is moving toward or away from a particular lead. So different leads may have waves pointing in different directions, e.g. in lead augmented vector right (aVR) (right shoulder/right arm/wrist) will always see the electrical stimulus travelling away from it, therefore the

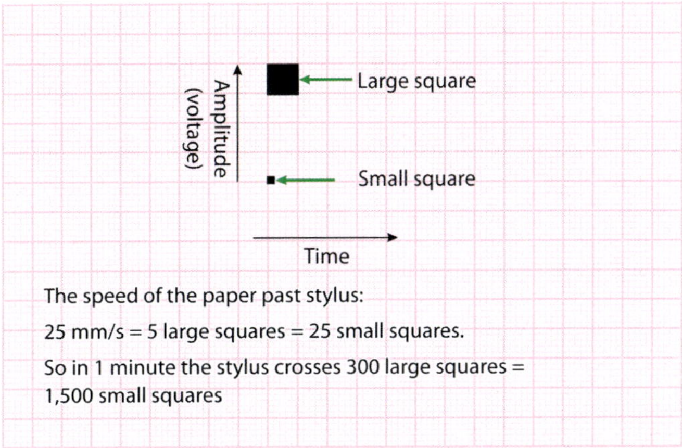

Fig. 3.1: Standard electrocardiogram (ECG) recording paper showing large and small squares.

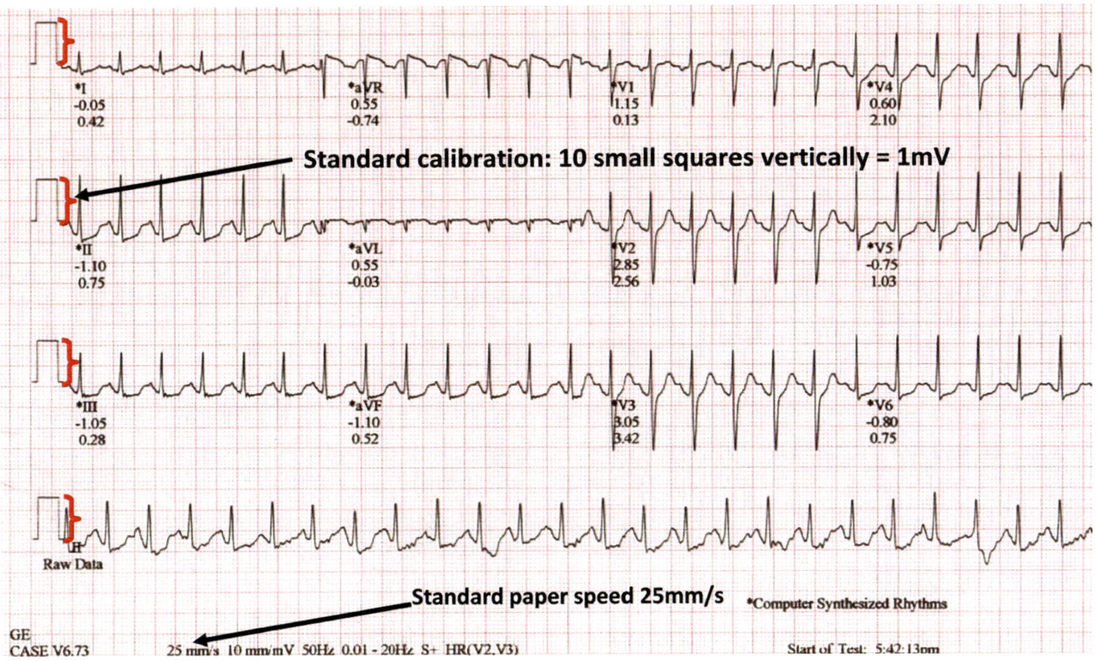

Fig. 3.2: Electrocardiogram showing standard calibration. Normal ECG machine calibration is 1 mV = 2 large squares = 10 small squares. Before interpreting ECG, calibration must be checked. Because, if machine calibration is wrong then calculation of the amplitude of all the waves will be also wrong. If paper speed is wrong (standard paper speed 25 mm/s) then time calculation will be also wrong. So, proper calibration signal along with standard paper speed should be included with every ECG record.

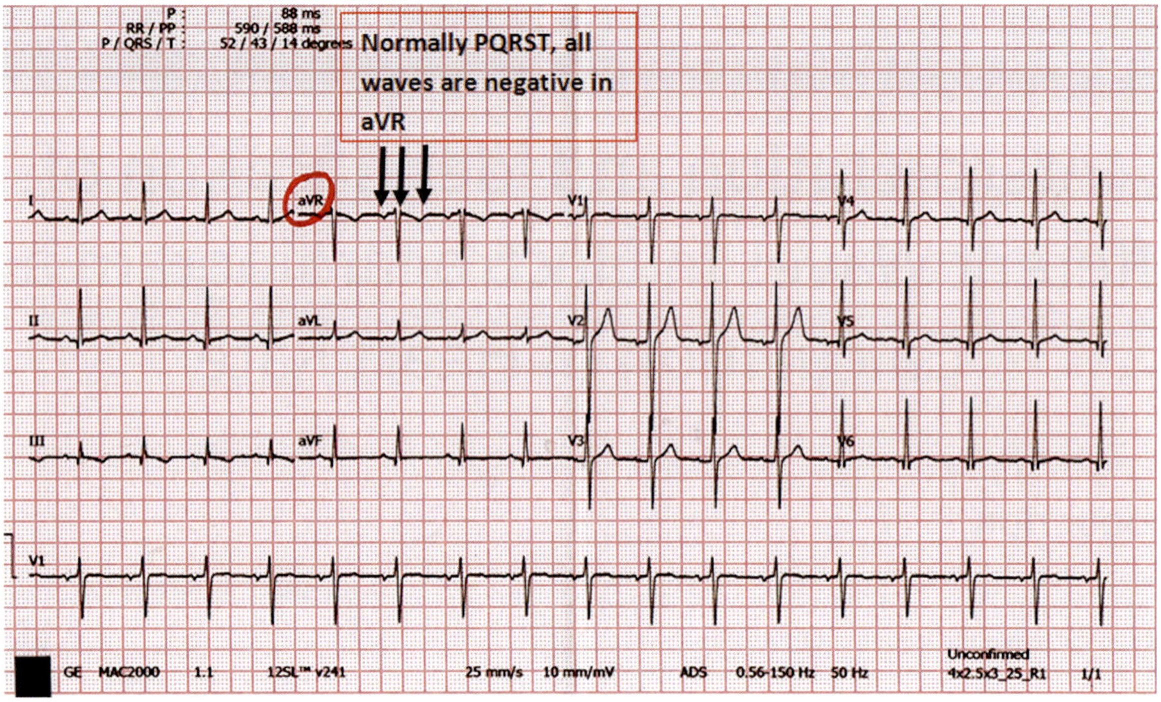

Fig. 3.3: In normal ECG, PQRST, all the waves are negative in lead aVR (*arrows*).

waves expressed in aVR for sinus rhythm, PQRST, will all point downward and negative (Fig. 3.3). Before interpreting ECG the calibration information on the ECG paper must be checked. A standard signal of 1 mV should move the stylus of the ECG machine vertically 1 cm (equal to two large squares). If machine calibration is wrong then calculation of the amplitude of all the waves will be also wrong (Figs. 3.4A to C). So, proper calibration signal should be included with every ECG record and before starting interpretation of ECG clinician must check that whether the calibration is correct or not.

Typically an ECG has five deflections, arbitrarily named "P" to "T" waves. The Q, R, and S waves occur in rapid succession, do not appear in all leads, and reflect a single event, and thus are usually considered together. A *Q wave* is any downward deflection after the *P wave*. An *R wave* follows as an upward deflection, and the *S wave* is any downward deflection after the R wave. The *T wave* follows the *S wave*, and in some cases an additional *U wave* follows the *T wave* (Fig. 3.5A).

During each cardiac cycle the first structure to be depolarized during normal sinus rhythm is the right atrium, closely followed by the left atrium. So the first electrical signal on a normal ECG originates from the atria and is known as the *P wave*. Although there is usually only one P wave in most leads of an ECG, the P wave is in fact the sum of the electrical signals from the two atria, which are usually superimposed. There is then a short, physiological delay as the atrioventricular (AV) node slows the electrical depolarization before it proceeds to the ventricles. This delay is responsible for the *PR interval*, a short period where no electrical activity is seen on the ECG, represented by a straight horizontal or "isoelectric" line. Depolarization of the ventricles results in usually the largest part of the ECG signal (because of the greater muscle mass in the ventricles) and this is known as the *QRS complex*. The Q wave is the first initial downward or "negative" deflection. The R wave is then the next upward deflection (provided it crosses the isoelectric line and becomes "positive"). The S wave is then the next deflection downward, provided it crosses the isoelectric line to become briefly negative before returning to the isoelectric baseline. In the case of the ventricles, there is also an electrical signal reflecting repolarization of the myocardium. This is shown as the *ST segment* and the *T wave*. The ST segment is normally isoelectric, and the T wave in most leads is an upright deflection of variable amplitude and duration (Fig. 3.5B).

P WAVE

Atrial activity, the P wave is usually apparent in most ECG leads. However, sometimes the P wave is of low amplitude and it may be necessary to inspect all leads of the ECG to establish the rhythm as sinus. Atrial depolarization wave spreads from the sinus node, which lies at the junction of the superior vena cava and right atrium, in an inferior direction toward the AV junction. The P wave, therefore, is upright in leads I, II, III, and augmented vector foot (aVF), which face the inferior surface of the heart, and is inverted in aVR, which faces the superior surface of the heart. In a 12-lead ECG, the small and rounded P wave is clearly visible

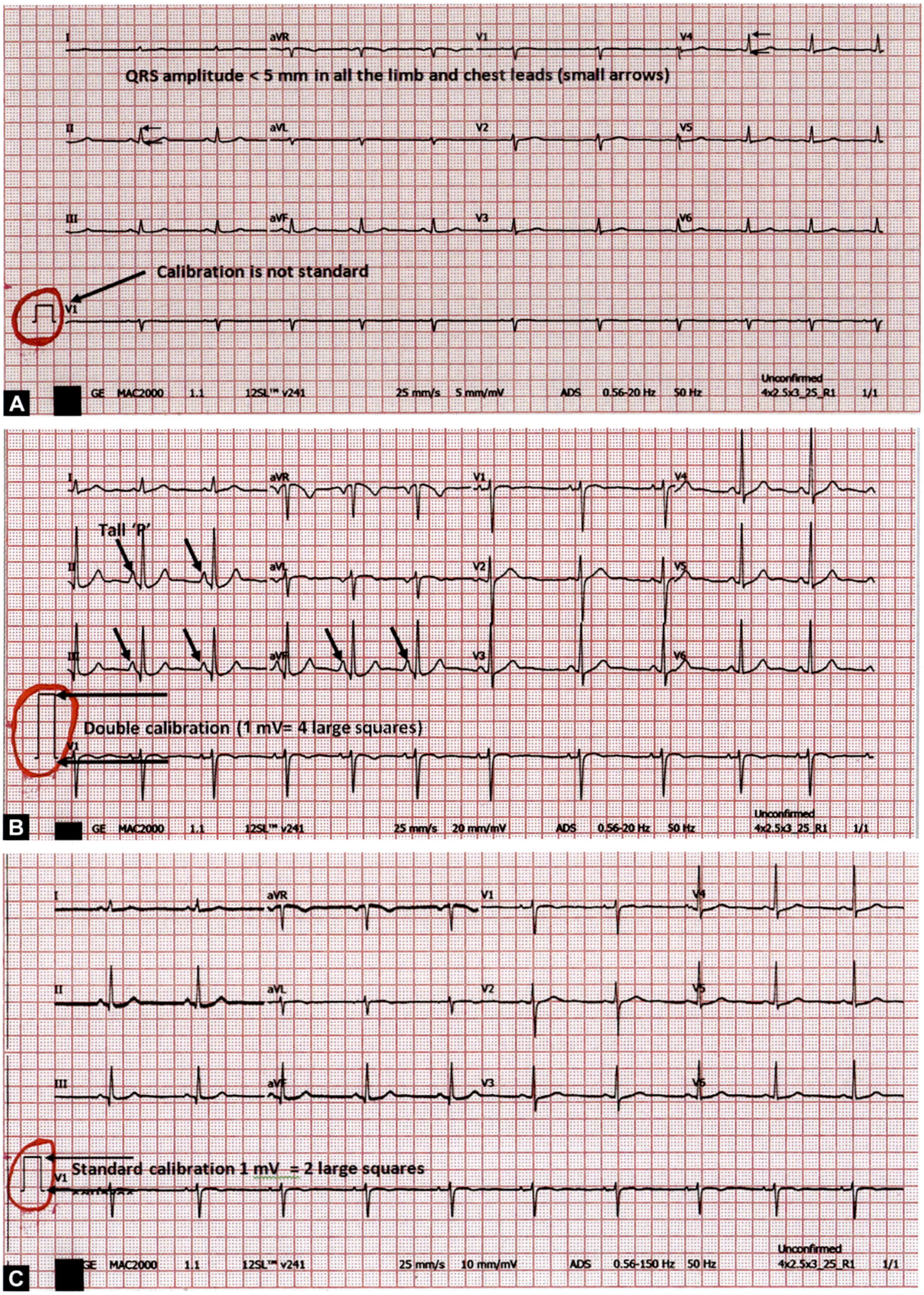

Figs. 3.4A to C: (A) Apparently this electrocardiogram is suggestive of low voltage ECG. But if you look at the calibration signal (red circle, *large arrow*), you can easily detect that the standardization of the machine is not proper. Machine calibration was not set at standard 1 mV (2 large squares), rather it was set at half of standard calibration (1 mV = 1 large square). So, the ECG is wrongly depicting low voltage, QRS amplitudes less than 5 mm in all the leads (*small arrows*). (B) In the same patient (A) this ECG suggests *P*-pulmonale [Tall and peak "P" waves >2.5 mm in height in LII, LIII, and augmented vector foot (aVF)]. But if you look at the calibration signal (red circle), you can easily detect that the standardization of the machine is not proper. Machine calibration was not set at standard 1 mV (2 large squares), rather it was set at double of the standard calibration, 1 mV = 4 large squares (*large arrows*). So, in this tracing all the waves appearing bigger and the ECG is wrongly depicting P-pulmonale (*small arrows*). (C) In the same patient with standard calibration (1 mV = 2 large squares) of the machine, the ECG appears normal (*red circle with arrows*).

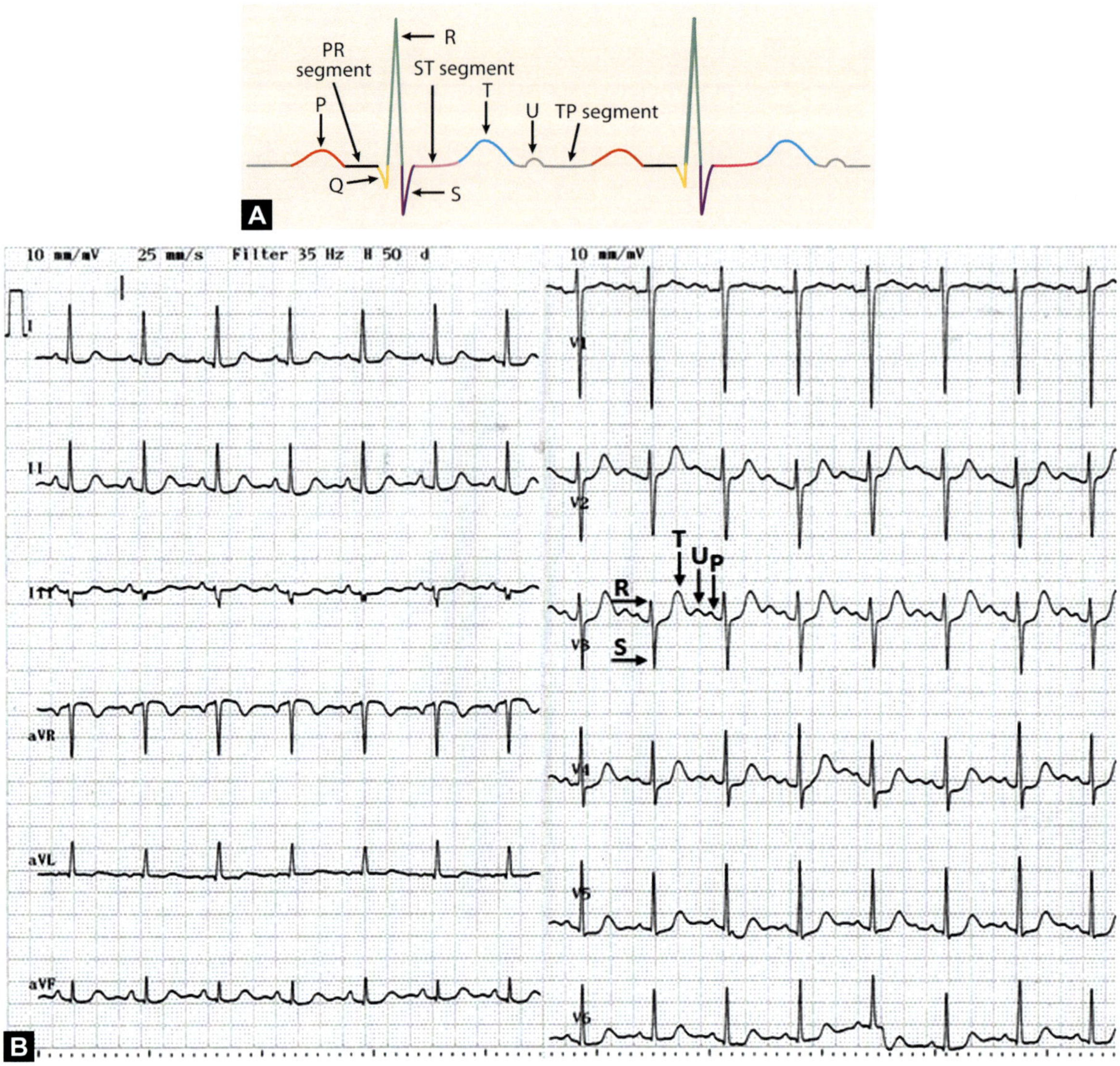

Figs. 3.5A and B: (A) Waves of the normal ECG. (B) Waves of the normal ECG. In this ECG "q" wave is not clearly discernible in any lead. "q" wave may be absent in normal tracing.

just before the taller, more peaked QRS complex. But if the heart rate (HR) is very fast, the P wave may merge with the preceding T wave and becomes difficult to identify.

Atrial depolarization proceeds sequentially from right to left, with the right atrium activated before the left atrium. The right and left atrial waveforms summate to form the P wave. The first one-third of the P wave corresponds to right atrial activation, the final one-third corresponds to left atrial activation; the middle one-third is a combination of the two (Fig. 3.6). In most leads (e.g. lead II), the right and left atrial waveforms move in the same direction, forming a monophasic P wave except in lead V1. In lead V1 the right and left atrial waveforms move in opposite directions (Fig. 3.7). This produces a biphasic P wave with the initial positive deflection corresponding to right atrial activation and the subsequent negative deflection denoting left atrial activation (Fig. 3.8).

Characteristics of Normal P wave

1. P wave precedes each QRS complex.
2. Upright in leads LI, LII, LIII, and aVF and inverted in lead aVR.
3. The P-wave contour is normally smooth.
4. P duration less than 0.12 seconds (120 ms)
5. P amplitude less than 2.5 millimeter (less than 0.25 mV)
6. Frontal plane P-wave axis: 0° to +75°
7. May see notched P waves in frontal plane.
8. The P waves in leads I and II must be upright (positive) if the rhythm is coming from the sinus node.

PR INTERVAL

The AV node delays conduction of the atrial impulse to the ventricles. The PR interval, which is measured from the

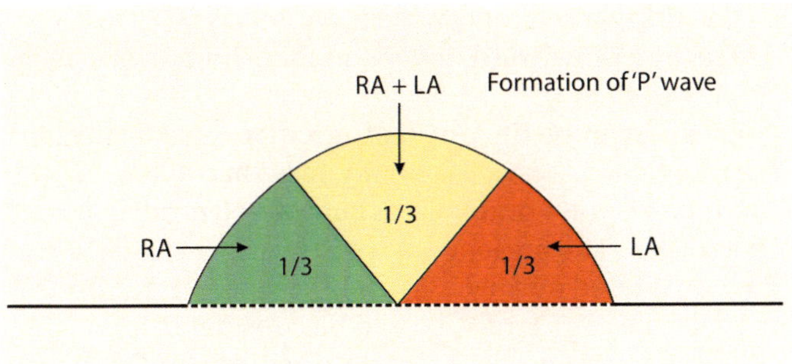

Fig. 3.6: The right atrial (RA) and left atrial (LA) waveforms summate to form the P-wave. The first one-third of the P-wave corresponds to RA activation, the final one-third corresponds to LA; the middle one-third is a combination of the two.

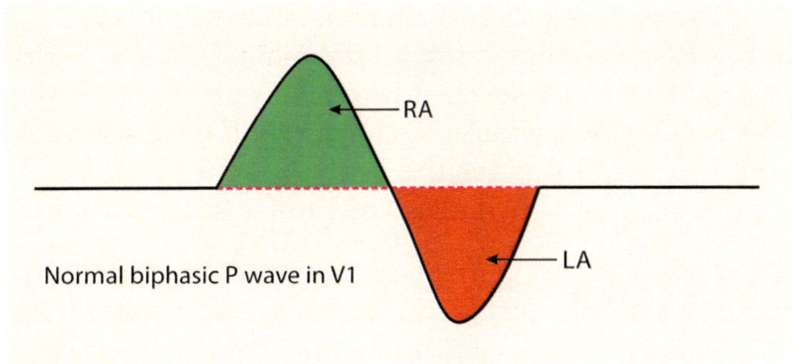

Fig. 3.8: Contribution of right and left atrium in the formation of biphasic P-wave in V1. The part of the wave above the isoelectric line is contributed by the RA and the part below the isoelectric line is by LA (*arrows*).

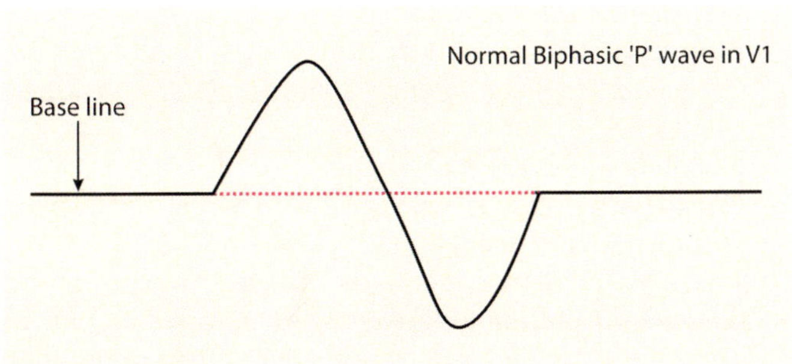

Fig. 3.7: Normal biphasic "P" wave in V1.

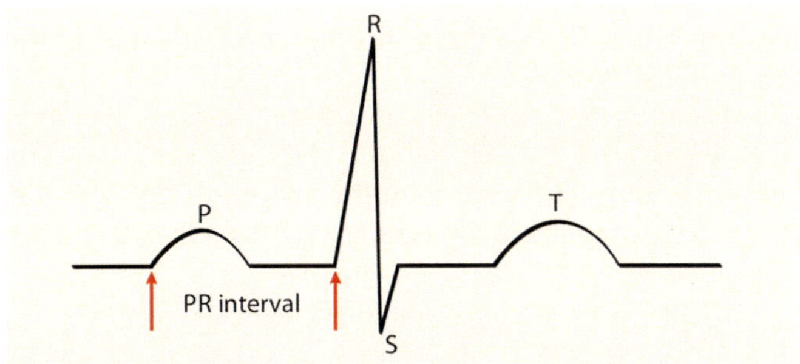

Fig. 3.9: The PR interval, which is measured from the onset of the P-wave to the onset of the QRS complex (*arrows*).

onset of the P wave to the onset of the ventricular complex (QRS), indicates the time taken for an atrial impulse to reach the ventricles (Fig. 3.9). If a Q wave is present then the PR interval is termed as PQ interval. So PR interval and PQ interval are synonymous.

The normal PR interval ranges from 0.12 seconds to 0.20 seconds (120–200 ms) or 3–5 small squares in duration. But the duration of PR interval depends on the HR, being shorter at faster HR [sinus tachycardia, HR greater than 100 beats/min (bpm)] and widens during slower HR (sinus bradycardia, HR less than 60 bpm). PR interval appears shorter during childhood and adolescence and tends to increase with age.[1-4] The PR interval is longer with high vagal tone. A prolonged PR interval corresponds to impaired AV conduction. Prolonged PR interval, or first degree AV block, has been traditionally regarded as a benign electrocardiographic finding in healthy individuals. In the middle-aged general population, prolonged PR interval normalizes in a substantial proportion of subjects during the time course, and it is not associated with an increased risk of all-cause or cardiovascular mortality.[3]

Causes of Prolonged PR Interval

PR interval greater than 0.20 seconds (greater than 200 ms, greater than 5 small squares)[4-6]

- Intrinsic AV nodal disease
- Enhanced vagal tone
- Acute myocardial infarction (MI), particularly acute inferior wall MI
- Myocarditis
- Electrolyte disturbances (e.g. hypokalemia and hypomagnesemia)
- Drug induced (beta-blockers, calcium channel blockers, digoxin, quinidine, procainamide, disopyramide, etc.).

Causes of Short PR Interval

PR interval less than 0.12 seconds (less than 120 ms, less than 3 small squares)[7-9]

1. Normal variant
2. Atrioventricular junctional rhythm
3. Wolff-Parkinson-White syndrome
4. Lown-Ganong-Levine syndrome.

PR SEGMENT

The *PR segment* is the flat, usually isoelectric segment between the end of the P wave and the start of the QRS complex (Fig. 3.10). PR segment is also called PQ segment or PTa segment. The PR segment is different than the PR interval which is measured in units of time (ms). Abnormalities of the PR segment are not very common, however, can indicate certain cardiac disease states. PR segment depression can indicate pericarditis or atrial infarction. PR segment elevation occurs in lead aVR in the setting of pericarditis.

PR segment elevation or depression in patients with MI indicates concomitant atrial ischemia or infarction. This finding has been associated with poor outcome following ST-elevation myocardial infarction (STEMI) and associated with increased risk for the development of AV block, supraventricular arrhythmias, and cardiac free-wall rupture.

QRS COMPLEX

On 12 lead ECG ventricular activation is represented by the QRS complex (Fig. 3.11) which is normally less than 0.10 seconds (less than 100 ms). Normal range in adults varies from 0.06 seconds to 0.10 seconds (60–100 ms). A duration of 0.11 seconds (110 ms) is sometimes observed in healthy subjects. After traversing the AV node, the impulse reaches the bundle of His and right and left bundles which rapidly conduct it to the ventricular myocardium through the distal part of the bundles and Purkinje fibers.

The amplitude of QRS complex is much larger than that of the atrial P wave, because the muscle mass of the ventricles is much larger than the atriums. QRS complex consists of three distinct waves, each of which has a name (Fig. 3.11):

1. The first downward deflection is called "Q" wave.

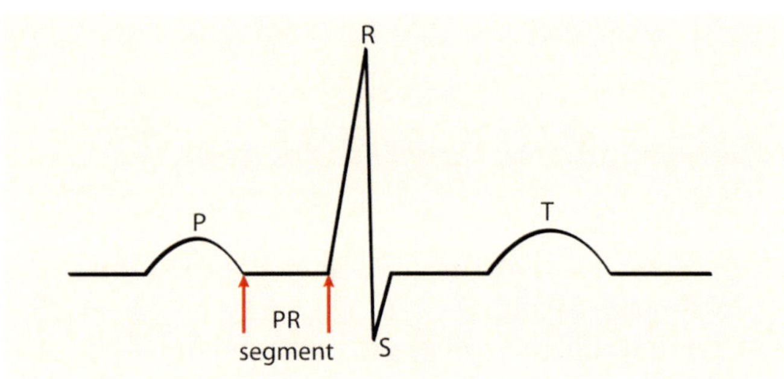

Fig. 3.10: The PR segment extends between the end of the P-wave and the start of the QRS complex (*arrows*).

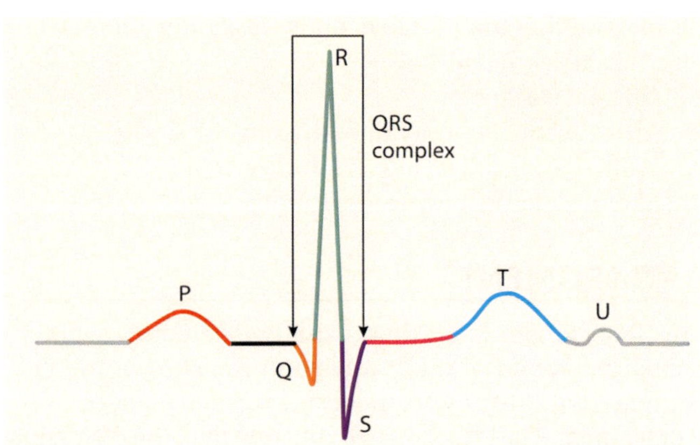

Fig. 3.11: QRS complex consists of three distinct waves, each of which has a name. The first downward deflection is called "Q" wave, the first positive wave after Q-wave is named as "R" wave and the first downward deflection following R-wave is the "S" wave (*arrows*).

2. The first wave after Q wave is named as "R" wave.
3. The first downward deflection following R wave is the "S" wave.

Q wave may be physiological or pathological. Physiological Q wave is usually less than 0.03 seconds duration. A Q wave of any size is considered normal in leads LIII and aVR. The presence of small Q wave in leads V5 and V6 is considered normal. But in some leads V1, V2, and V3, the presence of a Q wave should be considered abnormal.

The presence of a Q wave does not indicate any specific electrophysiological mechanism. To the contrary, Q waves can be related to one or more of the following four factors.[10,11]

1. Physiologic and positional effects (physiological Q wave)
2. Myocardial injury or infarction
3. Ventricular enlargement
4. Altered ventricular conduction.

Clinicians should be aware of three principles with respect to Q waves[11,12]

1. Not all Q waves are pathologic.
2. Not all pathologic Q waves are due to MI caused by fixed coronary artery occlusion.
3. There is no firm consensus on the criteria for the diagnosis of pathologic Q waves. But pathologic Q waves are usually defined as duration greater than or equal to 0.04 seconds or greater than 25% of R-wave amplitude.

R wave (Fig. 3.5) normally increases in amplitude and duration from lead V1 to V5 (V6) as during each cardiac cycle electrical activity progress from the thinner right ventricle towards the thicker left ventricle. So in normal 12-lead ECG "R" waves are smaller in amplitude in leads V1, V2 and larger in leads V4, V5. But reversal of this sequence occurs in presence of ventricular hypertrophy. Tall "R" waves are produced in leads V1 and V2 by right ventricular hypertrophy (RVH) and tall "R" waves are present in leads V5 and V6 in presence of left ventricular hypertrophy (LVH). Loss of R wave or poor progression of R wave from leads V1 to V5 may indicate previous myocardial infarction.

The *S wave* is the first downward deflection of the QRS complex that occurs after the R wave (Fig. 3.5). An S wave may not be present in all ECG leads in a given patient. In the normal ECG, there is a large S wave in V1 which progressively becomes smaller to the point where almost no S wave is present in V6. A large slurred S wave is seen in lead I and V6 in the setting of a right bundle branch block (RBBB).

The duration of QRS complex is termed as "QRS interval" and normally ranges from 0.06 seconds to 0.10 seconds. It tends to be slightly longer in males than females. The QRS interval has no lower limit that indicates abnormality. But QRS prolongation is usually caused by ventricular hypertrophy, arrhythmia, and conduction abnormalities. The QRS complex is often used to determine the axis of the ECG, although it is also possible to determine a separate P-wave axis. The duration, amplitude, and morphology of the QRS complex are useful in diagnosing cardiac arrhythmias, conduction abnormalities, ventricular hypertrophy, MI, electrolyte derangements, and other disease states.

J-POINT

The point at which the QRS complex meets the ST segment is known as the J-point. The J-point is easy to identify when the ST segment is horizontal and forms a sharp angle with the last part of the QRS complex (Figs. 3.12A and B). However, when the ST segment is sloped or the QRS complex is wide, the two features do not form a sharp angle and the location of the J-point is less clear. There is no consensus on the precise location of the J-point in these circumstances.[13,14]

ST SEGMENT

The ST segment is the flat, isoelectric section of the ECG between the end of the S wave (the J-point) and the beginning of the T wave. It represents the interval between ventricular depolarization and repolarization. The most important causes of ST segment abnormalities (elevation or depression) are myocardial ischemia/infarction, bundle branch block, ventricular hypertrophy, and pericarditis.

An ST elevation is considered significant if the vertical distance inside the ECG trace and the baseline greater than 1 mm or 1 small square in a limb lead or 2 mm or 2 small squares in a precordial lead. The baseline is either the PR segment or the TP segment. Significant ST depression is defined as depression of the ST segment level greater than 0.1 mV (1.0 mm) compared with the baseline.

Common Causes of ST Segment Elevation (Figs. 3.13A and B)

- Acute MI

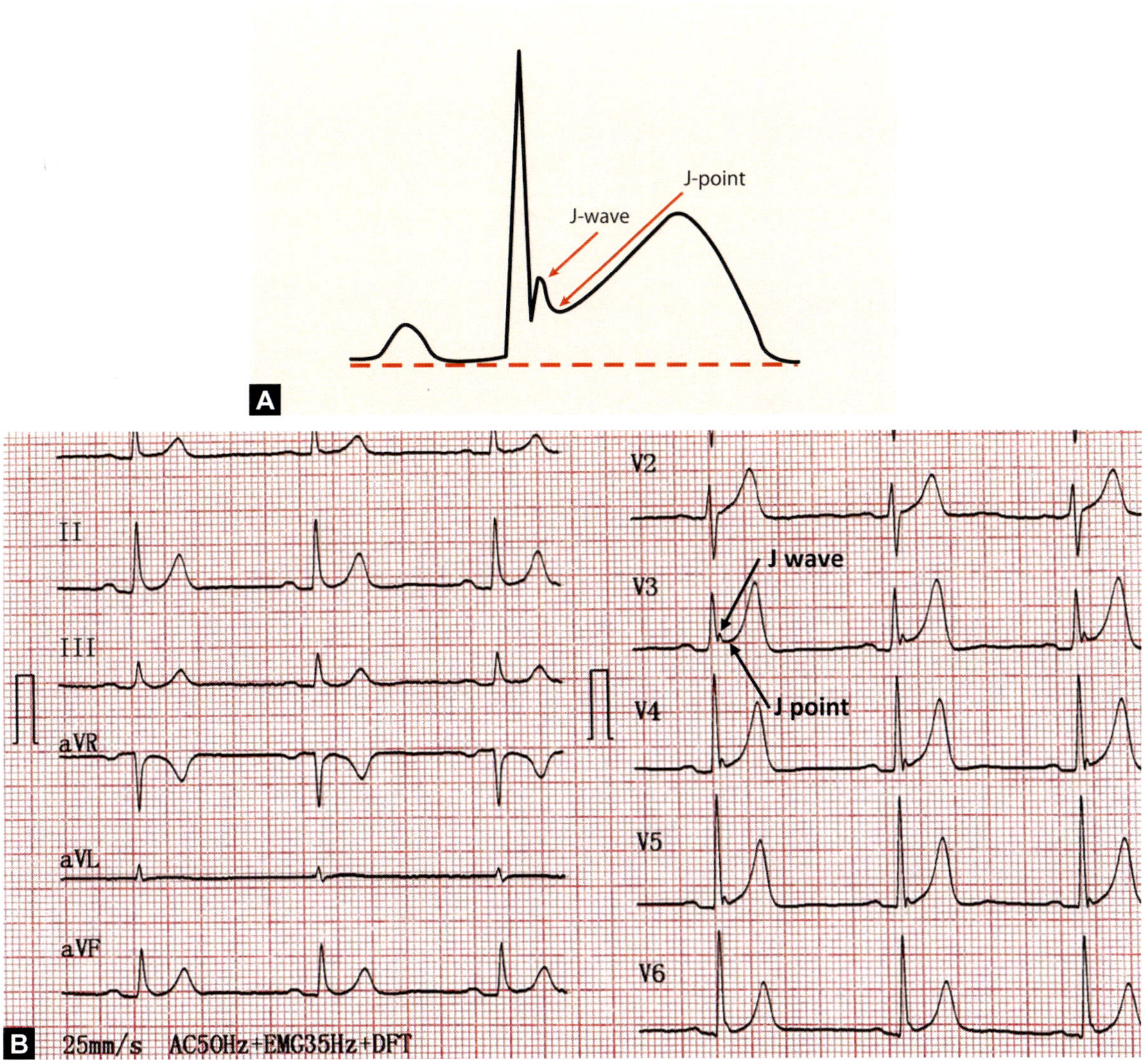

Figs. 3.12A and B: (A) J-point, the point at which the QRS complex meets the ST segment (*arrows*). (B) J-point elevation in leads V3 to V6 suggestive of early repolarization pattern, usually normal variant.

- Pericarditis
- Coronary vasospasm (Prinzmetal's angina)
- Early repolarization pattern (normal variant)
- Left bundle branch block
- Hyperkalemia
- Ventricular aneurysm
- Ventricular paced rhythm
- Raised intracranial pressure.

Less Common Causes of ST Segment Elevation

- Pulmonary embolism
- Acute aortic dissection
- Brugada syndrome
- Hypothermia
- Hypercalcemia
- Following electrical cardioversion.

Rare Causes of ST Segment Elevation

- Cardiac tumor
- Pancreatitis/gallbladder disease
- Myocarditis
- Septic shock
- Anaphylaxis.

Common Causes of ST Segment Depression

- Acute coronary syndrome (Non-STEMI/unstable angina)
- Left ventricular hypertrophy
- Physiologic J-junctional depression with sinus tachycardia
- Digoxin effect
- Subendocardial ischemia
- Reciprocal changes in STEMI.

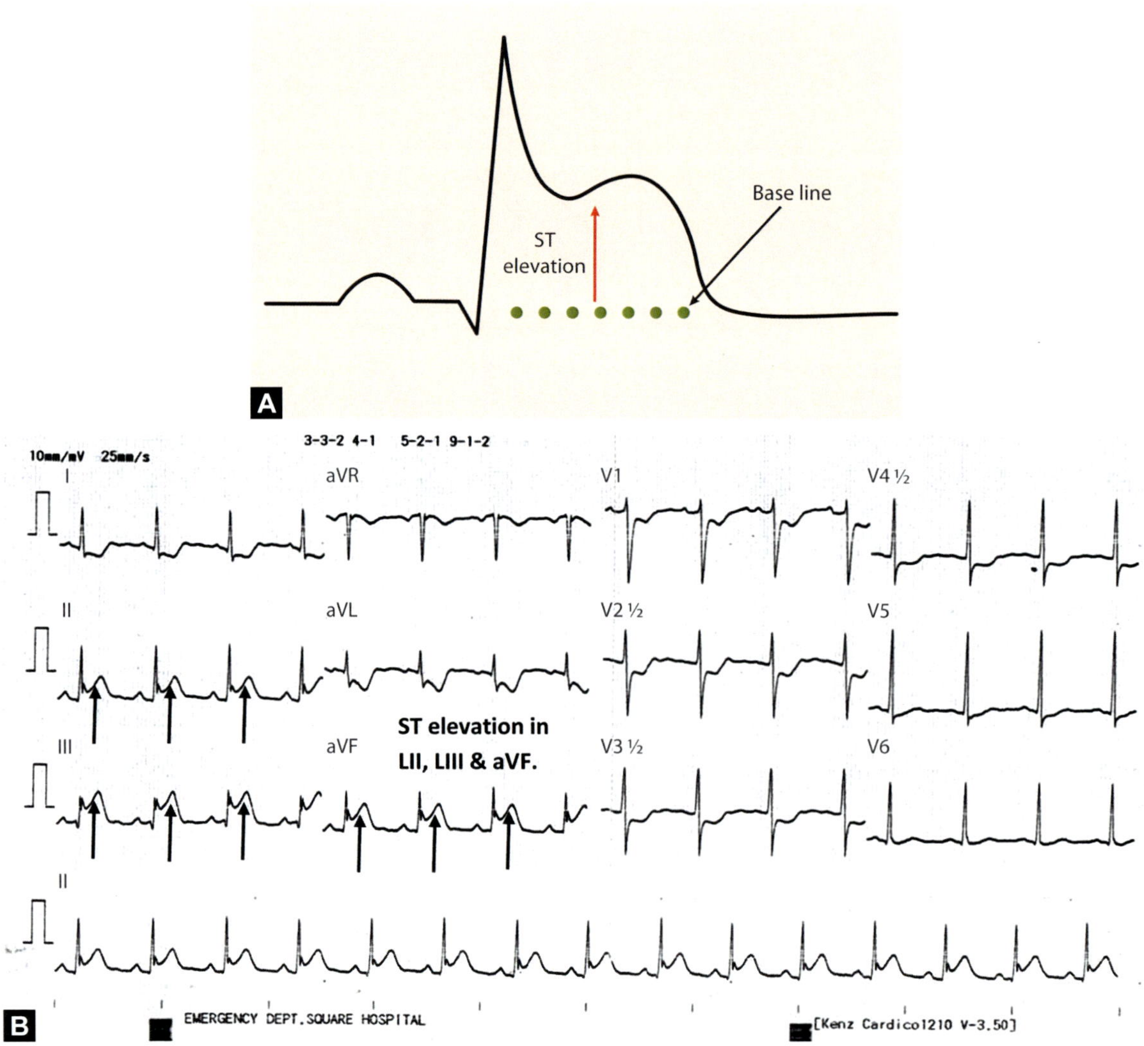

Figs. 3.13A and B: (A) ST segment elevation with convexity upwards suggestive of ST-elevation myocardial infarction (STEMI). (B) ST elevation with convexity upwards in LII, LIII, and aVF suggestive of acute inferior myocardial infarction.

Uncommon Causes of ST Segment Depression

- Hypokalemia
- Hyperventilation
- Hypothermia
- Mitral valve prolapse.

Heightened awareness of the characteristic patterns of ST-segment depression and T-wave inversion is paramount to quickly identify life-threatening disorders. Depression of the ST segment and inversion of the T wave are common electrocardiographic abnormalities. Knowing the various ischemic and nonischemic morphologic features is critical for a timely diagnosis of high-risk myocardial ischemia and electrolyte or drug-related abnormalities. ST-segment depression may be primary or secondary. ST segment and T-wave abnormalities may be unrelated to any QRS abnormality, in which case they are called primary repolarization abnormalities. These are caused by ischemia, pericarditis, myocarditis, drugs (digoxin and antiarrhythmic drugs), and electrolyte abnormalities, particularly potassium abnormalities. ST-T abnormalities concordant to the QRS complex suggest ischemia.[15] In secondary ST segment or T-wave abnormalities, QRS criteria for LVH or RVH or LBBB or RBBB or preexcitation are usually present. In secondary ST-segment depression the ST segment and T wave are directed opposite to the QRS—this is called discordance between the QRS complex and the ST-T abnormalities.[15] ST segment depression is often characterized as "upsloping" (Figs. 3.14A and B),

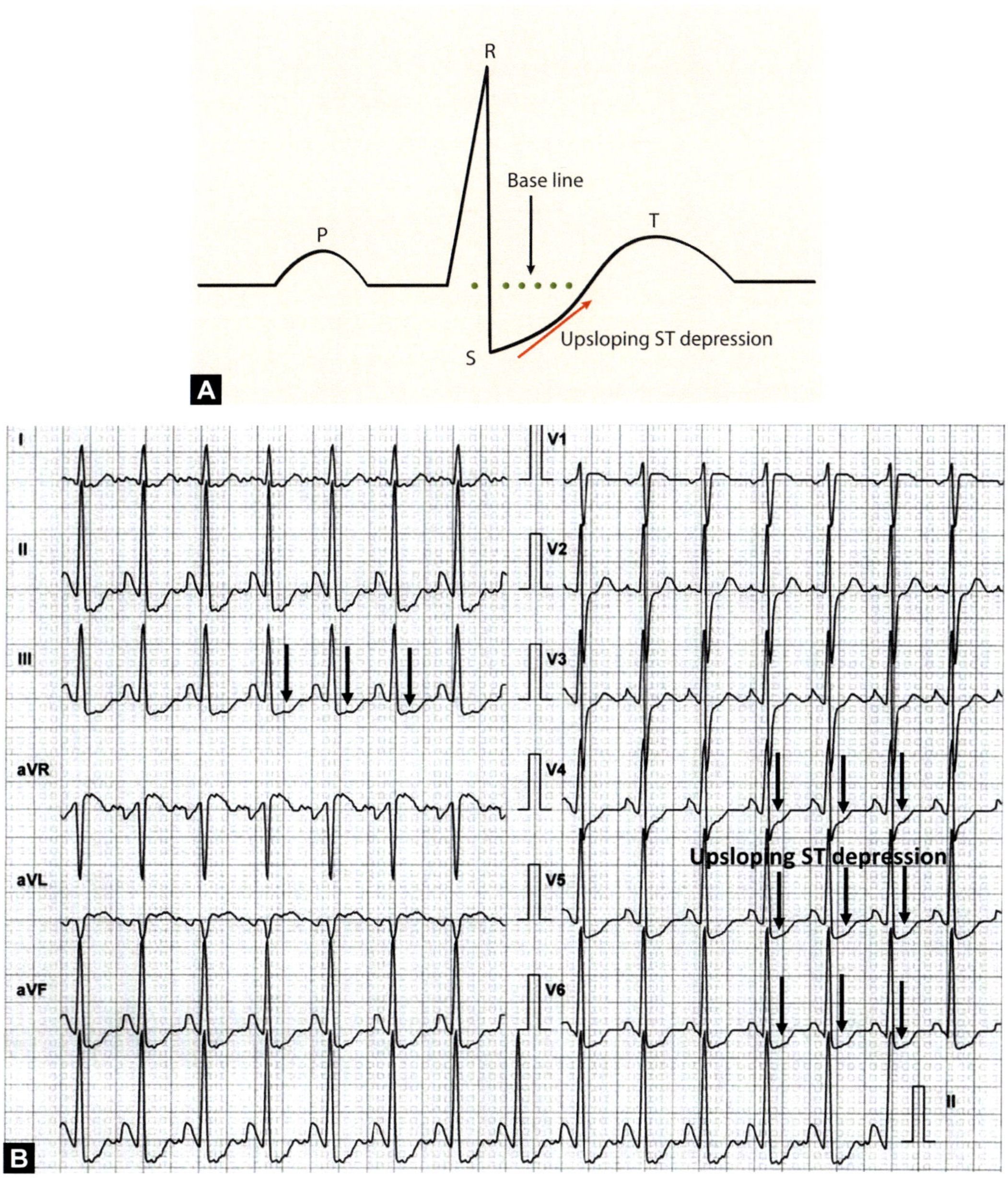

Figs. 3.14A and B: (A) Upsloping ST segment depression. (B) ECG showing widespread upsloping ST segment depression.

"horizontal" (Figs. 3.15A and B), or "downsloping" (Figs. 3.16A and B). Horizontal or downsloping ST segment depression is always significant.

ST depression attributable to ischemia is often diffuse and can be located in both anterior and inferior leads, and is not necessarily localizing. Extensive experience from cardiac stress testing shows that the actual configuration of the ST-segment depression influences the specificity of this finding, with a downsloping segment more specific for the diagnosis of ischemia than horizontal depression. A depressed but upsloping ST segment lacks adequate specificity for ischemia. At least 0.10 mV (1.0 mm) depression at the J-point and either horizontal or downward sloping ST segment depression is suggestive of myocardial ischemia.

T WAVE

The T wave reflects ventricular repolarization. This is the most labile wave in the ECG. T wave changes including low-

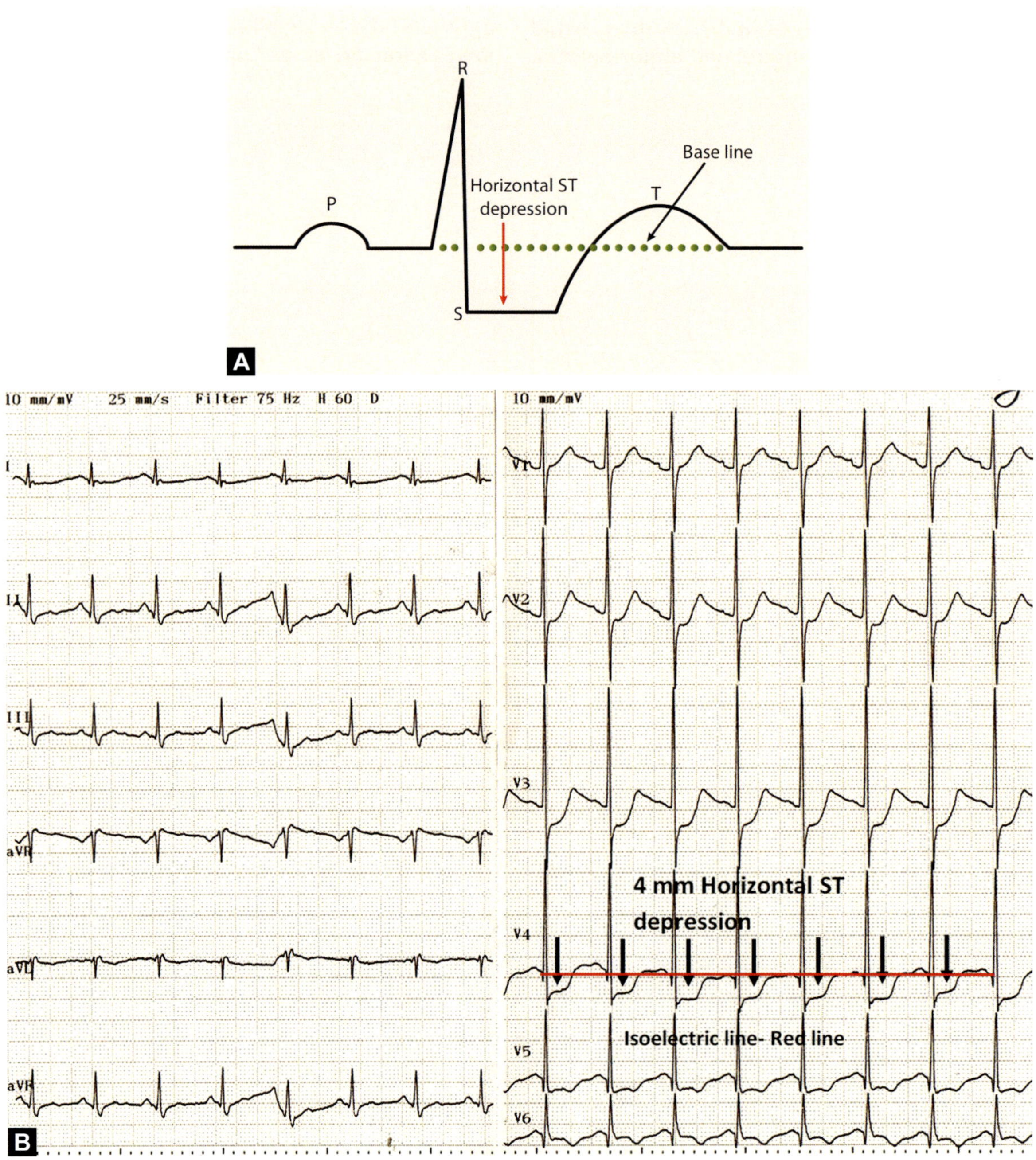

Figs. 3.15A and B: (A) Horizontal ST segment depression. (B) ECG showing 4 mm horizontal ST segment depression (*black arrows*). Red line indicates isoelectric line.

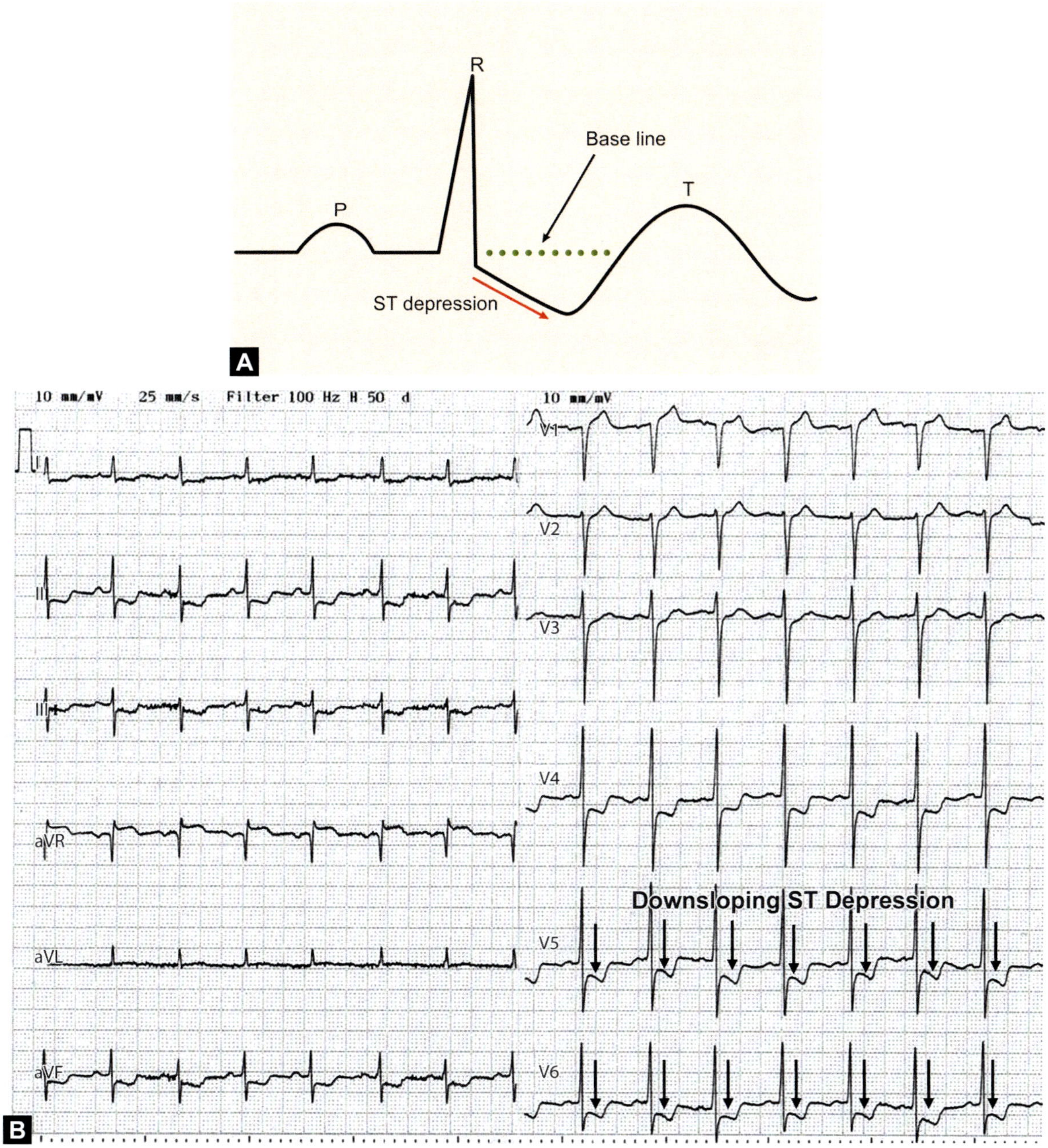

Figs. 3.16A and B: (A) Downsloping ST depression (*red arrow*). (B) Downsloping ST depression in lead V5, V6 (*black arrows*).

amplitude T waves and abnormally inverted T waves may be the result of many cardiac and noncardiac conditions. The normal T wave is usually in the same direction as the QRS except in the right precordial leads. Also, the normal T wave is slightly asymmetric with the first half moving more slowly than the second half. In the normal ECG the T wave is always upright in leads I, II, V3 to V6, and always inverted in lead aVR. The other leads are variable depending on the direction of the QRS and the age of the patient.

It usually takes the same direction as the QRS complex (concordance); opposite polarity (discordance) may indicate past or current infarction. The T wave is usually smooth and rounded but may be of low amplitude in hypokalemia and hypomagnesemia and may be tall and peaked in hyperacute MI, hyperkalemia and LVH.

The T-wave amplitude tends to vary with QRS complex amplitude and should always be greater than that of the U wave, if it is present. T waves do not normally exceed 5 mm in limb leads or greater than 10 mm in any precordial leads.

Patterns of Different "T" waves (Fig. 3.17)

- Normal T wave (Fig. 3.17A)
- Inverted T wave (Fig. 3.17B) may be symmetric or asymmetric

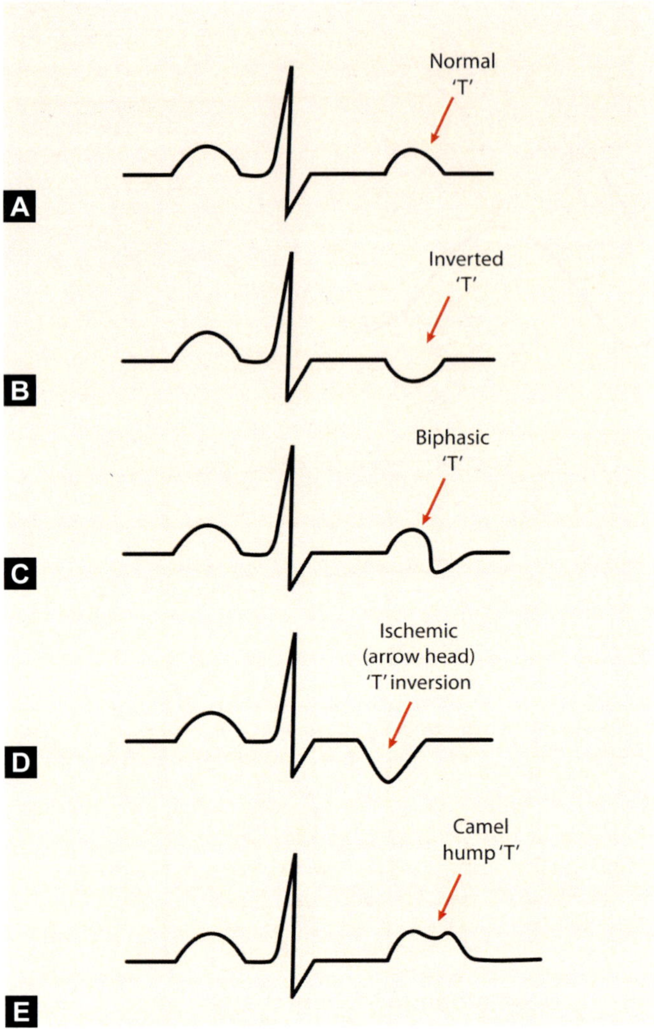

Figs. 3.17A to E: Patterns of different "T" waves. (A) Normal "T" wave, (B) inverted "T" wave, (C) biphasic "T" wave, (D) ischemic arrow head "T" wave inversion, (E) camel hump "T" wave.

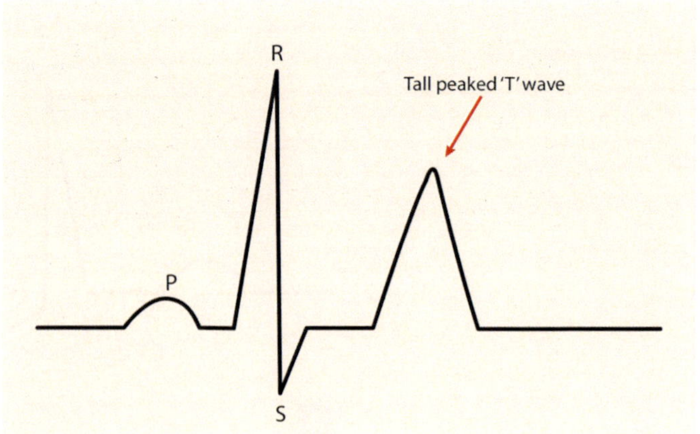

Fig. 3.18: Tall peaked "T" wave. This T wave is tall, narrow, and symmetrically peaked. This pattern of T waves is characteristically seen in hyperkalemia.

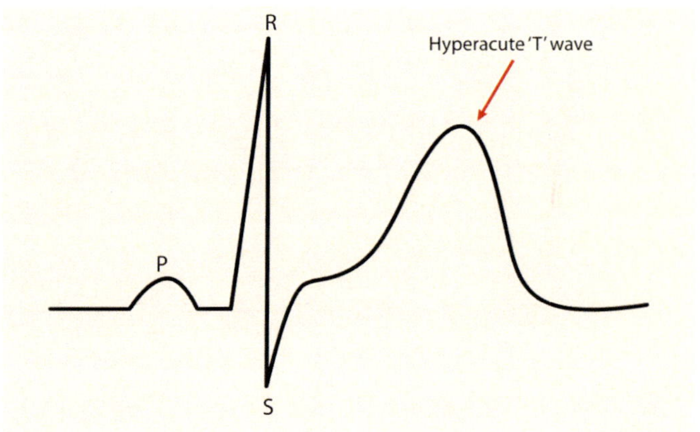

Fig. 3.19: Hyperacute "T" wave. This pattern of broad and asymmetrically peaked "T" waves are sometimes seen in the early phase of STEMI.

- Biphasic T wave (Fig. 3.17C)
- Ischemic (arrow head) T-wave inversion (Fig. 3.17D)
- Camel hump "T" wave (Fig. 3.17E)
- Tall peaked T wave (T waves taller than 5 mm in limb leads and taller than 10 mm in chest leads) (Fig. 3.18)
- Hyperacute T wave (Fig. 3.19).

Inverted T waves are mostly seen in ischemia and hypertrophy of the ventricles. Biphasic T waves are mostly seen in myocardial ischemia and hypokalemia. Biphasic T waves of ischemic origin or due to hypokalemia can be differentiated from the morphology of the waves, as the two waves go in opposite directions:

- Ischemic T waves go up then down (Fig. 3.20A)
- Hypokalemic T waves go down then up (Fig. 3.20B).

Tall, narrow, and symmetrically peaked T waves are characteristically seen in hyperkalemia (Fig. 3.21). Broad, asymmetrically peaked or "hyperacute" T waves are sometimes seen in the early stages of STEMI (Fig. 3.22) and often precede the appearance of ST elevation and Q waves. But hyperacute T waves of STEMI are usually broad based, tall and symmetrical. They are also seen with Prinzmetal angina (vasospastic angina). "Camel hump" T waves have a double peak or "camel hump" appearance (Fig. 3.23). There are two causes for camel hump T waves: Prominent U waves fused to the end of the T wave, as seen in severe hypokalemia and hidden P waves embedded in the T wave, as seen in sinus tachycardia and various types of heart block. Flattened T waves are a nonspecific finding and usually considered as normal variant, but this pattern of T wave changes may represent ischemia (if dynamic or in contiguous leads) or electrolyte abnormality, e.g. hypokalemia (if generalized).

Causes of T wave Inversion

- Myocardial infarction
- Myocardial ischemia
- Subacute or old pericarditis
- Myocarditis
- Central nervous system (CNS) disease causing long QT interval (especially subarachnoid hemorrhage)

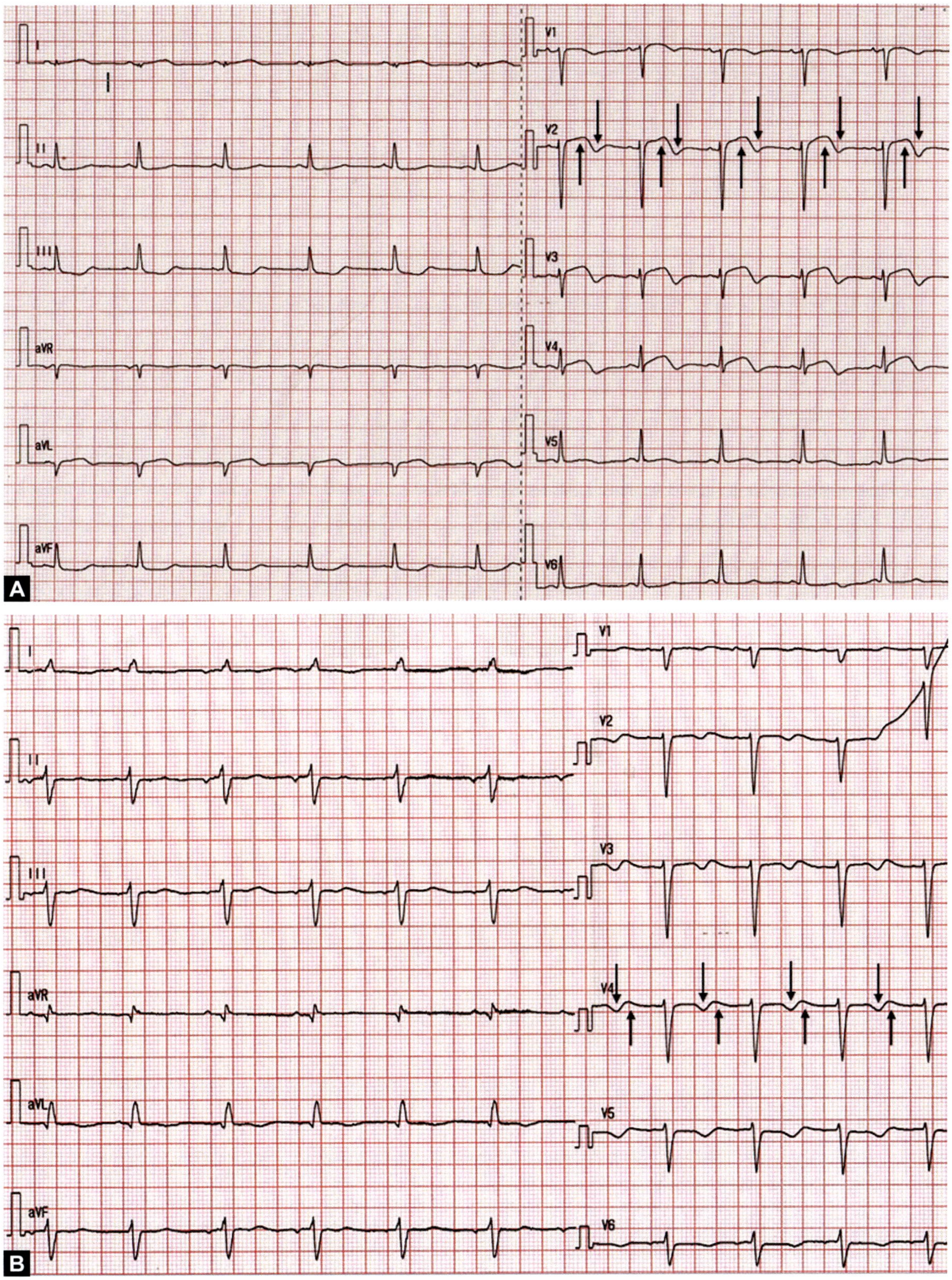

Figs. 3.20A and B: (A) Electrocardiogram shows biphasic "T" waves of ischemic origin. Ischemic T waves go up then down (*arrows*). (B) ECG shows biphasic "T" waves due to hypokalemia. In hypokalemia, T waves go down then up (*arrows*).

- Hypertrophic cardiomyopathy
- Mitral valve prolapse
- Digoxin effect.
- Right ventricular hypertrophy
- LVH with "strain".

Normally in females, the T wave in V3 may be shallowly inverted. But in adult males, it is considered pathologic if the T wave is inverted in V3 to V6. The T wave

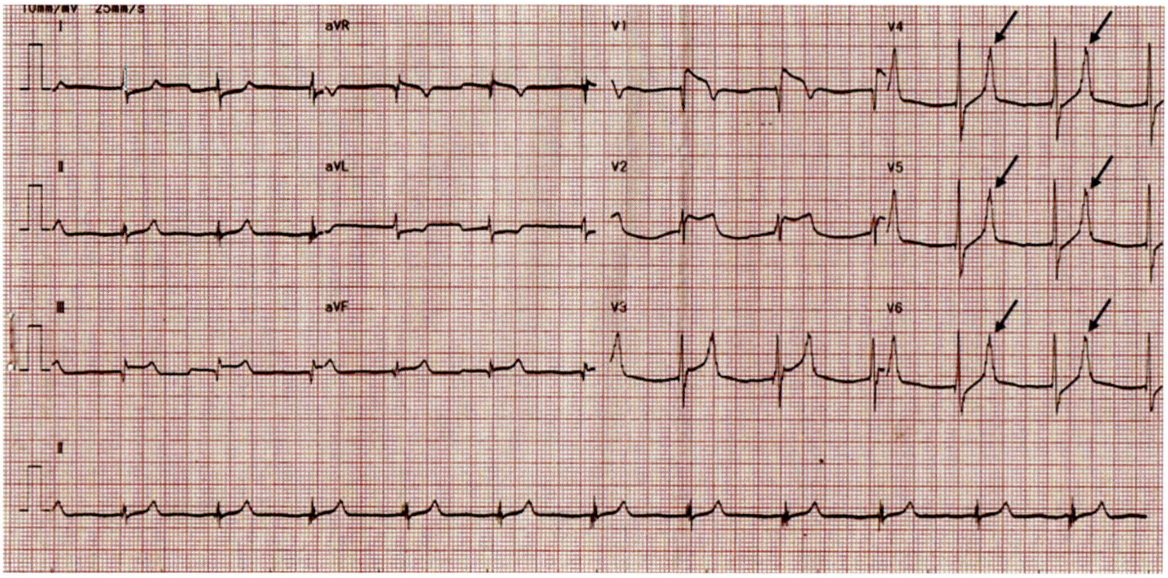

Fig. 3.21: Electrocardiogram shows tall peak (T amplitude >10 mm), narrow based, symmetric and pointed 'T' waves (*arrows*) in leads V4, V5 & V6 suggestive of early stage of hyperkalemia.

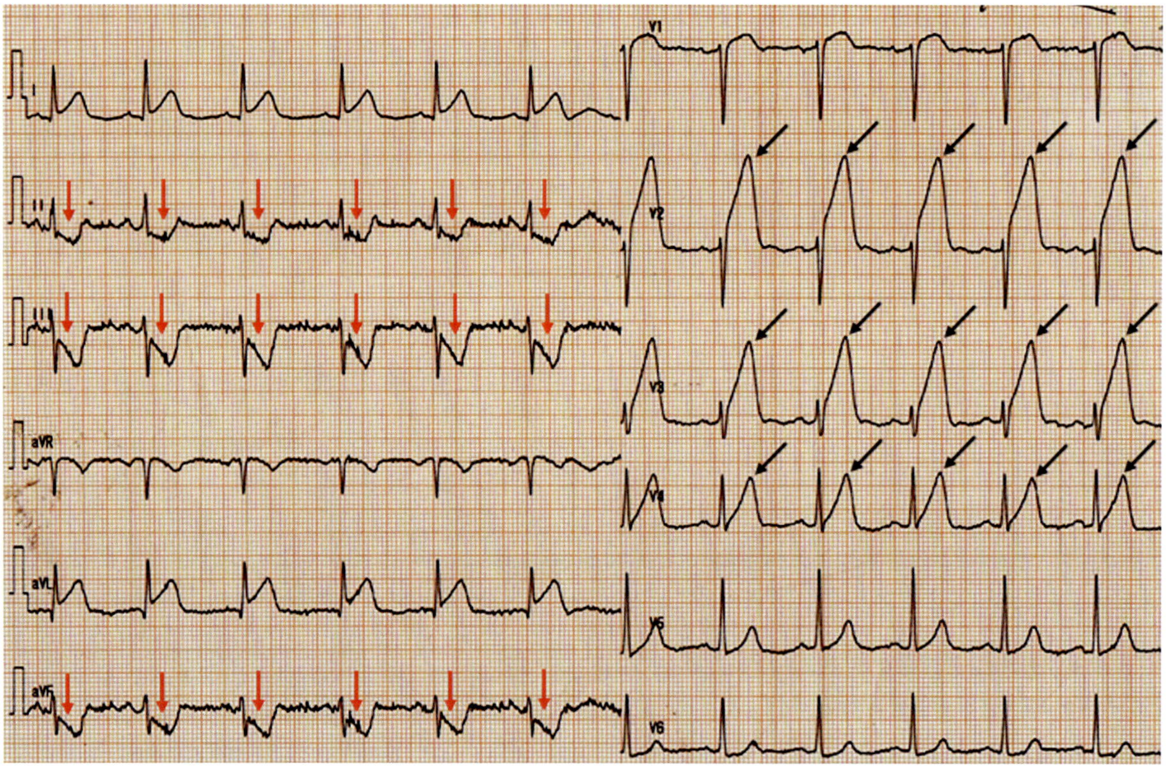

Fig. 3.22: Electrocardiogram shows broad based, asymmetrically peaked or 'hyperacute' T-waves (*black arrows*) in leads V2-V4 associated with reciprocal ST depression in inferior leads, LII,LIII & aVF (*red arrows*) suggestive of hyperacute anterior STEMI. But remember hyperacute T waves of STEMI are usually broad-based and symmetrical.

in V1 may be inverted normally at any age and in V2 it is sometimes normally negative.[16] T-wave inversion may be symmetrical or asymmetrical. The method of measuring the symmetry of the T-wave inversion is judged by assessing the ratio between the angle of descent (a) and the angle of ascent (b)[17] (Figs. 3.24 and 3.25). In general, inverted T waves related to acute coronary syndrome are symmetric in shape; this symmetry means that the downsloping limb is a mirror image of the upsloping limb and the angle of descent and the angle of ascent are almost same, so called arrowhead "T" wave (Fig. 3.26). T waves those are deep and symmetrically inverted strongly suggest myocardial ischemia (Figs. 3.27A and B). But T inversions due to ventricular hypertrophy or hypertrophic cardiomyopathy are usually asymmetrical (Figs. 3.28A and B).

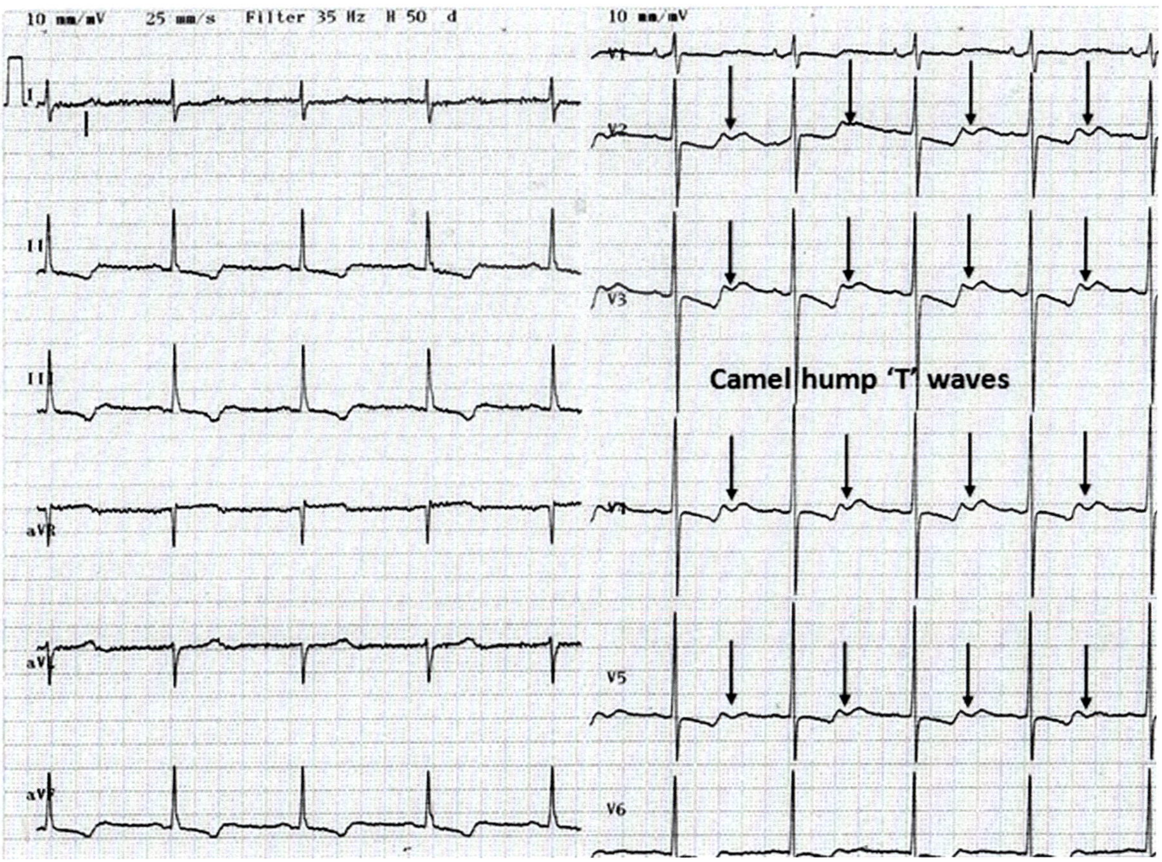

Fig. 3.23: Camel hump "T" waves showing double peak (*arrows*).

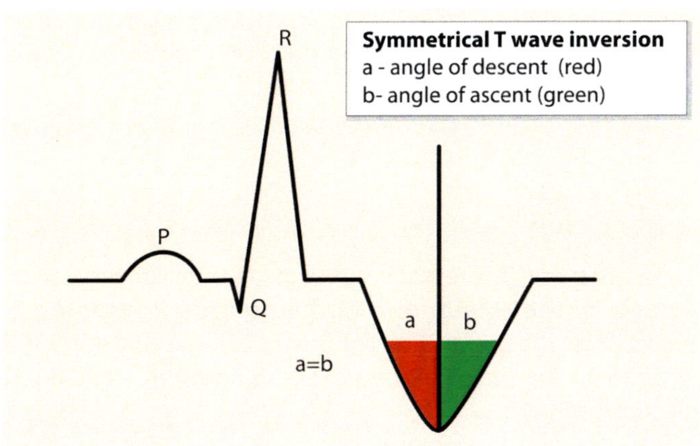

Fig. 3.24: Symmetrical "T" wave inversion. Angle (a) of descent (red) is equal to angle (b) of ascent (green).

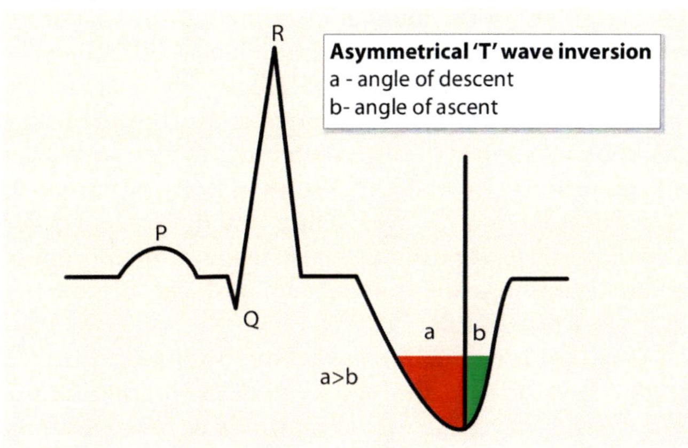

Fig. 3.25: Asymmetrical "T" wave inversion. Angle (a) of descent (red) is greater than angle (b) of ascent (green).

QT INTERVAL

The QT interval is measured from the start of the QRS complex to the end of the T-wave—the end of the T wave is defined as the point of return to the isoelectric line (Fig. 3.29). When a U wave is present, the QT interval is measured to the nadir of the curve between the T wave and U wave.[16]

- Represents the duration of activation and recovery of the ventricular myocardium, so it represents the time taken for ventricular depolarization and repolarization.
- In the normal adult, it should be between 0.35 seconds (350 ms) and 0.44 seconds (440 ms).
- A QT interval in excess of 0.44 seconds is a marker of myocardial electrical instability—prolongation of QT interval is associated with possible development of ventricular arrhythmia, syncope, and sudden death.[16]

The QT interval should be measured in either lead II or V5 to V6 (Fig. 3.30). Several successive beats should be measured, with the maximum interval taken. The QT shortens at faster HR. The QT lengthens at slower HR.

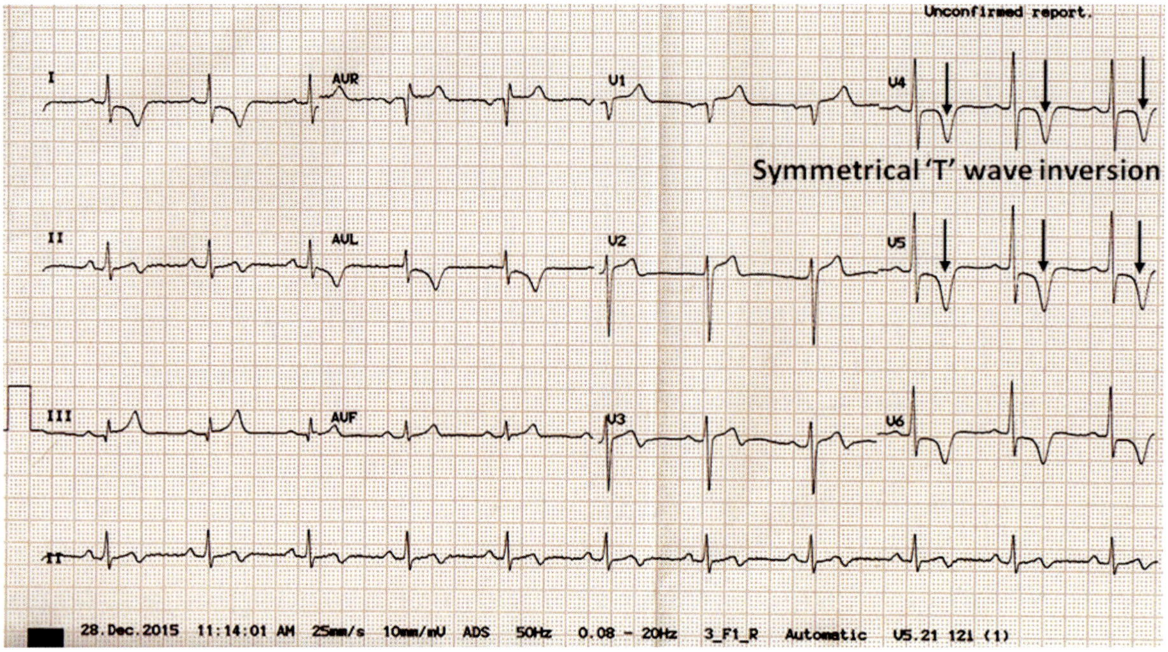

Fig. 3.26: Symmetrical "T" wave inversions (*arrows*), downsloping limb of each "T" wave is a mirror image of the upsloping limb.

Abnormally long and short QT intervals have been shown to be associated with an increased risk for life-threatening ventricular arrhythmias and sudden cardiac death.[17]

In the clinical setting, it is now widely recognized that typical measurement of the QT interval is subject to substantial variability, which can cloud interpretation.[18,19] This variability in QT interval measurement results from biological factors, such as diurnal effects, differences in autonomic tone, electrolytes, and drugs; technical factors, including the environment, the processing of the recording, and the acquisition of the ECG recording; and intraobserver and interobserver variability, resulting from variations in T-wave morphology, noisy baseline, and the presence of U waves. Interobserver variability also results from the lack of agreement among experts about standardizing approaches to measure the QT interval.[18-20]

Although it is standard practice to measure the QT interval from the beginning of the QRS complex to the end of the T wave, the actual methods of measurement have not been standardized. Because the QT interval is prolonged at slower HR and shortened at faster HR, many formulas have been proposed to adjust for these variations. Yet differences of opinion exist regarding the most useful correction for HR.[21-24] One of the commonly used formulas is the Bazett formula, in which the QT interval is adjusted for HR by dividing it by the square root of the R-R interval. However, this formula has been criticized for being inaccurate at fast HR.[25-27] Other formulas are the Fridericia cube-root correction (QT interval divided by the cube root of the R-R interval) and the Framingham linear regression equation.[20-22] From an epidemiological perspective, the Framingham approach is the most sound because it is based on empirical data from a large population sample rather than on hypothetical reasoning. Unfortunately, none of these corrections has been examined comparatively to determine the most effective formula in predicting which patients are at the greatest risk for torsades de pointes.[20]

Out of all the approaches Bazett's formula of QT interval determination is the most popular one (Fig. 3.31). According to this approach *corrected QT interval* (*QT_c*) is calculated by dividing the QT interval by the square root of the preceding R-R interval.

Bazett's formula is as follows:

$$QT_c = \frac{QT}{\sqrt{RR}}$$

Corrected QT interval is equal to QT interval in seconds divided by the square root of the preceding RR interval in seconds. RR is the interval from the onset of one QRS complex to the onset of the next QRS complex, measured in seconds.

Other formulas include:[24-25]

- *Fridericias formula*: $QT_c = QT/RR^{1/3}$
- *Framingham formula*: $QT_c = QT + 0.154\ (1 - RR)$
- *Hodges formula*: $QT_c = QT + 1.75\ (HR - 60)$.

Bazett's formula is the most commonly used due to its simplicity but it over-corrects at HR greater than 100 bpm and under-corrects at HR less than 60 bpm. This formula provides an adequate correction for HR ranging from 60 bpm to 100 bpm. At HR outside of the 60–100 bpm range, the Fridericia or Framingham corrections are more accurate.

Corrected QT interval is considered prolonged if it is greater than 0.44 seconds (440 ms) in men or greater than 0.46 seconds (460 ms) in women. QT_c greater than 0.50 seconds (500 ms) is associated with increased risk of torsades de pointes.

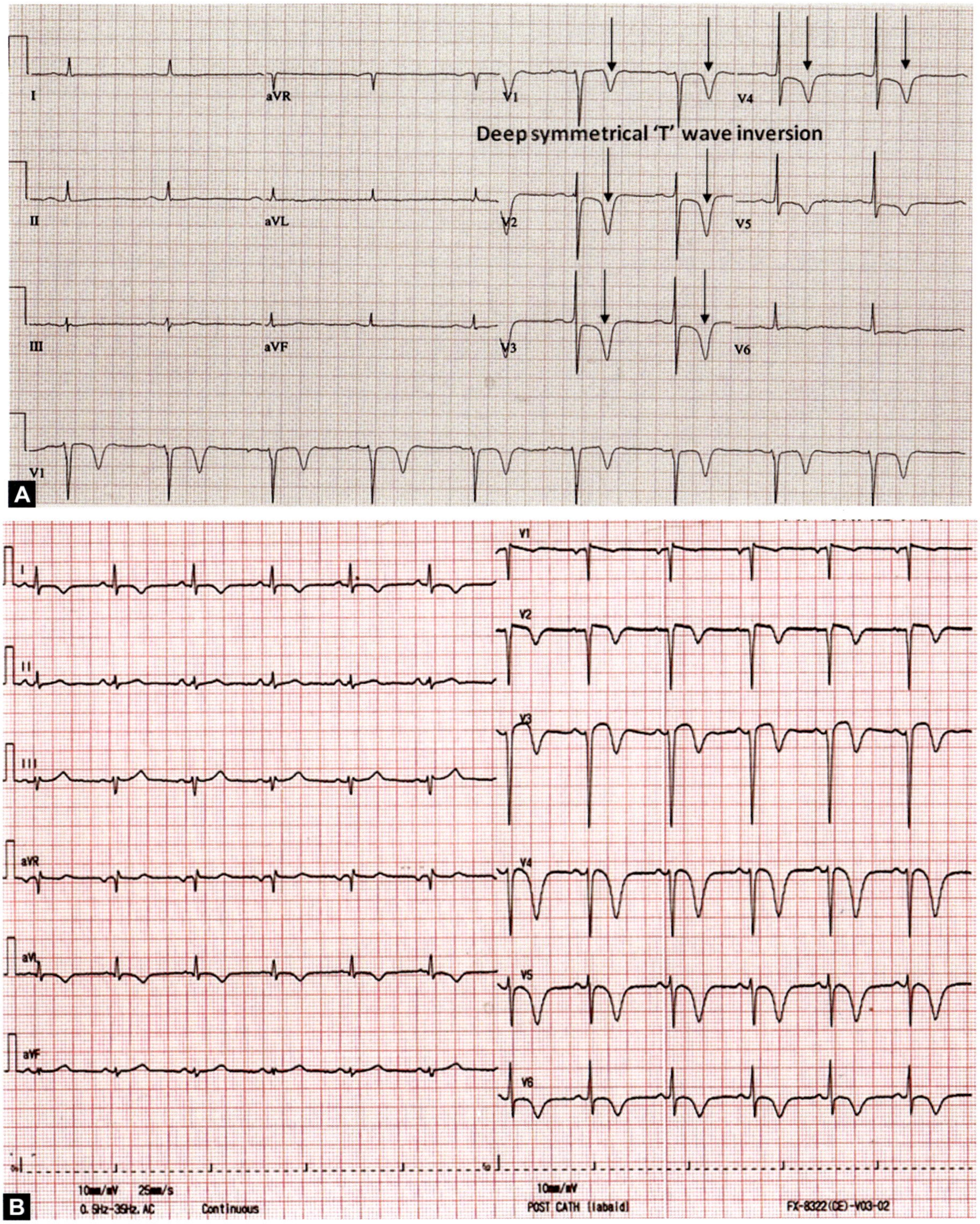

Figs. 3.27A and B: (A) Deep symmetrical "T" wave inversions in chest leads V1 to V4, suggestive of ischemic "T" waves (*arrows*). (B) Deep symmetrical "T" wave inversions in leads V4 to V6, suggestive of ischemic heart disease.

Causes of a Prolonged QT_c Greater than 0.44 Seconds (440 Milliseconds)

- Hypokalemia
- Hypomagnesemia
- Hypocalcemia
- Hypothermia
- Myocardial ischemia
- Postcardiac arrest
- Raised intracranial pressure
- Congenital long QT syndrome
- Drugs.

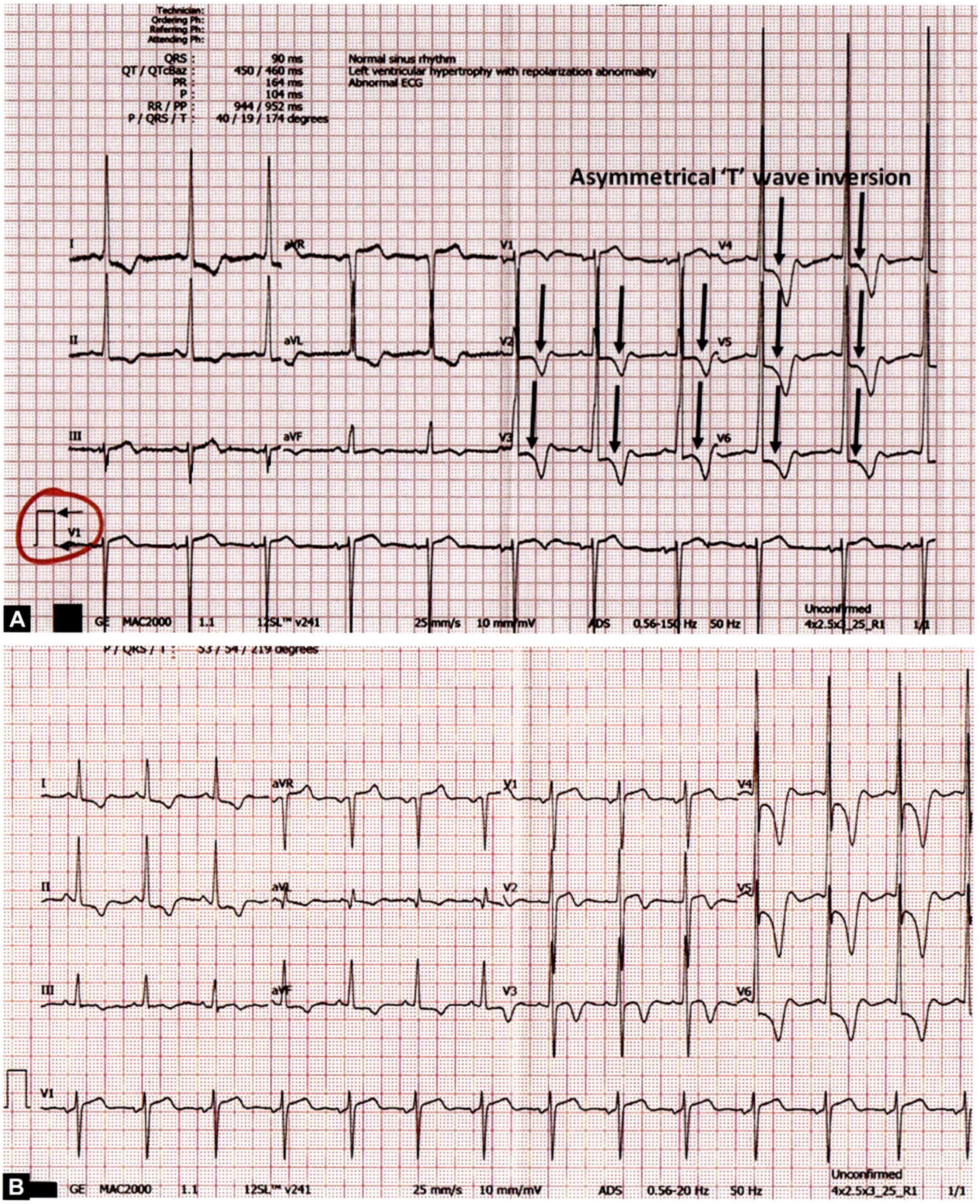

Figs. 3.28A and B: (A) Deep asymmetrical "T" wave inversions in chest leads V2 to V6 (*arrows*), suggestive of left ventricular hypertrophy or hypertrophic cardiomyopathy. (B) Deep asymmetrical "T" wave inversions in leads V4 to V6, suggestive of left ventricular hypertrophy.

Drugs Causing QT Prolongation[20,26,27]

Very Probable

- *Antiarrhythmics*
  - Amiodarone
  - Disopyramide
  - Dofetilide
  - Ibutilide
  - Quinidine
  - Sotalol
- *Antipsychotics*
  - Thioridazine

Probable

- *Antipsychotics*
  - Pimozide
  - Ziprasidone

Possible in High-risk Patients

- *Antiinfectives*
  - Clarithromycin
  - Erythromycin
  - Gatifloxacin
  - Pentamidine
  - Sparfloxacin
- *Antipsychotics*
  - Chlorpromazine
  - Haloperidol
  - Olanzapine
  - Risperidone
- *Antidepressants*
  - Amitriptyline
  - Desipramine
  - Imipramine
  - Sertraline
  - Venlafaxine.

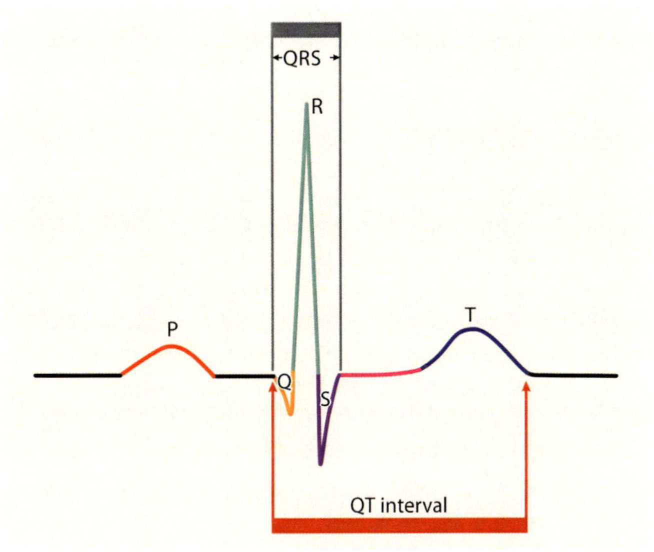

Fig. 3.29: QT interval measurement. QT interval is measured from the start of the QRS complex to the end of the T wave (*red arrows*).

Causes of a Short QT_c Less Than 0.35 Seconds (Less Than 350 Milliseconds)

- Hyperkalemia
- Hypercalcemia
- Hyperthermia
- Acidosis
- Effects of drugs such as digitalis
- Effect of catecholamine.

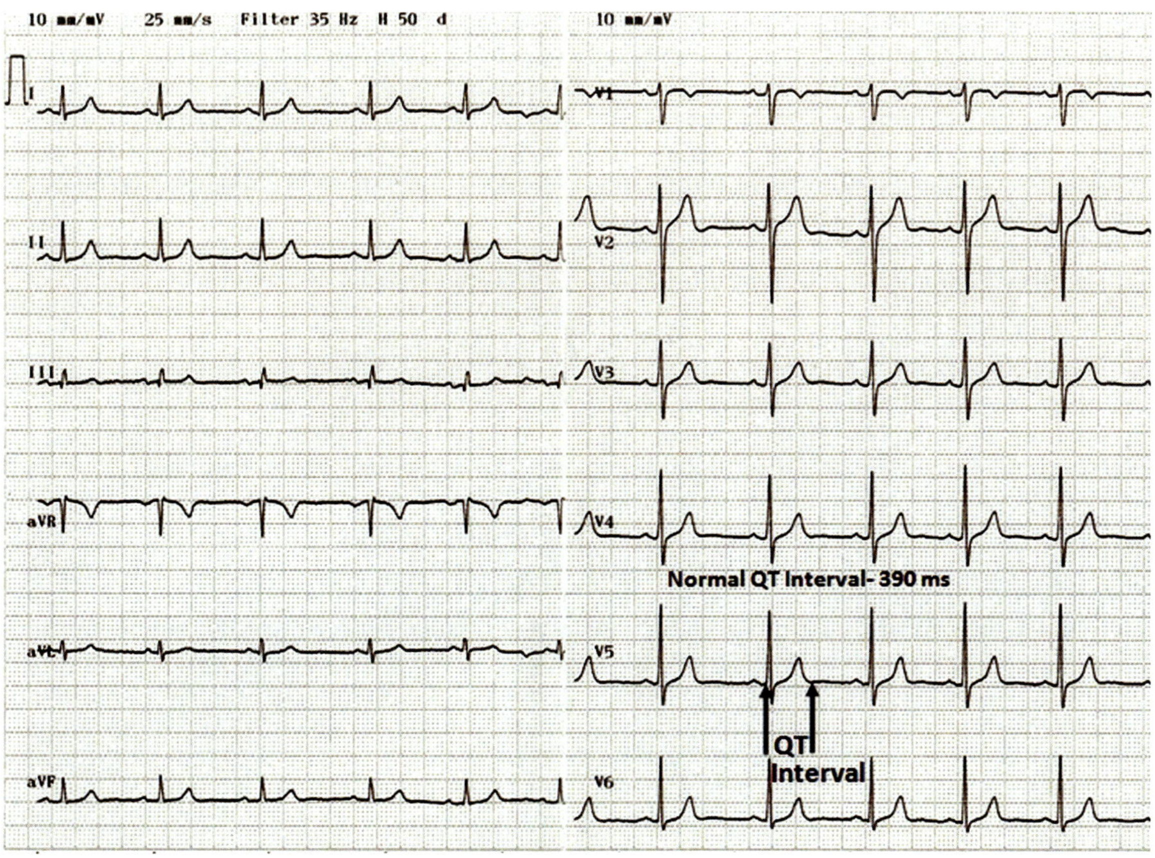

Fig. 3.30: Normal QT interval. In this ECG, QT interval is normal (390 ms).

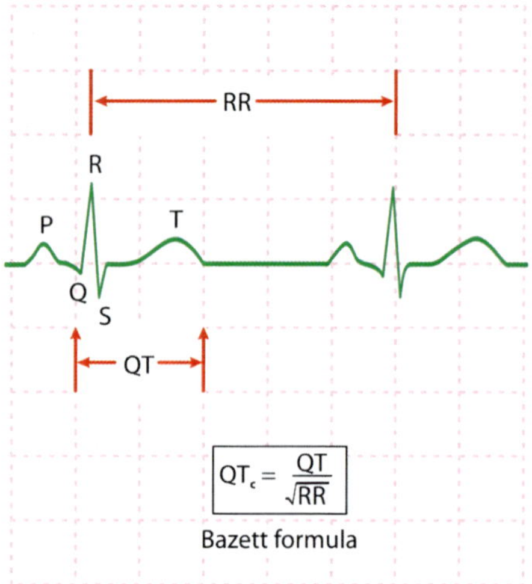

Fig. 3.31: Bazett's formula for calculating QT interval. According to this approach, corrected QT interval (QTc) is calculated by dividing the QT interval by the square root of the RR interval.

U WAVE

U wave is the most neglected of the ECG waveforms. The U wave is a wave on an ECG that is not always seen. This wave could normally be seen in younger, athletic individuals. It is typically small and, by definition, follows the T wave (Fig. 3.5A). U wave was thought to represent repolarization of the papillary muscles or Purkinje fibers.

- U-wave amplitude is usually less than one-third of T-wave amplitude in same lead.
- U-wave direction is the same as T-wave direction in that lead.
- U waves are more prominent at slow HR and usually best seen in the right precordial leads.
- Origin of the U wave is thought to be related to after depolarizations which interrupt or follow repolarization.

The significance of this wave and the reason for its inconstancy are not known with surety. Today a satisfactory explanation of its origin is still outstanding despite the U-wave's well-known clinical relevance in conditions like cooling, electrolyte disturbances, and drug-induced or congenital long-QT syndromes.[28] Three hypotheses are being entertained about the underlying mechanism. They are based on: (1) the tardy repolarization of the subendocardial Purkinje fibers; (2) the prolonged repolarization reported to exist in the cells of the mid-myocardium (M cells); and (3) after-potentials, possibly caused by mechanical forces in the ventricular wall. However, none of these hypotheses has received general acceptance.[28-30]

U wave is usually most prominent in leads V2 and V3. U wave usually appears larger in amplitude during slower HR and may merge with the following P wave during faster HR.

Causes of Prominent U waves

Prominent U waves are most often seen in hypokalemia, but may be present in hypercalcemia, thyrotoxicosis, or exposure to digitalis, epinephrine, and Class 1A and 3 antiarrhythmics, as well as in congenital long QT syndrome, and in the setting of intracranial hemorrhage. An inverted U wave may represent myocardial ischemia or left ventricular volume overload.[31,32]

TP SEGMENT

The portion of the ECG from the end of the T wave to the beginning of the P wave is termed as TP segment (Fig. 3.5A). This segment should always be at baseline and is used as a reference to see if the ST segment is elevated or depressed since there are no specific disease conditions which elevate or depress the TP segment. During states of tachycardia the TP segment is shortened and may be difficult to visualize altogether. It is good to examine the TP segment closely for the presence of U waves or atrial activity that could indicate pathology.[33-35]

Calculation of Heart Rate

The ECG paper which moves at a speed of 25 mm/sec moves 60 × 25 = 1,500 mm/min. Heart rate is the number of cardiac cycles per minute or more correctly the number of times the heart beats per minute.

The ECG is recorded on to standard paper travelling at a rate of 25 mm/sec. The paper is divided into large squares, each measuring 5 mm wide and equivalent to 0.2 seconds (200 ms). Each large square is five small squares in width, and each small square is 1 mm wide and equivalent to 0.04 seconds (40 ms).

Electrocardiogram paper is a grid where time is measured along the horizontal axis.

- Each small square is 1 mm in length and represents 0.04 seconds.
- Each larger square is 5 mm in length and represents 0.2 seconds.

Voltage is measured along the vertical axis.

- 10 mm is equal to 1 mV in voltage.

There are different short-cut methods that can be used to calculate rate, all of which assume a recording speed of 25 mm/sec.

One method is to divide 1,500 by the number of small squares between two R waves. For example, if the number of small squares in between two R waves is 15 then the HR will be 100 bpm (1,500 ÷ 15 = 100) (Fig. 3.32). Another method, which gives a rough approximation, is the "count off" method. Simply count the number of large squares between two R waves and divide 300 by the large square number. For example, if there are two large squares between two R waves, then the rate is 150 bpm,

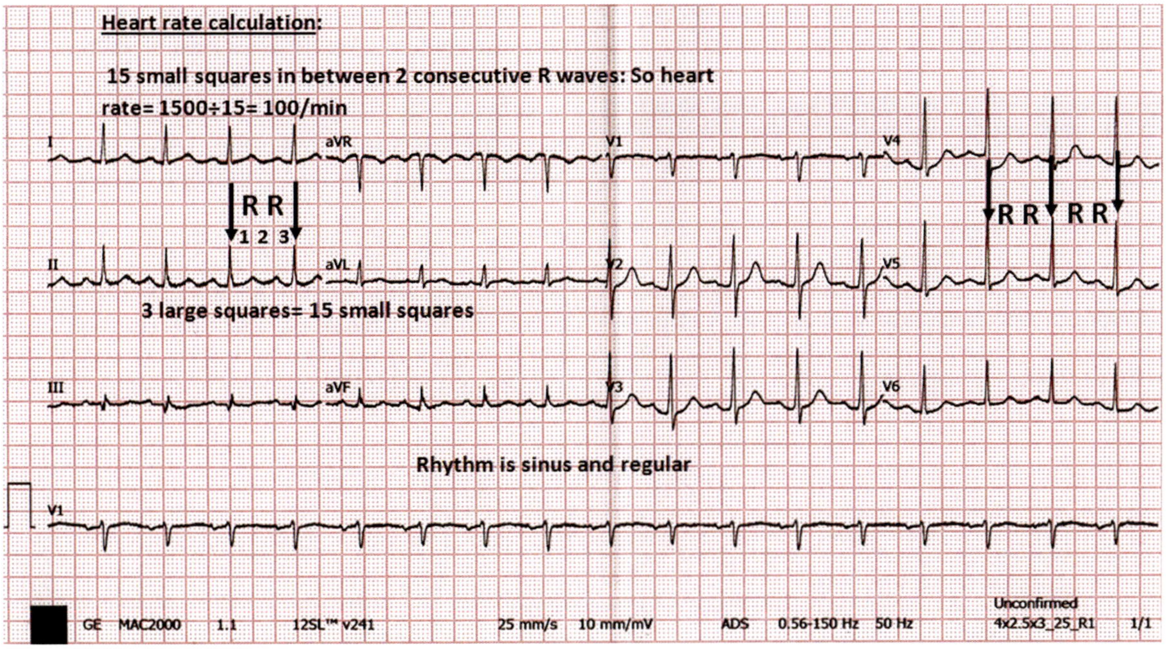

Fig. 3.32: Heart rate calculation by 1,500 small squares method. If rhythm is regular then divide 1,500 by the number of small squares between two R waves. In this ECG, 15 small squares are present in between two R waves, so heart rate = 1,500 ÷ 15 = 100 beats/min.

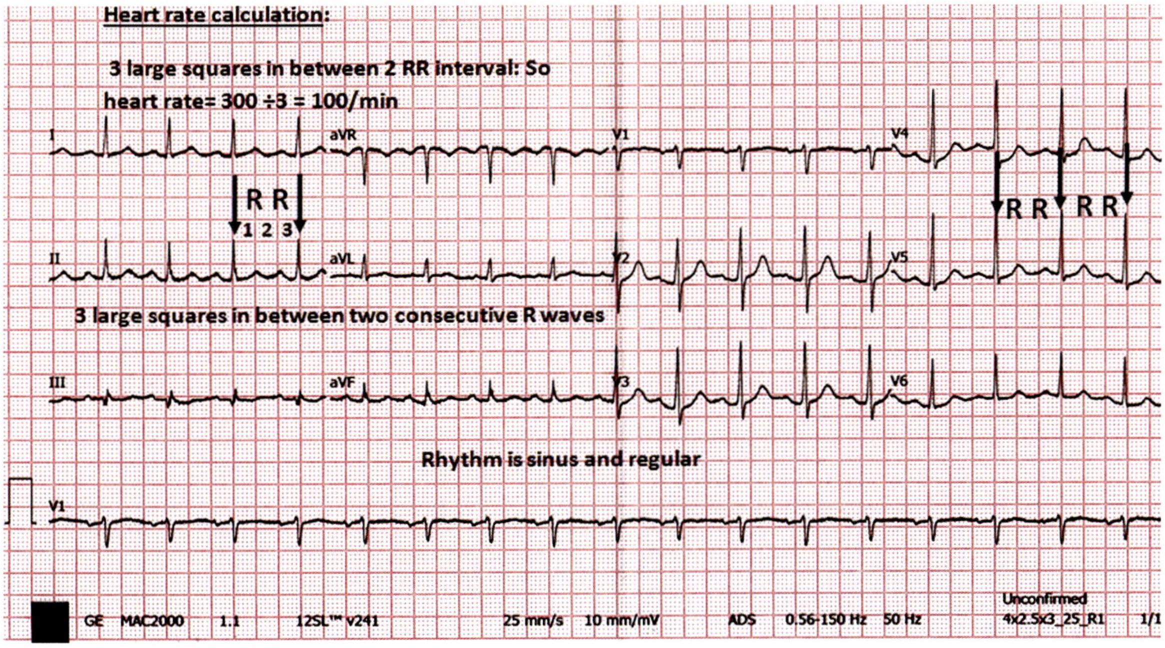

Fig. 3.33: Heart rate calculation by 300 large squares method. If rhythm is regular then divide 300 by the number of large squares between two R waves. In this ECG, three large squares are present in between two R waves, so heart rate = 300 ÷ 3 = 100 beats/min.

if there are three large squares between R waves, then the rate is 100 bpm (Fig. 3.33), and if there are four large boxes between R waves then the rate is 75 bpm. Atrial rate can be determined like the ventricular rate, but using the P waves. Remember, if the heart is in sinus rhythm and there is a one-to-one correspondence between P waves and QRS complex, then the atrial rate will be the same as ventricular rate.

But in presence of irregularly irregular QRS complexes, e.g. atrial fibrillation (AF) the above-mentioned methods are not valid. Using those two methods to determine HR would not be accurate since the R-R intervals vary significantly in AF. In this situation, the best way to determine the HR would be to simply count the QRS complexes for 6 seconds (30 large squares) in rhythm strip and multiple by 10 (Fig. 3.34).

So, heart rate can be calculated by using the following standard formulas (Box 3.1).

Box 3.1: Standard formulas for calculating heart rate.

1. 300 ÷ Number of large squares between two consecutive R waves
2. 1,500 ÷ Number of small squares between two consecutive R waves
3. If rhythm is irregular then use 6-second strip. Count the number of QRS complexes in 6 seconds (30 large squares) and then multiply the number by 10 (6 seconds × 10 = 60 seconds = 1 minute).

The normal human HR ranges from 60 bpm to 100 bpm. Sinus bradycardia refers to a slow HR, defined as below 60 bpm. Tachycardia refers to a fast HR, defined as above 100 bpm. When the heart is not beating in a regular pattern, this is referred to as an arrhythmia. These abnormalities of HR sometimes, but not always, indicate disease.

Sinus Bradycardia (Fig. 3.35)

Sinus bradycardia occurs in normal children and adults, particularly during sleep, which is regarded physiological when rates may transiently drop as low as of 30 bpm and pauses of up to 2 seconds are not uncommon.[34-36] It may

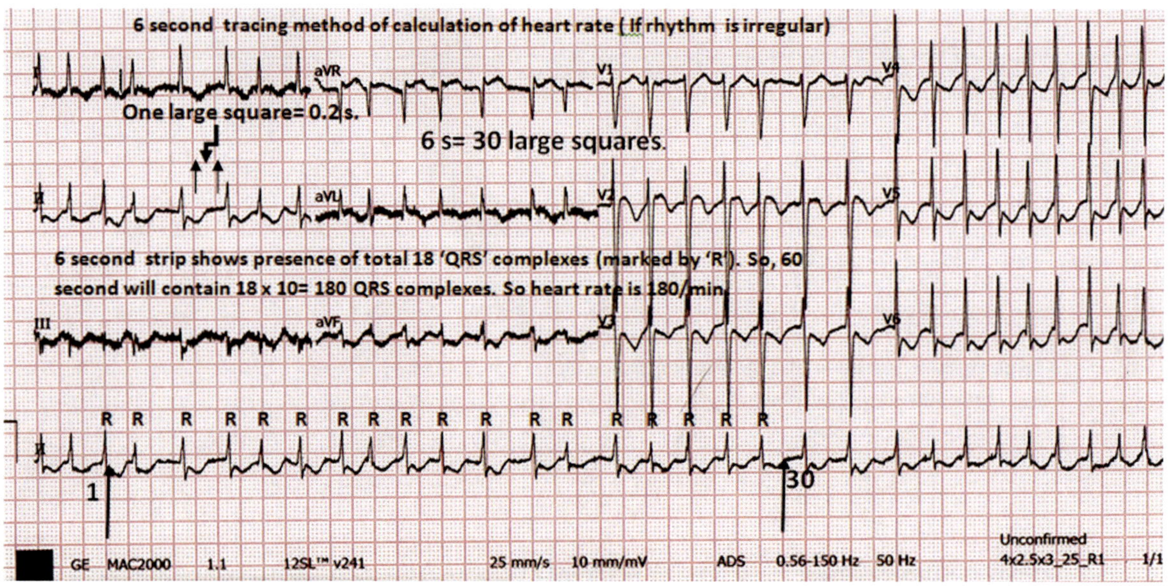

Fig. 3.34: Calculation of heart rate if rhythm is irregular (6 sec tracing method). ECG shows fast atrial fibrillation (AF). Six seconds ECG strip contains 18 QRS complexes. So, 1 minute (60 s) will contain 18 × 10 = 180 QRS complexes. So, in this ECG strip heart rate is 180 beats/min.

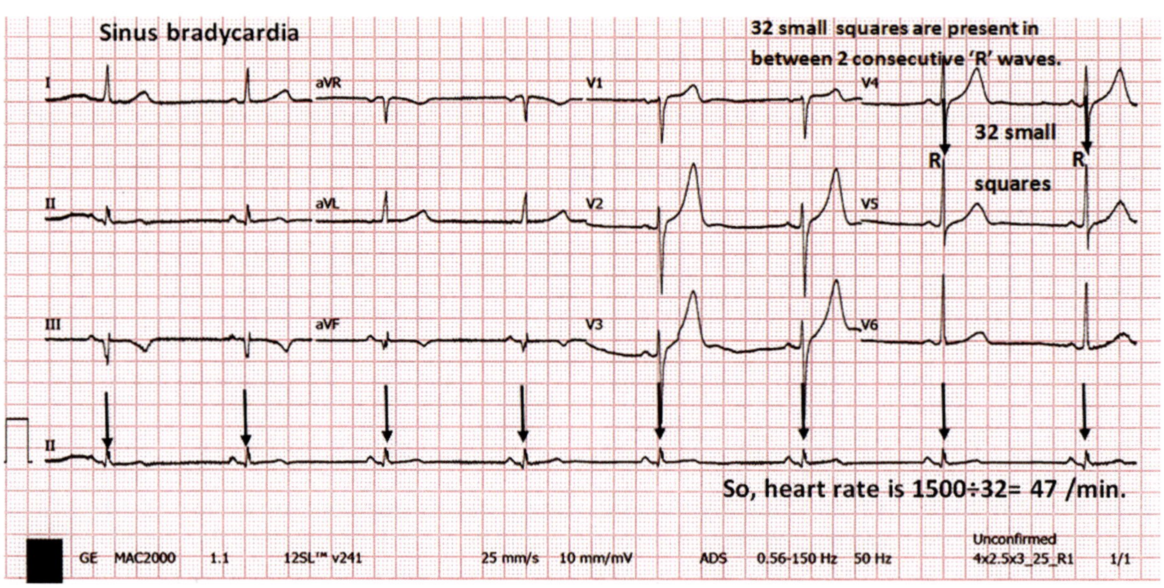

Fig. 3.35: Electrocardiogram shows sinus bradycardia. Thirty-two small squares are present in between two consecutive R waves. So, heart rate is 1,500 ÷ 32 = 47 beats/min (approx.).

also be seen in the absence of heart disease in the following settings[37-39]

- At rest, in 25–35% of asymptomatic individuals under 25 years of age.
- Athletes
- In some elderly patients
- Familial
- Hypothermia
- Hypothyroidism
- Vasovagal reaction
- Jaundice
- Raised intracranial pressure
- Electrolyte imbalance, e.g. hyperkalemia.

Sinus bradycardia may be the manifestation of intrinsic disease of the sinoatrial (SA) node (e.g. sick sinus syndrome). But commonly sinus bradycardia is caused by medication or by coronary artery disease. Digitalis, beta-blockers, quinidine, adenosine, calcium channel blockers diltiazem or verapamil frequently causes sinus bradycardia. There is no prognostic significance to sinus bradycardia in otherwise healthy subjects.

Sinus Tachycardia (Fig. 3.36)

The most common causes of sinus tachycardia are the normal response to exercise and conditions in which catecholamine release is physiologically enhanced: flight, fright, anger, or stress. A long list of other factors may be responsible in selected cases including:

- Fever
- Hyperthyroidism
- Hypotension with shock
- Anxiety
- Pheochromocytoma
- Sepsis
- Anemia
- Acute coronary syndrome
- Pulmonary embolism
- Rheumatic carditis
- Heart failure
- Chronic pulmonary disease
- Hypoxia
- Exposure to stimulants (nicotine and caffeine) or illicit drugs
- Tea and drinking
- Pregnancy.

SUMMARY

The diagnosis of the normal ECG is made by excluding any recognized abnormality. ECG must be interpreted along with history and clinical examination. A single normal ECG is not enough to exclude significant coronary artery disease. In presence of clinical suspicion serial ECGs are more important. Dynamic ECG changes are more significant than the permanent ECG abnormality.

Waves of the normal 12-Lead Electrocardiogram

P Wave

P wave is the first positive deflection on the ECG and it represents atrial depolarization. Each P wave is followed by a QRS complex. P wave is usually of smooth contour and monophasic in lead II and biphasic in V1.

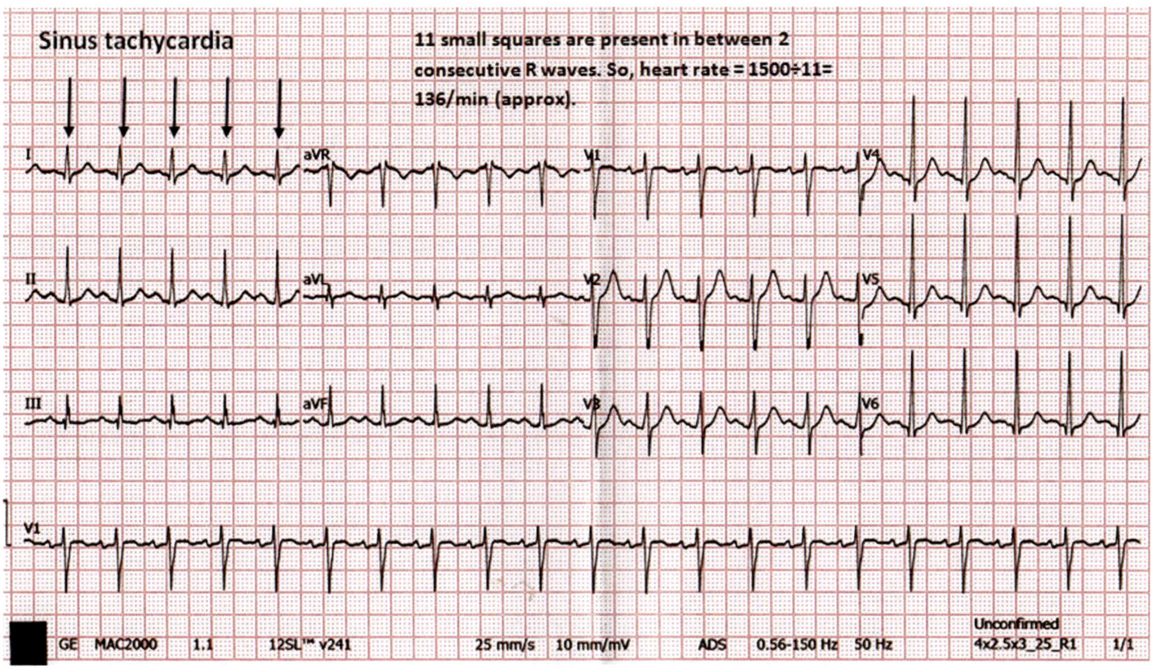

Fig. 3.36: Electrocardiogram shows sinus tachycardia. Eleven small squares are present in between two consecutive R waves. So, heart rate is 1,500 ÷ 11 = 136 beats/min (approx.).

Normal P waves:

- Height less than 2.5 mm
- Width less than 0.12 seconds (120 ms)

Tall or biphasic P waves are seen in atrial hypertrophy.

Normal PR interval: 0.12–0.20 seconds = 120–200 ms (3–5 small squares).

The PR interval is the period, measured, that extends from the beginning of the P wave (the onset of atrial depolarization) until the beginning of the QRS complex (the onset of ventricular depolarization). The PR interval varies with the HR, being shorter at faster rates when sympathetic component predominates, and vice versa. The PR interval tends to increase with age.

For short PR interval consider Wolff–Parkinson–White syndrome or Lown–Ganong–Levine syndrome.

For long PR interval consider the possibility of acute MI, particularly acute inferior wall MI, myocarditis, and electrolytes disturbance. Possibility of drug-induced prolongation of PR interval must be excluded by proper history.

PR segment: The PR segment is the flat, usually isoelectric segment between the end of the P wave and the start of the QRS complex. Remember that segments are different than intervals.

PR segment abnormalities occur in two main conditions:

1. Pericarditis
2. Atrial ischemia.

Q Wave

Small Q waves are normal in most leads. Deeper Q waves (greater than 2 mm) may be seen in leads III and aVR as a normal variant. Normally, Q waves are not seen in the right-sided leads (V1 to V3).

Characteristics of pathological Q waves include:

1. Greater than 0.04 seconds (40 ms) wide
2. Greater than 2 mm deep
3. Greater than 25% of depth of the corresponding R wave.

Normal QRS complex: Less than 0.10 seconds (less than 100 ms), usually less than 3 small squares.

For abnormally wide QRS consider right or left bundle branch block, ventricular ectopics, hyperkalemia, etc.

QT Interval

The QT interval is the time from the start of the Q wave to the end of the T wave. It represents the time taken for ventricular depolarization and repolarization. The QT interval should be measured in either lead II or V5 to V6. Several successive beats should be measured, with the maximum interval taken.

Normal QT interval: Calculate the QT_c dividing the QT interval by the square root of the preceding R-R interval. Normal QT interval in adult should be between 0.35 seconds and 0.44 seconds (350–440 ms).

Corrected QT interval is considered prolonged if it is greater than 0.44 seconds (440 ms) in men or greater than 0.46 seconds (460 ms) in women. QT_c greater than 0.50 seconds (500 ms) is associated with increased risk of torsades de pointes.

Bazett's formula is still considered as the standard way to calculate QT_c.

Bazett's formula:

$$QT_c = QT / \sqrt{(\text{RR in seconds})}$$

QT_c is equal to QT interval in seconds divided by the square root of the preceding RR interval in seconds.

Causes of long QT interval are:

- Myocardial infarction, myocarditis, and diffuse myocardial disease
- Hypokalemia, hypomagnesemia, hypocalcemia, and hypothermia
- Hypothyroidism
- Subarachnoid hemorrhage and intracerebral hemorrhage
- Drugs (e.g. sotalol and amiodarone)
- Hereditary.
  - Romano–Ward syndrome (autosomal dominant)
  - Jervell and Lange-Nielsen syndrome (autosomal recessive) associated with sensorineural deafness.

Normal ST Segment

Normally no elevation or depression.

An ST elevation is considered significant if the elevation is greater than 1 mm or 1 small square in a limb lead or 2 mm or two small squares in a precordial lead. Significant ST depression is defined as depression of the ST segment level greater than 0.1 mV (1.0 mm) compared with the baseline.

- Causes of ST segment elevation include acute MI (e.g. anterior and inferior), left bundle branch block, normal variants (e.g. athletic heart, Edeiken pattern, high-take off), and acute pericarditis.
- Causes of depression include myocardial ischemia, digoxin effect, ventricular hypertrophy, acute posterior MI, pulmonary embolus, and left bundle branch block.

Normal T Wave

The T wave reflects ventricular repolarization. This is the most labile wave in the ECG. T waves do not normally exceed 5 mm in limb leads or greater than 10 mm in any precordial leads.

- Causes of tall T waves include hyperkalemia, hyperacute MI, and left bundle branch block.
- Causes of small, flattened or inverted T waves are numerous and include ischemia, age, race, hyper-

ventilation, anxiety, drinking iced water, LVH, drugs (e.g. digoxin), pericarditis, intraventricular conduction delay (e.g. RBBB), and electrolyte disturbance.

T wave inversion in lead III is a normal variant. New T-wave inversion (compared with prior ECGs) is always abnormal. Pathological T-wave inversion is usually deep (greater than 3 mm) but may be symmetrical or asymmetrical.

Inverted T waves are mostly seen in ischemia and hypertrophy of the ventricles. Biphasic T waves are mostly seen in myocardial ischemia and hypokalemia. In general, inverted T waves related to acute coronary syndrome are symmetric in shape; this symmetry means that the downsloping limb is a mirror image of the upsloping limb. T waves those are deep and symmetrically inverted (arrowhead) strongly suggest myocardial ischemia. T inversions due to ventricular hypertrophy or hypertrophic cardiomyopathy are usually asymmetrical. Tall, narrow, symmetrically peaked T waves are characteristically seen in hyperkalemia. Broad, asymmetrically peaked or "hyperacute" T waves are sometimes seen in the early stages of STEMI and often precede the appearance of ST elevation and Q waves.

Normal U Wave

The U wave is a wave on an ECG that is not always seen. But when present this wave is usually best seen in the right precordial leads and smaller than the amplitude of the T wave. U-wave direction is the same as T-wave direction in that lead. U waves are more prominent at slow HR and usually best seen in the right precordial leads.

Prominent U waves are most often seen in hypokalemia. An inverted U wave may represent myocardial ischemia or left ventricular volume overload.

Determination of Heart Rate From Electrocardiogram

The ECG paper is usually heat sensitive. The smallest division on the paper is a 1 mm box. The largest division on the paper is a 5 mm box. By international convention, the speed of the paper moves at a rate of 25 mm/sec past the stylus. Because the speed of the paper is 25 mm/sec, a small 1 mm box is traversed in 0.04 seconds (40 ms) and a large 5 mm box is traversed in 0.2 seconds (200 ms). Because of the predictable ECG paper speed, we can count the number of boxes traversed over a period of time between heart beats to determine HR.

Method 1: The 300 Method

If the HR is regular, count the number of large boxes/squares between two "R" waves and divide this number into 300 to obtain the HR/min.

Example: If there were 2.5 large boxes/squares between two successive "R" waves, then the HR would be: 300 ÷ 2.5 large boxes = 120 bpm.

Method 2: The 1,500 Method

If the HR is regular, count the number of small boxes/squares between two "R" waves and divide this number into 1,500 to obtain the HR/min.

Example: If there were 12.5 small boxes between two successive "R" waves, then the HR would be: 1,500 ÷ 12.5 small boxes = 120 bpm.

Method 3: The Six Second Tracing Method

This method is valuable if the HR is irregular particularly in presence of AF.

Obtain a 6-second tracing (30 large 5 mm boxes) and count the number of "R" waves that appear within that 6-second period and multiply by 10 to obtain the HR/min.

Example: If there are 12 "R" waves in the 6-second tracing then the HR would be: 12 × 10 = 120 bpm.

Methods 1 and 2 are applicable if the HR is regular and method 3 is applicable if HR is irregular.

Sinus bradycardia is a common condition found in young healthy individual, during sleep and also among athletes. Noncardiac causes like hypothermia, hypothyroidism, and hyperkalemia may also cause sinus bradycardia. It can be a manifestation of sick sinus syndrome, acute coronary syndrome or may be drug induced.

Physiological sinus tachycardia is very common, and many factors affect HR, such as postural changes, physical activity, food digestion, emotional anxiety, pregnancy, excitement, fear, drinking, smoking, tea, etc. Pathologic systemic diseases, such as: high fever, anemia, hypoxia, infections, hyperthyroidism, pain, acute rheumatic fever, beriberi, and neurosis can cause tachycardia. Cardiac causes like acute MI, hypotension and shock, heart failure, myocarditis, cardiomyopathy, pericarditis, etc., can result in sinus tachycardia.

REFERENCES

1. Wagner GS, Strauss DG. Marriott's Practical Electrocardiography, 12th edition. Philadelphia, PA: Lippincott Williams & Wilkins; 2013.
2. Bennett DH. Cardiac Arrhythmias, 4th edition. Oxford: Butterworth-Heinemann Ltd.; 1993.
3. Aro AL, Anttonen O, Kerola T, et al. Prognostic significance of prolonged PR interval in the general population. Eur Heart J. 2014;35(2):123-9.
4. John AD, Fleisher LA. Electrocardiography: the ECG. Anesthesiol Clin. 2006;24(4):697-715.
5. Barold SS, Ilercil A, Leonelli F, et al. First-degree atrioventricular block. Clinical manifestations, indications for pacing, pacemaker management and consequences during cardiac resynchronization. J Interv Card Electrophysiol. 2006;17(2):139-52.
6. Berger PB, Ruocco NA, Ryan TJ, et al. Incidence and prognostic implications of heart block complicating inferior myocardial infarction treated with thrombolytic therapy: results from TIMI II. J Am Coll Cardiol. 1992;20(3): 533-40.

7. Kulig J, Koplan BA. Wolff-Parkinson-White syndrome and accessory pathways. Circulation. 2010;122:e480-3.
8. Mark DG, Brady WJ, Pines JM. Preexcitation syndromes: diagnostic consideration in the ED. Am J Emerg Med. 2009;27(7):878-88.
9. Eisenberger M, Davidson NC, Todd DM, et al. A new approach to confirming or excluding ventricular pre-excitation on a 12-lead ECG. Europace. 2010;12(1):119-23.
10. Goldberger AL. Clinical Electrocardiography: A Simplified Approach, 7th edition. St. Louis, MO: Mosby; 2006.
11. Mirvis DM, Goldberger AL. Electrocardiography. In: Bonow RO, Mann DL, Zipes DP, Libby P (Eds). Braunwald's Heart Disease: A Textbook of Cardiovascular Medicine, 9th edition. Philadelphia, PA: W.B. Saunders Company; 2011.
12. Delewi R, Ijff G, van de Hoef TP, et al. Pathological Q waves in myocardial infarction in patients treated by primary PCI. JACC Cardiovasc Imaging. 2013;6(3):324-31.
13. Junttila MJ, Sager SJ, Tikkanen JT, et al. Clinical significance of variants of J-points and J-waves: early repolarization patterns and risk. Eur Heart J. 2012;33(21):2639-43.
14. Brownfield J, Herbert M. EKG criteria for fibrinolysis: what's up with the J point? West J Emerg Med. 2008;9(1) 40-2.
15. Hanna EB, Glancy DL. ST-segment depression and T-wave inversion: Classification, differential diagnosis, and caveats. Cleve Clin J Med. 2011;78(6):404-14.
16. Said SAM, Bloo R, de Nooijer R, et al. Cardiac and non-cardiac causes of T-wave inversion in the precordial leads in adult subjects: A Dutch case series and review of the literature. World J Cardiol. 2015;7(2):86-100.
17. Short D, Weir J. Significance of asymmetrically inverted T wave. Br Heart J. 1983;49(6):564-7.
18. Barr CS, Naas A, Freeman M, et al. QT dispersion and sudden unexpected death in chronic heart failure. Lancet. 1994;343(8893):327-9.
19. Goldenberg I, Moss AJ, Zareba W. QT interval: how to measure it and what is "normal". J Cardiovasc Electrophysiol. 2006;17(3):333-6.
20. Morganroth J, Brozovich FV, McDonald JT, et al. Variability of the QT measurement in healthy men, with implications for selection of an abnormal QT value to predict drug toxicity and proarrhythmia. Am J Cardiol. 1991;67(8):774-6.
21. Molnar J, Zhang F, Weiss J, et al. Diurnal pattern of QT_c interval: how long is prolonged? possible relation to circadian triggers of cardiovascular events. J Am Coll Cardiol. 1996;27(1):76-83.
22. Al-Khatib SM, LaPointe NMA, Kramer JM, et al. What Clinicians Should Know About the QT Interval. JAMA. 2003;289(16):2120-7.
23. Funck-Brentano C, Jaillon P. Rate-corrected QT interval: techniques and limitations. Am J Cardiol. 1993;72(6):17B-22B.
24. Hodges M, Salerno D, Erlien D. Bazett's QT correction reviewed. Evidence that a linear QT correction for heart is better. J Am Coll Cardiol. 1983;1(2):694.
25. Sagie A, Larson MG, Goldberg RJ, et al. An improved method for adjusting the QT interval for heart rate (the Framingham Heart Study). Am J Cardiol. 1992;70:797-801.
26. Malik M. Problems of heart rate correction in assessment of drug-induced QT interval prolongation. J Cardiovasc Electrophysiol. 2001;12(4):411-20.
27. Milne JR, Ward DE, Spurrell RA, et al. The ventricular paced QT interval: the effects of rate and exercise. Pacing Clin Electrophysiol. 1982;5(3):352-8.
28. van Eck HJR, Kors JA, van Herpen G. The U wave in the electrocardiogram: A solution for a 100-year-old riddle. Cardiovasc Res. 2005;67(2):256-62.
29. Di Bernardo D, Murray A. Origin on the electrocardiogram of U-waves and abnormal U-wave inversion. Cardiovasc Res. 2002;53:202-8.
30. Wu J, Wu J, Zipes DP. Early after depolarisations, U waves, and torsade de pointes. Circulation. 2002;105(6): 675-6.
31. Perez Riera AR, Ferreira C, Filho CF, et al. The enigmatic sixth wave of the electrocardiogram: the U wave. Cardiol J. 2008;15(5):408-21.
32. Conrath C, Opthof T. The patient U wave. Cardiovasc Res. 2005;67(2):184-6.
33. Rautaharju PM, Surawicz B, Gettes LS, et al. AHA/ACCF/HRS recommendations for the standardization and interpretation of the Electrocardiogram. Part IV: the ST segment, T and U Waves, and the QT interval: a scientific statement from the American Heart Association Electrocardiography and Arrhythmias Committee, Council on Clinical Cardiology; the American College of Cardiology Foundation; and the Heart Rhythm Society. Endorsed by the International Society for Computerized Electrocardiology. Circulation. 2009;119(10):e241-50.
34. Scott O, Williams GJ, Fiddler GI. Results of 24 hour ambulatory monitoring of electrocardiogram in 131 healthy boys aged 10 to 13 years. Br Heart J. 1980;44(3):304-8.
35. Bjerregaard P. Mean 24 hour heart rate, minimal heart rate and pauses in healthy subjects 40-79 years of age. Eur Heart J. 1983;4(1):44-51.
36. Hilgard J, Ezri MD, Denes P. Significance of ventricular pauses of three seconds or more detected on twenty-four-hour Holter recordings. Am J Cardiol. 1985;55(8): 1005-8.
37. Abdon NJ, Landin K, Johansson BW. Athlete's bradycardia as an embolising disorder? Symptomatic arrhythmias in patients aged less than 50 years. Br Heart J. 1984;52(6):660.
38. Milanesi R, Baruscotti M, Gnecchi-Ruscone T, et al. Familial sinus bradycardia associated with a mutation in the cardiac pacemaker channel. N Engl J Med. 2006;354(2):151-7.
39. Tresch DD, Fleg JL. Unexplained sinus bradycardia: clinical significance and long-term prognosis in apparently healthy persons older than 40 years. Am J Cardiol. 1986;58(10): 1009-13.

Chapter

4

Axis Determination and Rotation of the Heart

INTRODUCTION

The cardiac electrical axis refers to the general direction of the heart's depolarization wave front (or mean electrical vector) in the frontal plane. With a healthy conducting system, the cardiac axis is related to where the major muscle bulk of the heart lies. Normally, this is the left ventricle, with some contribution from the right ventricle. It is usually oriented in a right shoulder to left leg direction, which corresponds to the left inferior quadrant of the hexaxial reference system, although –30° to +90° is considered to be normal. If the left ventricle increases its activity or bulk, then there is said to be "left axis deviation (LAD)" as the axis swings round to the left beyond –30°; alternatively, in conditions where the right ventricle is strained or hypertrophied, then the axis swings round beyond +90° and "right axis deviation (RAD)" is said to exist (Figs. 4.1A to C). Disorders of the conduction system of the heart can disturb the electrical axis without necessarily reflecting changes in muscle bulk. Cardiac axis may be age-dependent.[1]

Axis is the direction of an electrocardiogram (ECG) waveform in the frontal plane measured in degrees. ECG always records the instantaneous vector of electrical forces at any given moment, and using this norm we can represent the complete depolarization of a chamber by drawing all these instantaneous vectors. The first vector represents septal depolarization, and each successive vector represents progressive depolarization of the ventricles. The average vector of all these instantaneous vectors is called the mean vector and the direction of the mean vector is called the mean electrical axis.[2]

The axis of the ECG is the major direction of the overall electrical activity of the heart. It can be normal, leftward (LAD), rightward (RAD), or indeterminate (northwest axis) (Fig. 4.2). The QRS axis is the most important to determine, however, the P-wave or T-wave axis can also be measured. To determine the QRS axis, the limb leads need to be examined (not the precordial leads).

In hexaxial reference system the lead I is at 0°, lead II is at +60°, and lead III is at +120°. Lead augmented vector left (aVL) is at -30°, lead augmented vector foot (aVF) is at +90°, and the negative of lead augmented vector right (aVR) is at +30°. The positive of lead aVR is actually at -150°. The normal QRS axis should be between -30° and +90°. Left axis deviation is defined as the major QRS vector falling between -30° and -90°. Right axis deviation occurs with the QRS axis is between +90° and +180°. Indeterminate axis is between ± 180° and -90° (Figs. 4.2 and 4.3).

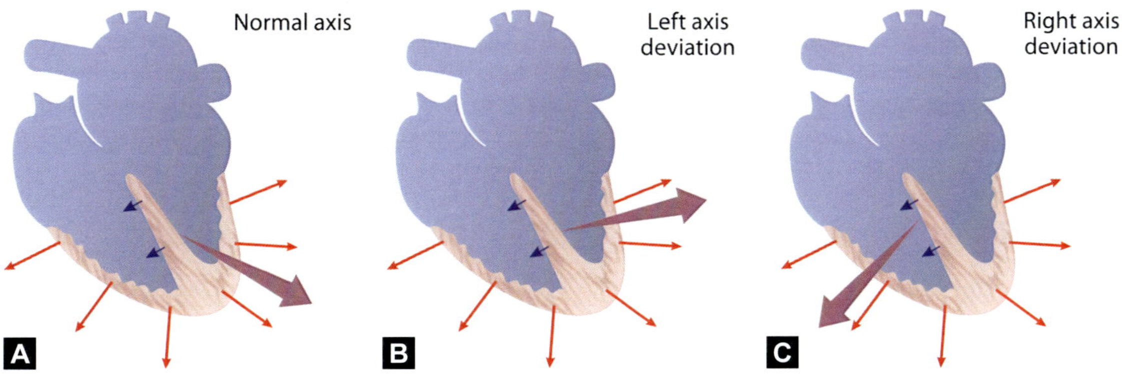

Figs. 4.1A to C: Cardiac electrical axis: showing direction of the depolarization waves of heart. (A) Normal axis. (B) Left axis deviation (LAD). (C) Right axis deviation (RAD).

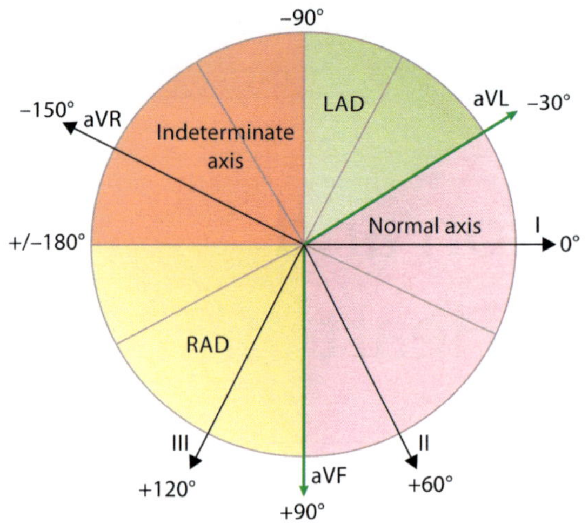

Fig. 4.2: Determination of electrocardiogram (ECG) axis. Normal axis ranges from –30° to +90° (inside green arrows).
(aVR: augmented vector right, aVL: augmented vector left, aVF: augmented vector foot, LAD: left axis deviation, RAD: right axis deviation)

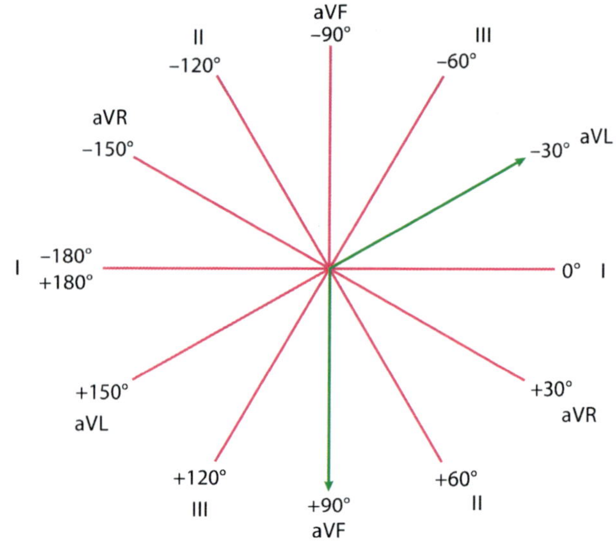

Fig. 4.3: Hexaxial reference system for calculation of cardiac axis. Normal axis varies from –30° to +90° (inside green arrows).

If the QRS complex is upright (positive) in both lead I and lead aVF, then the axis is normal. If the QRS is upright in lead I (positive) and downward in lead aVF (negative), then the axis is between 0° and -90°. However, recall that LAD is defined as between -30° and -90° and thus this scenario is not always technically LAD. In this scenario, the QRS axis could fall between 0° and -30° which is within normal limits. To further distinguish normal from LAD in this setting, look at lead II. If lead II is downward (negative), then the axis is more toward -120° and LAD is present. If the QRS complex in lead II is upright (positive), then the axis is more toward +60° and the QRS axis is normal. If the QRS is predominantly negative in leads I and positive in lead aVF, then the axis is rightward (RAD). If the QRS is downward (negative) in lead I and downward (negative) in lead aVF, then the axis is indeterminate.

The *hexaxial reference system*, also known as the *Cabrera system* is a convention to present the extremity leads of the 12-lead ECG that provides an illustrative logical sequence that helps interpretation of the ECG, especially to determine the heart's electrical axis in the frontal plane (Fig. 4.2). The hexaxial reference system allows calculation of cardiac QRS vector/axis, summation of all electrical activity throughout the ventricular myocardium and gives a final direction of electrical activity.

The most practical way of using this is by arranging extremity leads according to the Cabrera system, reversing polarity of lead aVR and presenting ECG complexes in the order (aVL, I, -aVR, II, aVF, III). Then determine the direction the maximal ECG vector is "pointing," i.e. in which lead there are most positive amplitude—this direction is the electrical axis. *Example*: If lead I has the highest amplitude (higher than aVL or -aVR), the axis is approximately 0°. Conversely, if lead III has the most negative amplitude it means the vector is pointing away from this lead, i.e. towards -60°.

An alternative use is to locate the most isoelectric (or equiphasic) lead (I, II, III, aVR, aVL, or aVF) on a diagnostic quality ECG with proper lead placement. Then find the corresponding spoke on the hexaxial reference system. The perpendicular spoke will point to the heart's electrical axis (Fig. 4.4). To determine which numerical value should be used, observe the polarity of the perpendicular lead on the ECG.[3-7]

A three step process can be used when determining axis:

1. Out of leads I, II, III, aVF, aVL, and aVR, determine which lead has roughly equal amplitude of positive and negative deflections. This is the equiphasic "isoelectric" lead.
2. Find the lead that is perpendicular to this isoelectric lead.
3. Identify the direction of the QRS axis in the lead identified in Step 2. If the QRS deflection is positive, then the axis is the same as the positive pole of that lead. If negative, then the axis is the same as the negative pole.

For example, if the most isoelectric (or equiphasic) lead is aVL, the perpendicular lead on the hexaxial reference system is lead II. If lead II is positively deflected on the ECG, the heart's electrical axis in the frontal plane will be approximately +60°.

Example 1 (Fig. 4.5): In this ECG the small and equiphasic QRS complex among the leads (I, II, III, aVR, aVL, or aVF) is LII. Equiphasic QRS complex means "R" wave height is almost equal to "S" wave depth. In hexaxial reference system the lead perpendicular to LII is aVL. Now determine whether the QRS is predominantly positive or negative in lead aVL. In this ECG, QRS is positive in aVL, so the axis is -30°.

Example 2 (Fig. 4.6): In this ECG the small and equiphasic QRS complex among the first six leads is in LI. In hexaxial reference system the lead perpendicular to LI is aVF. Now determine whether the QRS is predominantly positive or negative in lead aVF. In this ECG, QRS is positive in aVF, so the axis is +90°.

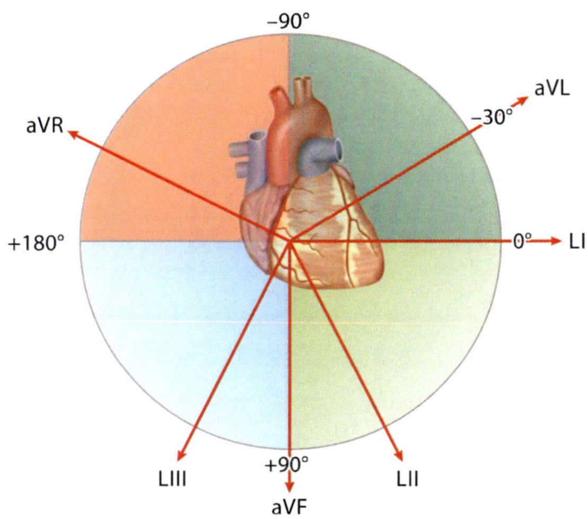

Fig. 4.4: Determination of electrical axis from hexaxial reference system. Locate the most isoelectric (or equiphasic) lead [I, II, III, augmented vector right (aVR), augmented vector left (aVL), or augmented vector foot (aVF)] on ECG. Then find the corresponding spoke on the hexaxial reference system. The perpendicular spoke will point to the heart's electrical axis.

NORMAL AND ABNORMAL AXIS ON ELECTROCARDIOGRAM

- *Normal axis*: –30° to +90°
- *Left axis deviation*: –30° to –90°
- *Right axis deviation*: +90° to +180°
- *Extreme axis deviation*: –90° to ±180°.

AXIS DETERMINATION FROM QRS CONFIGURATION IN LI, LII, AND LIII

The key is to look at the limb leads (leads I, II, and III). If QRS is positive in all the three leads LI, LII, and LIII then axis is normal (Figs. 4.7A and B). If QRS is positive in LI, negative in LIII, and biphasic or indeterminate in LII then axis lies between 0° and –30° (physiological LAD) (Figs. 4.8A and B). If QRS is positive in LI and negative in LII and LIII, then it is LAD (Figs. 4.9A and B). If QRS is negative in LI and positive in LII and LIII, then it is RAD (Figs. 4.10A and B). If QRS is negative in all the three leads LI, LII, and LIII, then it is called extreme or indeterminate axis deviation (Figs. 4.11A and B).

AXIS CALCULATION FROM LEAD I AND aVF

The simplest method of identifying gross deviations in axis is to look at the QRS complexes in *leads I and aVF*. Lead I is a left-sided lead, and as aVF is perpendicular to lead I, it can be considered as a right-sided lead.

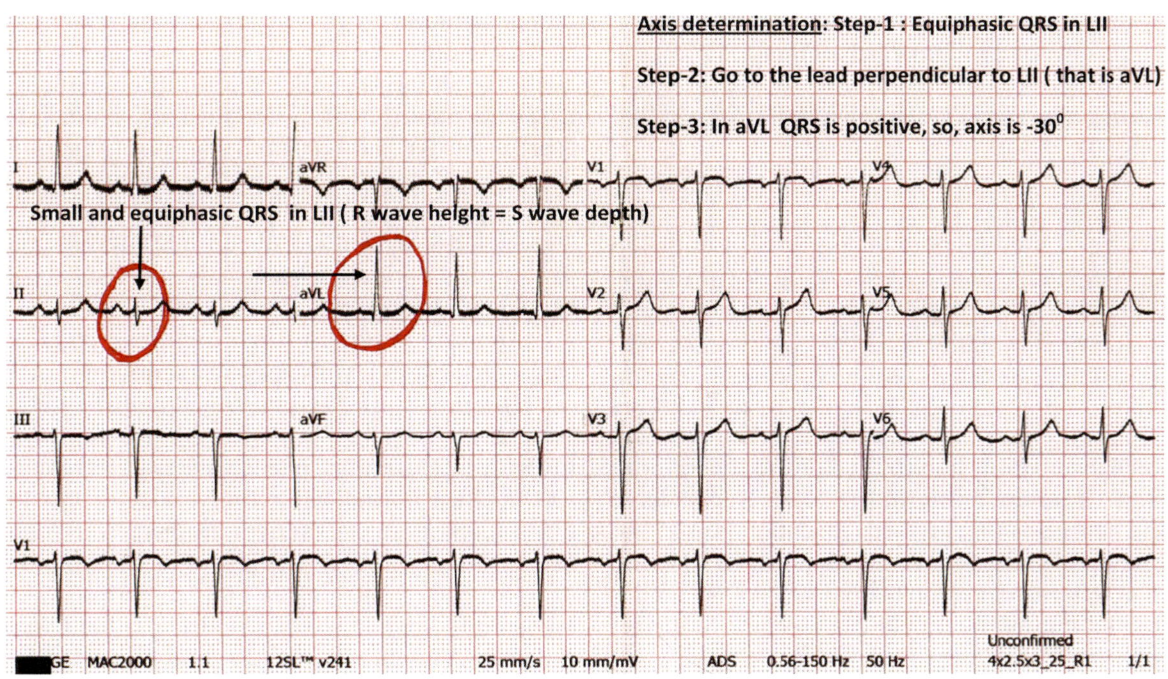

Fig. 4.5: In this ECG (Example-1) small and equiphasic QRS complex is in lead LII (short black arrow with red circle). In hexaxial reference system the lead perpendicular to LII is aVL (long arrow with red circle). As the major deflection of QRS in aVL is positive, the axis of this ECG is -30°.

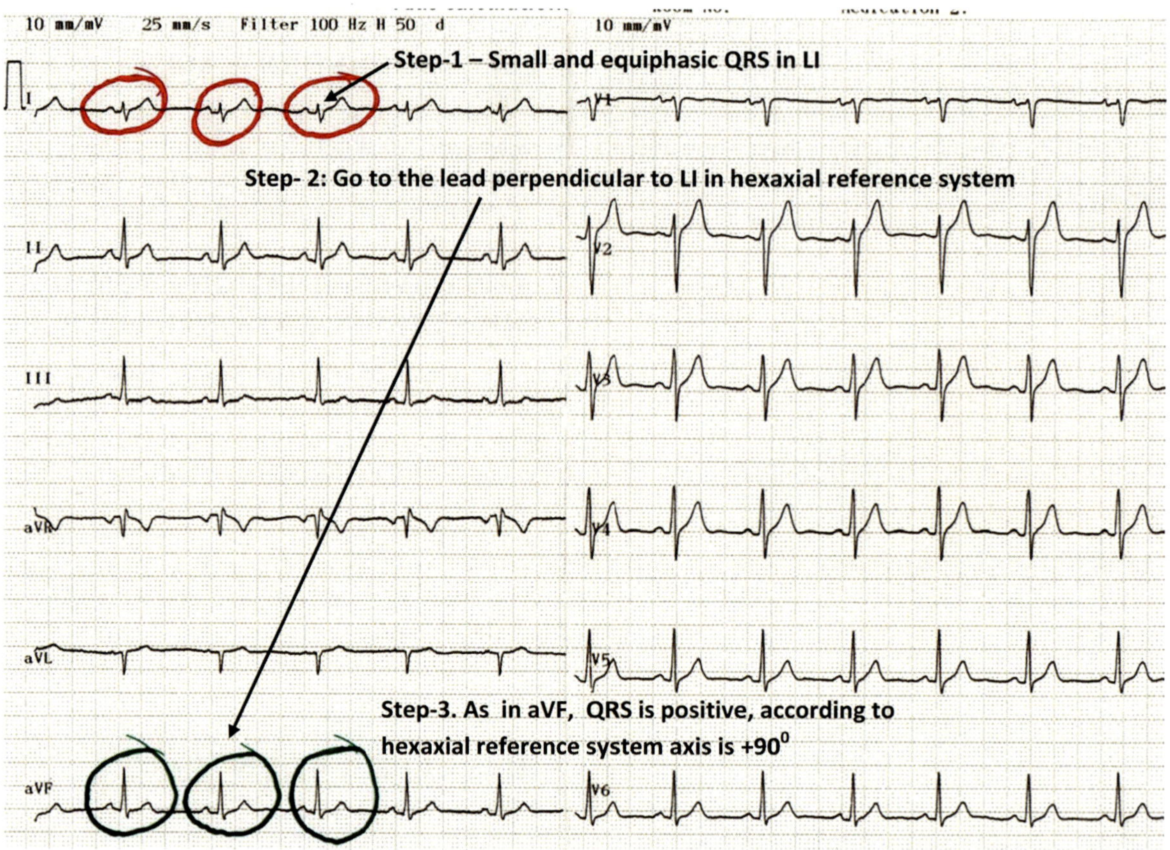

Fig. 4.6: In this ECG (Example-2) small and equiphasic QRS complex is in lead LI (short black arrow with red circle). In hexaxial reference system the lead perpendicular to LI is aVF (long arrow with green circle). As the major deflection of QRS in aVF is positive, the axis of this ECG is +90°.

- Both leads I and aVF have mainly positive QRS complexes equal to normal axis (Figs. 4.12A and B).
- Lead I is positive and aVF is negative equal to LAD (Figs. 4.13A and B).
- Lead I is negative and aVF is positive equal to RAD (Figs. 4.14A and B).
- Both leads negative equal to extreme RAD or "North-West" axis (Figs. 4.15A and B).

Another rapid method is to look at leads I and II. A positive QRS in lead I puts the axis in roughly the same direction as lead I. A positive QRS in lead II similarly aligns the axis with lead II. Therefore, if leads I and II are both positive, the axis is between –30° and +90° (i.e. normal axis).

The mean frontal plane electrical axis, determined by the vector of the maximal (dominant) QRS deflection, depends on age and body habitus. It shifts to the left with increasing age. In adults, the normal QRS axis is considered to be within –30° and +90°. Left-axis deviation is –30° and beyond. Moderate left-axis deviation is between –30° and –45°. Marked left-axis deviation is from –45° to –90° and is often associated with left anterior fascicular block. Moderate right-axis deviation in adults is from +90° to +120°, and marked right-axis deviation, which is often associated with left posterior fascicular block, is between +120° and +180°. In the absence of a dominant QRS deflection, as in an equiphasic QRS complex, the axis is said to be indeterminate.[8–10]

In children, there is normally a rightward QRS axis at birth that shifts gradually leftward throughout childhood. In the neonate, the mean electrical axis in the frontal plane is between +60° and +180° and is termed "marked right axis' deviation. Normally, the axis then shifts to the left, and by ages 1–5 years, it is generally between 10° and 110°. Between 5 years and 8 years of age, the normal QRS axis may extend to 140°, and between ages 8 years and 16 years, the range of QRS axis may extend upto +120°.[10,11]

Common causes of LAD include normal variation (physiologic, often with age), left ventricular hypertrophy (LVH), left bundle branch block (LBBB), left anterior hemiblock (LAHB), ventricular ectopic rhythms, inferior myocardial infarction, pacemaker rhythm, etc. Causes of RAD include normal variation (vertical heart with an axis of +90°), right ventricular hypertrophy (RVH), right bundle branch block (RBBB), left posterior hemiblock (LPHB), dextrocardia, ventricular ectopic rhythms, lateral wall myocardial infarction, right ventricular load, for example pulmonary embolism or cor pulmonale [as in chronic obstructive pulmonary disease (COPD)], emphysema, etc. Pre-excitation syndromes may produce both LAD and RAD according to the position of the accessory bypass tract.

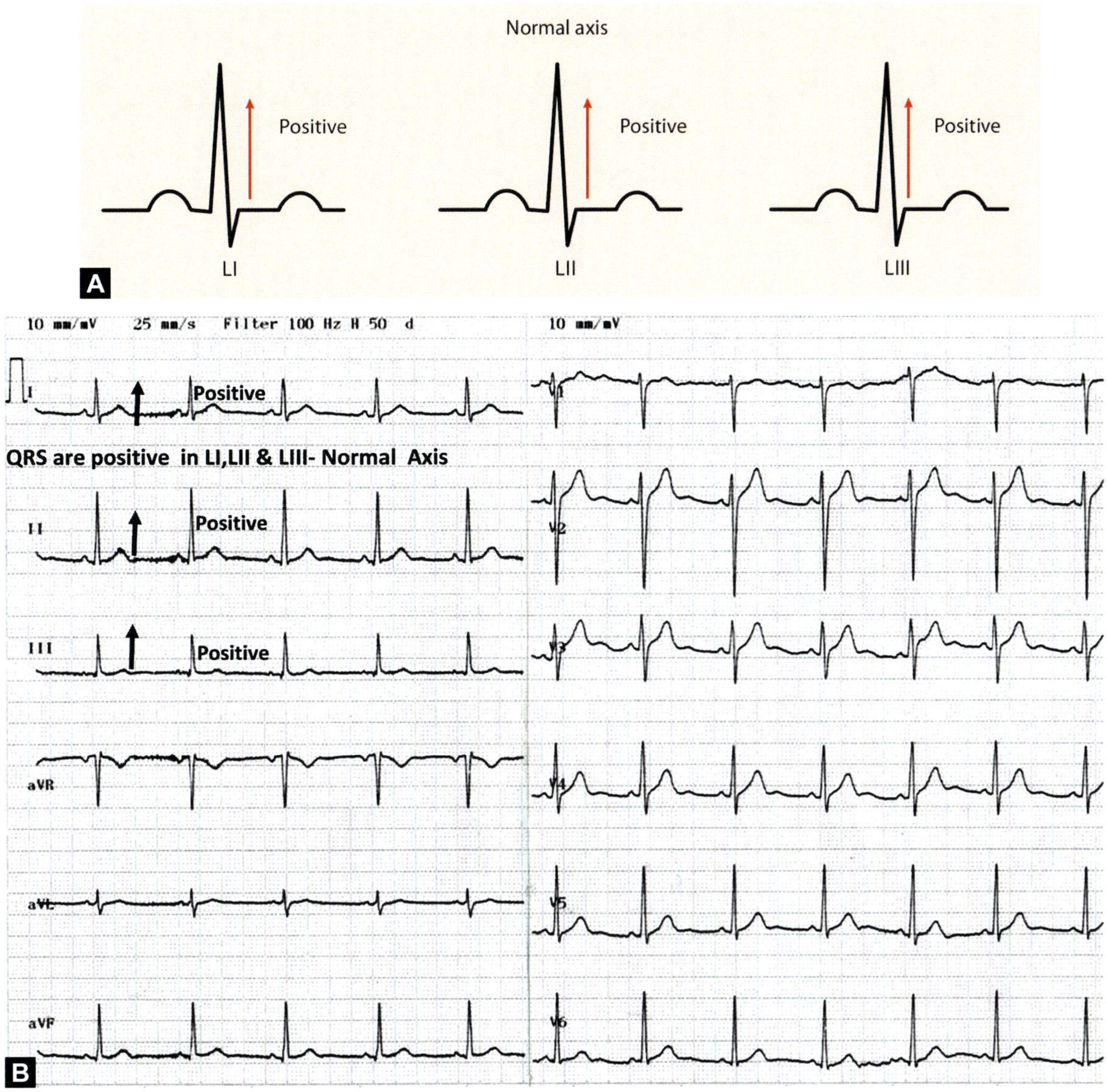

Figs. 4.7A and B: (A) Diagrammatic representation of normal axis. All three complexes in LI, LII, and LIII are positive, so axis is normal. (B) In this ECG, QRS complexes in leads LI, LII, and LIII are positive, so axis is normal.

ROTATION OF HEART

Deviation from normal horizontal rotation is a common ECG finding in individuals free of cardiovascular disease (CVD). Clockwise and counterclockwise rotation refers to a change in the electrical activity in a horizontal plane through the heart. If the electrical activity of the heart has turned more to the right side of the patient this is called *counterclockwise rotation*. If the electrical activity of the heart has turned more to the left side of the patient this is called *clockwise rotation* (Figs. 4.16A to C). Heart always rotates toward hypertrophy and away from infarction.[12,13]

Clockwise and counterclockwise rotation can be assessed only in the chest-leads (V1 to V6). Normally the R-wave amplitude increases from V1 to V5. Around V3 or V4 the R waves become larger than the S waves and this is called the *"transitional zone."* Normal transition zone could be easily recognized from standard 12-lead ECG by observing V3 and V4 where a dominant of S-wave in lead V3 and a dominant of R-wave in lead V4 should be present (Fig. 4.17). Transition outside of the normal zone is referred to as either clockwise or counterclockwise rotation. If the transition occurs before V3, this is called counterclockwise rotation (Fig. 4.18). If the transition occurs after V4, this is called clockwise rotation (Fig. 4.19).[12-14]

Although electrocardiographic rotation has been recognized since the addition of precordial leads and use of 12 ECG leads in clinical practice but little is known about its prognostic significance. But, several studies documented that when compared with normal rotation, clockwise rotation is associated with increased risk of all-cause and CVD mortality while counterclockwise rotation was associated with lower risk of all-cause mortality and nonsignificant association with CVD mortality.[12-17]

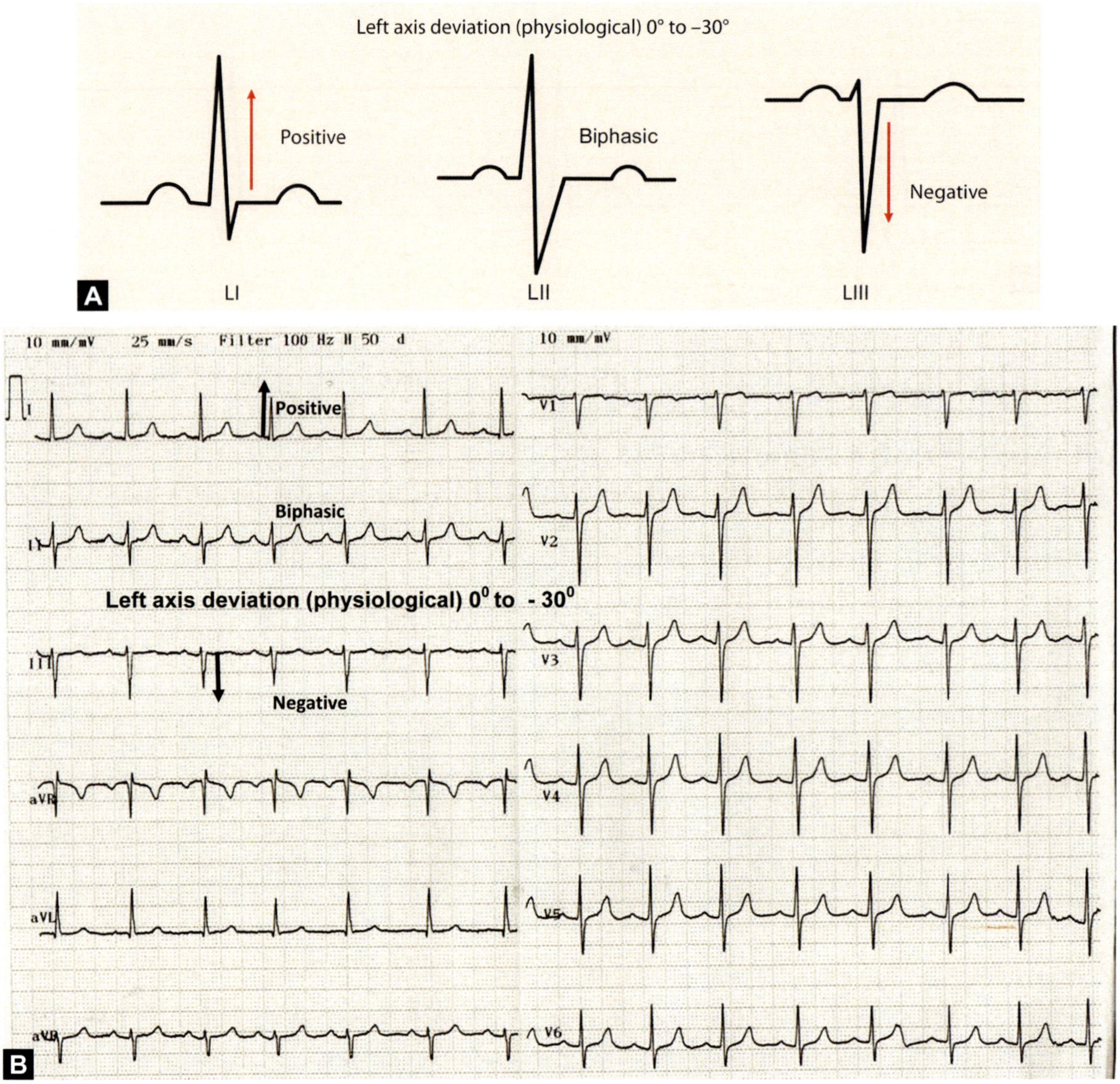

Figs. 4.8A and B: (A) Diagrammatic representation of left axis deviation (physiological), range 0° to –30°. QRS complex is positive in LI, biphasic in LII, and negative in LIII. (B) In this ECG, QRS complex is positive in LI, biphasic in LII, and negative in LIII, so axis will be around 0° to –30°.

Approximately two-thirds of clockwise rotation and counterclockwise rotation can be explained by anatomic rotation of the heart in the horizontal plane around the long axis, and in the remaining one third of cases, other factors may be contributory.[13,14] It is also known that counterclockwise rotation is more common in healthy young individuals.[14,18] Common causes of clockwise rotation include intraventricular conduction abnormalities secondary to myocardial degeneration, dilated cardiomyopathy, COPD, acute massive pulmonary thromboembolism, and vertical heart (usually thin and tall persons).[13,19,20] Causes of counterclockwise rotation include RVH, Wolff-Parkinson-White (WPW) syndrome, posterior myocardial infarction, left septal fascicular block, hypertrophic cardiomyopathy, right pneumonectomy, etc.[13,21]

SUMMARY

- The term "axis" refers to the direction of the mean electrical vector, and represents the average direction of the current flow. It actually refers to the direction of the depolarization wave as it passes through the heart. It is termed as "electrical axis." The direction in which depolarization is moving is termed as "vector." The QRS complex represents the depolarization of the ventricular myocardium.
- The "axis" of the heart is simply the mean QRS vector (direction).
- It is usually defined in the frontal plane only.
- The thicker left ventricular wall has larger vector compared to thin right ventricular wall, so that the mean QRS vector points more towards the left.

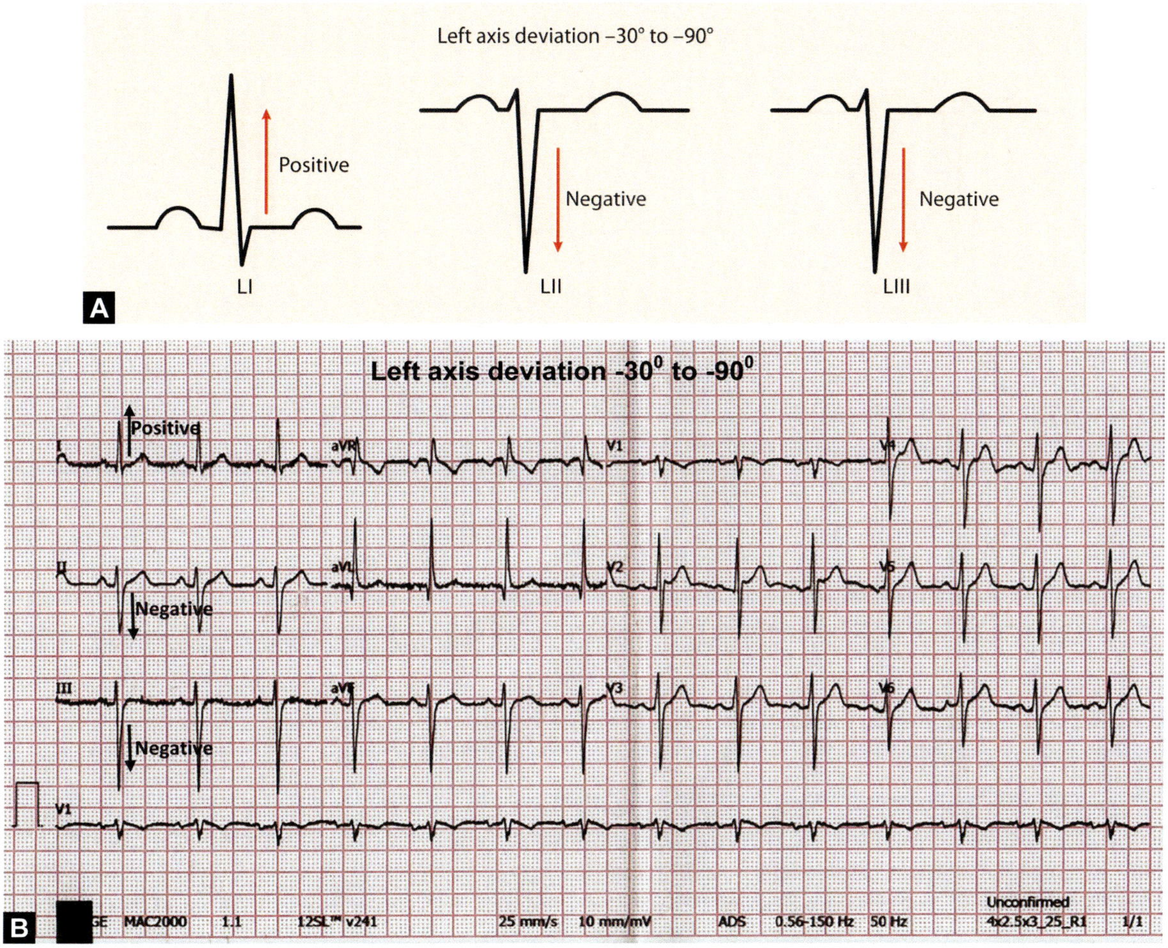

Figs. 4.9A and B: (A) Diagrammatic representation of pathological left axis deviation. QRS complex is positive in LI and negative in LII and LIII. (B) In this ECG, QRS complex is positive in LI and negative in LII and LIII, so axis will be around -30° to -90°.

To determine the axis, find the lead in which the QRS complex is most nearly equiphasic (biphasic). The QRS axis must lie approximately perpendicular to it. An equiphasic (biphasic) QRS where R-wave height is almost equal to Q or S-wave depth.

Interpretation of QRS Axis

- *Normal axis:* –30° to +90°
- *Left axis deviation:* –30° to –90°
- *Right axis deviation:* +90° to +180°
- *Indeterminate* (*extreme*) *axis deviation:* –90° to ±180°.

Axis Determination by Isoelectric (Equiphasic) Lead Method

Step 1: Find the isoelectric (equiphasic/biphasic QRS) lead. The QRS is isoelectric in any given lead (positive deflection equal to negative deflection), the axis is at 90° to this lead.

Step 2: The QRS axis is at 90° to the isoelectric lead, pointing in the direction of the positive leads.

Example:
- If QRS is most equiphasic (R-wave height equal to S-wave depth) in lead aVL.
- Then go to the lead perpendicular to lead aVL, that is lead II. The QRS axis is at 90° to the isoelectric lead.
- If in lead II, QRS is positive then axis is +60°
- If in lead II, QRS is negative then axis is –120°.

Axis Determination From LI, LII, and LIII

The axis determination from leads I, II, and III is shown in Table 4.1.

Axis Determination From QRS Morphology in Lead I and aVF

The most easy and effective way to estimate axis is to look QRS morphology at leads I and aVF, and is given in Table 4.2.

Quick and Easy Determination of Electrocardiogram Axis

Method 1

- If QRS complex is positive both in lead I and lead aVF-normal axis (0 to +90°).

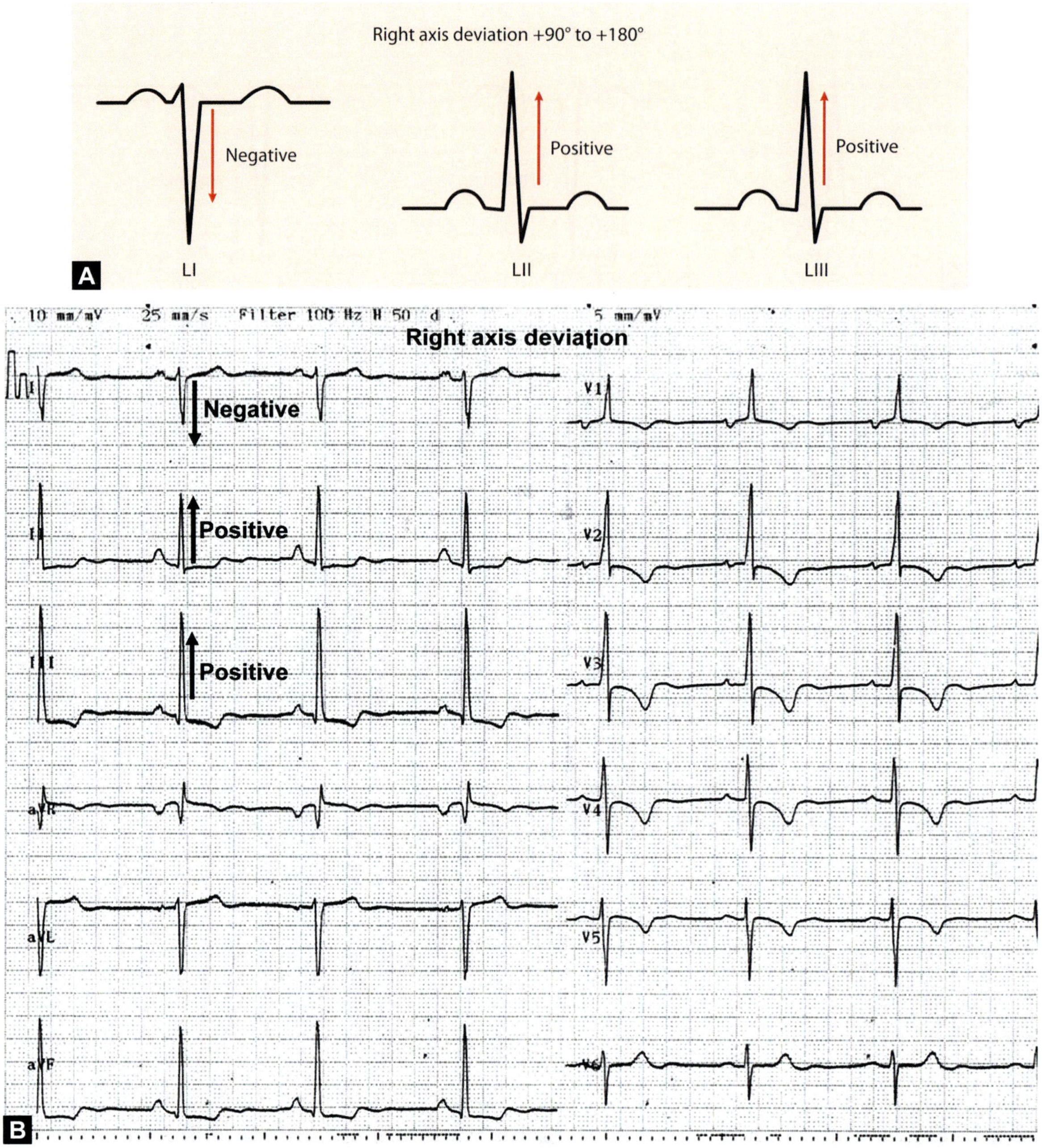

Figs. 4.10A and B: (A) Diagrammatic representation of right axis deviation. QRS complex is negative in LI and positive in LII and LIII. (B) In this ECG, QRS complex is negative in LI and positive in both LII and LIII, so axis will be around +90° to +180° (right axis deviation).

Table 4.1: Axis determination from Leads I, II, and III.

Lead I	*Lead II*	*Lead III*	*Axis*
Positive	Positive	Positive	Normal (axis 0° to +90°)
Positive	Biphasic or indeterminate	Negative	Left axis deviation (physiological) (axis 0° to −30°)
Positive	Negative	Negative	Left axis deviation (axis −30° to −90°)
Negative	Positive	Positive	Right axis deviation (axis +90° to +180°)
Negative	Negative	Negative	Extreme axis deviation

Table 4.2: Axis determination from QRS morphology in lead I and augmented vector foot (aVF).

Lead I	*aVF*	*Axis*
Positive	Positive	Normal (0° to +90°)
Positive	Negative	Possible LAD (0° to –90°)
Negative	Positive	RAD (+90° to +180°)
Negative	Negative	Extreme axis deviation

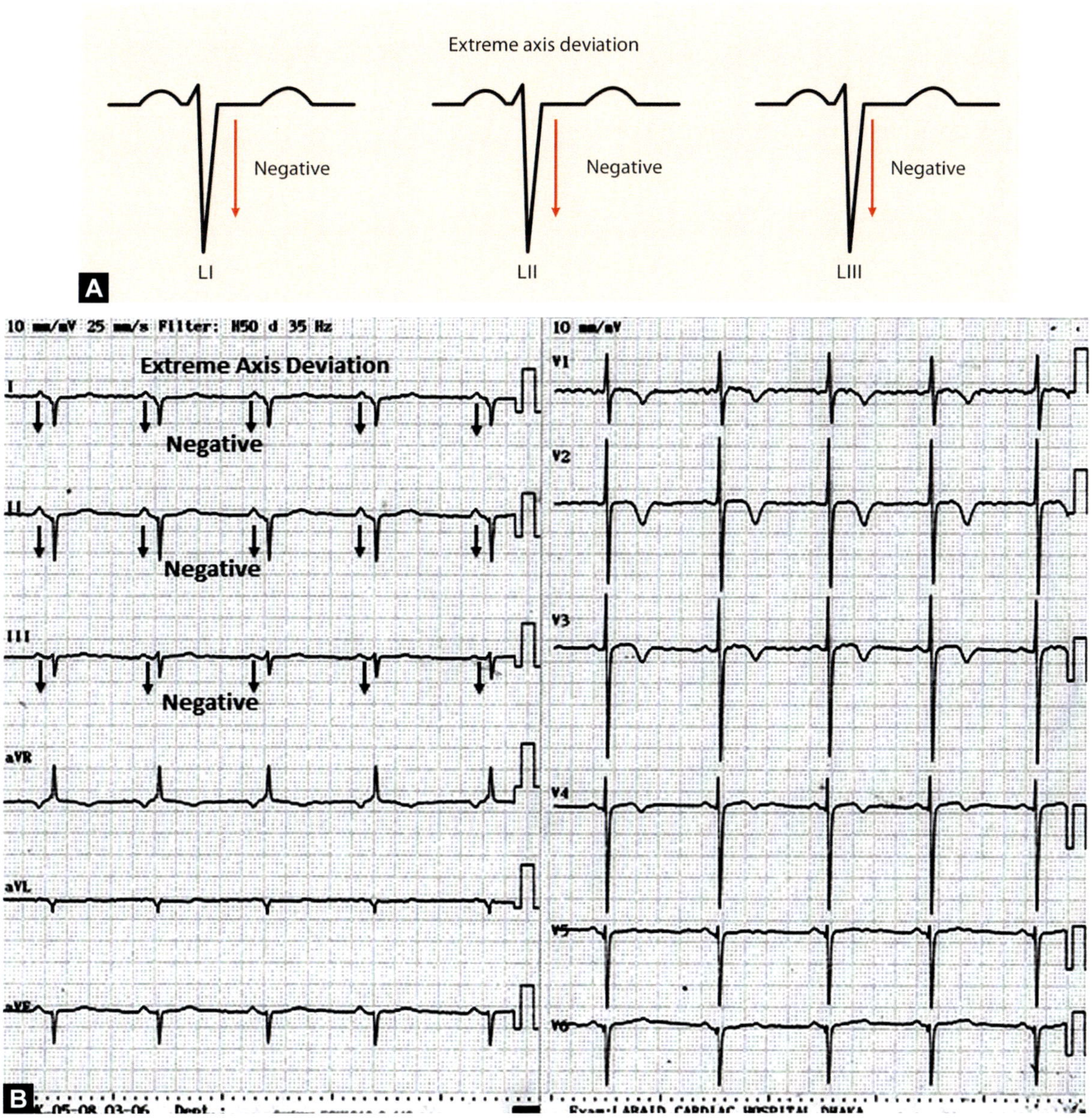

Figs. 4.11A and B: (A) Diagrammatic representation of extreme axis deviation. QRS complexes are negative in all the three leads LI, LII, and LIII. (B) In this ECG, QRS complexes are negative in LI, LII, and LIII suggesting extreme or indeterminate axis deviation.

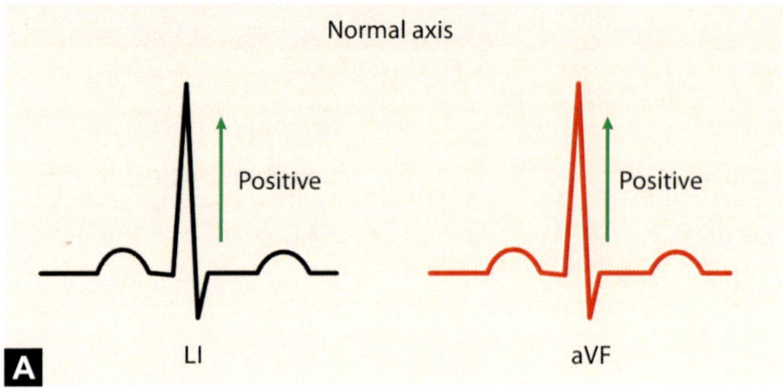

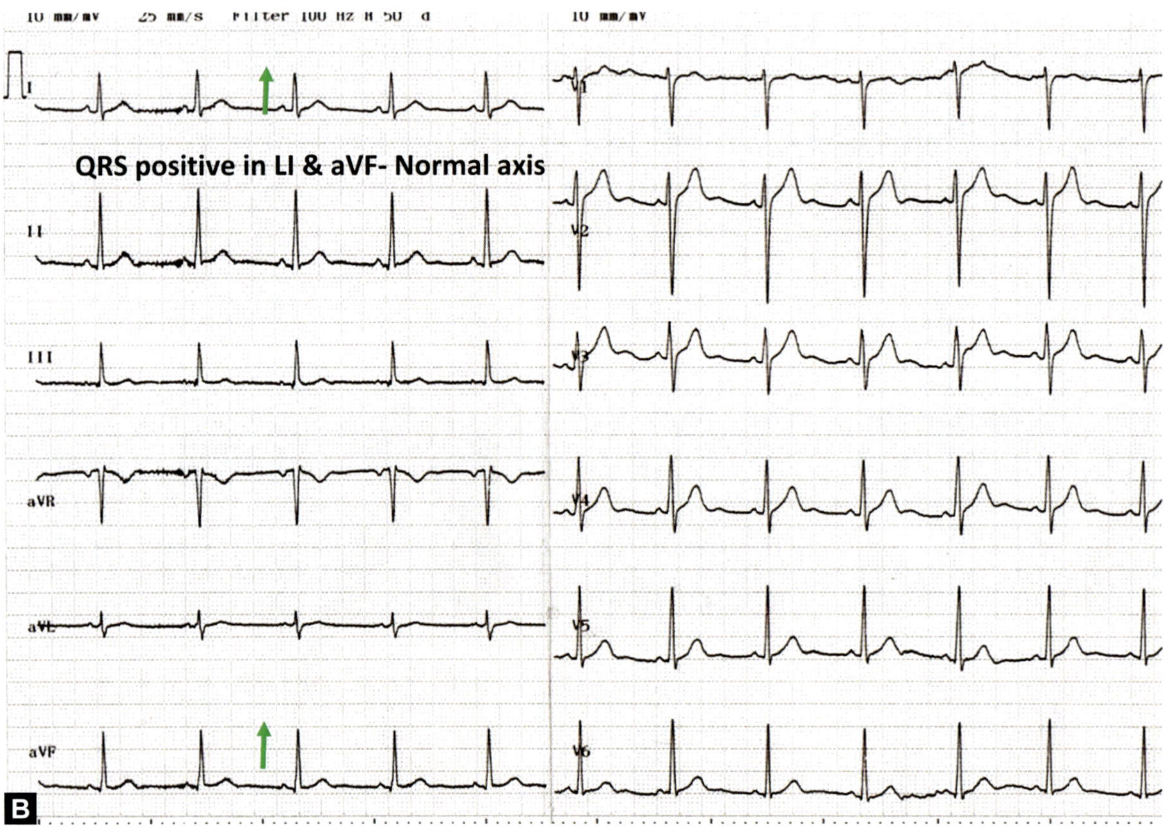

Figs. 4.12A and B: (A) Both leads I and aVF have mainly positive QRS complexes equal to normal axis. (B) In this ECG, QRS complexes are positive in both LI and aVF, so axis is normal.

- If QRS complex is positive in lead I and negative in lead aVF:

Then look at the Lead II QRS morphology,

- If lead II QRS is positive-normal axis (0 to –30°).
- If lead II QRS is negative-LAD (–30° to –90°).

Method 2

Another rapid method is to look at QRS morphology in leads I and II.

- A positive QRS in lead I puts the axis in roughly the same direction as lead I.
- A positive QRS in lead II similarly aligns the axis with lead II.
- If QRS in leads I and II are both positive, the axis is normal and lies between –30° and +90°.

Left Axis Deviation

Causes of Left Axis Deviation

- Normal variation (physiologic, often with age)
- Left ventricular hypertrophy
- Left bundle branch block
- Left anterior hemiblock
- Ventricular ectopic rhythms
- Inferior myocardial infarction
- Pacemaker rhythm.

Right Axis Deviation

Causes of Right Axis Deviation

- Normal variation (vertical heart)

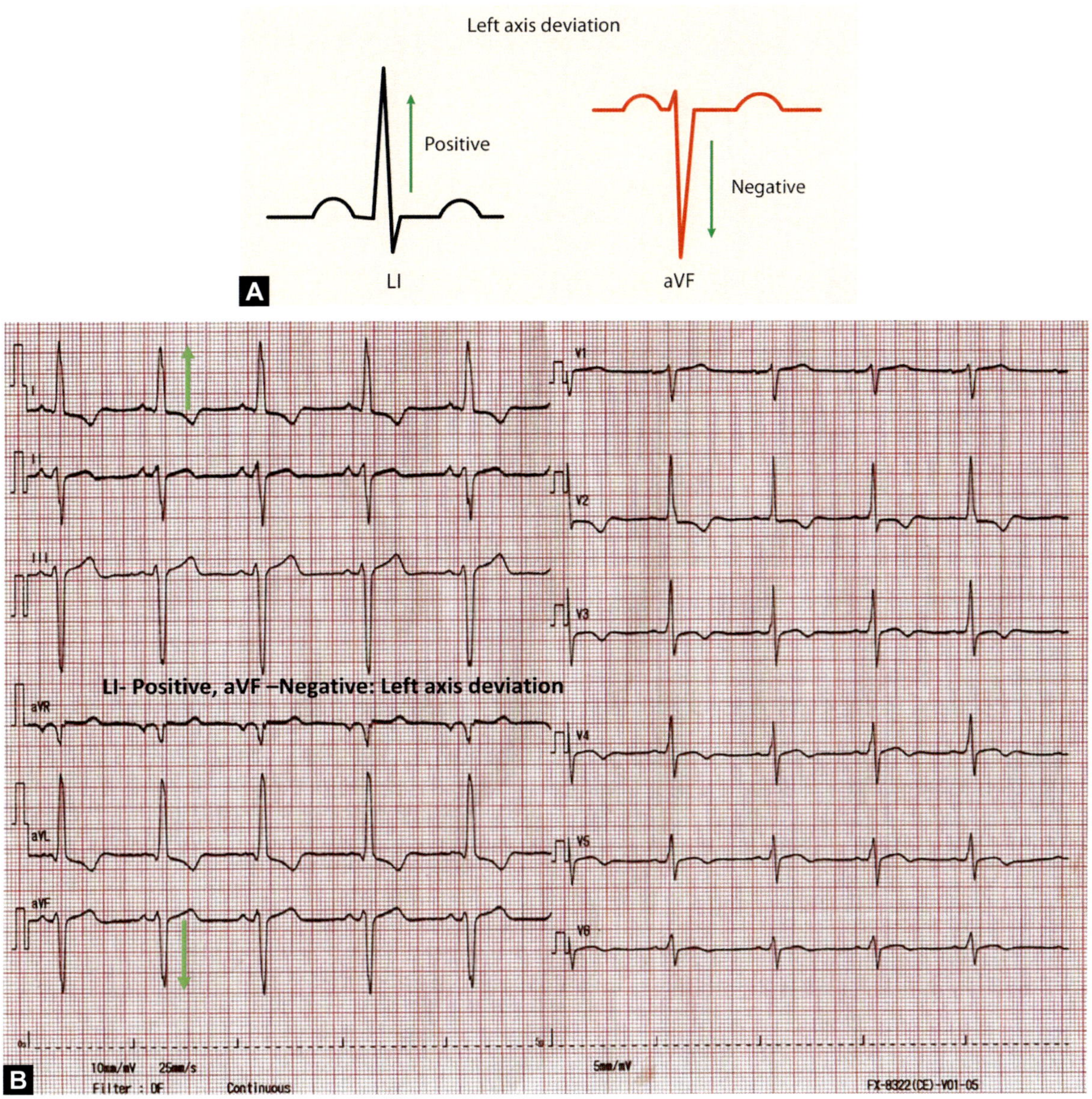

Figs. 4.13A and B: (A) Lead I is positive and aVF is negative equal to left axis deviation (LAD). (B) In this ECG, QRS complex is positive in LI but negative in aVF, so it is suggestive of left axis deviation.

- Right ventricular hypertrophy
- Right bundle branch block
- Left posterior hemiblock
- Dextrocardia
- Ventricular ectopic rhythms
- Lateral wall myocardial infarction
- Right ventricular load, for example pulmonary embolism or cor pulmonale (as in COPD)
- Emphysema.

Clockwise and Counterclockwise Rotation of Heart

In a "normal" ECG, the transition of the QRS axis in the precordial leads occurs between leads V3 and V4 (i.e. there is a dominant S in V3 and a dominant R in V4). The *transition zone* is where the QRS complex changes from predominantly negative to predominantly positive (R/S ratio becoming greater than 1), and this usually occurs at V3 or V4.

"Counterclockwise rotation" refers to a variant in which the transition is "early," occurring before lead V3, whereas "clockwise rotation" is a variant in which the transition occurs late, after lead V4. Clockwise rotation of the heart give rise to delayed R/S transition point in the precordial leads ± persistent S-wave in V6. There may be complete absence of R waves in leads V1 to 3.

Although clockwise rotation and counterclockwise rotation are distinct findings on ECG, their clinical values and their prognostic significance have not been well-defined. But few recently published data suggest that clockwise rotation

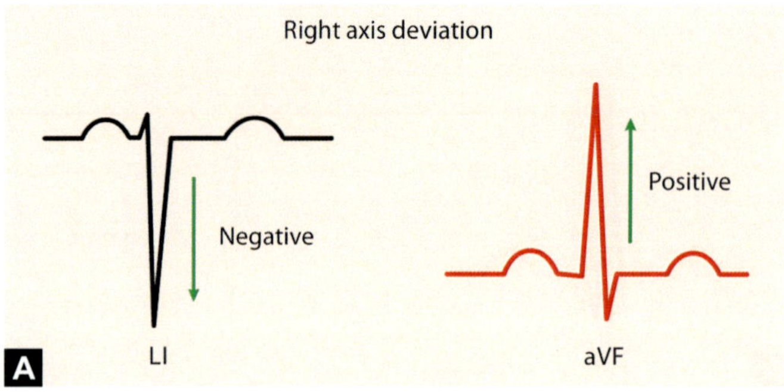

A

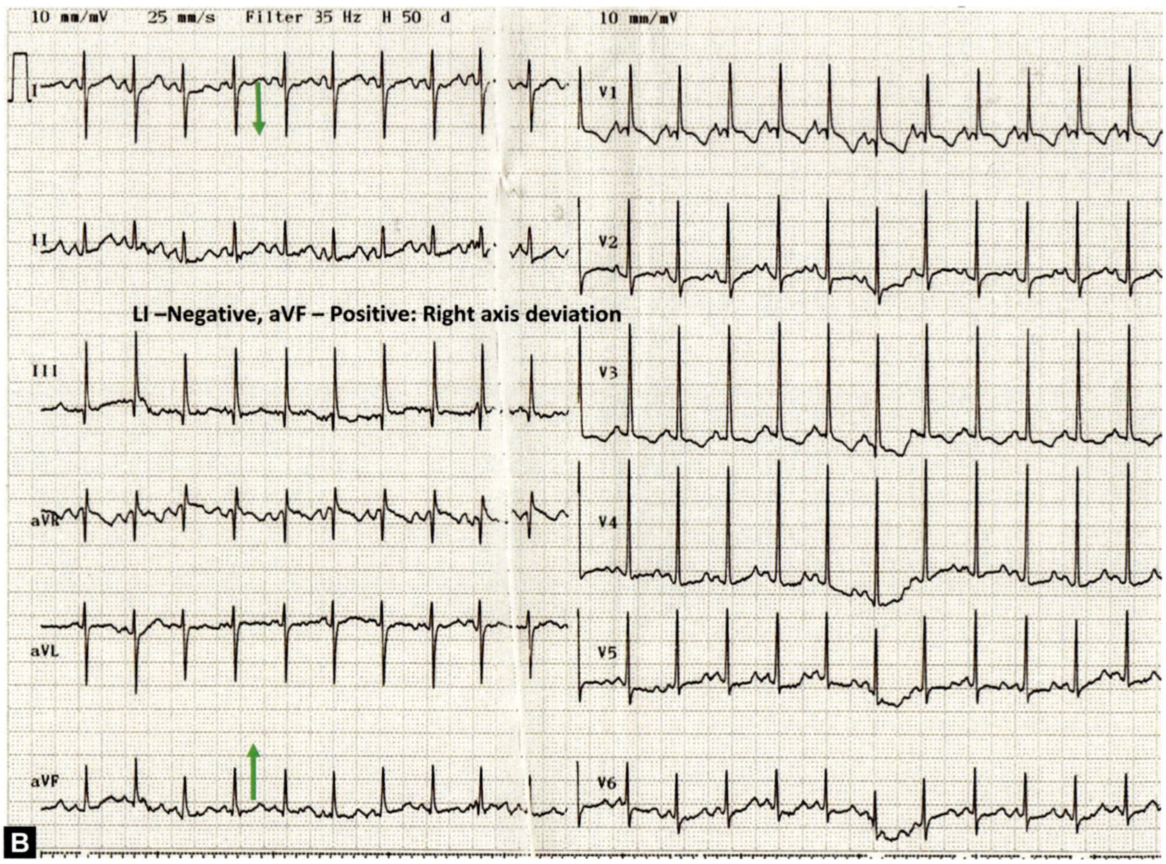

B

Figs. 4.14A and B: (A) Lead I is negative and aVF is positive equal to right axis deviation (RAD) (B) In this ECG strip, QRS is negative in LI and positive in aVF, suggestive of right axis deviation.

is associated with a substantial increase in all-cause mortality and CVD mortality compared with normal rotation. On the other hand, counterclockwise rotation has no significant association with cardiovascular mortality.

Causes of Clockwise Rotation

- Chronic obstructive pulmonary disease
- Intraventricular conduction abnormalities secondary to myocardial degeneration
- Dilated cardiomyopathy
- Vertical heart (usually thin and tall persons)
- Acute massive pulmonary thromboembolism.

Causes of Counterclockwise Rotation

- Right ventricular hypertrophy
- Wolff-Parkinson-White syndrome
- Posterior myocardial infarction
- Hypertrophic cardiomyopathy
- Right pneumonectomy, etc.

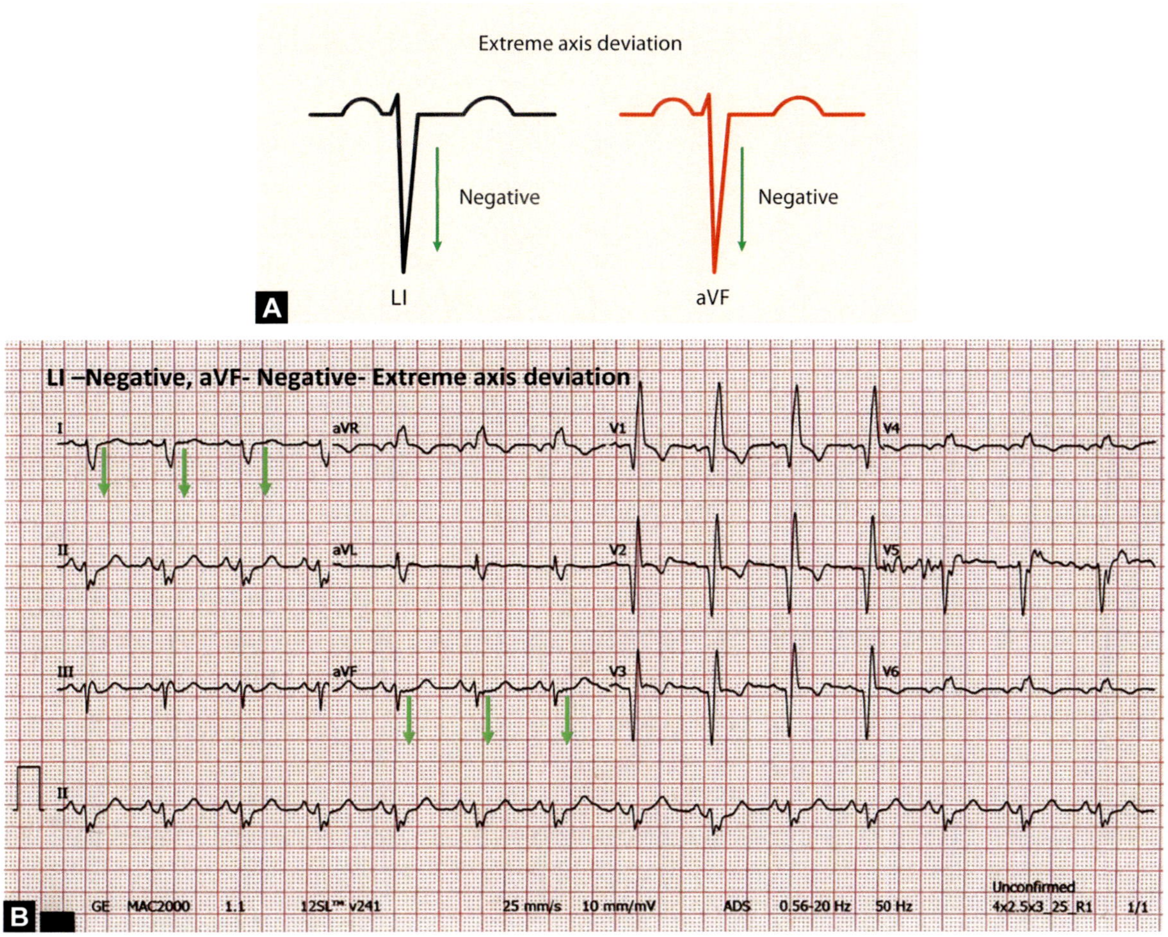

Figs. 4.15A and B: (A) QRS complexes are negative in both leads, LI and aVF equal to extreme axis deviation or "North-West" axis. (B) In this ECG strip, QRS complexes are predominantly negative both in leads LI and aVF, suggestive of extreme axis deviation or "North-West" axis.

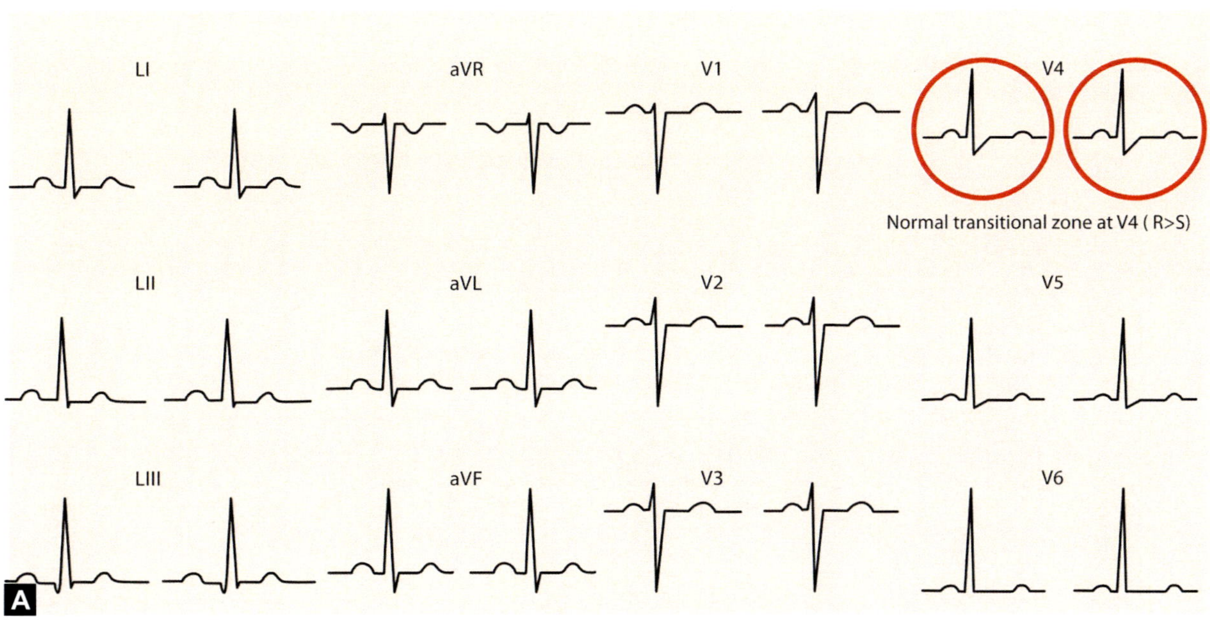

Fig. 4.16A: Diagrammatic representation of normal and abnormal rotations of heart. (A) Normal position without any significant rotation, with transitional zone at V4 (red circle).

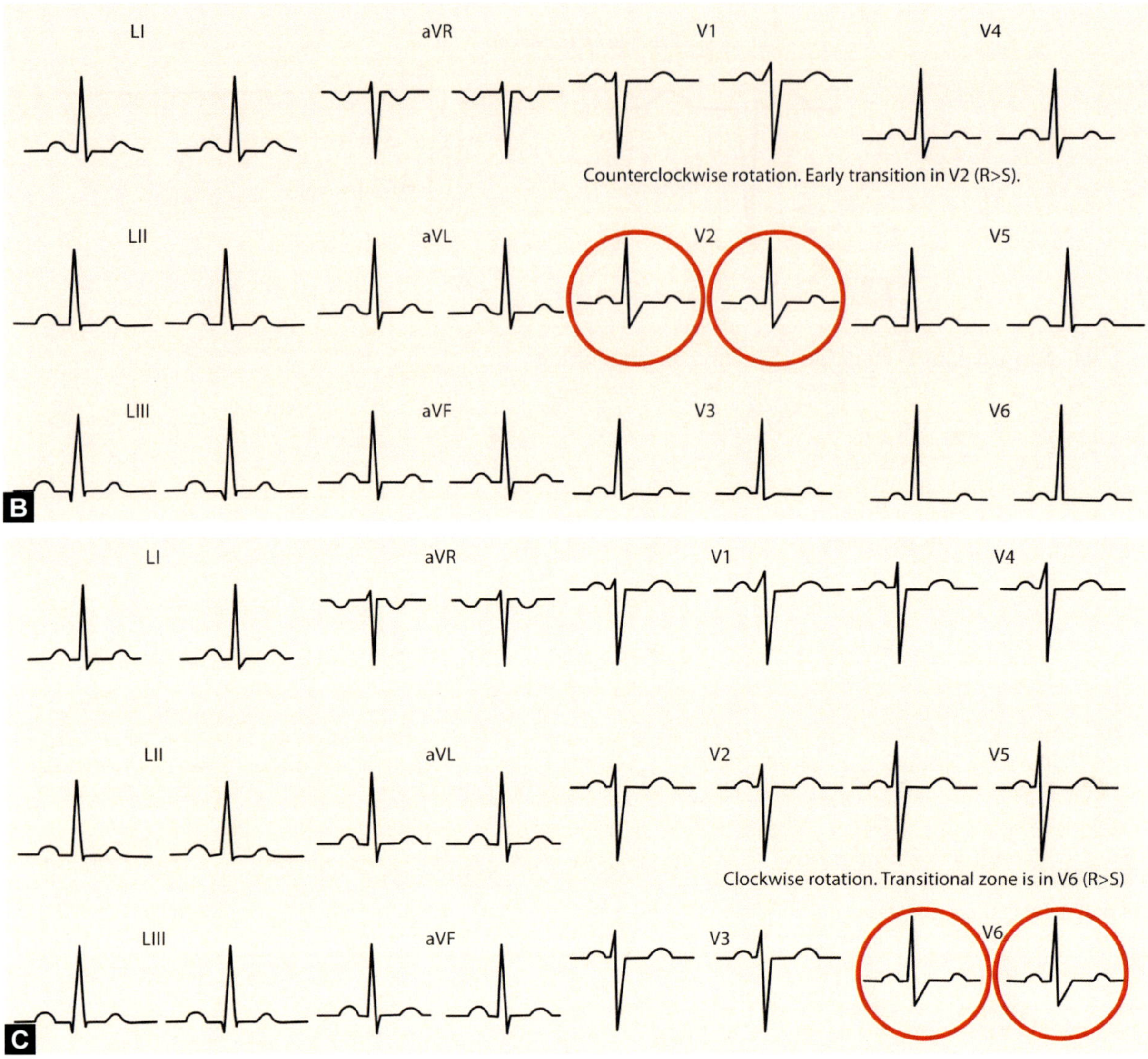

Figs. 4.16B and C: (B) Early transition at V2 (R > S), (red circle) suggestive of counterclockwise rotation. (C) Late transition at V6 (R > S), (red circle) suggestive of clockwise rotation.

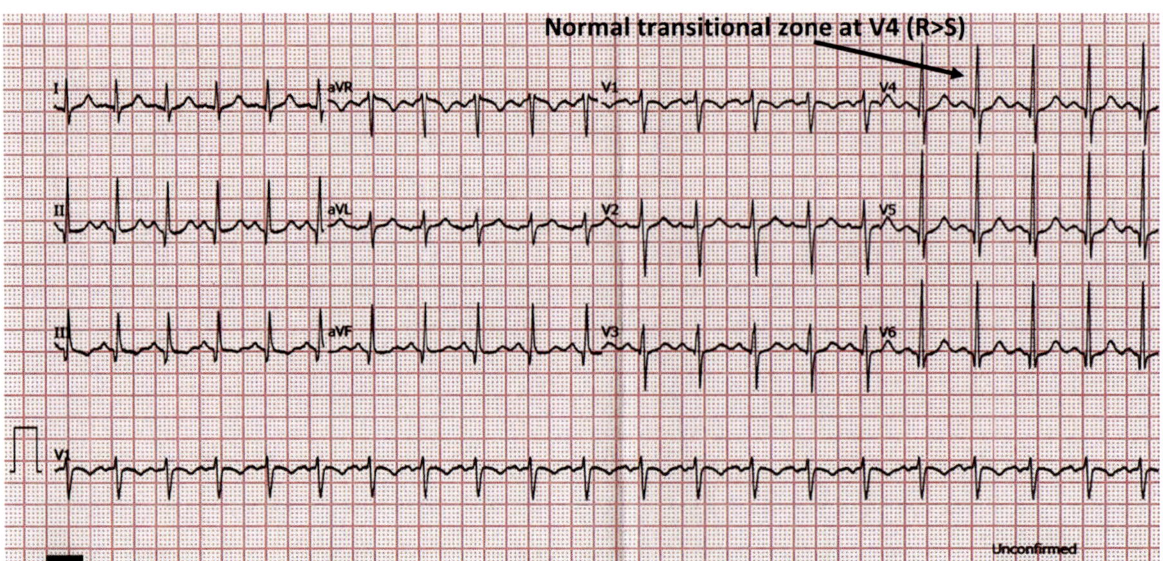

Fig. 4.17: Electrocardiogram shows normal transitional zone in lead V4 (R > S) (arrow).

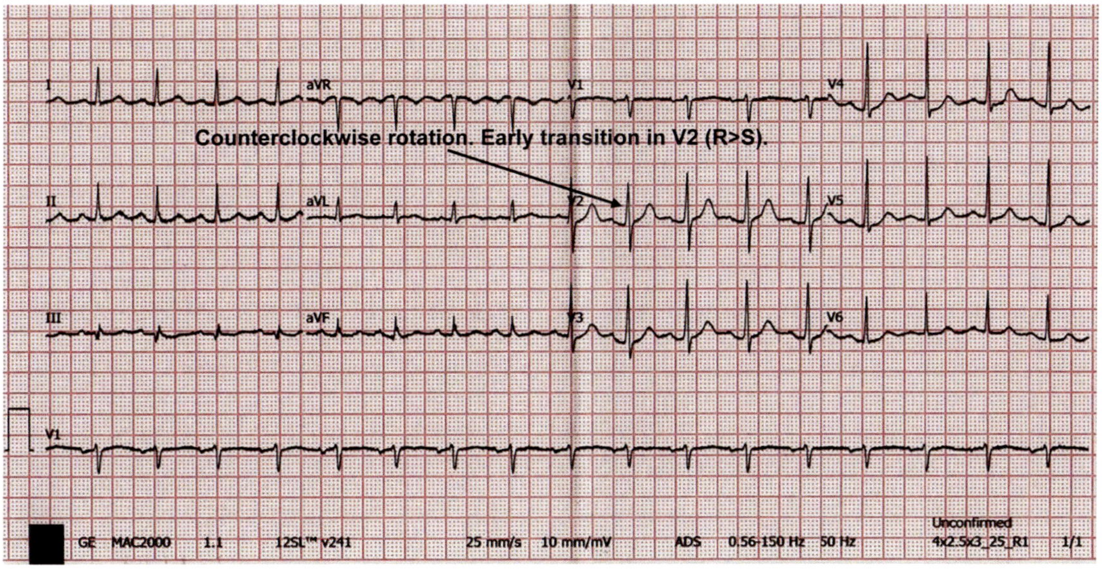

Fig. 4.18: Electrocardiogram shows early transition in lead V2 (R > S) suggestive of counterclockwise rotation.

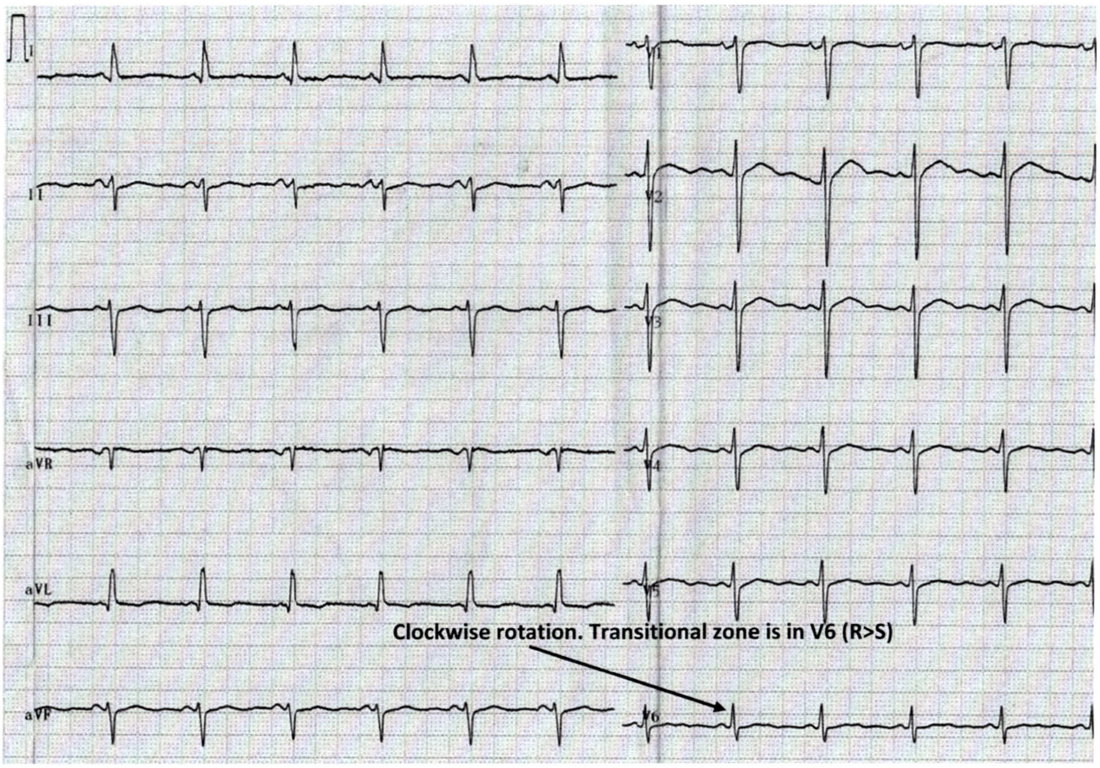

Fig. 4.19: Electrocardiogram shows late transition in lead V6 (R > S) suggestive of clockwise rotation.

REFERENCES

1. Stephen JM, Dhindsa H, Browne B, et al. Interpretation and clinical significance of the QRS axis of the electrocardiogram. J Emerg Med. 1990;8(6):757-63.
2. Thaler MS. The Only EKG Book You'll Ever Need. Philadelphia: LB Lippincott Company; 1988.
3. Lam A, Wagner GS, Pahlm O. The classical versus the Cabrera presentation system for resting electrocardiography: Impact on recognition and understanding of clinically important electrocardiographic changes. J Electrocardiol. 2015;48(4):476-82.
4. Sgarbossa EB, Barold SS, Pinski SL, et al. Twelve-lead electrocardiogram: the advantages of an orderly frontal lead display including lead-aVR. J Electrocardiol. 2004;37(3):141-7.
5. Dower GE, Nazzal SB, Pahlm O, et al. Limb leads of the electrocardiogram: sequencing revisited. Clin Cardiol. 1990;13(5):346-8.

6. Einthoven W, Fahr GE, DeWaart A. On the direction and manifest size of the variations of potential in the human heart and on the influence of the position of the heart on the form of the electrocardiogram (translation). Am Heart J. 1950;40(2):163.
7. Cabrera E. Electmcanliographie clinique: theorie et pratique. Paris: Masson; 1959.
8. Surawicz B, Childers R, Deal BJ, et al. AHA/ACCF/HRS recommendations for the standardization and interpretation of the electrocardiogram, part III: intraventricular conduction disturbances. A scientific statement from the American Heart Association Electrocardiography and Arrhythmias Committee, Council on Clinical Cardiology; the American College of Cardiology Foundation; and the Heart Rhythm Society. Endorsed by the International Society for Computerized Electrocardiology. Circulation. 2009;119(10):e235-40.
9. Mason JW, Hancock EW, Gettes L, et al. Recommendations for the standardization and interpretation of the electrocardiogram, part II: electrocardiography diagnostic statement list. A scientific statement from the American Heart Association Electrocardiography and Arrhythmias Committee, Council on Clinical Cardiology; the American College of Cardiology Foundation; and the Heart Rhythm Society. Circulation. 2007;115(10):1325-32.
10. MacFarlane PW, Lawrie TDV. The normal electrocardiogram and vector cardiogram. In: Macfarlane PW, Lawrie TDV (Eds). Comprehensive Electrocardiology: Theory and Practice in Health Disease. New York, NY: Pergamon Press; 1989. pp. 424-49.
11. Davignon A, Rautaharju P, Boiselle E, et al. Normal ECG standards for infants and children. Pediatr Cardiol. 1980;1:123-31.
12. Yanagisawa N. Counterclockwise rotation of the heart; correlation of electrocardiography and chest radiography and their clinical significance. J Electrocardiol. 1981;14(3): 233-8.
13. Tahara Y, Mizuno H, Ono A, et al. Evaluation of the electrocardiographic transitional zone by cardiac computed tomography. J Electrocardiol. 1991;24(3):239-45.
14. Nakamura Y, Okamura T, Higashiyama A, et al. Prognostic values of clockwise and counterclockwise rotation for cardiovascular mortality in Japanese subjects. A 24-Year follow-up of the National Integrated Project for Prospective Observation of Noncommunicable Disease and Its Trends in the Aged, 1980-2004 (NIPPON DATA80). Circulation. 2012;125(10):1226-33.
15. Rajala S, Haavisto M, Kaltiala K, et al. Electrocardiographic findings and 5-year cardiovascular mortality in very old people. Ann Clin Res. 1987;19:324-7
16. Horibe H, Kasagi F, Kagaya M, et al. A nineteen-year cohort study on the relationship of electrocardiographic findings to all-cause mortality among subjects in the national survey on circulatory disorders, NIPPON DATA80. J Epidemiol. 2005;15(4):125-34.
17. Bradford N, Shah AJ, Usoro A, et al. Abnormal electrocardiographic QRS transition zone and risk of mortality in individuals free of cardiovascular disease. Europace. 2015;17(1):131-6.
18. James FW, Kaplan S. The normal electrocardiogram in the infant and child. Cardiovasc Clin. 1973;5:294-311.
19. Yoshinaga T, Ikeda S, Shikuwa M, et al. Relationship between ECG findings and pulmonary artery pressure in patients with acute massive pulmonary thromboembolism. Circ J. 2003;67(3):229-32.
20. Stein PD, Dalen JI, Mclntyre KM, et al. The electrocardiogram in acute pulmonary embolism. Prog Cardiovasc Dis. 1975;17:247-57.
21. Frye DM, Sahn AS. Acute electrocardiographic changes after pneumonectomy. South Med J. 2000;93:977-81.

Chapter

5

Normal Variant Electrocardiogram

INTRODUCTION

It is important to remember that there is a wide range of normal variability in the 12-lead electrocardiogram (ECG). It takes considerable ECG reading experience to discover all the normal variants. Only by following a structured method and correlating the various ECG findings with the particular patient's clinical status will ensure proper diagnosis. Sinus arrhythmia, sinus tachycardia, sinus bradycardia, low atrial rhythm, isolated pathological Q-wave in single lead, ectopic atrial rhythm, indeterminate axis, first-degree atrioventricular (AV) block, Mobitz type I second degree AV block (Wenckebach phenomenon), few premature ventricular contraction or atrial contraction on a 12-lead ECG, incomplete RBBB (right bundle branch block), intraventricular conduction delay, early repolarization, left ventricular hypertrophy (LVH) by voltage criteria only, low voltage in limb leads (may be a sign of obesity or hypothyroidism), left axis deviation (less than or equal to -30°), wandering atrial pacemaker, rSR in leads VI or V2, R greater than S-wave in VI without other evidence of right ventricular hypertrophy are usually considered as normal variant ECG.[1] But these so called benign and normal variant ECGs should be interpreted cautiously.

SINUS ARRHYTHMIA

Sinus arrhythmia is a normal type of variation in sinus node discharge associated with the breathing cycle.[1] Heart rate changes during respiration due to Bainbridge reflex (Figs. 5.1A and B). In this benign arrhythmia P-wave morphology is normal; however, PP intervals change to more than 0.16 seconds (4 small squares). Respiration affects the frequency of impulses originating from the sinus node: the heart rate increases during inspiration and decreases during expiration. Since the impulses originate from the sinus node, P waves look like each other and are positive in leads I and II while negative in lead augmented vector right (aVR). Each P-wave is followed by a QRS complex. Since PP intervals are not equal, the RR intervals also are not equal. Sinus arrhythmia can be observed more frequently when sinus rate is slow. Since it is affected by vagal tone, sinus arrhythmia cannot be observed in patients who have received atropine or who have undergone vagotomy. It is more prevalent in children and adolescents. Sinus arrhythmia has no clinical significance.[2]

INVERTED P WAVES

Inverted P-wave usually denotes a low atrial rhythm. As the sinus node depolarizes slowly, a subsidiary atrial pacemaker has taken over. As it rises in the low atrium, the P waves are inverted. P-wave inversion in the inferior leads indicates a nonsinus origin of the P waves (Fig. 5.2). It is a benign condition and with exercise, the normal sinus rhythm with upright P-wave resumes.[3]

PR INTERVAL VARIATION

Short PR interval less than 0.12 seconds is usually considered normal. Short PR interval is probably due to shortened conduction time down the AV node. But occasionally this abnormality is associated with supraventricular tachycardia. PR interval may be prolonged normally in vagotonia, in young persons, and also in athletes. But possibility of rheumatic carditis, infective endocarditis, myocardial ischemia, fibrosis or drug-induced phenomenon need to be excluded.[4]

QRS DURATION: BUNDLE BRANCH BLOCK PATTERN

Partial right bundle branch block pattern (RSR) of the QRS complex in lead V1 not exceeding 0.12 seconds (120 ms) is usually considered as a normal variant (Fig. 5.3). But possibility of atrial septal defect needs to be excluded. Right bundle branch block with QRS duration of 0.12 seconds is also occasionally seen in normal individual without any significant cardiac abnormality but a new onset of RBBB is always a significant abnormality. Left bundle branch block (LBBB) is always considered abnormal.[4]

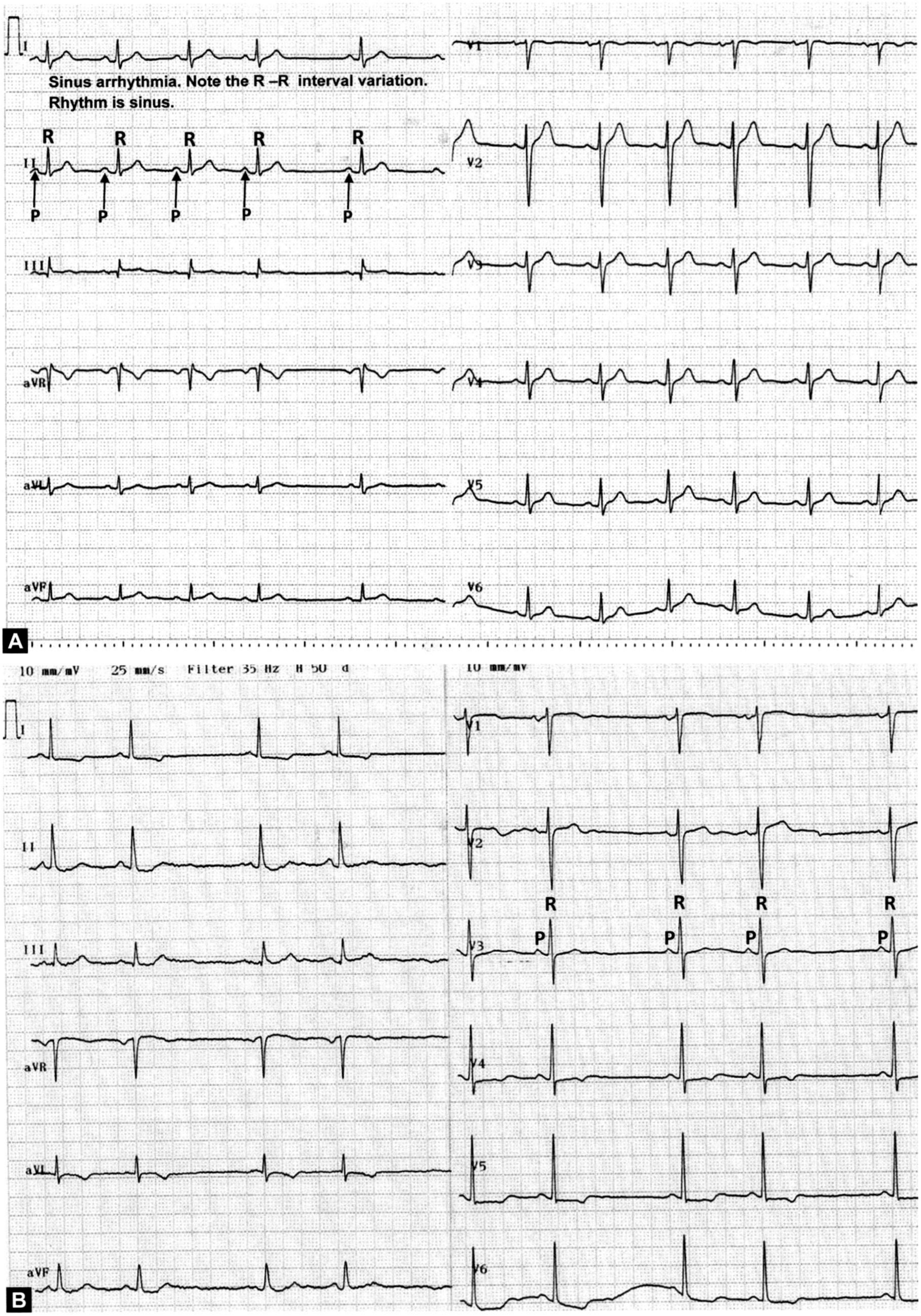

Figs. 5.1A and B: (A) Electrocardiogram (ECG) showing respiratory variation of cardiac rhythm (sinus arrhythmia). Rhythm is sinus. Note the RR interval variation. (B) ECG illustrates severe sinus arrhythmia. Note that all the QRS complexes are preceded by P waves of normal morphology, so the rhythm is sinus.

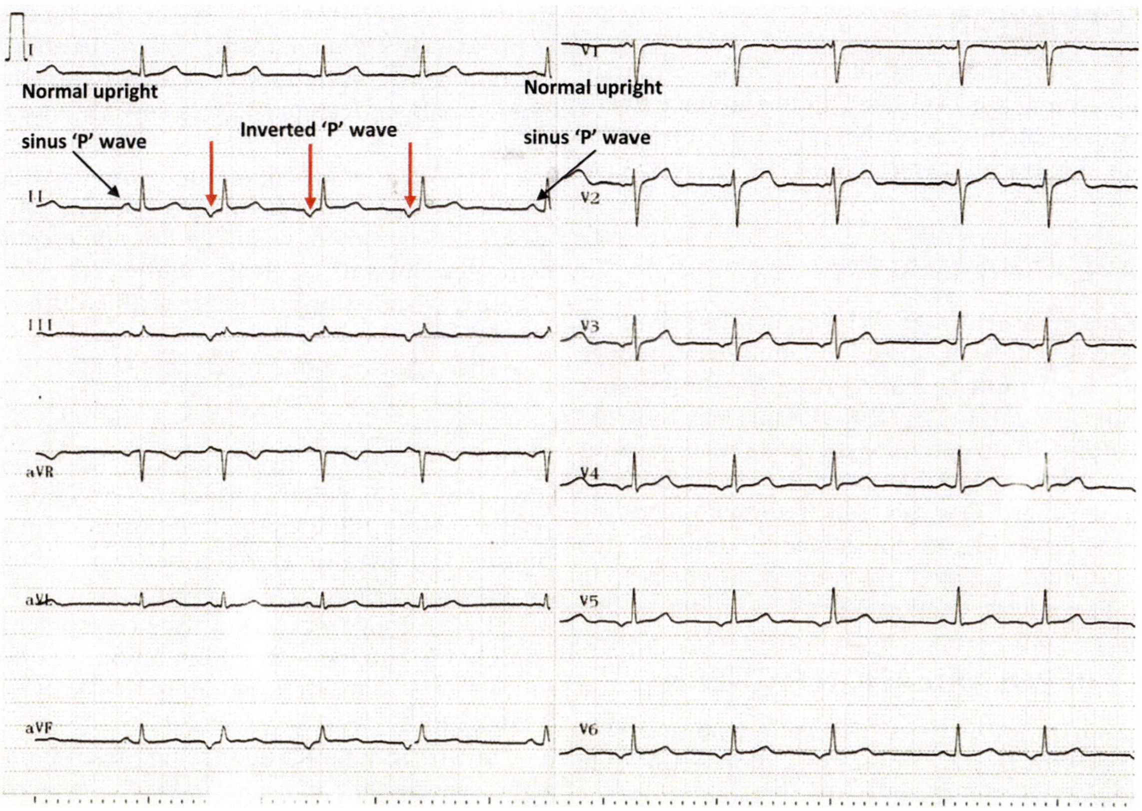

Fig. 5.2: Electrocardiogram (ECG) shows intermittent nodal rhythm. P waves are inverted (red arrows) along with normal sinus conducted beat in the same ECG strip (black arrows).

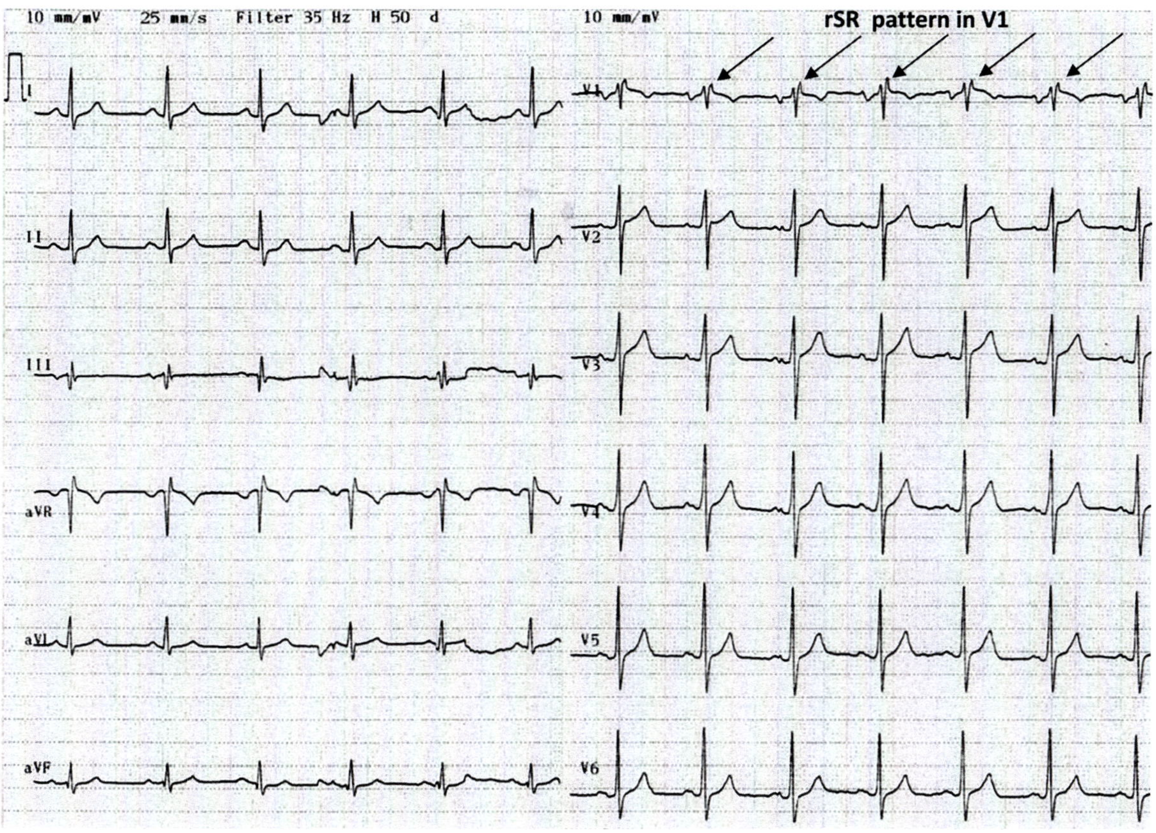

Fig. 5.3: Electrocardiogram shows rSR pattern in V1 without other ECG signs of right bundle branch block. Note that QRS duration in V1 is less than 0.12 seconds (120 ms). This pattern is occasionally seen in normal individual without any significant cardiac abnormality.

AXIS DEVIATION

Mild left axis deviation up to -30° is considered normal variation. Left anterior hemiblock in the absence of any cardiac disease can be a normal variant but left posterior hemiblock of axis shift greater than +110° is considered abnormal.[4]

Q-WAVE ABNORMALITY

A Q-wave, in limb lead III, even if it is very deep, is a common finding (Fig. 5.4). It is attenuated or abolishes with deep inspiration. It is a normal variant Q-wave. But the presence of associated Q waves in limb lead II, especially if greater than 25% of the QRS amplitude or greater than 0.04 seconds in duration, indicates old inferior myocardial infarction.[4] Lead III often shows Q waves, which are not pathologic as long as Q waves are absent in leads II and aVF (the contiguous leads).[5] Isolated Q-wave may also be seen in lead aVL in a vertically oriented heart.

EARLY REPOLARIZATION PATTERN

Early repolarization pattern (ERP) is a common ECG variant, characterized by J-point elevation manifested either as terminal QRS slurring (the transition from the QRS segment to the ST segment) or notching (a positive deflection inscribed on terminal QRS complex) associated with concave upward ST segment elevation and prominent T waves in at least two contiguous leads (Fig. 5.5).[6,7] Notched J-point elevation in V4 with a "fish hook" morphology, is characteristic of ERP. The American College of Cardiology (ACC)/American Heart Association (AHA)/Heart Rhythm Society (HRS) recommendations for the standardization and interpretation of the ECG include a statement that the term "early repolarization" is used frequently to characterize a normal QRS-T variant with J-point elevation (Fig. 5.6). In that sense, early repolarization is mostly benign.[8] Incidentally a detected ERP is very common in young athletes.

Truly ERP is an enigmatic common ECG finding, occurring in 1–2% of the general population with preponderance in men, young adults, adolescent Africans, Afro-descendants (African Americans), and athletes. There is a decreasing prevalence of ERP with an advancing age.[9,10]

There are two distinct varieties of ERP:

1. Grusin type II variant
2. Edeiken pattern.

In 1954, Grusin from South Africa described few distinctive ECG patterns which differed from the usual ECGs seen in the white population and considered as normal variant ECGs. He described two different patterns of normal variant ECGs. Grusin type I variant shows deeply inverted T waves, mostly in right precordial leads simulating subendocardial infarction. But this pattern is very rare in Asian population. Grusin type II is also called ERP.

In Grusin type II variant there is an initial, narrow Q-wave with tall R in leads V5, V6; ST segment is slightly elevated with concavity upward, especially in leads V4–V6; there is a tendency to counterclockwise rotation and sinus bradycardia; presence of a definite J-wave in descending limb of QRS complex, best seen in leads V4, V5. T-wave appears tall and asymmetric and U-wave is prominent in V2 and V4 (Fig. 5.7). In contrast to ST segment elevation acute myocardial infarction, in this pattern of ERP there is no reciprocal ST depression or T-wave changes in other leads and no dynamic evolving changes are reflected over

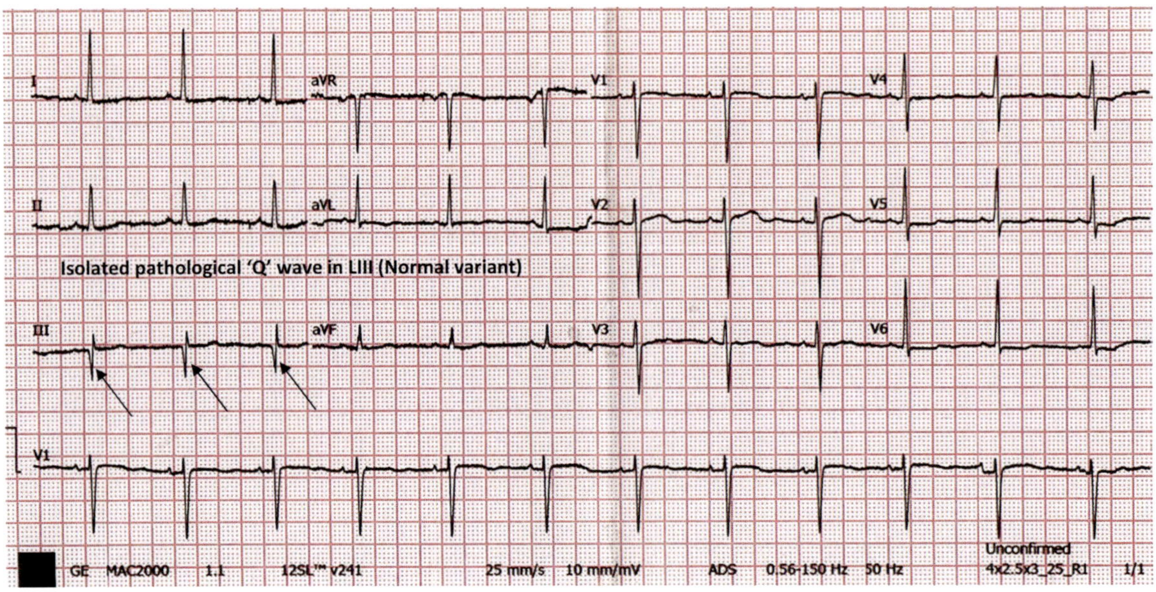

Fig. 5.4: Electrocardiogram shows isolated pathological "Q" wave in LIII (arrows). But there is no "Q" wave in LII and augmented vector foot (aVF). So, it is normal variant ECG.

serial ECG recording. The ECG changes are always static.[11] The Edeiken pattern is an ECG finding when leads V2 and V3 are placed too high. This results in upwardly concave ST segment elevation in these leads and can mimic ischemic ST elevation (Figs. 5.8 and 5.9). When the leads are lowered one intercostal space, the changes disappear.[11]

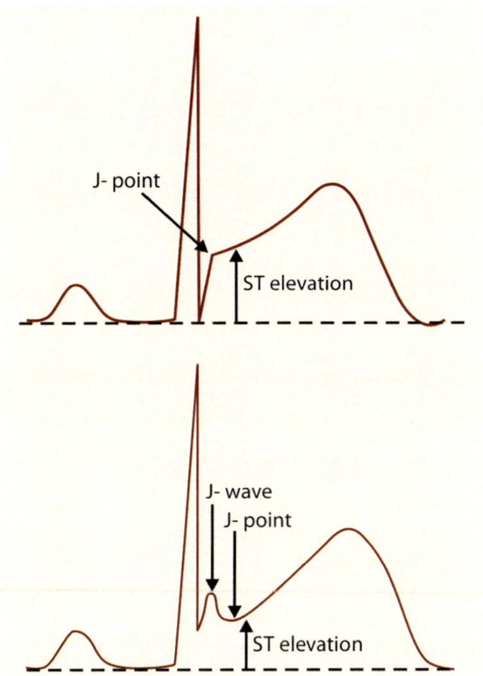

Fig. 5.5: Classic early repolarization pattern with or without J-wave.

Early repolarization pattern has generally been considered a normal ECG variant with good long-term prognosis. However, this long-held concept has been challenged, and recently published population-based studies and reports of associations with ventricular fibrillation and sudden death continue to fuel more momentum.[12-15] In the seminal article by Haissaguerre et al. cases of ERP associated with cardiac arrest had at least 0.1-mV J-point elevation manifested as QRS slurring or notching in the two contiguous inferior or lateral leads.[12] ERP has also emerged as a marker of increased long-term mortality (cardiac and arrhythmic) in the general population.[16,17] Thus, ERP is probably not as benign as traditionally believed.[16-18]

Antzelevitch et al. described early repolarization syndrome into three subtypes: [17]

- *Type 1*: Early repolarization pattern predominantly in the lateral precordial leads (Fig. 5.10). This form is very prevalent among healthy male athletes and is rarely seen in VF survivors.
- *Type 2*: Early repolarization pattern predominantly in the inferior or inferolateral leads (Fig. 5.11). Numerous cases of otherwise idiopathic VF have this ECG pattern; this is also prevalent in healthy young males.
- *Type 3*: Early repolarization pattern globally in the inferior, lateral, and right precordial leads (Fig. 5.12) and is associated with the highest level of risk for development of malignant arrhythmia. It is often associated with VT/VF storms.

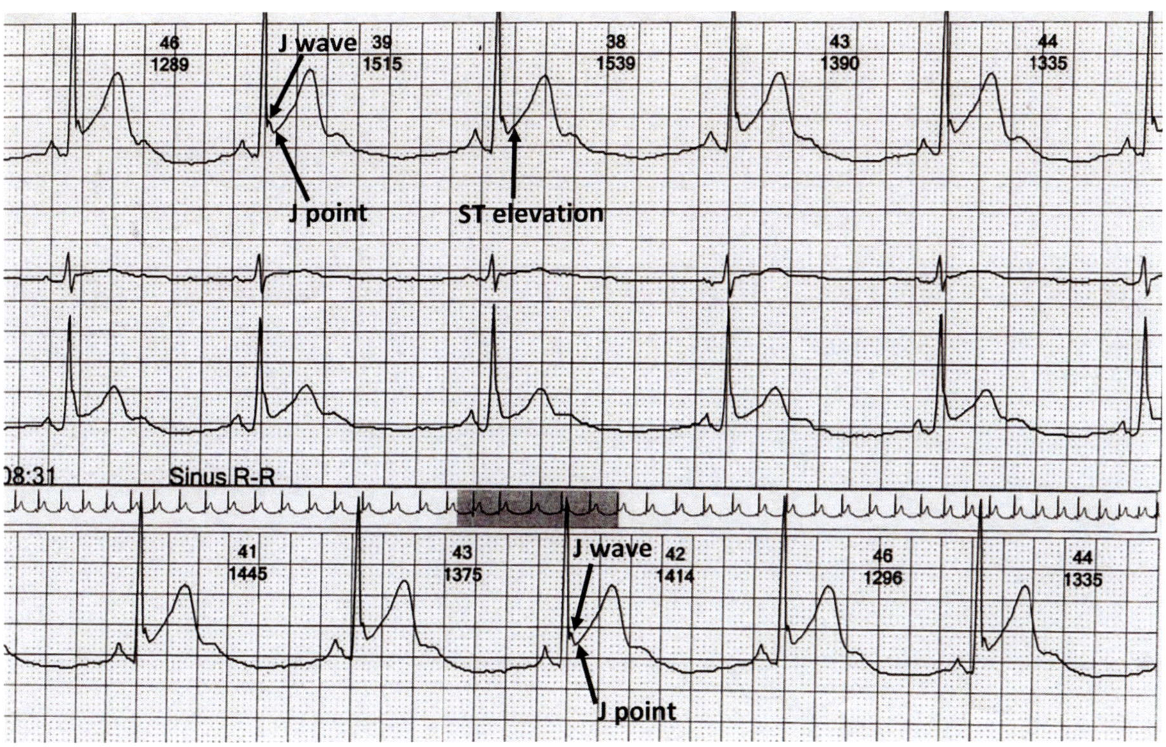

Fig. 5.6: Electrocardiogram showing typical J-wave and J-point elevation (*arrows*).

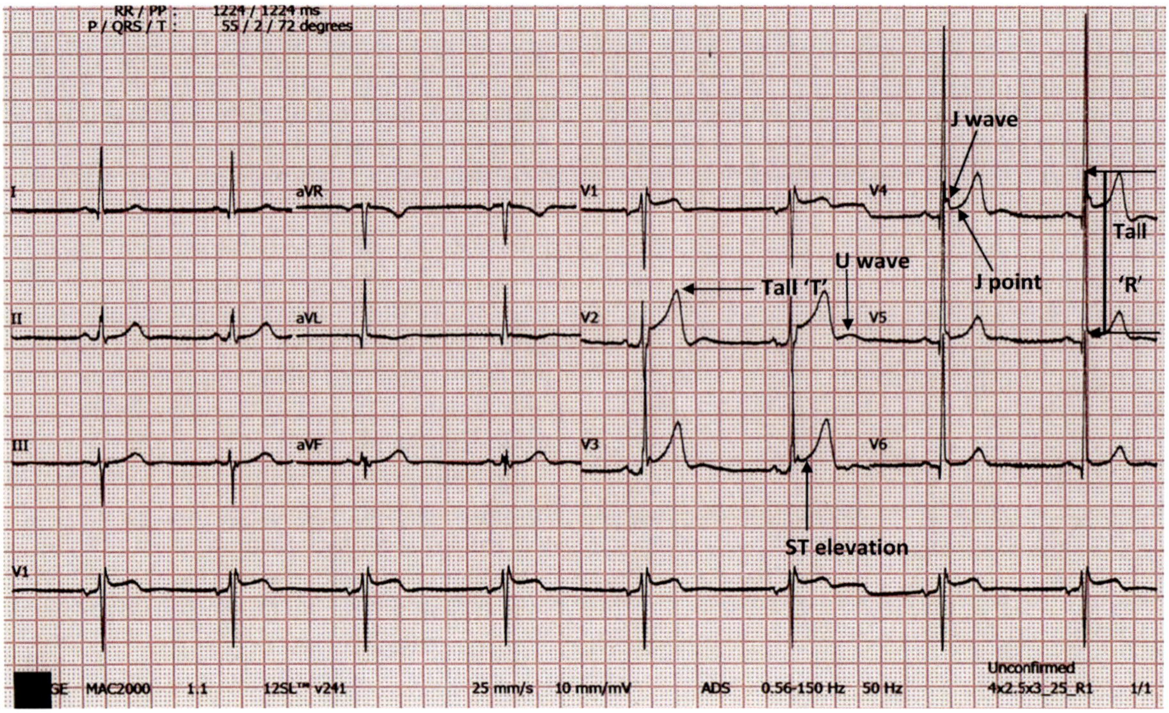

Fig. 5.7: Electrocardiogram showing typical features of Grusin type II normal variant (early repolarization pattern), e.g. (1) sinus bradycardia (heart rate 48/min), (2) presence of J-wave and J-point in chest leads (arrows), (3) tall "R" wave in V5 and V6, (4) > 1 mm ST elevation in chest leads, and (5) tall "T" waves.

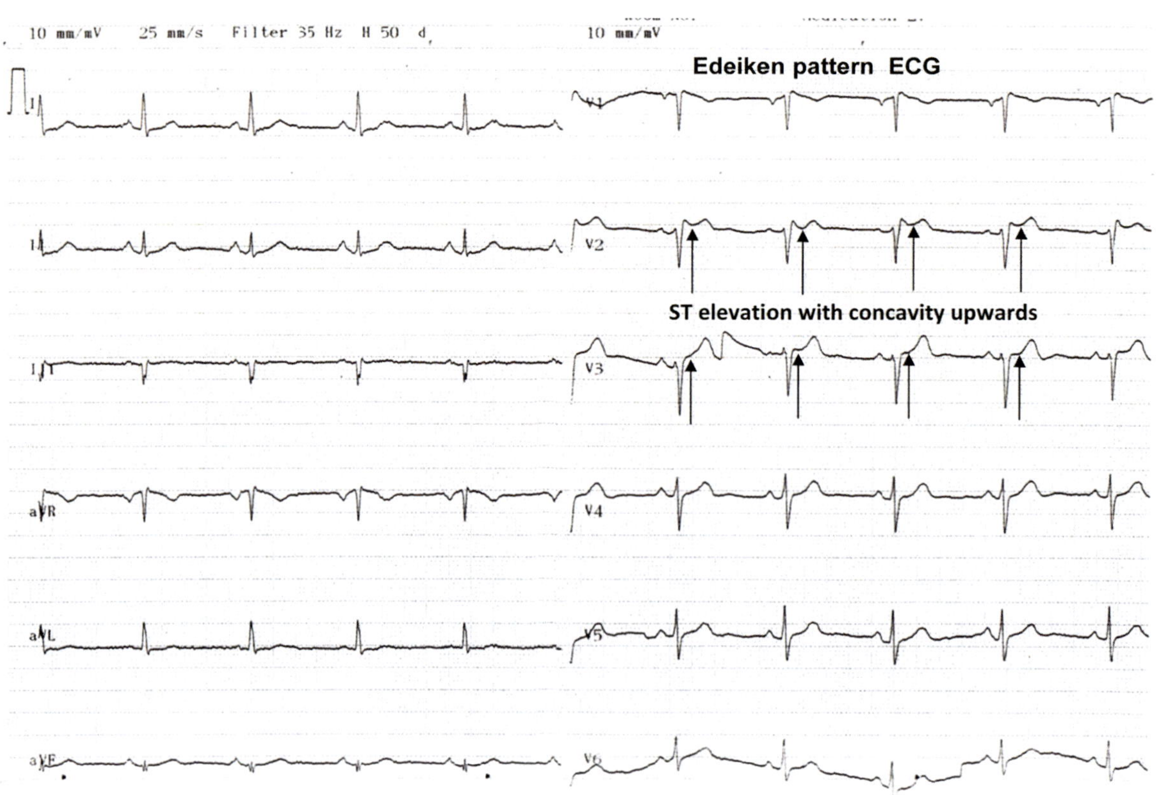

Fig. 5.8: Normal variant ECG of Edeiken pattern showing upwardly concave ST elevation in leads V2 and V3 (arrows).

Tikkanen et al. proposed another classification.[16] This classification is based on the presence of J-point and ST segment elevation (>1 mm) in two or more contiguous leads. Two types of J-point elevation are described:

1. J-point with a rapidly ascending ST segment, which is considered as a benign form.
2. J-point with a horizontal or descending ST segment, which is considered as a malignant form.

The difference between early repolarization pattern and acute myocardial infarction is given in Table 5.1.

NONSPECIFIC T-WAVE INVERSION

A common occurrence that may mimic pathologic condition is the nonspecific T-wave inversion (Fig. 5.13). Diagnosis is then made by exclusion of clinically suspected conditions.

Table 5.1: Difference between early repolarization pattern and acute myocardial infarction.

Early repolarization pattern (ERP)	*Acute myocardial infarction (STEMI)*
An upward concave ST segment elevation	An upward convex ST elevation
No reciprocal ST depression	Associated with reciprocal ST segment depression
ST segment elevation is commonly encountered in the precordial leads and more distinct in these leads	ST elevation in acute myocardial infarction is surface oriented. In inferior myocardial infarction ST elevation is noted in leads LII, LIII, and augmented vector foot (aVF) and in anterior myocardial infarction ST elevation is noted in LI, augmented vector left (aVL), and chest leads
ST segment changes are static	ST segment changes are dynamic
Tall peak T waves are usually seen without any dynamic change	Dynamic T-wave changes are usually present
Usually distinct J waves are present	No such J-wave is present

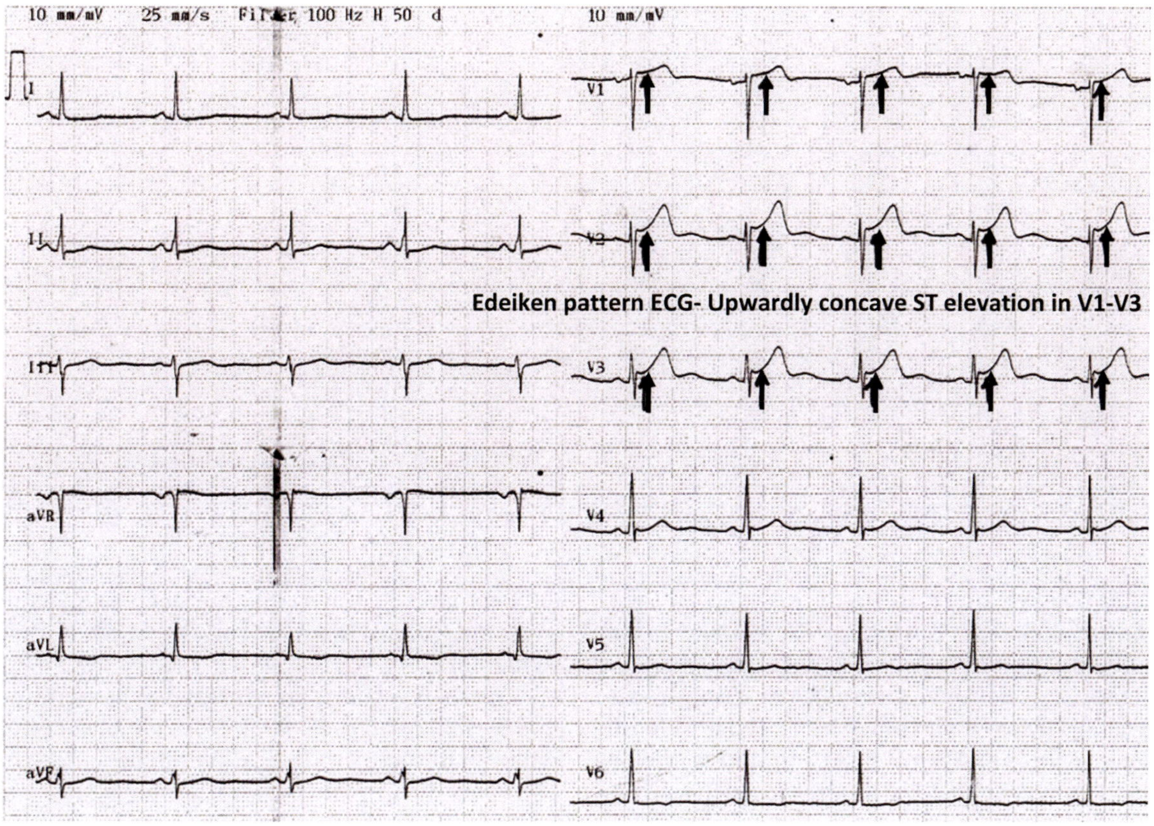

Fig. 5.9: Early repolarization with Edeiken pattern features. Upwardly concave ST elevation in leads V1 to V3 (arrows). There is no reciprocal ST depression in inferior leads. There is no other feature of ST elevation myocardial infarction (STEMI) in this ECG strip. Edeiken pattern is considered as a normal variant ECG.

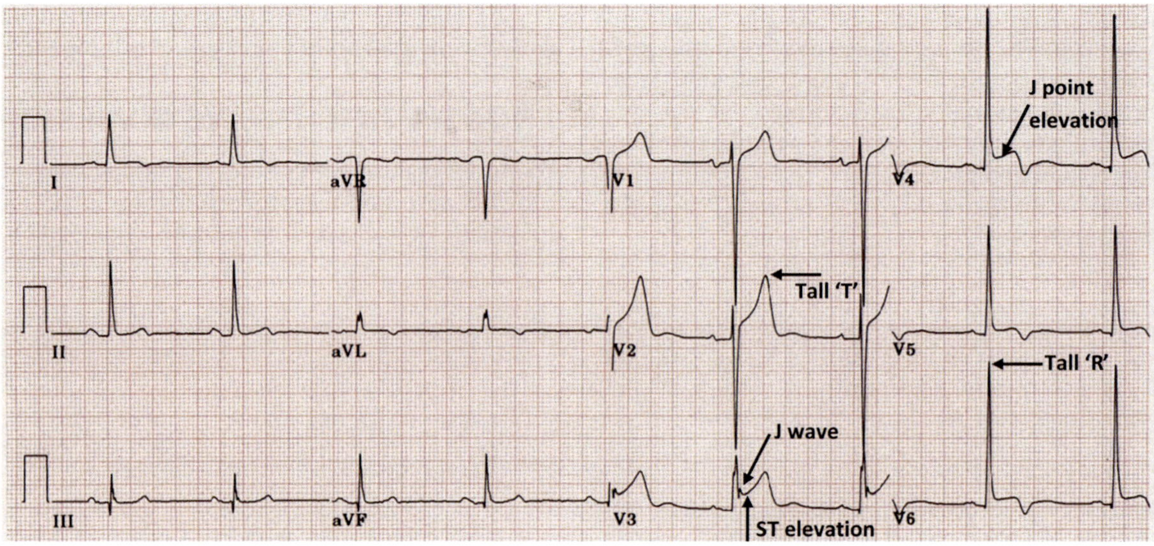

Fig. 5.10: Early repolarization pattern (Type 1). J-wave and J-point elevation with tall "R" and tall "T" waves in lateral precordial leads (arrows).

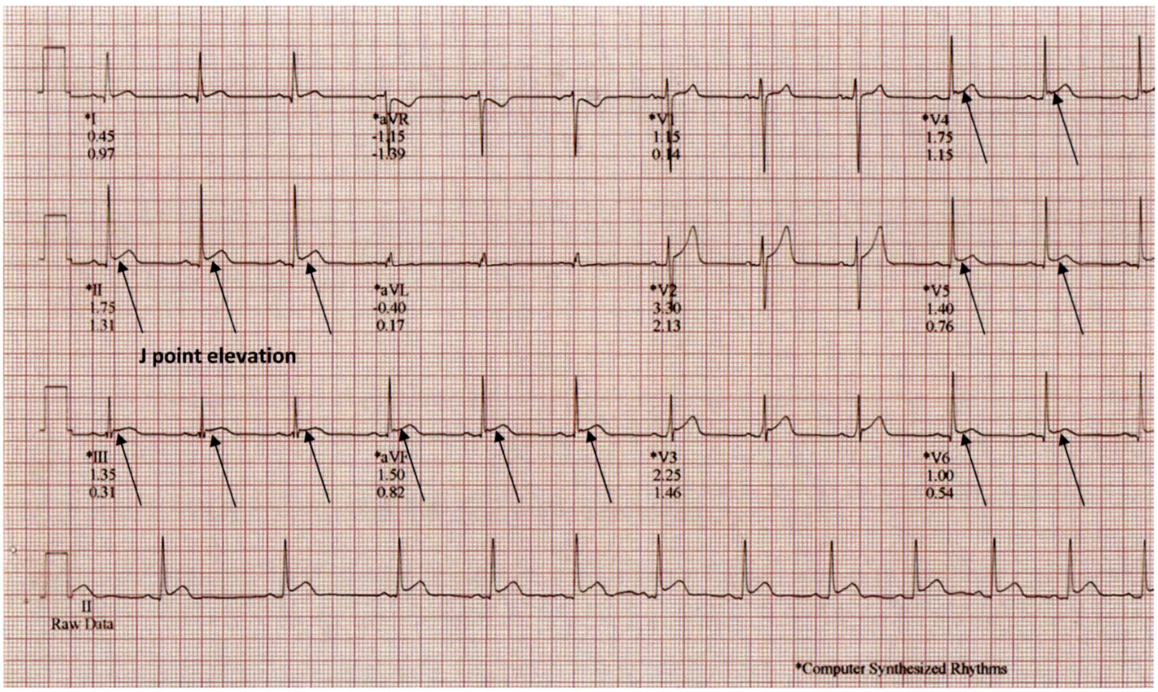

Fig. 5.11: Early repolarization pattern (Type 2). J-wave and ST elevation in inferior (LII, LIII, and aVF) and lateral precordial leads (V4 to V6) (arrows).

Nonspecific T-wave inversion may be seen in fever, anxiety, postural change, postprandial state and during hyperventilation. Sometimes post-tachycardia state and acute or chronic abdominal disorder may also give rise to nonspecific T-wave inversion.[11] Myocardial ischemia commonly gives rise to T-wave inversion, but it must be remembered that inverted T waves are normal in leads III, aVR, and V1 in association with a predominantly negative QRS complex. T waves that are deep and symmetrically inverted (arrowhead) strongly suggest myocardial ischemia.[19]

T-wave inversions are regarded to be representative of the normal spectrum of cardiovascular adaptation in a minority of highly trained adult athletes. The prevalence of T-wave inversions in adult athletes is 3–4%.[19-21] The interpretation of the ECG in young, asymptomatic adolescent

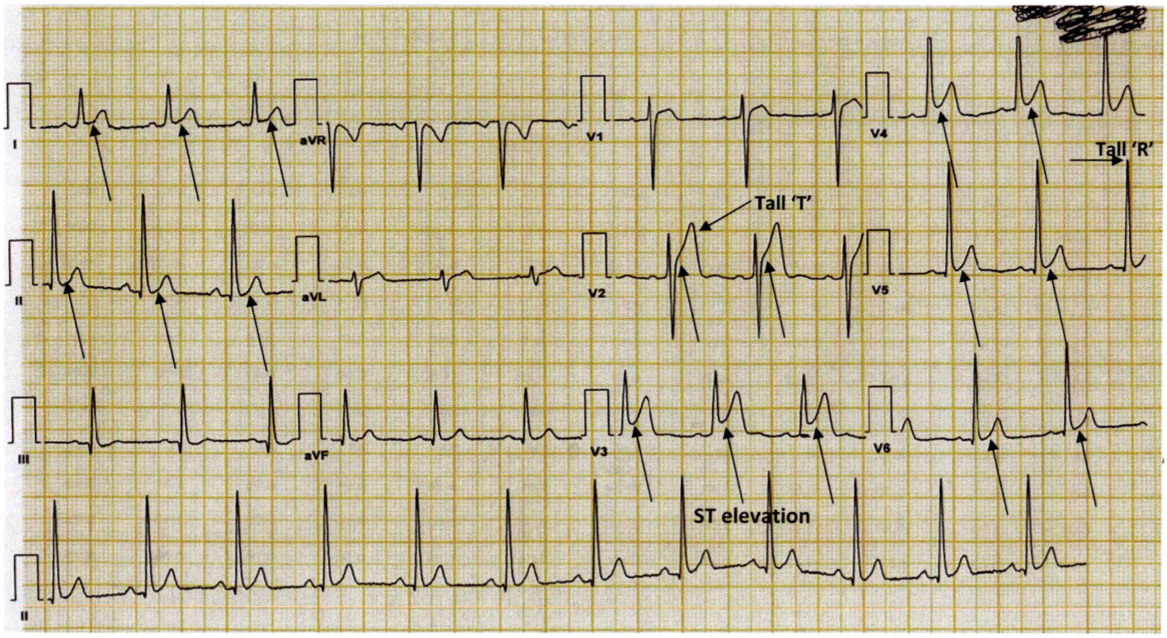

Fig. 5.12: Early repolarization pattern (Type 3). This ECG shows ST elevation with concavity upwards along with prominent "J" point in almost all the leads. Also note the tall "T" waves and tall "R" waves in lateral precordial leads (arrows).

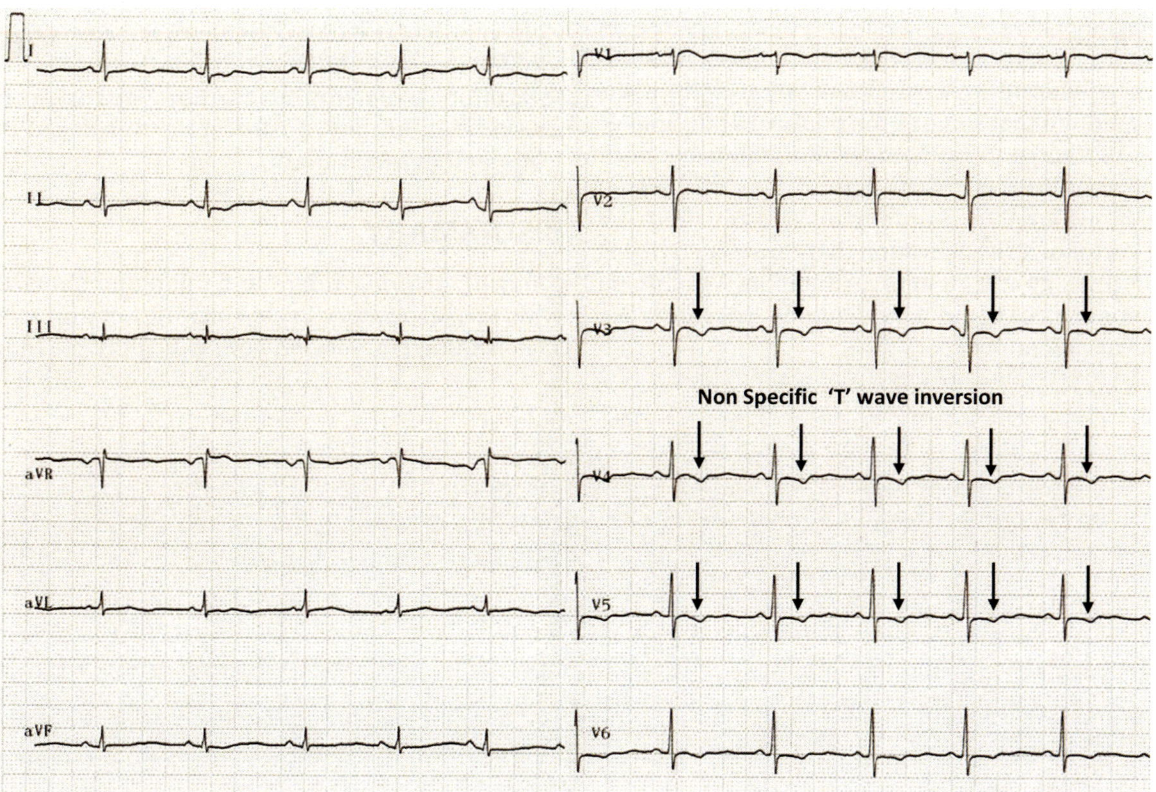

Fig. 5.13: This ECG shows diffuse nonspecific "T" wave inversion in precordial leads. Note that these "T" wave inversions are not deep and are not of arrow head appearance.

athletes can be challenging, since they often exhibit T-wave inversions in the right precordial leads (V1–V3).[22]

PERSISTENT JUVENILE PATTERN

Inverted T-wave in V1 to V4 (Fig. 5.14), commonly seen in childhood but may persist into adulthood. Persistent juvenile pattern of T-wave inversion is seen in 0.4–4.2% of normal adult population.[11] These T-wave inversions may disappear with deep inspiration.

WANDERING PACEMAKER

This is completely harmless, totally insignificant variation of sinus rhythm. The shape of the P-wave changes from beat to beat, but the timing of the beats does not. The rhythm is usually regular and uninterrupted even though the P waves look different. But sometimes the rhythm may be slightly irregular. This phenomenon is important only because it is sometimes confused with significant arrhythmias. The peculiar change in P-wave shape is a result of "wandering" of the impulse in the region around the sinoatrial (SA) node.[1]

Wandering pacemaker is usually caused by varying vagal tone. With increased vagal tone the SA node slows, allowing a pacemaker in the atria or AV nodal area, which may briefly become slightly faster. After vagal tone decreases, the SA node assumes its natural pace. A wandering pacemaker is present when there are three or more ectopic foci within the atrial myocardium that serve as the dominant pacemaker. Since they discharge in random fashion, the pacemaker location is continuously shifting and may be located anywhere in the atrial myocardium. As a result, there is a changing vector of atrial activation that causes a changing P wave morphology and PR interval duration. A dominant P wave (sinus or atrial) cannot be identified. The rate is less than 100 beats per minute.

In the presence of wandering pacemaker the rhythm may be regular but may be irregularly irregular mimicking atrial fibrillation (Figs. 5.15A and B). In such situation it can be confused with atrial fibrillation. However, in contrast to atrial fibrillation, distinct P waves are present in presence of wandering pacemaker (Fig. 5.15B). Ventricular conduction is normal with wandering pacemaker, and thus the QRS complex is normal. Wandering pacemaker rhythm is sometimes confused with multifocal atrial tachycardia (MAT). Multifocal atrial tachycardia is defined as multiple distinct P-wave morphologies, irregular P-P intervals, and a rapid ventricular rate. The normal heart rate in wandering atrial pacemaker differentiates this condition from MAT.[23]

TALL R IN V1

Tall R in lead V1 (tall RV1), is defined as an R/S ratio equal to or greater than 1, is not an infrequent occurrence (Fig. 5.16). This electrocardiographic finding exists as a normal variant in 1% of normal subjects. Physicians should therefore be familiar with the differential diagnosis for this important QRS configuration.[24,25] The electrocardiographic entities which can present with this finding include RBBB, left ventricular ectopy, right ventricular hypertrophy, acute right ventricular dilation (acute right heart strain), type A Wolff-Parkinson-White syndrome, posterior myocardial infarction, hypertrophic cardiomyopathy, progressive muscular dystrophy, dextrocardia, misplaced precordial leads, and normal variant.

SUMMARY

Sinus arrhythmia refers to a changing sinus node rate with the respiratory cycle (inspiration and expiration). This is quite common in young, healthy individuals, and

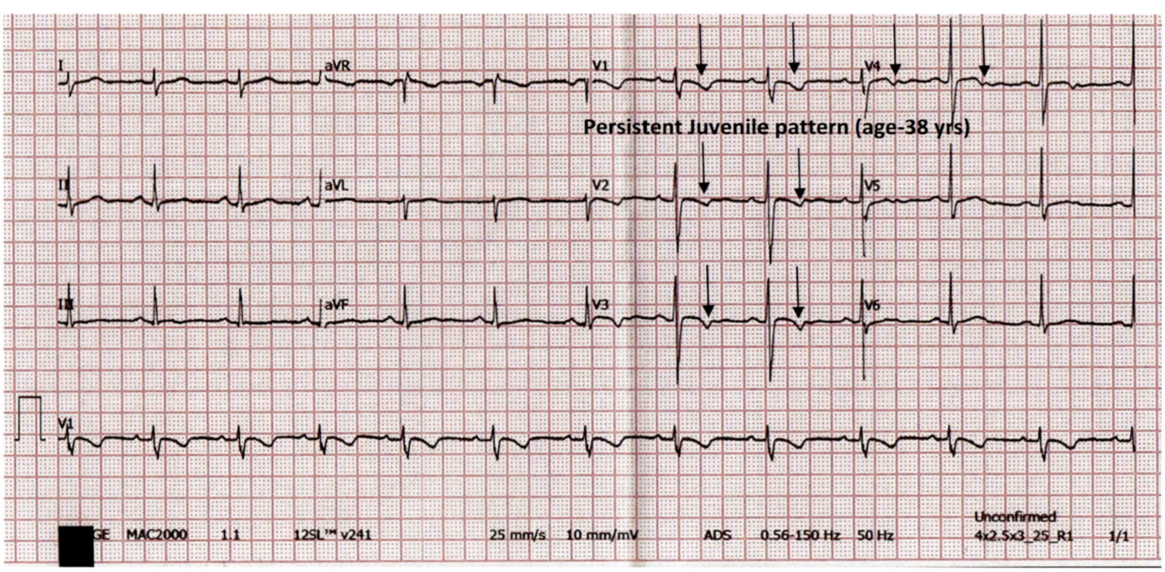

Fig. 5.14: Electrocardiogram shows "T" wave inversion in leads V1 to V4 in a man of 38 years age, suggestive of persistent juvenile pattern.

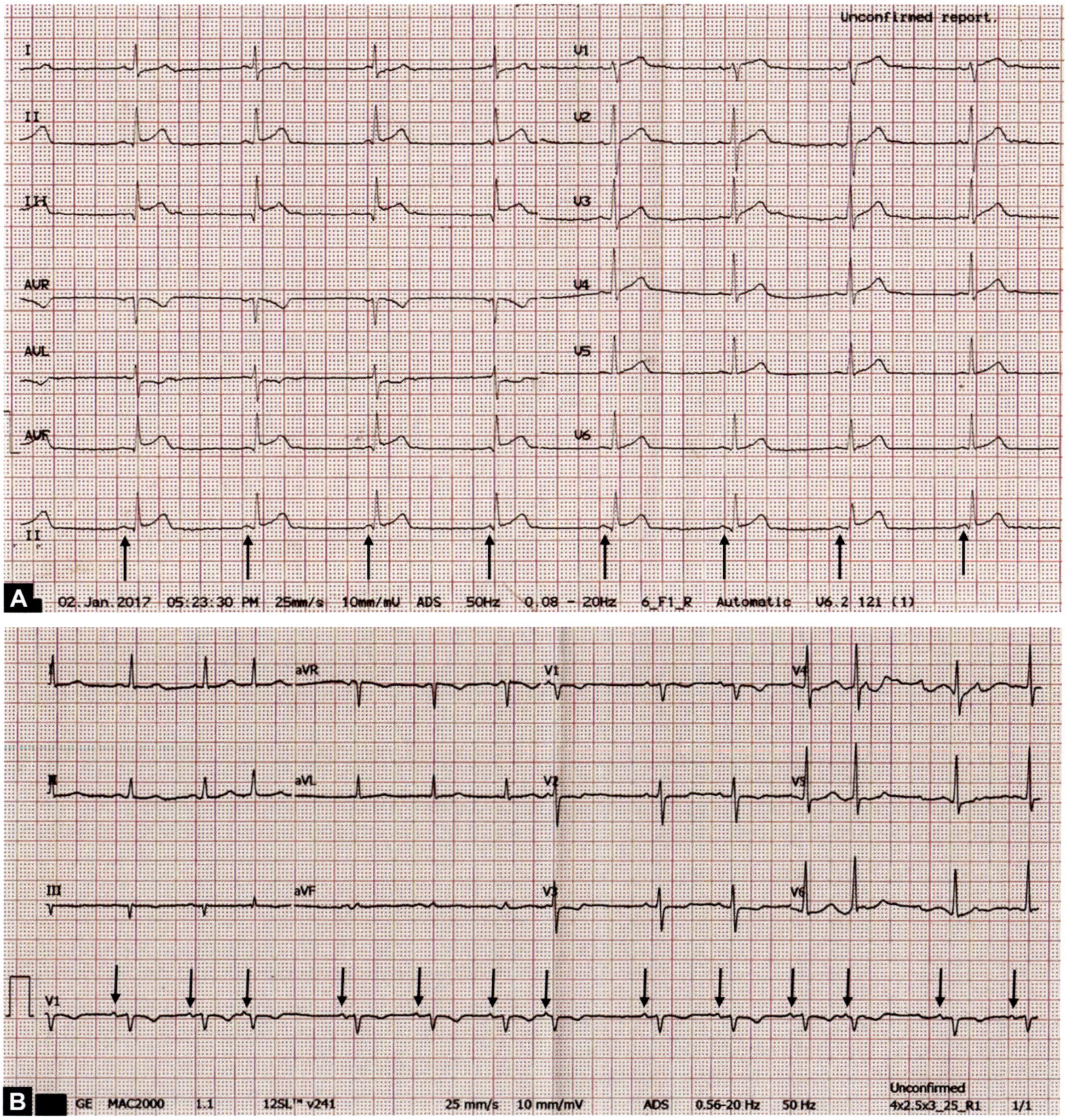

Figs. 5.15A and B: (A) This ECG is suggestive of wandering pacemaker. Each QRS complex is preceded by a P-wave but P waves varies in morphology (arrows) and the rhythm is regular. P waves consisting of greater than three distinct morphologies are seen in this ECG. Note changing P-wave morphology along with variation of PR intervals (Source: Dr. Ziaul Kabir, Labaid Cardiac Hospital). (B) This ECG illustrates the features of wandering pacemaker. Each QRS complex is preceded by a P-wave but P waves varies in morphology (arrows). P waves of three distinct morphologies are seen in this ECG. This ECG mimics atrial fibrillation but note each QRS complex is preceded by a distinct P-wave. ECG of wandering atrial pacemaker is similar to multifocal atrial tachycardia (MAT) except the heart rate. In wandering pacemaker heart rate is normal (less than 100 beats/min) but in MAT greater than 100 beats/min.

has no clinical significance. The heart rate increases with inspiration and decreases with expiration.

Inverted P-wave usually denotes a low atrial rhythm. It is a benign condition and disappears with exercise.

Short PR interval of less than 0.12 seconds (120 ms) is usually considered normal. PR interval may be prolonged normally in vagotonia, in young persons and also in athletes.

A *Q-wave*, in limb lead III, even if it is very deep, is a common finding. It is attenuated or abolishes with deep inspiration. Isolated Q-wave may also be seen in lead aVL, which is considered as nonpathological.

Significant Q waves (greater than 0.04 seconds in duration and at least one-fourth of the height of the corresponding R-wave) suggest myocardial infarction. Isolated small Q waves in leads II, III, and aVF (in the electrically vertical heart) and leads I and aVL (in the electrically horizontal heart) frequently are normal. These small Q waves are known as "septal Q waves" because of the origin of the initial vector in ventricular depolarization.

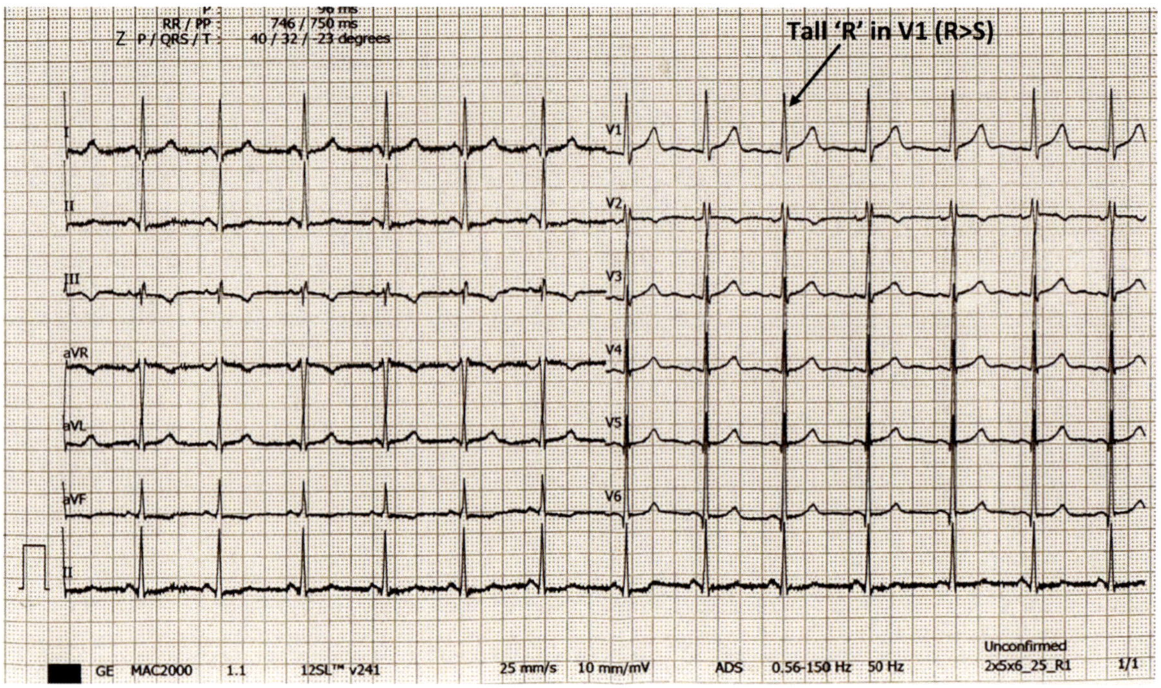

Fig. 5.16: This is a normal variant ECG showing tall "R" in V1 without any other ECG evidence of right ventricular hypertrophy or ST and T-wave changes.

Nonspecific T-wave inversion is a common finding in ECG. Presence of T-wave inversion does not always mean that the individual has coronary artery disease or any other cardiac abnormality. They can occur with hyperventilation, anxiety, drinking hot or cold beverages, positional changes, and also among the athletes.

Early Repolarization pattern (ERP) is a term used classically for ST segment elevation without underlying disease. It probably has nothing to do with actual early repolarization. It is commonly seen in young men. Early repolarization pattern of ST elevation is sometimes confused with acute ST elevation myocardial infarction (STEMI). So recognition of this relatively benign ECG condition is of paramount clinical significance.

Diagnostic criteria of ERP include the following:

- Widespread concave ST elevation, which is most prominent in the mid- to left precordial leads (V2–5).
- Notching or slurring at the J-point.
- Presence of J-wave.
- Tall peak asymmetrical T waves that are concordant with the QRS complexes (pointing in the same direction).
- Tall R waves in V5, V6 along with voltage criteria of LVH.

It is important to recognize the ERP because it may be mistaken for the hyperacute phase of STEMI. But differentiation of these two conditions is not very difficult. ST segment elevation with convexity upward with reciprocal changes is suggestive of STEMI and ST elevation with concavity upward without any reciprocal changes is suggestive of ERP. In STEMI, ECG changes are dynamic but in ERP, ECG changes are static.

T-wave Inversion

- T-wave inversion can be normal
- It occurs in leads III, aVR, and V1 (and in V2, but only in association with T-wave inversion in lead V1).

Wandering pacemaker occurs when multiple areas (ectopic foci) within the atrium generate consecutive action potentials that are all conducted to the ventricles.

Criteria for diagnosis of wandering pacemaker:

- Each QRS complex will be preceded by a P-wave
- P-waves will have different morphologies.
- QRS complex is of normal morphology
- By definition, wandering pacemaker has to have at least three distinctly different P-wave morphologies
- Ventricular rate of less than 100 beats per minute
- Rhythm is usually regular but may be irregular and sometimes mimics AF.

Wandering atrial pacemaker has to have at least three distinctly different P-wave morphologies and a ventricular rate of less than 100 beats per minute. The ECG of wandering atrial pacemaker is similar to multifocal atrial tachycardia (MAT) except the heart rate. In a wandering pacemaker heart rate is normal (less than 100 beats/min) but in MAT greater than 100 beats per minute.

Tall R in V1

Tall R wave in lead V1 is defined as an R/S ratio equal to or greater than 1, which is not an infrequent occurrence. This electrocardiographic finding exists as a normal variant in 1% of general population.

REFERENCES

1. Phibbs RP. Advanced ECG, 2nd edition. Philadelphia: Elsevier; 2009.
2. Engel G, Beckerman JG, Froelicher VF, et al. Electrocardiographic arrhythmia risk testing. Curr Probl Cardiol. 2004;29:357-432.
3. Silberman WS. Electrocardiogram problems. Fed Air Surg Med Bull. 2009;49:4.
4. Hai KT, Wah LK. The normal electrocardiogram and its variants. In: The Electrocardiogram, 3rd revision course. Bukit Merah: Singapore General Hospital; 1990. pp. 5-7.
5. Thygesen K, Alpert JS, White HD, et al. Universal definition of myocardial infarction. Circulation. 2007;116(22):2634-53.
6. Mehta M, Jain AC, Mehta A. Early repolarization. Clin Cardiol. 1999;22:59-65.
7. Klatsky AL, Oehm R, Cooper RA, et al. The early repolarization normal variant electrocardiogram: correlates and consequences. Am J Med. 2003;115(3):171-7.
8. Rautaharju PM, Surawicz B, Gettes LS, et al. AHA/ACCF/HRS recommendations for the standardization and interpretation of the electrocardiogram: part IV: the ST segment, T and U waves, and the QT interval: a scientific statement from the American Heart Association Electrocardiography and Arrhythmias Committee, Council on Clinical Cardiology; the American College of Cardiology Foundation; and the Heart Rhythm Society: endorsed by the International Society for Computerized Electrocardiology. Circulation. 2009;119(10):e241-50.
9. Di Paolo FM, Schmied C, Zerguini YA. The athlete's heart in adolescent Africans: An electrocardiographic and echocardiographic study. J Am Coll Cardiol. 2012;59(11):1029-36.
10. Perez-Riera AR, de Abreu LC, Yanowitz F, et al. "Benign" early repolarization versus malignant early abnormalities: Clinical-electrocardiographic distinction and genetic basis. Cardiol J. 2012;19(4):337-46.
11. Siong CT. Normal variant ECG. The Electrocardiogram, 4th Basic and Advanced Course on ECG. Bukit Merah: Singapore General Hospital; 1993. pp. 9-13.
12. Haissaguerre M, Derval N, Sacher F, et al. Sudden cardiac arrest associated with early repolarization. N Engl J Med. 2008;358(19):2016-23.
13. Nam GB, Kim YH, Antzelevitch C. Augmentation of J waves and electrical storms in patients with early repolarization. N Engl J Med. 2008;358:2078-9.
14. Rosso R, Kogan E, Belhassen B, et al. J-point elevation in survivors of primary ventricular fibrillation and matched control subjects: incidence and clinical significance. J Am Coll Cardiol. 2008;52(15):1231-8.
15. Derval N, Simpson CS, Birnie DH, et al. Prevalence and characteristics of early repolarization in the CASPER registry: cardiac arrest survivors with preserved ejection fraction registry. J Am Coll Cardiol. 2011;58:722-8.
16. Tikkanen JT, Anttonen O, Junttila MJ, et al. Long-term outcome associated with early repolarization on electrocardiography. N Engl J Med. 2009;361(26):2529-37.
17. Antzelevitch C. Yan GX. J wave syndromes-contemporary review. Heart Rhythm. 2010;7(4):549-59.
18. Derval N, Shah A, Jais P. Definition of early repolarization: a tug of war. Circulation. 2011; 124(20):2185-6.
19. Pelliccia A, Maron BJ, Culasso F, et al. Clinical significance of abnormal electrocardiographic patterns in trained athletes. Circulation. 2000;102(3):278-84.
20. Marcus FI. Prevalence of T-wave inversion beyond V1 in young normal individuals and usefulness for the diagnosis of arrhythmogenic right ventricular cardiomyopathy/dysplasia. Am J Cardiol. 2005;95(9):1070-1.
21. Pelliccia A, Culasso F, Di Paolo FM, et al. Prevalence of abnormal electrocardiograms in a large, unselected population undergoing pre-participation cardiovascular screening. Eur Heart J. 2007;28(16):2006-10.
22. Papadakis M, Basavarajaiah S, Rawlins J, et al. Prevalence and significance of T-wave inversions in predominantly Caucasian adolescent athletes. Eur Heart J. 2009;30(14):1728-35.
23. Aburawi EH, Narchi H, Souid AK. Persistent wandering atrial pacemaker after epinephrine overdosing-a case report. BMC Pediatr. 2013;13:1.
24. Mattu A, Brady WJ, Perron AD, et al. Prominent R wave in lead V1: electrocardiographic differential diagnosis. Am J Emerg Med. 2001;19(6):504-13.
25. MacKenzie R. Tall R wave in lead V1. J Insur Med. 2004;36(3):255-9.

Chapter 6

Chamber Enlargement

INTRODUCTION

Cardiac chamber hypertrophy/enlargement has important prognostic implications and ECG is the technique most often recommended in the diagnosis of cardiac hypertrophy or enlargement.

Left ventricular hypertrophy (LVH) can be diagnosed in ECG with good specificity. When the myocardium is abnormally thickened and electrical activity takes longer to traverse throughout the whole heart, thus QRS amplitude increases and the duration of the QRS complex may be widened. In LVH, the repolarization process may be affected which can result in abnormal ST segments or T waves. This is referred to as "LVH with strain" or "LVH with repolarization abnormality". At times these repolarization abnormalities can mimic ischemic ST changes, so distinguishing them from those during acute coronary syndrome (ACS) is important, though often difficult. The typical pattern with LVH includes deviation of the ST segment in the opposite direction of the QRS complex (discordance) and a typical T-wave inversion pattern is present. Electrocardiographic signs of LVH are accepted as independent cardiovascular risk factors and indicators of target organ damage but these signs are strongly criticized for their low sensitivity. A broad spectrum of changes are seen in ECG in LVH, including increased QRS voltage, prolonged duration of QRS complex, left axis deviation, prolonged intrinsicoid deflection, left bundle branch block (LBBB), and left anterior hemiblock (LAHB) patterns, as well as pseudo-normal ECG findings.[1]

The detection and assessment of cardiac chamber hypertrophy has long been an important objective of clinical electrocardiography. Its importance has increased in recent years with the recognition that hypertrophy can be reversed with therapy, and that by doing so, adverse clinical outcomes can be prevented or delayed.[2,3] Two terms "hypertrophy" and "enlargement" are often used interchangeably. The 1978 Bethesda Conference favored use of the term enlargement, but hypertrophy is more commonly used in recent research reports and clinical practice. Enlargement may be taken to imply an increase in chamber dimension, which may not be present in concentric hypertrophy. It is doubtful whether enlargement occurs without hypertrophy, at least in chronic stable syndromes.[4]

ELECTROCARDIOGRAPHIC CRITERIA FOR THE DIAGNOSIS OF LEFT VENTRICULAR HYPERTROPHY

Electrocardiographic criteria for the diagnosis of left ventricular hypertrophy consist of:

- Increased QRS amplitude (voltage criteria)
- Delayed intrinsicoid deflection [increase ventricular activation time (VAT)]
- Widened QRS/T angle
- Left axis deviation
- Secondary ST-T abnormalities
- Left atrial (LA) abnormalities.

Increased QRS Amplitude (Voltage Criteria)

The increased voltage is attributed to one or more of the following factors: Increased left ventricular mass, increased left ventricular surface, increased intracavitary blood volume, and closer proximity of the ventricle to the chest wall (Figs. 6.1A and B).

An increase in voltage may be due to the increase in the number or the size of fibers in the hypertrophied ventricle. The enlarged cells and increased number of intercalated discs in the hypertrophied myocardium are believed to facilitate the intercellular current flow, and this may be expected to increase the strength of the equivalent dipole generated by the excitation of muscle layers.[5] Hypertrophy increases the area of ventricular muscle in relation to the short-circuiting fluid surrounding the heart. Increased surface area and greater wall thickness may be expected to increase the amplitude of R wave.

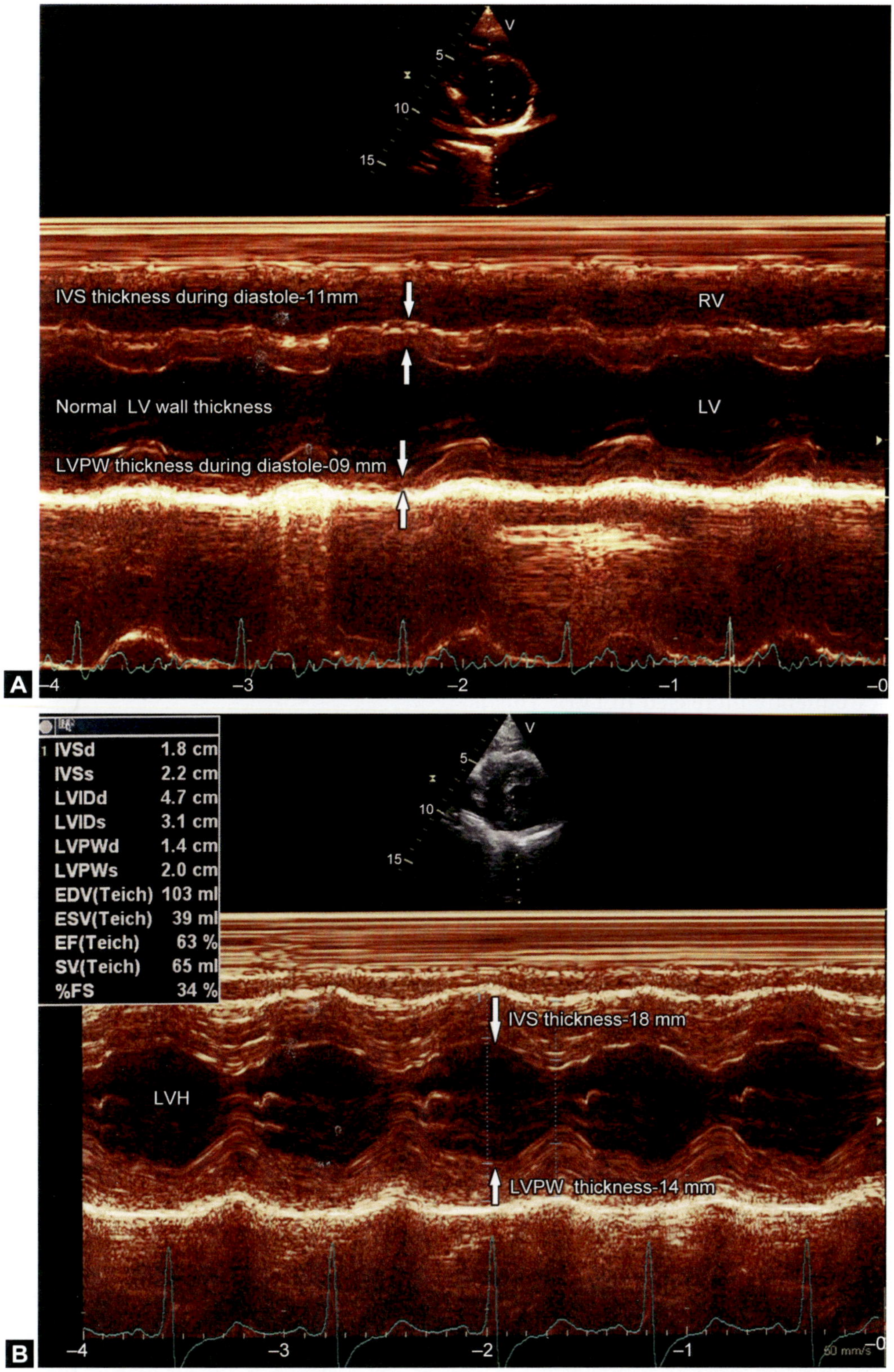

Figs. 6.1A and B: (A) Echocardiogram showing normal left ventricular wall thickness. Normal wall thickness is less than 12 mm. In this picture, the thickness of interventricular septum (IVS) during diastole is 11 mm and left ventricular posterior wall (LVPW) is 09 mm (*arrows*). (B) Echocardiogram showing left ventricular hypertrophy with increase in wall thickness. In this picture, the thickness of interventricular septum during diastole is 18 mm and left ventricular posterior wall is 14 mm (*arrows*).
(*Courtesy:* Dr AHM Abul Monsur)

The most commonly used ECG criteria of LVH are voltage criteria which include:

Precordial leads (Fig. 6.2):

- R wave in V5 or V6 + S wave in V1 > 35 mm.
- R wave in V5 or V6 >26 mm.

Limb leads (Fig. 6.3):

- R wave in lead I + S wave in lead III > 25 mm.
- R wave in aVL > 11 mm.

Delayed Intrinsicoid Deflection (Increase Ventricular Activation Time)

In the ECG, the time of the onset of the intrinsicoid deflection, also referred to as the R-wave peak time, is measured from the beginning of the QRS complex to the peak of the R wave (Fig. 6.4). The intrinsicoid deflection reflects the depolarization vector from the endocardium to the epicardium. The terms ventricular activation time (VAT) and the intrinsicoid deflection are used synonymously. An interval of 50 ms (0.05 second) in a left precordial lead (in the absence of LBBB) is a highly specific criterion for LVH.

Widened QRS/T Angle

QRS duration is frequently increased in LVH. This is manifested by a diffuse increase in QRS duration or an increase in the time from onset of QRS to the R-wave peak in V5 or V6 (increased VAT) (Fig. 6.5). The increased QRS duration may be attributed to the increased thickness of the left ventricular wall and to intramural fibrosis, which distorts and prolongs transmural impulse propagation. When the electrocardiographic pattern of LVH with a widened QRS is present, there may be loss of the septal Q-wave, often with a slurred R-wave upstroke. Deviation of the ST segment and the T wave in the direction opposite to the main QRS vector in the horizontal and frontal planes *causes widening* of the *QRS/T angle*. The combination of increased QRS amplitude and a wide QRS/T angle results LVH with strain pattern.[4]

Left Axis Deviation

Left axis deviation may be associated with LVH (Fig. 6.6). However, it is not known whether left axis deviation results from hypertrophy itself, a degree of left anterior fascicular block (LAFB), or other factors that may underlie the tendency toward a more leftward axis with increasing age, even in the absence of hypertrophy. Thus, this ECG finding may be used to support a diagnosis of LVH rather than to make the diagnosis.[4]

Secondary ST-T Abnormalities

Typical repolarization changes seen in LVH are ST segment depression and T-wave inversion. This "strain" pattern

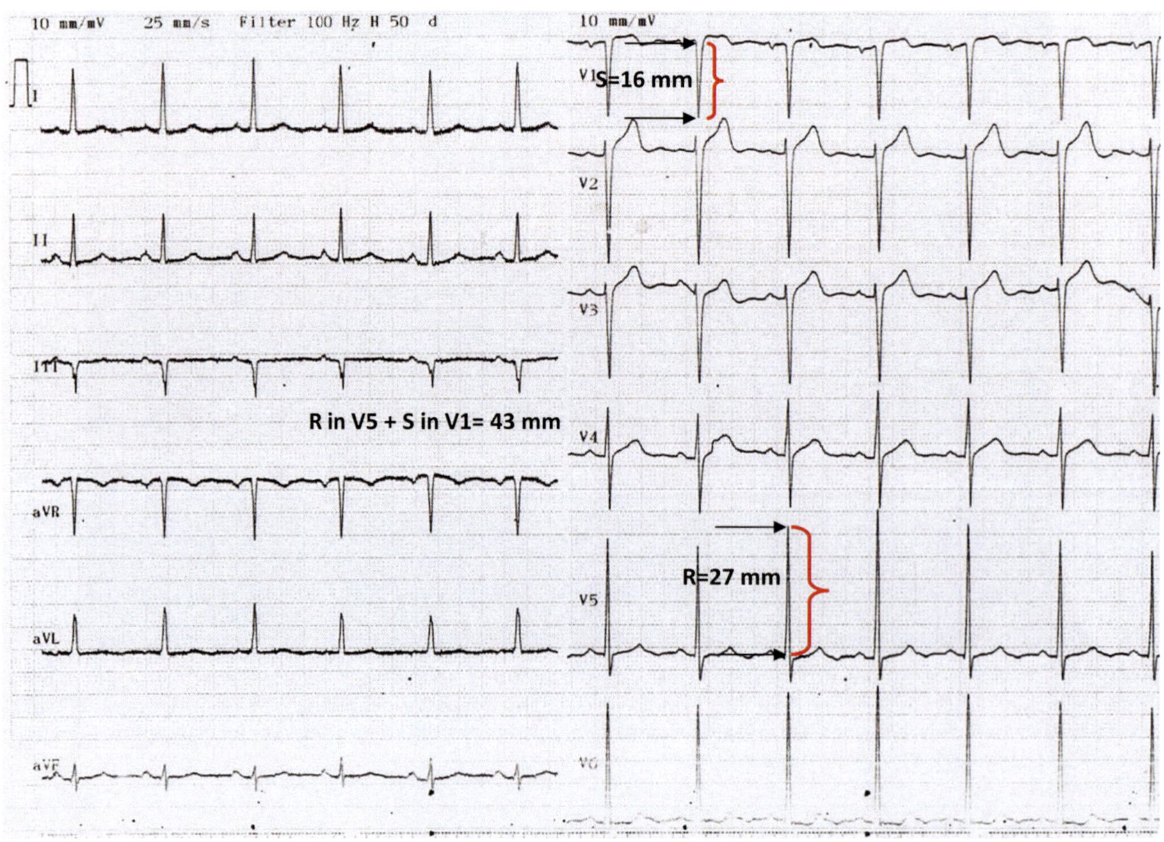

Fig. 6.2: Left ventricular hypertrophy with voltage criteria. In this electrocardiogram, amplitude of R wave in V5 is 27 mm and S depth in V1 is 16 mm. As the sum of RV5 + SV1 (43 mm) is greater than 35 mm, on voltage criteria, left ventricular hypertrophy is present.

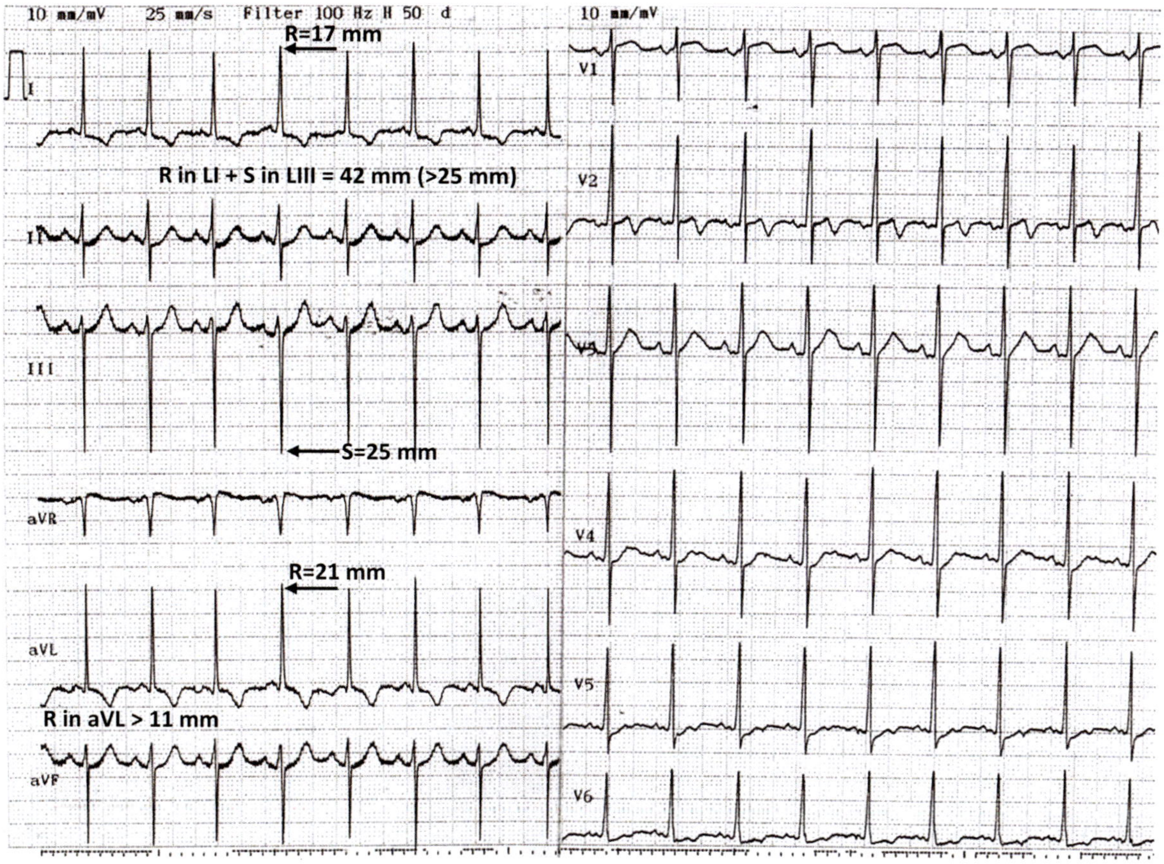

Fig. 6.3: Left ventricular hypertrophy with voltage criteria. In this electrocardiogram, amplitude of R wave in LI is 17 mm and S depth in LIII is 25 mm. As the sum of RLI + SLIII (42 mm) is greater than 25 mm, on voltage criteria, left ventricular hypertrophy is present. In the same electrocardiogram, R-wave height in aVL is 21 mm (>11 mm), so left ventricular hypertrophy is present on voltage criteria.

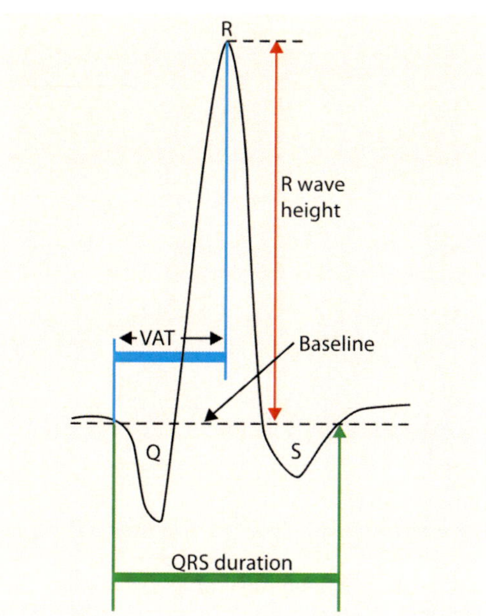

Fig. 6.4: Schematic representation of ventricular activation time.

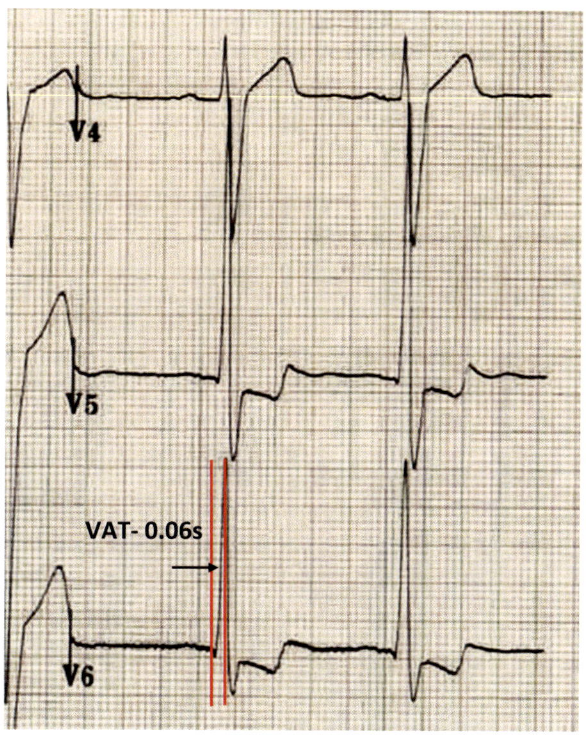

Fig. 6.5: Electrocardiogram documentation of ventricular activation time. In this electrocardiogram, ventricular activation time is 0.06 second. Normal ventricular activation time is less than 0.05 second in leads V5 and V6.

is seen in the left precordial leads and is associated with reciprocal ST segment elevation in the right precordial leads. Furthermore, in patients known to have LVH it can be difficult to diagnose confidently acute ischemia on the basis of ST segment changes in the left precordial leads (Fig. 6.7). It is an advantage to have old ECGs for comparison. Other nonvoltage criteria are common in LVH. Left atrial enlargement (LAE)/hypertrophy or prolonged atrial depolarization and left axis deviation are often present; and poor R-wave progression is commonly seen. The electrocardiogram is abnormal in almost 50% of patients with hypertension, with minimal changes in 20% and obvious features of LVH in 30%. There is a linear correlation between the ECG changes and the severity and duration of the hypertension. High amplitude QRS complexes are seen first, followed by the development of nonvoltage criteria.[6] The presence of these ST segment changes can cause diagnostic difficulty in patients complaining of ischemic type chest pain; failure to recognize the features of LVH can lead to the inappropriate administration of thrombolytic therapy or coronary angiography with a view to perform percutaneous coronary intervention (PCI). LVH systolic

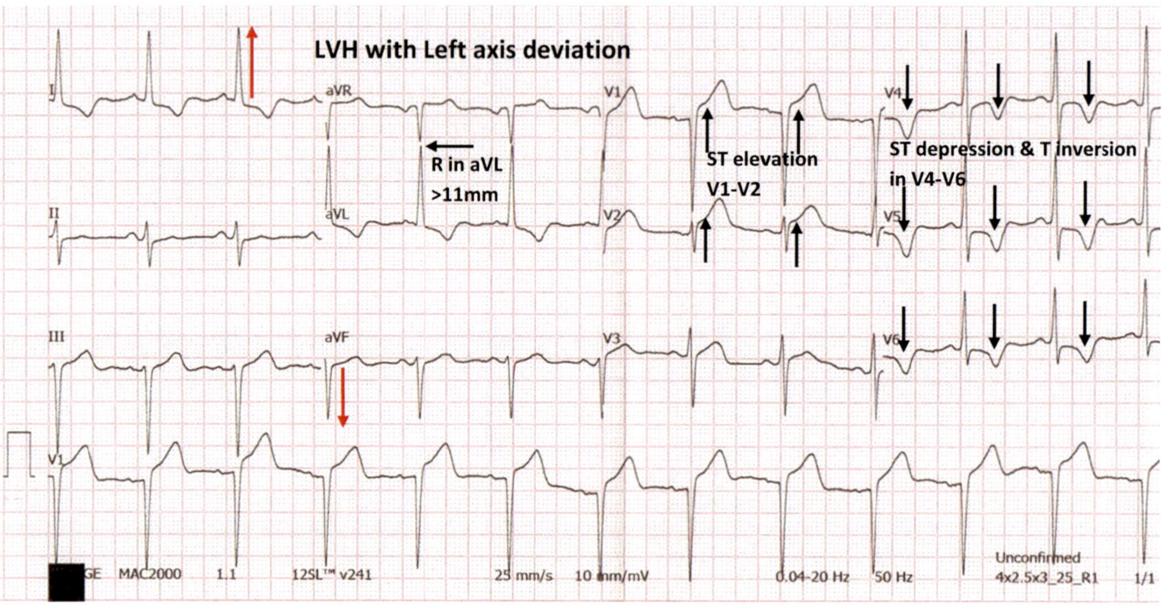

Fig. 6.6: Electrocardiogram shows left ventricular hypertrophy with left axis deviation (Tall R in LI and dominant S in aVF) (*red arrows*). This electrocardiogram also shows other evidences of left ventricular hypertrophy (R in aVL > 11 mm, ST elevation in right precordial leads and ST segment depression and T-wave inversions in left precordial leads (*black arrows*).

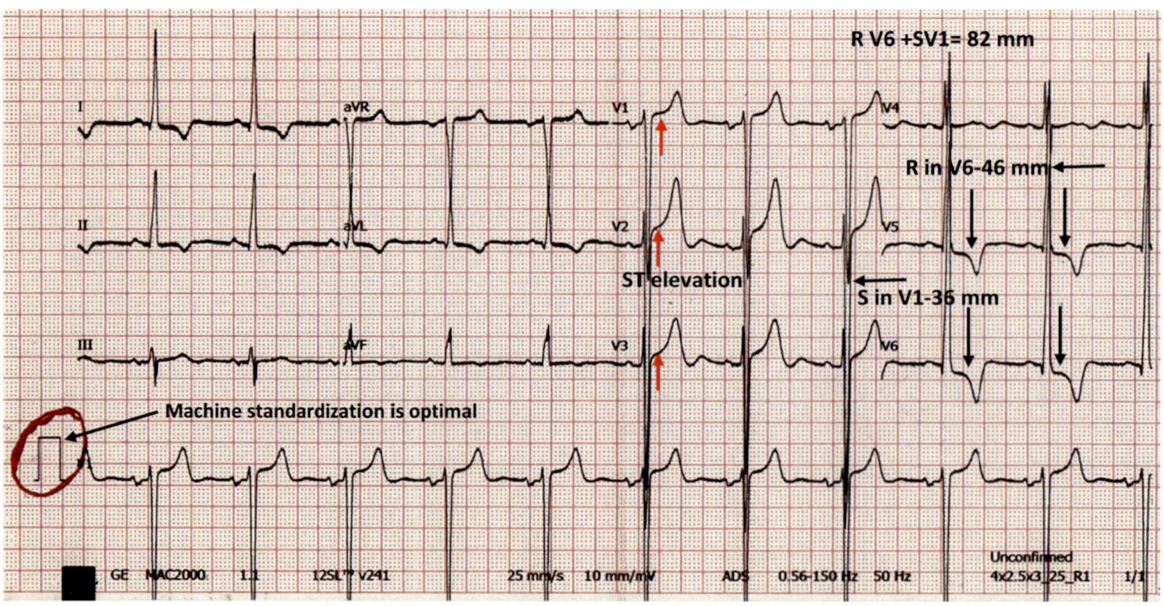

Fig. 6.7: Electrocardiogram of left ventricular hypertrophy strain pattern. RV6 + SV1 = 82 mm suggestive of left ventricular hypertrophy. Electrocardiogram also reveals ST segment depression with asymmetrical T-wave inversions in lateral chest leads most marked in leads V5, V6 (*inverted black arrows*) and ST elevation in right precordial leads V1–V3 (*red arrows*).

overload pattern (LVH strain) may produce ST elevation in right precordial leads (V1–V3) mimicking anteroseptal STEMI (Fig. 6.8) and sometimes it becomes so confusing that serial ECGs or bedside echocardiogram are needed to confirm the diagnosis.

Left Atrial Abnormalities

P-wave abnormalities that are known to be associated with LA dilatation, hypertrophy, conduction delay, or elevated pressure are frequently associated with LVH and have been used as diagnostic criteria (Fig. 6.9). P-wave changes occur frequently in patients with hypertension, and they may be the earliest ECG sign of hypertensive heart disease. However, similar P-wave abnormalities often occur in the absence of LVH. For this reason, P-wave abnormalities should only be used as a supporting criterion for the ECG diagnosis of LVH.

DIAGNOSTIC CRITERIA OF LEFT VENTRICULAR HYPERTROPHY BASED ON QRS VOLTAGE

The most commonly used diagnostic criteria for LVH are based on measurements of QRS voltages. Criteria were

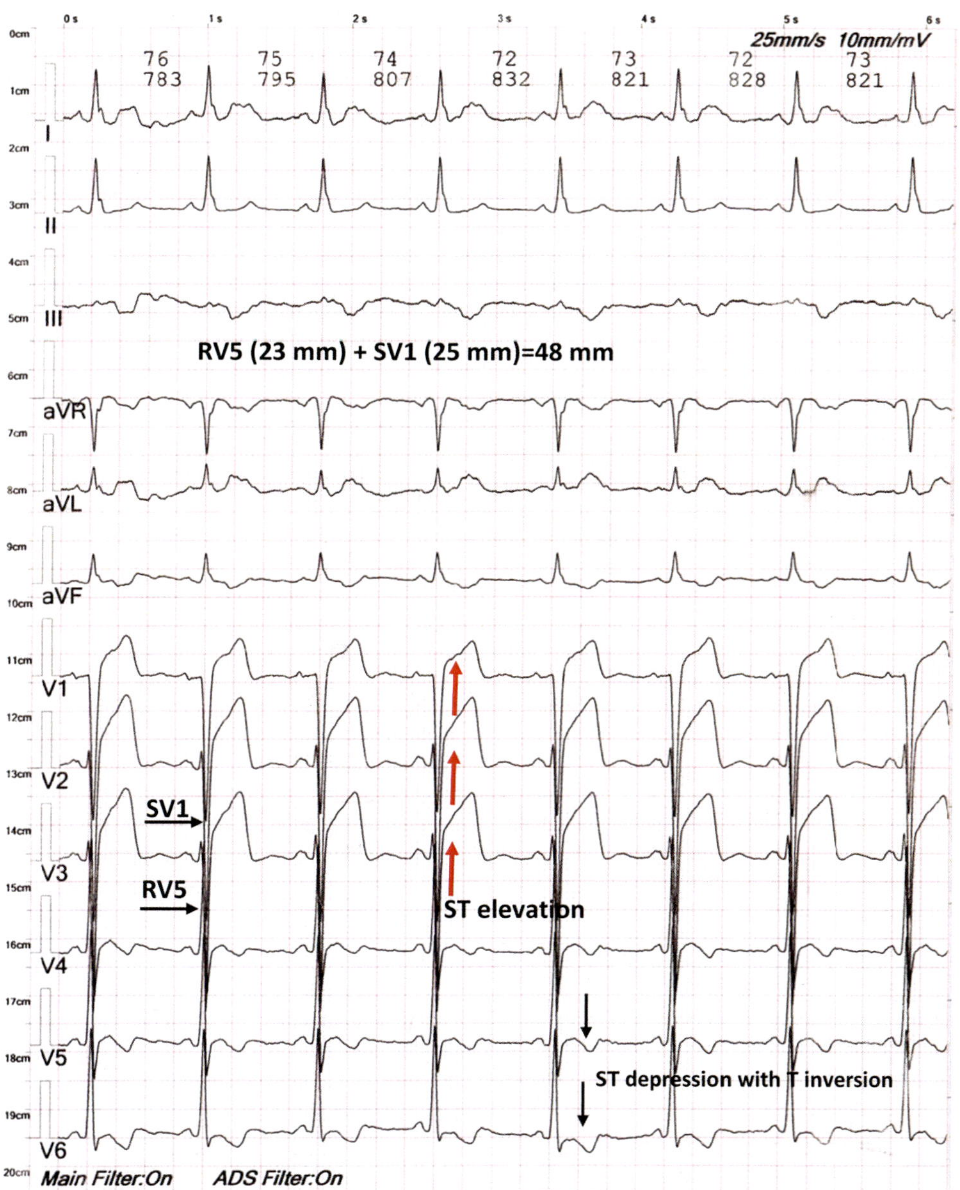

Fig. 6.8: Left ventricular hypertrophy strain pattern electrocardiogram showing ST segment elevation with tall peak T waves in leads V1–V3 (*red arrows*) mimicking anterior STEMI. In this electrocardiogram, RV5 (23 mm) + SV1 (25 mm) = 48 mm suggesting left ventricular hypertrophy and note ST depression and T wave inversions in lead V5 and V6. Also note there is no significant reciprocal ST depression in inferior leads which is usually present in the setting of anterior STEMI. Sometimes history and initial electrocardiogram is so confusing that serial electrocardiograms or bedside echocardiogram may help to exclude the diagnosis of STEMI.

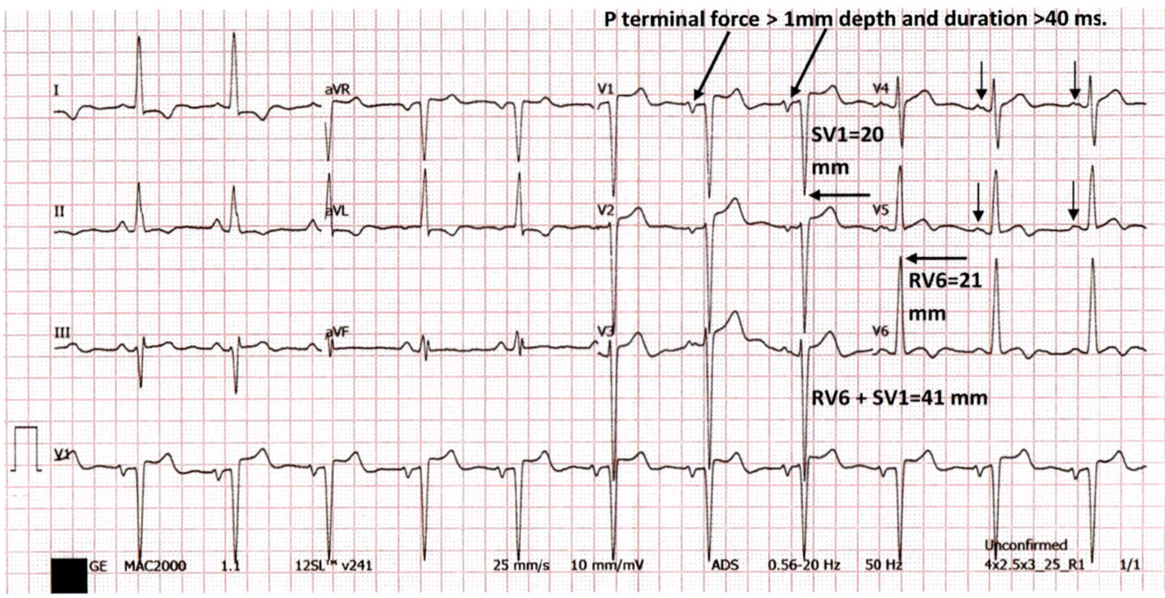

Fig. 6.9: Left ventricular hypertrophy with electrocardiogram evidence of left atrial enlargement. Note terminal P negativity in lead V1 (P-terminal force) is greater than 1 mm depth and is greater than 40 ms duration and also note upright and notched P waves in leads V4 and V5.

originally based on R and S amplitudes in standard limb leads I and III, using clinical and autopsy data as reference standards. (Amplitudes of ECG complexes are referred to in millimeters, rather than millivolts. Using normal standardization, 10 mm equals 1 mV; 1 mm equals 0.1 mV.) Many other voltage criteria were introduced after the general acceptance of the standard 12-lead ECG, most notably by Sokolow and Lyon, who in 1949 introduced the widely used criterion based on the sum of SV1 and RV5 or RV6.[7] More recently, the sum of SV3 and RaVL, referred to as the "Cornell voltage," has been used.[8] The point score of Romhilt and Estes, introduced in 1968, incorporates abnormalities in QRS axis and duration, QRS onset-to-peak time, and P and ST-T morphology, in addition to QRS amplitude.[9]

Factors Influencing QRS Voltage

QRS voltages are influenced by a variety of factors other than left ventricular size or mass. These factors include age, gender, race, and body habitus. Their effects may contribute to the limited accuracy of the ECG criteria. Apart from the wide variation in the normal limits of QRS voltage in infants and children of various ages, there are important differences between adults of various ages, with QRS voltages tending to decline with increasing age. In general, the commonly used QRS voltage criteria apply to adults older than 35 years.[10] Adult women have a slightly lower upper limit of QRS voltage than men do. The difference persists after adjustment for body size and cardiac mass. Some criteria have been shown to improve their performance with gender adjustment, but the adjustment is not the same for all criteria.[11-13] Normal values of QRS voltages vary by race. African-Americans have a higher upper normal limit of QRS voltage than Euro-Americans; whereas Hispanic Americans have lower limits.[4] Obesity is associated with increased left ventricular mass by echocardiographic measurement but not with increased QRS voltage. This may be attributed to the insulating effect of adipose tissue and the greater distance from heart to the chest wall electrodes. The effect of obesity differs among the various ECG criteria.[4] The QRS voltage tends to be greater in persons with a thin chest. The voltage is markedly reduced in obese individuals or persons with large breasts.[5] It can also be attenuated by increased resistivity of the lungs.[14] A significant increase in R-wave amplitude in leads VI to V5 occurred after left mastectomy, and in leads V3R and VI after right mastectomy.[15]

The existence of many different criteria for diagnosing LVH makes clinical application more complex. The sensitivity of the various criteria is generally quite low (usually less than 50%), whereas the specificity is quite high (often in the range of 85–90%).[10,16] However, the sensitivity and specificity of each criterion is different. Thus, the diagnostic accuracy will depend on the specific criterion used. Because of these differences in sensitivity and specificity, patients who meet one set of criteria for LVH commonly do not meet the other criteria. In a large group of patients with mild or moderate hypertension, only 11.2% of patients with LVH by either the Cornell voltage criteria or the Sokolow–Lyon criteria had LVH diagnosed by both criteria.[17] In addition, the various criteria have different positive and negative predictive values in different patient populations, suggesting that the value of multiple criteria may be additive.[4,18]

Sokolow–Lyon Criteria

Sokolow–Lyon voltage criteria are very easy to employ in the assessment of LVH.[7,19] Despite the high specificity, the ability of Sokolow–Lyon ECG voltage criteria to detect anatomical echo LVH or the increased left ventricular mass measured by autopsy is relatively low compared with several different ECG criteria.[20] Although there are surprisingly few studies concerning the prognostic effect of employing only the ECG method, in guidelines, Sokolow–Lyon ECG voltage criteria are still on the list of routine tests to determine target organ damage, together with the Cornell index.[21]

The Sokolow–Lyon index[19]

- S in V1 + R in V5 or V6 (whichever is larger) >35 mm (>7 large squares)
- R in aVL ≥ 11 mm.

Cornell Criteria to Detect Left Ventricular Hypertrophy

Cornell criteria is based upon echocardiographic correlative studies designed to detect a left ventricular mass index >132 g/m² in men and >109 g/m² in women. The Cornell voltage criteria for the ECG diagnosis of LVH involve measurement of the sum of the R wave in lead aVL and the S wave in lead V3.[8,22,23]

For men: S in V3 + R in aVL >2.8 mV (28 mm)

For women: S in V3 + R in aVL >2.0 mV (20 mm).

Its sensitivity is around 41% and specificity 98%.[23,24] Based on The Losartan Intervention For Endpoint reduction (LIFE) study the Cornell product criterion may be more accurate to detect LVH than the voltage criteria only.[25] Cornell product criterion is based on the product of the Cornell voltage, with the addition of a 8-mm adjustment for females, and the QRS duration [(RaVL + SV3) × QRS duration] > 2,440 mm.ms. Based on the LIFE study, many professional guidelines recommend the use of the Sokolow-Lyon voltage and the Cornell product criteria for the assessment of LVH. In the Losartan Intervention For Endpoint study, ECG-LVH defined by Cornell product was more frequently observed in women; in contrast, the Sokolow–Lyon voltage criteria was more frequently positive in men.[26]

Romhilt–Estes Score

The Romhilt–Estes score is a unique composite ECG criterion which includes not only QRS complex amplitude but also the ST-T segment. The Romhilt–Estes score, which is based on a point system where six different criteria are awarded a different number of points with a maximum of 13 points and two cut-off values of four and five points, with the five-point cut-off value being more specific. Romhilt–Estes scores include excessive amplitude: three points (largest R or S wave in limb leads ≥20 mm or S wave in V1 or V2 ≥30 mm or R wave in V5 or V6 ≥ 30 mm). ST-T segment pattern of LV strain: three points (ST-T segment vector shifted in direction opposite to mean QRS vector). LA involvement: three points (terminal negativity of P wave in V1 ≥ 1 mm with duration ≥0.04 second). Left axis deviation: two points (left axis ≥ –30° in frontal plain). Prolonged QRS duration: one point (≥0.09 second). Intrinsicoid deflection: one point (intrinsicoid deflection in V5 or V6 ≥ 0.05 second). Two thresholds in use: positive, if greater than or equal to four points or greater than or equal to five points.[9] ST-T abnormalities were commonly observed in patients with LVH by aortic valve disease as compared with much lower prevalence in hypertensive patients with LVH.

Perugia Score

Perugia score requires positivity of one or more of the following three criteria: SV3 + RaVL > 2.4 mV (24 mm) (men) or > 2.0 mV (20 mm) (women), left ventricular strain or a Romhilt–Estes score of five or more points.[27] When compared with traditional criteria for ECG diagnosis of LVH, the Perugia score showed the highest sensitivity (34%) at the expense of a slight decrease in specificity (93%).[28] In one study, the prognostic value of Perugia score for diagnosis of LVH was compared with five standard methods (Cornell voltage, Framingham criterion, Romhilt–Estes point score, left ventricular strain, and Sokolow–Lyon voltage) and the Perugia score carried the highest population-attributable risk for cardiovascular morbidity and mortality compared with classic methods for detection of LVH.[28]

Framingham Electrocardiographic Score and Other System

Framingham ECG score for detection of LVH needs the presence of a strain pattern and at least one of the following voltage criteria: RI + SIII ≥ 2.5 mV (25 mm), SV1/V2 + RV5/V6 ≥ 3.5 mV (35 mm), the S wave on the right precordial lead ≥ 2.5 mV (25 mm) and the R wave on the left precordial lead ≥ 2.5 mV (25 mm).[29,30] The Lewis index voltage criterion is based on voltage amplitudes in leads LI and LIII [(RI – RIII) + (SIII – SI) ≥ 17 mm] and the Gubner and Ungerleider voltage detects LVH, if RI + SIII ≥ 2.2 mV (22 mm).[31,32]

A systematic review of 21 studies, published in 2007, found that all the criteria were less sensitive than specific: Cornell voltage—median sensitivity 15%, median specificity 96%, Cornell product—median sensitivity 19.5%, median specificity 91%, Sokolow-Lyon voltage—median sensitivity 21%, median specificity 89%, and Romhilt-Estes point score—median sensitivity 17%, median specificity 95%.[33]

Electrocardiography is insensitive for diagnosing LVH because it relies on measuring the electrical activity of the heart by electrodes on the surface of the skin to predict the left ventricular mass. The intracardiac electrical activity is problematic to measure externally because the measurements are affected by everything between the myocardium and the electrodes, most notably fat, fluid, and air.[34] Because of this effect, ECG underdiagnoses LVH in patients with obesity, pleural effusions, pericardial effusions, anasarca, or chronic obstructive pulmonary disease (COPD). In addition, the diagnosis of LVH by electrocardiography is strongly influenced by age and ethnicity.[35,36]

Left Ventricular Strain Pattern

The term "left ventricular strain pattern" was introduced in 1941 and referred to a specific ST-T abnormality, which was attributed to an increased hemodynamic burden. It consisted of (1) J-point depression, (2) upwardly convex down-sloping depression of the ST segment, and (3) asymmetrical inversion of the T wave (Fig. 6.10).[4] It is now appreciated that electrocardiographic LVH with ST-segment and T-wave abnormalities occurs in conditions that are not necessarily caused by increased hemodynamic work, as in patients with dilated or hypertrophic cardiomyopathies. Thus, the terms "strain" and "typical strain" are discouraged, and the term "secondary ST-T abnormalities" is preferred. The presence of ST-T-wave abnormalities provides major support to a diagnosis of LVH that would otherwise be based only on increased QRS voltage, and there is evidence to suggest that the presence of ST-T abnormalities are associated with larger values for left ventricular mass and higher risks of cardiovascular complications and mortality than an increase in QRS voltage alone.[37,38] This LVH strain pattern can be encountered in approximately 70% of LVH cases. This strain pattern by itself has 52% sensitivity in the recognition of LVH with a specificity nearing 95%. Identifying this strain pattern is consistent with LVH repolarization changes and could easily be confused with ACS. The strain pattern, however, has a relative permanence and should not change over the short-term as compared with the dynamic changes seen in ACS.[39] ST segment and T wave changes are usually relatively static in LVH strain pattern but these changes are usually dynamic in ACS patients. In contrast to voltage-only LVH, LVH defined by a combination of voltage and repolarization abnormalities has been consistently shown to predict cardiovascular mortality irrespective of adjustment for clinical covariates, suggesting stronger risk associations with the LVH strain pattern.[40,41]

Differentiation between Left Ventricular Hypertrophy with Strain and Ischemia

Left ventricular hypertrophy with strain pattern can produce ST depression in leads LI, aVL, V4–V6 ± II and aVF, asymmetric T-wave inversions in same leads, ST elevation in V1–V3 (±aVR) along with QRS widening possibly due to nonspecific intraventricular conduction delay. These similar

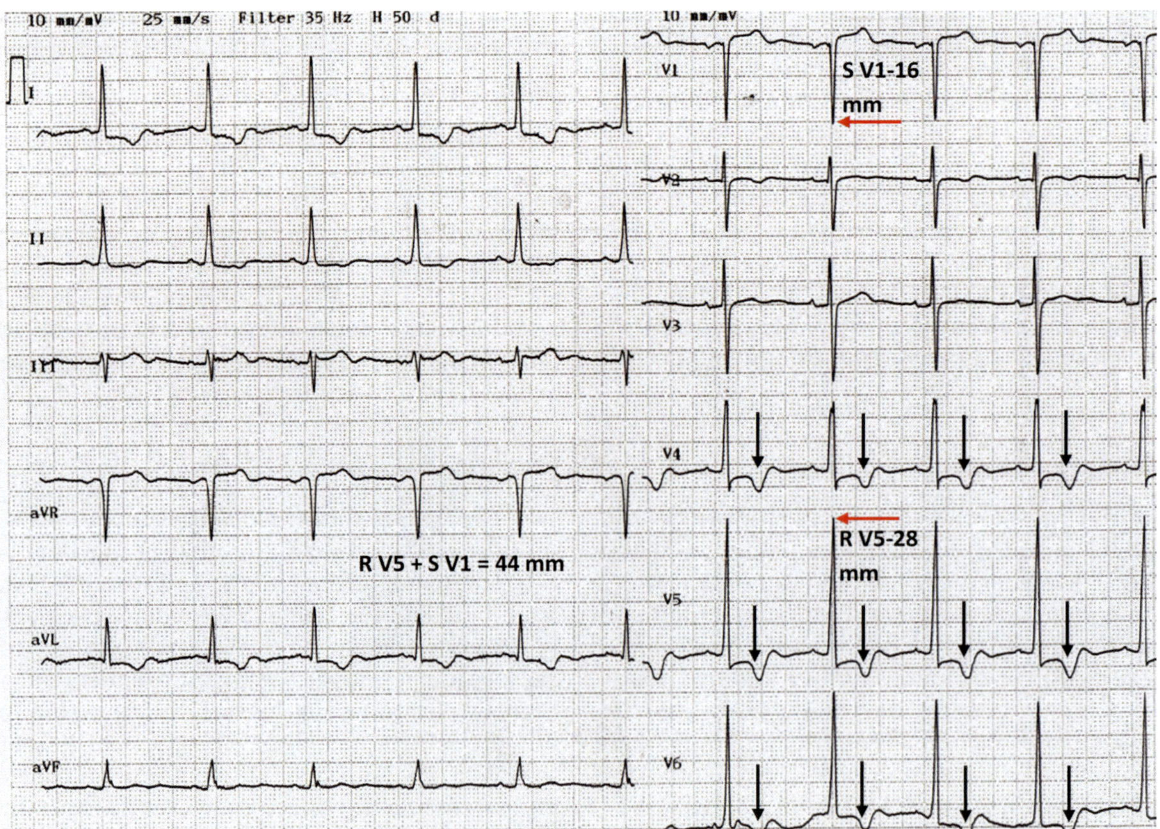

Fig. 6.10: Electrocardiogram of left ventricular hypertrophy strain pattern. RV5 (28 mm) + SV1 (16 mm) = 44 mm suggestive of left ventricular hypertrophy. Electrocardiogram also reveals ST-segment depression with asymmetrical T-wave inversions in leads V4–V6 (*black arrows*).

ECG changes may occur in ACS and sometimes it become problematic in differentiating these two conditions. No reliable way to distinguish between ACS vs. LVH with strain. But horizontal ST depression along with symmetric T-wave inversions are associated with ischemia and downsloping ST depression and asymmetric T-wave inversions are in favor of LVH with strain pattern. Serial ECGs and bed side echocardiogram can differentiate these two conditions.

Diagnosis of Left Ventricular Hypertrophy in the Presence of Left Bundle Branch Block

Although ECG is the technique most often recommended in the diagnosis of LVH, its diagnostic accuracy is hampered in the presence of a LBBB. Studies of the electrocardiographic diagnosis of LVH in the presence of complete LBBB have yielded conflicting results. Some have concluded that the diagnosis should not be attempted in this setting, whereas others believe that the diagnosis can be made.[42-48] Estimations of specificity are affected by the relatively high prevalence of anatomic LVH in patients with LBBB, especially in autopsy series, where it may be 90% or more. LA enlargement type P-wave abnormality [45,46,48] and a QRS duration greater than approximately 155 ms, as well as precordial lead voltage criteria, tend to have relatively high specificity for LVH in the presence of LBBB (Fig. 6.11).[42,45,49,50] While some authors have demonstrated that voltage criteria cannot be utilized for the diagnosis of LVH in LBBB and recommend the use of complementary data[51,52], others have found no significant limitations.[52-55] The sensitivity and specificity of the ECG in patients with LBBB can vary depending on the leads considered, and the precordial leads are those that have a reduced sensitivity.[56] Thus, it has been proposed that a set of criteria that combines precordial leads and limb leads, or the combination of QRS voltage and duration with LAE, may be more accurate in cases of LBBB.[53,57,58] In patients meeting these specific criteria, it is reasonable to diagnose LVH, even though the sensitivity is low. Otherwise, the ECG diagnosis of LVH should not be attempted when LBBB is present.[4]

Electrocardiographic Diagnosis of Left Ventricular Hypertrophy in Presence of Right Bundle Branch Block

Right bundle branch block (RBBB) reduces the amplitude of the S wave in the right precordial leads and tends to reduce the sensitivity of ECG criteria for LVH.[4] The ancillary features of LA abnormality and left axis deviation have enhanced value for the diagnosis of LVH in the presence of RBBB.[59-63] Several criteria have been proposed for use specifically in the presence of RBBB, including SV1 greater than 2 mm (0.2 mV), RV5,6 greater than 15 mm (1.5 mV), and QRS axis to the left of –30°, with S in LIII + largest R+S in a precordial lead greater than 30 mm (3.0 mV). These criteria were reported to have sensitivities of 46–68% and specificities of 57–71%.[62]

Left Ventricular Hypertrophy in Presence of Left Anterior Fascicular Block

In LAFB, also called LAHB, the QRS vector shifts in a posterior and superior direction, resulting in larger R waves in leads I and aVL and smaller R waves but deeper S waves in leads V5 and V6. R-wave amplitude in leads I and

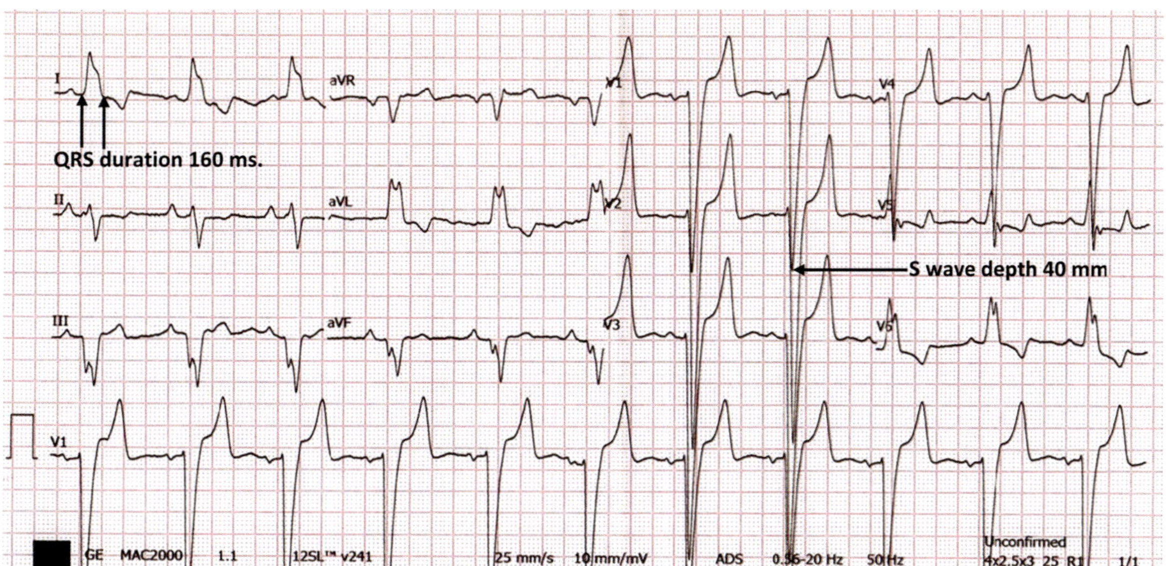

Fig. 6.11: Electrocardiogram evidence of possible left ventricular hypertrophy in the presence of left bundle branch block. Note very deep S wave in V1 (40 mm) and QRS duration 160 ms. Very high voltage and QRS duration more than 155 ms are indirect evidence of left ventricular hypertrophy in the presence of concurrent left bundle branch block. It must be noted that the diagnosis of left ventricular hypertrophy is always hampered in the presence of left bundle branch block.

aVL are not reliable criteria for LVH in this situation. Criteria that include the depth of the S wave in left precordial leads improve detection of LVH in the presence of LAHB.[64-66] In LAHB, LVH is diagnosed whenever the sum of S wave in lead III plus the maximal R + S in a precordial lead is greater than or equal to 30 mm. Further criteria are SV1 + (R + S) in V5 or V6 is greater than or equal to 25 mm, and the presence of secondary ST-T changes.[63]

Left Ventricular Hypertrophy: Pressure versus Volume Overload

When the heart faces a hemodynamic burden, it can do the following to compensate: (1) Use the Frank–Starling mechanism to increase cross-bridge formation; (2) augment muscle mass to bear the extra load; and (3) recruit neurohormonal mechanisms to increase contractility.[67] Increasing mass assumes a key role in the compensation for hemodynamic overload. This increase in mass is due to the hypertrophy of existing myocytes rather than hyperplasia, because cardiomyocytes become terminally differentiated soon after birth. In response to pressure overload in conditions such as aortic stenosis (AS) or hypertension, the parallel addition of sarcomeres causes an increase in myocyte width, which in turn increases wall thickness. This remodeling results in concentric hypertrophy (increase in ratio of wall thickness/chamber dimension).[67] According to Laplace's law, the load on any region of the myocardium is given as follows: (pressure × radius)/(2 × wall thickness); thus, an increase in pressure can be offset by an increase in wall thickness. Because systolic stress (afterload) is a major determinant of ejection performance, the normalization of systolic stress helps to maintain a normal ejection fraction even when needing to generate high levels of systolic pressure.[68] Volume overload in conditions such as chronic aortic regurgitation (AR), mitral regurgitation (MR), or anemia engenders myocyte lengthening by sarcomere replication in series and increase in ventricular volume. This pattern of eccentric hypertrophy (cavity dilatation with a decrease in ratio of wall thickness/chamber dimension) is also initially compensatory, such that the heart can meet the demand to sustain a high stroke volume.[67]

Depending on pressure or volume overload, LVH may be characterized by increased wall thickness (concentric LVH), increased chamber volume (eccentric LVH) or both.[69,70] In order to identify LVH, the ECG is widely used as a primary screening tool. LV pressure overload is usually due to hypertension, AS, coarctation of aorta, hypertrophic cardiomyopathy, etc. When there is pressure or systolic overload the LV becomes concentrically hypertrophied. The walls of the LV are thickened but the size of the LV cavity remains normal. LVH due to pressure overload is reflected in ECG with tall R in V4, V5, and V6 associated with ST segment depression and T-wave inversion. These ST-T-wave changes are often described as LVH strain pattern (Fig. 6.12). Causes of LVH volume overload include AR, MR, peripheral arteriovenous shunts, anemia, and thyrotoxicosis.

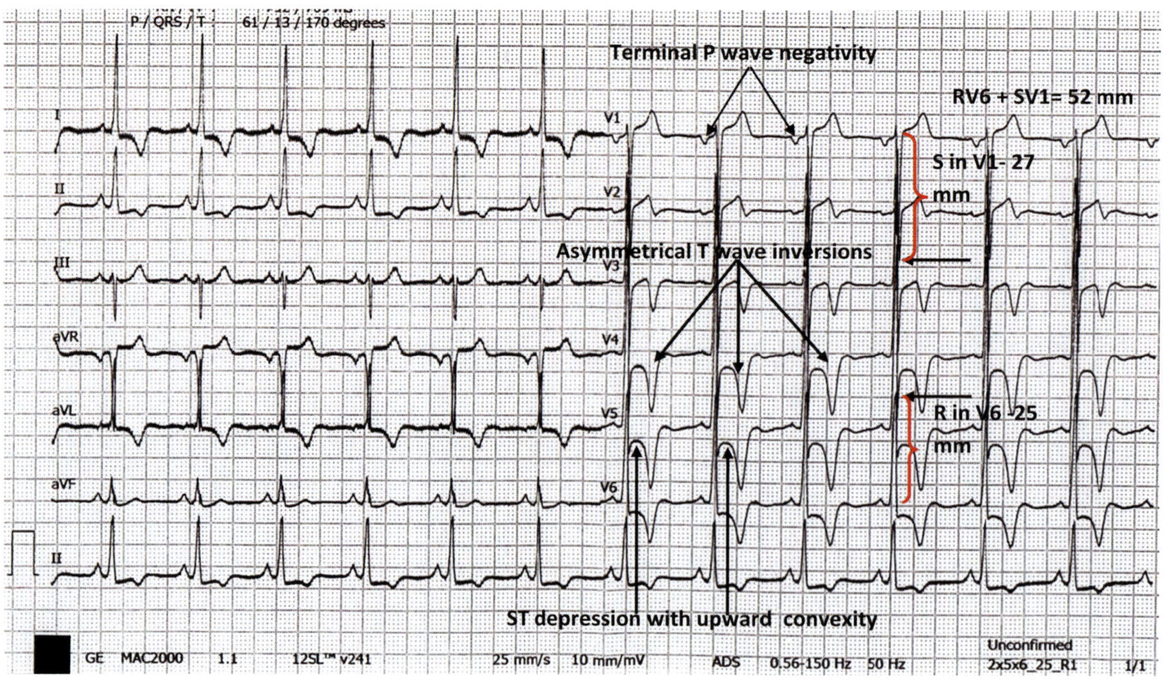

Fig. 6.12: Electrocardiogram is suggestive of left ventricular hypertrophy systolic overload pattern. R in V6 (25 mm) + S in V1 (27 mm) = 52 mm. ST-segment depression with upward convexity along with deep asymmetrical T-wave inversions in lateral chest leads are suggestive of left ventricular hypertrophy systolic overload pattern. Note also terminal P negativity in lead V1 (P-terminal force) is greater than 1 mm depth, which further suggests the presence of left ventricular hypertrophy. This pattern of left ventricular hypertrophy is synonymous with left ventricular hypertrophy strain pattern.

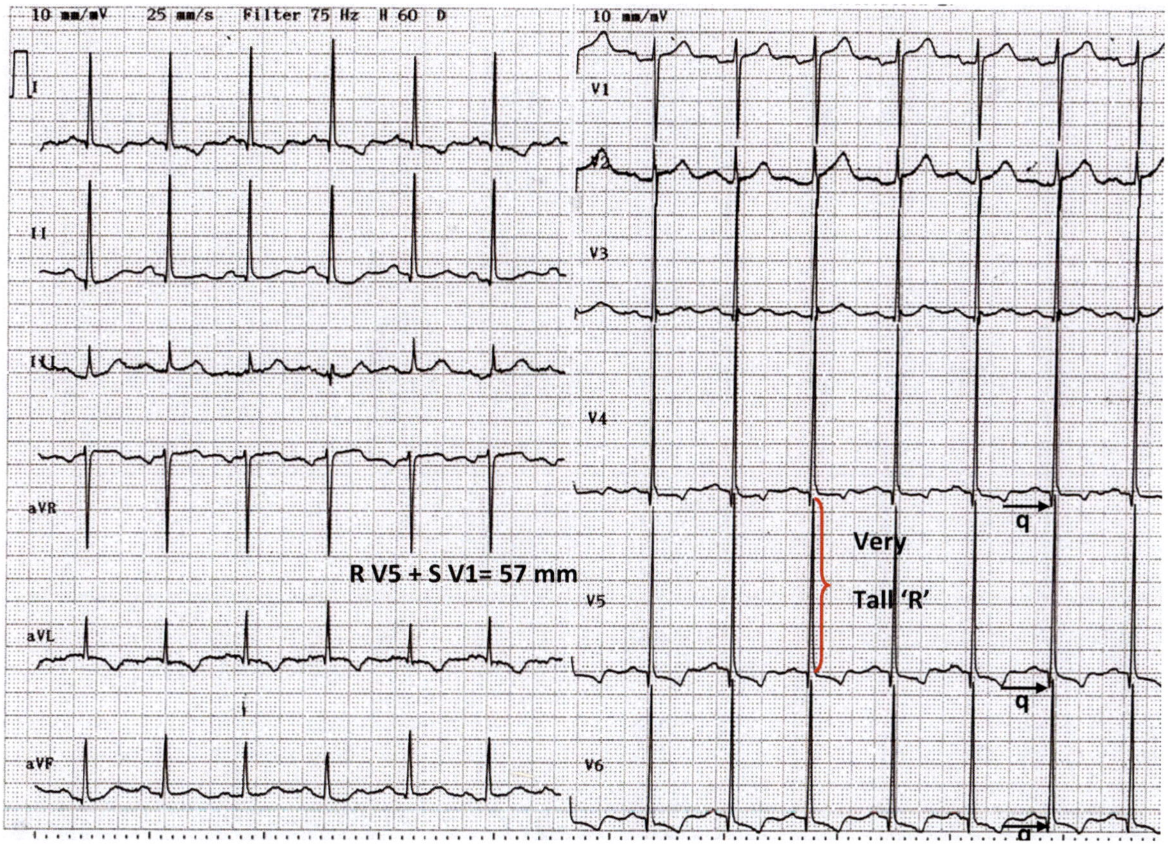

Fig. 6.13: Electrocardiogram is suggestive of left ventricular hypertrophy diastolic overload pattern. Note very tall R waves in lateral leads (V4–V6) along with narrow q waves (*arrows*). R in V5 (38 mm) + S in V1 (19 mm) = 57 mm. Also note there is no significant ST depression or deep asymmetrical T-wave inversions in these leads, which are usually present in the electrocardiogram of left ventricular hypertrophy systolic overload pattern. Narrow q waves are usually present in V4–V6 in the electrocardiogram of left ventricular hypertrophy diastolic overload which is usually absent in the electrocardiogram of left ventricular hypertrophy systolic overload pattern.

When there is volume or diastolic overload LV becomes eccentrically hypertrophied, and LV cavity becomes dilated. In volume overload ECG shows lateral precordial (V4–V6) narrow Q waves due to septal depolarization along with very tall R waves. The ST segment and T waves are often normal or nearly normal (Fig. 6.13). The QRS complex vector may demonstrate left axis deviation, but this is not absolute. A negative U wave, best identified in leads V4–V6, is a common finding in left ventricular volume overload.[71]

RIGHT VENTRICULAR HYPERTROPHY

Right ventricular dilation and hypertrophy occurs from either volume overload or hypertrophy from pressure overload. Normally, the thicker-walled left ventricle predominates resulting in a small R wave in V1 and a large S wave. However, when the RV begins to thicken, a prominent R wave can be seen in V1. The differential diagnosis of tall R wave in V1 includes acute RV dilation, posterior myocardial wall infarction, dextrocardia, misplaced precordial leads, RBBB, and rarely normal variant. Right axis deviation is also seen in RVH or with right heart dilation.

The typical right ventricular hypertrophy (RVH) pattern is a mirror image of the LVH pattern with right axis deviation in the frontal plane, tall R waves in the right precordial leads (V1–V3), deep S waves in the left precordial leads (V5 and V6) and normal or slight increases in the QRS duration (Fig. 6.14). This pattern is characteristically present in patients with congenital pulmonary stenosis, tetralogy of Fallot, primary pulmonary hypertension and other conditions in which the right ventricular mass tends to approach or exceed the left ventricular mass.[5] The earliest portion of the QRS complex is usually unchanged because the septal activation is normal. The anterior displacement of the main QRS vector manifested by a tall R wave in the right precordial leads is attributed to a longer activation time of the hypertrophied right ventricular free wall.[5,72] However, the resulting lengthening of the QRS complex is usually slight and the intrinsicoid deflection is seldom sufficiently delayed to be of diagnostic use.[73] The T waves are directed opposite to the main QRS vector, and therefore are inverted in the right precordial lead and upright in the left precordial lead. These secondary T wave abnormalities may be accompanied by secondary deviations of the ST segment. In some cases of severe RVH, the R wave in the right precordial leads is preceded by a Q wave. In such cases, the right atrium is frequently enlarged and tricuspid regurgitation is commonly present. The incomplete RBBB causing the "rSR" pattern

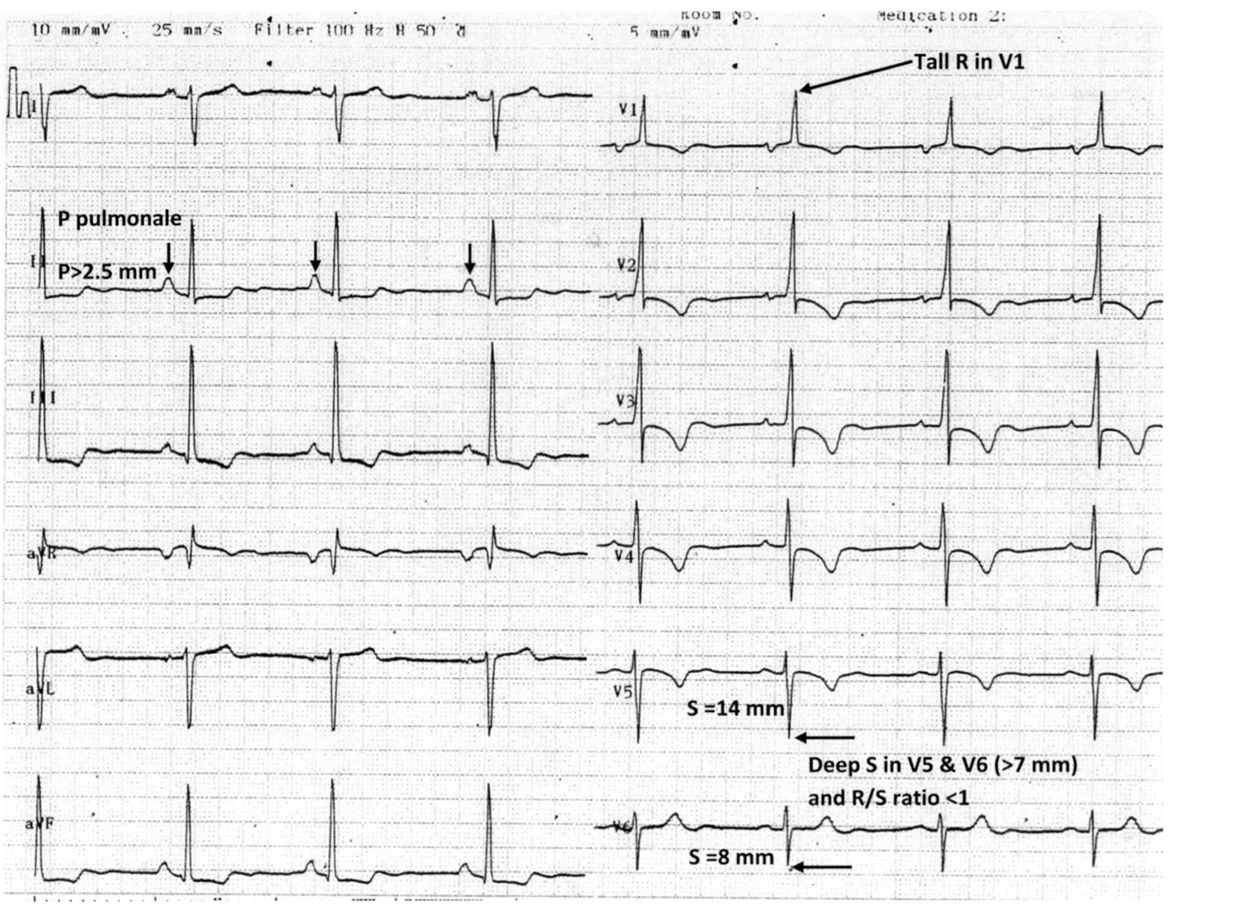

Fig. 6.14: Electrocardiogram showing typical features of right ventricular hypertrophy. (1) Tall R wave in V1. (2) Right axis deviation. (3) Dominant S wave in V5 and V6 (>7 mm deep and R/S ratio < 1). (4) Right atrial enlargement (P pulmonale).

in the right precordial leads is attributed to the delayed activation of the hypertrophied right ventricular outflow tract. This pattern is most frequently due to factors other than RVH. However, it can signify hypertrophy, dilation or overload of the right ventricle; perhaps most commonly in mitral valve disease with pulmonary hypertension and atrial septal defect (ASD).[5] A "right heart strain" pattern is seen with delayed repolarization of the right ventricular myocardium producing negative ST segments and T wave pattern. Tall R wave in V1 along with ST depression and inverted T waves in V1–V3 suggests right heart strain (Fig. 6.15).

Numerous criteria mostly derived from the amplitude of R and S in leads I, V1, V6, and the R-wave peak time in V1 have been proposed. They have been correlated primarily with autopsy data, although some are based on clinical and hemodynamic identification of conditions that impose increased workloads on the right ventricle.[74-77] The echocardiogram has also been used as a reference standard, but it is less definitive than in LVH because of the complex 3-dimensional shape of the right ventricle and the frequent difficulty of measuring the thickness of the right ventricular free wall.[4]

Sensitivity and specificity of various criteria for ECG diagnosis of RVH vary inversely with each other.[5] The early criteria of Sokolow and Lyon included: (1) R amplitude in V1 greater than 0.7 mV (7mm); (2) S amplitude in VI less than 0.2 mV (2 mm); (3) S amplitude in V5 and V6 greater than 0.7 mV (7 mm); (4) sum of R amplitude in V1 and S amplitude in V5 and V6 greater than 1.05 mV (10.5 mm); (5) R amplitude in V5 and V6 less than 0.5 mV (5 mm); (6) R/S ratio in V5 and V6 less than 1; (7) R amplitude in aVR greater than 0.5 mV (5 mm); (8) R/S ratio in V5 divided by R/S ratio in V1 less than 0.4; (9) R/S ratio in V1 greater than I; (10) intrinsicoid deflection in V1 = 0.04 second; (11) negative T wave in V1 in the presence of R greater than 0.5 mV (5 mm); and (12) right axis deviation greater than 110°.[78] These criteria have high specificity but low sensitivity.[79,80]

Myers criteria of RVH include Tall R V1 > 6 mm, increased R:S ratio V1 >1.0, deep S in V5 >10 mm, deep S in V6 > 3 mm, small S in V1 < 2 mm, small R in V5, V6 <3 mm, etc.[81]

Milnor simplified the Sokolow and Lyon criteria and limited the ECG criteria of RVH. These criteria include:[82]

- R/S or R'/S ratio in V1 greater than 1.0
- R or R' amplitude greater than 0.5 mV (5 mm) in V1
- Right axis deviation with frontal plane axis from +110° to ±180°
- QRS duration is less than 0.12 second.

Although, the sensitivity of the electrocardiographic criteria for RVH is generally low, some criteria have high specificity and can be used to advantage in diagnostic schemes or to derive continuous variables. The greatest accuracy is in congenital heart disease, with intermediate accuracy in acquired heart disease and primary pulmonary hypertension in adults. The lowest accuracy occurs in chronic lung disease.[4,77,83]

Electrocardiographic RVH may be of two types:

1. Volume overload pattern (Fig. 6.16).
2. Pressure overload pattern (Fig. 6.17).

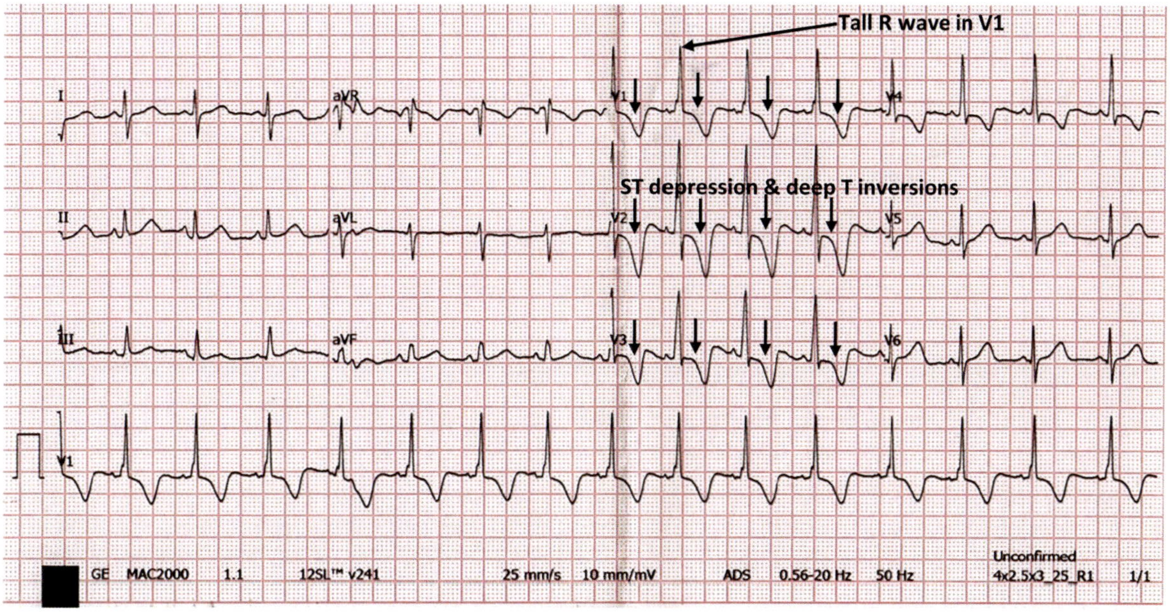

Fig. 6.15: Electrocardiogram is suggestive of right ventricular hypertrophy strain pattern and shows tall R wave in V1, ST segment depression with deep T-wave inversions in leads V1–V3 along with right axis deviation.

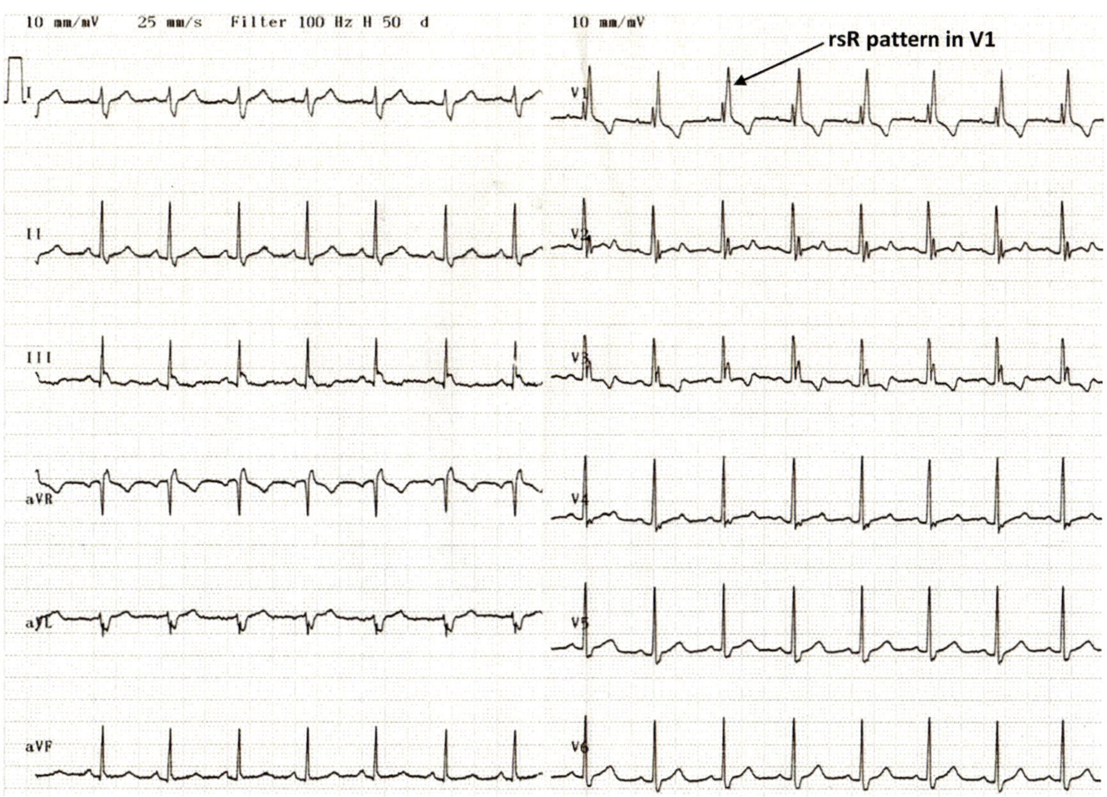

Fig. 6.16: Electrocardiogram of right ventricular hypertrophy volume overload. rsR pattern (QRS < 0.12 second) in lead V1 along with right axis deviation. Electrocardiogram features of right ventricular hypertrophy volume overload is similar to that of incomplete right bundle branch block.

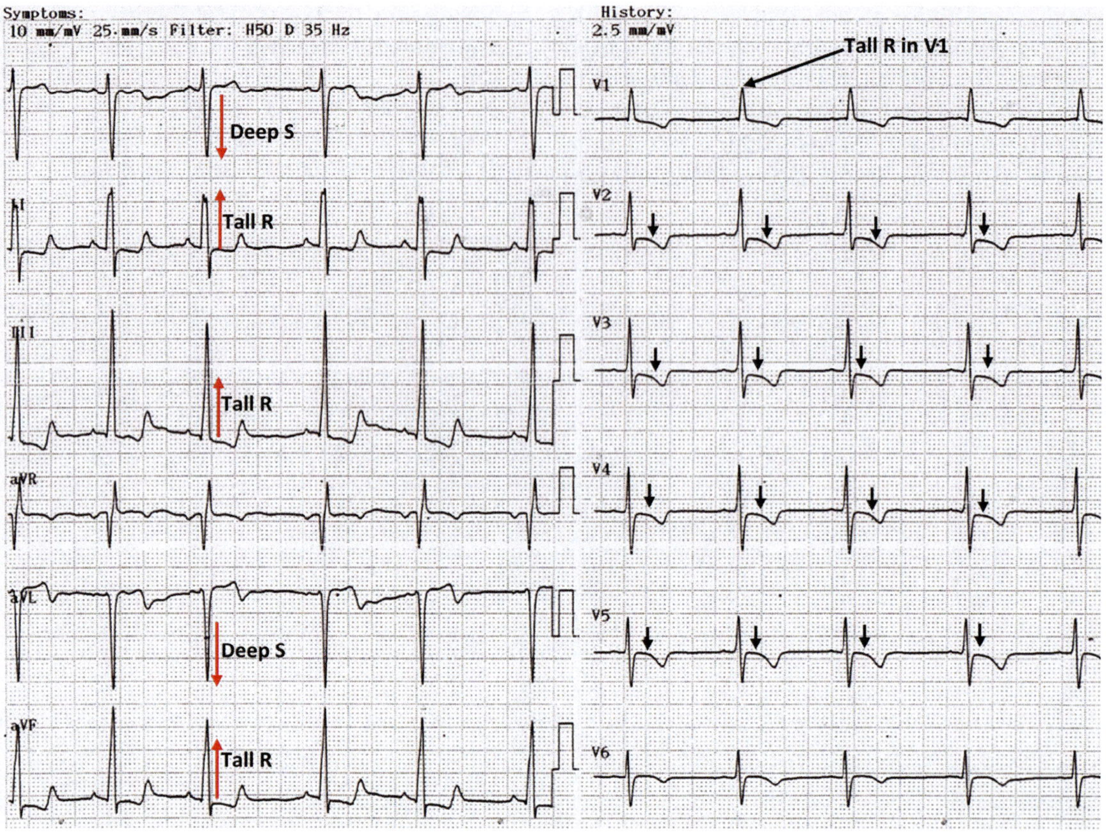

Fig. 6.17: Electrocardiogram is suggestive of right ventricular hypertrophy systolic overload pattern. Electrocardiogram shows tall R wave in V1 with ST-segment depression with T-wave inversions in leads V1–V5 (*small arrows*) along with right axis deviation, tall R waves in LII, LIII, and aVF and predominant S waves in leads L1 and aVL (*red arrows*).

Volume overload pattern is similar to that of incomplete RBBB and is associated with mitral valve disease with pulmonary hypertension and ASD. Pressure overload pattern is manifested in ECG with predominantly tall R waves (as part of Rs, R, or Qr complexes) in right precordial leads particularly in lead V1. Both patterns are associated with right axis deviation. Typical RVH with pressure overload pattern is seen in pulmonary stenosis.

Both volume overload and pressure overload pattern are also frequently associated with ST depression and T-wave inversion in right precordial leads; as with LVH, these ST-T abnormalities are better referred to as "secondary ST-T abnormality" than as "strain".[4]

BIVENTRICULAR HYPERTROPHY

An opposite direction of the forces generated by LVH and RVH may result in a normal pattern due to partial cancellation. For example, the development of RVH due to pulmonary hypertension may sometimes obscure the established LVH pattern. However, the concurrent presence of LVH and RVH is sometimes recognizable because of the asynchrony of ventricular depolarization and also because the precordial leads are semidirect and exaggerate the electromotive force in proximity to the electrodes. A right axis in the frontal plane in the presence of a LVH pattern suggests an associated right ventricular enlargement. A less reliable indicator of a possible right ventricular dilation in the presence of a LVH pattern is the shift to the left of the transition zone in the precordial leads.[5]

Hypertrophy of both the right and left ventricle, as called biventricular hypertrophy (BVH) is relatively common in patients with heart disease of many types, e.g. ventricular septal defect (VSD), patent ductus arteriosus (PDA), Eisenmenger syndrome, etc.

Its recognition by ECG has a particularly low sensitivity, explained at least in part by the cancellation of increased QRS vectors of both RVH and LVH. In the presence of ECG criteria for LVH, the following conditions suggest associated RVH.[84,85]

- Presence of prominent S waves in V5 or V6
- Right axis deviation
- Unusually tall biphasic R/S complexes in several leads (Katz-Wachtel sign) (Fig. 6.18).
- ECG signs of right atrial (RA) abnormality.

In patients with electrocardiographic criteria of RVH, the presence of combined tall R waves and deep S waves in leads V2–V4, with combined amplitude greater than 50 mm (5.0 mV), suggests the presence of associated LVH.[4]

Katz–Wachtel Sign

The Katz-Wachtel sign is tall diphasic RS complexes at least 50 mm in height in lead V2, V3, or V4—mid precordial leads (Fig. 6.19A). The sign has been described in VSD with BVH in children. It can be seen with isolated VSD as well as complex VSD.[86,87] In BVH tall R waves may be present in both left and right precordial leads with a tall diphasic QRS complex in the midprecordial leads (Katz-Wachtel sign) (Fig. 6.19B).

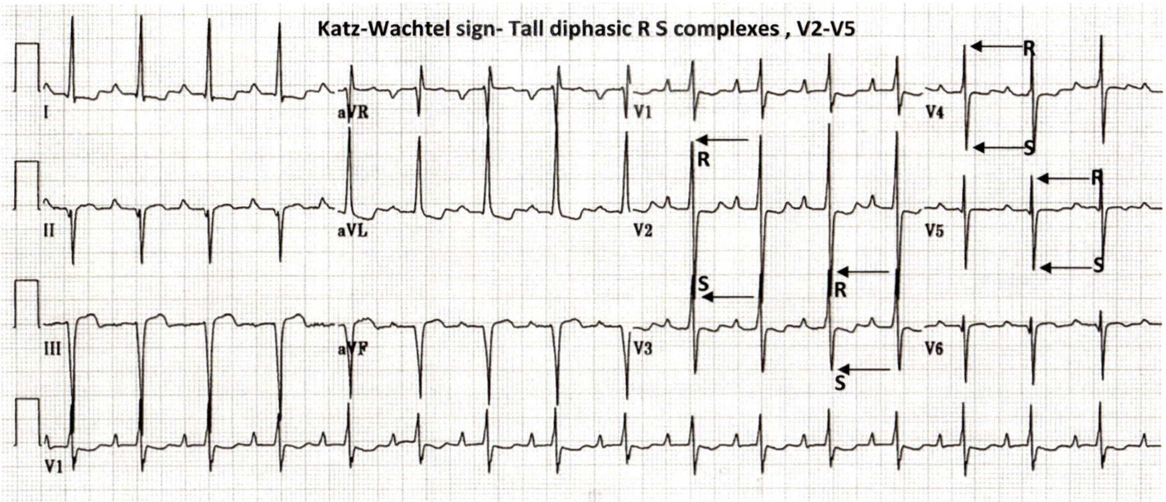

Fig. 6.18: Electrocardiogram is suggestive of biventricular hypertrophy. Electrocardiogram shows evidence of Katz–Wachtel sign (tall biphasic or diphasic R/S complexes in leads V2–V5).

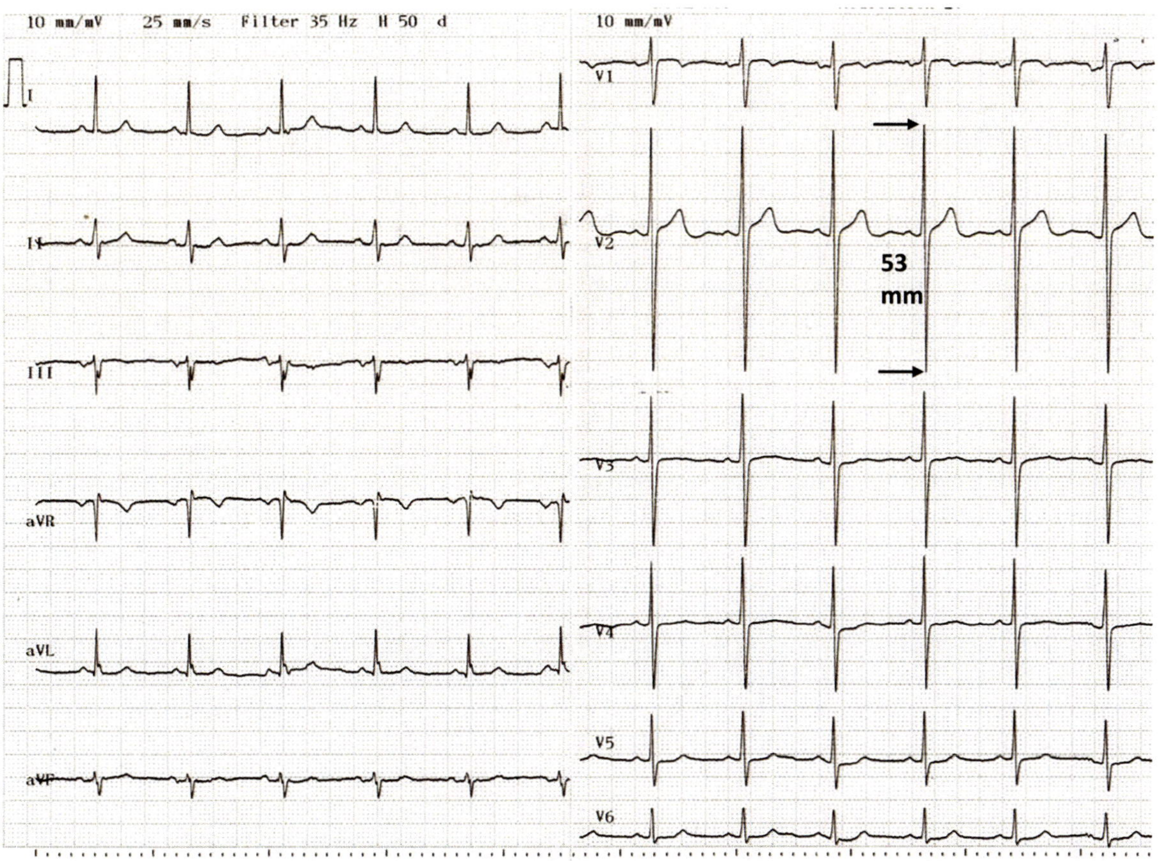

Fig. 6.19A: Electrocardiogram showing Katz–Wachtel phenomenon on the electrocardiogram of a patient with ventricular septal defect. Note tall diphasic RS complexes in leads V2–V4. Also note very tall RS complex >50 mm in V2.

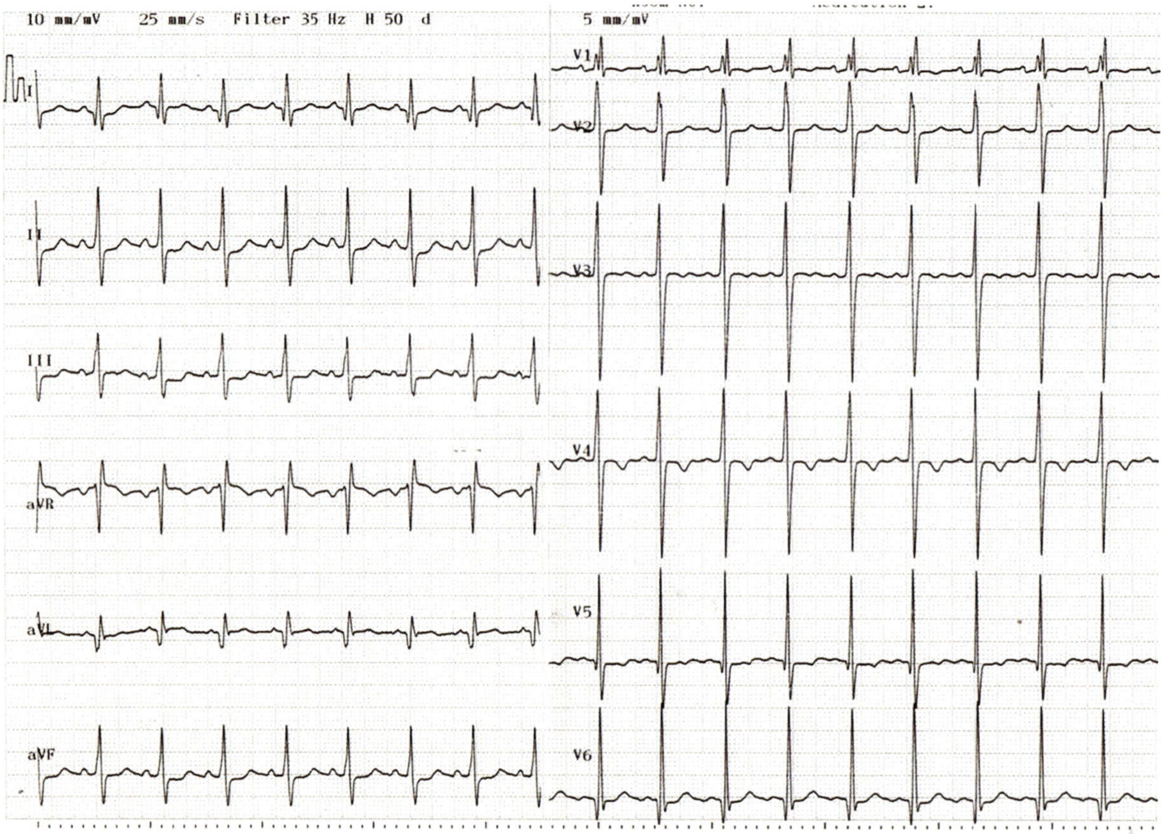

Fig. 6.19B: Electrocardiogram illustrating Katz–Wachtel phenomenon in a patient with biventricular hypertrophy. In biventricular hypertrophy tall R waves may be present in both left and right precordial leads with a tall diphasic QRS complex in the midprecordial leads, V2–V4 (Katz–Wachtel sign).

ATRIAL ABNORMALITIES

Normal P wave is usually upright in LII and biphasic in lead V1 (Fig. 6.20). Abnormalities in the P wave that are related to anatomic or physiological abnormalities in the right or left atrium have been recognized since the early years of electrocardiography. The terms P-mitrale, P-congenitale, and P-pulmonale were later replaced by the terms left atrial enlargement (LAE) and right atrial enlargement (RAE), as it was realized that different clinical conditions caused similar abnormalities. However, other terms such as atrial hypertrophy, atrial overload, atrial strain, and interatrial (or intraatrial) conduction defect have also been used, reflecting the fact that atrial dilatation, atrial muscular hypertrophy, elevated atrial pressure, impaired ventricular distensibility, and delayed intraatrial conduction all seem to play a role in causing P-wave abnormalities. Because the effects of these several factors on the P wave may often appear in combination and may not be distinguishable, the less specific terms LA abnormality and RA abnormality are preferable.[4]

Left Atrial Abnormality/Enlargement

This can be suspected when a wide P wave is due to an increased duration of the terminal, posteriorly directed P-wave component. The wide separation between the anteriorly and posteriorly directed P-wave components results in a prolonged interval between the peak of the initial upright portion and the nadir of the following inverted P-wave portion in the right precordial leads. Such P waves are usually upright and notched in leads I, II, and V4–V6, and either positive-negative or negative in leads III and aVF. Because the pattern associated with LAE indicates an intraatrial conduction disturbance rather than hypertrophy or dilation, the preferred term is LA abnormality rather than enlargement.[88]

Left atrial abnormality usually involves prolongation of the total atrial activation time, because LA activation begins and ends later than RA activation. Delay in the LA activation tends to cause a double-peaked or notched P wave, because the RA and LA peaks that are normally nearly simultaneous and fused into a single peak become more widely separated. Activation of the left atrium has a more leftward and posterior vector than that of the right atrium. The product of the amplitude and the duration of the terminal negative component of the P wave in lead V1 (the P terminal force) (Fig. 6.21) has been used most frequently of the various criteria for LA abnormality, but the P-wave duration (120 ms or more) and widely notched P wave (40 ms or more) appear to have equal value.

Electrocardiographic features of LAE include (1) Terminal P negativity in lead V1 (i.e., "P-terminal force") duration $\geq$ 40 ms, depth $\geq$ 1 mm. (2) Notched P wave in limb leads and V4–V6 with the inter-peak duration >40 ms, and (3) P-wave duration >120 ms (usually lead II) (Figs. 6.22A

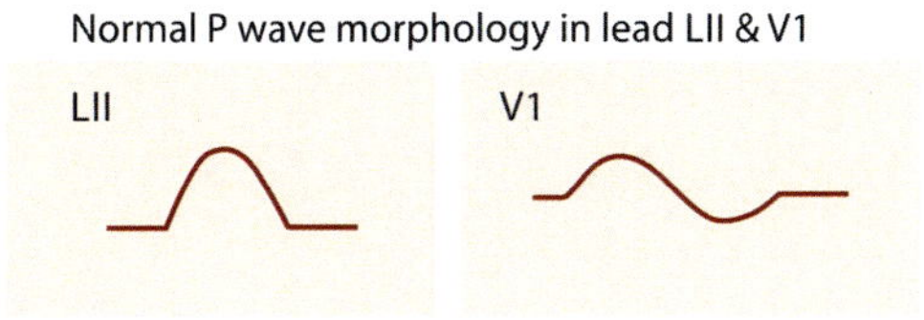

Fig. 6.20: Normal P wave morphology. Amplitude of normal P wave is less than 2.5 mm in the limb leads, it is upright and monophasic in LII and biphasic in V1.

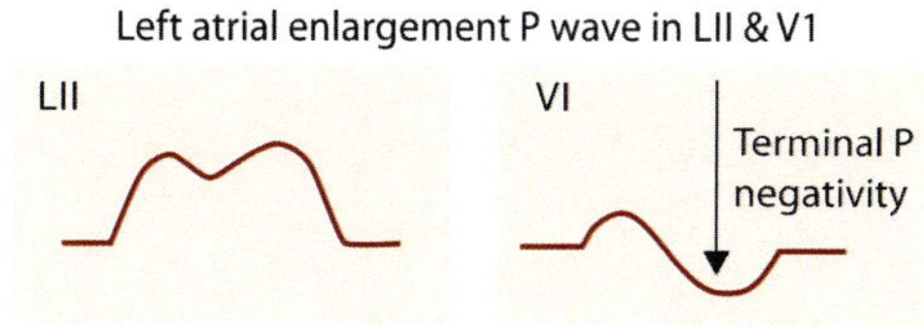

Fig. 6.21: Terminal P negativity in lead V1 (P-terminal force) duration ≥ 40ms and depth ≥ 1 mm is suggestive of left atrial enlargement

and B). Several other criteria, including left axis of the terminal P wave (–30° to –90°), and possibly the P-wave area, are also useful.[89,90] A purely negative P wave in V1 is suggestive of LA enlargement (Fig. 6.22B), but can occur without an increased P terminal force.[4]

P-wave terminal force in lead V1 (PTFV1), a consistently used marker of LAE on a 12-lead electrocardiogram is also known as Morris index. Normally the depth of the terminal P wave in V1 is less than 1 mm and duration is less than 0.04 second (<40 ms). *Morris index* is derived from multiplying the depth of terminal P-wave deflection in V1 in millimeter (mm) by duration in second (s) and expressed in mm s. Normally the depth of terminal P wave in V1 is less than 1 mm and duration is less than 0.04 seconds. So maximum Morris index is around: $1 \times 0.04 = 0.04$ mm s (Figs. 6.22C and D). If the P terminal force (Morris index) exceeds 0.04 mm s, it is suggestive of LAE. [91-94] Morris index is found to be the best criterion for ECG diagnosis of LAE in many studies with high degree of sensitivity and specificity.[92-94] *Macruz index* can also be used for the ECG documentation of LAE. The ratio of the duration of the P wave to that of the P-R segment (The P-R segment is the flat, isoelectric segment between the end of the P wave and the start of the QRS complex. P-R segment = P-R interval–P-wave duration), reflects the relative balance of the RA and LA excitation forces and is known as Macruz index. Normal range in adults to be 1.0–1.6; the value <1.0 is suggestive of RAE and values >1.6 indicative of LAE.[95]

In LA abnormality, LA depolarization lasts longer than normal but its amplitude remains unchanged. Therefore, the height of the resultant P wave remains within normal limits but its duration is longer than 120 ms. A notch (broken line) near its peak may or may not be present (so called "P mitrale") (Fig. 6.23).

Right Atrial Abnormality/Enlargement

Right atrial abnormality/enlargement is typically manifested as an increase in amplitude of the P wave (Fig. 6.24) and a tendency to rightward shift of the P-wave vector.[96] ECG criteria of RA enlargement include: (1) A tall upright P wave in lead II (greater than 2.5 mm) is characteristic (Fig. 6.25), often with a peaked or pointed appearance that presumably reflects summation of the enhanced RA component with the simultaneous LA component. (2) Prominent initial positivity of the P wave in V1 or V2 [1.5 mm (0.15 mV) or more] also indicates RA abnormality. (3) Rightward axis of the P wave and a peaked form are supportive signs. (4) Total P-wave duration is usually normal.[4] Because RAE is so frequently seen in chronic pulmonary disease, the peaked P wave is often called "P pulmonale" (Fig. 6.26).

Pseudo-P Pulmonale

Right atrial abnormality increases the amplitude of the initial P-wave forces, contrasting with increase in the later P-wave forces that can result from LA abnormality sometimes referred as pseudo-P pulmonale.[4]

A pseudo-P pulmonale pattern may be seen in patients with LA enlargement due to mitral valve disease. In a pseudo-P pulmonale pattern, as seen in LA enlargement, analyzing lead V1 for the presence of a negative P terminal force may help in the differential diagnosis of true versus pseudo-P pulmonale.

Tall P waves (pseudo-P pulmonale) may be seen associated with severe hypokalemia and combined electrolyte depletion. After the treatment, P waves decrease in amplitude with the normalization of serum potassium.

Biatrial Abnormality/Enlargement

Biatrial abnormality is indicated essentially by the presence of some of the features of both RA and LA abnormality (Fig. 6.27). Biatrial enlargement (BAE) include (1) Features of both RAE and LAE in same ECG. (2) P wave in lead II >2.5 mm tall and ≥0.12 second in duration. (3) Initial positive component of P wave, RA component (P1) in V1 >1.5 mm tall and terminal negative deflection, LA component (P2) ≥1 mm deep and ≥40 ms duration (Figs. 6.28A and B and 29). However, little evidence is available regarding the accuracy of ECG criteria for combined atrial abnormality. Common causes of BAE include restrictive cardiomyopathy, rheumatic heart disease, and constrictive pericarditis.[97]

SUMMARY

Left ventricular hypertrophy can be detected by ECG, echocardiography, or cardiac magnetic resonance imaging (MRI). Each has unique advantages and disadvantages. ECG is specific, but not sensitive but it is the cheapest and most readily available of the three tests for LVH. While its specificity is acceptably high, its clinical utility is limited by its very low sensitivity.

Many different criteria for electrocardiographic LVH have been proposed over the years. Most of the criteria use the voltage in one or more leads, with or without additional

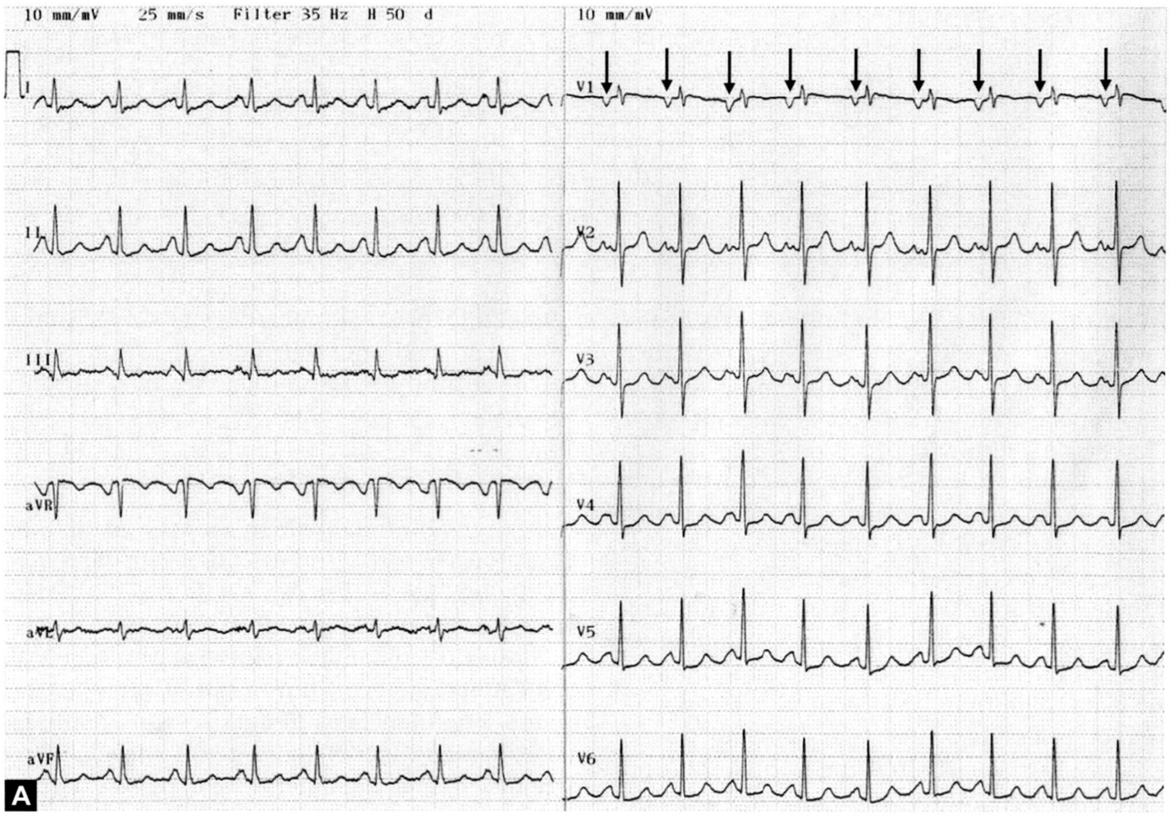

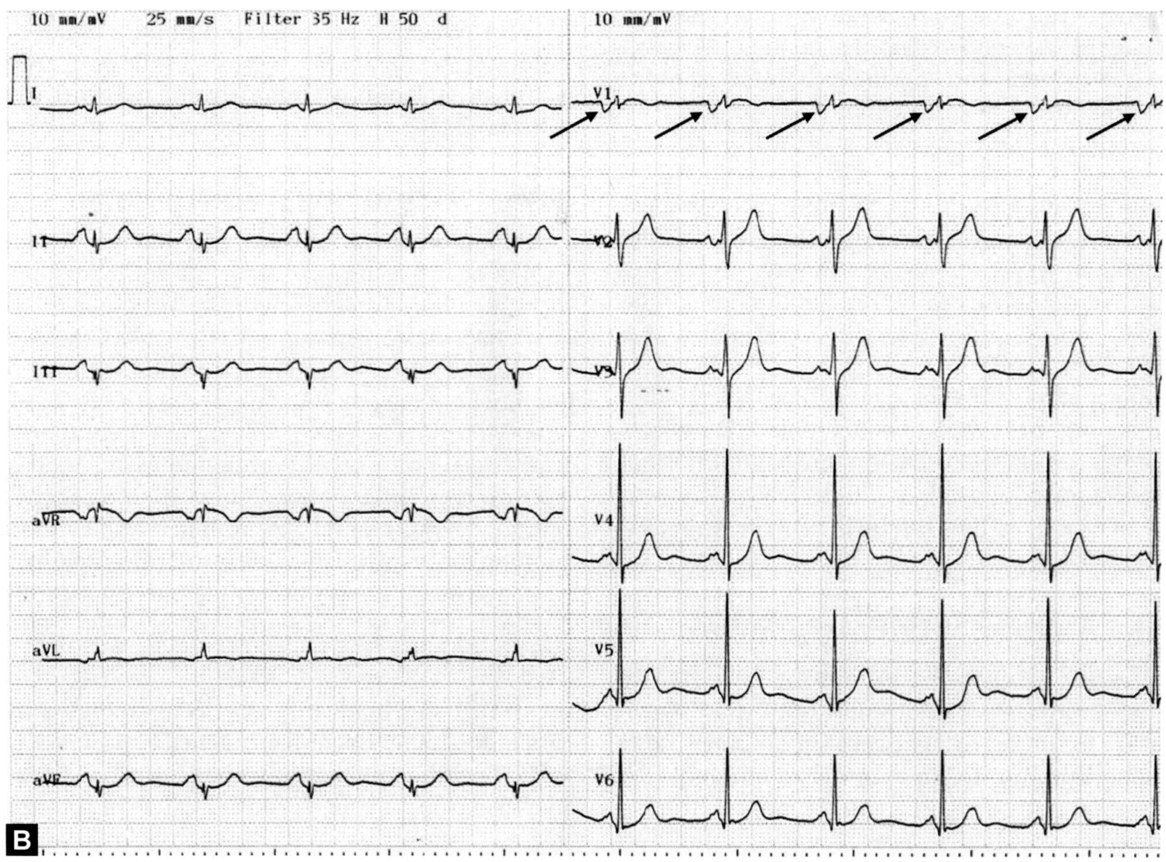

Figs. 6.22A and B: (A) Electrocardiogram shows features of left atrial enlargement with broad and bifid P wave in LI and LII and terminal P negativity in V1 (P duration > 40 ms and depth > 1 mm) (*arrows*). Also note broad and notched P waves in leads V2–V4 and tall R wave in V1. (B) Electrocardiogram is consistent with features of left atrial enlargement with broad (P duration 120 ms) and bifid P wave in lead II. Electrocardiogram also shows other evidences of left atrial enlargement with terminal P negativity in lead V1 with P terminal force duration is greater than 40 ms and depth is greater than 1 mm (*arrows*). Also note notched P waves in lead I, V3–V6.

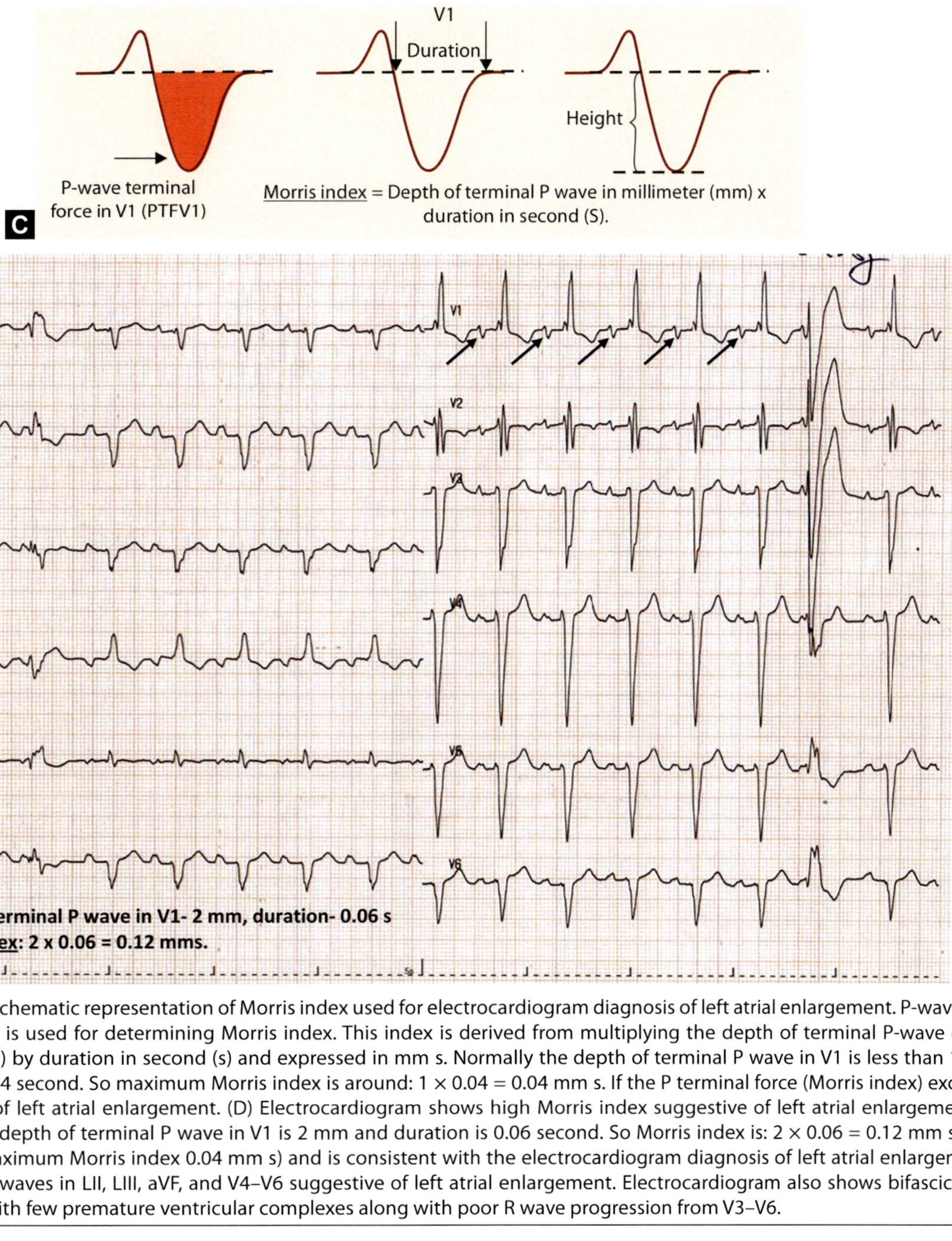

Figs. 6.22C and D: (C) Schematic representation of Morris index used for electrocardiogram diagnosis of left atrial enlargement. P-wave terminal force in lead V1 (*arrow*) is used for determining Morris index. This index is derived from multiplying the depth of terminal P-wave deflection in V1 in millimeter (mm) by duration in second (s) and expressed in mm s. Normally the depth of terminal P wave in V1 is less than 1 mm and duration is less than 0.04 second. So maximum Morris index is around: 1 × 0.04 = 0.04 mm s. If the P terminal force (Morris index) exceeds 0.04 mm s, it is suggestive of left atrial enlargement. (D) Electrocardiogram shows high Morris index suggestive of left atrial enlargement. In this electrocardiogram, the depth of terminal P wave in V1 is 2 mm and duration is 0.06 second. So Morris index is: 2 × 0.06 = 0.12 mm s (which is greater than normal maximum Morris index 0.04 mm s) and is consistent with the electrocardiogram diagnosis of left atrial enlargement. Also note broad and bifid P waves in LII, LIII, aVF, and V4–V6 suggestive of left atrial enlargement. Electrocardiogram also shows bifascicular block pattern (RBBB + LAD) with few premature ventricular complexes along with poor R wave progression from V3–V6.

factors such as QRS duration, secondary ST-T-wave abnormalities, or LA abnormalities. The most well-known electrocardiographic criteria are the Sokolow–Lyon index, Cornell voltage, the Cornell product, and the Romhilt–Estes point score system.

Left Ventricular Hypertrophy—Electrocardiographic Criteria

Through many studies, multiple criteria have been developed to diagnose LVH on an ECG but the Sokolow–Lyon index is possibly the most widely utilized ECG score for LVH.

Sokolow–Lyon criteria: Add the S wave in V1 plus the R wave in V5 or V6. If the sum is >35 mm, then LVH is present.

Cornell criteria: Add the R wave in aVL and the S wave in V3. If the sum is >28 mm in males or is >20 mm in females, then LVH is present.

Modified Cornell criteria: Examine the R wave in aVL. If the R wave is >12 mm in amplitude, then LVH is present.

Romhilt–Estes Point Score System

The Romhilt–Estes criteria for LVH is shown in Box 6.1.

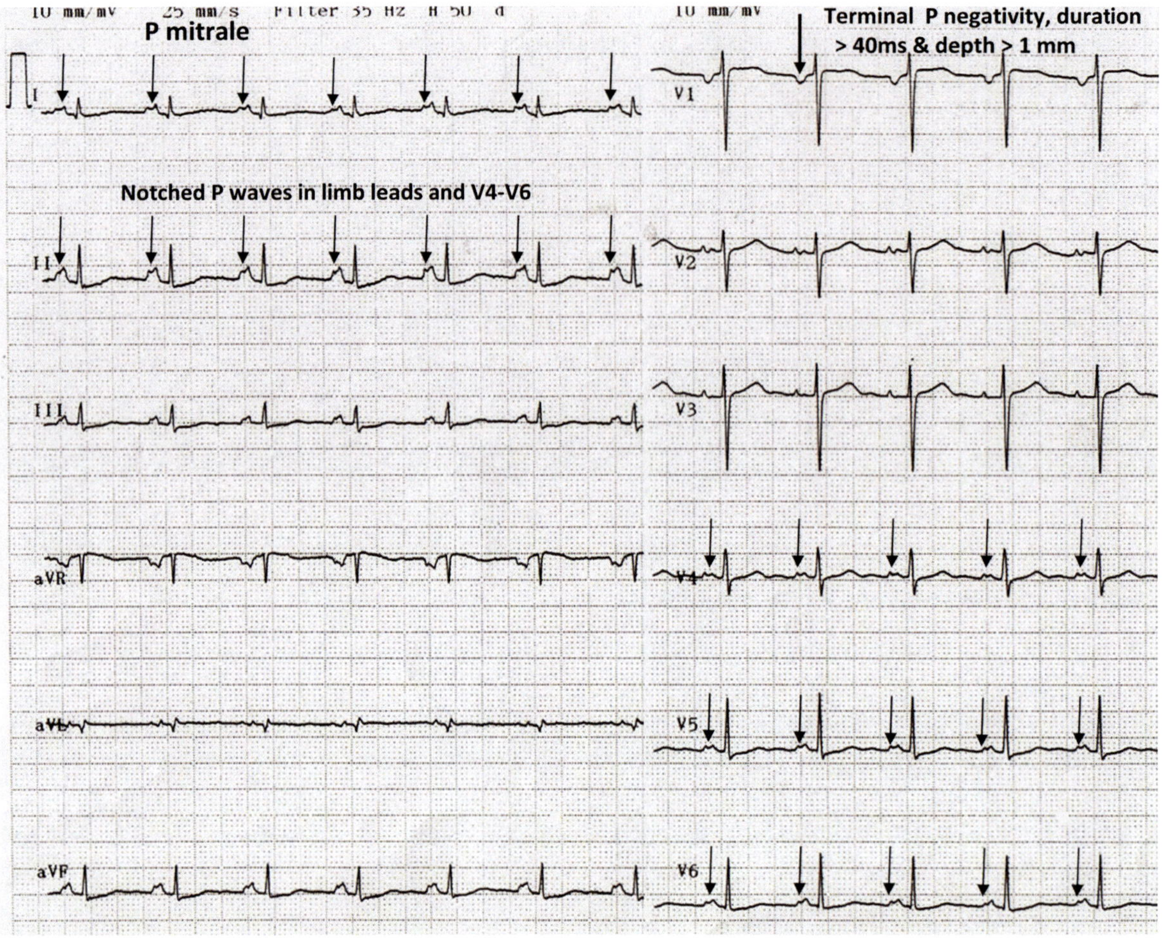

Fig. 6.23: ECG of P-mitrale, showing evidence of left atrial enlargement. Note terminal P negativity in lead V1 with P terminal force duration > 40ms and depth > 1 mm. Also note notched P waves in limb leads and V4-V6 (*small arrows*).

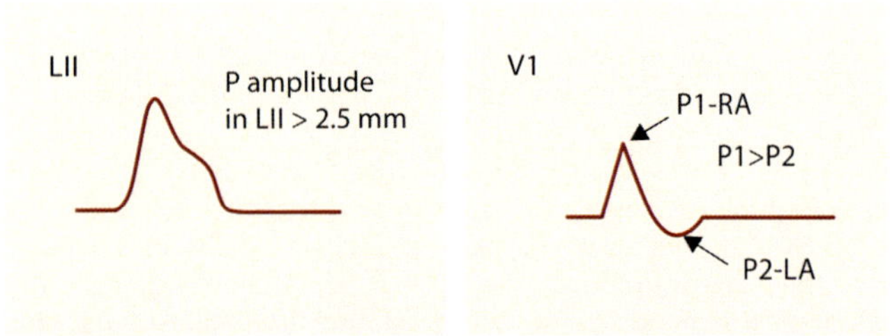

Fig. 6.24: P-wave morphology in right atrial enlargement in lead LII and V1. Tall peak P (>2.5 mm) in amplitude and initial positive component of P wave in V1 is >1.5 mm and P1 (right atrial component) is >P2 (left atrial component) are suggestive of right atrial enlargement.

Box 6.1: Romhilt–Estes Criteria for LVH (diagnostic, ≥5 points; probable, 4 points).

ECG Criteria	*Points*
Voltage criteria (any of):	3 points
• R or S in limb leads ≥ 20 mm	
• S in V1 or V2 ≥ 30 mm	
• R in V5 or V6 ≥ 30 mm	
ST–T Abnormalities:	
• Without digitalis	3 points
• With digitalis	1 point
Left atrial enlargement in V1	3 points
Left axis deviation	2 points
QRS duration ≥0.09 second	1 point
Delayed intrinsicoid deflection in V5 or V6 (>0.05 second)	1 point

Left Ventricular Hypertrophy Strain

Left ventricular hypertrophy strain is usually associated with hypertensive heart disease. It is a type of ECG pattern seen in ECGs consistent with ventricular hypertrophy. It usually indicates a compensatory response to uncontrolled hypertension and may indicate underlying ischemia. Electrocardiographic criteria for LVH strain includes:

- Voltage criteria of LVH (R in V5 or V6 + S in V1 >35 mm)
- ST depression greater than or equal to 1 mm in lateral leads I, aVL and V4–V6
- Downsloping ST-T segment, rapid upslope
- Asymmetrical T-wave inversions
- Direction of the T wave usually opposite to the upright QRS complex
- U-wave inversion in left precordial leads.

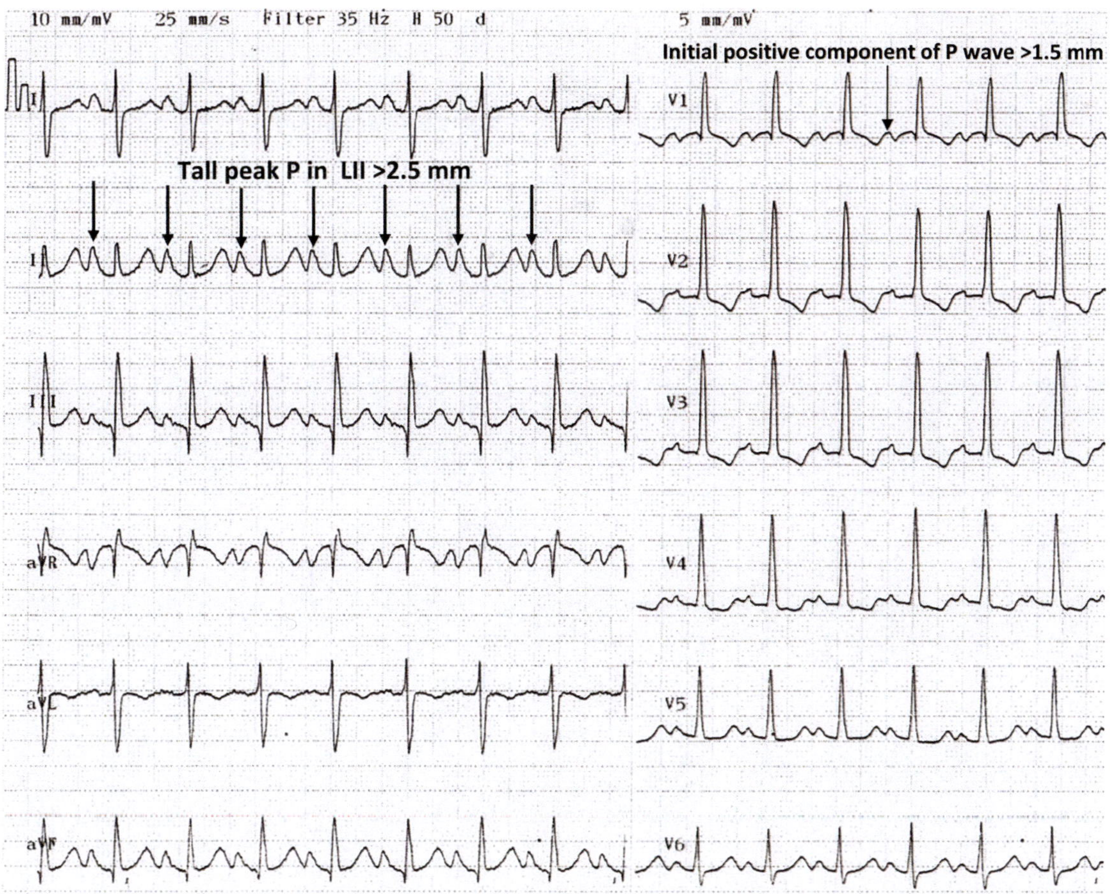

Fig. 6.25: Electrocardiogram is suggestive of right atrial enlargement. Note tall peak P (4 mm) in amplitude in LII and initial positive component of P wave in V1 = 2 mm (>1.5 mm) are suggestive of right atrial enlargement. Electrocardiogram also has evidence of right ventricular hypertrophy (tall R in V1).

Table 6.1: Electrocardiogram differentiation between left ventricular hypertrophy strain and ischemia.

ECG change	*LVH*	*Ischemia*
ST change	Usually downsloping ST depression, mostly seen in LI, aVL, and V4–V6	Usually horizontal ST depression
T waves	Asymmetrical T wave inversions	Symmetrical T wave inversions
ST elevation	LVH strain is usually associated with ST elevation in leads V1–V3	ST elevation is only present in case of STEMI
Serial ECG change	ST and T wave changes are static.	ST and T wave changes are dynamic. Serial ECG change can differentiate these two conditions.

(LVH: left ventricular hypertrophy)

Left Ventricular Hypertrophy Versus Ischemia

No reliable way to distinguish between ACS versus LVH with strain. Horizontal ST depression and symmetric T-wave inversions are associated with ischemia. When in doubt it is better to get serial ECGs or to compare it with old ECGs.

The ECG differentiation between LVH strain and ischemia is shown in Table 6.1.

Left Ventricular Hypertrophy in the Presence of Left Bundle Branch Block

Diagnosis of LVH in presence of LBBB is difficult. But the following ECG features may give a clue to the diagnosis of LVH in presence of LBBB.

- LA enlargement type P-wave abnormality
- QRS duration greater than approximately 155 ms
- Precordial lead voltage criteria of LVH.

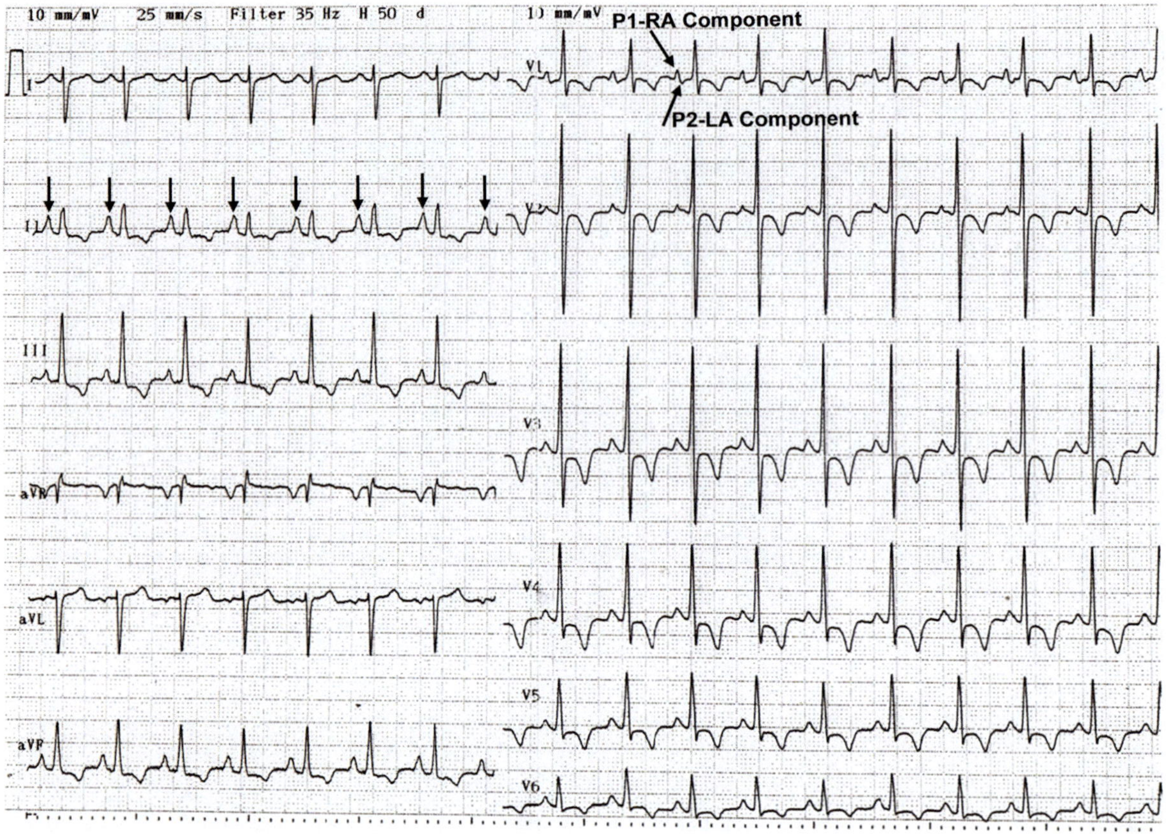

Fig. 6.26: Electrocardiogram of P-pulmonale (right atrial enlargement). Note tall peak P (3.0 mm) in amplitude in LII (*arrows*) and initial positive component of P wave (P1) in V1 = 2.0 mm (>1.5 mm) suggestive of right atrial enlargement. In this electrocardiogram, P wave is biphasic in V1 but negative component of P in V1 (P2) is very narrow, so it is not suggestive of concurrent left atrial enlargement. Electrocardiogram also has evidence of right ventricular hypertrophy strain pattern with tall R in V1, ST segment depression with T-wave inversions in leads V1–V6 with right axis deviation.

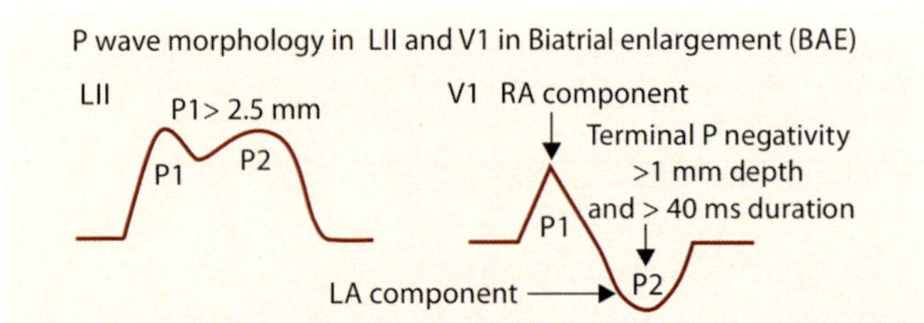

Fig. 6.27: P-wave morphology in LII and V1 in biatrial enlargement. P wave (P1) in LII is greater than 2.5 mm and terminal P negativity in lead V1 (P2) duration is greater than 40 ms and depth is greater than 1 mm.

Traditionally, it is believed that the ECG diagnosis of LVH should not be attempted when LBBB is present.

Left Ventricular Hypertrophy in the Presence of Right Bundle Branch Block

In RBBB, LVH is suggested by a LAE pattern, secondary repolarization changes, and a sum of S wave in lead III plus the maximal R + S in a precordial lead $\geq$ 30 mm.

Left ventricular hypertrophy is a compensatory mechanism in response to both pressure and volume overload. The most commonly used criteria for diagnosis of LVH is the Sokolow–Lyon criteria (S wave depth in V1 + tallest R-wave height in V5–V6 >35 mm). Voltage criteria must be accompanied by nonvoltage criteria to be considered diagnostic of LVH. Nonvoltage criteria include ST segment depression and T-wave inversion in the left-sided leads, LAE, left axis deviation, and ST elevation in the right precordial leads V1-3, discordant to the deep S waves etc.

The common causes of LVH pressure overload are:

- Hypertension
- Aortic stenosis
- Coarctation of aorta
- Hypertrophic cardiomyopathy.

Electrocardiographic features of LVH pressure overload include:

- Tall R in V4, V5, and V6
- ST segment depression in lateral precordial leads (V4–V6)
- T-wave inversion in lateral precordial leads.

Causes of LVH volume overload are:

- Aortic regurgitation

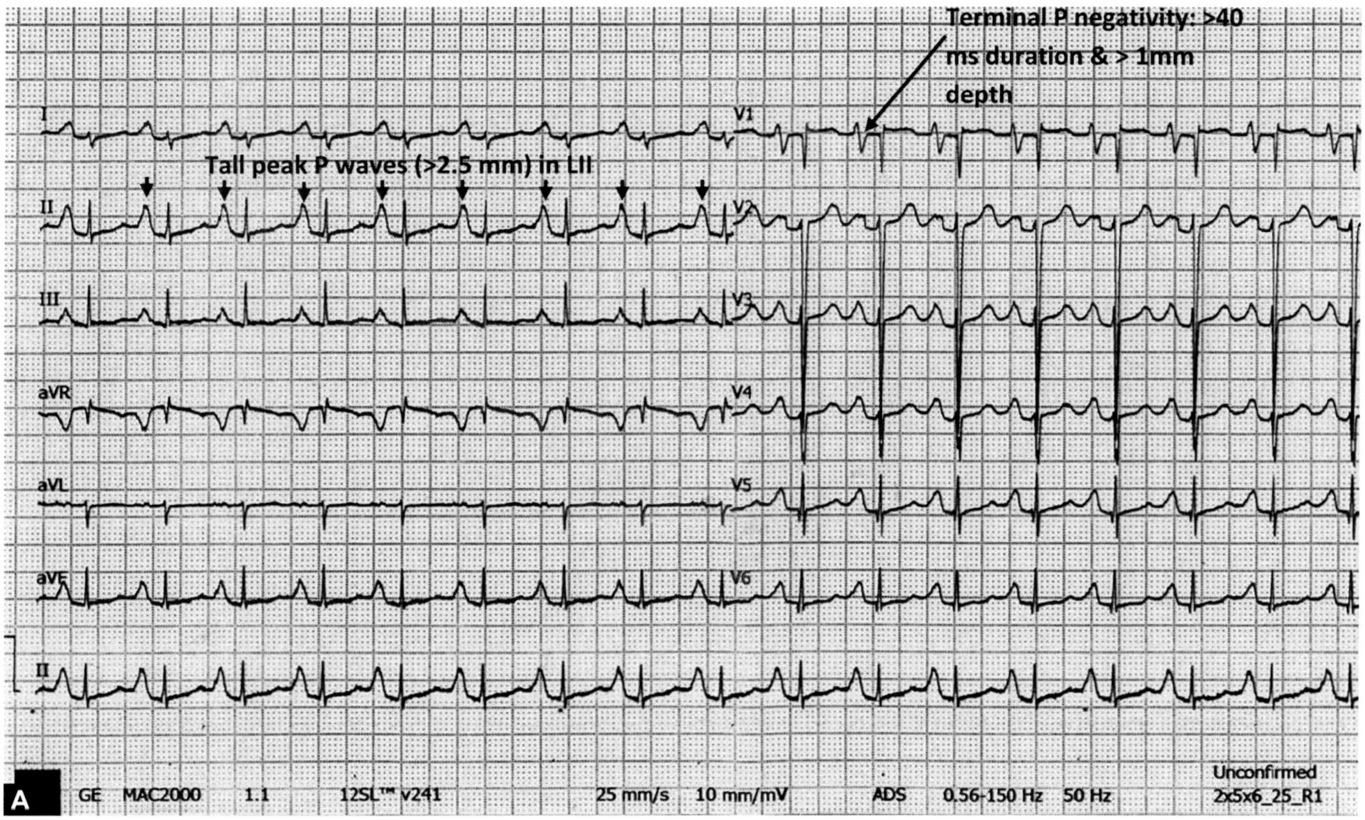

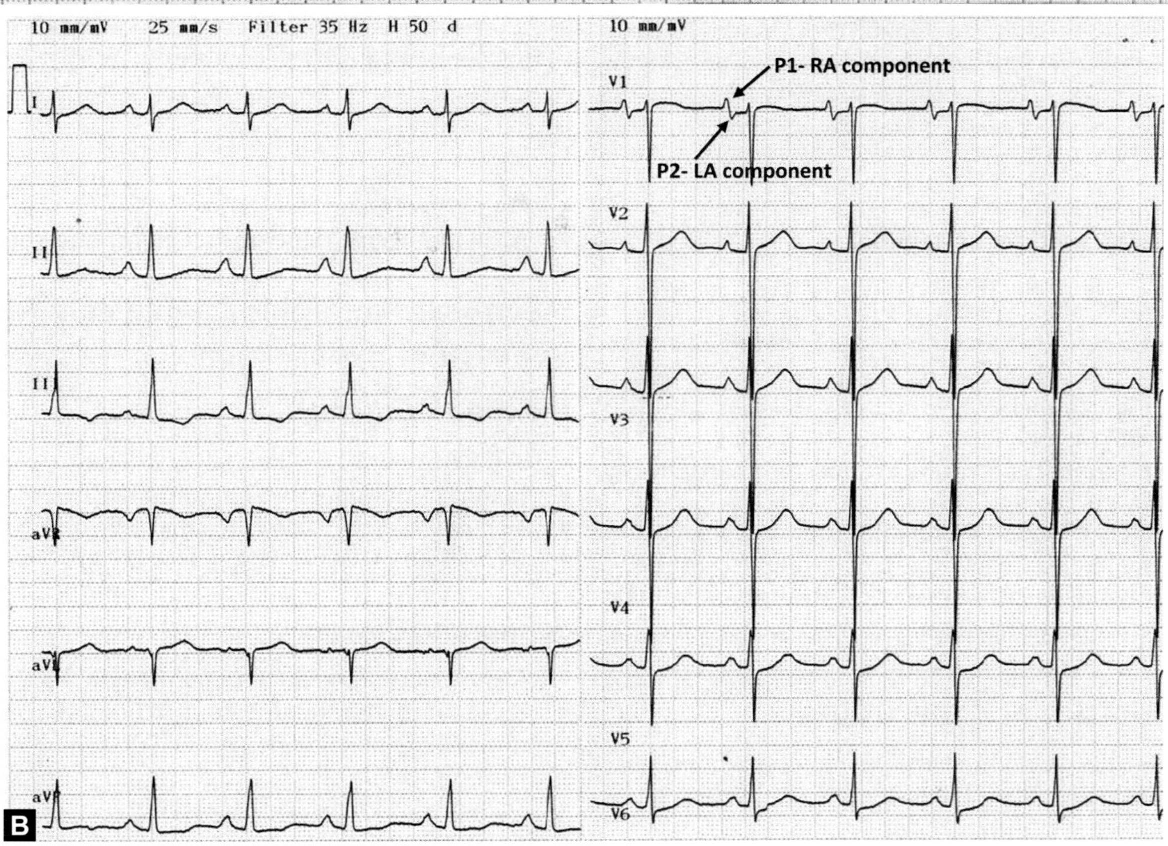

Figs. 6.28A and B: (A) Electrocardiogram is suggestive of biatrial enlargement showing tall peak P wave (3.5 mm) in LII and terminal P negativity in lead V1 of duration 55 ms (>40 ms) and depth 3 mm (>1 mm). (B) Electrocardiogram shows typical biphasic P wave in V1 suggestive of biatrial enlargement. Note initial positive deflection, right atrial component (P1) of the biphasic P wave is greater than 1.5 mm tall and terminal negative deflection, LA component (P2) is more than 1 mm deep and more than 40 ms duration (*arrows*).

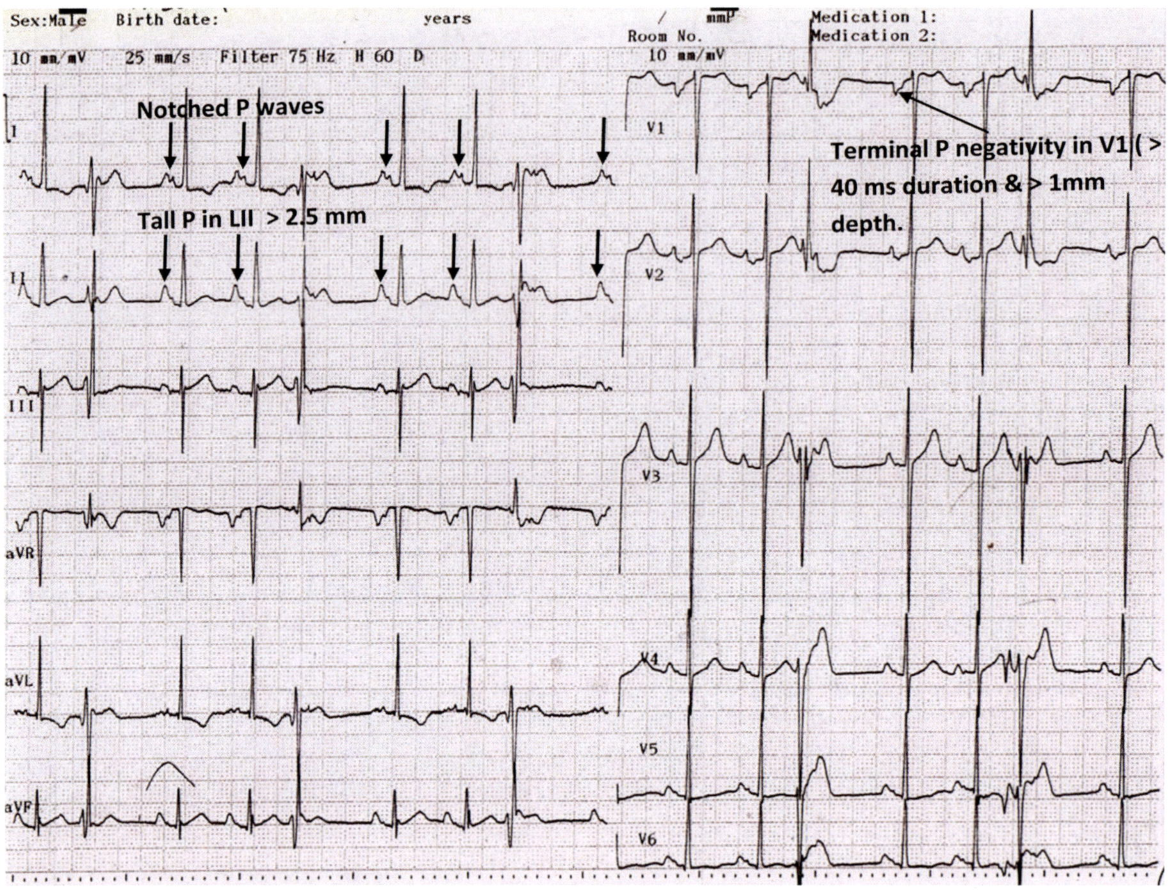

Fig. 6.29: Electrocardiogram is suggestive of biatrial enlargement with features of both P-pulmonale (tall P wave 3 mm in LII) and P-mitrale (notched P wave in LI and terminal P negativity in lead V1 of duration (80 ms) and depth (3 mm). Note few PVCs.

- Mitral regurgitation
- Peripheral arteriovenous shunts
- Anemia
- Thyrotoxicosis.

Electrocardiographic features of LVH volume overload include:

- Lateral precordial (V4–V6) narrow Q waves and with very tall R waves.
- The ST segment and T wave are often normal or nearly normal.
- A negative U wave, best identified in leads V4–V6, is a common finding in left ventricular volume overload.

The ECG differences between LVH pressure and volume overload is shown in Table 6.2.

Right Ventricular Hypertrophy

Right ventricular dilation and hypertrophy occurs from either volume overload or hypertrophy from pressure overload.

Important causes of RVH include:

- Mitral stenosis with pulmonary hypertension
- Pulmonary stenosis
- Primary pulmonary hypertension
- Chronic lung disease (cor pulmonale)
- Pulmonary embolism
- Tetralogy of Fallot
- Arrhythmogenic right ventricular cardiomyopathy.

Electrocardiographic Diagnosis of Right Ventricular Hypertrophy

Diagnostic Criteria

- Tall R wave in V1 (>7 mm tall or R/S ratio > 1).
- Right axis deviation of +110° or more
- Deep S wave in V5 or V6 (>7 mm deep or R/S ratio < 1)
- QRS duration usually is less than 120 ms.

Supporting Criteria

- Right atrial enlargement (P pulmonale)
- Right ventricular strain pattern (ST depression/T-wave inversion in the right precordial (V1-3) and inferior (II, III, aVF) leads.
- Deep S waves in leads I, II, and III.

There are no universally accepted criteria for diagnosing RVH in the presence of RBBB; the standard voltage criteria do not apply. However, the presence of incomplete or complete RBBB with a tall R wave in V1, right axis deviation of +110° or more and supporting criteria (such as RV strain pattern or P pulmonale) would be considered suggestive of RVH.

Table 6.2: Electrocardiographic differences between left ventricular hypertrophy pressure and volume overload.

ECG change	*LVH pressure overload*	*LVH volume overload*
R waves in lateral precordial leads (V4–V6).	Tall	Very tall
ST segment change	ST segment depression with slight convexity upwards are usually present in V4–V6	Very minimal change in ST segment in leads V4–V6. ST segment may be minimally elevated in leads V4–V6 with concavity upwards.
Initial narrow Q waves in leads V4–V6.	Usually absent	Usually present
T-wave inversions in anterolateral leads	Asymmetrical deep T-wave inversions are usually present in leads LI, aVL, V5–V6.	Usually upright T waves are present in left precordial leads.
Change in ventricular activation time (VAT).	VAT is increased due to hypertrophied ventricle.	VAT remains usually normal.
Presence of inverted U waves in leads V4–V6	Usually not present	May be present

(LVH: left ventricular hypertrophy)

Biventricular Hypertrophy

The ECG has a low sensitivity for the diagnosis of BVH, as the opposing left and right ventricular forces tend to cancel each other out. There may be signs of both LVH and RVH on the same ECG—e.g. positive diagnostic criteria for LVH with some additional features suggestive of RVH. The *Katz-Wachtel sign* large diphasic QRS complexes in mid precordial leads (V2-4) is suggestive of BVH. This is the classic ECG pattern of BVH, most commonly seen in children with VSD.

The typical ECG feature of BVH is the presence of electrocardiographic sign of LVH with right axis deviation.

In the presence of ECG criteria of LVH,

Additional signs indicating RVH:

- Right atrial enlargement
- Right axis deviation
- Tall biphasic QRS complexes in multiple leads
- Deep S waves in V5-6.

In the presence of ECG criteria of RVH,

Additional signs indicating LVH:

- Tall R waves and deep S waves in V2-5.
- QRS amplitude is greater than 50 mm.

Atrial Abnormalities

Abnormal P waves should usually be referred to as right or left "atrial abnormality" rather than enlargement, overload, strain, or hypertrophy. But in clinical practice the terms "LAE/hypertrophy" or "RAE/hypertrophy" are very popular and frequently used by the clinicians during interpretation of the ECGs.

Left Atrial Abnormality/Enlargement

Dilation or hypertrophy of the LA may increase the duration of the P wave. In LA enlargement, LA depolarization lasts longer than normal but its amplitude (height) remains unchanged. The P wave is normally less than 120 ms of duration. The long or abnormally shaped P wave occurs because of delay in electrical activation of the enlarged left atrium. A P wave longer than 120 ms is diagnostic of LAE.

Two other abnormalities indicate LAE. A "double hump" or "notched P" wave is diagnostic of LAE. A biphasic P wave indicates LAE, if the downward portion of the P wave is one box or larger in both depth and length. LA enlargement often occurs in mitral valve disease (either stenosis or insufficiency). Because of this association, a broad notched P wave is often called "P mitrale." In addition, LAE often occurs with any cause of LVH.

Electrocardiographic features of LAE are:

- P-wave duration $\geq$120 ms (usually lead II).
- Notched P wave in limb leads with the inter-peak duration $\geq$40 ms.
- Terminal P negativity in lead V1 (i.e. "P-terminal force") duration $\geq$40 ms and depth $\geq$1 mm.

Morris index: P-wave terminal force in lead V1 (PTFV1), also known as Morris index can be used as a marker of LAE on a 12-lead ECG. Normally the depth of the terminal P wave in V1 is less than 1 mm and duration is less than 0.04 s (<40 ms). Morris index is derived from multiplying the depth of terminal P-wave deflection in V1 in millimeter (mm) by duration in second (s) and expressed in mm s. Normally the depth of terminal P wave in V1 is less than 1 mm and duration is less than 0.04 s. So the maximum Morris index is around: $1 \times 0.04 = 0.04$ mm s. If the P terminal force (Morris index) exceeds 0.04 mm s, it is suggestive of LAE.

Right Atrial Abnormality/Enlargement

Right atrial enlargement is diagnosed by the presence of a P wave 2.5 mm or greater in height. The P wave often has a sharp, peaked appearance. The increased voltage is best seen in the "inferior" leads L II, III, and aVF. The lead most likely to show the RAE is lead II. Causes of RAE include COPD, Ebstein's anomaly, atrial septal defect (ASD) and pulmonary embolism. Because RAE is so frequently seen in chronic pulmonary disease, the peaked P wave is often called "P pulmonale."

Right atrial abnormality/enlargement produces a peaked P wave (P pulmonale) with amplitude:

- Greater than 2.5 mm in the inferior leads, usually best seen in LII.
- P1 amplitude greater than 1.5 mm in V1 and V2.

Box 6.2: Quick ECG diagnosis of hypertrophy and enlargement

Left ventricular hypertrophy (LVH)

- S in V1 + R in V5 or V6 >35 mm
- Electrocardiographic evidence of left atrial enlargement
- Left axis deviation
- ST segment depression and T-wave inversion in the left-sided leads.

Right ventricular hypertrophy (RVH)

- Tall R wave in V1 (R/S ratio >1)
- Right axis deviation of +110° or more
- Dominant S wave in V5 or V6 (> 7 mm deep or R/S ratio < 1)
- Right atrial enlargement (P pulmonale).

Biventricular hypertrophy (BVH)

The ECG has a low sensitivity for the diagnosis of BVH.

- There may be signs of both LVH and RVH on the same ECG.

or

- Electrocardiographic criteria of LVH with right axis deviation.

or

- Electrocardiographic criteria of RVH with tall R waves and deep S waves in V2-5.

or

- Katz–Wachtel phenomenon, large diphasic QRS complexes (tall R waves + deep S waves) in mid precordial leads (V2-4).

Left atrial enlargement (LAE)

- Left atrial enlargement produces a broad, bifid P wave in lead II (P mitrale).
- Biphasic P wave with terminal negative portion >1 mm deep in V1.

Right atrial enlargement (RAE)

Right atrial enlargement produces a peaked P wave (P pulmonale) with amplitude:

- Greater than 2.5 mm in the inferior leads (best seen in lead LII)
- Greater than 1.5 mm in V1 and V2.

Biatrial enlargement (BAE)

The diagnosis of biatrial enlargement requires criteria for LAE and RAE to be met in either lead II, lead V1, or a combination of leads.

- *In lead II, bifid P wave with*: Amplitude ≥ 2.5 mm and duration ≥120 ms.
- In V1, biphasic P waves with: Initial deflection >1.5 mm tall and terminal negative deflection ≥1 mm deep and ≥40 ms duration.

The other causes of RA enlargement are:

- Chronic lung disease (cor pulmonale)
- Tricuspid stenosis
- Congenital heart disease (pulmonary stenosis, tetralogy of Fallot)
- Primary pulmonary hypertension.

Right atrial abnormality/enlargement causes an increase in the height or amplitude of the P wave (P-wave amplitude > 2.5 mm) but LA abnormality causes increased duration of P wave (>120 ms).

Biatrial Enlargement

- Features of both RA enlargement and LA enlargement in same ECG
- P wave in lead II is greater than 2.5 mm tall and is greater than or equal to 0.12 second (≥120 ms) in duration
- Initial positive component of P wave in V1 is greater than 1.5 mm tall and terminal negative deflection ≥1 mm deep and ≥40 ms duration.

Quick Electrocardiographic Diagnosis of Hypertrophy And Enlargement

The quick ECG diagnosis of hypertrophy and enlargement are shown in Box 6.2.

REFERENCES

1. Bacharova L, Estes EH. Electrocardiographic diagnosis of left ventricular hypertrophy: depolarization changes. J Electrocardiol. 2009;42(3):228-32.
2. Mathew J, Sleight P, Lonn E, et al. Reduction of cardiovascular risk by regression of electrocardiographic markers of left ventricular hypertrophy by the angiotensin-converting enzyme inhibitor ramipril. Circulation. 2001;104(14): 1615-21.
3. Okin PM, Devereux RB, Jern S, et al. Regression of electrocardiographic left ventricular hypertrophy by losartan versus atenolol: the Losartan Intervention for Endpoint Reduction in Hypertension (LIFE) Study. Circulation. 2003;108(6):684-90.
4. Hancock EW, Deal BJ, Mirvis DM, et al. AHA/ACCF/HRS recommendations for the standardization and interpretation of the electrocardiogram: part V: electrocardiogram changes associated with cardiac chamber hypertrophy: a scientific statement from the American Heart Association Electrocardiography and Arrhythmias Committee, Council on Clinical Cardiology; the American College of Cardiology Foundation; and the Heart Rhythm Society. Endorsed by the International Society for Computerized Electrocardiology. Circulation. 2009;119(10): e251-e261.
5. Surawicz B. Electrocardiographic diagnosis of chamber enlargement. J Am Coll Cardiol. 1986;8(3):711-24.
6. Edhouse J, Thakur RK, Khalil JM. ABC of clinical electrocardiography: Conditions affecting the left side of the heart. BMJ. 2002;324(7348):1264-7.
7. Sokolow M, Lyon TP. The ventricular complex in left ventricular hypertrophy as obtained by unipolar and limb leads. Am Heart J. 1949;37(2):161-86.

8. Casale P, Devereux R, Kligfield P, et al. Electrocardiographic detection of left ventricular hypertrophy: development and prospective validation of improved criteria. J Am Coll Cardiol. 1985;6(3):572-80.
9. Romhilt DW, Estes EH. A point score system for the ECG diagnosis of left ventricular hypertrophy. Am Heart J. 1968;75(6):752-8.
10. MacFarlane PW, Lawrie TD. Comprehensive Electrocardiography: Theory and Practice in Health and Disease. Oxford: Pergamon Press; 1988.
11. Alfakih K, Walters K, Jones T, et al. New gender-specific partition values for ECG criteria of left ventricular hypertrophy: recalibration against cardiac MRI. Hypertension. 2004;44(2):175-9.
12. Casale PN, Devereux RB, Alonso DR, et al. Improved sex-specific criteria of left ventricular hypertrophy for clinical and computer interpretation of electrocardiograms: validation with autopsy findings. Circulation. 1987;75(3):565-72.
13. Norman JE Jr, Levy D. Improved electrocardiographic detection of echocardiographic left ventricular hypertrophy: results of a correlated data base approach. J Am Coll Cardiol. 1995;26(4):1022-9.
14. Baxley WA, Dodge HT, Sandler H. A quantitative angiocardiographic study of left ventricular hypertrophy and the electrocardiogram. Circulation. 1968;37(4):509-17.
15. LaMonte CS, Frieman AH. The electrocardiogram after mastectomy. Circulation. 1965;32(5):746-54.
16. Ogah OS, Adebiyi AA, Oladapo OO, et al. Association between electrocardiographic left ventricular hypertrophy with strain pattern and left ventricular structure and function. Cardiology. 2006;106(1):14-21.
17. Okin PM, Devereux RB, Jern S, et al. Baseline characteristics in relation to electrocardiographic left ventricular hypertrophy in hypertensive patients: the Losartan Intervention for Endpoint Reduction (LIFE) in hypertension study: the Life Study Investigators. Hypertension. 2000;36(5):766-73.
18. Murphy ML, Thenabadu PN, de Soyza N, et al. Sensitivity of electrocardiographic criteria for left ventricular hypertrophy according to type of cardiac disease. Am J Cardiol. 1985;55(5):545-9.
19. Molloy TJ, Okin PM, Devereux RB, et al. Electrocardiographic detection of left ventricular hypertrophy by the simple QRS voltage-duration product. J Am Coll Cardiol. 1992, 20: 1180-1186.
20. Antikainen RL, Grodzicki T, Palmer AJ, et al. Left ventricular hypertrophy determined by Sokolow–Lyon criteria: a different predictor in women than in men? J Hum Hypertens. 2006;20:451-9.
21. 2003 European Society of Hypertension-European Society of Cardiology. Guidelines for the management of arterial hypertension. J Hypertens. 2003;21:1011-53.
22. Carey MG, Pelter MM. Cornell voltage criteria. Am J Crit Care. 2008;17(3):273-4.
23. Hanna EB, Glancy L, Oral E. Sensitivity and specificity of frequently used electrocardiographic criteria for left ventricular hypertrophy in patients with anterior wall myocardial infarction. Proc (Bayl Univ Med Cent). 2010;23(1):15-8.
24. Julien J, Tranche C, Souchet T. Left ventricular hypertrophy in hypertensive patients. Epidemiology and prognosis. Arch Mal Coeur Vaiss. 2004;97(3):221-7.
25. Dahlof B, Devereux R, de Faire U, et al. The Losartan Intervention For Endpoint reduction (LIFE) in Hypertension study: rationale, design, and methods. The LIFE Study Group. Am J Hypertens. 1997;10(7):705-13.
26. Benjamin EJ, Levy D. Why is left ventricular hypertrophy so predictive of morbidity and mortality? Am J Med Sci. 1999;317(3):168-75.
27. Schillaci G, Verdecchia P, Borgioni C, et al. Improved electrocardiographic diagnosis of left ventricular hypertrophy. Am J Cardiol. 1994;74(7):714-19.
28. Verdecchia P, Schillaci G, Borgioni C, et al. Prognostic value of a new electrocardiographic method for diagnosis of left ventricular hypertrophy in essential hypertension. J Am Coll Cardiol. 1998;31(2):383-90.
29. Levy D, Labib SB, Anderson KM, et al. Determinants of sensitivity and specificity of electrocardiographic criteria for left ventricular hypertrophy. Circulation. 1990;81(3):815-20.
30. Jain A, Tandri H, Dalal D, et al. Diagnostic and prognostic utility of ECG for left ventricular hypertrophy defined by MRI in relationship to ethnicity: The Multi-Ethnic Study of Atherosclerosis (MESA). Am Heart J. 2010;159(4):652-8.
31. Erice B, Romero C, Anderiz M, et al. Diagnostic value of different electrocardiographic voltage criteria for hypertrophic cardiomyopathy in young people. Scand J Med Sci Sports. 2009;19(3):356-63.
32. Hsieh BP, Pham MX, Froelicher VF. Prognostic value of electrocardiographic criteria for left ventricular hypertrophy. Am Heart J. 2005;150(1):161-7.
33. Pewsner D, Juni P, Egger M, et al. Accuracy of electrocardiography in diagnosis of left ventricular hypertrophy in arterial hypertension: systematic review. BMJ. 2007;335(7622):711.
34. Bauml MA. Left ventricular hypertrophy: An overlooked cardiovascular risk factor. Cleve Clin J Med. 2010;77(6): 381-7.
35. Levy D, Labib SB, Anderson KM, et al. Determinants of sensitivity and specificity of electrocardiographic criteria for left ventricular hypertrophy. Circulation. 1990;81(3):815-20.
36. Okin PM, Wright JT, Nieminen MS, et al. Ethnic differences in electrocardiographic criteria for left ventricular hypertrophy: the LIFE study. Losartan Intervention For Endpoint. Am J Hypertens. 2002;15(8):663-71.
37. Kannel WB, Gordon T, Castelli WP, et al. Electrocardiographic left ventricular hypertrophy and risk of coronary heart disease. The Framingham study. Ann Intern Med. 1970;72(6):813-22.
38. Okin PM, Devereux RB, Nieminen MS, et al. Electrocardiographic strain pattern and prediction of cardiovascular morbidity and mortality in hypertensive patients. Hypertension. 2004;44(1):48-54.
39. Brady WJ, Chan TC, Pollack M. Electrocardiographic manifestations: patterns that confound the EKG diagnosis of acute myocardial infarction-left bundle branch block, ventricular paced rhythm, and left ventricular hypertrophy. J Emerg Med. 2000;18(1):71-8.
40. Larsen CT, Dahlin J, Blackburn H, et al. Prevalence and prognosis of electrocardiographic left ventricular hypertrophy, ST segment depression and negative T-wave; the Copenhagen City Heart Study. Eur Heart J. 2002;23(4): 315-24.

41. Hsieh BP, Pham MX, Froelicher VF, et al. Prognostic value of electrocardiographic criteria for left ventricular hypertrophy. Am Heart J. 2005;150(1):161-7.
42. Petersen GV, Tikoff G. Left bundle branch block and left ventricular hypertrophy: electrocardiographic-pathologic correlations. Chest. 1971;59(2):174-7.
43. Havelda CJ, Sohi GS, Flowers NC, et al. The pathologic correlates of the electrocardiogram: complete left bundle branch block. Circulation. 1982;65(3):445-51.
44. Fragola PV, Autore C, Ruscitti G, et al. Electrocardiographic diagnosis of left ventricular hypertrophy in the presence of left bundle branch block: a wasted effort. Int J Cardiol. 1990;28(2):215-21.
45. Klein RC, Vera Z, DeMaria AN, et al. Electrocardiographic diagnosis of left ventricular hypertrophy in the presence of left bundle branch block. Am Heart J. 1984;108(3 Pt 1):502-6.
46. Noble LM, Humphrey SB, Monoghan GB. Left ventricular hypertrophy in left bundle branch block. J Electrocardiol. 1984;17(2):157-60.
47. Kafka H, Burggraf GW, Milliken JA. Electrocardiographic diagnosis of left ventricular hypertrophy in the presence of left bundle branch block: an echocardiographic study. Am J Cardiol. 2000;55(1):103-6.
48. Mehta A, Jain AC, Mehta MC, et al. Usefulness of left atrial abnormality for predicting left ventricular hypertrophy in the presence of left bundle branch block. Am J Cardiol. 2000;85(3):354-9.
49. Haskell RJ, Ginzton LE, Laks MM. Electrocardiographic diagnosis of left ventricular hypertrophy in the presence of left bundle branch block. J Electrocardiol. 1987;20(3):227-32.
50. Devereux RB, Reichek N. Left ventricular hypertrophy. Cardiovasc Rev Rep. 1980;3:155-68.
51. Romhilt DW, Bove KE, Norris RJ, et al. A critical appraisal of the electrocardiographic criteria for the diagnosis of left ventricular hypertrophy. Circulation. 1969;40(2):185-95.
52. Kafka H, Burggraf GW, Milliken JA. Electrocardiographic diagnosis of left ventricular hypertrophy in the presence of left bundle branch block: an echocardiographic study. Am J Cardiol. 1985;55(1):103-6.
53. Yamaki M, Ikeda K, Kubata I, et al. Improved diagnostic performance on the severity of left ventricular hypertrophy with body surface mapping. Circulation, 1989;79(2):312-23.
54. Hugenholtz PG, Ellison RC, Micttinen OS. Spatial voltages in the assessment of left ventricular hypertrophy. J Electrocardiol. 1968;1(1):7-90.
55. Cokkinos DV, Demopoulos JN, Heimonas ET, et al. Electrocardiographic criteria of left ventricular hypertrophy in left bundle-branch block. Br Heart J. 1978;40(3): 320-4.
56. Vandenberg BF, Romhilt DW. Electrocardiographic diagnosis of left ventricular hypertrophy in the presence of bundle branch block. Am Heart J. 1991;122(3 Pt 1):818-22.
57. Oreto G, Saporito F, Messina F, et al. Electrocardiographic diagnosis of left ventricular hypertrophy in the presence of intraventricular conduction disturbances. G Ital Cardiol. 2007;8(3):161-7.
58. Rodríguez-Padial L, Rodríguez-Picon B, Jerez-Valero M, et al. Diagnostic accuracy of computer-assisted electrocardiography in the diagnosis of left ventricular hypertrophy in left bundle branch block. Rev Esp Cardiol. 2012;65(1):38-46.
59. Holt JH Jr, Barnard AC, Kramer JO Jr. A study of the human heart as a multiple dipole source. IV. Left ventricular hypertrophy in the presence of right bundle branch block. Circulation. 1977;56(3):391-4.
60. Murphy ML, Thenabadu PN, de Soyza N, et al. Left atrial abnormality as an electrocardiographic criterion for the diagnosis of left ventricular hypertrophy in the presence of right bundle branch block. Am J Cardiol. 1983;52(3):381-3.
61. De Leonardis V, Goldstein SA, Lindsay J Jr. Electrocardiographic diagnosis of left ventricular hypertrophy in the presence of complete right bundle branch block. Am J Cardiol. 1988;62(9):590-3.
62. Vandenberg B, Sagar K, Paulsen W, et al. Electrocardiographic criteria for diagnosis of left ventricular hypertrophy in the presence of complete right bundle branch block. Am J Cardiol. 1989;63(15):1080-4.
63. Oreto G, Saporito F, Messina F, et al. Electrocardiographic diagnosis of left ventricular hypertrophy in the presence of intraventricular conduction disturbances. G Ital Cardiol. 2007;8(3):161-7.
64. Gertsch M, Theler A, Foglia E. Electrocardiographic detection of left ventricular hypertrophy in the presence of left anterior fascicular block. Am J Cardiol. 1988;61(3):1098-101.
65. Bozzi G, Figina A. Left anterior hemiblock and electrocardiographic diagnosis of left ventricular hypertrophy. Adv Cardiol. 1976;16:495-500.
66. Fragola P, Autore C, Magni G, et al. Limitations of the electrocardiographic diagnosis of left ventricular hypertrophy: the influence of left anterior hemiblock and right bundle branch block. Int J Cardiol. 1992;34(1):41-8.
67. Lorell BH, Carabello BA. Left ventricular hypertrophy: pathogenesis, detection, and prognosis. Circulation. 2000;102(4):470-9.
68. Gunther S, Grossman W. Determinants of ventricular function in pressure-overload hypertrophy in man. Circulation. 1979;59(4):679-88.
69. Opie LH, Commerford PJ, Gersh BJ, et al. Controversies in ventricular remodelling. Lancet. 2006;367(9507):356-67.
70. Buchner S, Deb K, Haimer J, et al. Electrocardiographic diagnosis of left ventricular hypertrophy in aortic valve disease: evaluation of ECG criteria by cardiovascular magnetic resonance. J Cardiovasc Magn Reson. 2009;11:18.
71. Venkatachalam S, Rimmerman CM. Electrocardiography in aortic regurgitation: It's in the details. Cleve Clin J Med. 2011;78(8):505-6.
72. Kyriacopoulos JD, Conrad LL, Cuddy TE, et al. Activation of the free wall of the right ventricle in experimental right ventricular hypertrophy with and without right bundle branch block. Am Heart J. 1964;67(1):81-7.
73. Milnor WR. Electrocardiogram and vectorcardiogram in right ventricular hypertrophy and right bundle-branch block. Circulation. 1957;16(3):348-67.
74. Butler PM, Leggett SI, Howe CM, et al. Identification of electrocardiographic criteria for diagnosis of right ventricular hypertrophy due to mitral stenosis. Am J Cardiol. 1986;57(8):639-43.
75. Scott RC. The electrocardiographic diagnosis of right ventricular hypertrophy in the adult. Heart Bull. 1967;16:65-7.
76. Murphy M, Hutcheson F. The electrocardiographic diagnosis of right ventricular hypertrophy in chronic obstructive pulmonary disease. Chest. 1974;65(6):622-7.

77. Murphy ML, Thenabadu PN, de Soyza N, et al. Reevaluation of electrocardiographic criteria for left, right, and combined cardiac ventricular hypertrophy. Am J Cardiol. 1984;53(8):1140-7.
78. Antikainen R, Grodzicki T, Palmer AJ, et al. The determinants of left ventricular hypertrophy defined by Sokolow-Lyon criteria in untreated hypertensive patients. J Hum Hypertens. 2003;17(3):159-64.
79. Murphy ML, Thenabadu PN, Blue LR, et al. Descriptive characteristics of the electrocardiogram from autopsied men free of cardiopulmonary disease-a basis for evaluating criteria for ventricular hypertrophy. Am J Cardiol. 1983;52(10):1275-80.
80. Walker JC Jr, Helm RA, Scott Re. Right ventricular hypertrophy, correlation of isolated right ventricular hypertrophy at autopsy with the electrocardiographic findings. Circulation. 1955;11(2):215-22.
81. Myers GB, Klein HA, Stofer BE. Electrocardiographic diagnosis of right ventricular hypertrophy. Am Heart J. 1948;35(1):1-40.
82. Milnor WR. Electrocardiogram and vectorcardiogram in right ventricular hypertrophy and right bundle-branch block. Circulation. 1957;16(3):348-67.
83. Lehtonen J, Sutinen S, Ikaheimo M, et al. Electrocardiographic criteria for the diagnosis of right ventricular hypertrophy verified at autopsy. Chest. 1988;93(4):839-42.
84. Nunez BD, Messerli FH, Amodeo C, et al. Biventricular hypertrophy in essential hypertension. Am Heart J. 1987;114(4 Pt 1):813-8.
85. Jain A, Chandna H, Silber EN, et al. Electrocardiographic patterns of patients with echocardiographically determined biventricular hypertrophy. J Electrocardiol. 1999;32(3): 269-73.
86. Katz LN, Wachtel H. The diphasic QRS type of electrocardiogram in congenital heart disease. Am Heart J. 1937;13(2):202-6.
87. Elliott LP, Anderson RC, Tuna N, et al. Complete transposition of the great vessels: II. An electrocardiographic analysis. Circulation. 1963;27:1118-27.
88. Thomas P, Dejong D. The P wave in the electrocardiogram in the diagnosis of heart disease. Br Heart J. 1954;16(3):241-54.
89. Alpert MA, Munuswamy K. Electrocardiographic diagnosis of left atrial enlargement. Arch Intern Med. 1989;149(5): 1161-5.
90. Lee KS, Appleton CP, Lester SJ, et al. Relation of electrocardiographic criteria for left atrial enlargement to two-dimensional echocardiographic left atrial volume measurements. Am J Cardiol. 2007;99(1):113-8.
91. Hazen MS, Marwick TH, Underwood DA. Diagnostic accuracy of the resting electrocardiogram in detection and estimation of left atrial enlargement: an echocardiographic correlation in 551 patients. Am Heart J. 1991;122(3 Pt 1):823-8.
92. Munuswamy K, Alpert MA, Martin RH, et al. Sensitivity and specificity of commonly used electrocardiographic criteria for left atrial enlargement determined by M-mode echocardiography. Am J Cardiol. 1984;53(6):829-32.
93. Bureekam S, Boonyasirinant T. Accuracy of left atrial enlargement diagnosed by electrocardiography as compared to cardiac magnetic resonance in hypertensive patients. J Med Assoc Thai. 2014;97(Suppl 3):S132-8.
94. Alingandula A, Ramana Murthy PSV, Komma S. Detection of left atrial enlargement by echocardiography and electrocardiogram correlation in cardiac and non-cardiac diseases. Int J Sci Stud. 2016;4(5):1-5.
95. Valimaki I. Macruz index and measurement errors: A critical evaluation. J Electrocardiogr. 1972;5(1):96-8.
96. Reeves WC, Hallahan W, Schwiter EJ, et al. Two-dimensional echocardiographic assessment of electrocardiographic criteria for right atrial enlargement. Circulation. 1981;64(2): 387-91.
97. Sethi T, Singh AP, Singla V, et al. Biatrial enlargement: an unusual cause of massive cardiomegaly. BMJ Case Reports 2013; 2013.

Chapter 7

Myocardial Ischemia

INTRODUCTION

Electrocardiogram (ECG) is the most commonly used diagnostic tool to exclude or to establish the diagnosis of coronary artery disease (CAD). But ECG has limitations. ECG may appear normal or near normal even in the presence of severe CAD. So, the clinical history of the patient is very important. Electrocardiography is not sufficiently specific or sensitive to be used without a patient's clinical history.

The whole spectrum of CAD is divided into two broad groups: (1) stable angina, and (2) acute coronary syndromes (ACS). A typical presentation of stable angina is that of chest discomfort and associated symptoms precipitated by some activity (running, walking, etc.) with minimal or nonexistent symptoms at rest or with administration of sublingual nitroglycerin (NTG). ACS encompasses a spectrum of unstable CAD from unstable angina (UA) to ST-elevation myocardial infarction (STEMI). All have a common etiology in the formation of thrombus on an inflamed and complicated atheromatous plaque. The leading symptom of ACS is typically chest pain. The clinical presentation of ACS includes a wide variety of symptoms. Traditionally, several clinical presentations have been distinguished: (1) prolonged (>20 min) anginal pain at rest, (2) new onset (de novo) angina, (3) recent destabilization of previously stable angina to crescendo angina, and (4) postmyocardial infarct angina.[1-5]

ECG FEATURES OF STABLE ANGINA

A resting ECG is often normal in stable angina pectoris. During pain, the ECG may show transient ST-segment depression, T-wave inversion or both. Abnormal ECG changes are more common with UA pectoris.

All patients with suspected angina pectoris based on symptoms should have a resting 12-lead ECG recorded. It should be emphasized that a normal resting ECG is not uncommon even in patients with severe angina and does not exclude the diagnosis of ischemia. However, the resting ECG may show signs of CAD, such as previous MI or an abnormal repolarization pattern. The ECG may assist in clarifying the differential diagnosis if taken in the presence of pain, allowing detection of dynamic ST-segment changes in the presence of ischemia, or by identifying features of pericardial disease. An ECG during pain may be particularly useful if vasospasm is suspected.[6] The ECG may also show other abnormalities such as left ventricular hypertrophy (LVH), bundle branch block, preexcitation, arrhythmias, or conduction defects. Such information may be helpful in defining the mechanisms responsible for chest pain, in selecting appropriate further investigation or in tailoring individual patient treatment. There is little direct evidence to support routinely repeating the resting ECG at frequent intervals, unless to obtain an ECG during pain or if there has been a change in functional class.[6]

ECG FEATURES OF ACUTE CORONARY SYNDROMES

The leading symptom that initiates the diagnostic and therapeutic cascade is chest pain, but the classification of patients is based on the ECG. Two categories of patients may be encountered:

1. Patients with typical acute chest pain and persistent (>20 min) ST-segment elevation. This is termed ST-elevation-ACS (STE-ACS) and generally reflects an acute total coronary occlusion. Most of these patients will ultimately develop STEMI. STEMI is defined as new or presumed new ST elevation in two or more contiguous leads that is greater than or equal to 0.2 mV (≥2 mm) in leads V1, V2, and V3 and greater than 0.1 mV (>1 mm) in other leads or the occurrence of new onset LBBB. The therapeutic objective is to achieve rapid, complete, and sustained reperfusion by primary angioplasty or fibrinolytic therapy.[5,7]
2. Patients with acute chest pain but without persistent ST-segment elevation have rather persistent or transient ST-segment depression or T-wave inversion,

flat T waves, pseudonormalization of T waves, or no ECG changes at presentation. At presentation, the working diagnosis of non-ST elevation-ACS (NSTE-ACS), based on the measurement of troponins, will be further qualified into non-ST elevation MI (NSTEMI) or UA. If cardiac markers, troponins are raised the diagnosis of NSTEMI is confirmed and if troponins are not raised the diagnosis of UA is established. ECG features of NSTEMI or UA are similar and only cardiac markers elevation can differentiate between these two conditions. The resting 12-lead ECG is the first-line diagnostic tool in the assessment of patients with suspected NSTE-ACS.[5,6]

The characteristic ECG abnormalities of NSTE-ACS are ST-segment depression or transient elevation and/or T wave changes.[8,9] The finding of persistent (>20 min) ST-elevation suggests STEMI, which mandates different treatment.[6] If the initial ECG is normal or inconclusive, additional recordings should be obtained if the patient develops symptoms and these should be compared with recordings obtained in an asymptomatic state.[9] Comparison with a previous ECG, if available, is valuable, particularly in patients with coexisting cardiac disorders, such as LVH or a previous MI. ECG recordings should be repeated at least at 3 hours, 6–9 hours and 24 hours after first presentation and immediately in the case of recurrence of chest pain or symptoms. It should be appreciated that a completely normal ECG does not exclude the possibility of NSTE-ACS. In particular, ischemia in the territory of the circumflex artery or isolated right ventricular ischemia frequently escapes the common 12-lead ECG, but may be detected in leads V7–V9 and in leads V3R and V4R, respectively.[8] Transient episodes of bundle branch block occasionally occur during ischemic attacks.[8,10]

Findings on ECG associated with UA include ST-segment depression, transient ST-segment elevation, T-wave inversion, or some combination of these changes and depending on the severity of the clinical presentation, these findings are present in 30–50% of patients.[11,12] New ST-segment deviation, even of only 0.05 mV (0.5 mm), is an important and specific measure of ischemia and prognosis.[11,13] T-wave inversion is sensitive for ischemia but is less specific, unless it is marked as greater than or equal to 0.3 mV (3 mm).[11,14]

Because the process of myocardial ischemia is quite dynamic and a single 12-lead ECG provides only a snapshot view of this process, so it is recommended that patients hospitalized for UA/NSTEMI should undergo serial ECG tracings or continuous ST-segment monitoring.[11]

ST-segment depression is the most common findings in patients presenting with features of ACS (UA or NSTEMI). According to the result of GUSTO-IIb trial, the following ECG changes are usually present in patients with ACS:[15]

- ST depression (35%)
- T-wave inversion (22%)
- Transient ST-elevation (28%)
- A combination of ST-elevation and depression (15%).

Patients presenting with ST depression are more likely to have severe disease than that of T inversion group. ST depression (>2 mm in two contiguous leads) is associated with an almost six- to ten-fold hazard of 1-year death.[16,17]

Unstable angina and NSTEMI differ primarily in whether the ischemia is severe enough to cause sufficient myocardial damage to release detectable quantities of a marker of myocardial injury. UA is considered to be present in patients with ischemic symptoms suggestive of an ACS and no elevation in troponin or creatine kinase-MB (CK-MB), with or without ECG changes indicative of ischemia (e.g. ST-segment depression or transient elevation or new T-wave inversion). Since an elevation in troponin and/or CK-MB may not be detectable for up to 12 hours after presentation, UA and NSTEMI are frequently indistinguishable at initial evaluation. ST-segment and/or T wave changes are often persistent in NSTEMI while, if they occur in UA, they are usually transient.

Changes in the ST-segment and T waves are not specific for ischemia; they also occur in association with several other disease processes, such as LVH, hypokalemia, and digoxin therapy.[18]

ST-SEGMENT DEPRESSION

Causes of ST Depression

The causes of ST depression are:

- Unstable angina/NSTEMI
- Reciprocal change in STEMI
- Digoxin effect
- Hypokalemia
- Supraventricular tachycardia
- Right bundle branch block
- Right ventricular hypertrophy
- Left bundle branch block
- Left ventricular hypertrophy
- Ventricular paced rhythm.

Patterns of ST-segment Depression

Typically, myocardial ischemia gives rise to ST-segment depression. The normal ST-segment usually blends with the T wave smoothly, making it difficult to determine where the ST-segment ends and the T wave starts. One of the first and most subtle changes in the ST-segment is flattening of the segment, resulting in a more obvious angle between the ST-segment and T wave. ST-segment depression may be transient, and its resolution with treatment is reassuring. The degree of ST-segment depression in any given lead is related to the size of the R wave. Thus, ST-segment depression is usually most obvious in leads V4–V6 of the 12-lead ECG. Moreover, because the height of the R wave varies with respiration, the degree of ST depression in any one lead may vary from beat to beat. ST-segment depression is usually not as marked in the inferior leads because here the R waves tend to be smaller. Substantial (>2 mm) and widespread (>7 leads) ST depression is a grave prognostic finding as it implies widespread myocardial ischemia from extensive CAD (Figs. 7.1 and 7.2).

Abnormalities in the ST-segment and T wave, which are the result of changes in the shape and/or duration of the repolarization phases of the transmembrane action potential and occur in the absence of changes in depolarization, are referred to as primary repolarization abnormalities. They may be localized or diffuse and may be caused by a variety of events, including ischemia, myocarditis, drugs, toxins, and electrolyte abnormalities, particularly abnormalities of serum calcium and potassium. An abrupt change in heart rate, hyperventilation, changes in body position, catecholamines, sympathetic stimulation or ablation of the stellate ganglion, and temperature changes also can cause primary repolarization abnormalities.[19,20]

Abnormalities in the ST-segment and T wave that occur as the direct result of changes in the sequence and/or duration of ventricular depolarization, manifested electrocardiographically as changes in QRS shape and/or duration, are referred to as secondary repolarization abnormalities. These changes do not require changes in the shape or duration of phase 2 and phase 3 of ventricular action potential of individual cells. Rather, they may be due to voltage gradients that are normally largely cancelled but become manifested when the changes in the sequence of depolarization alter the repolarization sequence. The ST-segment and T wave changes that occur in association with bundle branch blocks, ventricular hypertrophy, preexcitation, and ectopic and paced ventricular complexes are examples of secondary repolarization abnormalities.[20]

Primary and Secondary ST Depression

Primary ST Depression[21]

ST-segment and T-wave abnormalities may be unrelated to any QRS abnormality, in which case they are called primary ST-segment depression (Fig. 7.3). These are caused by ischemia, pericarditis, myocarditis, drugs (digoxin, antiarrhythmic drugs), and electrolyte abnormalities, particularly potassium abnormalities.

ST-segment depression or T-wave inversion is consistent with ischemia if any of the following is true:

- The ST-segment depression or T-wave inversion is directed in the same direction as the QRS complex, this is called concordance between the QRS complex and the ST or T abnormality.
- The ST-segment is depressed but the T wave is upright.

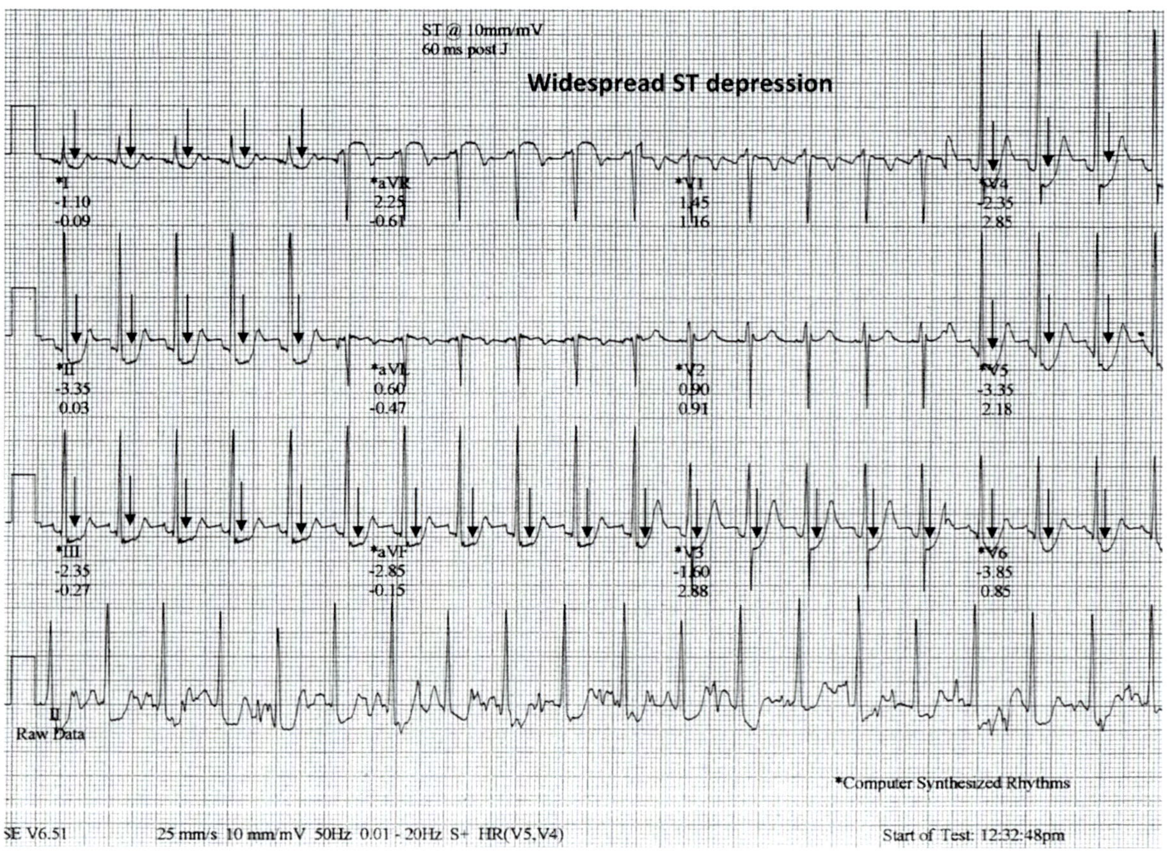

Fig. 7.1: Electrocardiogram shows widespread ST-segment depression (>2 mm) in LI, LII, LIII, aVF, and V3–V6.

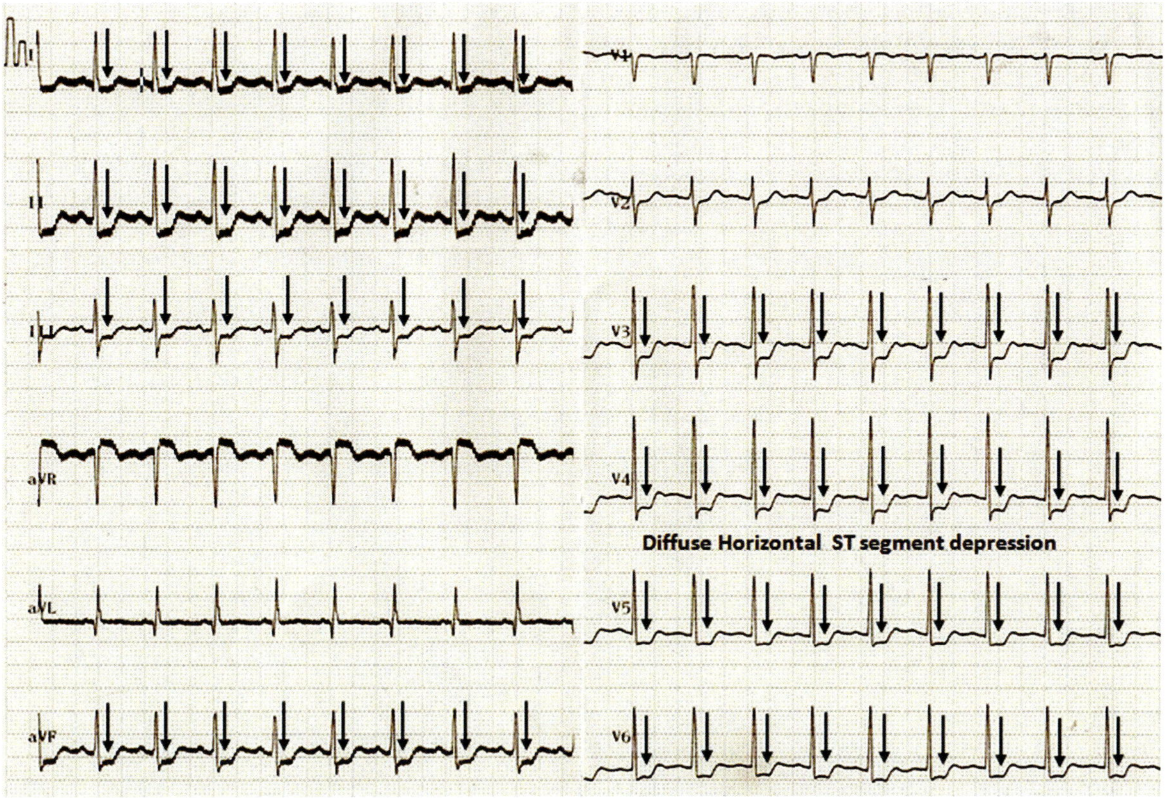

Fig. 7.2: Diffuse horizontal ST-segment depression in both anterior and inferior leads.

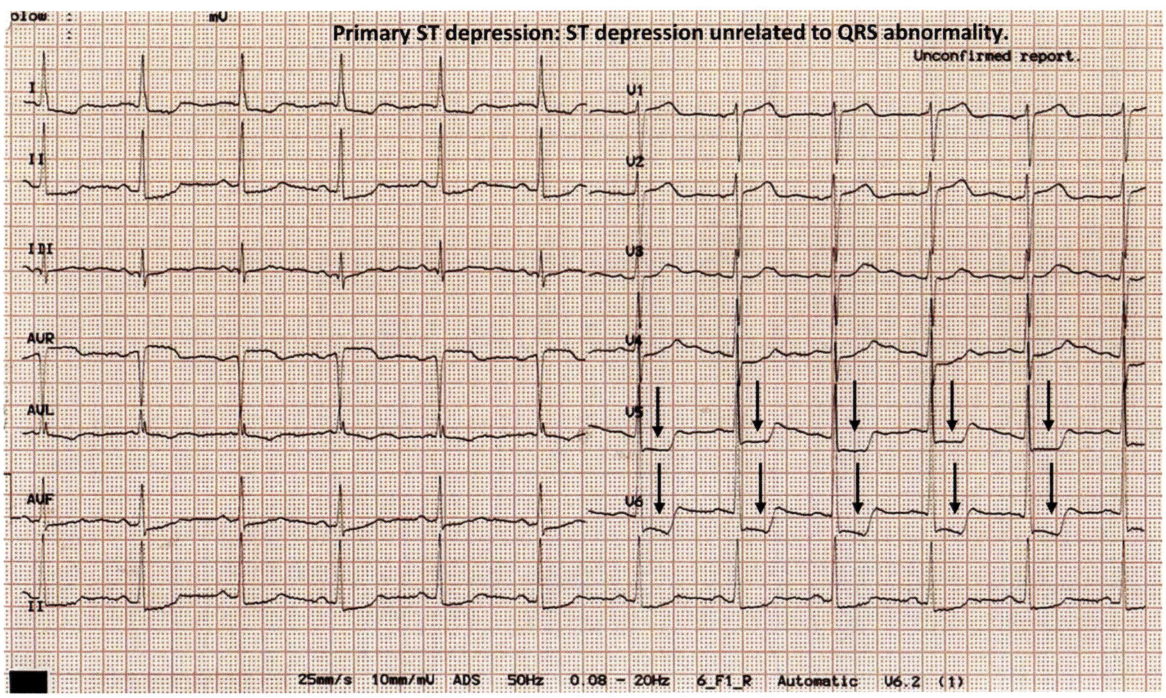

Fig. 7.3: Electrocardiogram showing marked degree of ST-segment depression in leads V5 and V6, suggestive of primary ST-segment depression. Note there is no electrocardiogram evidence of ventricular hypertrophy or bundle branch block pattern.

- The T wave has a positive–negative biphasic pattern.
- The T wave is symmetrically inverted and has a pointed configuration, while the ST-segment is not deviated or is upwardly bowed (coved) or horizontally depressed.
- The magnitude of ST-segment depression progresses or regresses on serial tracings, or ST-segment depression progresses to T-wave abnormality during ischemia-free intervals (dynamic ST-segment depression).

Secondary ST Depression[20,21]

In secondary ST-segment or T-wave abnormalities, QRS criteria for left or right ventricular hypertrophy (Fig. 7.4) or left or right bundle branch block (Figs. 7.5 and 7.6) or preexcitation are usually present, and the ST-segment and T wave have all of the following morphologic features:

- The ST-segment and T wave are directed opposite to the QRS, this is called discordance between the

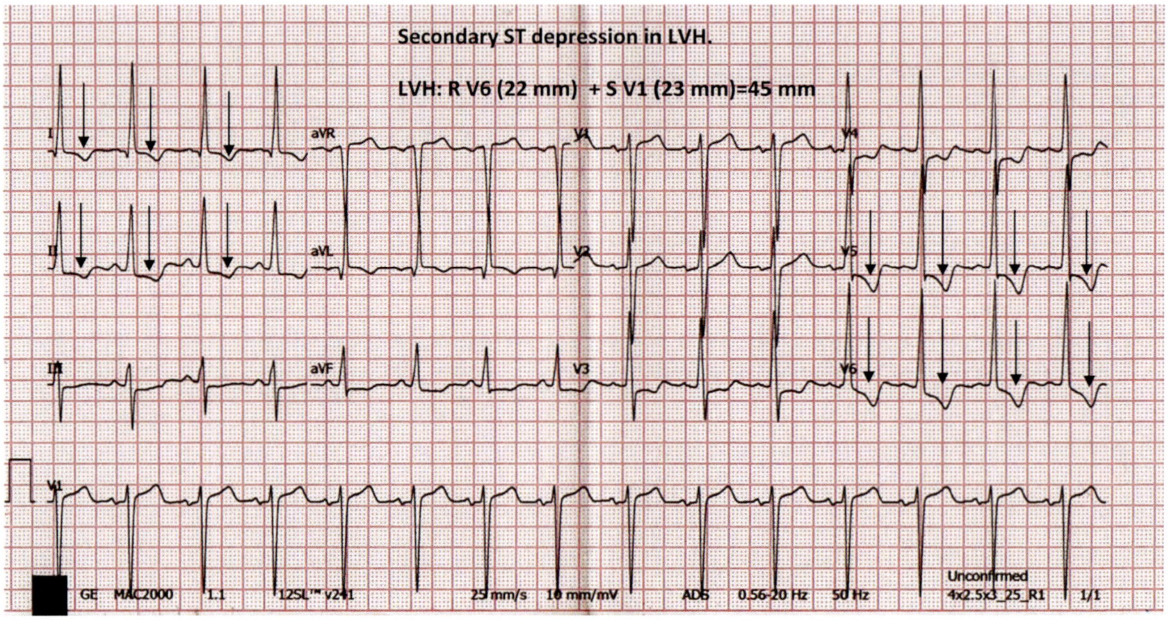

Fig. 7.4: Electrocardiogram showing secondary ST-segment depression and T-wave inversions in left ventricular hypertrophy (arrows). Note R V6 (22 mm) + S V1 (23 mm) = 45 mm suggestive of LVH. Note also discordance between the QRS complex and the ST-T abnormalities (the ST-segment depression and T waves are directed opposite to the QRS).

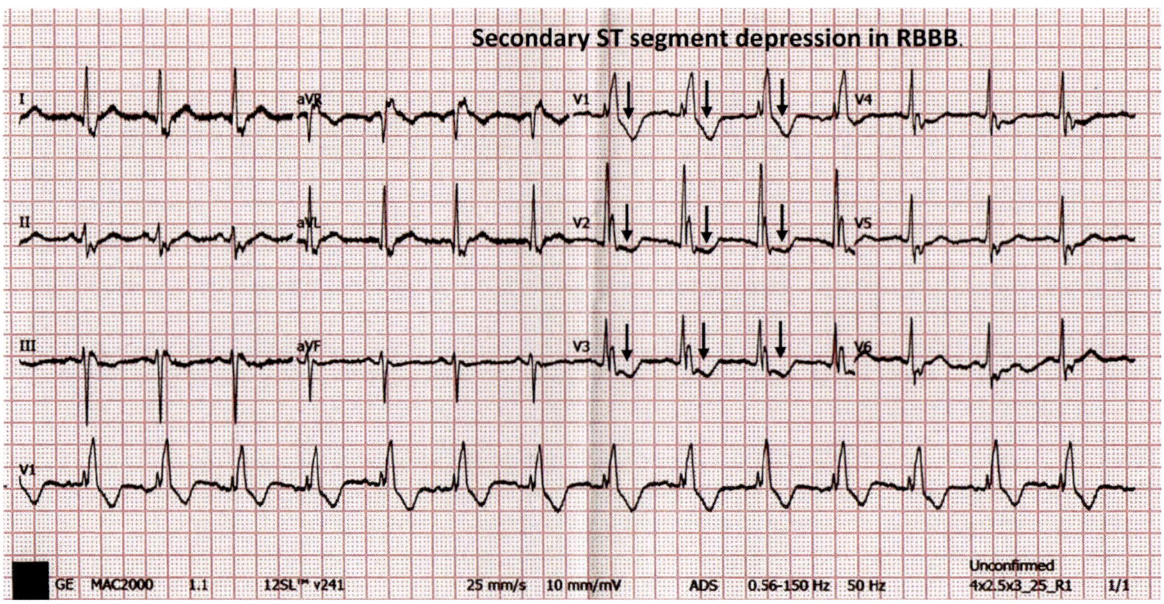

Fig. 7.5: Electrocardiogram showing secondary ST-segment depression and T-wave inversions (arrows) in right bundle branch block (rsR pattern in V1 and slurred S wave in V5 and V6).

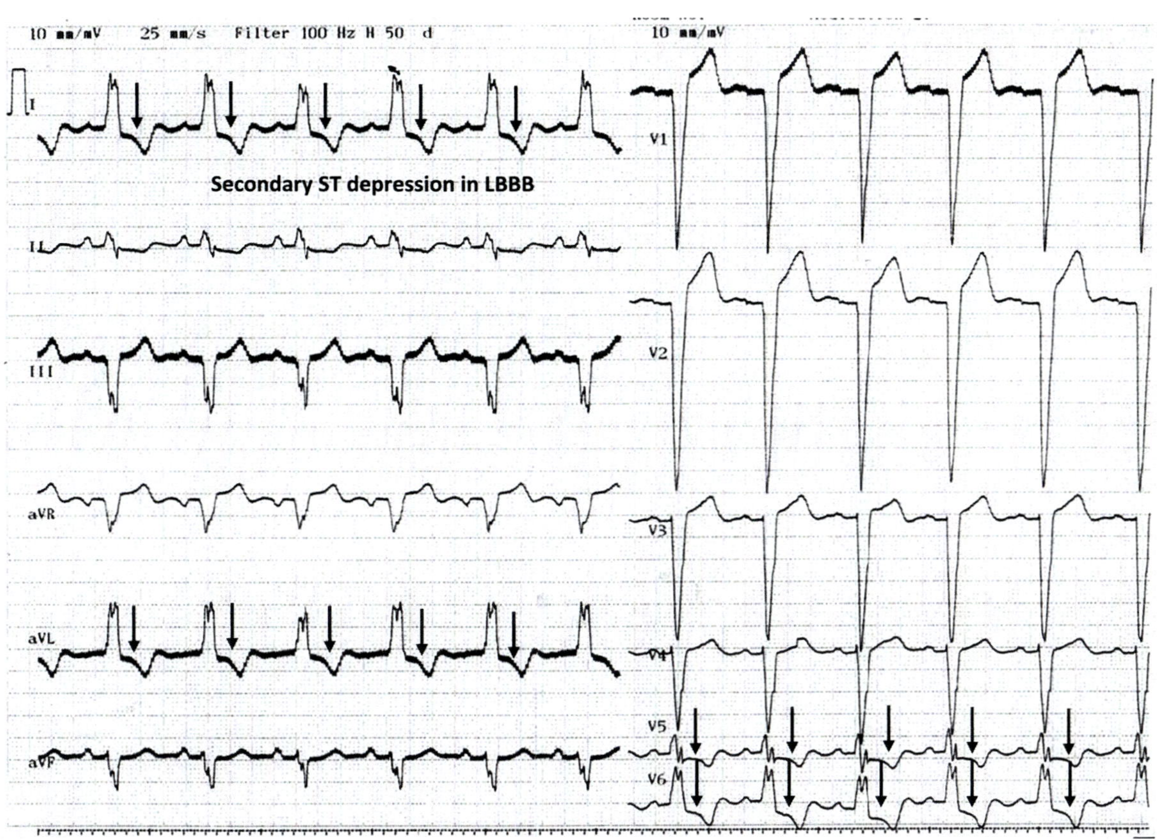

Fig. 7.6: Electrocardiogram showing secondary ST-segment depression and T-wave inversions in LI, aVL, V5, and V6 (*arrows*) in left bundle branch block. Note "M" pattern morphology of QRS complex in LI, aVL, V5, and V6, and QRS duration 0.14 seconds (140 ms).

QRS complex and the ST-T abnormalities. In the case of right bundle branch block, the ST and T are directed opposite to the terminal portion of the QRS, i.e. the part of the QRS deformed by the conduction abnormality.

- The ST-segment and T wave are both abnormal and deviate in the same direction, i.e. the ST-segment is downsloping and the T wave is inverted in leads with an upright QRS complex, which gives the ST-T complex a "reverse checkmark" asymmetric morphology.
- The ST and T abnormalities are not dynamic, i.e. they do not change in the course of several hours to several days.

ST depression attributable to ischemia is often diffuse and can be located in both anterior and inferior leads, and is not necessarily localizing.[22] So unlike the ST-segment elevation, the ST-segment depression does not localize ischemia. However, the extent and the magnitude of ST-segment depression correlate with the extent and the severity of ischemia.[22,23]

Types of ST-segment Depression (Figs. 7.7A to D)

ST-segment depression may be of three types:

1. Upsloping ST depression (Fig. 7.8)
2. Horizontal ST depression (Fig. 7.9)
3. Downsloping ST depression (Fig. 7.10).

Extensive experience from cardiac stress testing shows that the actual configuration of the ST-segment depression influences the specificity of this finding, with a downsloping segment more specific for the diagnosis of ischemia than horizontal depression.[24-26] But it must be mentioned that downsloping ST depression is also found in association with LVH and in patients taking digoxin. A depressed but upsloping ST-segment lacks the adequate specificity for ischemia. A combination of two diagnostic criteria have typically been required in at least one electrocardiographic lead to diagnose, myocardial ischemia—at least 1.0 mm (0.10 mV) depression at the J-point and either horizontal or downsloping ST-segment depression.[22,24-26]

Reciprocal ST-segment Depression

Reciprocal ST depression, also known as reciprocal change, is defined as a horizontal or downsloping ST depression in leads that are separate and distinct from leads manifesting ST elevation (Fig. 7.11). The causes of reciprocal change are thought to be secondary to the coexisting distant ischemia, a manifestation of infarct extension, or an electrophysiological phenomenon caused by displacement of the injury current vector away from the noninfarcted myocardium. Reciprocal change can be identified in about one-third of patients with acute anterior wall MI and up to 80% of patients with acute

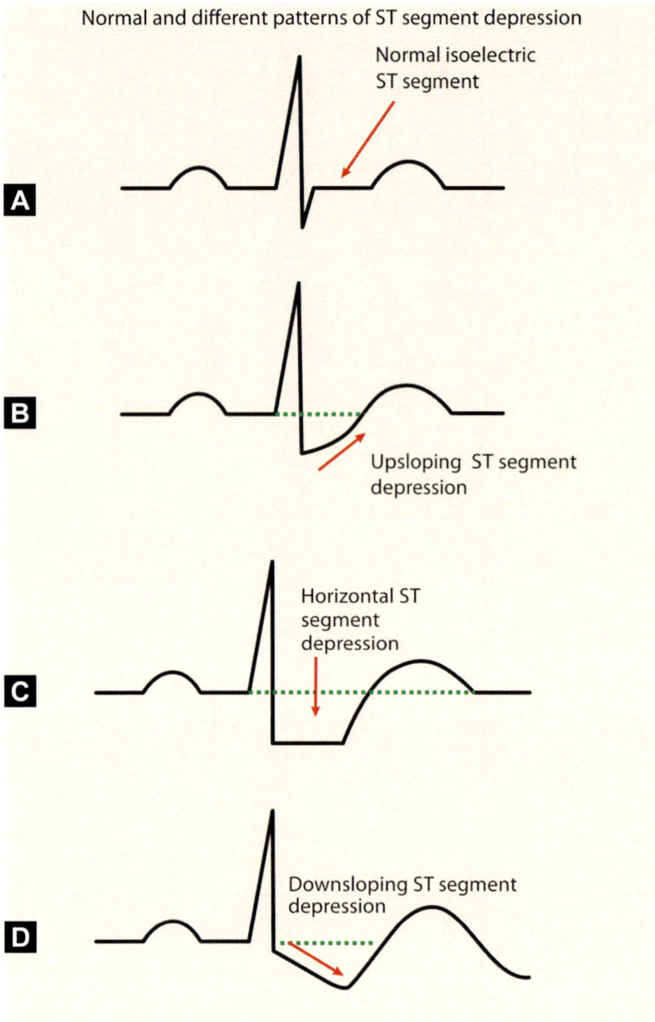

Figs. 7.7A to D: Normal and different patterns of ST-segment depression. (A) Normal isoelectric ST-segment. (B) Upsloping ST-segment depression. (C) Horizontal ST-segment depression. (D) Downsloping ST-segment depression.

inferior MI will demonstrate anterior ST-segment depression in leads V1, V2, or V3. The presence of reciprocal change increases the positive predictive value for a diagnosis of acute MI to greater than 90%.[27]

True Posterior ST-segment Elevation Myocardial Infarction

When accompanied by inferior STEMI, posterior infarction is easily recognized (Fig. 7.12), but it can be difficult to diagnose when it occurs alone, the so-called true posterior STEMI. ST-segment depression that is most prominent in leads V1 through V3 often indicates posterior STEMI rather than non-ST-segment elevation ischemia which indicates the need for emergency revascularization.[27-30]

T-wave Changes

Myocardial ischemia can affect T-wave morphology in a variety of ways: T waves may become tall, flattened, inverted, or biphasic. Tall T waves are one of the earliest changes seen in acute MI, most often seen in the anterior chest leads. Isolated tall T waves in leads V1–V3 may also be due to ischemia of the posterior wall of the left ventricle (the mirror image of T-wave inversion).[18] Myocardial ischemia may also give rise to T-wave inversion, but it must be remembered that inverted T waves are normal in leads III, aVR, and V1 in association with a predominantly negative QRS complex. T waves that are deep and symmetrically inverted (arrowhead) strongly suggest myocardial ischemia (Fig. 7.13). In some patients with partial thickness ischemia the T waves show a biphasic pattern. This occurs particularly in the anterior chest leads and is an acute phenomenon. Biphasic T wave changes usually evolve and are often followed by symmetrical T-wave inversion. These changes occur in patients with ACS and strongly suggest myocardial ischemia.[18]

Pseudonormalization of T Waves

In some patients with severe CAD, during the episodes of angina, the initial abnormal terminal negative T waves convert to normal positive T waves. This phenomenon is called pseudonormalization of T waves. Pseudonormalization of T waves is directly related to transmural myocardial ischemia and is a bad prognostic sign. After reperfusion therapy, if the inverted T waves become suddenly upright, this is diagnostic of reocclusion of the infarct-related artery (IRA).

Wellens' Syndrome

Wellens' syndrome is an electrocardiographic manifestation of critical proximal left anterior descending (LAD) coronary artery stenosis in patients with UA. This syndrome is characterized by two patterns of T wave changes. In 25% of cases, the T wave has a characteristic positive–negative biphasic morphology in leads V2 through V4 (Type A pattern) (Fig. 7.14). In 75% of cases, T waves are deeply (≥5 mm) and symmetrically inverted in leads V2 through V4 (Type B pattern) (Fig. 7.15).[31] The T waves in Wellens' syndrome may evolve over time from a Type A to a Type B pattern. In both patterns, the ST-segment is isoelectric or minimally elevated (<1 mm) with a straight or convex morphology, the downslope of the T wave is sharp, and the QT interval is often prolonged. These abnormalities are characteristically seen hours to days after the ischemic chest pain resolves. In fact, the ischemic episode is usually associated with transient ST-segment elevation or depression that progresses to the T-wave abnormality after the pain subsides.[32] This ECG sign may be the only indication of an impending large anterior infarction in a chest-pain-free patient.[33]

Nonspecific ST- and T-Wave Changes

Nonspecific ST- and T-wave changes may represent CAD, other cardiac pathology or be a normal variant.

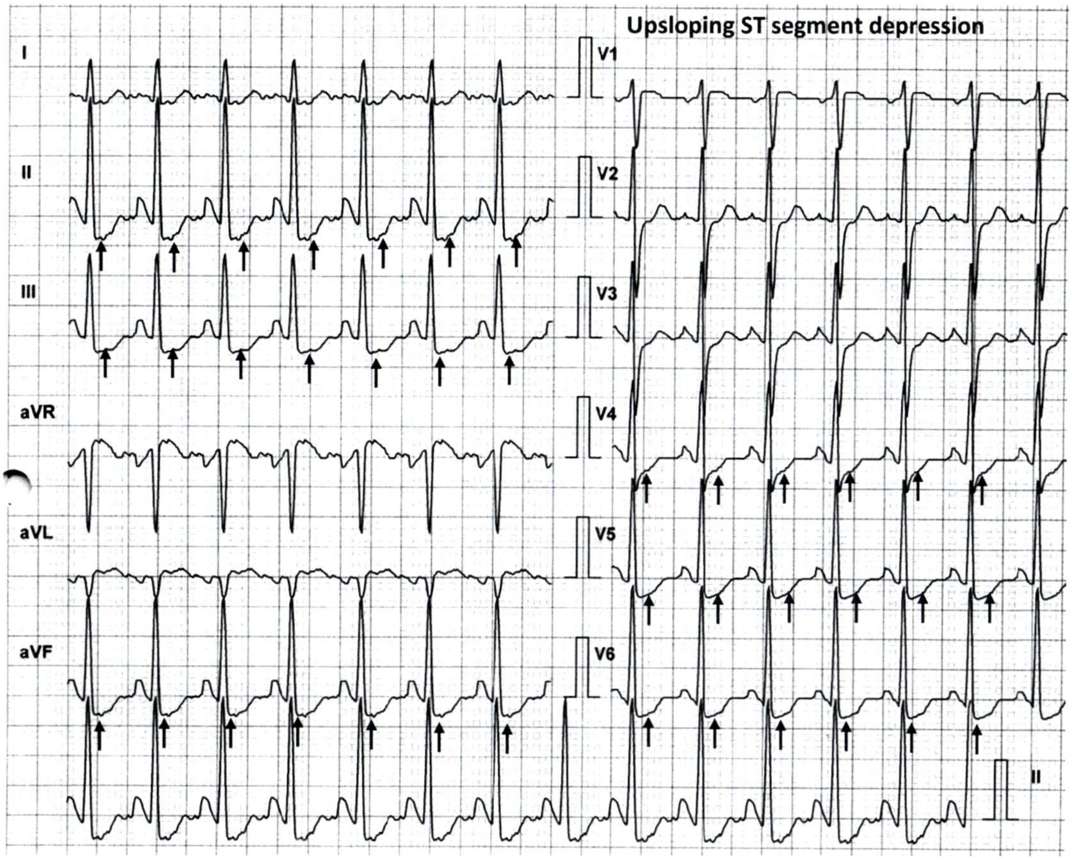

Fig. 7.8: Electrocardiogram shows sinus tachycardia (heart rate 136/min) with upsloping ST-segment depression in leads LII, LIII, aVF, and V4–V6 (arrows).

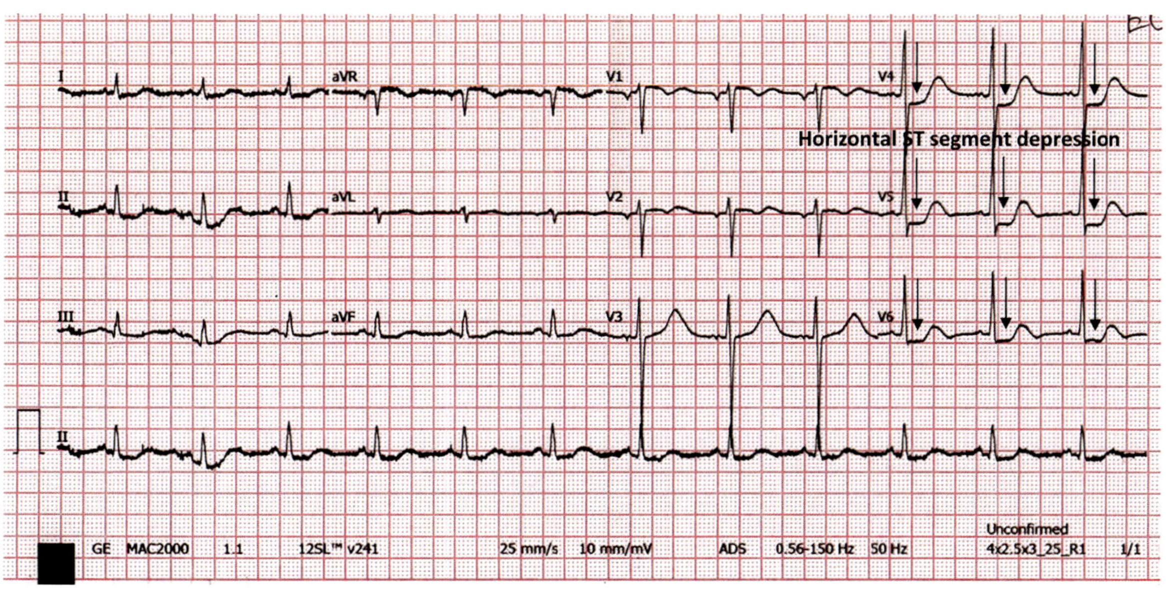

Fig. 7.9: Electrocardiogram showing horizontal ST-segment depression in leads V4–V6 (arrows).

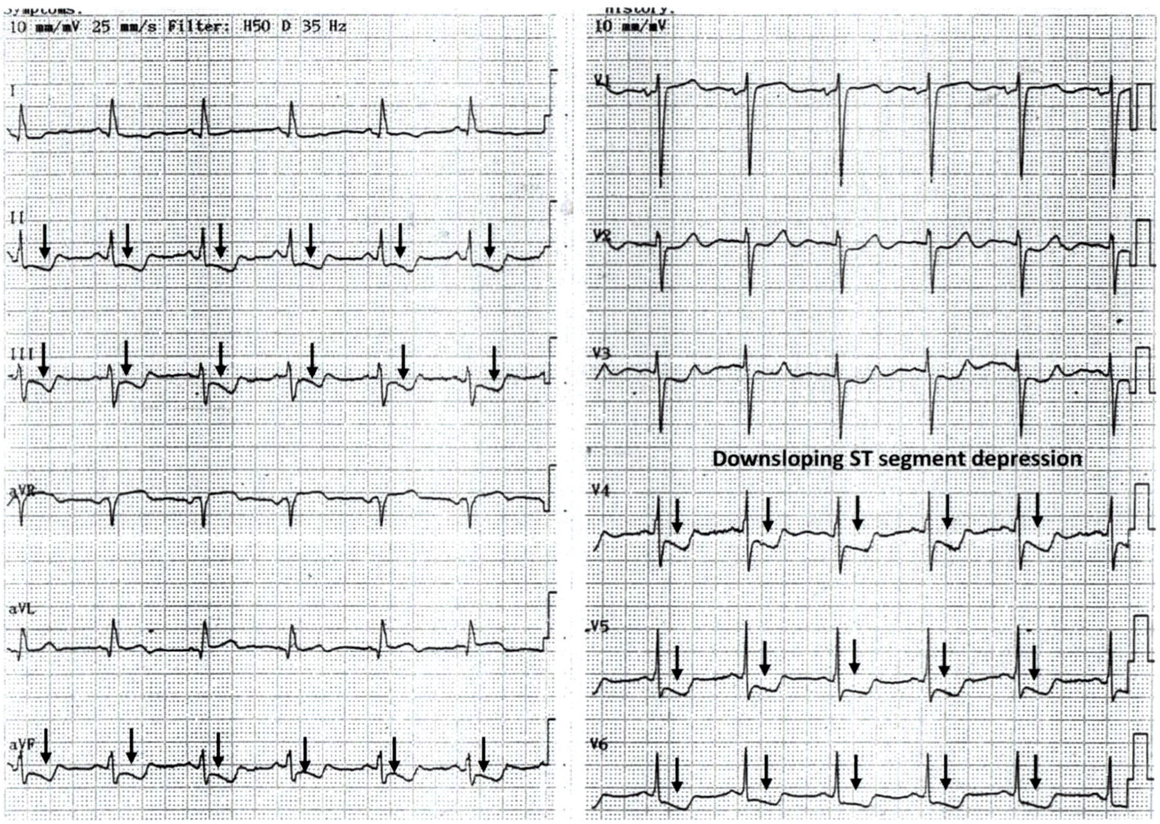

Fig. 7.10: Electrocardiogram shows significant downsloping ST-segment depression in inferior and lateral chest leads (arrows).

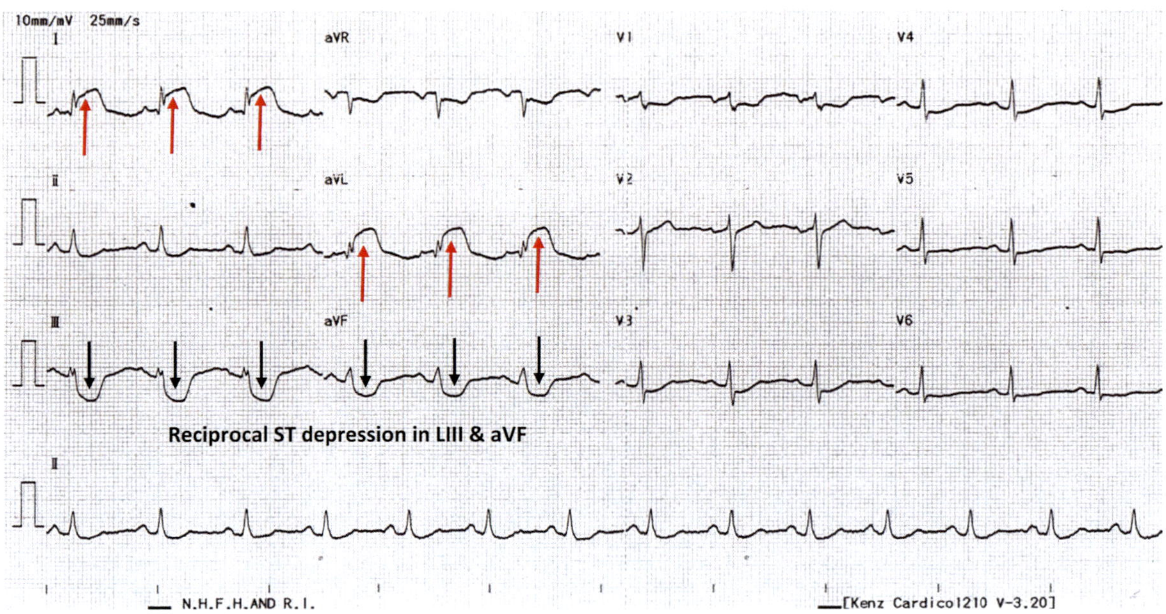

Fig. 7.11: This electrocardiogram shows ST elevation in LI and aVL (red arrows) suggestive of acute high lateral myocardial infarction. Note marked reciprocal ST-segment depression in LIII and aVF (black arrows).

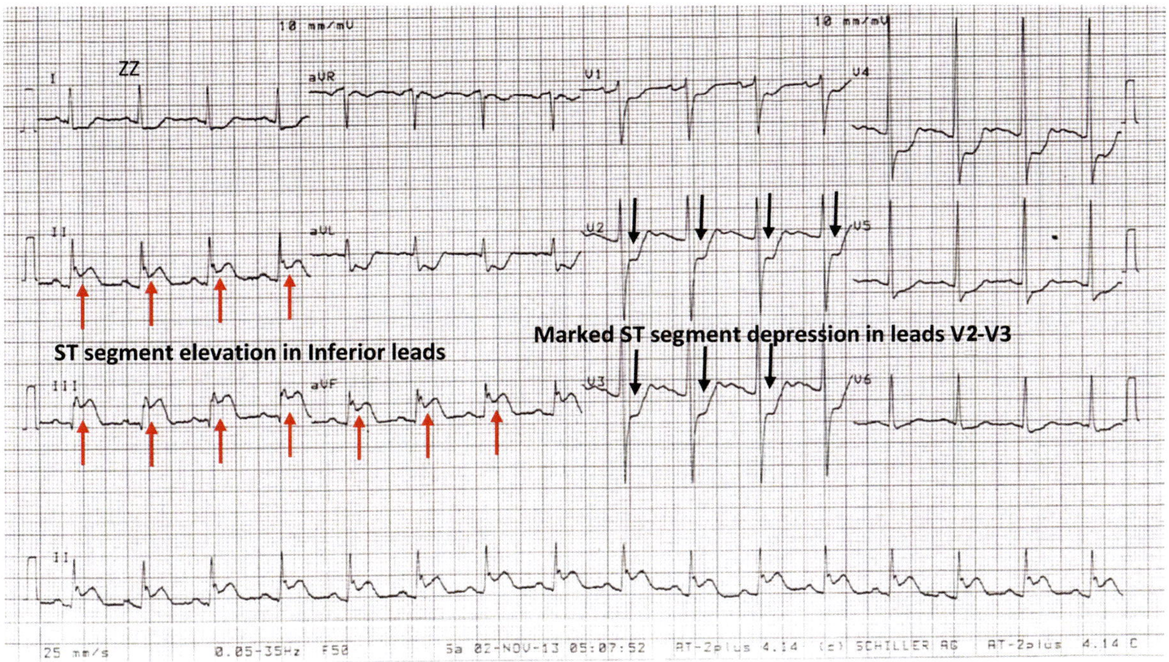

Fig. 7.12: Electrocardiogram shows ST-segment elevation (red arrows) in inferior leads (LII, LIII, and aVF) suggestive of acute inferior myocardial infarction. Also note marked ST-segment depression in leads V2–V3 (black arrows), suggestive of concomitant posterior myocardial infarction.

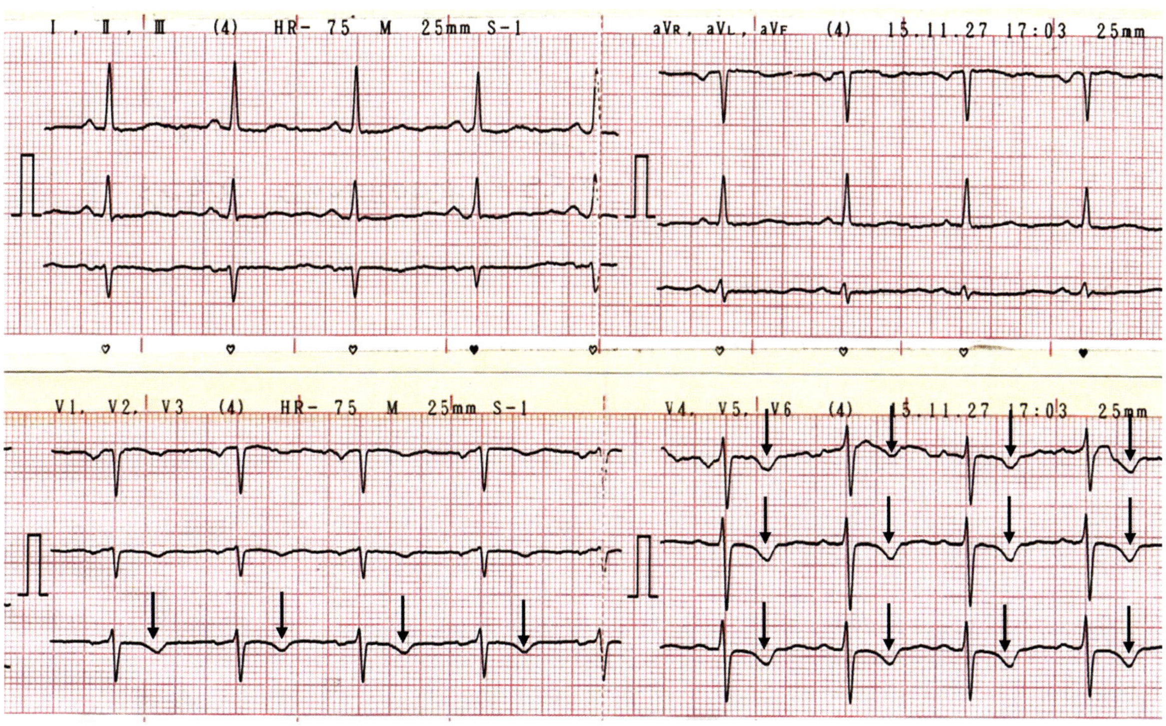

Fig. 7.13: Electrocardiogram shows symmetrical T-wave inversions (arrow head T inversion) in chest leads most marked in leads V4–V6 (arrows). Also note concordance between the QRS complex and the ST and T abnormality (the ST-segment depression and T-wave inversions are directed in the same direction as the QRS complex).

Interpretation of the findings, therefore, depends on the clinical context and presence of similar findings on prior ECGs. Nonspecific ST-T wave changes are very common and may be seen in any lead of the electrocardiogram. The changes may be seen in all or most of the leads or they may be present in contiguous leads, such as the inferior, lateral, or anterior leads. The types of abnormalities are varied and include subtle straightening of the ST-segment, actual ST-segment depression or elevation, flattening of the T wave, biphasic T waves, or T-wave inversion

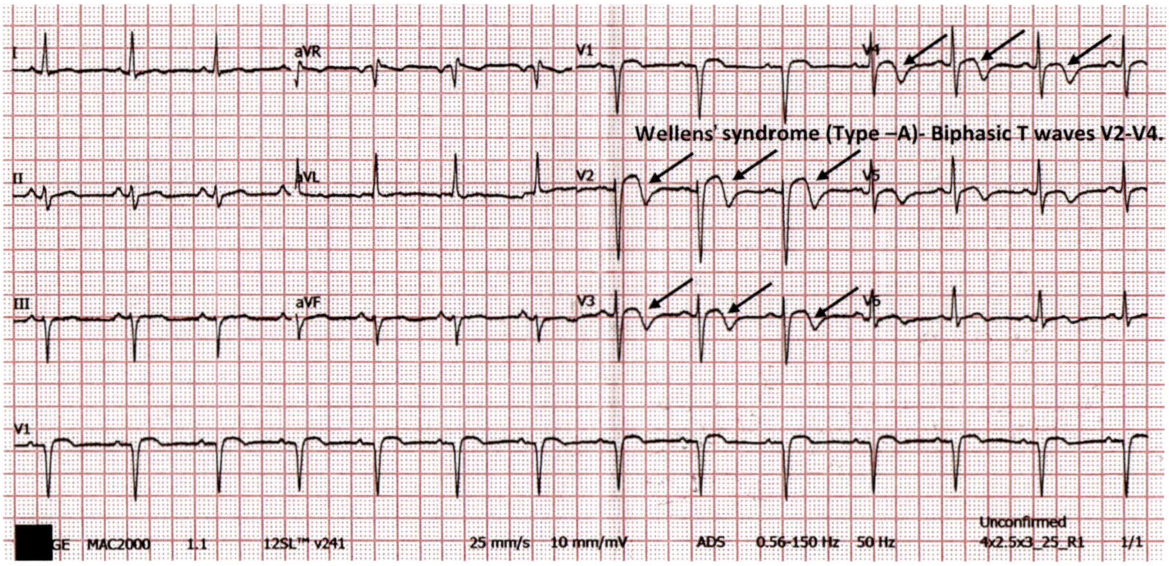

Fig. 7.14: Electrocardiogram is suggestive of Wellens' syndrome (Type A): Biphasic T waves V2–V4. Also note minimal precordial ST elevation with preserved R wave progression (R wave in V3 > 3 mm) which are usually present in the ECG of Type A Wellens' syndrome.

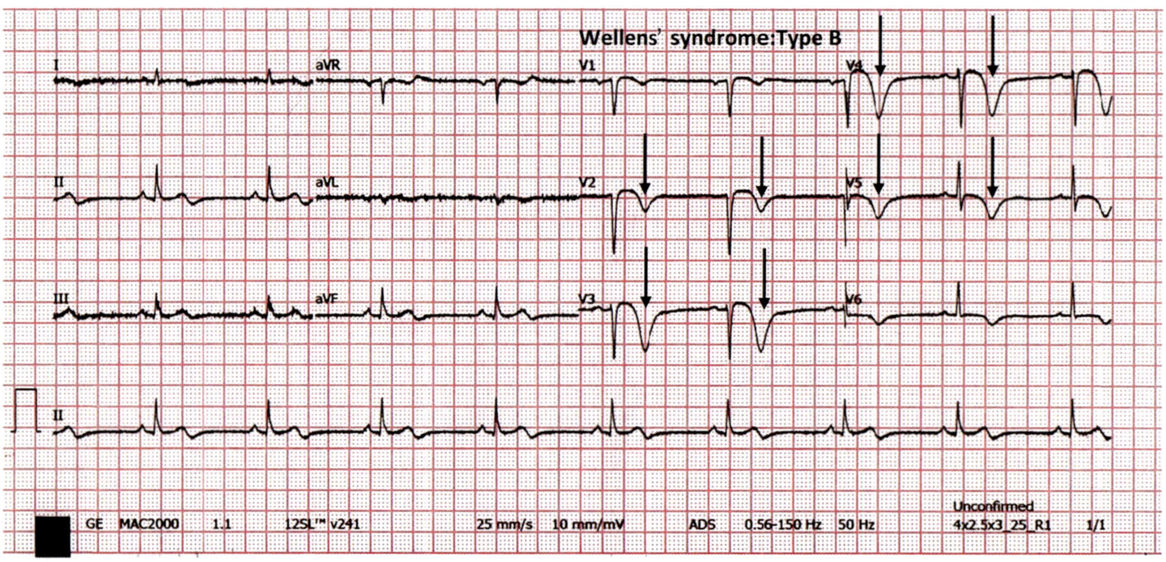

Fig. 7.15: Electrocardiogram is suggestive of Wellens' syndrome (Type B): Deep and almost symmetrical T-wave inversions (>5 mm) are present in leads V3–V4. Also note T-wave inversions in other chest leads. This ECG pattern is suggestive of critical proximal left anterior descending artery stenosis in patients with acute coronary syndrome.

(Fig. 7.16). In the absence of a clinical history or symptoms, T-wave abnormalities and flattened and depressed ST-segment changes are nonspecific. Causes of these changes include functional and physiologic variants (e.g. postprandial), electrolyte abnormalities, postcardiac surgical state, anemia, fever, acidosis or alkalosis, drugs, such as digoxin, acute abdominal process, endocrine abnormalities, cerebrovascular accidents, etc. Flat T waves and mild ST-segment changes may also be seen in healthy individuals, including well-trained athletes, leading to mistaken diagnosis of CAD.

Diffuse ST-segment Depression

Diffuse ST-segment depression in the inferior + anterolateral leads with ST-segment elevation in lead aVR has been described as characteristic of diffuse circumferential subendocardial ischemia caused by acute subtotal occlusion of the left main coronary artery (LMCA). ST-segment depression in >7 leads combined with ST elevation in aVR and V1 is predictive of LMCA stenosis or left main equivalent disease (Figs. 7.17 to 7.19).[34-36]

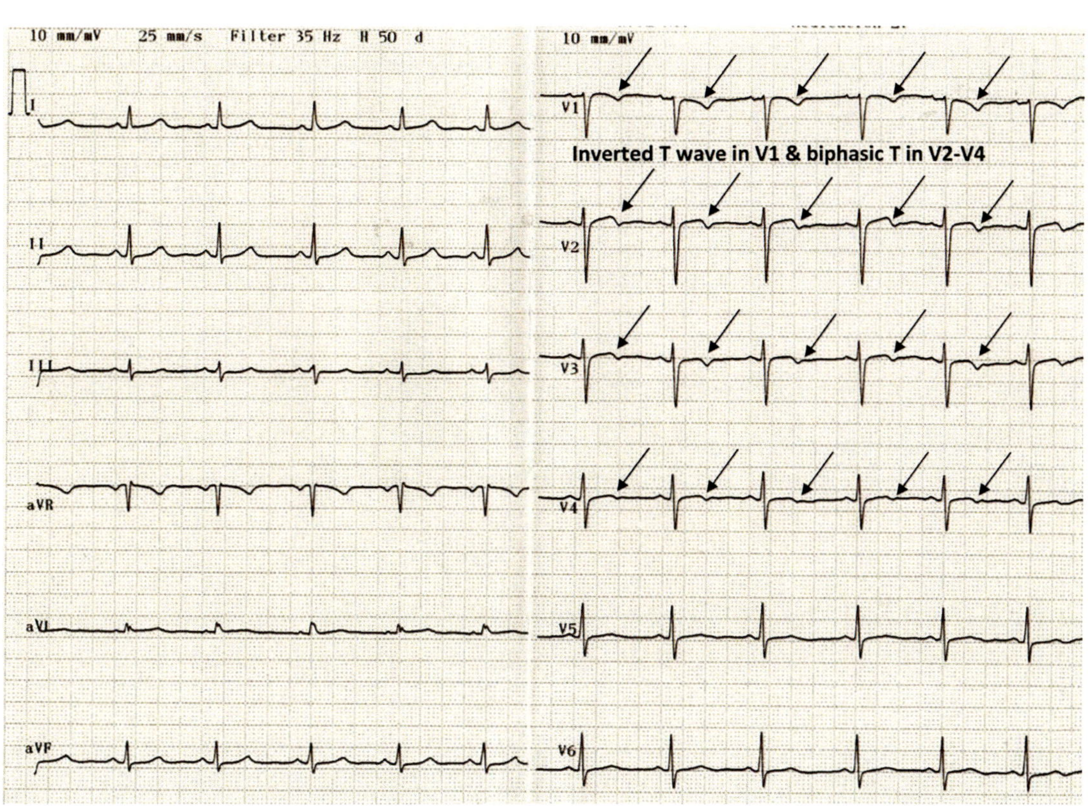

Fig. 7.16: Electrocardiogram shows nonspecific T wave changes in leads V1–V4. T wave appears inverted in V1 and biphasic in leads V2–V4. These changes are not specific for the diagnosis of myocardial ischemia. These electrocardiogram changes may be due to other noncoronary cardiac pathology or normal variant electrocardiogram.

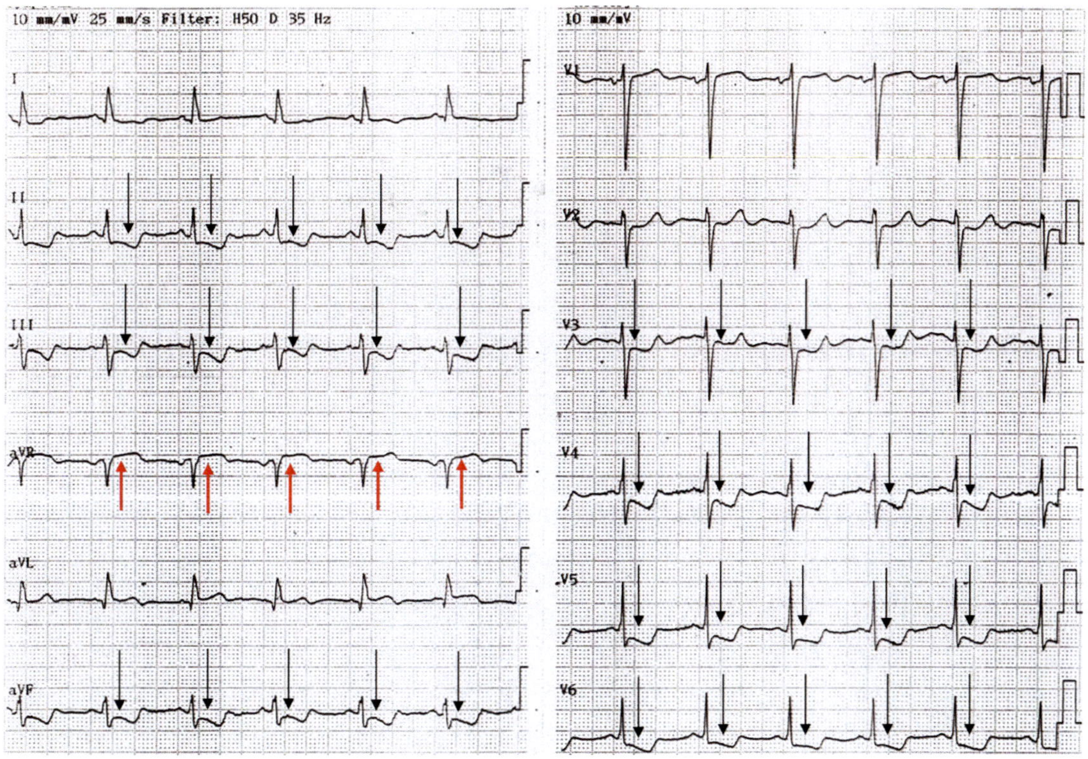

Fig. 7.17: Electrocardiogram shows diffuse ST-segment depression more than 2.0 mm in leads LII, LIII, aVF, and V3–V6 (*black arrows*). Also note ST-segment elevation in lead aVR (*red arrows*). This pattern of diffuse ST-segment depression along with ST elevation in lead aVR is suggestive left main coronary artery stenosis.

(*Source:* Dr Ziaul Kabir, Labaid Cardiac Hospital)

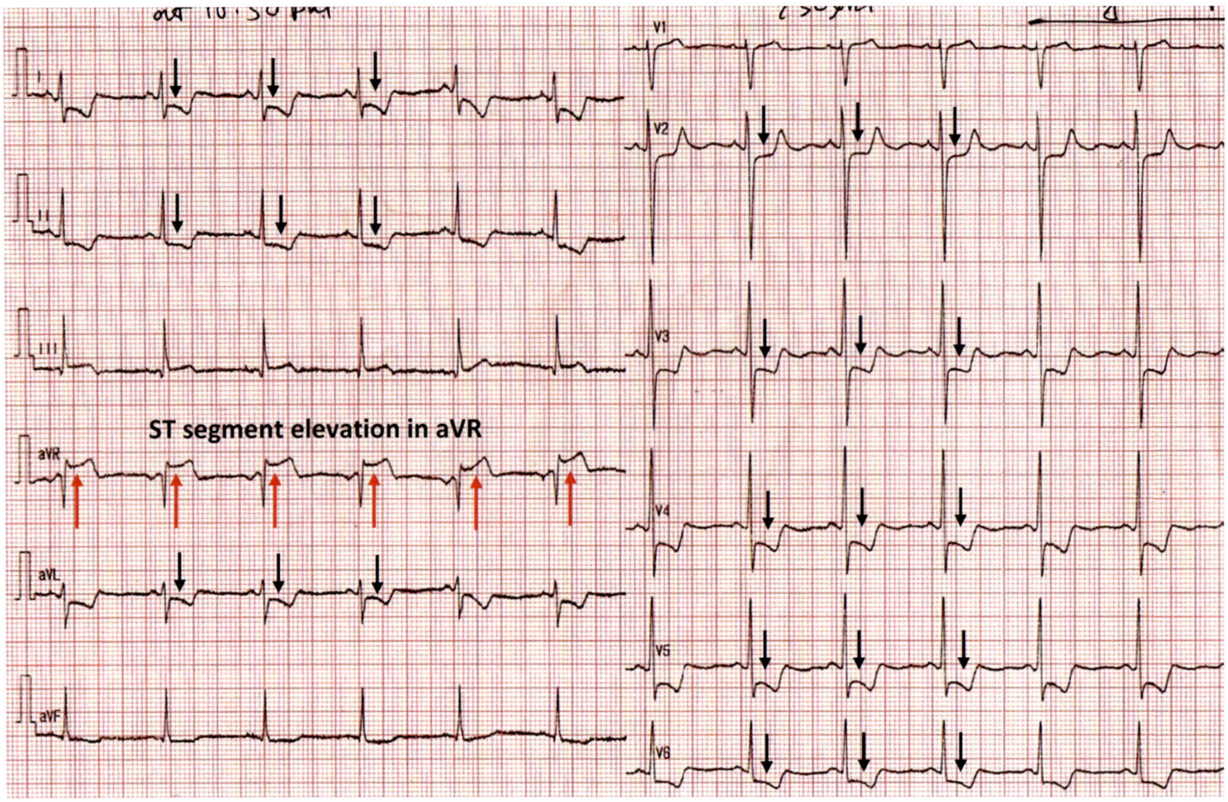

Fig. 7.18: Electrocardiogram shows diffuse down sloping ST-segment depression in leads LI, LII, aVL, and V2–V6 (black arrows). Also note ST-segment elevation in lead aVR (red arrows). This electrocardiogram finding is highly suggestive to left main coronary artery stenosis.

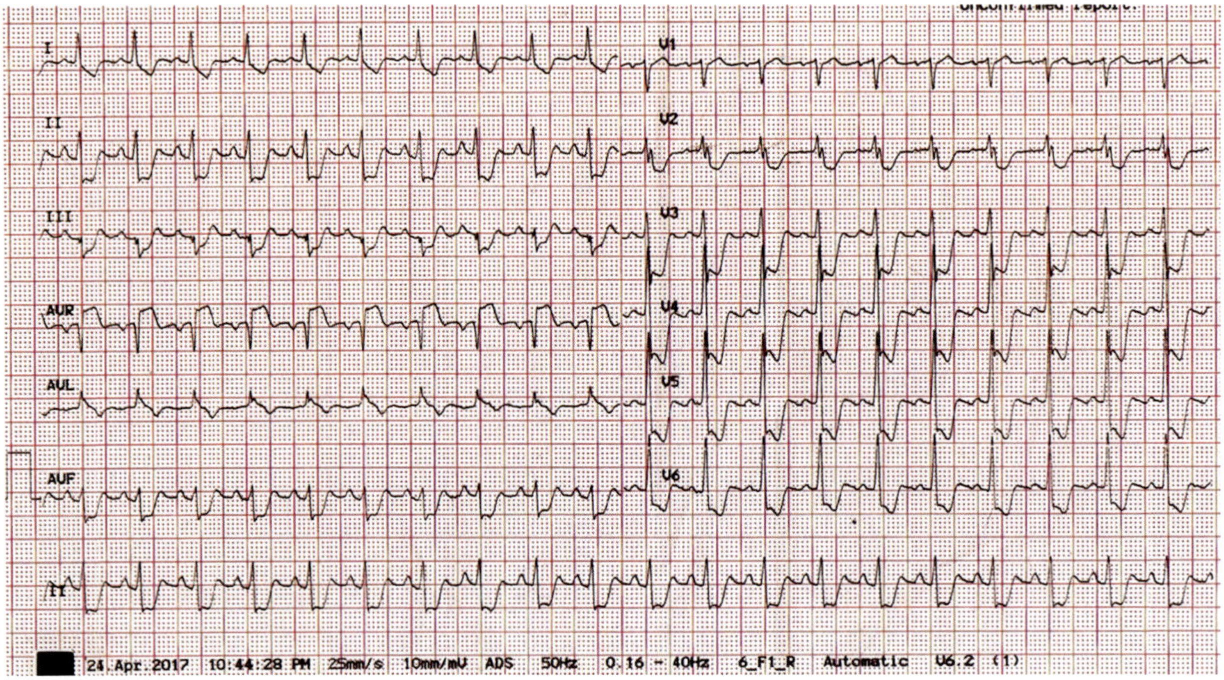

Fig. 7.19: Electrocardiogram shows diffuse down sloping ST-segment depression in both inferior and anterior leads (>7 leads) along with marked ST-segment elevation in lead aVR suggestive of left main coronary artery stenosis. Note greater than 5 mm ST-segment depression in leads V3–V5 and 4 mm ST-segment elevation in lead aVR.

(*Source:* Dr M Jalaluddin, Labaid Cardiac Hospital)

PRINZMETAL ANGINA

Prinzmetal angina [also known as variant angina (VA), vasospastic angina, angina inversa] is a form of angina pectoris that shows transient ST-segment elevation on ECG during an attack of chest pain. These symptoms happen at rest and often may wake up the patient during the night.[37,38] This angina is named after Myron Prinzmetal (1908–1987), who worked for most of his life in Los Angeles and published 165 medical publications during his brilliant career.[39] This is a form of UA that usually occurs spontaneously and is characterized by transient ST-segment elevation that spontaneously resolves or resolves with sublingual NTG use, without progression to MI, usually in the presence of CAD (Figs. 7.20A and B). Clinically, the patient presents with chest discomfort, mostly at rest without any preceding increase in myocardial oxygen demand. The pathogenesis relies upon focal coronary artery spasm, in a single or multiple vessels, leading to transient severe transmural myocardial ischemia.[40,41]

The most important ECG change during a focal proximal coronary spasm is in around 50% of cases the appearance of peaked and symmetrical T wave that is followed, if the spasm persists, by progressive ST-segment elevation that lasts for a few minutes, and later it is progressively resolved. The most frequent ECG changes associated with ST-segment elevation are: (1) increased height of the R wave, (2) coincident S-wave diminution, (3) upsloping TQ in many cases, and (4) alternans of the elevated ST-segment and negative T-wave deepness in 20% of cases. The presence of arrhythmias is very frequent during Prinzmetal angina, especially ventricular arrhythmias. The prevalence and importance of ventricular arrhythmias are related to: (1) duration of episodes, 2) degree of ST-segment elevation, (3) presence of ST-T wave alternans, and (4) the presence of greater than 25% increases of the R wave.[42]

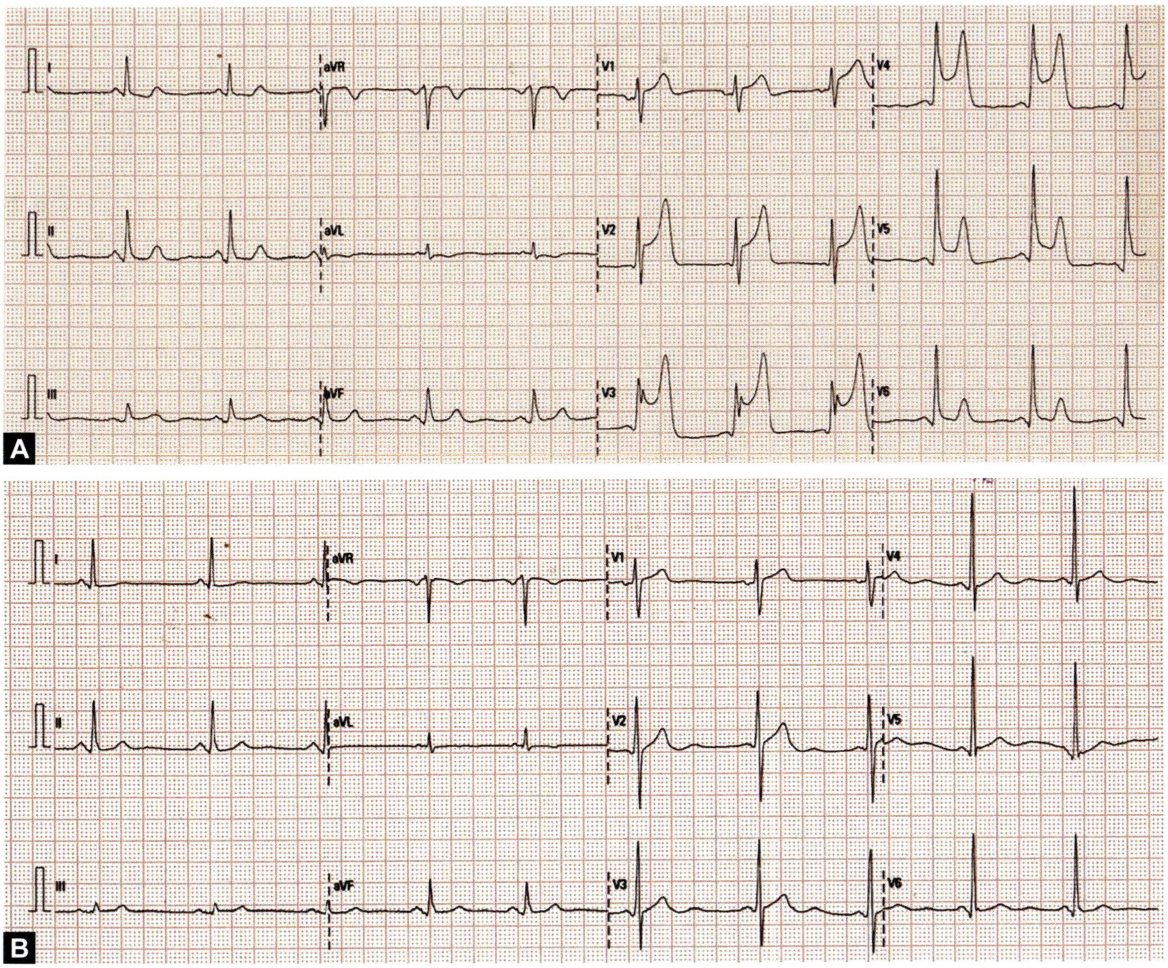

Figs. 7.20A and B: (A) Electrocardiogram of a patient with Prinzmetal angina during chest pain. Note ST-segment elevation with tall and peaked T waves in leads V2–V5. (B) Electrocardiogram of the patient with Prinzmetal angina (A) after giving sublingual (S/L) nitroglycerin. Note the electrocardiogram changes after giving sublingual nitroglycerin. ST elevation in the electrocardiogram (A) has resolved and ST-segment now appears isoelectric. Also note the disappearance of the tall and peaked T waves in leads V2–V5 and T-wave morphology now appear normal.

(*Source:* Dr Abul Khayer, Labaid Cardiac Hospital)

MINOCA (MYOCARDIAL INFARCTION WITH NONOBSTRUCTIVE CORONARY ARTERIES)

Early coronary angiography performed during acute MI (AMI) identifies an occluded vessel in most patients with ST-elevation MI (STEMI) and less frequently in those with non-STEMI; however, more than or equal to 90% of patients with AMI have evidence of obstructive coronary artery disease (CAD). In up to 10% of patients with clinical diagnostic features of AMI, early angiography does not reveal an occluded vessel or possibly any evidence of CAD. These patients constitute an intriguing subgroup referred to as MI with nonobstructive coronary arteries (MINOCA).[43-46]

The following criteria are needed for a diagnosis of MINOCA (Box 7.1): A positive cardiac biomarker such as cardiac troponin I, with a serial rise and fall, along with clinical evidence of ischemia (symptoms, ST-T wave changes, development of pathologic Q waves, development of new left bundle branch block, imaging evidence of new loss of viable myocardium or new wall motion abnormality), intracoronary thrombus evident on angiography or at autopsy, or nonobstructive coronary arteries on angiography (Fig. 7.21).[44-46]

Nonobstructive coronary arteries on angiography are defined as the absence of obstructive CAD on angiography (i.e. no coronary artery stenosis ≥50%) in any potential infarct-related artery. While males outnumber females for AMI with obstructive CAD, the number of males is only slightly higher than females among patients with MINOCA.[46]

The mechanism responsible for AMI in this group of patients involves an interaction between atheroma,

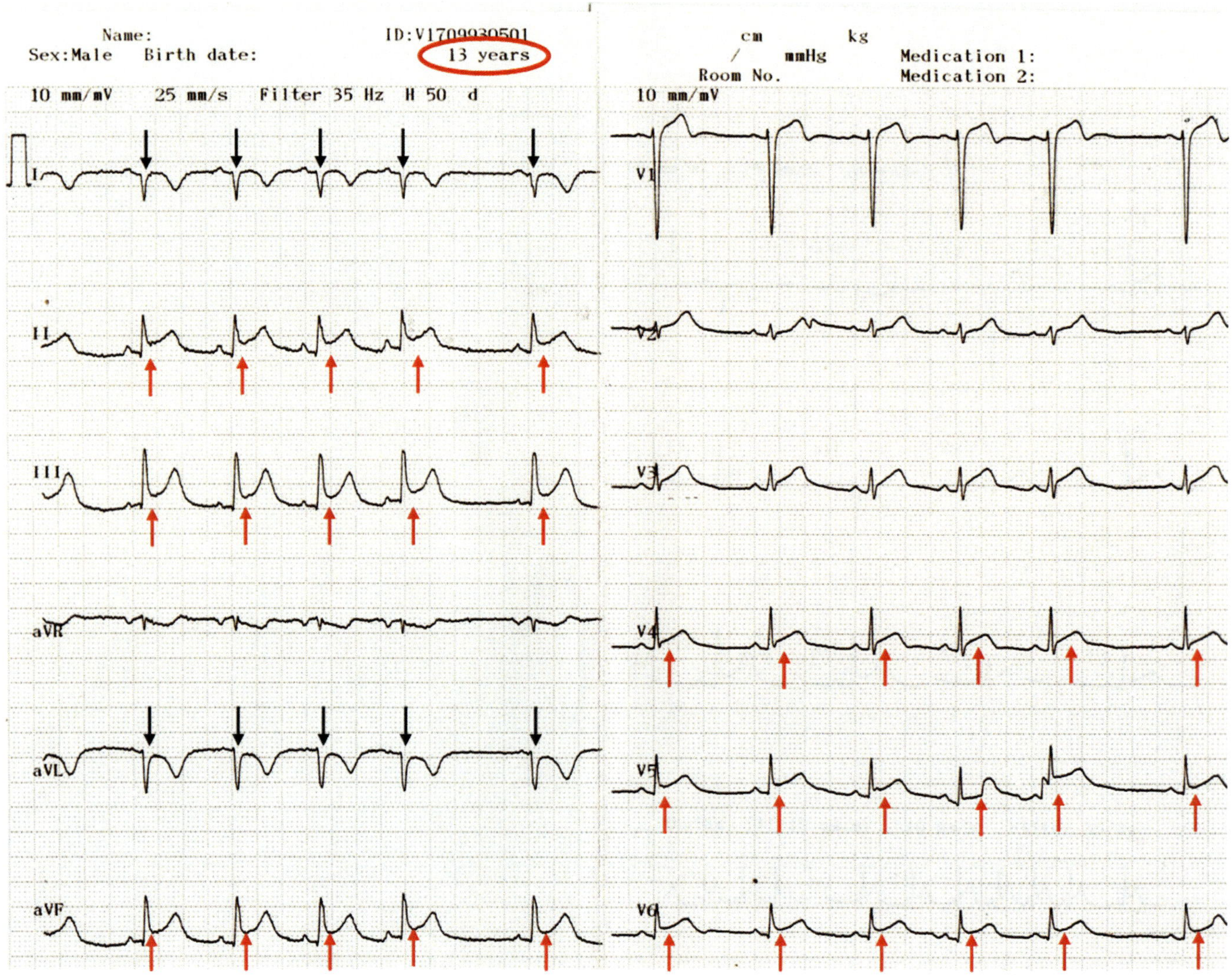

Fig. 7.21: A 13-year-old boy was admitted in a hospital with history of recurrent chest pain with sweating for 2 days. His initial ECG in emergency department showed pathological Q waves in LI and aVL (*black arrows*) with T-wave inversions suggestive of recent high lateral infarction with ST-segment elevation in LII, LIII, aVF and V4-V6 (*red arrows*). His troponin I level was very high but echocardiogram did not show any regional wall motion abnormality. In view of his ongoing ischemic chest pain, he was scheduled for coronary angiogram but his coronary angiogram was normal. He was diagnosed as a case of myocardial infarction with nonobstructive coronary arteries (MINOCA). Also note marked sinus arrhythmia on this ECG. (*Courtesy*: Dr APM Sohrabuzzaman, Labaid Cardiac Hospital).

Box 7.1: Diagnosis of myocardial infarction with nonobstructive coronary arteries (MINOCA)

Diagnosis of MINOCA
- *Acute myocardial infarction (AMI) criteria:* Clinical evidence of AMI (positive troponin test) including any of the following:
  - *Symptom:* typical ischemic chest pain.
  - ECG:
    - ST-segment changes, elevation or depression
    - Development of pathological Q waves
    - New appearance of left bundle branch block (LBBB)
  - Myocardial perfusion imaging—new loss of viable myocardium
  - *Echocardiogram:* New regional wall motion abnormality.
- No stenosis more than or equal to 50% on coronary angiogram
- No other clinically overt cause for AMI presentation.

thrombosis and vascular dysfunction. Previous studies have implicated spasm, microvascular dysfunction and thrombophilic states (Factor V Leiden, protein C deficiency and malignancy-associated thrombophilia).[45-50] DaCosta et al. reported that a third of patients with MINOCA had evidence of coronary spasm or thrombotic disorders.[49] Other potential causes include spontaneous coronary dissection, spontaneous coronary thrombosis–thrombophilia disorders, coronary emboli, sympathomimetic agents (such as cocaine, or methamphetamines), and *noncoronary causes* such as myocarditis, takotsubo cardiomyopathy, cardiomyopathies, cardiac trauma, strenuous exercise, tachyarrhythmias, cardiotoxins (such as chemotherapeutic agents) associated with extracardiac disorders, stroke, pulmonary embolism, sepsis, adult respiratory distress syndrome, and end-stage renal failure.[46]

SUMMARY

Electrocardiogram Criteria of Stable Angina

- Resting ECG is often normal.
- Sometimes ECG may show transient ST-segment depression, T-wave inversion or both.
- Electrocardiogram taken during chest pain may show ST-segment depression.
- Diagnosis of CAD is usually established by stress test.

Acute Coronary Syndromes

The ACS is used to describe the spectrum of conditions that include UA, NSTEMI, and STEMI.

The classification of patients is based on ECG findings. Patients are divided into two categories:

1. Chest pain with persistent ST-segment elevation on ECG; classified as STEMI.
2. Chest pain with ST-segment depression, transient ST-segment elevation or T wave changes, or no ECG changes at presentation; classified as non-ST elevation ACS.

Further categorization of non-ST elevation ACS is by measurement of cardiac biomarkers, troponins/CK-MB (two or more blood samples collected at least 6–9 hours apart):

- *Elevated*: NSTEMI
- *Not-elevated*: UA.

Distinction between NSTEMI and UA is based on the presence (non-STEMI) or absence (UA) of a rise in cardiac enzymes or troponin. ECG may or may not show any change in both the conditions.

Electrocardiogram Findings of Acute Coronary Syndromes (Unstable Angina and Non-ST Elevation Myocardial Infarction)

The following changes may be noted in ECG during ACS:

- ST depression
- T-wave inversion
- Transient ST elevation.

But normal ECG findings do not exclude the possibility of ACS.

ST depression may be primary or secondary. In "primary" ST depression, ST-T wave changes are independent of changes in ventricular activation but in "secondary" ST depression, ST-T wave changes are solely due to alterations in the sequence of ventricular activation and generally the ST-T polarity is opposite to the major or terminal deflection of the QRS.

Causes of Primary ST Depression

The causes of primary ST depression are:

- Myocardial ischemia
- Electrolyte abnormalities (e.g. hypokalemia)
- Drug effects (e.g. digoxin, quinidine, etc.).

Causes of Secondary ST Depression

The causes of secondary ST depression are:

- Bundle branch blocks
- Ventricular hypertrophy
- Preexcitation syndromes
- Premature ventricular complex (PVC), ventricular arrhythmias, and ventricular paced beats.

There are three patterns of ST-segment depression: horizontal ST depression, downsloping ST depression, and upsloping ST depression. Horizontal (flat) or downsloping ST-segment depression is associated more often with ACS. Upsloping ST-segment may be having nonspecific changes and lacks adequate specificity for myocardial ischemia. Horizontal or downsloping ST depression ≥ 1.0 mm at the J-point in ≥ 2 contiguous leads indicates myocardial ischemia.

There are two main ECG abnormalities seen with ACS:

1. ST-segment depression
2. T-wave flattening or inversion

While there are numerous conditions that may simulate myocardial ischemia (e.g. LVH and digoxin effect), dynamic ST-segment and T wave changes on serial ECGs over time, are strongly suggestive of myocardial ischemia.

ST depression due to myocardial ischemia may be present in a variable number of leads and with variable morphology—ST depression due to subendocardial ischemia is usually widespread—typically present in leads I, II, V4-V6 and a variable number of additional leads.

A pattern of widespread ST depression plus ST elevation in aVR > 1 mm is suggestive of left main coronary artery (LMCA) occlusion. ST depression localized to a particular territory (especially inferior or high lateral leads only) is more likely to represent reciprocal change due to STEMI. The corresponding ST elevation may be subtle and difficult to see, but should be sought.

Reciprocal ST Depression

ST elevation during acute STEMI is associated with simultaneous ST depression in the electrically opposite leads:

1. Inferior STEMI produces reciprocal ST depression in aVL (±lead I).
2. Lateral or anterolateral STEMI produces reciprocal ST depression in III and aVF (±lead II).
3. Reciprocal ST depression in V1-3 occurs with posterior infarction.

T-wave Inversion

T-wave inversion may be regarded to be evidence of myocardial ischemia but possibility of normal variant T inversion must be considered. Presence of T-wave inversion is a normal variant in leads III, aVR, and V1. T-wave inversion is only significant if seen in leads with upright QRS complexes (dominant R waves). T-wave inversion reflects the evidence of myocardial ischemia if T inversion is:

- At least 3 mm deep
- Present in ≥ 2 contiguous leads that have dominant R waves (R/S ratio > 1)
- If its morphology is dynamic. New appearance, not present on old ECG or changing configuration over time.

Diagnostic Electrocardiogram Criteria of Wellens' Syndrome

An ECG manifestation of critical proximal LAD coronary artery stenosis in patients with ACS shows the following:

- Symmetrical deep T-wave inversion in leads V2–V4 or the T wave has characteristic positive-negative biphasic morphology in leads V2 through V4.
- Mild or no ST-segment elevation
- No loss of precordial R waves.

There are two patterns of T-wave abnormality which are seen in Wellens' syndrome:

1. *Type A*: Biphasic T, with initial positivity and terminal negativity in leads V2–V4 (25% of cases).
2. *Type B*: Deeply (>5 mm) and symmetrically inverted T waves in leads V2–V4 (75% of cases).

The T waves evolve over time from a Type A to a Type B pattern.

Electrocardiogram Evidence of Left Main Stenosis

Diffuse ST-segment depression in the inferior and anterolateral leads with ST-segment elevation in lead aVR is considered as an ECG criteria of left main CAD.

Prinzmetal Angina

Prinzmetal angina or variant angina (VA) is characterized by a transient reduction in the luminal diameter of a coronary artery resulting in spontaneous and often recurrent episodes of chest pain with transient ST elevation on electrocardiogram. The attack of Prinzmetal angina occurs at rest or during ordinary activity and is not precipitated by strenuous exercise.

- This causes a pattern of ST elevation that is very similar to acute STEMI. ST elevation in Prinzmetal angina may or may not be associated with reciprocal ST depression.
- However, unlike acute STEMI the ECG changes in Prinzmetal angina are transient, reversible with vasodilators and not usually associated with myocardial necrosis.
- It may be impossible to differentiate these two conditions based on the ECG alone. Prompt resolution of chest pain and ST elevation by sublingual NTG may differentiate Prinzmetal angina from STEMI.

ECG Features of Prinzmetal Angina

Transient ST-segment elevation is the hallmark sign of Prinzmetal angina. Other features include:

- Appearance of peaked and symmetrical T wave
- Increased height of the R wave
- S-wave diminution
- Alternans of the elevated ST-segment
- Ventricular arrhythmias.

MINOCA (Myocardial Infarction with Nonobstructive Coronary Arteries)

Approximately 10% of patients presenting with acute myocardial infarction (AMI) have no significant obstructive coronary artery disease (CAD). A diagnosis of MINOCA can be made in patients presenting with features consistent with AMI with positive troponin test and a coronary angiogram demonstrating nonobstructive CAD (No stenosis ≥50% on coronary angiogram).

ECG features of MINOCA include:

- ST-segment changes, elevation or depression
- Development of pathological Q waves
- New appearance of left bundle branch block (LBBB).

Common causes of MINOCA include coronary vasospasm, microvascular dysfunction, thrombophilic states, spontaneous coronary dissection, spontaneous coronary thrombosis, coronary embolization, sympathomimetic agents (such as cocaine, or methamphetamines), and *noncoronary causes* such as myocarditis, takotsubo cardiomyopathy, etc.

REFERENCES

1. Campeau L. Grading of angina pectoris. Circulation. 1976;54(3):522-3.
2. van Domburg RT, van Miltenburg-van Zijl AJ, Veerhoek RJ, et al. Unstable angina: good long-term outcome after a complicated early course. J Am Coll Cardiol. 1998;31(7): 1534-9.
3. Canto JG, Fincher C, Kiefe CI, et al. Atypical presentations among Medicare beneficiaries with unstable angina pectoris. Am J Cardiol. 2002;90(3):248-53.
4. Culic V, Eterovic D, Miric D, et al. Symptom presentation of acute myocardial infarction: influence of sex, age, and risk factors. Am Heart J. 2002;144(6):1012-7.
5. Bassand JP, Hamm CW, Ardissino D, et al. Guidelines for the diagnosis and treatment of non-ST-segment elevation acute coronary syndromes. The Task Force for the Diagnosis and Treatment of Non-ST-Segment Elevation Acute Coronary Syndromes of the European Society of Cardiology. Eur Heart J. 2007;28(13):1598-660.
6. Fox K, Garcia MAA, Ardissino D, et al. Guidelines on the management of stable angina pectoris—executive summary: the Task Force on the Management of Stable Angina Pectoris of the European Society of Cardiology. Eur Heart J. 2006;27(11):1341-81.
7. Van de Werf F, Bax J, Betriu A, et al. Management of acute myocardial infarction in patients presenting with persistent ST-segment elevation: the Task Force on the Management of ST-Segment Elevation Acute Myocardial Infarction of the European Society of Cardiology. Eur Heart J. 2008;29(23):2909-45.
8. Bacquer DD, Backer GD, Kornitzer M, et al. Prognostic value of ischemic electrocardiographic findings for cardiovascular mortality in men and women. J Am Coll Cardiol. 1998;32(3):680-5.
9. Thygesen K, Alpert JS, White HD, et al. Universal definition of myocardial infarction. Circulation. 2007;116(22):2634-53.
10. Hamm CW, Bassand JP, Agewall S, et al. ESC Guidelines for the management of acute coronary syndromes in patients presenting without persistent ST-segment elevation; The Task Force for the management of acute coronary syndromes (ACS) in patients presenting without persistent ST-segment elevation of the European Society of Cardiology (ESC). Eur Heart J. 2011;32(23):2999-3054.
11. Kumar A, Cannon CP. Acute coronary syndromes: diagnosis and management, Part I. Mayo Clin Proc. 2009;84(10):917-38.
12. Cannon CP, McCabe CH, Stone PH, et al. The electrocardiogram predicts one-year outcome of patients with unstable angina and non-Q wave myocardial infarction: results of the TIMI III Registry ECG Ancillary Study. J Am Coll Cardiol. 1997;30(1):133-40.
13. Hyde TA, French JK, Wong CK, et al. Four-year survival of patients with acute coronary syndromes without ST-segment elevation and prognostic significance of 0.5-mm ST-segment depression. Am J Cardiol. 1999;84(4):379-85.
14. Platelet Receptor Inhibition for Ischemic Syndrome Management in Patients Limited by Unstable Signs and Symptoms (PRISM-PLUS) Trial Investigators. Inhibition of the platelet glycoprotein IIb/IIIa receptor with tirofiban in unstable angina and non-Q-wave myocardial infarction. N Engl J Med. 1998;338(21):1488-97.
15. Savonitto S, Ardissino D, Granger CB, et al. Prognostic value of the admission electrocardiogram in acute coronary syndromes. JAMA. 1999;281(8):707-13.
16. Kaul P, Fu Y, Chang WC, et al. Prognostic value of ST segment depression in acute coronary syndromes: insights from PARAGON-A applied to GUSTO-IIb. PARAGON-A and GUSTO IIb investigators. Platelet IIb/IIIa antagonism for the reduction of acute global organization network. J Am Coll Cardiol. 2001;38(1):64-71.
17. Gurm HS, Topol EJ. The ECG in acute coronary syndromes: new tricks from an old dog. Heart. 2005;91(7):851-53.
18. Channer K, Morris F. Myocardial ischaemia. BMJ. 2002;324:1023-6.
19. Surawicz B, Knilans TK. Chou's Electrocardiography in Clinical Practice. Philadelphia: WB Saunders Co.; 2001. pp. 540-53.
20. Rautaharju PM, Surawicz B, Gettes LS, et al. AHA/ACCF/HRS recommendations for the standardization and interpretation of the electrocardiogram: part IV: the ST segment, T and U waves, and the QT interval: a scientific statement from the American Heart Association Electrocardiography and Arrhythmias Committee, Council on Clinical Cardiology; the American College of Cardiology Foundation; and the Heart Rhythm Society. Endorsed by the International Society for Computerized Electrocardiology. J Am Coll Cardiol. 2009;53:982-91.
21. Hanna EB, Glanacy DL. ST-segment depression and T-wave inversion: classification, differential diagnosis, and caveats. Cleve Clin J Med. 2011;78(6):404-14.
22. Pollehn T, Brady WJ, Perron AD, et al. The electrocardiographic differential diagnosis of ST segment depression. Emerg Med J. 2002;19(2):129-35.
23. Li D, Li CY, Yong AC, et al. Source of electrocardiographic ST changes in subendocardial ischemia. Circ Res. 1998;82(9):957-70.
24. Aufderheide TD, Brady WJ. Electrocardiography in the patient with myocardial ischemia or infarction. In: Gibler WB, Aufderheide TP (Eds). Emergency cardiac care, 1st edition. St Louis: Mosby, 1994. pp. 69-216.
25. Wagner, GS. Marriott's practical electrocardiography, 9th edition. Baltimore: Williams and Wilkins, 1994.

26. Goldschlager N, Selzer A, Cohn K. Treadmill stress tests as indicators of the presence and severity of coronary artery disease. Ann Intern Med. 1976;85(3):277-86.
27. Brady WJ. Mastering the electrocardiogram: state-of-the-art techniques for evaluating ST segment elevation in acute myocardial infarction and other clinical syndromes. Emergency Medicine Rep. 1998;19:78-93.
28. Boden WE, Spodick DH. Diagnostic significance of precordial ST-segment depression. Am J Cardiol. 1989;63(5):358-61.
29. Shah A, Wagner GS, Green CL, et al. Electrocardiographic differentiation of the ST-segment depression of acute myocardial injury due to the left circumflex artery occlusion from that of myocardial ischemia of nonocclusive etiologies. Am J Cardiol. 1997;80(4):512-3.
30. Krishnaswamy A, Lincoff AM, Menon V. Magnitude and consequences of missing the acute infarct-related circumflex artery. Am Heart J. 2009;158:706-12.
31. de Zwaan C, Bär FW, Wellens HJ. Characteristic electrocardiographic pattern indicating a critical stenosis high in left anterior descending coronary artery in patients admitted because of impending myocardial infarction. Am Heart J. 1982;103(4 Pt 2):730-6.
32. de Zwaan C, Bar FW, Janssen JH, et al. Angiographic and clinical characteristics of patients with unstable angina showing an ECG pattern indicating critical narrowing of the proximal LAD coronary artery. Am Heart J. 1989;117(3):657-65.
33. Lilaonitkul M, Robinson K, Roberts M. Wellens' syndrome: significance of ECG pattern recognition in the emergency department. Emerg Med J. 2009;26(10):750-1.
34. Knotts RJ, Wilson JM, Kim E, et al. Diffuse ST depression with ST elevation in aVR: Is this pattern specific for global ischemia due to left main coronary artery disease? J Electrocardiol. 2013;46(3):240-8.
35. Nough H, Jorat MV, Varasteravan HR, et al. The value of ST-segment elevation in lead aVR for predicting left main coronary artery lesion in patients suspected of acute coronary syndrome. Rom J Intern Med. 2012;50(2):159-64.
36. Kim E, Birnbaum Y. Acute coronary syndromes presenting with transient diffuse ST segment depression and ST segment elevation in lead aVR not caused by "acute left main coronary artery occlusion": description of two cases. Ann Noninvasive Electrocardiol. 2013;18(2):204-9.
37. Slavich M, Patel RS. Coronary artery spasm: current knowledge and residual uncertainties. Int J Cardiol Heart Vasc. 2016;23(10):47-53.
38. Yasue H, Nakagawa H, Itoh T, et al. Coronary artery spasm--clinical features, diagnosis, pathogenesis, and treatment. J Cardiol. 2008;51(1):2-17.
39. Roguin A. Myron Prinzmetal 1908-1987: the man behind the variant angina. Int J Cardiol. 2008;123(2):129-30.
40. Kusama Y, Kodani E, Nakagomi A, et al. Variant angina and coronary artery spasm: the clinical spectrum, pathophysiology, and management. J Nippon Med Sch. 2011;78(1):4-12.
41. Nakad G, Bayeh, H. Unusual vasospastic angina: a documented asymptomatic spasm with normal ECG—a Case Report and a Review of the Literature. Case Rep Cardiol. 2012;2013:407242.
42. de Luna AB, Cygankiewicz I, Baranchuk A, et al. Prinzmetal angina: ECG changes and clinical considerations: a consensus paper. Ann Noninvasive Electrocardiol. 2014;19(5):442-53.
43. Pasupathy S, Tavella R, McRae S, et al. Myocardial Infarction With Non-obstructive Coronary Arteries—Diagnosis and Management. European Cardiology Review. 2015;10(2):79-82.
44. DeWood MA, Stifter WF, Simpson CS, et al. Coronary arteriographic findings soon after non-Q-wave myocardial infarction. N Engl J Med. 1986;315:417-23.
45. Pasupathy S, Air T, Dreyer RP, et al. Systematic review of patients presenting with suspected myocardial infarction and nonobstructive coronary arteries. Circulation. 2015;131:861-70.
46. Agewall S, Beltrame JF, Reynolds HR, et al. ESC working group position paper on myocardial infarction with non-obstructive coronary arteries. Eur Heart J. 2017;38(3):143-53.
47. Ong P, Athanasiadis A, Hill S, et al. Coronary artery spasm as a frequent cause of acute coronary syndrome: The CASPAR (coronary artery spasm in patients with acute coronary syndrome) study. J Am Coll Cardiol. 2008;52:523-7.
48. Mansourati J, Da Costa A, Munier S, et al. Prevalence of factor V Leiden in patients with myocardial infarction and normal coronary angiography. Thromb Haemost. 2000;83:822-5.
49. Da Costa A, Isaaz K, Faure E, et al. Clinical characteristics, aetiological factors and long-term prognosis of myocardial infarction with an absolutely normal coronary angiogram:

Chapter 8

ECG Diagnosis of ST-Elevation Myocardial Infarction

INTRODUCTION

ST-elevation myocardial infarction (STEMI) is a clinical syndrome defined by characteristic symptoms of myocardial ischemia in association with persistent electrocardiographic ST elevation and subsequent release of biomarkers of myocardial necrosis. Acute myocardial infarction (AMI) resulting from an occlusive thrombus is recognized on an electrocardiogram (ECG) by ST-segment elevation. Early reperfusion therapy has proved beneficial in such infarctions. The earlier the reperfusion, the greater the benefit, and the time to treatment is now considered to indicate the quality of care.[1-3] The ECG remains a crucial tool in the identification and management of AMI. A detailed analysis of patterns of ST-segment elevation may influence decisions regarding the use of reperfusion therapy. The early and accurate identification of the infarct-related artery on the ECG can help to predict the amount of myocardium at risk and guide decisions regarding the urgency of revascularization. Electrocardiographic signs of reperfusion represent an important marker of microvascular blood flow and consequent prognosis. The ECG is also crucial for identifying new conduction abnormalities and arrhythmias that influence both short- and long-term outcome.[4] The ECG is the most important diagnostic tool in the diagnosis of STEMI, and therefore it should be accomplished immediately at hospital admission. In fact, it represents an important step not only for STEMI diagnosis, but also and more importantly for the therapeutic plan.

In the clinical assessment of chest pain, electrocardiography is an essential adjunct to the clinical history and physical examination. A rapid and accurate diagnosis in patients with AMI is vital, as expeditious reperfusion therapy can improve prognosis. The most frequently used ECG criterion for identifying AMI is ST segment elevation in two or more anatomically contiguous leads. The ST-segment elevation associated with an evolving myocardial infarction is often readily identifiable, but a knowledge of the common "pseudo" infarct patterns is essential to avoid the unnecessary use of thrombolytic treatment or early coronary angiogram with a view to perform primary percutaneous coronary intervention (PPCI). In the early stages of AMI the ECG may be normal or near normal; less than half of patients with AMI have clear diagnostic changes on their first ECG tracing. About 10% of patients with a proved AMI (on the basis of clinical history and enzymatic markers) fail to develop ST-segment elevation or depression.[5] In most cases, however, serial ECGs show evolving changes that tend to follow well-recognized patterns.

Typically, the ECG in the evolving STEMI shows five sequential changes, which develop in turn (Fig. 8.1):

1. Hyperacute T-waves
2. ST-segment elevation
3. Appearance of pathological Q-waves
4. T-waves inversion
5. Normalization of the ST segment.

HYPERACUTE T WAVES

The earliest signs of AMI are subtle and include increased T-wave amplitude over the affected area. T waves become more prominent, tall, broad based, usually symmetrical and not pointed. Classically hyperacute T waves have been described as tall-amplitude, primary T-wave abnormalities sometimes seen in the early phases of transmural MI. Despite numerous human and animal studies addressing the presence and significance of hyperacute T, there are no widely held, reliable ECG criteria for their accurate identification. T-wave amplitudes greater than accepted standards: limb leads, greater than 0.5 mV (>5 mm); precordial leads, greater than 1.0 mV (>10 mm) are considered as hyperacute T waves (Fig. 8.2).

Hyperacute T-waves are most evident in the anterior chest leads and are more readily visible when an old ECG is available for comparison. These changes in T-waves are usually present for only 5–30 minutes after the onset of the infarction and are followed by ST-segment changes.[5] The T-waves represent the period of ventricular repolarization on the surface ECG. During the first minutes of coronary

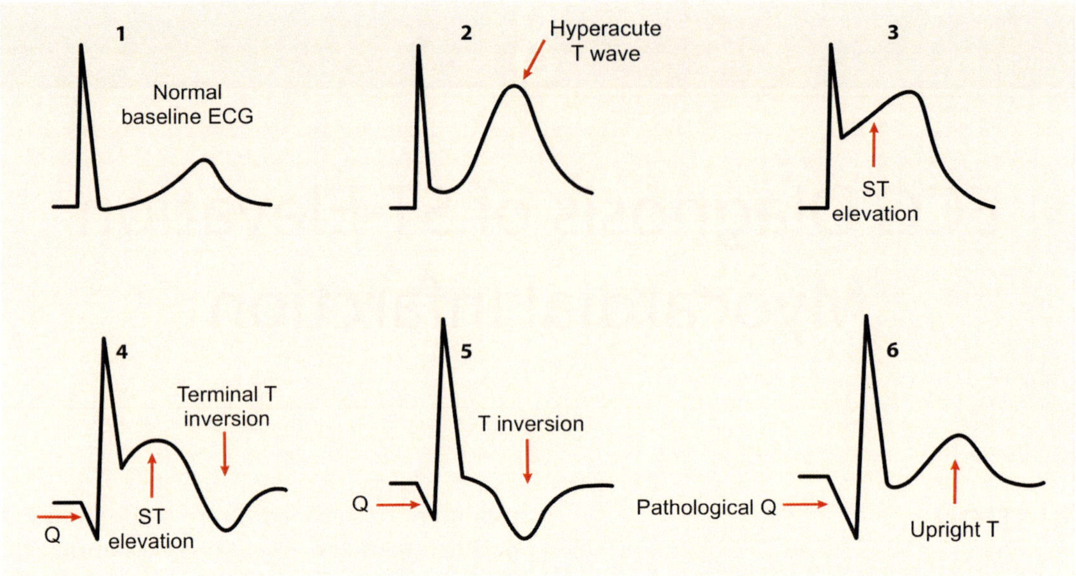

Fig. 8.1: Stages of evolution of STEMI. 1. Normal ECG prior to acute chest pain. 2. Hyperacute T-wave changes- tall peak T with broad base. 3. Marked ST-segment elevation. 4. Appearance of Q-wave, less ST elevation with terminal T-wave inversion. 5. Pathologic Q-wave and T is still inverted. 6. Persistence of Q-wave and T is now upright. ST elevation normalized.

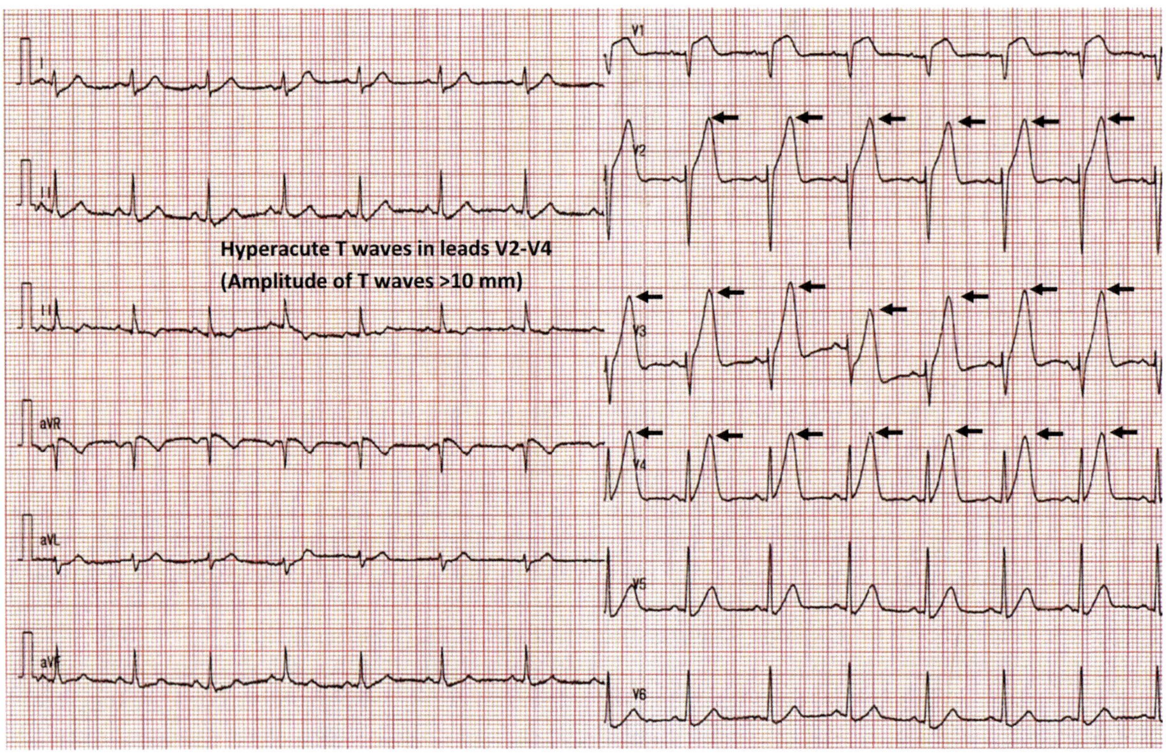

Fig. 8.2: Electrocardiogram (ECG) showing hyperacute T-wave changes in leads V2–V4 (arrows) suggesting acute anterior myocardial infarction. Note T-wave amplitude greater than 10 mm in leads V2–V4.

arterial occlusion, the earliest ECG changes are represented by an increase in the amplitude of the T-wave, the so-called "hyperacute T-waves." The morphologic characteristics of hyperacute T-wave are typical of ischemic event: they are usually symmetrical with a broad base and may or may not be associated with reciprocal ST-segment depression (Figs. 8.3A and B). In the evolving STEMI the hyperacute T-waves turn into giant R-wave. Hyperacute T-waves represent the electrocardiographic expression of ischemia before the beginning of necrosis; for this reason they are considered as the most significant phase during which the reperfusion therapy may achieve the greatest benefit in term

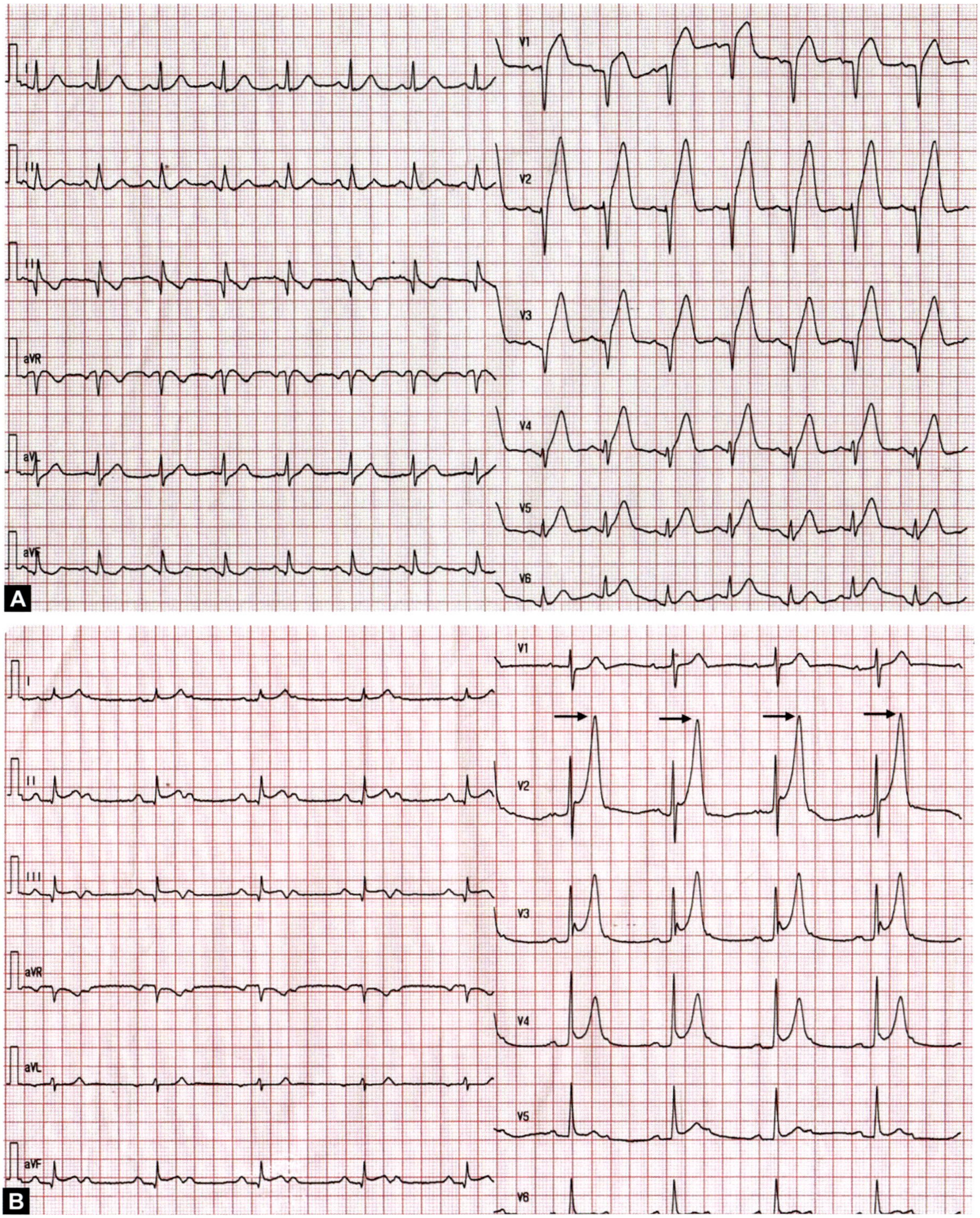

Figs. 8.3A and B: (A) Electrocardiogram (ECG) showing hyperacute T-wave changes in leads V2–V4, suggesting acute anterior myocardial infarction. Note T-wave amplitude greater than 10 mm in leads V2–V4. (B) Electrocardiogram (ECG) showing hyperacute T-wave changes in leads V2–V4, suggesting acute anterior myocardial infarction. Note T-wave amplitude in V2 (arrows) is 23 mm. Also note 2:1 AV block with, heart rate 55 bpm. (*Source:* Dr Reyan Anis, Labaid Cardiac Hospital.)

of myocardial salvage.[6] Prominent T-waves, however, are also associated with other diagnoses, including hyperkalemia, early repolarization and left ventricular (LV) hypertrophy.[7] Thus in the differential diagnosis, the clinicians must consider additional features related to patient, including age, comorbidity and current medical status.

ST-SEGMENT ELEVATION

ST-segment elevation is often the earliest recognized sign of AMI and is usually evident within hours of the onset of symptoms. Initially the ST segment may straighten, with loss of the ST-T wave angle. Then the T-wave becomes broad and the ST segment elevates, losing its normal concavity. As further elevation occurs, the ST segment tends to become convex upwards. The degree of ST segment elevation varies between subtle changes of less than 1 mm and gross elevation of greater than 10 mm. The definition of "significant" ST elevation varies considerably with respect to both the required minimum height (mm) of ST elevation, and the numbers of leads with ST elevation. The Minnesota code 9-2 requires 1 mm ST elevation in one or more of leads I, II, III, aVL, aVF, V5, V6, or 2 mm ST elevation in one or more of leads V1–V4 (Fig. 8.4).[8] But different definitions of "significant" ST elevation led to marked variations in sensitivity and specificity for diagnosis of AMI.[9] Minnesota criteria have 94% of specificity and 56% sensitivity for diagnosing STEMI.[9]

Though initial ST elevation is considered as a part of the classic evolutionary pattern of AMI, however, ST-segment elevation can also be attributed to other causes, different from AMI—a normal variant, frequently referred as early repolarization, commonly characterized by J-point elevation and rapidly upsloping or normal ST-segment; ventricular aneurysm, often characterized by persistent ST elevation; pericarditis, in which usually the ST elevation can be detected in more than one discrete region, as the inflammation involves a large portion of the epicardial surface, and reciprocal ST-depression is absent; elevated serum potassium; acute myocarditis; cardiac tumors or intrathoracic mass. An additional ECG criteria in diagnosis of evolving STEMI is represented by the morphology of ST-segment elevation.[10]

There are three patterns of ST-segment morphology can be identified, according to the direction of the ST slope:

1. Convex morphology
2. Concave morphology
3. Saddle-shaped morphology.

The convex morphology (upwardly convex ST-elevation) is usually consistent with STEMI; on the other hand concave morphology is usually not consistent with AMI diagnosis. The concave morphology ST elevation (upwardly concave ST-elevation) rather related to other conditions, such as benign early repolarization, acute pericarditis.[11-14] But it must be remembered that acute STEMI may produce ST elevation with either convex, concave, or obliquely straight morphology.

The assessment of ST-segment elevation during AMI is also useful to evaluate the extension of the myocardium at risk, and then the prognosis. In fact the number of leads with ST-segment elevation and the sum of the total ST deviation have been related to the extension of area of myocardium at risk, defined as the extent of jeopardize ischemic myocardium, and consequently to the extent of necrotic area if reperfusion is not undertaken.[15] The normal ST segment should not be flat. It should have little upward concavity sometimes referred to as a "take-off." When an ST segment becomes upwardly convex, it can indicate AMI. ST elevation whether convexity upwards or concavity upwards can be recognized by drawing an imaginary line between the J-point and the apex of the T-wave. If the ST segment is below that line, then it is upwardly concave. If it is even with or above that line, then it is "non-concave" (straight or

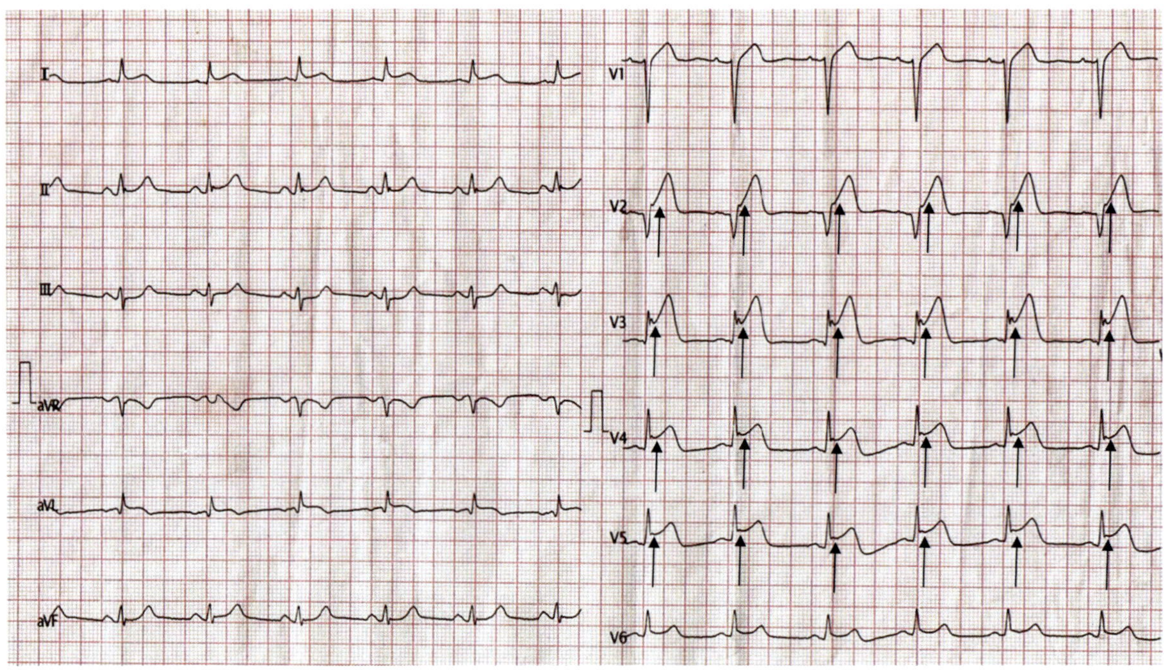

Fig. 8.4: Electrocardiogram (ECG) showing ST elevation in leads V2–V5 (arrows) suggesting acute anterior wall myocardial infarction.

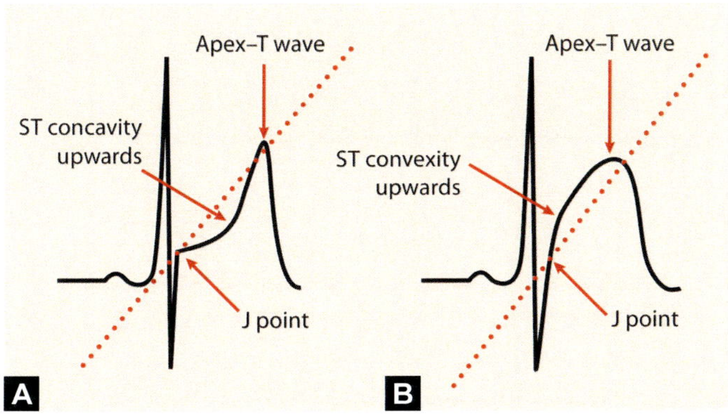

Figs. 8.5A and B: (A) ST elevation whether convexity upward or concavity upward can be recognized by drawing an imaginary line between the J-point and the apex of the T-wave. If the ST segment is below that line, then it is upwardly concave. (B) If above that line, then it is upwardly convex, which is suggestive of acute ST-elevation myocardial infarction.

upwardly convex) which is suggestive of acute ST elevation MI (Figs. 8.5A and B).[16]

Cause of ST Elevation with Convexity Upward

- Acute STEMI.

Causes of ST Elevation with Concavity Upward

- Early repolarization defect
- Pericarditis.

Cause of Saddle-shaped ST Elevation in Lead V1–V3

- Brugada Syndrome

Anterior STEMI can be difficult to differentiate from early repolarization on the ECG. But the following ECG features suggest early repolarization:[17]

1. Widespread ST-segment elevation (precordial greater than limb leads)
2. J-point elevation
3. Concavity of initial upsloping portion of ST segment
4. Notching or irregular contour of J-point
5. Prominent, concordant T-waves (large amplitude).

Few other criteria can also differentiate these two conditions. R-wave amplitude is lower, ST-segment elevation greater, and QT_c longer favor the diagnosis of anterior MI versus early repolarization.[18]

Sometimes the QRS complex, the ST segment, and the T-wave fuse to form a single monophasic deflection, called a giant R-wave or "tombstone." ST-segment elevation surpassing the R-wave exhibits such a morphological appearance that it reminds a tombstone. Wilmalaratna was the first to term this characteristic as tombstone-like and convex ST segment elevation in MI patients as tombstoning.[19] Later on, Guo et al. modified the tombstoning criteria. The criteria of tombstoning ST-segment elevation are as follows:[20]

1. Absent R-wave or R-wave duration less than 0.04 seconds with minimal amplitude.
2. Convex upward ST segment merging with the descending R.
3. The peak of the ST segment is higher than the R-wave.
4. The ST segment merges with the T-wave.

Acute myocardial infarction accompanied by tombstoning ST-segment elevation is associated with extensive myocardial damage, reduced left ventricle function, serious hospital complications and poor prognosis.[21]

APPEARANCE OF PATHOLOGICAL Q-WAVES

Small Q-wave is commonly present in normal ECG. Abnormal Q-wave suggesting myocardial necrosis has greater negative deflection and longer duration. Small septal Q waves in the LV leads result from depolarization of the septum from left to right. A Q-wave in lead III may represent a normal finding. Pathological Q-waves occur if they are 25% or more of the height of the succeeding R-wave and/or they are greater than 0.04 seconds in width (one small square) and greater than 2 mm (two small squares) in depth. Q waves are a marker of electrical silence, which, when pathological, implies full thickness death of myocardium. They are negative because they are effective windows through which the opposite side of the heart can be seen. Here depolarization will be moving away from the electrode.

As AMI evolves, changes to the QRS complex include loss of R-wave height and the development of pathological Q-waves (Fig. 8.6). Both of these changes develop as a result of the loss of viable myocardium beneath the recording electrode, and the Q-waves are the only firm electrocardiographic evidence of myocardial necrosis. Q-waves may develop within 1–2 hours of the onset of symptoms of AMI, though often they take 12 hours and occasionally up to 24 hours to appear. The presence of pathological Q waves, however, does not necessarily indicate a completed infarct. If ST-segment elevation and Q-waves are evident on the ECG and the chest pain is of recent onset, the patient may still benefit from thrombolysis or direct intervention. When there is extensive MI, Q-waves act as a permanent marker of necrosis. With more localized infarction the scar tissue may contract during the healing process, reducing the size of the electrically inert area and causing the disappearance of the Q-waves.[5]

Q-wave should not be used exclusively as a marker of late presentation of acute coronary occlusion, denying patients potentially beneficial reperfusion therapy either thrombolysis or PCI.[10] It is also important to note that, in the

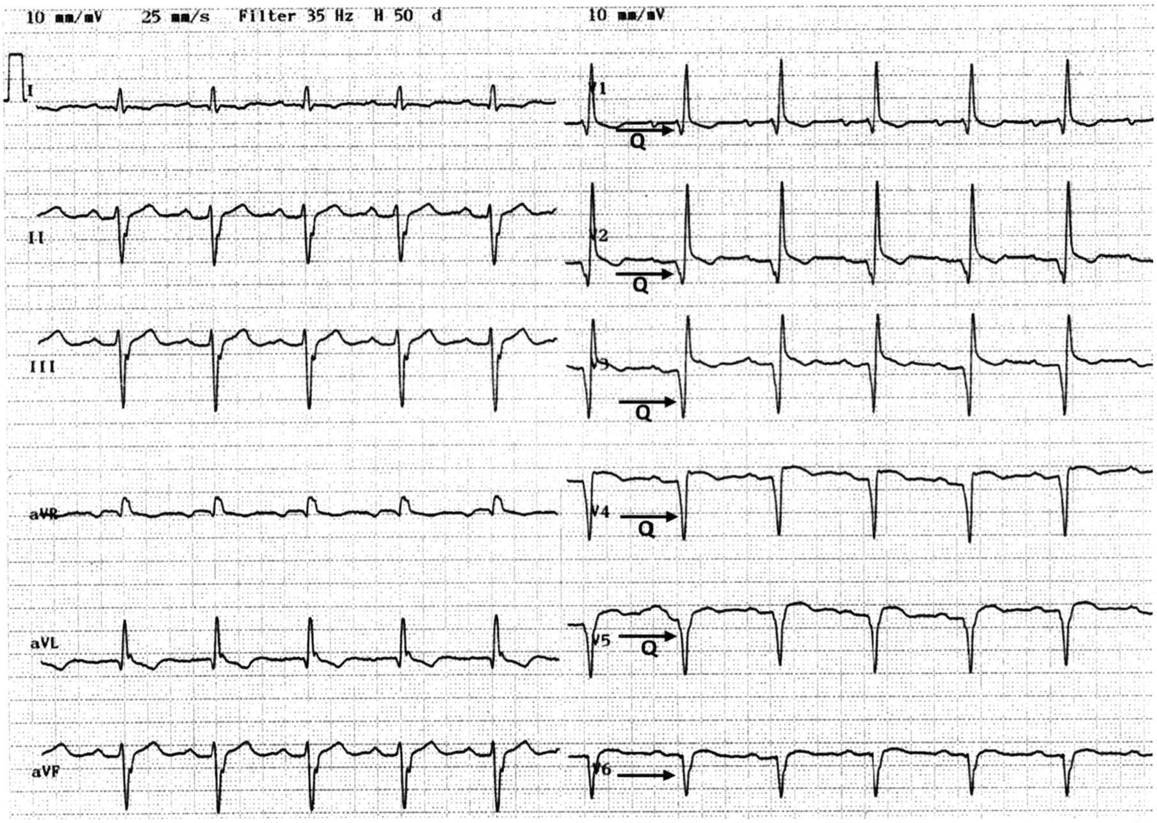

Fig. 8.6: Electrocardiogram (ECG) shows pathological Q waves in leads V1–V6 (arrows), suggestive of old anterior myocardial infarction.

Global Utilization of Streptokinase and Tissue Plasminogen Activator for Occluded Coronary Arteries (GUSTO-I) trial patients who did not develop Q-wave after fibrinolysis for STEMI had a lower mortality rate when compared to those who did develop Q-wave at 30 days postinfarction and 1 year postinfarction.[22] Thus, the absence of Q-wave after reperfusion therapy is a powerful marker of non-transmural necrosis and then of favorable prognosis.

In the presence of right bundle branch block (RBBB), Q waves have the same significance as when associated with normal intraventricular conduction. This is because the advent of RBBB does not affect the initial QRS vector. But in the presence of left bundle branch block (LBBB), Q waves in leads V5, V6 indicate septal infarction because the Q-waves should disappear from these leads due to abnormal septal activation.

Absence of Q-waves in lateral leads (I, V5–V6) is important ECG criteria for diagnosing LBBB. If Q waves of whatever size are present in these leads in presence of LBBB, indicate septal infarction.

T-WAVES INVERSION

Within hours to days, an evolving STEMI will typically demonstrate T-wave inversion. The inverted T-wave appears generally in the same leads showing ST-segment elevation (Fig. 8.7).[23] The morphology of inverted T-wave tends to be symmetric.[24] In the course of an evolving STEMI, T-wave inversion occurs when ischemia involves the epicardium. T-wave inversion is hypothesized to occur because of delayed depolarization in ischemic tissue.[10,25] T-wave inversion occurs in approximately three-fourths of all patients with a completed myocardial necrosis.[24] Indeed, a deepening T-wave soon after reperfusion therapy may then determine successful reperfusion. However, normalization of T-waves may also predict a lower morbidity months after STEMI. It has been found that patients with T-wave normalization within 6 months of infarction had higher LV ejection fraction than those who did not, indicating that patients with normalization of inverted T-waves had improved myocardial recovery.[26] T-wave inversion may also persist for many months and occasionally remains as a permanent sign of infarction.[5]

NORMALIZATION OF THE ST-SEGMENT

As the infarct evolves, the ST-segment elevation diminishes and the T-waves begin to invert. The ST-segment elevation associated with an inferior MI may take up to 2 weeks to resolve. ST-segment elevation associated with anterior MI may persist for even longer, and if a LV aneurysm develops it may persist indefinitely.[5] Nowadays the normalization

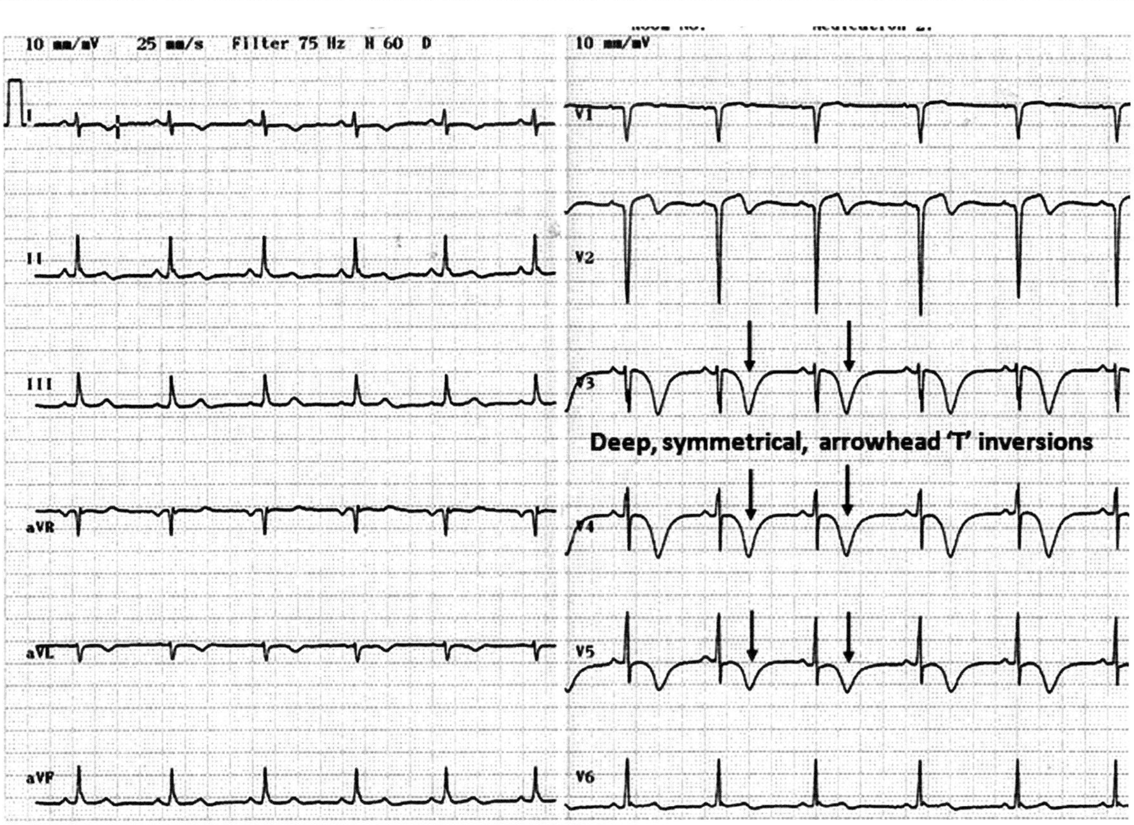

Fig. 8.7: Electrocardiogram (ECG) shows deep, symmetrical and arrowhead T-wave inversions in leads V3–V5. Note presence of pathological Q-wave in leads V1 and V2 and poor progression of R-wave in leads V3 and V4. These findings are suggestive of previous anterior myocardial infarction. These patterns of inverted T waves usually appear in the same leads showing ST-segment elevation during acute episode. These T-wave inversions may persist permanently or normalize over time.

of the ST-segment can be observed in the majority of patients as a result of successful reperfusion therapy. In fact, after successful thrombolysis or mechanical reopening of infarct-related artery, abrupt changes occur in ECG as a result of recovery in depolarization currents across the myocytes membrane. Thus a prompt decrease in ST-segment elevation is a powerful predictor of reperfusion, whereas the persistence of ST-segment elevation represent a marker of unsuccessful reperfusion therapy and is an independent determinant of major adverse cardiac event.[27,28] Interestingly, a decrease in ST-segment elevation > 70% seems to be associated with 94% positive predictive value for complete reperfusion.[29]

ECG CRITERIA FOR THE DIAGNOSIS OF ST-ELEVATION MYOCARDIAL INFARCTION

The universal definition of acute STEMI is stated as new ST elevation at the J-point in at least 2 contiguous leads of greater than or equal to 2 mm (0.2 mV) in men or greater than or equal to 1.5 mm (0.15 mV) in women in leads V2–V3 and/or of greater than or equal to 1 mm (0.1 mV) in other contiguous chest leads or the limb leads in the absence of LV hypertrophy or LBBB.[30]

The earliest manifestations of myocardial ischemia are typically T-wave and ST-segment changes. Increased T-wave amplitude, with prominent symmetrical T-waves in at least two contiguous leads, is an early sign that may precede the elevation of the ST-segment. "Contiguous leads" refers to lead groups such as anterior leads (V1–V6), inferior leads (II, III, and aVF) or lateral/apical leads (I, aVL). Supplemental leads such as V3R and V4R reflect the free wall of the right ventricle and V7–V9 the posterior wall.[30] In anterior MI, ST elevation appears in LI, aVL and chest leads, V1–V6 (Figs. 8.8A and B).

The majority of patients will evolve ECG evidence of Q-wave infarction. New or presumably new LBBB has been considered a STEMI equivalent.[31] Most cases of LBBB at time of presentation, however, are "not known to be old" because of prior ECG is not available for comparison. New or presumably new LBBB at presentation occurs infrequently, may interfere with ST-elevation analysis, and should not be considered diagnostic of AMI in isolation.[32] Baseline ECG abnormalities other than LBBB (e.g. paced rhythm, LV hypertrophy, Brugada syndrome) may obscure interpretation.[31] In addition, ST depression in ≥2 precordial leads (V1–V4) may indicate transmural posterior injury; multilead ST depression with coexistent ST elevation in lead aVR has been described in patients

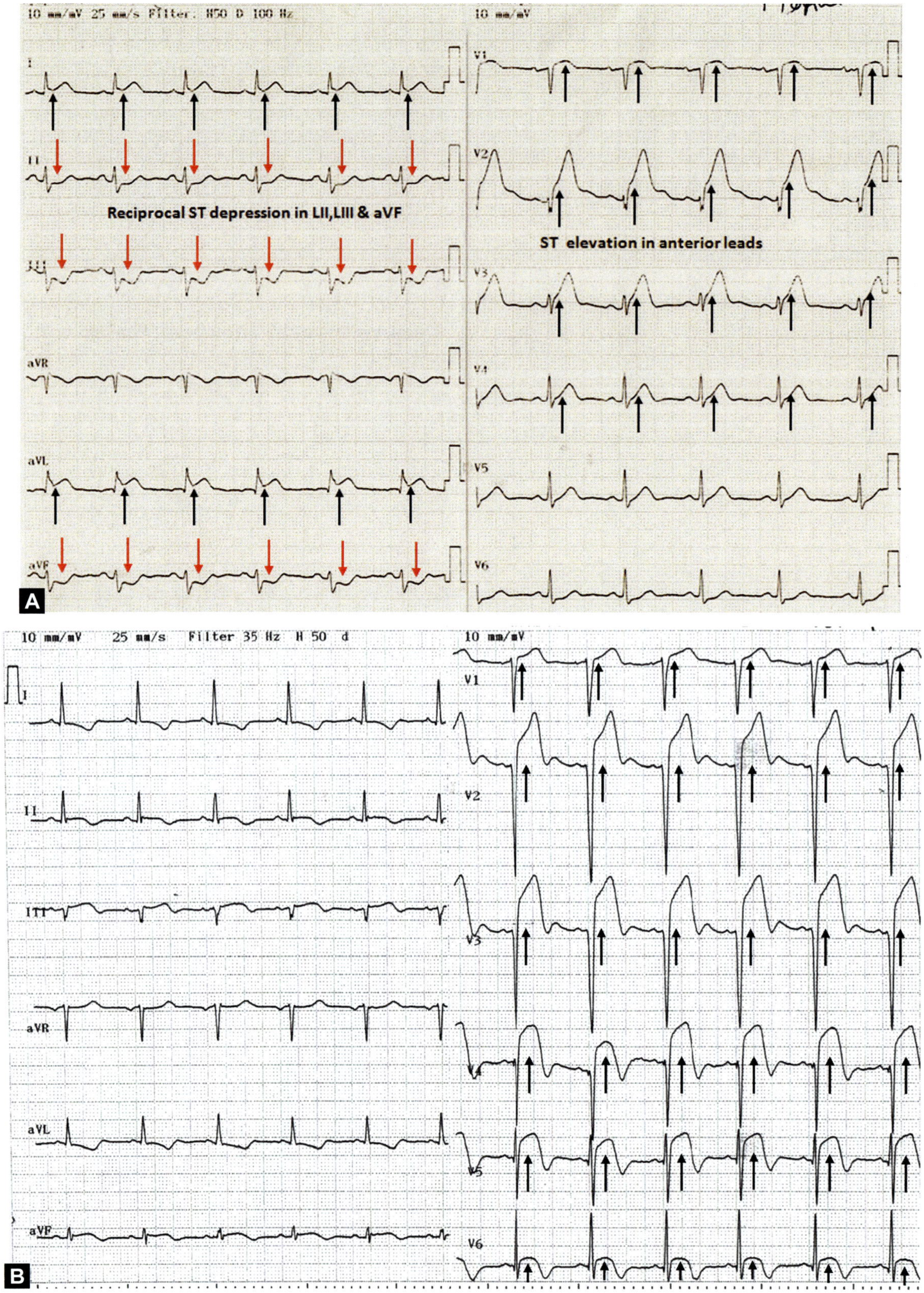

Figs 8.8A and B: (A) Electrocardiogram (ECG) is suggestive of acute anterior myocardial infarction showing ST-segment elevation in anterior leads (LI, aVL, V1–V4) (black arrows). Also note remarkable reciprocal ST-segment depression in inferior leads, LII, LIII, and aVF (red arrows). (B) Electrocardiogram (ECG) is suggestive of acute anterior myocardial infarction showing ST segment elevation in anterior leads V1–V6 (arrows). Also note there is no reciprocal ST-segment depression in inferior leads.

with left main or proximal left anterior descending (LAD) artery occlusion.[33-35] Rarely, hyperacute T-wave changes may be observed in the very early phase of STEMI, before the development of ST elevation. Transthoracic echocardiography may provide evidence of focal wall motion abnormalities and facilitate triage in patients with ECG findings that are difficult to interpret. If doubt persists, immediate referral for invasive angiography may be necessary to guide therapy in the appropriate clinical context.[34,35] Cardiac troponin is the preferred biomarker for diagnosis of MI.

Significance of Reciprocal ST-segment Depression in STEMI

Patients who have ST elevation in one territory often have ST depression in other territories. Reciprocal ST-segment depression in leads remote from the site of an acute infarct is known as reciprocal change and is a highly sensitive indicator of AMI (Fig. 8.9). Typically, the depressed ST segments tend to be horizontal or downsloping. The presence of reciprocal change is particularly useful when there is doubt about the clinical significance of ST-segment elevation.

This additional ST deviation may represent ischemia in a myocardial region other than the area of infarction or may represent pure reciprocal changes.[36] Most of the common patterns of remote ST depression probably represent reciprocal changes and not "ischemia at a distance".[37,38]

Reciprocal change strongly indicates acute infarction, with a sensitivity and positive predictive value of over 90%, though its absence does not rule out the diagnosis. Reciprocal changes are most frequently seen when the infarct is large, and they may reflect an extension of the infarct or occur as a result of coexisting remote ischemia. Alternatively, it may be a benign electrical phenomenon. The positive potentials that are recorded by electrodes facing the area of acute injury are projected as negative deflections in leads opposite the injured area, thus producing a "mirror image" change. Extensive reciprocal ST-segment depression in remote regions often indicates widespread arterial disease and consequently carries a worse prognosis.

In anterior STEMI, ST depression in the inferior leads is reciprocal to involvement of the basal anterolateral region, and represented by ST elevation in leads I and aVL.[39,40] In patients who have inferior STEMI, ST depression in lead aVL is a pure reciprocal change and is found in almost all patients and ST depression in leads V1-V3 probably does not represent ischemia at a distance but rather reciprocal changes caused by more posterior, inferoseptal, apical, or lateral LV involvement.[41-43] In contrast, among patients who have inferior STEMI, ST depression in leads V4-V6 is associated with concomitant multivessel disease, LAD coronary artery stenosis or three-vessel disease.[44-46] Thus, presence of an atypical pattern of ST depression and especially ST depression in leads V4-V6 in inferior STEMI may signify ischemia at a distance.[37]

LOCALIZATION OF SITE OF INFARCTION

The distribution of changes recorded in AMI allows the area of infarction to be localized, thus indicating the site of arterial disease. Proximal arterial occlusions tend to produce the most widespread electrocardiographic abnormalities. The anterior and inferior aspects of the heart are the areas most commonly subjected to infarction.

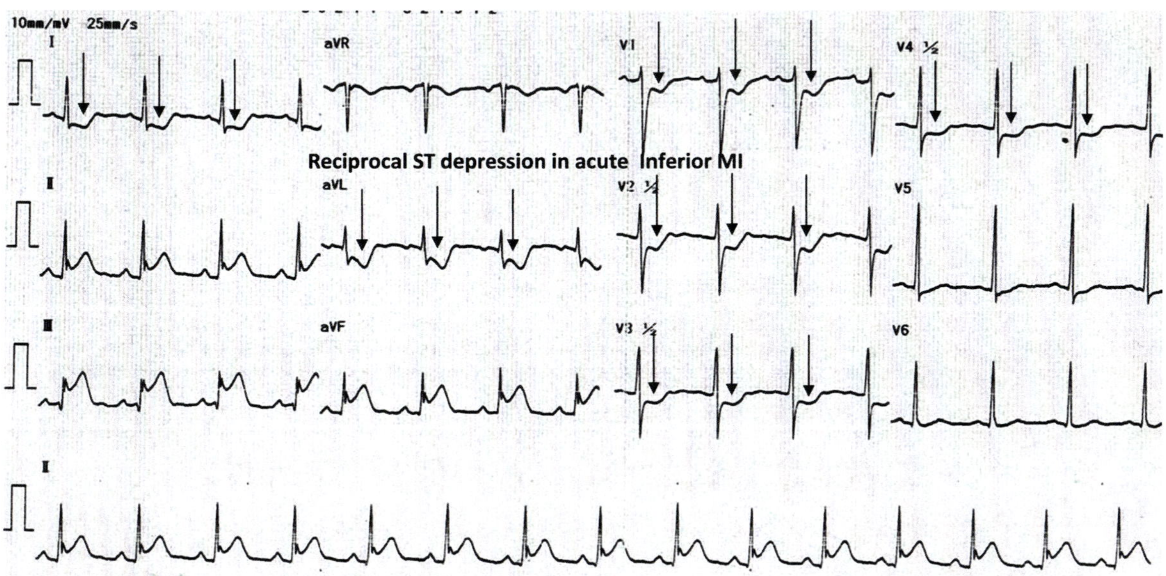

Fig. 8.9: Electrocardiogram (ECG) reveals reciprocal ST segment depression in leads LI, aVL, V1–V4 (arrows) in the setting of acute inferior myocardial infarction (ST elevation in leads LII, LIII, and aVF).

ECG Criteria of Acute Anterior Myocardial Infarction

The classic pattern of acute anterior MI causes ST elevation in the precordial leads V1–V4. Aldrich and colleagues reported the frequency of ST elevation in patients who have acute STEMI caused by LAD coronary artery occlusion to be, in descending order: V2, V3, V4, V5, aVL, V1, and V6.[47,48] In extensive anterior MI, ST elevation is noted in leads L1, aVL, and V1–V6, the injury extends to the distal anterolateral wall and cardiac apex (Fig. 8.10), whereas patients who have an anteroseptal pattern of STEMI, ST elevation is confined to leads V1–V4 with or without any reciprocal ST depression in inferior leads (Fig. 8.11). Later pathological Q-wave appears in the precordial leads V2–V6 (Fig. 8.12).[49]

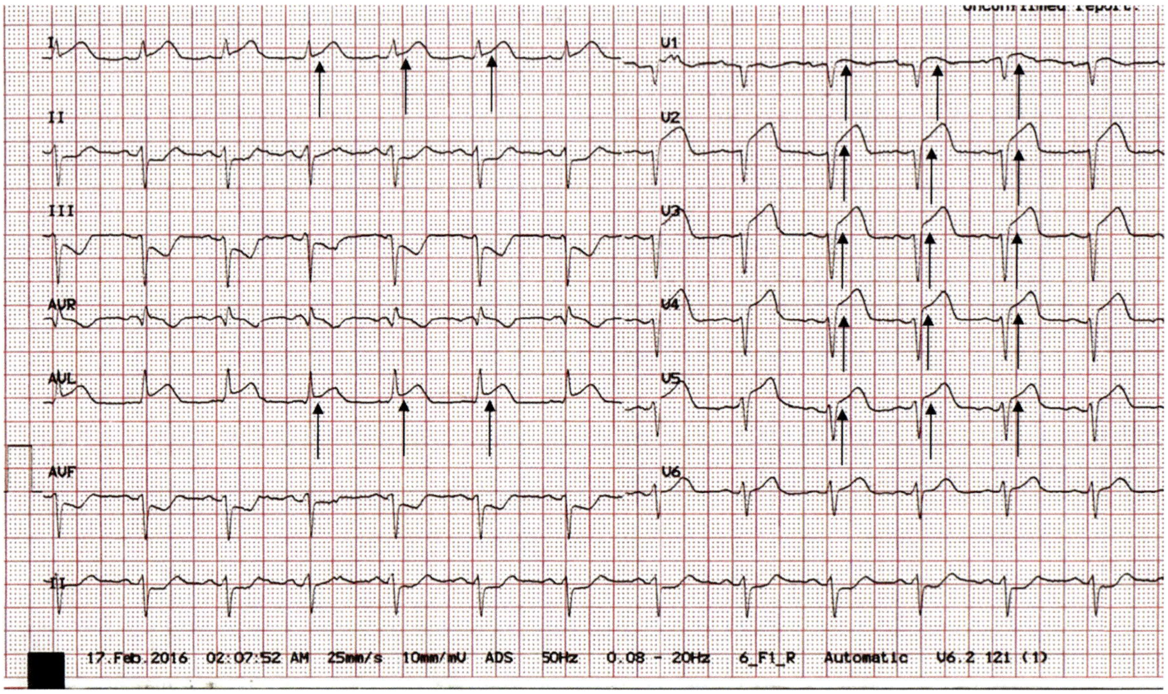

Fig. 8.10: Electrocardiogram (ECG) is suggestive of acute extensive anterior myocardial infarction showing ST-segment elevation in leads LI, aVL, V1–V5) (arrows). Note also reciprocal ST-segment depression in inferior leads, LII, LIII, and aVF.

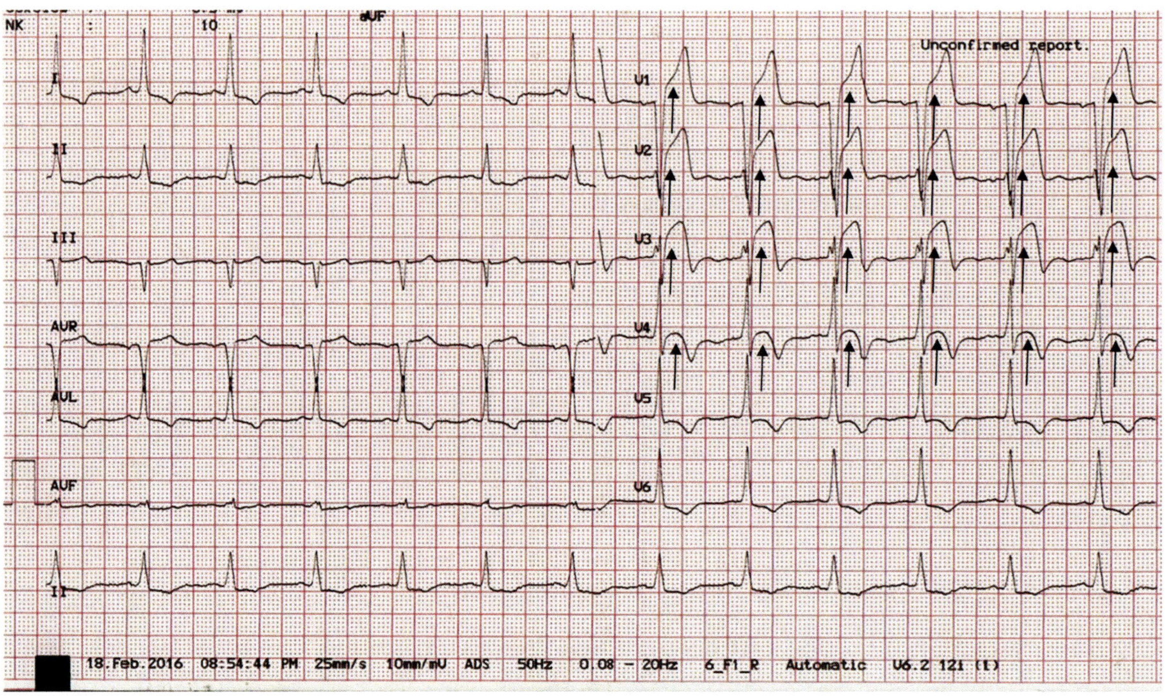

Fig. 8.11: Electrocardiogram (ECG) is suggestive of acute anteroseptal myocardial infarction showing upwardly convex ST segment elevation in leads V1–V4 (arrows). There is no significant reciprocal ST segment depression in inferior leads, LII, LIII, and aVF.

ECG Criteria of Acute Inferior Myocardial Infarction

In inferior STEMI, ST elevation is noted in leads II, III, and aVF. In addition to ST elevation in the inferior leads II, III, and aVF, reciprocal ST depression in lead aVL is seen in almost all patients who have acute inferior STEMI (Figs. 8.13A to C). Most patients who have ST elevation in these inferior leads (80%–90%) have an occlusion of the right coronary artery (RCA); however, in 10–20% cases an occlusion of the left circumflex (LCX) can produce almost similar ECG pattern. Also occasionally, inferior STEMI may result from occlusion of a "type III" or "wraparound" LAD artery. This produces the unusual pattern of concomitant inferior and anterior ST elevation.

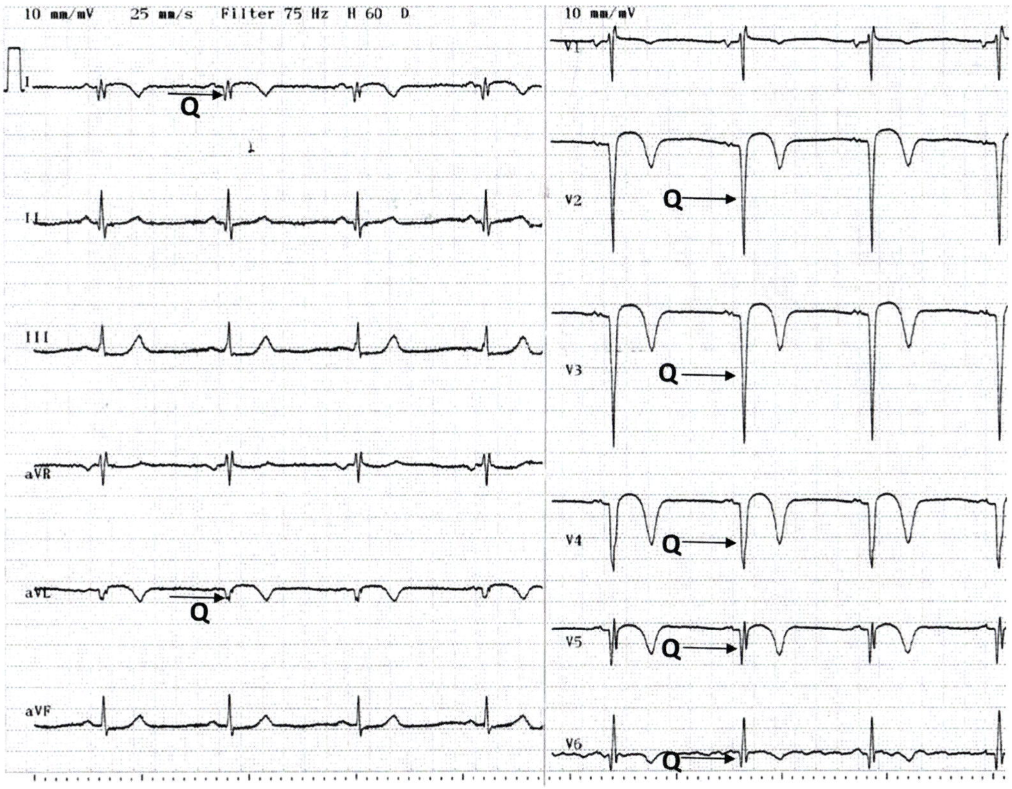

Fig. 8.12: Electrocardiogram (ECG) shows deep pathological Q waves in chest leads V2–V5 (arrows). Also note presence of Q waves in leads LI, aVL, and V6. These Q waves are evidences of past extensive anterior myocardial infarction.

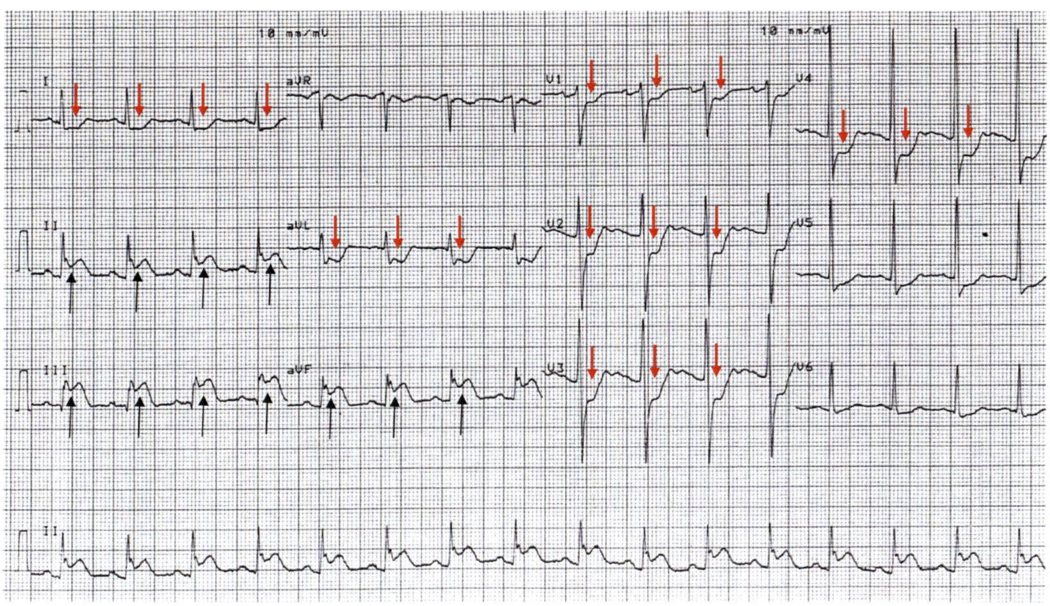

Fig. 8.13A: Electrocardiogram (ECG) findings are suggestive of acute inferior myocardial infarction, ST elevation in leads LII, LIII, and aVF (black arrows). Also note reciprocal ST segment depression in leads aVL, LI, and V1–V4 (red arrows).

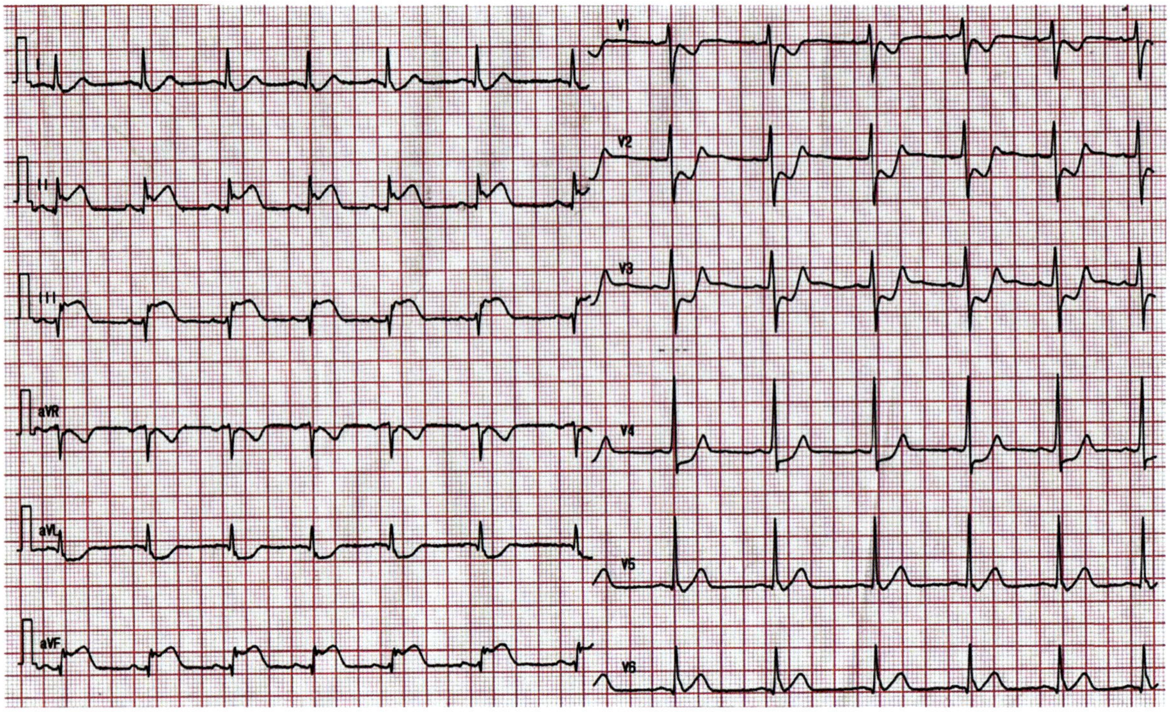

Fig. 8.13B: Electrocardiogram (ECG) findings are suggestive of acute inferior myocardial infarction, ST elevation in leads LII, LIII, and aVF with reciprocal ST-segment depression in leads aVL, LI, and V1–V4.

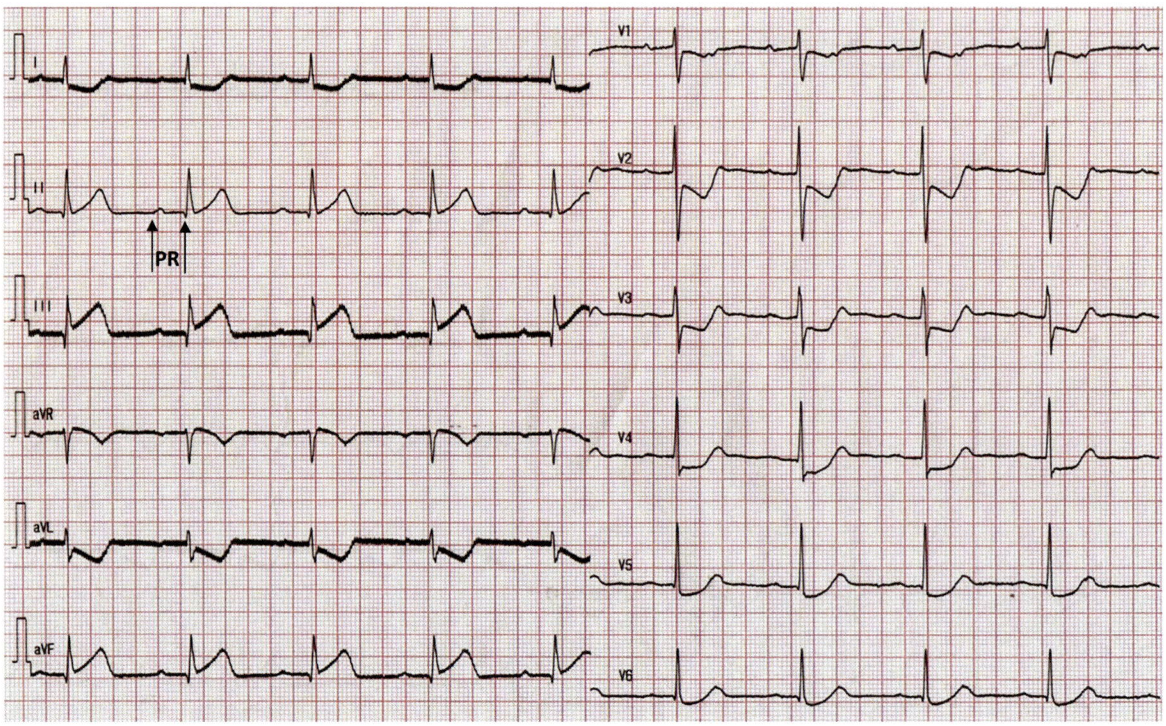

Fig. 8.13C: Electrocardiogram (ECG) findings are suggestive of acute inferior myocardial infarction, ST-elevation in leads LII, LIII, and aVF with reciprocal ST-segment depression in leads in LI, aVL, and V2–V6. Also note first degree heart block, PR interval 260 ms (arrows).

Left anterior descending artery is graded into three types:

- *Type 1*: Falls short of apex
- *Type 2*: Reach up to the LV apex
- *Type 3*: Wraps around LV apex and travels some distance in the posterior Inter-ventricular groove.

Left anterior descending artery should descend only in anterior aspect but in about 15% population it can take a posterior descending course as well. When LAD wraps around the LV apex, anterior MI due to LAD occlusions can show changes in inferior leads (anteroinferior MI) (Fig. 8.14).

Electrocardiogram pattern due to occlusion of RCA or LCX can be differentiated from classical surface ECG criteria.[37,38]

ECG Criteria of Right Ventricular Infarction

Right ventricular (RV) infarction is often overlooked, as a standard 12-lead electrocardiography is not a particularly sensitive indicator of right ventricular damage. Right ventricular MI is usually associated with occlusion of the proximal segment of the RCA and this type of infarction is associated with 40% of inferior infarctions. Less commonly, RV infarction is associated with occlusion of the circumflex artery, if this vessel is dominant. It may also complicate some anterior infarctions but rarely occurs as an isolated phenomenon. Isolated right ventricular MI accounts for only 3% of all infarctions.

On the standard 12-lead ECG right ventricular infarction is indicated by signs of inferior infarction, associated with ST-segment elevation in lead V1 (Fig. 8.15). It is unusual for ST-segment elevation in lead V1 to occur as an isolated phenomenon. Right-sided chest leads, V3R–V6R are much

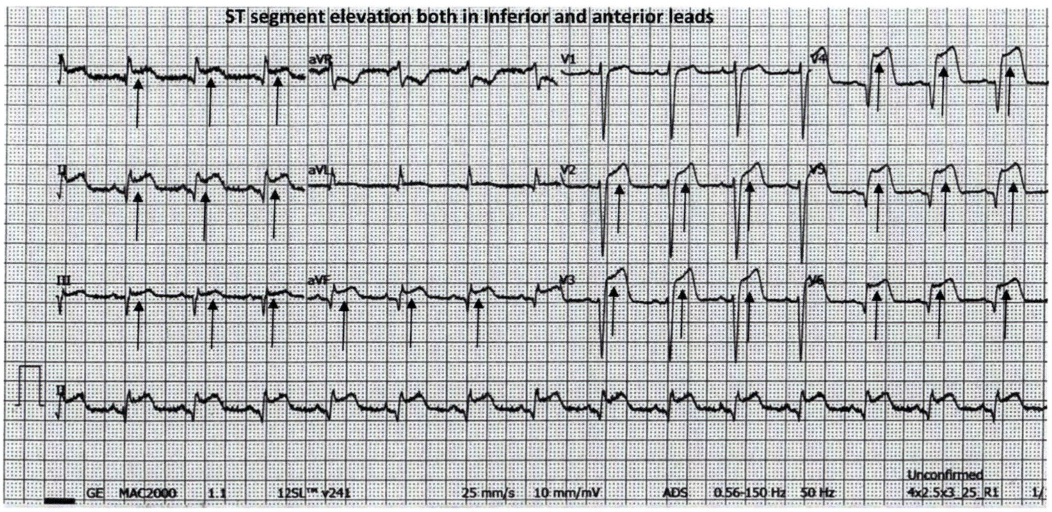

Fig. 8.14: Electrocardiogram (ECG) shows diffuse ST segment elevation in both inferior (LII, LIII, and aVF) and anterior leads (LI and V2–V6) (arrows). This type of unusual pattern of concomitant inferior and anterior STEMI is possible in presence of "wraparound" left anterior descending artery (LAD).

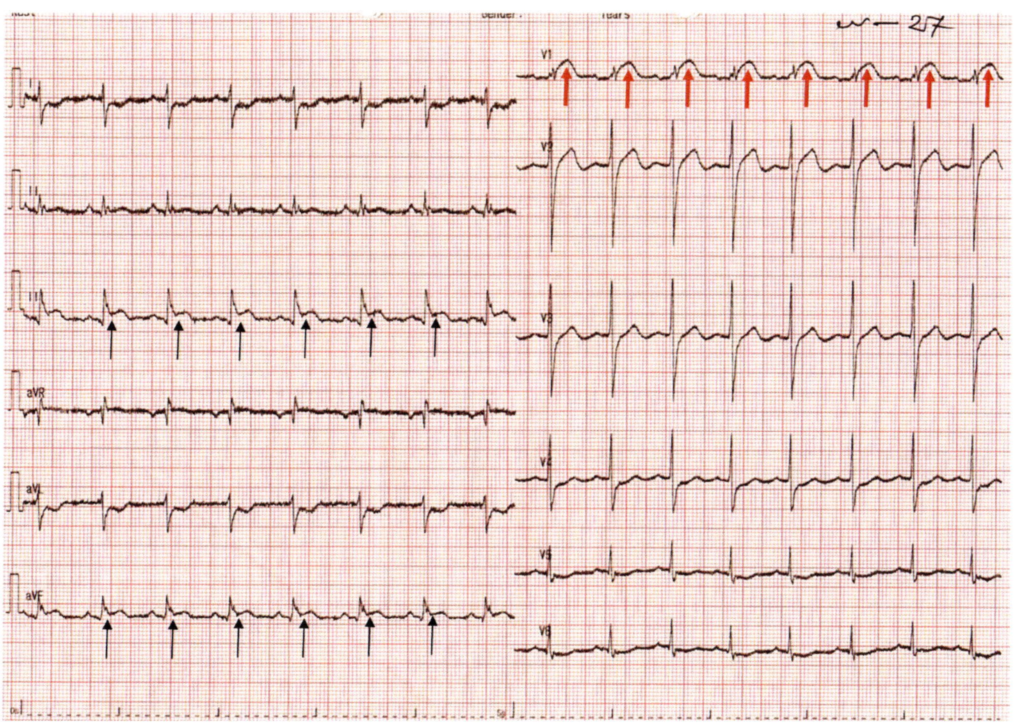

Fig. 8.15: Electrocardiogram (ECG) showing evidences of acute inferior myocardial infarction, ST elevation in LIII and aVF (black arrows) with simultaneous ST elevation greater than 1 mm in V1 (red arrows), suggestive of concomitant RV infarction.

more sensitive to the presence of right ventricular infarction (Fig. 8.16). The most useful lead is lead V4R (an electrode is placed over the right fifth intercostal space in the mid-clavicular line).[5]

The most sensitive electrocardiographic sign of RV infarction is ST-segment elevation of more than 1 mm in lead V4R with an upright T-wave in that lead (Fig. 8.17).[50] This sign is rarely present more than 12 hours after the infarction. Lead V4R should be recorded as soon as possible in all patients with inferior infarction, as ST-segment elevation in right ventricular infarction may be short lived.

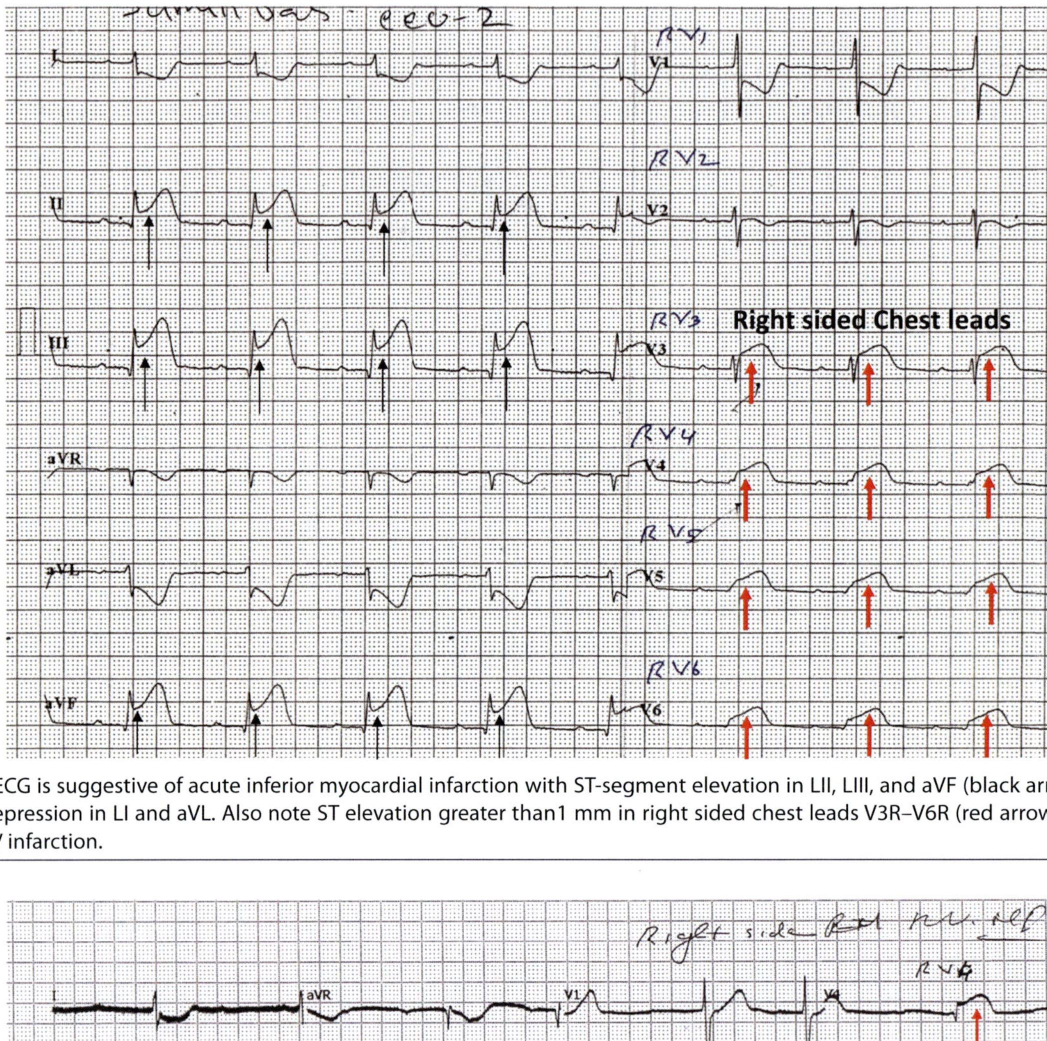

Fig. 8.16: This ECG is suggestive of acute inferior myocardial infarction with ST-segment elevation in LII, LIII, and aVF (black arrows) along with reciprocal ST depression in LI and aVL. Also note ST elevation greater than1 mm in right sided chest leads V3R–V6R (red arrows) suggestive of concomitant RV infarction.

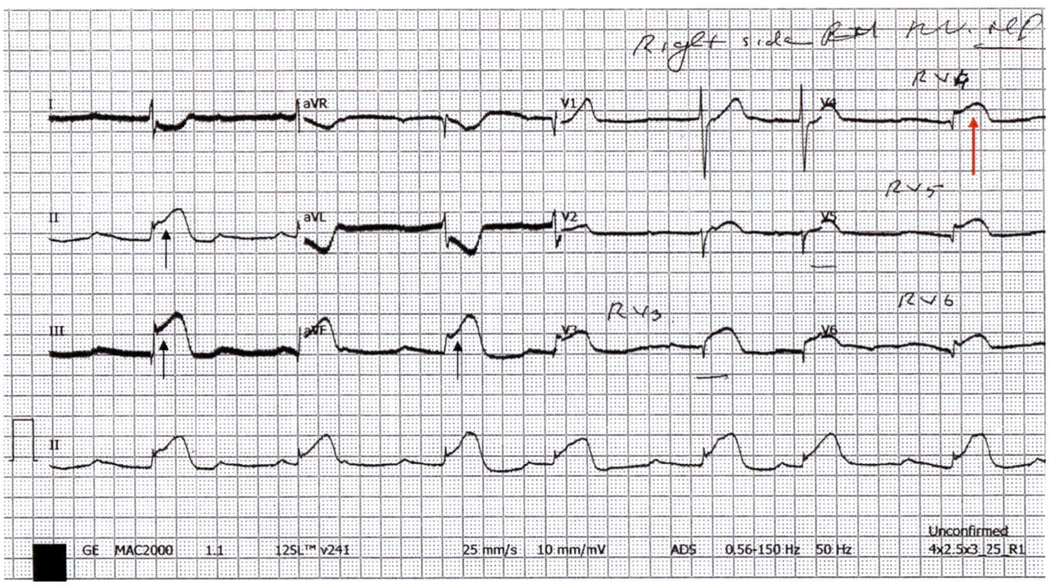

Fig. 8.17: This ECG is suggestive of acute inferior myocardial infarction with ST-segment elevation in LII, LIII, and aVF (black arrows) along with reciprocal ST depression in LI and aVL. Note marked ST segment elevation in lead V4R (red arrow). Also note ST elevation greater than 1 mm in other right sided chest leads V3R, V5R, and V6R. This ECG also reveals marked degree bradycardia due to associated high grade AV block.

ECG Criteria of Posterior Infarction

Posterior MI refers to infarction of the posterobasal wall of the left ventricle. Posterior infarction accompanies 15–20% of STEMIs, usually occurring in the context of an inferior or lateral infarction. Isolated posterior MI is less common (3–11% of infarcts). The diagnosis is often missed as the standard 12-lead electrocardiography does not include posterior leads. Early detection is important as expeditious thrombolytic treatment or primary percutaneous coronary intervention (PPCI) may improve the outcome for patients with posterior infarction. The changes of posterior MI are seen indirectly in the anterior precordial leads. Leads V1–V3 face the endocardial surface of the posterior wall of the left ventricle. As these leads record from the opposite side of the heart instead of directly over the infarct, the changes of posterior infarction are reversed in these leads. The R waves increase in size, becoming broader and dominant, and are associated with marked horizontal ST depression and upright T-waves in leads V1–V3 (Fig. 8.18). This contrasts with the Q-waves, ST-segment elevation, and T-wave inversion seen in acute anterior MI.[5]

In inferior STEMI caused by proximal RCA occlusion with concomitant RV infarction, however, posterior wall infarction may be masked because the two opposed electrical vectors may cancel each other (that is, ST elevation in leads V1–V3 with RV infarction and reciprocal ST depression in these same leads with concurrent posterior infarction) (Box 8.1).[51] A more direct sign of posterior wall injury is ST elevation in leads V7–V9.[52-54] Waveform amplitudes in these posterior leads are smaller than in standard precordial leads, however, there is preliminary evidence that ST elevation of 0.5 mm should be considered a sign of injury when analyzing the posterior leads.[55] Isolated ST elevation in leads V7–V9 without ST elevation in the inferior leads occurs in only 4% of patients who have AMI and usually is caused by LCX occlusion.[54-56] In patients who have acute inferior STEMI, ST elevation in leads V7–V9 is associated with a higher incidence of reinfarction, heart failure, and death.[52]

Box 8.1: Explanation of the ST-segment depression in V1–V3 in posterior ST elevation myocardial infarction.

ST elevation myocardial infarction is usually manifested by ST-segment elevation in the specific leads but true posterior STEMI is manifested by ST segment depression in leads V1–V3. As because during taking standard bedside 12 leads ECG, the posterior electrical activity is recorded from the anterior side of the heart, so the typical injury pattern of ST elevation and Q-waves becomes inverted:
- ST elevation becomes ST depression
- Q-waves become R-waves
- T-wave inversion becomes an upright T-wave.

Posterior electrical activity is recorded from the anterior side of the heart, the typical injury pattern of ST elevation and Q waves becomes inverted, so, ST elevation becomes ST depression, Q waves become R waves and terminal T-wave inversion becomes an upright T-wave. In presence of Inferior STEMI concomitant posterior MI is suggested by:
1. Horizontal or downsloping ST depression in V1–V3;
2. Tall R waves in V1–V3;
3. Dominant R-wave (R:S ratio greater than 1) in V1 or V2; and
4. Upright T waves in V1–V3 (Fig. 8.19). Old posterior MI is evidenced by tall R waves in V1, V2 (R:S ratio greater than 1) and upright T in leads V1, V2 (Fig. 8.20).

HIGH LATERAL ST-ELEVATION MYOCARDIAL INFARCTION

ST elevation primarily localized to leads I and aVL is referred to as a high lateral STEMI and usually results from the

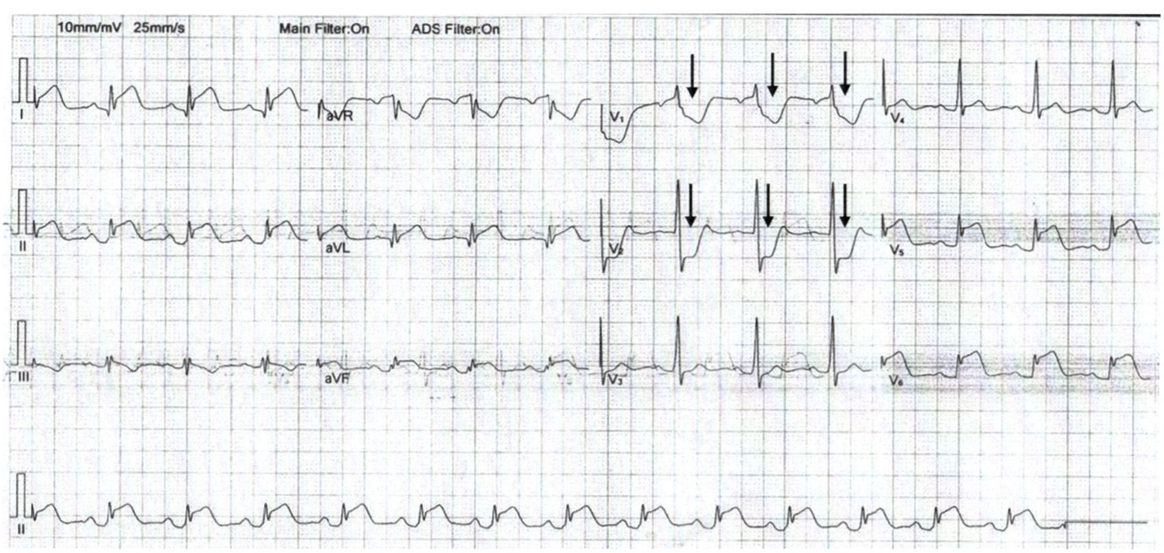

Fig. 8.18: This ECG findings are suggestive of posterior MI, evidenced by marked degree horizontal ST-segment depression greater than 5 mm in leads V1 and V2 (*arrows*), tall R waves in V1 and V2, dominant R-wave in V2 with R/S ratio greater than 1 and upright T waves in V1–3. Also note ST segment elevation in inferior and lateral leads suggesting inferior and lateral STEMI.

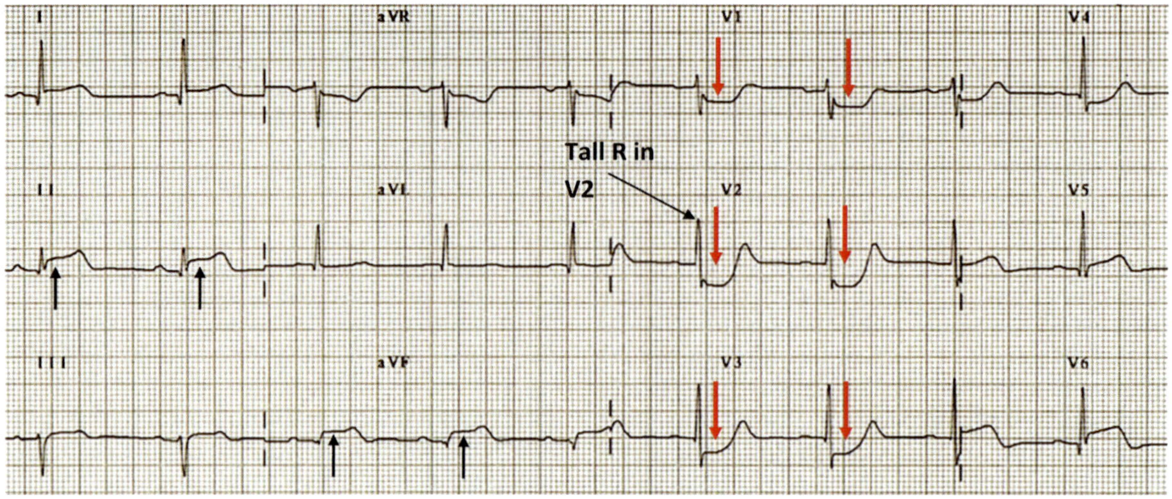

Fig. 8.19: In this ECG posterior MI is suggested by the following changes: horizontal ST depression greater than 1.5 mm in leads V1–V3 (red arrows), tall R waves in leads V1–V3, upright T waves in leads V1–V3 and dominant R-wave (R/S ratio > 1) in V1–V3. Note ST segment elevation in LII and aVF (black arrows), suggestive of concurrent inferior STEMI.

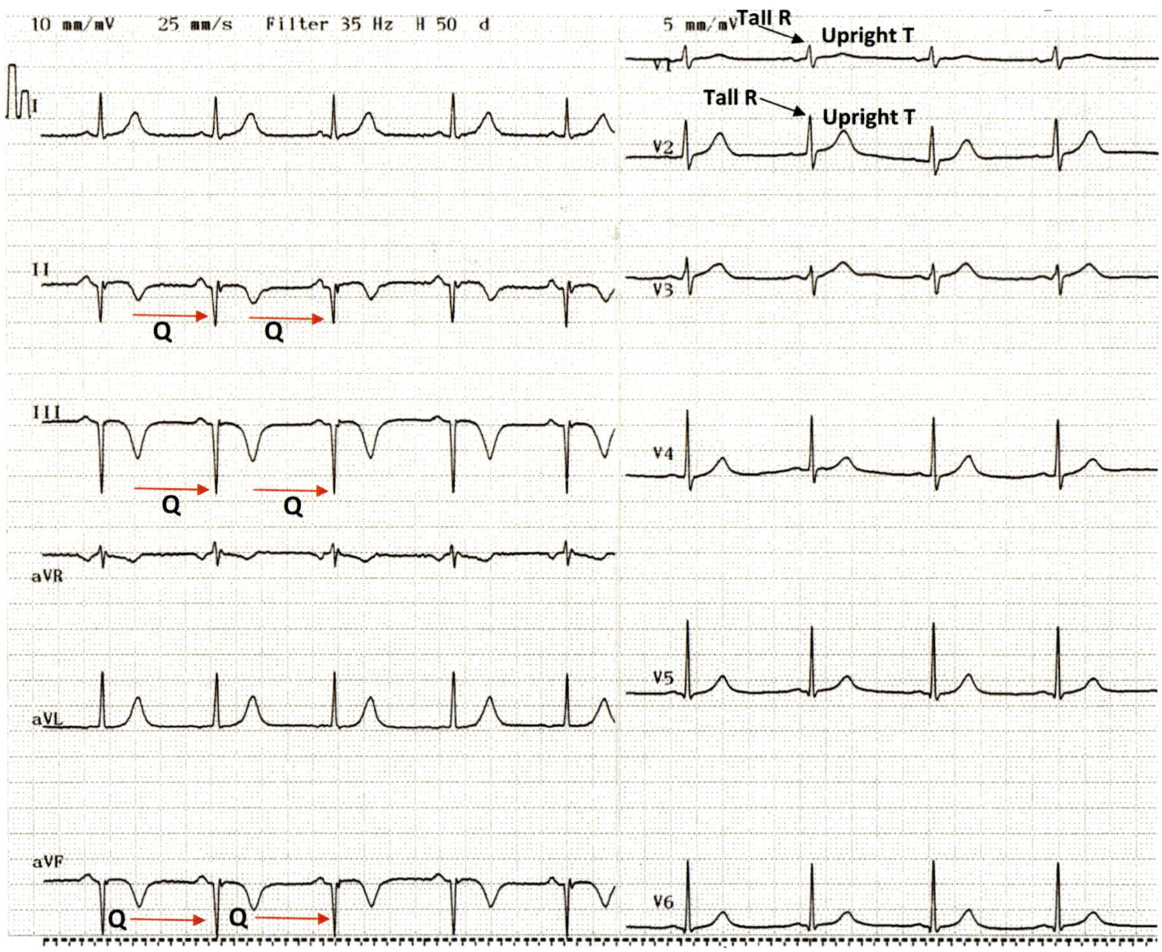

Fig. 8.20: This ECG is suggestive of old inferior and posterior myocardial infarction. Old inferior MI is suggested by the presence of deep Q waves in leads LII, LIII, and aVF. Old posterior MI is evidenced by tall R waves in V1, V2 (R:S ratio > 1) and upright T in leads V1, V2.

occlusion of first diagonal (D1) branch of the LAD. ECG criteria of high lateral STEMI include—ST elevation in LI and aVL. There may be subtle ST elevation with hyperacute T waves in V5-V6. High lateral infarction is usually associated with reciprocal ST depression in the inferior leads (III and aVF) (Fig. 8.21). This pattern is consistent with an acute infarction localized to the superior portion of the lateral wall of the left ventricle. After acute episode, Q-waves may appear in the same leads (LI and aVL) which showed ST-segment elevation during STEMI (Fig. 8.22).

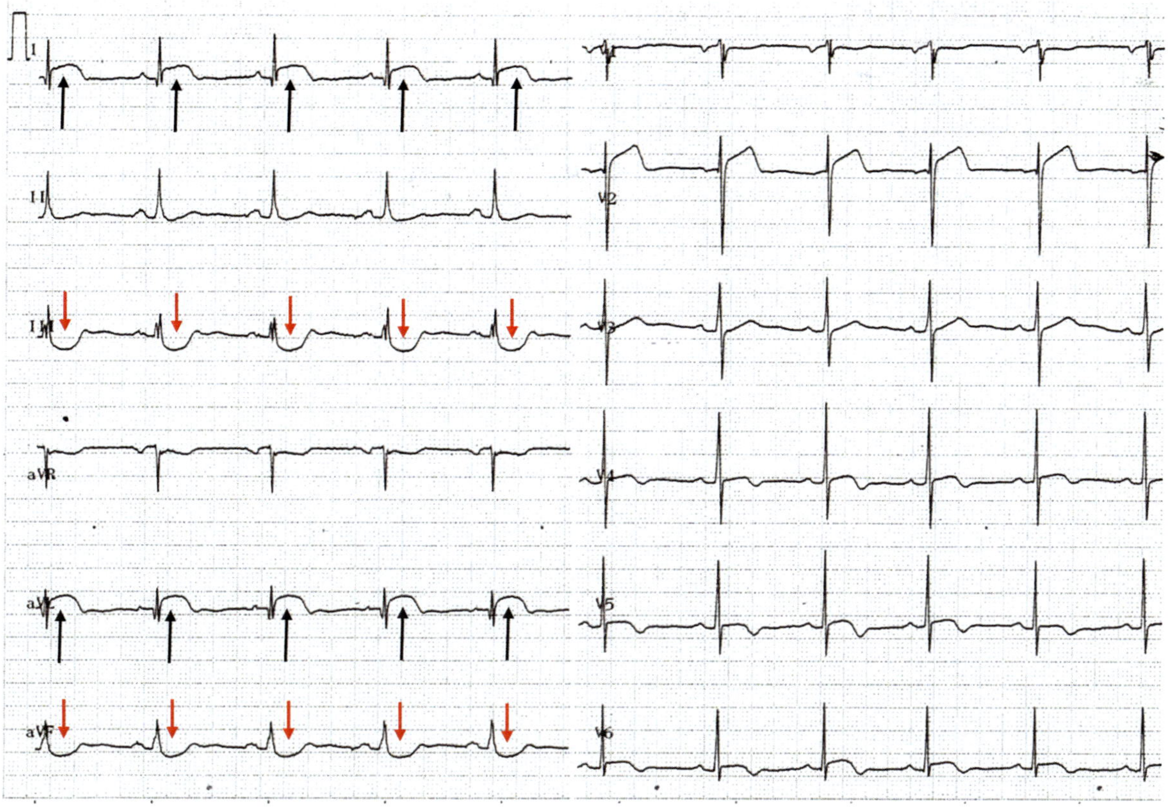

Fig. 8.21: Electrocardiogram (ECG) shows ST elevation with convexity upward in leads LI and aVL and reciprocal ST depression in leads LIII and aVF, suggestive of acute high lateral MI. Also note biphasic T waves in leads V4–V6.

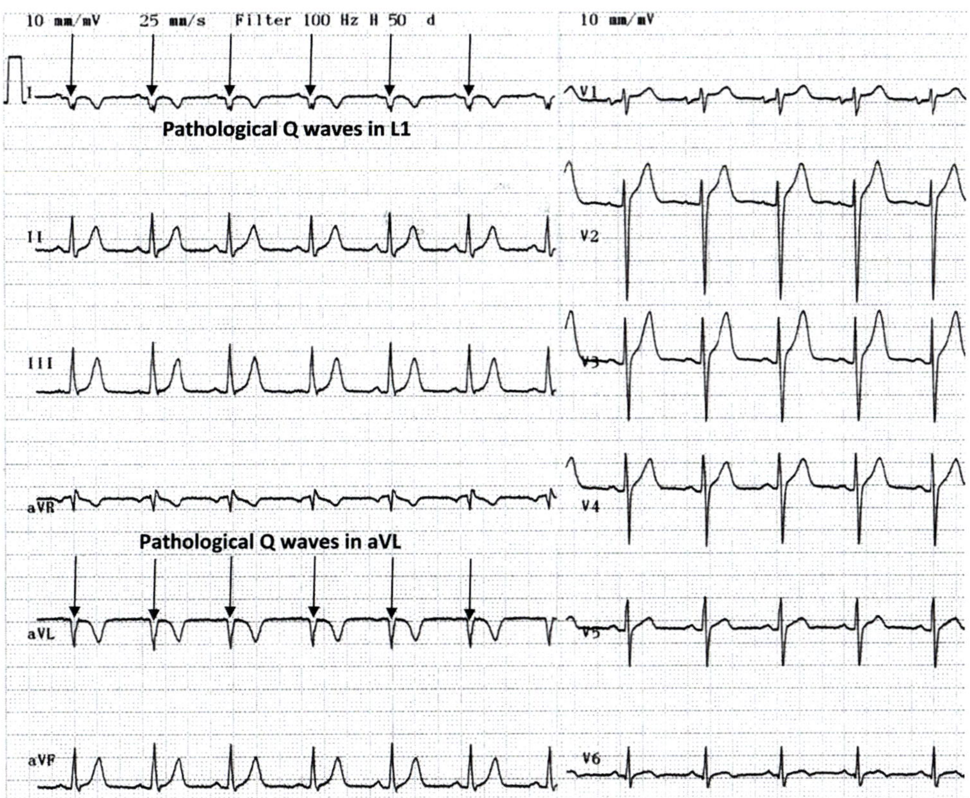

Fig. 8.22: Electrocardiogram (ECG) shows pathological Q waves in leads LI and aVL (arrows) with T-wave inversions suggestive of old high lateral MI.

TOMBSTONE ST ELEVATION

Tombstone ST elevation is an unusual morphological ECG appearance of AMI. The ST segment is convexed upwards and the peak of the convexed ST segment is often higher than the preceding R-wave, which is less than 0.04 second and small in amplitude (Fig. 8.23). This type of tombstone pattern is associated with polymorphous ventricular tachyarrhythmias and is thought to represent extensive and rapid myocardial damage after the ischemic episode. At coronary angiography, patients with tombstoning are likely to have high grade stenosis of the proximal LAD artery.

The criteria of tombstoning ST-segment elevation are as follows: (1) Absent R-wave or an R-wave duration less than 0.04 second with minimal amplitude, (2) convex upward ST segment merging with the descending R or the ascending QS/QR, (3) the peak of the ST segment is higher than the R-wave, and (4) the ST segment merges with the T-wave (Figs. 8.24A and B).

DIAGNOSIS OF ST-ELEVATION MYOCARDIAL INFARCTION IN PRESENCE OF BUNDLE-BRANCH BLOCK

Acute myocardial infarction in the presence of bundle-branch block carries a much worse prognosis than AMI with normal ventricular conduction. This is true both for patients whose bundle-branch block precedes the infarction and for those in whom bundle-branch block develops as a result of the acute event. It is therefore essential that the electrocardiographic identification of AMI in patients with bundle-branch block should be both timely and accurate because thrombolytic therapy or primary PCI produces dramatic reductions in mortality in these patients, and the greatest benefits are seen in those treated early.[57]

ECG Diagnosis of ST-Elevation Myocardial Infarction in Presence of Left Bundle-Branch Block

Making the diagnosis of acute infarction in the presence of LBBB can be problematic, since the ST segment is either elevated or depressed secondarily, simulating or masking an infarction pattern. These secondary ST–T changes are shifted to the opposite direction from the major component of the QRS complex (i.e. discordant). When these changes are concordant, they are specific for AMI. However, in LBBB, the QRS complexes are mostly negative in leads V1–V3, and the ST-segment elevation from an anteroseptal infarction cannot be manifested as a concordant ST-segment shift.[50]

Spontaneous or pacing-induced LBBB can obscure the electrocardiographic diagnosis of AMI. In the presence of LBBB or a right ventricular paced rhythm, right ventricular activation precedes LV activation; this activation of the infarcted left ventricle occurs later and is obscured within the QRS complex. Thus, Q-waves cannot be used to diagnose infarction. An indicator of MI in the presence

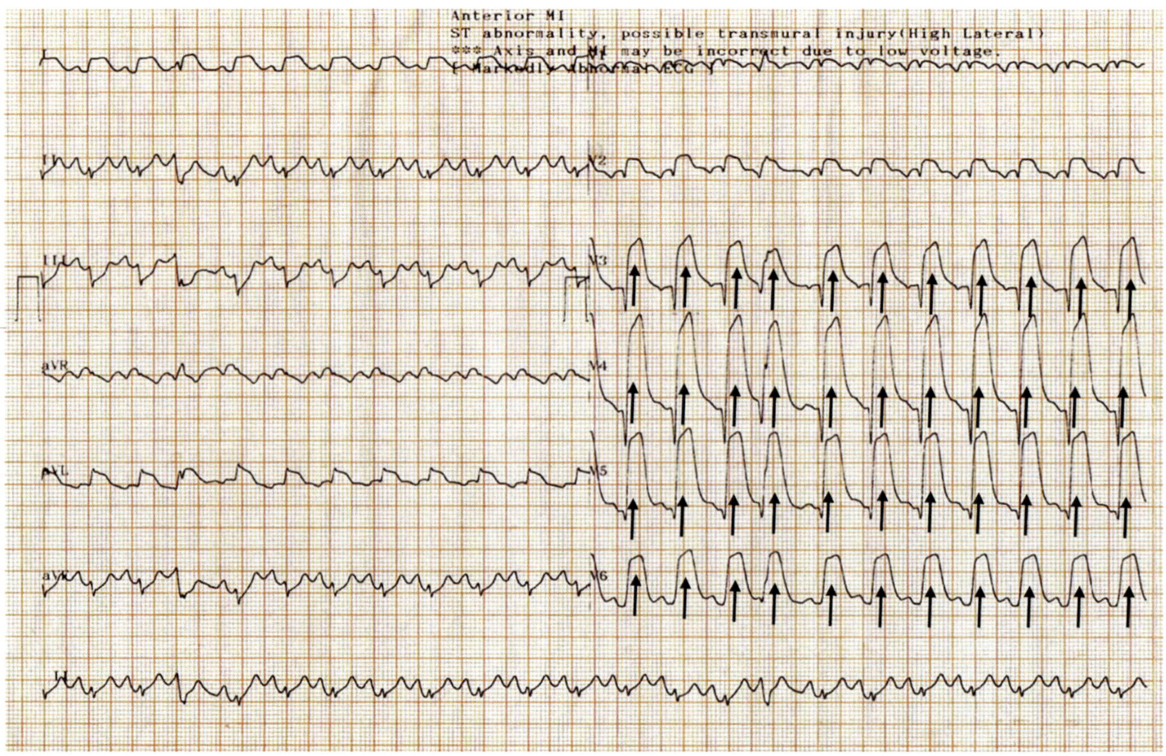

Fig. 8.23: Electrocardiogram (ECG) is suggestive of acute anterior myocardial infarction with tombstone pattern ST elevation (arrows) in chest leads V3–V6.

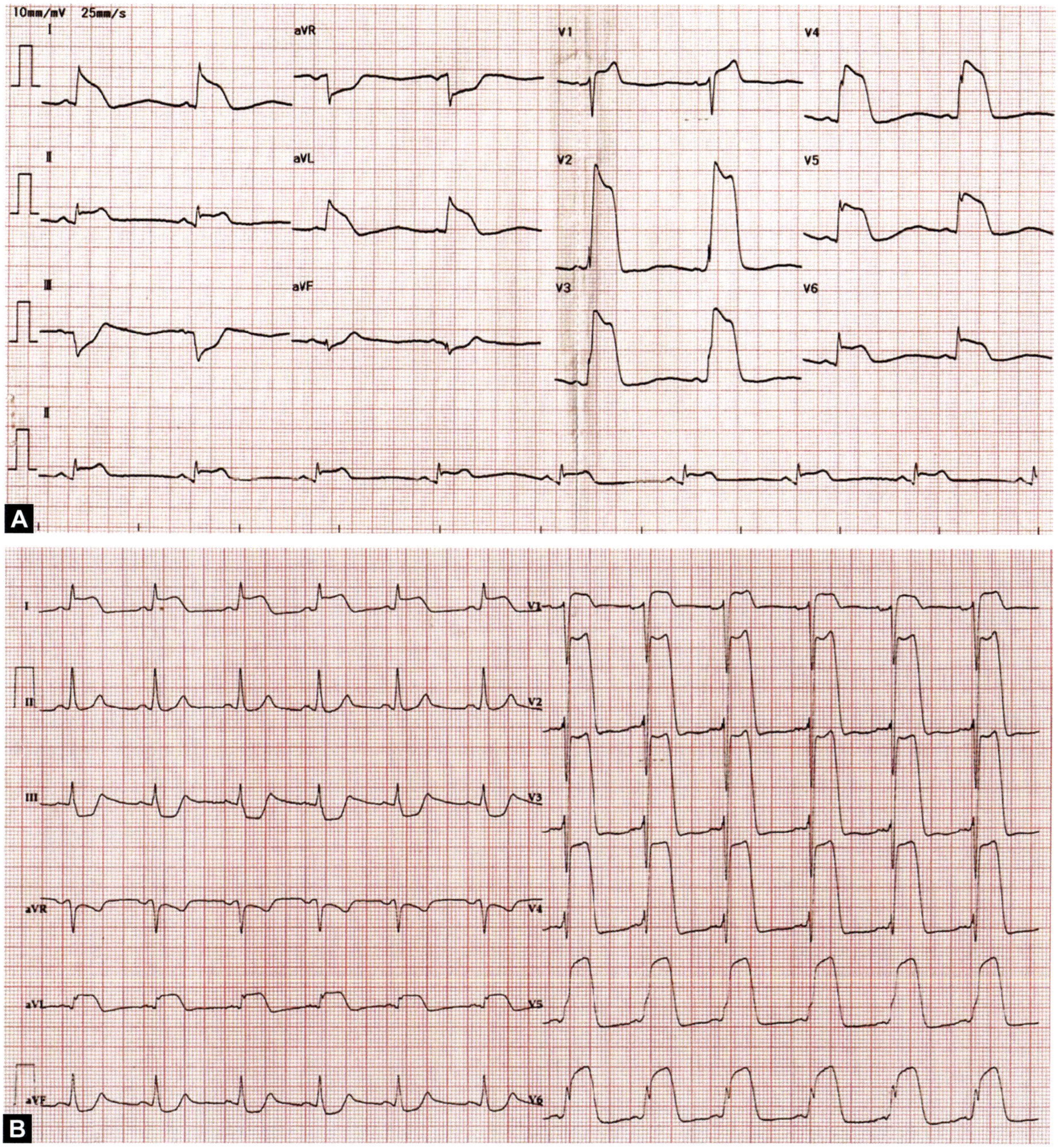

Figs. 8.24A and B: (A) Electrocardiogram (ECG) is suggestive of acute anterior MI showing tombstoning ST-segment elevation in leads V2–V5. Note the peak of the ST segment is very high and the ST segment merges with the T-wave. Also note reciprocal ST depression in leads LIII and aVF. (B) Electrocardiogram (ECG) is suggestive of acute extensive anterior MI showing tombstoning ST-segment elevation in leads V2–V6. Note the peak of the ST segment is very high (ST peak>R wave peak) and the ST segment merges with the T-wave. Also note ST segment elevation in LI, aVL, and V1 with reciprocal ST depression in leads LIII and aVF.

of LBBB is primary ST change, that is, ST deviation in the same (concordant) direction as the major QRS vector. So, in patients with LBBB or ventricular paced rhythm, infarct diagnosis based on the ECG is difficult. The baseline ST segments and T waves tend to be shifted in a discordant direction ("appropriate discordance"), which can mask or mimic AMI. However, serial ECGs may show dynamic ST segment changes during ischemia and a new LBBB is always pathological and can be a sign of MI. Few ECG criteria as suggested by Sgarbossa et al. may detect AMI in presence of LBBB. The three electrocardiographic criteria with independent value in the diagnosis of acute infarction in these patients are: ST-segment elevation of 1 mm or more that is concordant with (in the same direction as) the QRS complex; ST-segment depression of 1 mm or more in lead V1, V2, or V3; and ST-segment elevation of 5 mm or more that is discordant with (in the opposite direction from) the QRS complex (Fig. 8.25).[58] Presence of Q-wave in LI, aVL, V5, or V6 in the presence of LBBB usually indicates associated anterior MI.

Sgarbossa Scoring System for Diagnosis of ST-Elevation Myocardial Infarction in Presence of Left bundle branch block[58,59]

Three criteria are included in Sgarbossa's scoring system* (Fig. 8.26):

- ST elevation ≥1 mm in a lead with a positive QRS complex (i.e. concordance): 5 points
- ST depression ≥1 mm in lead V1, V2, or V3: 3 points
- ST elevation ≥5 mm in a lead with a negative (discordant) QRS complex: 2 points.

*≥3 points = 90% specificity of STEMI (sensitivity of 36%).

A Sgarbossa score of greater than or equal to 3 was specific but not sensitive (36%) in the validation sample in the original report. A subsequent meta-analysis of 10 studies consisting of 1,614 patients showed that a Sgarbossa score

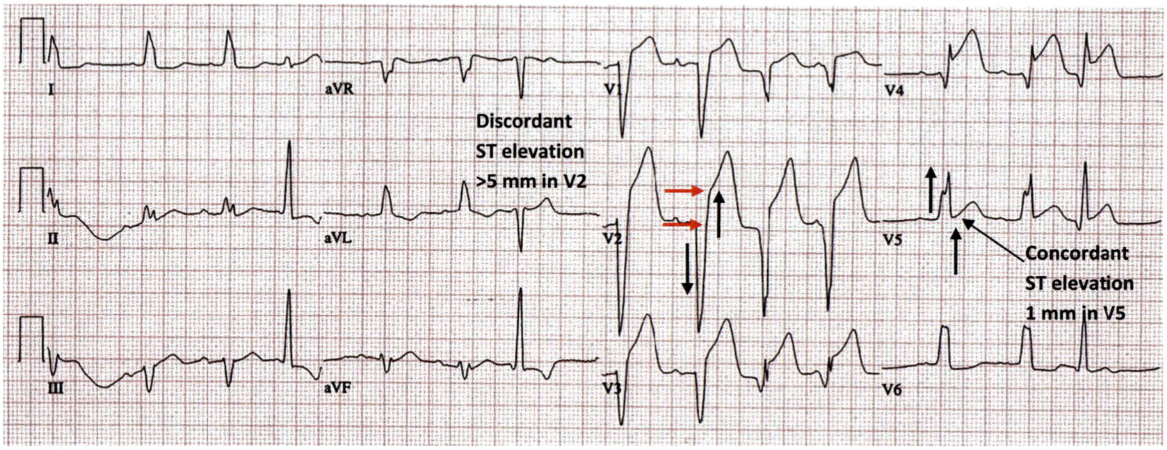

Fig. 8.25: This ECG is suggestive of STEMI in presence of LBBB. Note 1 mm concordant ST-segment elevation (ST deviation is in the same direction of major QRS vector) in V5 (score-5) and 7 mm (red arrows) discordant ST segment elevation (ST deviation is in the opposite direction of major QRS vector) in V2 (score-2). So in this ECG total Sgarbossa score is 7, which is suggestive of STEMI.

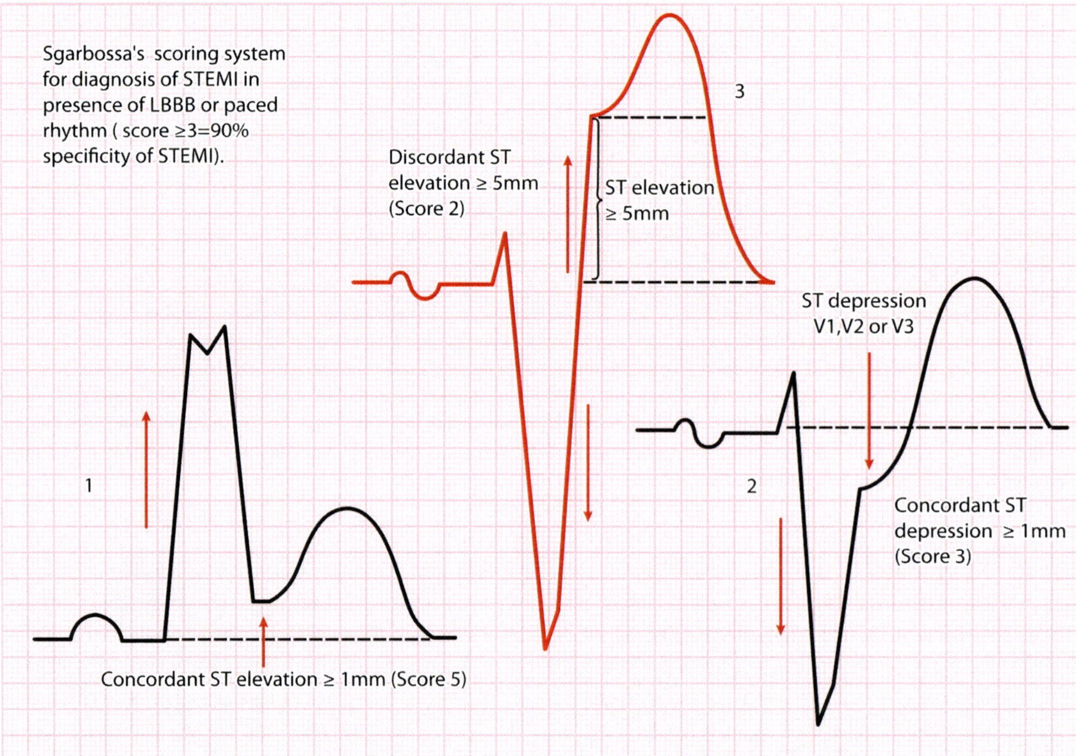

Fig. 8.26: Sgarbossa's scoring system for the diagnosis of STEMI in the presence of LBBB and paced rhythm: 1. ST elevation greater than or equal to 1 mm in a lead with a positive QRS complex (i.e. concordance: ST deviation is in the same direction of major QRS vector): 5 points. **2.** ST depression (concordant) greater than or equal to 1 mm in lead V1, V2, or V3: 3 points. 3. ST elevation greater than or equal to 5 mm in a lead with a negative (discordant, ST deviation is in the opposite direction of major QRS vector) QRS complex: 2 points. (≥3 points = 90% specificity of STEMI).

of greater than or equal to 3 had a specificity of 98% and sensitivity of 20%.[60] The sensitivity may increase if serial or previous ECGs are available.[61]

The Cabrera's sign and Chapman's sign have been used to diagnose AMI in the setting of a LBBB as well. Notching 0.04 second in duration in the ascending limb of the S-wave of leads V3 or V4 is termed as Cabrera's sign (Fig. 8.27) and notching of the upstroke of the R-wave in leads I, aVL, or V6 is known as Chapman's sign (Fig. 8.28).[62-64]

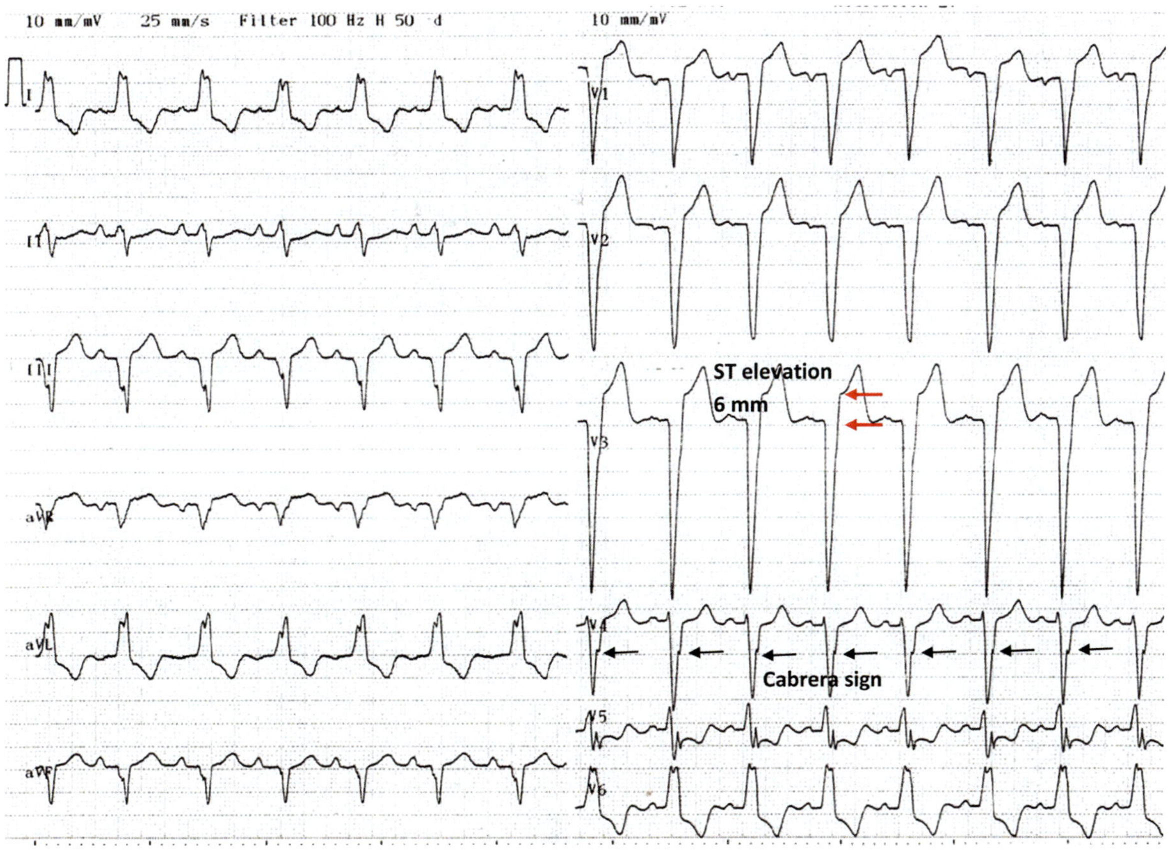

Fig. 8.27: Electrocardiogram (ECG) showing Cabrera's sign (notching in the ascending limb of the S-wave in lead V4) (black arrows). Also note discordant ST segment elevation around 6 mm (red arrows) in lead V3, suggestive of STEMI in the presence of LBBB.

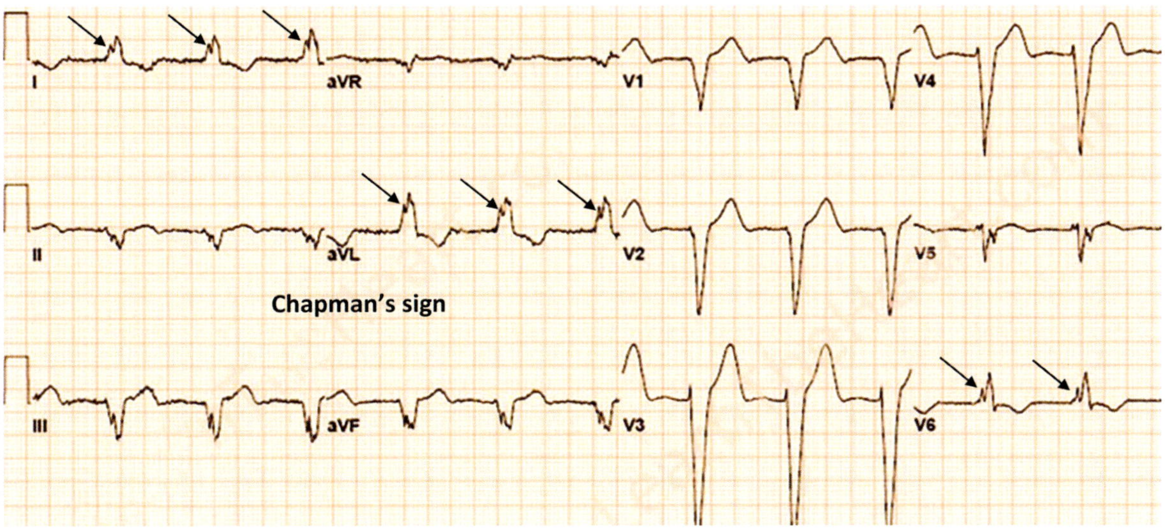

Fig. 8.28: Electrocardiogram (ECG) showing Chapman's sign (notching of the upstroke of the R-wave in LI, aVL and V6) (arrows). This sign is suggestive of acute myocardial infarction in the setting of a LBBB.

ECG Diagnosis of ST-Elevation Myocardial Infarction in Presence of Right Bundle Branch Block

Right bundle branch block may be seen in association with coronary artery disease, but in many cases no organic heart disease is present. Uncomplicated RBBB usually causes little ST segment displacement and neither causes nor masks Q waves. Thus it does not generally interfere with the diagnosis of AMI, though it may mask a posterior MI (Fig. 8.29).[57] In patients with RBBB, ST-T abnormalities in leads V1–V3 may create difficulty in assessing the presence of ischemia in these leads: however, when new ST elevation or Q waves are found, myocardial ischemia or infarction should be considered.[30]

Differential Diagnosis of ST-Segment Elevation

There are several causes of ST-segment elevation besides STEMI. Some of these conditions can be misdiagnosed as acute infarction, resulting in unwarranted thrombolytic therapy or emergency angiography. Many times, the shape of the ST-segment elevation, the leads involved, other features of the ECG, the clinical setting in which the elevation occurs, and most important, awareness of the conditions that mimic infarction can help to differentiate the conditions. In addition, echocardiography can sometimes be useful.

Causes of ST-Segment Elevation Other than ST-Elevation Myocardial Infarction

- Normal variant ST elevation
- Benign early repolarization
- Left bundle branch block
- Left ventricular hypertrophy
- Ventricular aneurysm
- Hyperkalemia
- Coronary vasospasm/Prinzmetal's angina
- Pericarditis
- Brugada syndrome
- Subarachnoid hemorrhage.

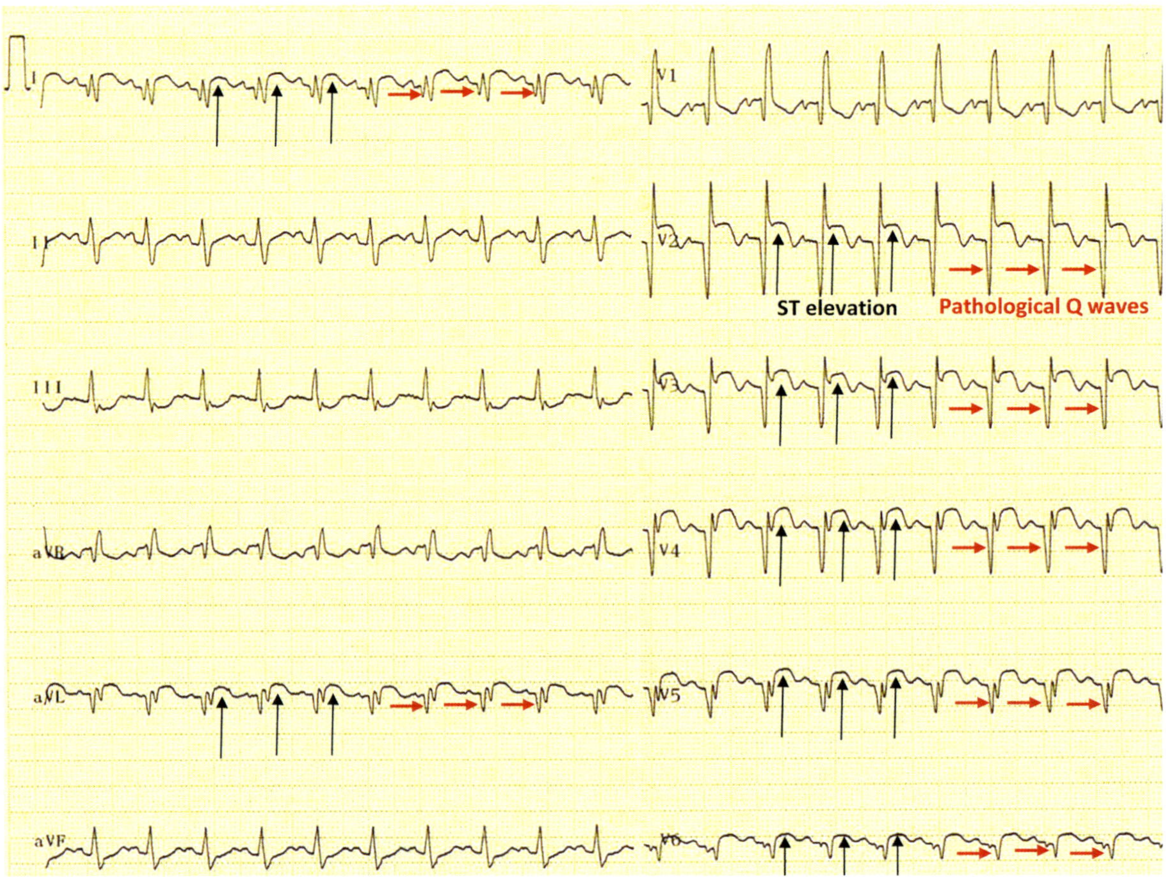

Fig. 8.29: Anterior STEMI in presence of right bundle branch block (RBBB). Note ST-segment elevation in LI, aVL, V2–V6 suggesting acute anterior myocardial infarction (black arrows). Also note pathological Q waves in the same leads (red arrows). Note also reciprocal ST-segment depression in LIII. RBBB usually does not interfere with the diagnosis of STEMI.

Normal Variant ST Elevation

In a study of 6,014 healthy men in the U.S. Air Force who were 16 to 58 years old, 91% had ST-segment elevation of 1–3 mm in one or more precordial leads. The elevation was most common and marked in lead V2. The prevalence declined gradually with increasing age, reaching 30% in men who were 76 years of age or older. In contrast, about 20% of normal ECGs from women had ST-segment elevation of 1 mm or more, and this prevalence remained unchanged regardless of the women's ages. Since the majority of men have ST elevation of 1 mm or more in precordial leads, it is a normal finding, and is designated as a male pattern; ST elevation of less than 1 mm is designated as a female pattern. In these patterns, the ST segment is concave.[50,65]

ST segment may appear elevated due to "high take-off." Care is required when interpreting ST-segment elevation in right-sided chest leads as the ST segments, particularly in leads V2 and V3, tend to be upsloping rather than flat. Isolated ST-segment elevation in these leads should be interpreted with caution.[57]

Benign Early Repolarization

In some healthy young people, especially in black men, the ST segment is elevated by 1–4 mm in the midprecordial leads as a normal variant. This pattern is commonly referred to as early repolarization pattern (ERP). In most instances of early repolarization, the ST-segment elevation is most marked in V4, there is a notch at the J-point (the junction between the QRS complex and the ST segment), and the ST segment is concave. The T waves are tall and are not inverted. Early repolarization of atrial tissue is also present, resulting in PR-segment depression. However, the PR-segment depression is not as marked as that in patients with acute pericarditis.[66]

Left Bundle-Branch Block

In LBBB the ST segment is either elevated or depressed secondarily, simulating or masking an infarction pattern. These secondary ST-T changes are shifted to the opposite direction from the major component of the QRS complex (i.e. discordant). In LBBB ST elevation is usually concave and ST-segment deviation discordant from the QRS.[50]

Left Ventricular Hypertrophy

The deeper the S-wave, the greater the ST-segment elevation: a relation that is often observed in patients with LV hypertrophy and often associated with a QS pattern in leads V1 through V3. In fact, LV hypertrophy is one of the conditions that is most frequently mistaken for acute infarction. However, the elevated ST segment is concave in a patient with uncomplicated LV hypertrophy as compared with convex in a patient with acute concomitant AMI. Concave ST elevation and presence of other ECG features of LV hypertrophy differentiate these two conditions.[50,57]

Ventricular Aneurysm

A LV aneurysm can be diagnosed on ECG when there is persistent ST segment elevation occurring 6 weeks after a known transmural MI (usually an anterior MI) (Fig. 8.30). Without knowing the past medical history, the ECG changes of an aneurysm may mimic an acute anterior MI. With an anterior or apical aneurysm, the persistent ST elevation is in lead V1 and V2 with associated Q-waves indicating the old anterior MI. In an inferior aneurysm it would be in lead II, III, and aVF, although this is less common. The only way to be sure that the ECG changes present are from a LV aneurysm (not ST elevation from STEMI) is to have the patient's history of a prior MI and echocardiography to document the presence of an aneurysm. The shape of the ST elevation is also relatively unique and has been described as "coving."[67,68]

Hyperkalemia

Hyperkalemia as a cause of ST-segment elevation is well recognized. Other electrocardiographic features of hyperkalemia that are often, but not always, present are widened QRS complexes; tall, pointed, and tented T waves; and low-amplitude or no P waves. Even though the pseudoinfarction pattern of hyperkalemia is well known, but at times the ST-segment elevation is so striking that, it becomes very difficult to exclude possibility of coexistent acute infarction. In patients with hyperkalemia, the elevated ST segment is often downsloping, a finding that is somewhat unusual in AMI, which is more likely to be characterized by an ST segment that has a plateau or a shoulder or is upsloping. An echocardiogram can be extremely useful in this situation.[50]

Coronary Vasospasm/Prinzmetal's Angina

When an epicardial artery is completely "pinched off" as a result of spasm, the ST segment becomes elevated in the leads facing the affected area, reflecting transmural ischemia. This condition is called Prinzmetal's angina, a form of coronary vasospasm, the spasm is usually brief and the ST segment returns to normal, with no resultant myocardial damage.[69,70] The ST-segment elevations in Prinzmetal's angina and in acute infarction are indistinguishable, since they reflect the same pathophysiological process: transmural ischemia from occlusion of an epicardial artery by transient spasm.[50] As the changes are due to coronary artery spasm rather than acute infarction, they may be completely reversible if treated promptly. ST segment abnormalities may be seen in association with cocaine use and are probably due to a combination of vasospasm and thrombosis.[57]

Pericarditis

Acute pericarditis is commonly mistaken for AMI as both cause chest pain and ST segment elevation. In pericarditis, however, the ST segment elevation is diffuse rather than

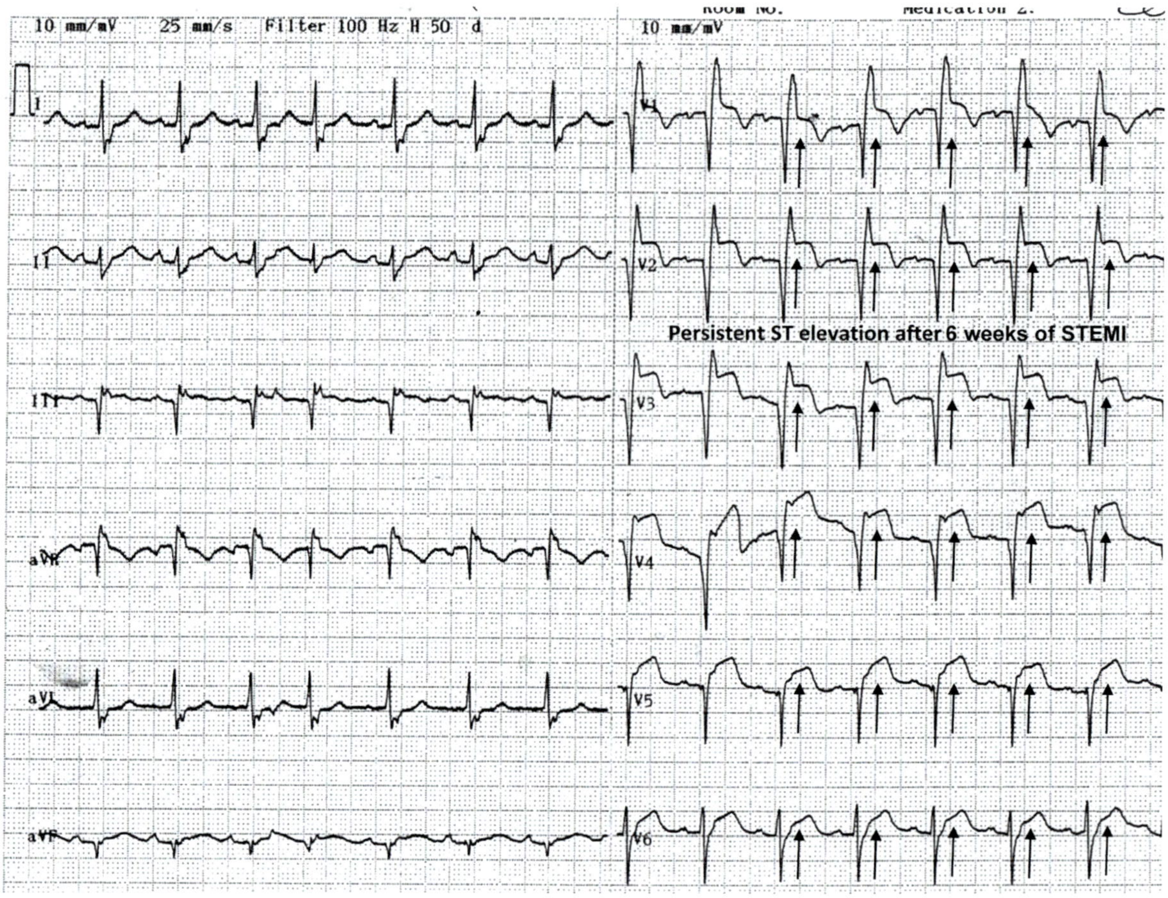

Fig. 8.30: Electrocardiogram (ECG) of left ventricular aneurysm with RBBB. Note persistent ST segment elevation in leads V1–V6 (arrows), 6 weeks after anterior STEMI. Also note that there is no reciprocal ST-segment depression in inferior leads suggestive of acute myocardial infarction.

localized, often being present in all leads except aVR and V1. The elevated ST segments are concave upwards, rather than convex upwards as seen in acute infarction. Depression of the PR segment may also be seen.[57] Acute myocarditis can cause diffuse ST-segment elevation, as does acute pericarditis. Furthermore, at times the prominent ST-segment elevation of acute myocarditis can simulate AMI.[71]

Brugada Syndrome

Right bundle branch block pattern and ST-segment elevation in the right precordial leads in the absence of long QT intervals and any structural heart disease is known as Brugada syndrome.[72] The ST-segment elevation is primarily limited to leads V1 and V2 and can have a saddleback shape, but in typical cases the ST segment begins from the top of the R-wave, is downsloping, and ends with an inverted T-wave. This pattern is so distinctive that it should not be mistaken for acute infarction.

Subarachnoid Hemorrhage

ST-segment abnormalities are seen in association with intracranial (particularly subarachnoid) hemorrhage. ST-segment elevation or depression may be seen; a putative explanation is that altered autonomic tone affects the duration of ventricular repolarization, producing these changes.[57]

IDENTIFICATION OF THE EXACT SITE OF THE INFARCT-RELATED ARTERY

Heart is supplied by two coronary arteries, left and right coronary artery. Left main coronary artery (LMCA) divides into two branches LAD coronary artery and left circumflex coronary artery. The LAD coronary artery and its branches usually supply the anterior and anterolateral walls of the left ventricle and the anterior two-thirds of the septum. The LCX coronary artery and its branches usually supply the posterolateral wall of the left ventricle. The RCA supplies the right ventricle, the inferior (diaphragmatic) and true posterior walls of the left ventricle, and the posterior-third of the septum. The RCA also gives off the AV nodal coronary artery in 85–90% of individuals; in the remaining 10–15%, this artery is a branch of the LCX.

ECG Criteria of Left Main Coronary Artery Occlusion

An acute obstruction of left main coronary artery (LMCA) is encountered approximately in only 0.5% of AMI cases.

Acute myocardial infarction due to acute obstruction of LMCA, which has poor prognosis, causes severe LV dysfunction and life-threatening malignant arrhythmias as a consequence of large infarction area.[73] Prediction of acute LMCA obstruction is important with regard to selecting the appropriate treatment strategy and estimating the prognosis. Both acute LMCA and LAD obstruction generally produce anterior wall ischemia, resulting in ST-segment elevation in the precordial leads. One can easily assume that LMCA, but not LAD, obstruction is ordinarily associated with posterior wall ischemia. Acute LMCA obstruction may show ST segment shifts in the precordial leads different from those found in acute LAD obstruction, due to concomitant posterior wall ischemia, which produces reciprocal changes in the precordial leads. The ST segment in lead aVR would be elevated in acute LMCA obstruction, and that the relationship between the ST segment elevation in lead aVR and that in the precordial leads would differ between acute LMCA and LAD obstruction.[74] In anterior STEMI, it has been reported that ST elevation in lead aVR is associated with left main occlusion and with MI in the presence of multivessel coronary artery disease. It also has been reported in anterior STEMI that aVR ST elevation greater than elevation in V1 is associated with occlusion of the left main artery and that elevation in aVR less than elevation in V1 is associated with proximal LAD occlusion (Fig. 8.31).[75] In lead aVR, ST-segment elevation is significantly higher in LMCA stenosis patients than in LAD or RCA stenosis patients. The finding of a higher ST elevation in lead aVR than in lead V1 distinguished LMCA lesions from LAD lesions with a sensitivity of 81% and a specificity of 80%.[76] The presence of RBBB with ST elevation in lead aVR increases the possibility that the LMCA is the culprit vessel in acute coronary syndrome.[76-78] Other than anterior STEMI, LMCA occlusion should be suspected in severely ill patients with widespread ST-segment depressions, especially in leads V4–V6 with inverted T-waves when accompanied with lead aVR ST elevation (Fig. 8.32).[79] ST elevation in aVR is not entirely specific to LMCA occlusion. It may also be seen with proximal LAD artery occlusion and severe triple-vessel disease.

ECG Criteria of Left Anterior Descending Artery Occlusion

The location of the occlusion within the left anterior descending coronary artery (LAD), that is, whether proximal or distal, is suggested by the chest leads in which the ST-segment elevation occurs and the presence of ST-segment elevation or depression in other leads. Occlusion of the proximal LAD above the first septal branch results in involvement of the basal portion of the left ventricle, as well as the anterior and lateral walls and the interventricular septum and associated with ST-segment elevation in leads V1 through V4, I, aVL, and often aVR. It will also be associated with reciprocal ST-segment depression in the LII, LIII, aVF, and often V5.[10] When the occlusion is located between the first septal and first diagonal branches the ST segment in lead V1 will not be elevated. When the occlusion is located more distally, that is, below both the first septal and first diagonal branches, the ST segment will not be elevated in leads V1, aVR, or aVL, and the ST segment will not be depressed in leads II, III, or aVF.[10]

Isolated occlusion of the first diagonal branch may also cause ST elevation in lead aVL. However, the ECG can be useful in distinguishing isolated diagonal branch (D1) occlusion from a LAD artery occlusion proximal to the first diagonal branch. Occlusion of the diagonal branch typically results in ST elevation in leads I, aVL, and V2 with ST segments in leads V3 and V4 either isoelectric or depressed. In contrast, a LAD occlusion proximal to the first diagonal branch results in ST elevation extending beyond lead V2–V3 and occasionally, to V4–V6.[37,38]

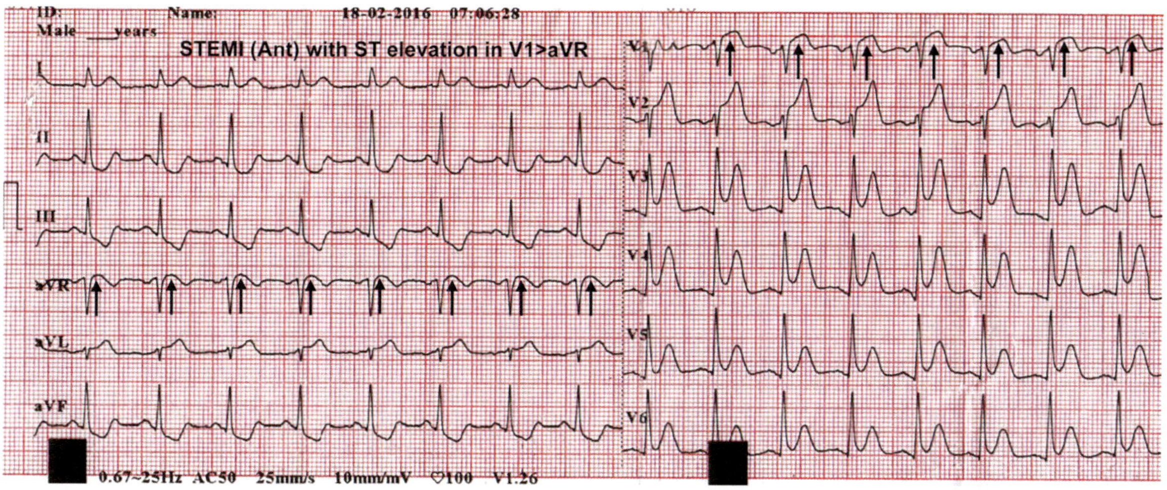

Fig. 8.31: Electrocardiogram (ECG) is suggestive of STEMI (anterior) showing ST elevation in leads LI, aVL, V1–V6 with reciprocal ST depression in inferior leads. Note ST elevation in V1>aVR, suggesting anterior MI due to possible proximal left anterior descending artery (LAD) occlusion. ECG of anterior STEMI due to left main coronary artery (LMCA) occlusion usually shows ST elevation in aVR > V1..

ECG Signs of Different Sites of Left Anterior Descending Occlusion in the Context of Anterior ST-Elevation Myocardial Infarction:[80]

- Before first septal branch (S1)
  - ST-elevation in lead V1 and aVR
  - Complete right bundle branch block
  - ST-depression in lead V5
  - ST elevation in lead V1>2.5 mm strongly predicted LAD occlusion proximal to S1.
- Distal to S1
  Abnormal Q-waves in V4-6 were associated with occlusion distal to S1.
- Proximal to First diagonal (D1)
  Abnormal Q-wave in lead aVL is associated with occlusion proximal to D1.
- Distal to D1
  ST depression in aVL is suggestive of occlusion distal to D1.
- Inferior reciprocal ST depression ≥1.0 mm strongly predicts proximal LAD occlusion (Fig. 8.33), whereas absence of inferior ST depression predicts mid or distal occlusion (Fig. 8.34).

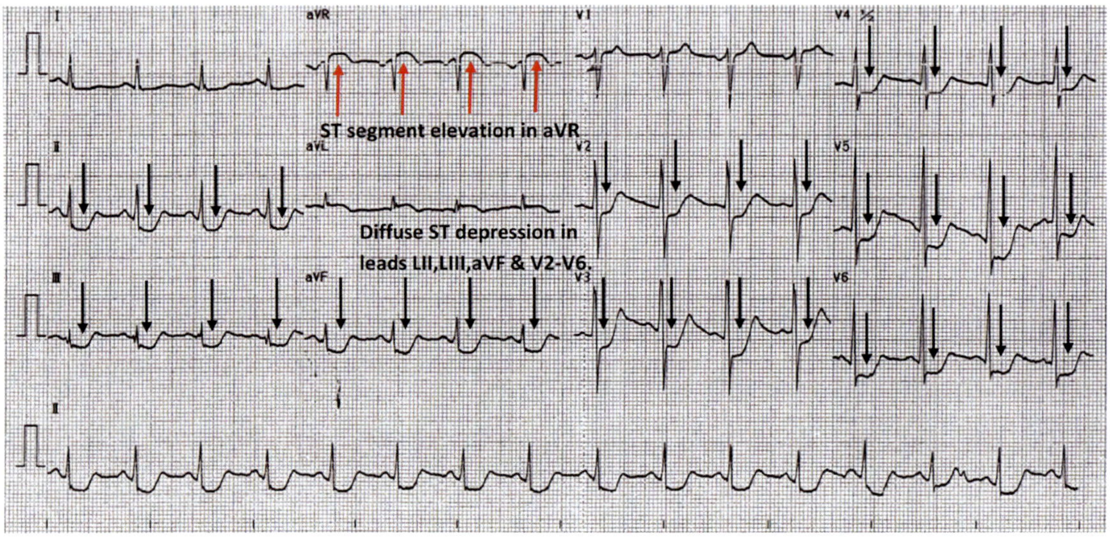

Fig. 8.32: Electrocardiogram (ECG) shows diffuse ST-segment depression in both anterior and inferior leads (black arrows) with ST segment elevation in lead aVR (red arrows), suggesting left main coronary artery (LMCA) occlusion.

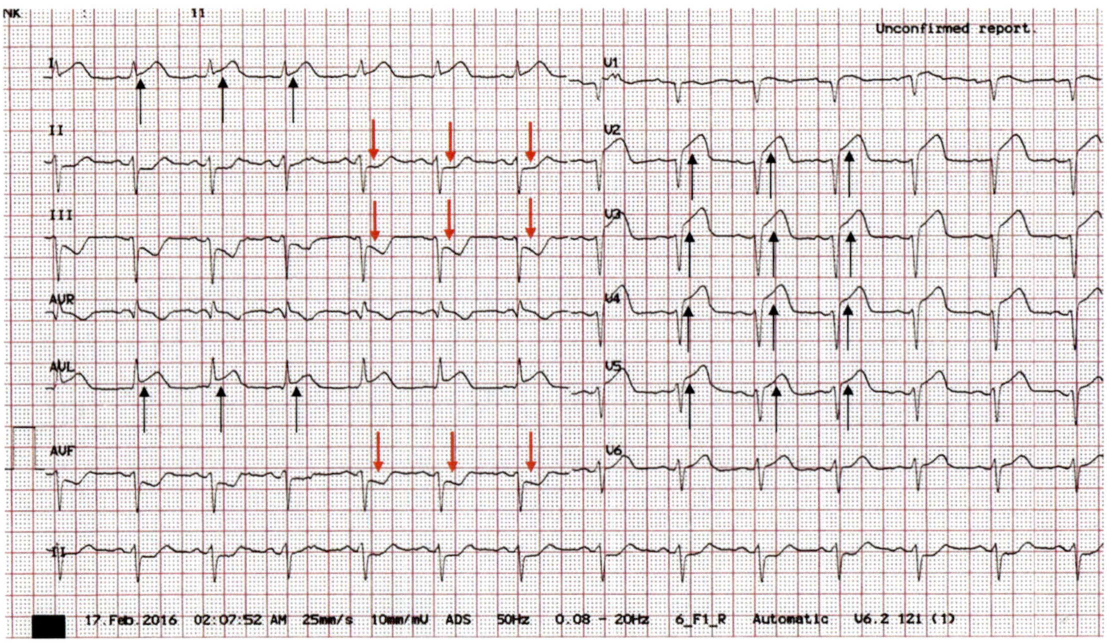

Fig. 8.33: Electrocardiogram (ECG) shows anterior STEMI with ST elevation in leads LI, aVL, and V2–V5 (black arrows). Also note greater than 1 mm reciprocal ST-segment depression in inferior leads (LII, LIII, and aVF) (red arrows) suggestive of proximal left anterior descending artery (LAD) occlusion.

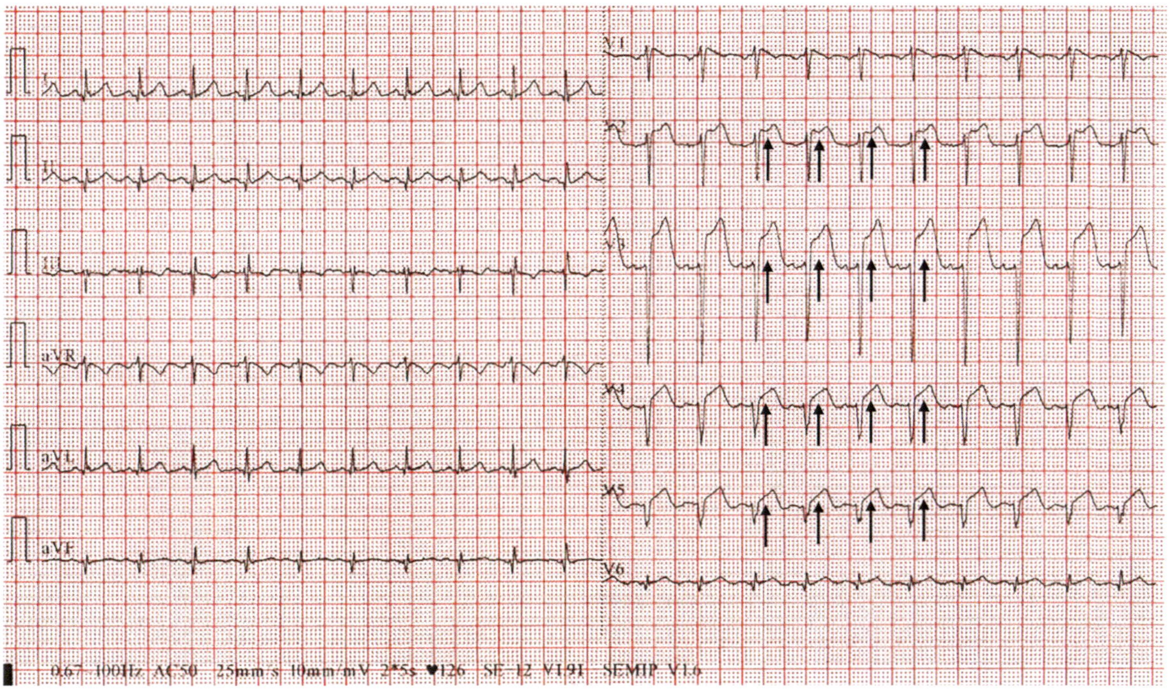

Fig. 8.34: Electrocardiogram (ECG) shows anterior STEMI with ST elevation in leads V2–V5 (black arrows) with sinus tachycardia (heart rate 125/min). Note no reciprocal ST-segment depression in inferior leads (LII, LIII, and aVF). This ECG is suggestive of possible mid or distal left anterior descending artery (LAD) occlusion.

In 2008, de Winter et al. described a novel STEMI-equivalent ECG pattern that signifies acute occlusion of the proximal LAD. Diagnostic criteria of "de Winter ST/T-wave" on ECG include 1–3 mm of ST-depression that is upsloping at the J-point in leads V2 through V6 and associated with persistently tall, upright, and symmetric precordial T waves (Figs 8.35A to C).[34,81] The ascending limb of the T-wave commence below the isoelectric baseline and the changes are dynamic. de Winter T represents approximately 2% of LAD occlusions and recognized as a STEMI equivalent.

Another morphology of T-waves is suggestive of LAD artery occlusion termed as Wellens' syndrome/sign and is evidenced by the appearance of deeply inverted or biphasic T-waves in V2–V4. This pattern is highly specific for a critical stenosis of the LAD and they are at extremely high risk for extensive anterior wall MI within the next few days to weeks. Electrocardiogram criteria include; (1) Deeply-inverted or biphasic T-waves in V2–V4 (may extend to V1–V6); (2) isoelectric or minimally-elevated ST segment (< 1 mm); (3)preserved precordial R-wave progression and no precordial Q waves (Fig. 8.36).

Electrocardiogram Criteria of Left Circumflex Occlusion

The vast majority of patients (93%) with an acute anterior MI due to LAD artery occlusion have an "anteroseptal" pattern (ST elevation in leads V1–V3) (Fig. 8.37). In contrast, isolated ST elevation in leads V4–V6, without ST elevation in leads V1–V3 is usually due to an occlusion of the LCX artery or distal diagonal branch rather than the main LAD.[37,48,82] ST elevation in leads I and aVL are due to occlusion of the LCX artery (Fig. 8.38), reciprocal ST depression is usually observed in leads V1–V3 because the vascular bed supplied by the LCX extends more posteriorly.[83] ST elevation in leads I and aVL may also be due to isolated diagonal branch (D1) occlusion. Proximal LCX obstruction may produce ST segment elevation in inferior (LII, LIII, and aVF) and leads V4–V6 and this pattern of ECG is called inferolateral STEMI (Figs. 8.39A and B). Left circumflex occlusion may be the cause of the inferior MI causing ST elevation in leads LII, LIII, and aVF.

ECG Criteria of Right Coronary Artery Occlusion

The vast majority (80–90%) of patients with ST elevation in the "inferior" leads have an occlusion of the RCA; however, an occlusion of the LCX artery can produce a similar ECG pattern. In addition to ST elevation in the inferior leads II, III, and aVF, reciprocal ST depression in lead aVL is seen in almost all patients with acute inferior MI (Fig. 8.40).[41,84] Because the right ventricular branch originates from the proximal RCA, criteria for right ventricular infarction, especially ST elevation in leads V3R and V4R, provide compelling evidence that the infarct-related artery in acute inferior MI is the RCA (Fig. 8.41).[37] In inferior MI due to proximal RCA occlusion with concomitant right ventricular infarction, posterior wall injury may be masked because the two opposed electrical vectors may cancel each other (that is, ST elevation in leads V1–V3 with right ventricular infarction and reciprocal ST depression in these same leads with concurrent posterior infarction). A more direct sign of posterior wall injury is ST elevation in leads V7–V9.[85]

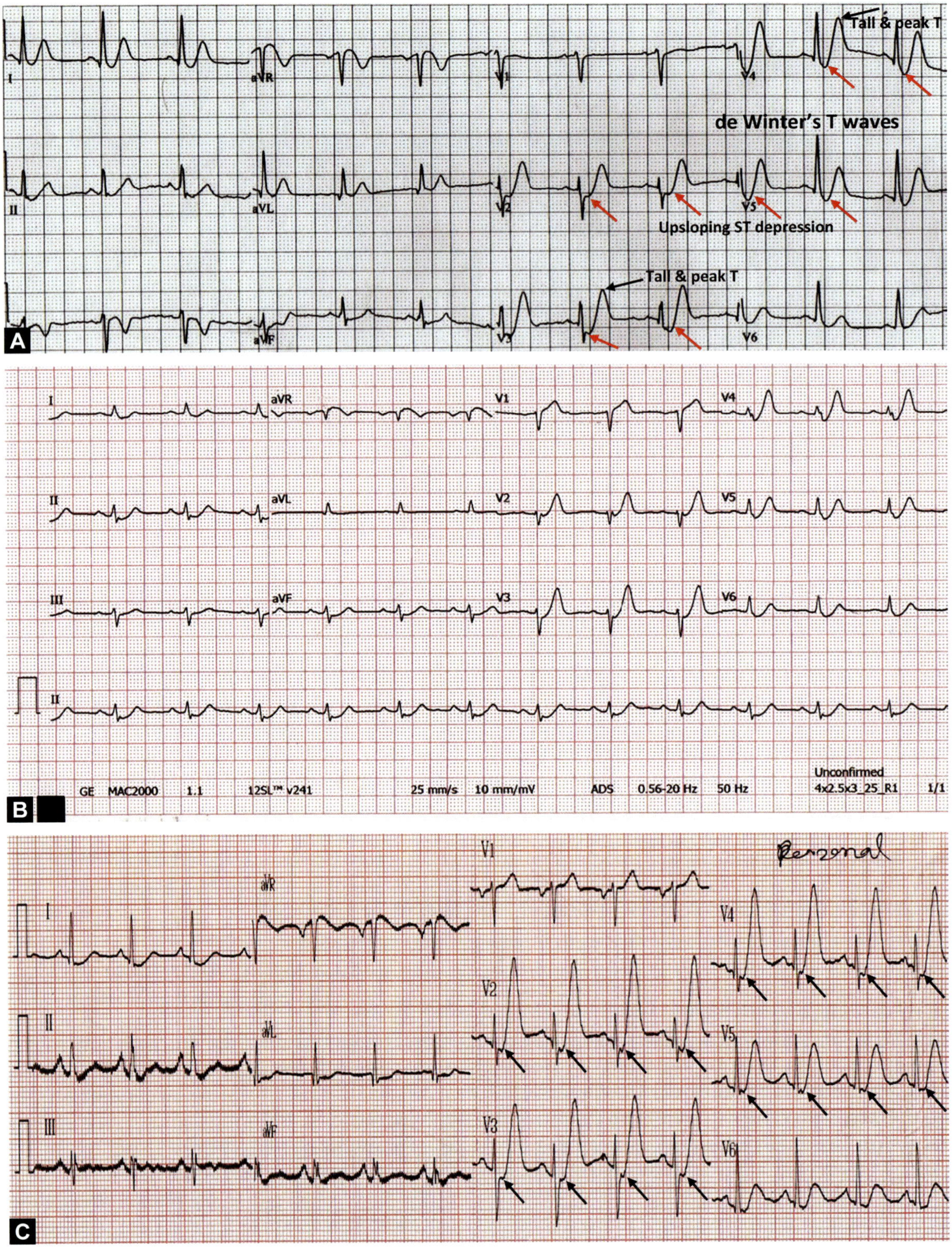

Figs. 8.35A to C: (A) Electrocardiogram (ECG) showing de Winter's T waves in chest leads suggestive of proximal left anterior descending artery (LAD) occlusion. ECG shows—1. Upsloping ST depression in the precordial leads V2–V5 (> 1 mm at J-point) (red arrows). 2. Tall and peaked T waves in leads V3 and V4 (black arrows). 3. Ascending limb of the T-wave commencing below the isoelectric baseline. (B) Electrocardiogram (ECG) showing de Winter's T waves in chest leads suggestive of proximal left anterior descending artery (LAD) occlusion. ECG shows upsloping ST depression greater than 1 mm in the precordial leads V2–V6 and peaked T waves in leads V2–V4 along with some ST depression in leads LII and aVF. Note ascending limb of the T-wave commencing below the isoelectric baseline. (*Source*: Dr Abduz Zaher, Labaid Cardiac Hospital.) (C) Electrocardiogram (ECG) illustrates de Winter's T waves in chest leads V2–V5. ECG shows upsloping ST depression greater than 1 mm in the precordial leads and peaked T waves in leads V2–V5 along with some ST elevation in lead aVR. Note ascending limb of the T-wave commencing below the isoelectric baseline (arrows). Coronary angiogram of this patient showed proximal LAD occlusion and he was treated with primary PCI. (*Source:* Dr Mahbubor Rahman, Labaid Cardiac Hospital.)

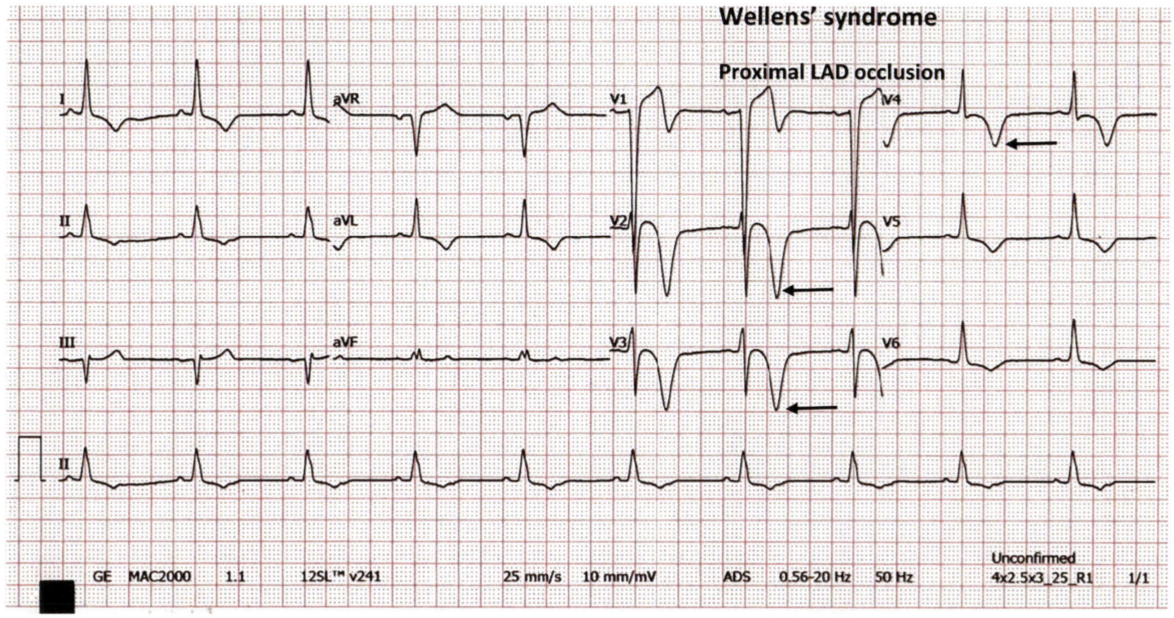

Fig. 8.36: Electrocardiogram (ECG) is suggestive of Wellens' syndrome (Type-B) showing—1. Deeply-inverted T waves (>5 mm) in leads V2–V4 (arrows); 2. Minimally-elevated ST segment in leads V1–V3; 3. Preserved precordial R-wave progression and no precordial Q waves. This pattern is highly specific for a critical stenosis of the LAD and they are at extremely high risk for extensive anterior wall MI within the next few days to weeks.

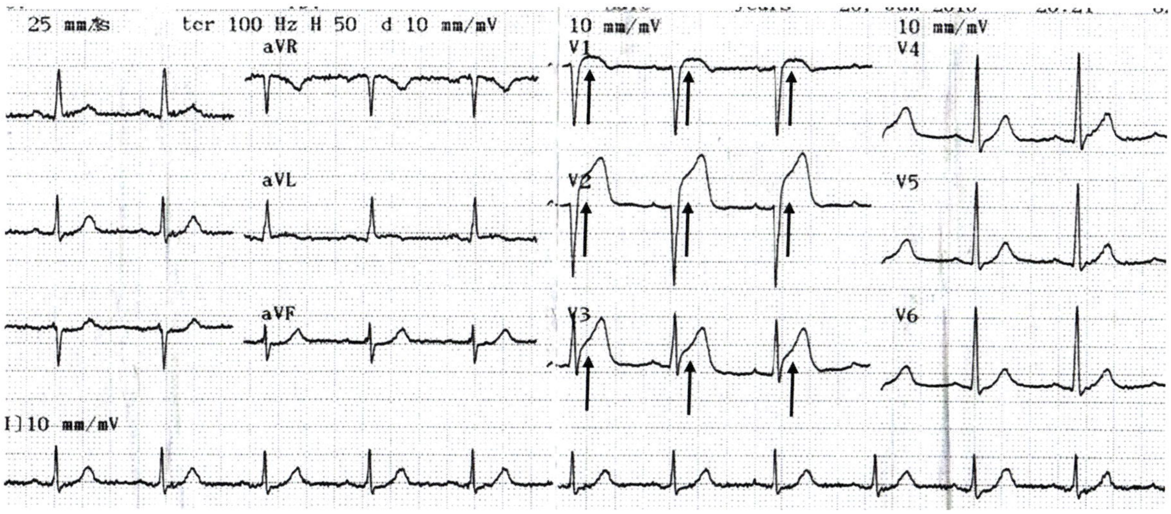

Fig. 8.37: Electrocardiogram (ECG) is suggestive of acute anteroseptal STEMI showing ST segment elevation (arrows) in leads V1–V3. Note no significant reciprocal ST depression in inferior leads.

ECG Distinction between Right Coronary Artery versus Left Circumflex Coronary Artery Related Acute Inferior Myocardial Infarction

1. Inferior wall infarction that results in ST-segment elevation in leads II, III, and aVF may be the result of occlusion of either the RCA or the LCX coronary artery, depending on which provides the posterior descending branch, that is, which is the dominant vessel. When the RCA is occluded, the spatial vector of the ST segment will usually be directed more to the right than when the LCX is occluded. This will result in greater ST-segment elevation in lead III than in lead II and will often is associated with ST-segment depression in leads I and aVL. In LCX occlusion ST elevation in LII is usually greater than the ST elevation in LIII (Figs. 8.42A and B).[10,37,38]
2. Because the right ventricular branch originates from the proximal RCA, criteria for right ventricular infarction, especially ST elevation in leads V3R and V4R, provide compelling evidence that the infarct-related artery in acute inferior MI is the RCA.[38]

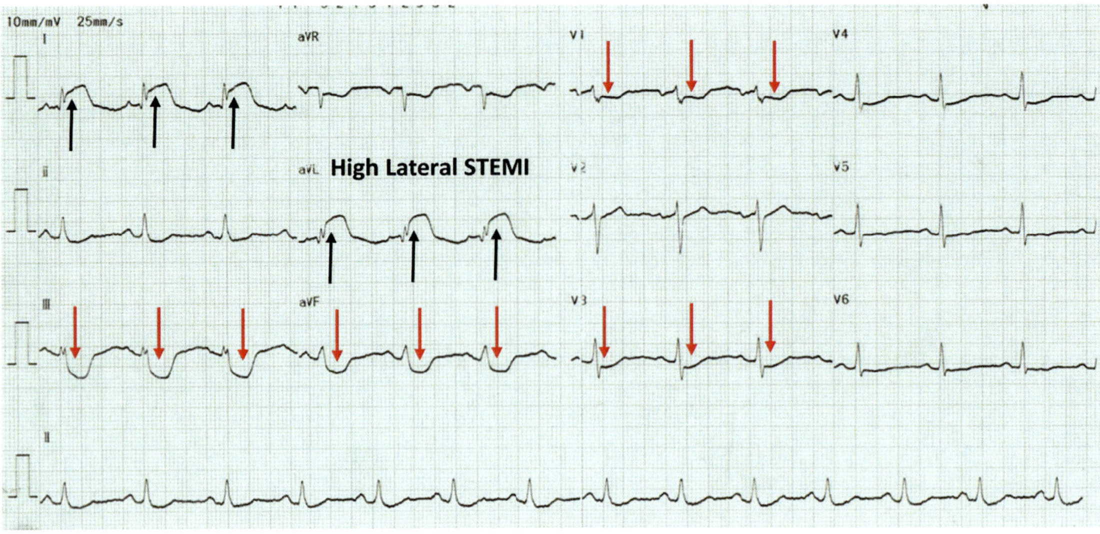

Fig. 8.38: Electrocardiogram (ECG) is suggestive of high lateral STEMI due to left circumflex artery (LCX) occlusion. Note ST elevation in leads LI and aVL (black arrows) and reciprocal ST-segment depression in leads LIII, aVF, V1, and V3 (red arrows).

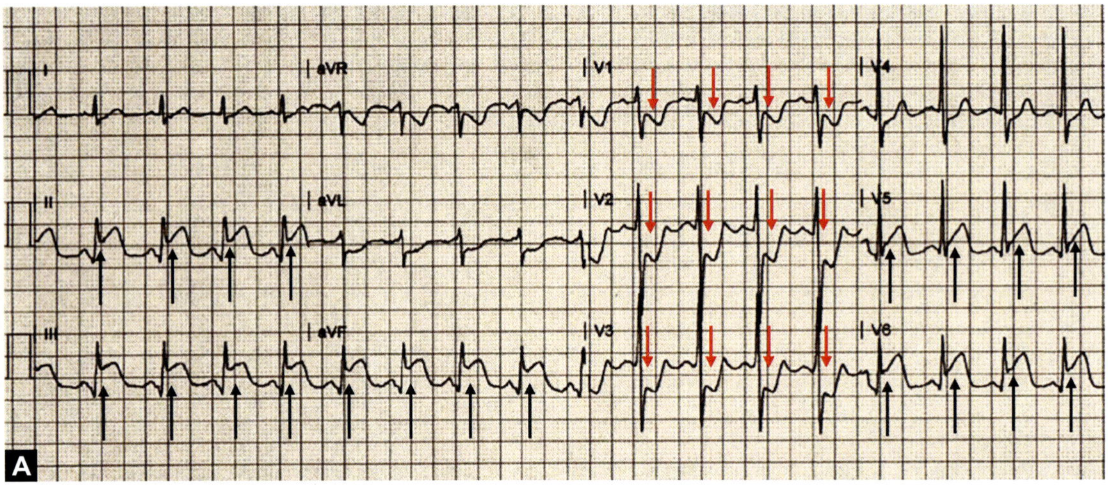

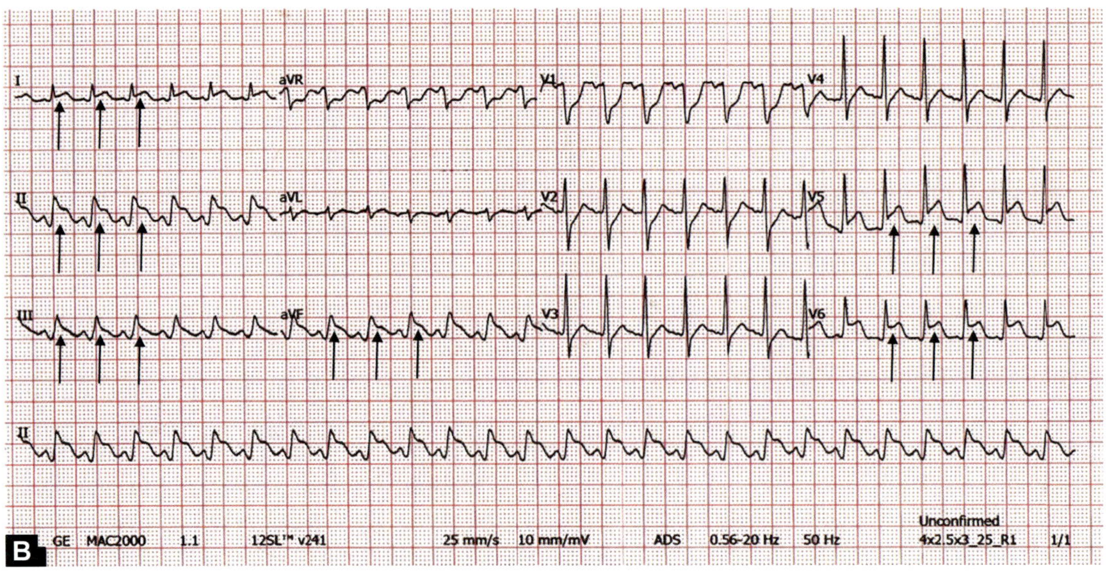

Figs. 8.39A and B: (A) Electrocardiogram (ECG) shows ST-segment elevation in leads LII, LIII, aVF, V5, and V6 (black arrows) with ST segment depression in leads V1–V3 (red arrows). Proximal LCX obstruction may produce ST-segment elevation in inferior (LII, LIII, and aVF) leads and V4–V6 and this pattern of ECG is called inferolateral STEMI. Marked ST depression in this ECG strip in leads V1–V3 are possibly due to associated posterior infarction. (B) Electrocardiogram (ECG) shows ST-segment elevation in leads LI, LII, LIII, aVF, V5, and V6 (arrows) and this ECG is suggestive of inferolateral STEMI possibly due to LCX obstruction. ECG also shows marked sinus tachycardia (heart rate 150/min).

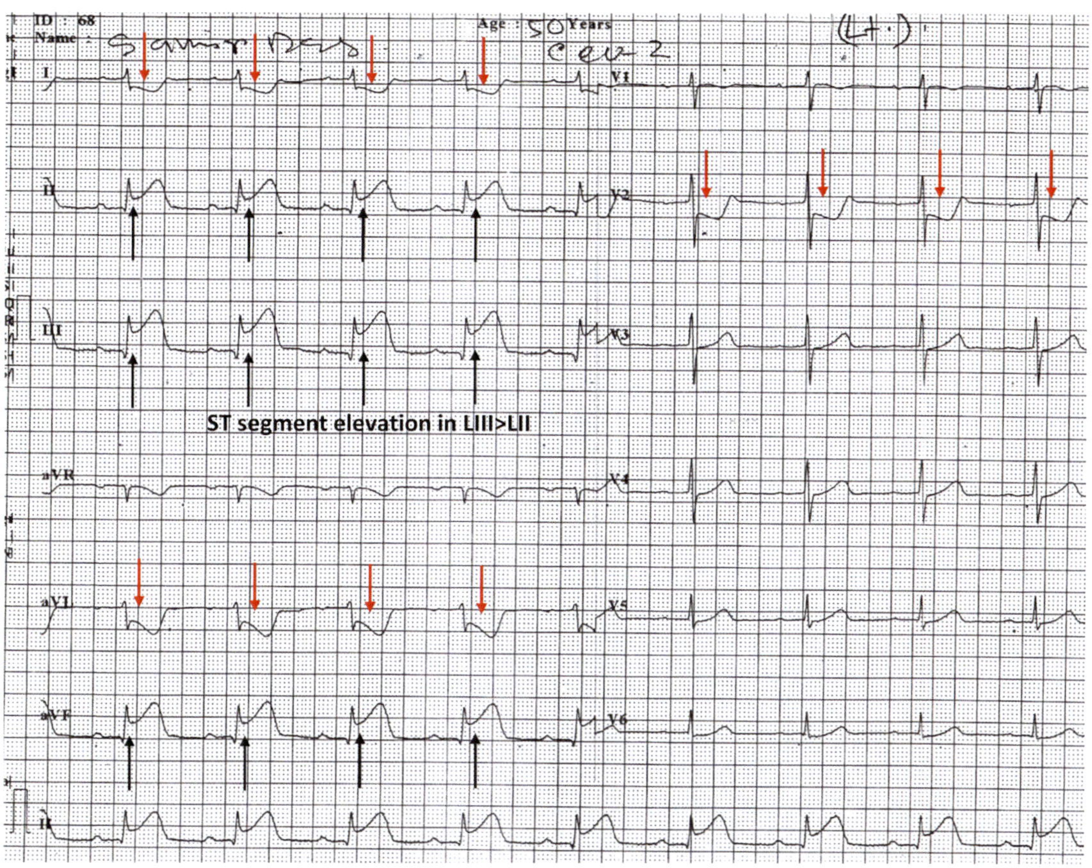

Fig. 8.40: Electrocardiogram (ECG) is suggestive of acute inferior myocardial infarction with ST segment elevation in LII, LIII, and aVF (black arrows) with reciprocal ST depression in LI and aVL (red arrows). Note also marked ST-segment depression in lead V2 with tall R wave, may be due to posterior extension. In this ECG, the ST elevation in LIII greater than LII, suggestive of right coronary artery (RCA) occlusion.

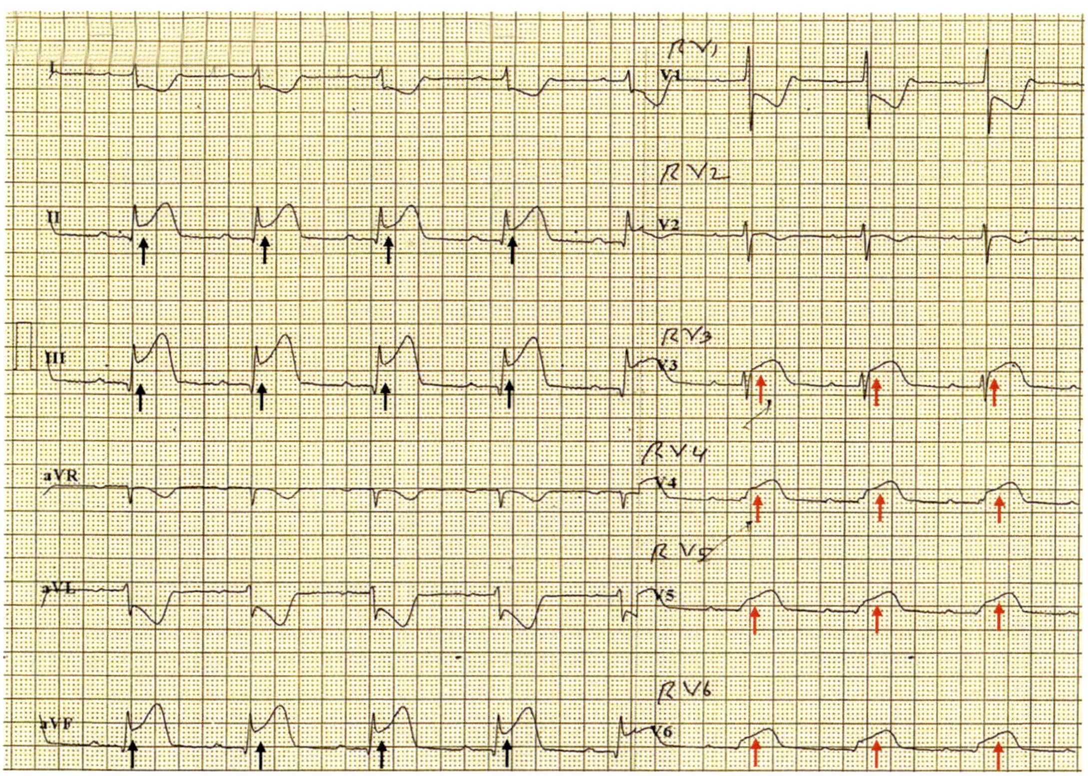

Fig. 8.41: Electrocardiogram (ECG) of acute inferior and right ventricular (RV) infarction. This ECG strip shows ST segment elevation in LII, LIII, and aVF (black arrows) with reciprocal ST-segment depression in LI and aVL. Note also ST-segment elevation in right sided leads from V3R–V6R (red arrows), most remarkable in leads V3R andV4R suggestive of RV infarction.

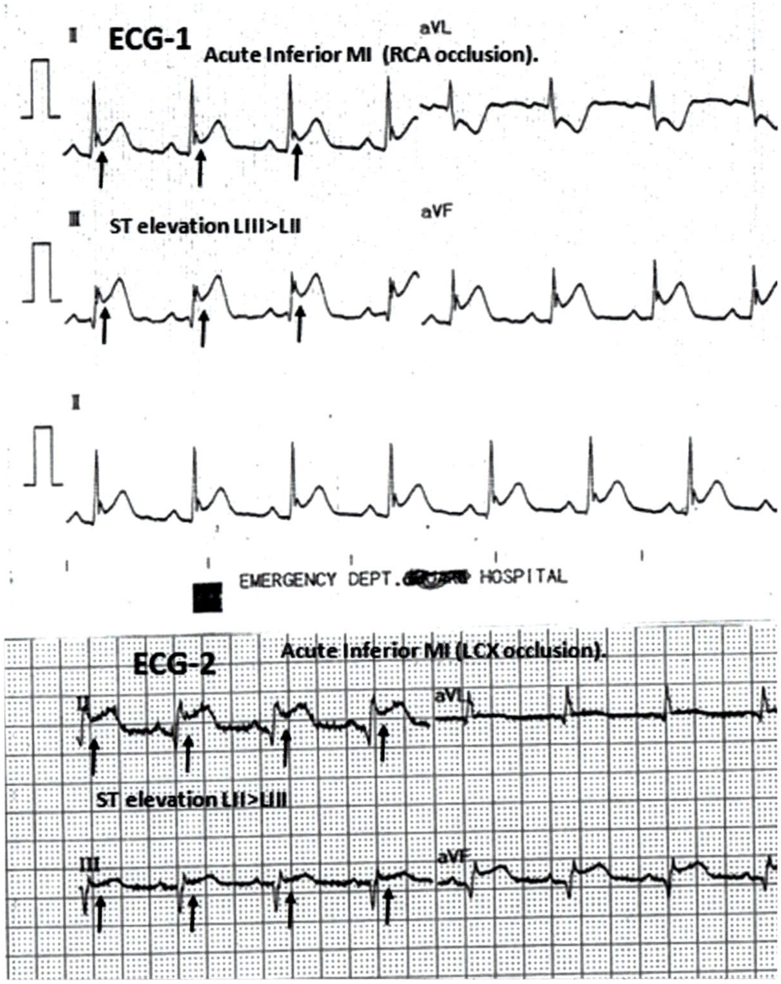

Fig. 8.42A: Both ECG 1 and 2 are suggestive of inferior STEMI but if you look carefully in ECG–1, ST segment elevation in LIII>LII, suggestive of right coronary artery (RCA) occlusion and in ECG–2, ST segment elevation in LII>LIII, suggestive of left circumflex artery (LCX) occlusion.

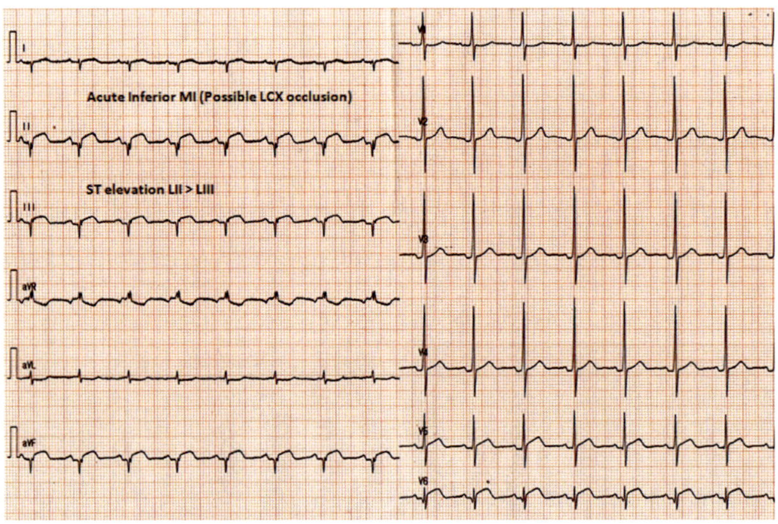

Fig. 8.42B: This ECG is suggestive of acute inferior myocardial infarction with ST segment elevation in LII,LIII and aVF. In this ECG, the ST elevation in LII > LIII, suggestive of left circumflex artery (LCX) occlusion. Also note tall R waves with upright T in V1 and V2 with some ST segment elevation in leads V5 and V6 suggestive of possible posterior and lateral wall involvement. Inferior wall infarction that results in ST-segment elevation in leads II, III, and aVF may be the result of occlusion of either the right coronary artery (RCA) or the left circumflex coronary artery (LCX). If RCA is occluded, this will result in greater ST-segment elevation in lead III than in lead II and will often be associated with ST-segment depression in leads I and aVL. But in LCX occlusion ST elevation in LII is usually greater than the ST elevation in LIII and reciprocal ST depression in LI and aVL may be absent. Note in this ECG there is no associated reciprocal ST segment depression in LI and aVL, and this ECG finding is also suggestive of LCX occlusion.

Table 8.1: Localization of site of occlusion in STEMI

Location of STEMI	*Leads showing ST elevation*	*Site of occlusion*
Extensive anterior MI	ST segment elevation in LI, aVL and, V1–V6	Proximal LAD
Anteroseptal MI	ST elevation V1–V3/V4	Mid LAD
Anterolateral MI	ST elevation in LI, aVL,V5 and V6	LAD/LCX
High lateral MI	ST elevation in LI and aVL	LCX (OM branch) or First diagonal (D1) branch of LAD or Ramus intermedius
Inferior MI	ST elevation in LII, LIII and aVF	RCA occlusion (80–90%), LCX occlusion 10–20%
Inferolateral MI	ST elevation in LII, LIII, aVF, V5 and V6	LCX
Posterior MI	ST elevation in V7–V9/ST segment depression in leads V1–V3 and dominant R-wave (R/S ratio > 1) in V1 or V2 in 12 leads ECG	RCA/LCX
Right ventricular infarction	1. 12 lead ECG: ST elevation in V1. 2. Right-sided leads: ST elevation V3R–V6R	RCA

(LAD: left anterior descending artery; LCX: left circumflex artery; RCA: right coronary artery; OM: obtuse marginal; STEMI: ST-elevation myocardial infarction; ECG: electrocardiogram; MI: myocardial infarction)

3. An additional criterion for identifying the culprit artery in acute inferior MI is the magnitude of ST depression in lead aVL compared to lead I. Greater reciprocal ST depression in lead aVL than in lead I suggests a RCA occlusion.[86,87]
4. The amplitude of the respective R and S waves in lead aVL may help to detect the culprit artery in acute inferior MI. A decrease in R-wave amplitude and an increase in S-wave amplitude with a S:R ratio of greater than 3 predicted RCA occlusion whereas a S:R ratio less than 3 predicted LCX occlusion.[88,89]

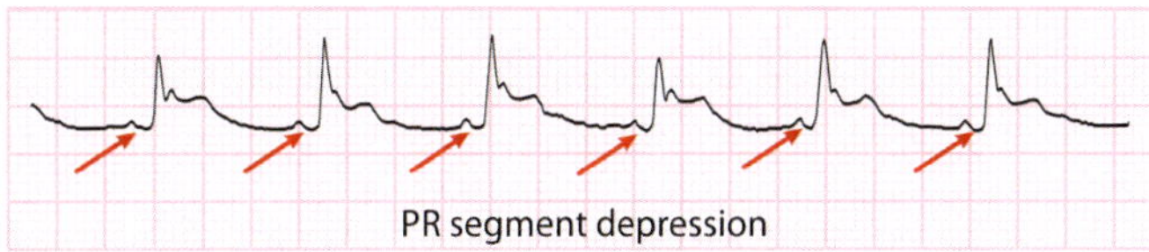

Fig. 8.43: Electrocardiogram (ECG) strip shows PR segment depression in atrial infarction (arrows).

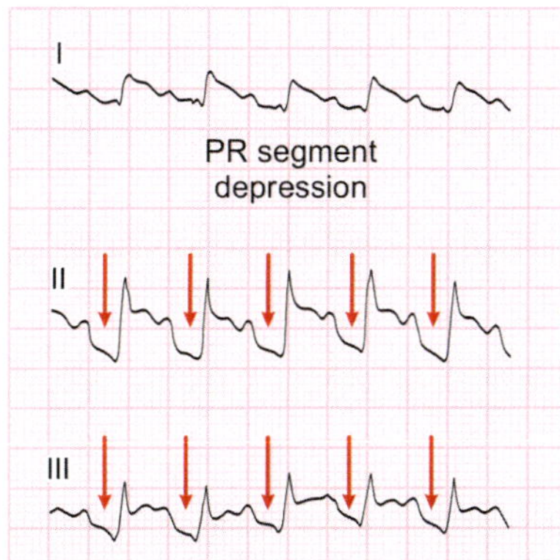

Fig. 8.44: Electrocardiogram (ECG) reveals PR segment depression in LII and LIII associated with inferior STEMI (red arrows).

LOCALIZATION OF SITE OF OCCLUSION IN ST-ELEVATION MYOCARDIAL INFARCTION (TABLE 8.1)

Atrial Infarction

Atrial infarction has been a relatively understudied entity. Its incidence by autopsy study has been widely variable, from 0.7% to 42%, with the largest series of 182 patients demonstrating an incidence of 17%. The right atrium is involved five times as often as the left, with the auricle the predominant site in either atria.[90] Gardin and Singer reviewed several larger series and found the right atrium involved in 81–98% of infarctions, the left atrium involved in 2–19% of infarctions and biatrial involvement in 19–24% of infarctions.[91] PR segment elevation or depression in patients with STEMI indicates concomitant atrial ischemia or infarction (Figs 8.43 and 8.44) (Box 8.2). This finding has been associated with poor outcomes following STEMI and is associated with, increased risk for the development of atrioventricular (AV) block, supraventricular arrhythmias and cardiac free-wall rupture.

Clinical atrial infarction may present with supraventricular arrhythmias, atrial rupture, and hemodynamic compromise from loss of atrial "kick," and thromboembolic phenomena.[90]

Box 8.2: Liu's diagnostic criteria of atrial infarction.[92]

- *Major criteria*
  - PR-segment elevation greater than 0.5 mm in leads V5 and V6 with reciprocal PR-segment depression in leads V1 and V2
  - PR-segment elevation greater than 0.5 mm in lead I with reciprocal depression in leads II and III
  - PR-segment depression greater than 1.5 mm in precordial leads and 1.2 mm in leads I, II, and III associated with any atrial arrhythmias.
- *Minor criteria*
  - Abnormal P waves: M-shaped, W-shaped, irregular, or notched P waves.

Other suggested criteria are PR segment prolongation, P-wave axis changes and abnormal atrial rhythms, including atrial flutter, AF, wandering atrial pacemaker, and AV nodal rhythm.[93,94] In approximately 10% of infarct patients, atrial infarct is suspected. An atrial infarct can manifest itself in atrial rhythm disturbances: atrial fibrillation (AF)/atrial flutter. Because the atria is hemodynamically of minor importance, the consequences of an atrial infarct are limited and therefore often missed.[94]

Arrhythmias and Conduction Disturbances in the Acute Phase

Arrhythmias are frequent complication in patients with AMI. Ventricular tachycardia (VT), ventricular fibrillation (VF), and complete atrioventricular block, may be the first manifestation of ischemia and requires immediate correction, since these arrhythmias may cause sudden cardiac death. VF and VT have been reported up to 20% of patients with STEMI.[95] Often arrhythmias are the manifestation of a serious underlying disorder, such as persisting ischemia, severe pump failure, or endogenous factors such as abnormal potassium levels, autonomic imbalances, hypoxia, and acid-base disturbances, that may require corrective measures. The need for arrhythmias treatment depends mainly upon the hemodynamic impact of the rhythm disorder.[10] Early ventricular arrhythmias are a serious complication of MI. However, if they are revealed and treated in time, they apparently do not represent a negative prognostic factor. Later occurred VF or VT is more a symptom of larger MI.[96]

Classification of Peri-Infarction Arrhythmias

Peri-infarction arrhythmias can be broadly classified into the following categories:

1. Supraventricular tachyarrhythmias, including sinus tachycardia, premature atrial contractions, paroxysmal supraventricular tachycardia, atrial flutter, and AF
2. Accelerated junctional rhythms
3. Bradyarrhythmias, including sinus bradycardia and junctional bradycardia
4. Atrioventricular (AV) blocks, including first-degree AV block, second-degree AV block, and third-degree AV block
5. Intraventricular blocks, including left anterior fascicular block, RBBB, and LBBB
6. Ventricular arrhythmias, including premature ventricular contractions (PVCs), accelerated idioventricular rhythm (AIVR), VT, and VF.
7. Reperfusion arrhythmias

Ventricular Ectopic Rhythms

Ventricular ectopic beats are common during the initial phase of STEMI. Irrespective of their complexity (multiform QRS complex beats, short runs of ventricular beats or the R-on-T phenomenon) their value, as predictor of VF, is questionable.[10]

Ventricular Tachycardia and Ventricular Fibrillation

Patients with AMI are prone to develop potentially life-threatening ventricular arrhythmias such as VT during the acute phase of the MI. Factors associated with the occurrence of ventricular activity in these patients are the presence of extensive myocardial damage, reduced LV function and formation of ventricular aneurysm.[97] Sustained and/or hemodynamically compromising VT occurs almost in 3% of cases of STEMI and requires suppressive therapy. Pulseless VT and VF should be managed according to the resuscitation guidelines.[98]

Accelerated Idioventricular Rhythm

Accelerated idioventricular rhythm appears similar to VT but is benign and doesn't need any treatment. It can most easily be distinguished from VT in that the rate is less than 120 and usually less than 100 beats per minute. Accelerated idioventricular rhythm has been considered a marker of successful reperfusion in fibrinolytic-treated patients. Accelerated idioventricular rhythm is the most frequent arrhythmia occurring during PPCI in patients with STEMI. However, AIVR is associated with extensive myocardial damage and delayed microvascular reperfusion.[99]

Supraventricular Arrhythmias

Atrial fibrillation, which complicates 10–20% of STEMI, is more prevalent in older patients and in those with severe LV damage and heart failure. Atrial fibrillation is associated with increased in-hospital mortality.[100] Atrial fibrillation, which is not directly life-threatening for the patients, frequently occurs in patients with larger MI and it is an independent predictor of a poor long-term prognosis of these patients. In many cases this arrhythmia is well-tolerated and no specific treatment is required. In other instances, the high ventricular response contributes to heart failure and prompt treatment is needed.

Sinus Bradycardia and High Grade Heart Block

Sinus bradycardia: is common (9–25%) in the first hour, particularly in inferior infarction.[101] If associated with hemodynamic compromise it should be treated. Data from four large, randomized trials suggest that AV block occurs in almost 7% and persistent LBBB in up to 5.3% of cases of STEMI.[102,103] Patients with peri-infarction AV block have an higher in hospital mortality than those with preserved AV conduction. The increased mortality seems related to the extensive myocardial damage required to develop heart block rather than to heart block itself. AV block associated with inferior wall infarction is usually transient, whereas AV block related to anterior wall infarction is more often located below the AV node and associated with an unstable, wide QRS escape rhythm due to extensive myocardial necrosis.

A new LBBB usually indicate extensive anterior infarction with high probability to develop complete AV block and pump failure.[102]

ECG Evidence of Prior Myocardial Infarction

Twelve-lead ECG is an integral part of the evaluation of an acute and a remote MI. Recognition of a prior MI is more difficult because once the repolarization abnormalities (ST-segment and T-wave changes) stabilize after an acute MI, then the Q-wave remains as the only universally recognized sign of MI. Q waves on a 12-lead ECG are markers of a prior MI (Figs. 8.45 and 8.46A and B). However, they may regress or even disappear over time. The fragmented QRS (fQRS) is another recently described sign of a remote MI (Box 8.3).[104-107] Fragmented QRS on 12-lead electrocardiography is defined by the presence of single or multiple notches in the R- or S-wave, without a typical bundle-branch block (Figs. 8.47A and B). Fragmented QRS developed in 51% patients with MI.[108] The specificity of fQRS is inferior to that of a Q-wave for an MI scar (89% vs 99%). However, fQRS has a superior sensitivity and a negative predictive value compared with a Q-wave. In addition, there is an incremental gain in the sensitivity up to 91.4% when these 2 signs (fQRS and Q-wave) are combined. The repolarization abnormalities of MI may also persist indefinitely as a sign of a remote MI in few patients. These abnormalities include persistent ST elevation, ST depression, nonspecific ST T-wave changes, and T-wave inversion.[104-108]

Poor R-wave Progression

Poor R-wave progression refers to the absence of the normal increase in size of the R-wave in the precordial leads as R-wave progress from lead V1 to V6. In lead V1, the R-wave should be small. The R-wave becomes larger throughout the precordial leads to the point where the R-wave is larger than the S-wave in lead V4. The S-wave then becomes quite small in lead V6. By definition poor R-wave progression means R-wave height is less than or equal to 3 mm in V3 (Fig. 8.48). It may be ECG sign of old anteroseptal MI. But it may be a normal variant ECG. Poor R-wave progression may also be due to LV hypertrophy, dilated cardiomyopathy, LBBB or left anterior fascicular block, WPW syndrome or due to inaccurate lead placement.

Significance of Persistently Elevated ST Segment after ST-Elevation Myocardial Infarction

A relative small number of patients after MI still show persistence of ST-segment elevation even days and months after the acute event. Historically, this late persistence of ST-segment elevation has been ascribed to LV aneurysm or impending rupture of free wall or ventricular septum, identifying patients at very high risk for heart failure and death.[10] However, this association is among the most controversial in electrocardiography, since previous studies, including echocardiography and angiography, clearly showed a more severe systolic dysfunction and

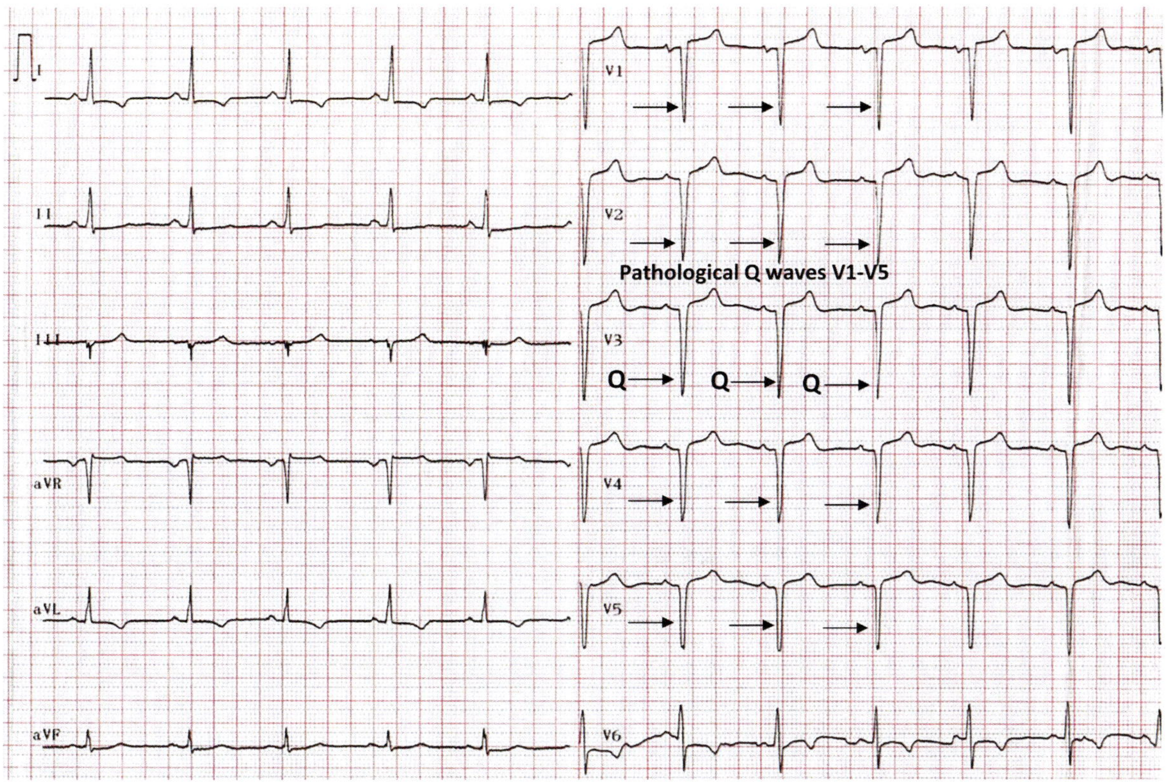

Fig. 8.45: Electrocardiogram (ECG) shows deep pathological Q waves (*arrows*) in leads V1–V5, suggestive of old anterior MI.

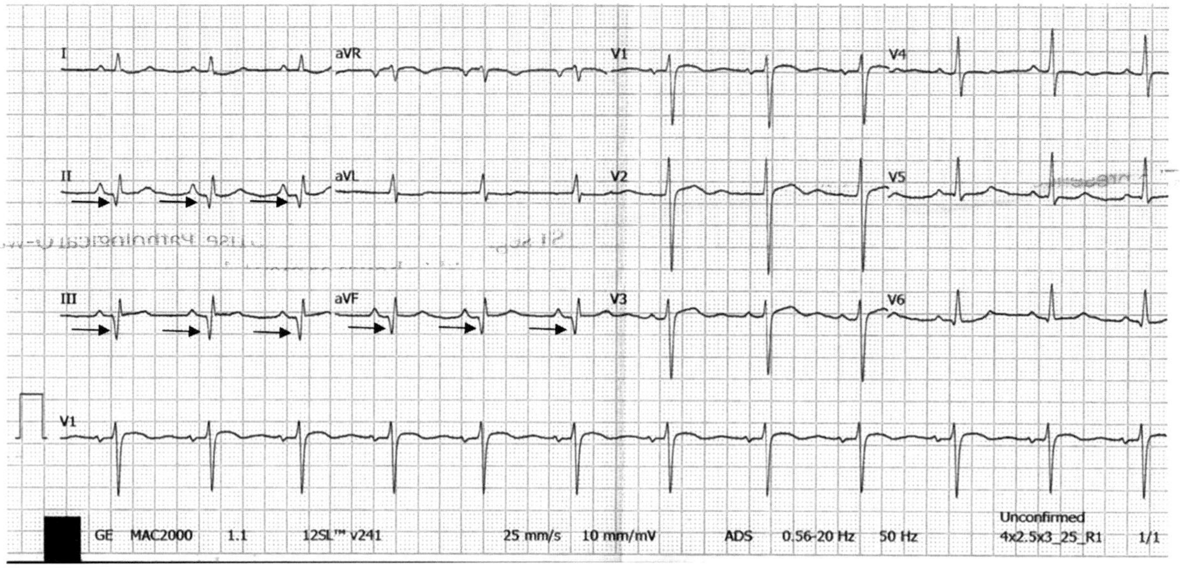

Fig. 8.46A: Electrocardiogram (ECG) shows deep pathological Q waves (*arrows*) in leads LII, LIII, and aVF suggestive of old inferior MI.

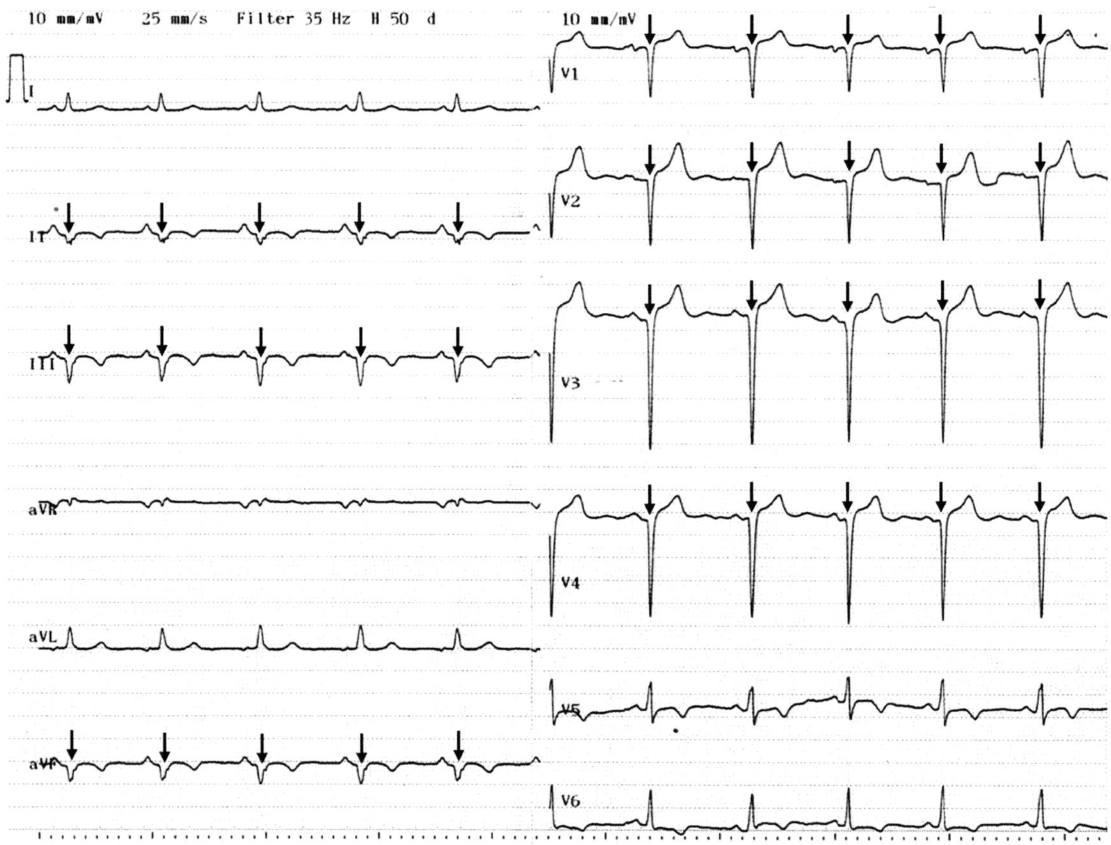

Fig. 8.46B: Electrocardiogram (ECG) shows deep pathological Q waves (*arrows*) in leads LII, LIII, and aVF and V1–V4 suggestive of old inferior and anterior MI.

wall motion abnormalities in patients with persistent ST elevation. Other than LV aneurysm the presence of persisting ST-elevation seems related to the presence of large microvascular damage in the context of transmural necrosis. Persistent ST-segment elevation may be associated with LV aneurysm formation (Fig. 8.49), but more likely to occur with regional contractile dysfunction.[109] In one study, persistent ST segment elevation was associated with LV aneurysm in 30% of patients.[110] In the pre-thrombolytic and thrombolytic eras, persistent ST-segment elevation on 12-lead ECG was found to be associated with the development of postinfarct LV aneurysm, often as a result of failure of reperfusion treatment. ST-segment elevation may still be found persistently raised after successful PPCI.

Box 8.3: Electrocardiogram evidence of fragmentation of QRS (fQRS) complex.

- *Fragmentation of narrow QRS is defined as:*
  - Presence of an additional R-wave (R') or
  - Notching in the nadir of the S-wave, or
  - The presence of more than 1 R' in two contiguous leads.
- *Fragmentation of wide complex QRS is defined as:*
  - Various RSR patterns, with more than two R waves or
  - More than two notches in the R-wave, or
  - More than two notches in the downstroke or upstroke of the S-wave.

SUMMARY

ST elevation myocardial infarction (STEMI) is a clinical syndrome defined by characteristic symptoms of myocardial ischemia in association with persistent ST elevation on ECG and subsequent release of biomarkers of myocardial necrosis.

An ST elevation is considered significant—

1. If the vertical distance between the ECG trace and the isoelectric line at a point 0.04 seconds after the J-point is at least 0.1 mV (usually representing 1 mm or 1 small square) in a limb leads.
2. 0.2 mV (2 mm or 2 small squares) in a precordial leads. The isoelectric line is either the PR segment or the TP segment.

So, ST-segment elevation greater than or equal to 1 mm in at least two contiguous limb leads and greater than or equal to 2 mm in chest leads are considered significant (Box 8.4).

The earliest presentation of AMI is the hyperacute T-wave, which is treated the same as ST-segment elevation. In practice this is rarely seen, because it only exists for up to 30 minutes after the onset of infarction. In the first few hours the ST segments usually begin to rise. Pathological Q-waves may appear within hours or may take greater than 24 hours. The T-wave will generally become inverted in the first 24 hours, as the ST elevation begins to resolve. Long-term changes of ECG include persistent Q-waves (in 90% of cases) and persistent inverted T-waves. Persistent ST elevation is rare except in the presence of a ventricular aneurysm.

The differential diagnosis of ST elevation includes STEMI, coronary artery spasm, acute pericarditis, J-point elevation as normal variant, LV hypertrophy, myocarditis, Brugada syndrome, hyperkalemia, pulmonary embolism, and repolarization abnormalities in the setting of bundle-branch blocks. ST elevation has also been reported in various intra-abdominal conditions, including acute pancreatitis, hiatal hernia.

More strictly diagnostic ST elevation in the absence of LV hypertrophy or LBBB is defined as new ST elevation in at least 2 contiguous leads of greater than or equal to 2 mm (0.2 mV) in men or greater than or equal to 1.5 mm (0.15 mV) in women in leads V2–V3 and/or of greater than or equal to 1 mm (0.1 mV) in other contiguous chest leads or the limb

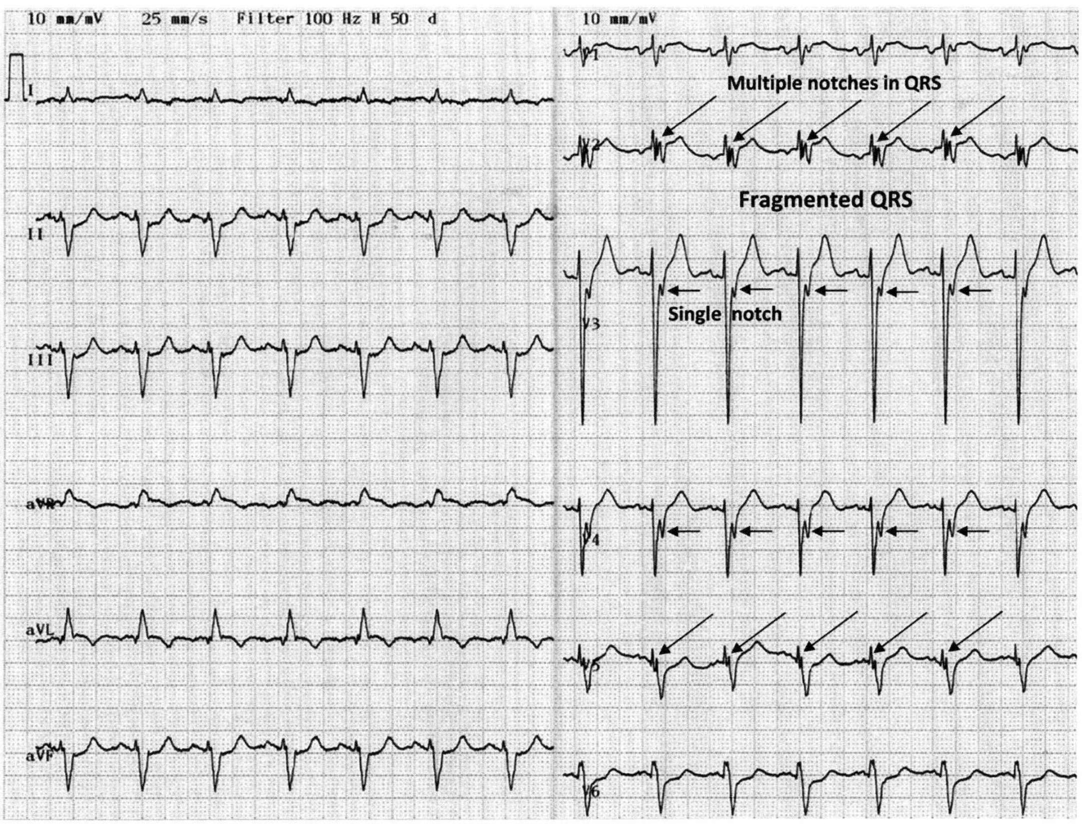

Fig. 8.47A: Electrocardiogram (ECG) reveals presence of fragmented QRS complexes in chest leads suggestive of old MI. Note multiple notches in the QRS complex in leads V2 and V5 (large arrows) and also note single notch in the ascending limb of S wave in V3 and V4 (small arrows).

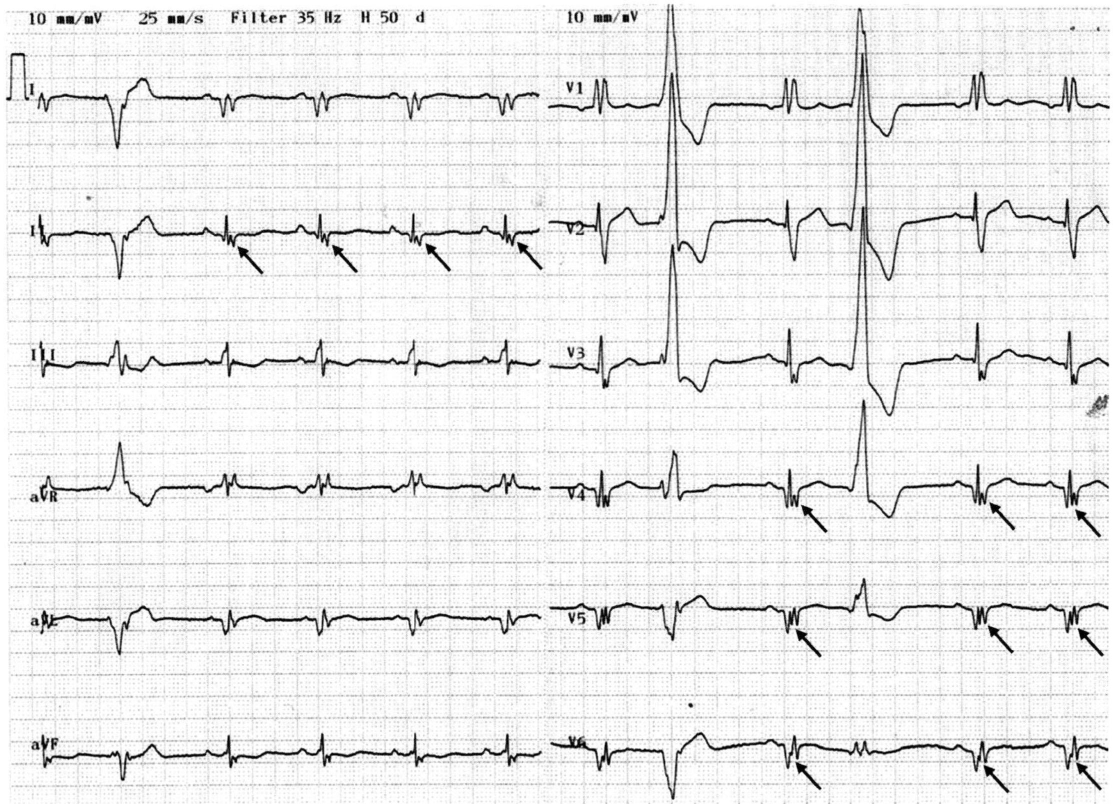

Fig. 8.47B: Electrocardiogram (ECG) shows presence of fragmentation of QRS complex (fQRS) in leads LII, V4–V6. Note more than 2 notches in the downstroke and upstroke of the S waves (arrows). Presence of pathological Q waves in leads L1, aVL, and V4–V6 is suggestive of old anterolateral MI. Also note few PVC.

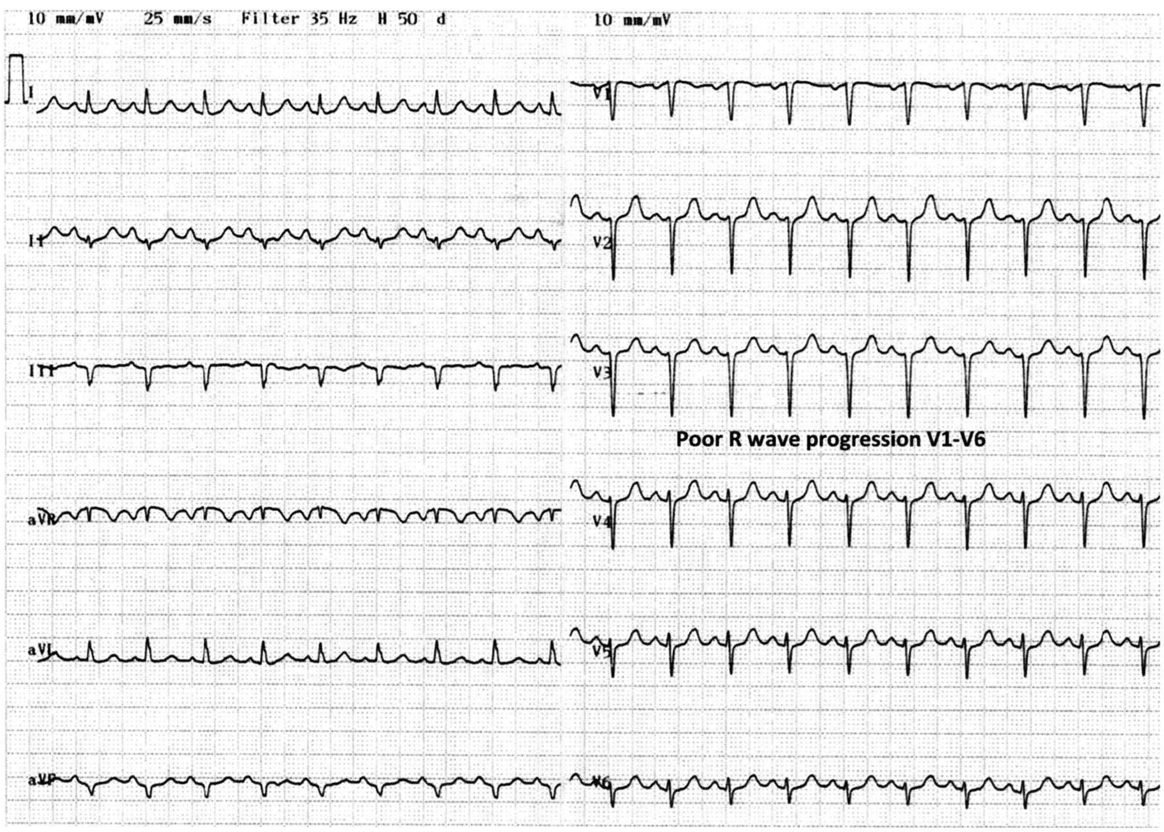

Fig. 8.48: Electrocardiogram (ECG) shows poor R wave progression in leads V1–V6 suggestive of old anterior myocardial infarction.

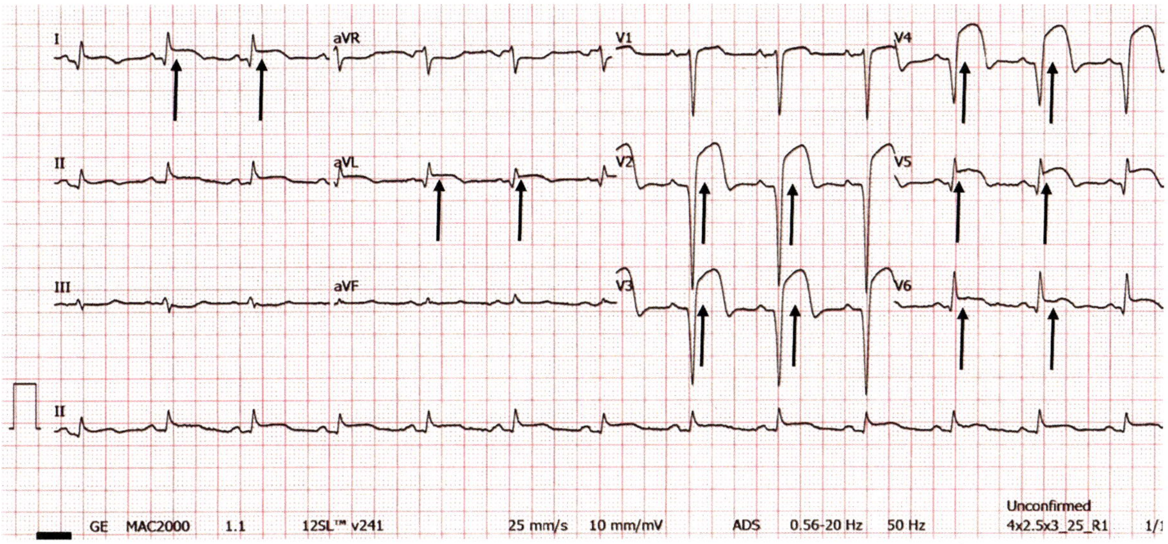

Fig. 8.49: Electrocardiogram (ECG) shows persistent coved ST elevation (arrows) in anterior leads even 3 months after anterior STEMI, suggestive of development of left ventricular aneurysm.

Box 8.4: The diagnosis of ST-elevation myocardial infarction.

The diagnosis of STEMI is established in the presence of—
- Chest pain lasting for >20 minutes associated with ECG changes:
  - ST-segment elevation of ≥1.0 mm in at least 2 extremity leads
    or
  - ≥2 mm in at least 2 contiguous precordial leads
    or
  - New onset of left bundle-branch block.

leads. The majority of patients will evolve ECG evidence of Q-wave infarction. New or presumably new LBBB has been considered a STEMI equivalent.

Typically, the ECG in the evolving STEMI shows five sequential changes, which develop in turn; hyperacute T waves > ST-segment elevation > appearance of pathological Q waves > T waves inversion > normalization of the ST-segment.

Reciprocal Change

ST elevation during acute STEMI is associated with simultaneous ST depression in the electrically opposite leads. Typically, the depressed ST segments tend to be horizontal or downsloping. The presence of reciprocal change is particularly useful when there is doubt about the clinical significance of ST-segment elevation. This additional ST deviation may represent ischemia in a myocardial region other than the area of infarction or may represent pure reciprocal changes.

Localization of ST-Elevation Myocardial Infarction From ST Elevation In Different Leads

- *Inferior wall MI*: Leads II, III, and aVF
- *Anterior wall MI*: Leads V1–V4
- *Lateral wall MI*: Leads I, aVL, V5, and V6
- *Extensive anterior MI*: Leads I, aVL, V1–V6
- *RV infarct*: Right-sided chest leads, best in V3R/V4R.The most useful lead is V4R.
- *Posterior wall*: Leads V7–V9.

ECG Criteria of Posterior Infarction

1. ST segment depression rather elevation in the septal leads V1–V3.
2. The ratio of the R-wave to the S-wave in leads V1 or V2 is greater than 1.
3. ST elevation in the posterior leads V7–V9.
4. ST elevation in the inferior leads (II, III, and aVF) may be seen if an inferior MI is also present. ST elevation may also be noted in lateral leads (Box 8.5).

Box 8.5: Posterior myocardial infarction.

How to spot posterior infarction
1. Posterior MI is usually associated with inferior or lateral MI. So, be vigilant for evidence of posterior MI in a patient presenting with inferolateral STEMI.
2. As the posterior myocardium is not directly visualized by the standard 12-lead ECG, reciprocal changes of STEMI are usually manifested in anteroseptal leads V1–V3.
3. In patients presenting with acute ischemic symptoms, horizontal ST depression in V1–V3 should raise the suspicion of posterior MI.
4. ECG diagnosis of posterior MI is suggested by the following changes in V1–V2 (V3):
   - Marked horizontal ST depression in V1 and V2 with tall R waves.
   - Upright T waves in leads V1–V2 (sometimes in V3)
   - Dominant R-wave in V2 (R/S ratio > 1)
5. Diagnosis of posterior MI is confirmed by the presence of ST elevation and Q waves in the posterior leads V7–V9.

ECG Criteria for Right Ventricular Myocardial Infarction

1. ST elevation in right-sided chest leads i.e. V3R–V6R can detect RV infarction. The most useful lead is V4R. ST-elevation greater than 1 mm in lead V4R is suggestive of RV infarction.
2. ST elevation greater than 1 mm in lead V1
3. Associated ECG evidence of inferior STEMI confirms the diagnosis.

ST elevation in the right-sided leads is a transient phenomenon, usually lasting less than 12 hours in 50% of patients with RV infarction.

Causes of ST-Segment Elevation

- Acute myocardial infarction
- Early repolarization pattern
- Left bundle-branch block
- Left ventricular hypertrophy
- Ventricular aneurysm
- Coronary vasospasm/Prinzmetal's angina
- Pericarditis
- Brugada syndrome
- Subarachnoid hemorrhage

Differential Diagnosis of ST-segment Elevation

Normal variant ST elevation in "early repolarization" usually concave upwards, ending with symmetrical, large, upright T waves.

In AMI, ST elevation is usually convex upwards, or straightened.

In pericarditis concave upwards ST elevation is reflected in most leads except aVR with no reciprocal ST-segment depression (except in aVR).Unlike "early repolarization", T waves are usually low amplitude, and heart rate is usually increased. ECG may manifest PR segment depression, a manifestation of atrial injury.

Persistent ST elevation after acute MI suggests ventricular aneurysm or severe systolic dysfunction with large microvascular damage.

The diagnosis of acute infarction in the presence of LBBB can be difficult. Three ECG criteria as suggested by Sgarbossa et al. may be of help in the detection of AMI in presence of LBBB (Box 8.6). The three electrocardiographic criteria are: (1) ST-segment elevation of 1 mm or more that is concordant with (in the same direction as) the QRS complex; (2) ST-segment depression of 1 mm or more in lead V1, V2, or V3; (3) ST-segment elevation of 5 mm or more that is discordant with (in the opposite direction from) the QRS complex.

A new onset of LBBB is always pathological and can be a sign of AMI. So the previous ECG of the patient is very important in this context. If previous ECG is not available during presentation serial ECGs may show dynamic ST segment changes during ischemia and may suggest acute MI. Presence of Q-wave in LI, aVL, V5 or V6 in the presence of LBBB usually indicates associated anterior MI.

Box 8.6: Sgarbossa's scoring system* for the diagnosis of ST-elevation myocardial infarction in the presence of LBBB.

- ST elevation ≥ 1 mm in a lead with a positive QRS complex (i.e. concordance): 5 points
- ST depression (concordant) ≥ 1 mm in lead V1, V2, or V3: 3 points
- ST elevation ≥5 mm in a lead with a negative (discordant) QRS complex: 2 points.

**Greater than or equal to 3 points = 90% specificity of STEMI.*

Uncomplicated RBBB usually causes little ST-segment displacement. Thus it does not generally interfere with the diagnosis of AMI,

Identification of the Culprit Artery

- Anterior STEMI with ST elevation in aVR: Left Main (LMCA) occlusion
- Anterior-STEMI with reciprocal changes in inferior leads: proximal LAD occlusion
- Anterior-STEMI without reciprocal changes in inferior leads: mid or distal LAD occlusion
- High-lateral STEMI: diagonal branch of LAD occlusion
- Lateral STEMI: LCX occlusion
- Inferior MI with ST elevation in LIII greater than LII: RCA occlusion
- Inferior MI with ST elevation in LII greater than LIII: LCX occlusion.

Inferior STEMI can result from occlusion of all three coronary arteries:

- The vast majority (80–90%) of inferior STEMIs are due to occlusion of the dominant RCA.
- Less commonly (around 10–20%), the culprit vessel is a dominant LCX.
- Occasionally, inferior STEMI may result from occlusion of a "type III" or "wraparound" LAD artery. This produces the unusual pattern of concomitant inferior and anterior ST elevation.

ECG manifestations of LMCA occlusion may be of two types:

1. Anterior STEMI with ST segment elevation in aVR. ST elevation in aVR>V1 is associated with occlusion of the left main artery
2. Other than anterior STEMI, LMCA occlusion should be suspected with widespread ST-segment depression >7 leads, with inverted T waves when accompanied with ST elevation in aVR.

de Winter's T and Wellens' syndrome/sign are suggestive of acute occlusion of the proximal left anterior descending (LAD) artery. Both the conditions are equivalent to anterior STEMI (Box 8.7)

Box 8.7: Significance of de Winter's T and Wellens' syndrome.

de Winter's T waves (represents approximately 2% of LAD occlusions)
- Upsloping ST depression in the precordial leads (1–3 mm at J-point).
- Tall and peaked anterior T waves (V2–6), with the ascending limb of the T-wave commencing below the isoelectric baseline.
- Subtle ST elevation in aVR greater than 0.5mm.
- Absence of ST elevation in the precordial leads
- Classical STEMI morphology may precede or follow the de Winter pattern

Wellens' syndrome: Diagnostic criteria
- Deeply-inverted or biphasic T-waves in V2–V4 (may extend to V1–V6)
- Isoelectric or minimally-elevated ST segment (< 1mm)
- No precordial Q-waves
- Preserved precordial R-wave progression
- Recent history of angina.

It is suggested that the de Winter ECG pattern and Wellens' syndrome are highly predictive of acute LAD occlusion. Both of them should be considered a "STEMI equivalent", and patients with chest pain and these ECG pattern should receive emergent reperfusion therapy.

Concomitant Inferior and Anterior ST Elevation

Concomitant inferior and anterior ST elevation suggestive of simultaneous both acute anterior and inferior MI is possible in presence of wrap around LAD. When LAD wraps around the LV apex, anterior MI due to LAD occlusion can show changes in inferior leads (Anteroinferior MI).

ECG Evidence of Prior Myocardial Infarction

1. Presence of Q-waves
2. The fragmented QRS (fQRS). Fragmented QRS is defined as an additional spike of QRS complexes without bundle-branch block.
3. Persistent ST elevation, ST depression, nonspecific ST T-wave changes, and T-wave inversion

Diagnostic Criteria for an Atrial Infarct

Major criteria: 1. PR-segment elevation >0.5 mm in leads V5 and V6 with reciprocal PR-segment depression in leads V1 and V2. 2. PR-segment elevation >0.5 mm in lead I with reciprocal depression in leads II and III. 3. PR-segment depression >1.5 mm in precordial leads and 1.2 mm in leads I, II, and III associated with any atrial arrhythmias.

Minor criteria: Abnormal P waves: M-shaped, W-shaped, irregular, or notched P waves.

REFERENCES

1. TIMI Study Group. The Thrombolysis in Myocardial Infarction (TIMI) trial: phase I findings. N Engl J Med. 1985;312(4):932-6.
2. Gruppo Italiano per lo Studio della Streptochinasi nell'Infarto Miocardico (GISSI). Effectiveness of intravenous thrombolytic treatment in acute myocardial infarction. Lancet. 1986;1(8478):397-402.
3. ISIS-2 Collaborative Group. Randomised trial of intravenous streptokinase, oral aspirin, both, or neither among 17,187 cases of suspected acute myocardial infarction: ISIS-2. Lancet. 1988;2(8607):349-60.
4. Zimetbaum PJ, Josephson ME. Use of the electrocardiogram in acute myocardial infarction. N Engl J Med. 2003;348(10): 933-40.
5. Morris F, Brady WB. Acute myocardial infarction—part I. BMJ. 2002;324:831-4.
6. Lee KL. Predictors of 30-day mortality in the era of reperfusion for acute myocardial infarction. Circulation. 1995;91:1659-68.
7. Somers MP. The prominant T wave: electrocardiographic differential diagnosis. Am J Emerg Med. 2002;20(3):243-51.
8. Prineas RJ, Crow RS, Blackburn H. The Minnesota code manual of electrocardiographic findings: standards and procedures for measurement and classification. Boston: John Wright, PSG Inc; 1982.
9. Menown BA, MacKenzie G, Adgey AAJ. Optimizing the initial 12-lead electrocardiographic diagnosis of acute myocardial infarction. Eur Heart J. 2000;21:275-83.
10. Napodano M, Paganelli C. ECG in acute myocardial infarction in the reperfusion. In: Richard Millis (Ed). Era, advances in electrocardiograms—clinical applications. Croatia: InTech; 2012.
11. Brady WJ, Perron A, Ullman E. Errors in emergency physician interpretation of ST-segment elevation in emergency department chest pain patients. Acad Emerg Med. 2000;7(11):1256-60.
12. Brady WJ, Peron AD, Chan T. Electrocardiographic ST-segment elevation: correct identification of acute myocardial infarction (AMI) and non-AMI syndromes by emergency physicians. Acad Emerg Med. 2001;8:349-60.
13. Brady WJ, Peron AD, Syverud SA, et al. Reciprocal ST segment depression: impact on the electrocardiographic diagnosis of ST segment elevation acute myocardial infarction. Am J Emerg Med. 2002;20:35-8.
14. Brady WJ, Perron AD, Ullman EA, et al. Electrocardiographic ST segment elevation: a comparison of AMI and non-AMI ECG syndromes. Am J Emerg Med. 2002;20:609-12.
15. Aldrich HR, Wagner NB, Boswick J, et al. Use of initial ST-segment deviation for prediction of final electrocardiographic size of acute myocardial infarcts. Am J Cardiol. 1988;61:749-53.
16. Brady WJ, Syverud SA, Beagle C, et al. Electrocardiographic ST-segment elevation: the diagnosis of acute myocardial infarction by morphologic analysis of the ST segment. Acad Emerg Med. 2001;8(10):961-7.
17. Brady WJ, Chan TC. Electrocardiographic manifestations: benign early repolarization. J Emerg Med. 1999;17:473-8.

18. Smith SW, Khalil A, Henry TD, et al. Electrocardiographic differentiation of early repolarization from subtle anterior ST-segment elevation myocardial infarction. Ann Emerg Med. 2012;60:45-56.
19. Wimalaratna HSK. Tombstoning of ST segment in acute myocardial infarction (letter). Lancet. 1993;342:96.
20. Guo XH, Yap YG, Chen LJ, et al. Correlation of coronary angiography with tombstoning electrocardiographic pattern in patients with after acute myocardial infarction. Clin Cardiol. 2000;23:347-52.
21. Balci B. Tombstoning ST-Elevation Myocardial Infarction. Curr Cardiol Rev. 2009;5(4):273-8.
22. Barbagelata A, Califf RM, Sgarbossa EB, et al. Thrombolysis and Q wave versus non-Q wave first acute myocardial infarction: a GUSTO-I substudy. J Am Coll Cardiol. 1997;29(4):770-7.
23. Oliva PB, Hammill SC, Edwards WD. Electrocardiographic diagnosis of postinfarction regional pericarditis. Ancillary observations regarding the effect of reperfusion on the rapidity and amplitude of T wave inversion after acute myocardial infarction. Circulation. 1993;88:896-904.
24. Goldschlager N. Principles of clinical electrocardiography, 13th edition. Norwalk: Appleton and Lange; 1989. pp. 110-2.
25. Smith SW. Acute coronary syndromes: acute myocardial infarction and ischemia. In: Chan TC, Brady WJ, Harrigan RA (Eds). ECG in emergency medicine and acute care, 1st edition. Philadelphia: Mosby; 2005. pp. 151-63.
26. Tamura A, Nagase K, Mikuriya Y, et al. Significance of spontaneous normalization of negative T waves in infarct related leads during healing of anterior wall acute myocardial infarction. Am J Cardiol. 1999;84:1341-4.
27. Richardson SG. Relation of coronary arterial patency and left ventricular function to electrocardiographic changes after streptokinase treatment during acute myocardial infarction. Am J Cardiol. 1988;61:0002-9149.
28. Claeys M, Bosmans J, Veenstra L, et al. Determinants and prognostic implications of persistent ST segment elevation after primary angioplasty for AMI. Importance of microvascular reperfusion injury on clinical outcome. Circulation. 1999;99:1972-7.
29. Krucoff MW, Croll MA, Pope JE, et al. Continuous 12-lead ST-segment recovery analysis in the TAMI 7 study. Performance of a noninvasive method for real-time detection of failed myocardial reperfusion. Circulation. 1993;88:437-46.
30. Thygesen K, Alpert JS, Jaffe AS, et al. Third universal definition of myocardial infarction. Circulation. 2012;126:2020-35.
31. O'Gara PT, Kushner FG, Ascheim DD, et al. 2013 ACCF/AHA guideline for the management of ST-elevation myocardial infarction: a report of the American College of Cardiology Foundation/American Heart Association Task Force on Practice Guidelines. J Am Coll Cardiol. 2013;61(4):e78-e140.
32. Jain S, Ting HT, Bell M, et al. Utility of left bundle branch block as a diagnostic criterion for acute myocardial infarction. Am J Cardiol. 2011;107:1111-6.
33. Go AS, Barron HV, Rundle AC, et al. National registry of myocardial infarction 2 investigators bundle-branch block and in-hospital mortality in acute myocardial infarction. Ann Intern Med. 1998;129(9):690-7.
34. de Winter RJ, Verouden NJ, Wellens HJ, et al. A new ECG sign of proximal LAD occlusion. N Engl J Med. 2008;359(19):2071-3.
35. Jong GP, Ma T, Chou P, et al. Reciprocal changes in 12-lead electrocardiography can predict left main coronary artery lesion in patients with acute myocardial infarction. Int Heart J. 2006;47:13-20.
36. Becker R, Alpert J. Electrocardiographic ST segment depression in coronary heart disease. Am Heart J. 1988;115:862-68.
37. Atar S, Barbagelata A, Birnbaum Y. Electrocardiographic diagnosis of ST-elevation myocardial infarction. Cardiol Clin. 2006;24(3):343-65.
38. Birnbaum Y, Drew BJ. The electrocardiogram in ST elevation acute myocardial infarction: correlation with coronary anatomy and prognosis. Postgrad Med J. 2003;79(935): 490-504.
39. Birnbaum Y, Solodky A, Herz I, et al. Implication of inferior ST segment depression in anterior acute myocardial infarction: electrocardiographic and angiographic correlation. Am Heart J. 1994;127:1467-73.
40. Sclarovsky S, Birnbaum Y, Solodky A, et al. Isolated mid-anterior myocardial infarction: a special electrocardiographic sub-type of acute myocardial infarction consisting of ST-elevation in non-consecutive leads and two different morphologic types of ST-depression. Int J Cardiol. 1994;46:37-47.
41. Birnbaum Y, Sclarovsky S, Mager A, et al. ST segment depression in aVL: a sensitive marker for acute inferior myocardial infarction. Eur Heart J. 1993;14(1):4-7.
42. Ruddy TD, Yasuda T, Gold HK, et al. Anterior ST segment depression in acute inferior myocardial infarction as a marker of greater inferior, apical, and posterolateral damage. Am Heart J. 1986;112:1210-6.
43. Ong L, Valdellon B, Coromilas J, et al. Precordial S-T segment depression in inferior myocardial infarction: evaluation by quantitative thallium-201 scintigraphy and technetium-99m ventriculography. Am J Cardiol. 1983;51:734-9.
44. Strasberg B, Pinchas A, Barbash GI, et al. Importance of reciprocal ST segment depression in leads V5 and V6 as an indicator of disease of the left anterior descending coronary artery in acute inferior wall myocardial infarction. Br Heart J. 1990;63(6):339-41.
45. Birnbaum Y, Wagner GS, Barbash GI, et al. Correlation of angiographic findings and right (V1 to V3) versus left (V4 to V6) precordial ST-segment depression in inferior wall acute myocardial infarction. Am J Cardiol. 1999;83:143-8.
46. Hasdai D, Birnbaum Y, Porter A, et al. Maximal precordial ST-segment depression in leads V4–V6 in patients with inferior wall acute myocardial infarction indicates coronary artery disease involving the left anterior descending coronary artery system. Int J Cardiol. 1997;58:273-8.
47. Blanke H, Cohen M, Schlueter GU, et al. Electrocardiographic and coronary arteriographic correlations during acute myocardial infarction. Am J Cardiol. 1984;54:249-55.
48. Aldrich HR, Hindman NB, Hinohara T, et al. Identification of the optimal electrocardiographic leads for detecting acute epicardial injury in acute myocardial infarction. Am J Cardiol. 1987;59(1):20-3.
49. Wung SF, Kahn DY. A quantitative evaluation of ST-segment changes on the 18-lead electrocardiogram during acute coronary occlusions. J Electrocardiology. 2006;39(3):275-81.
50. Wang K, Asinger RW. Marriott HJ. ST-segment elevation in conditions other than acute myocardial infarction. N Engl J Med. 2003;349:2128-35.

51. Lew AS, Maddahi J, Shah PK, et al. Factors that determine the direction and magnitude of precordial ST-segment deviations during inferior wall acute myocardial infarction. Am J Cardiol. 1985;55:883-8.
52. Matetzky S, Freimark D, Chouraqui P, et al. Significance of ST segment elevations in posterior chest leads (V7 to V9) in patients with acute inferior myocardial infarction: application for thrombolytic therapy. J Am Coll Cardiol. 1998;31:506-11.
53. Casas RE, Marriott HJ, Glancy DL. Value of leads V7–V9 in diagnosing posterior wall acute myocardial infarction and other causes of tall R waves in V1–V2. Am J Cardiol. 1997;80(4):508-9.
54. Matetzky S, Freimark D, Feinberg MS, et al. Acute myocardial infarction with isolated ST-segment elevation in posterior chest leads V7–9: "hidden" ST-segment elevations revealing acute posterior infarction. J Am Coll Cardiol. 1999;34:748-53.
55. Wung SF, Drew BJ. New electrocardiographic criteria for posterior wall acute myocardial ischemia validated by a percutaneous transluminal coronary angioplasty model of acute myocardial infarction. Am J Cardiol. 2001;87(8):970-4.
56. Agarwal JB, Khaw K, Aurignac F, et al. Importance of posterior chest leads in patients with suspected myocardial infarction, but nondiagnostic, routine 12-lead electrocardiogram. Am J Cardiol. 1999;83(3):323-6.
57. Edhouse J, Brady WJ, Morris F. Acute myocardial infarction—Part II. BMJ. 2002;324:963-6.
58. Sgarbossa EB, Pinski SL, Barbagelata A, et al. Electrocardiographic diagnosis of evolving acute myocardial infarction in the presence of left bundle-branch block. N Engl J Med. 1996;334:481-7.
59. Sgarbossa EB, Pinski SL, Gates KB, et al. Early electrocardiographic diagnosis of acute myocardial infarction in the presence of ventricular paced rhythm. GUSTO-I investigators. Am J Cardiol. 1996;77(5):423-4.
60. Jeffrey AT, Robert MR, Hilary KS, et al. Electrocardiographic criteria for detecting acute myocardial infarction in patients with left bundle branch block: a meta-analysis. Annals Emerg Med. 2008;52(4):329-336.e1.
61. Sgarbossa EB. Value of the ECG in suspected acute myocardial infarction with left bundle branch block. J Electrocardiology. 2000;33(Suppl):87-92.
62. Cabrera E, Friedland C. Wave of ventricular activation in left branch block with infarct; new electrocardiographic sign. Arch Inst Cardiol Mex. 1953;23(4):441-60.
63. Chapman MG, Pearce ML. Electrocardiographic diagnosis of myocardial infarction in the presence of left bundle-branch block. Circulation. 1957;16:558-71.
64. Deveci B, Ozeke O. Comparison of the electrocardiographic features of complete left bundle branch block in patients with ischemic and nonischemic left ventricular dysfunction. Indian Pacing Electrophysiol J. 2007;7(1):26-32.
65. Surawicz B, Parikh SR. Prevalence of male and female patterns of early ventricular repolarization in the normal ECG of males and females from childhood to old age. J Am Coll Cardiol. 2002;40:1870-6.
66. Spodick DH. Differential characteristics of the electrocardiogram in early repolarization and acute pericarditis. N Engl J Med. 1976;295:523-6.
67. Cokkinos DV, Hallman GL, Cooley DA, et al. Left ventricular aneurysm: analysis of electrocardiographic features and postresection changes. Am Heart J. 1971;82(2):149-57.
68. Graber JD, Oakley CM, Pickering BN, et al. Ventricular aneurysm. An appraisal of diagnosis and surgical treatment. Br Heart J. 1972;34(8):831-8.
69. Oliva PB, Potts DE, Pluss RG. Coronary arterial spasm in Prinzmetal angina: documentation by coronary arteriography. N Engl J Med. 1973;288:745-51.
70. Maseri A, Severi S, Nes MD, et al. "Variant" angina: one aspect of a continuous spectrum of vasospastic myocardial ischemia: pathogenetic mechanisms, estimated incidence and clinical and coronary arteriographic findings in 138 patients. Am J Cardiol. 1978;42:1019-35.
71. Spodick DH, Greene TO, Saperia G. Images in cardiovascular medicine: acute myocarditis masquerading as acute myocardial infarction. Circulation. 1995;91:1886-7.
72. Brugada P, Brugada J. Right bundle branch block, persistent ST segment elevation and sudden cardiac death: a distinct clinical and electrocardiographic syndrome: a multicenter report. J Am Coll Cardiol. 1992;20(6):1391-6.
73. Aygul N, Salamov E, Dogan U, et al. Acute occlusion of the left main trunk presenting as ST-elevation acute coronary syndrome. J Electrocardiol. 2010;43:76-8.
74. Yamaji H, Iwasaki K, Kusachi S, et al. Prediction of acute left main coronary artery obstruction by 12-lead electrocardiography ST segment elevation in lead aVR with less ST segment elevation in lead V1. J Am Coll Cardiol. 2001;38(5):1348-54.
75. Hennings JR, Fesmire FM. A new electrocardiographic criteria for emergent reperfusion therapy. Am J Emerg Med. 2012;30:994-1000.
76. Yamaji H, Iwasaki K, Kusachi S, et al. Prediction of acute left main coronary artery obstruction by 12-lead electrocardiography: ST segment elevation in lead aVR with less ST segment elevation in lead V1. J Am Coll Cardiol. 2001;38:1348-54.
77. Chen Y, Jao YTFN, Fang CC, et al. Recognition of left main occlusion in acute coronary syndrome. Acta Cardiol Sin. 2004;20:139-46.
78. Hori T, Kurosawa T, Yoshida M, et al. Factors predicting mortality in patients after myocardial infarction caused by left main coronary artery occlusion: significance of ST segment elevation in both aVR and aVL leads. Jpn Heart J. 2000;41:571-81.
79. Nikus KC, Eskola MJ. Electrocardiogram patterns in acute left main coronary artery occlusion. J Electrocardiol. 2008;41(6):626-9.
80. Engelen DJ, Gorgels AP, Cheriex EC, et al. Value of the electrocardiogram in localizing the occlusion site in the left anterior descending coronary artery in acute anterior myocardial infarction. J Am Coll Cardiol. 1999;34(2):389-95.
81. Sala MF, de Luna AB, Andres Carrillo Lopez AC, et al. The "De Winter Pattern" can progress to ST-segment elevation acute coronary syndrome. Revista Espanola de Cardiologia. 2015;68:1042-3.
82. Blanke H, Cohen M, Schlueter GU, et al. Electrocardiographic and coronary arteriographic correlations during acute myocardial infarction. Am J Cardiol. 1984;54:249-55.
83. Birnbaum Y, Hasdai D, Sclarovsky S, et al. Acute myocardial infarction entailing ST segment elevation in lead aVL: electrocardiographic differentiation among occlusion of the left anterior descending, first diagonal, and first obtuse marginal coronary arteries. Am Heart J. 1996;131:38-42.

84. Braat SH, Brugada P, den Dulk K, et al. Value of lead V4R for recognition of the infarct coronary artery in acute inferior myocardial infarction. Am J Cardiol. 1984;53:1538-41.
85. Lew AS, Maddahi J, Shah PK, et al. Factors that determine the direction and magnitude of precordial ST-segment deviations during inferior wall acute myocardial infarction. Am J Cardiol. 1985;55:883-8.
86. Kontos MC, Desai PV, Jesse RL, et al. Usefulness of the admission electrocardiogram for identifying the infarct-related artery in inferior wall acute myocardial infarction. Am J Cardiol. 1997;79:182-4.
87. Herz I, Assali AR, Adler Y, et al. New electrocardiographic criteria for predicting either the right or left circumflex artery as the culprit coronary artery in inferior wall acute myocardial infarction. Am J Cardiol. 1997;80:1343-5.
88. Assali AR, Herz I, Vaturi M, et al. Electrocardiographic criteria for predicting the culprit artery in inferior wall acute myocardial infarction. Am J Cardiol. 1999;84:87-9.
89. Birnbaum Y, Hale SL, Kloner RA. Changes in R wave amplitude: ECG differentiation between episodes of reocclusion and reperfusion associated with ST-segment elevation. J Electrocardiol. 1997;30:211-6.
90. Lazar EJ, Goldberger J, Peled H, et al. Atrial infarction: diagnosis and management. Am Heart J. 1988;116(4):1058-63.
91. Gardin JM, Singer DH. Atrial infarction. Importance, diagnosis, and localization. Arch Intern Med. 1981;141:1345-8.
92. Liu CK, Greenspan G, Piccirillo RT. Atrial infarction of the heart. Circulation. 1961;23:331-8.
93. Sivertssen E, Hoel B, Bay G, et al. Electrocardiographic atrial complex and acute atrial myocardial infarction. Am J Cardiol. 1973;31:450-6.
94. Shakir DK, Arafa SO. Right atrial infarction, atrial arrhythmia and inferior myocardial infarction form a missed triad: a case report and review of the literature. Can J Cardiol. 2007;23(12):995-7.
95. Henkel DM, Witt BJ, Gersh BJ. Ventricular arrhythmias after acute myocardial infarction: a 20 year community study. Am Heart J. 2006;151(4):806-12.
96. Osmancik PP, Stros P, Herman D. In-hospital arrhythmias in patients with acute myocardial infarction - the relation to the reperfusion strategy and their prognostic impact. Acute Card Care. 2008;10(1):15-25.
97. Timmer JR, Breet N, Zijlstra F. Predictors of ventricular tachyarrhythmia in high-risk myocardial infarction patients treated with primary coronary intervention. Neth Heart J. 2010;18(3):122-8.
98. Zipes DP, Camm AJ, Borggrefe M, et al. ACC/AHA/ESC 2006 guidelines for management of patients with ventricular arrhythmias and the prevention of sudden cardiac death—executive summary. Eur Heart J. 2006;27(17):2099-140.
99. Terkelsen CJ, Sorensen JT, Kaltoft AK, et al. Prevalence and significance of accelerated idioventricular rhythm in patients with ST-elevation myocardial infarction treated with primary percutaneous coronary intervention. Am J Cardiol. 2009;104(12):1641-6.
100. Fuster V, Rydén LE, Cannom DS, et al. ACC/AHA/ESC 2006 guidelines for the management of patients with atrial fibrillation. Circulation. 2006;114:e257-e354.
101. Goldstein JA, Lee DT, Pica MC, et al. Patterns of coronary compromise leading to bradyarrhythmias and hypotension in inferior myocardial infarction. Coron Artery Dis. 2005;16(5):265-74.
102. Meine TJ, Al-Khatib SM, Alexander JH, et al. Incidence, predictors, and outcomes of high-degree atrioventricular block complicating acute myocardial infarction treated with thrombolytic therapy. Am Heart J. 2005;149(4):670-4.
103. Newby KH, Pisano E, Krucoff MW, et al. Incidence and clinical relevance of the occurrence of bundle-branch block in patients treated with thrombolytic therapy. Circulation. 1996;94:2424-8.
104. Michael MA, El Masry H, Khan BR, et al. Electrocardiographic signs of remote myocardial infarction. Prog Cardiovasc Dis. 2007;50(3):198-208.
105. Das MK, Khan B, Jacob S, et al. Significance of a fragmented QRS complex versus a Q wave in patients with coronary artery disease. Circulation. 2006;113(21):2495-501.
106. Pietrasik G, Zaręba W. QRS fragmentation: diagnostic and prognostic significance. Cardiol J. 2012;19(2):114-21.
107. Erdogan T, Cetin M, Kocaman SA, et al. Relationship of fragmented QRS with prognostic markers and in-hospital MACE in patients undergoing CABG. Scand Cardiovasc J. 2012;46(2):107-13.
108. Das MK, Michael MA, Suradi H, et al. Usefulness of fragmented QRS on a 12-lead electrocardiogram in acute coronary syndrome for predicting mortality. Am J Cardiol. 2009;15;104(12):1631-7.
109. Bhatnagar SK. Observations of the relationship between left ventricular aneurysm and ST segment elevation in patients with a first acute anterior Q wave myocardial infarction. Eur Heart J. 1994;5(11):1500-4.
110. Galiuto L, Barchetta S, Crea F. Functional and structural correlates of persistent ST elevation after acute myocardial infarction successfully treated by percutaneous coronary intervention. Heart. 2007;93(11):1376-80.

Chapter 9

Electrocardiogram Documentation of Reperfusion in ST-Elevation Myocardial Infarction

INTRODUCTION

The most important step in the treatment of ST-elevation myocardial infarction (STEMI) is to sustain myocardial blood supply as soon as possible. The two main treatment methods used today to provide myocardial reperfusion are thrombolytic therapy (fibrinolytic therapy) and primary percutaneous coronary intervention (PPCI). It is recommended that reperfusion therapy should be administered to all eligible patients with STEMI with symptom onset within the prior 12 hours. This therapy is a class 1 indication with level of evidence A in the treatment of STEMI.[1] Primary PCI should be performed in patients with STEMI and ischemic symptoms of less than 12 hours duration. Primary PCI of the infarct related artery is preferred to fibrinolytic therapy when time-to-treatment delays are short and the patient presents to a high-volume, well-equipped center with experienced interventional cardiologists and skilled support staff. Compared with fibrinolytic therapy, PPCI produces higher rates of infarct artery patency.[1]

Both thrombolytic therapy and PPCI are widely used as the reperfusion strategy in the treatment of STEMI. The ECG remains a simple yet powerful tool in the assessment of reperfusion efficacy and prognosis following STEMI. Most of the professional guidelines advocate greater than 50% resolution of ST-segment elevation at 60–90 minutes following fibrinolysis as a marker of successful reperfusion.[2,3] This metric is also associated with enhanced myocardial perfusion, recovery of left ventricular function, reduced infarct size, and improved outcomes.[4,5] Contemporary studies have also affirmed the prognostic utility of ST-segment elevation resolution following PPCI independent of procedural outcome and restoration of flow in the culprit artery.[6-8] Failure of significant resolution of ST-segment elevation after reperfusion therapy indicates persistence of occlusion of the infarct-related artery (IRA) and failure of reperfusion therapy (Figs. 9.1A and B).

As a tool to identify epicardial reperfusion, ST-segment resolution is a valuable bed side guide. A resolution of ST-segment elevation of more than 70% of the initial value at 60–90 minutes after the initiation of therapy, is a powerful predictor of successful myocardial reperfusion and is, therefore, associated with enhanced recovery of LV function, reduced infarct size, and improved prognosis.[5] Thus patients with complete ST resolution at 90 minutes after fibrinolysis have a greater than 90% probability of a patent infarct-related artery associated with a successful reperfusion at the microvascular level. However, approximately 50% of patients with no ST-segment resolution after fibrinolysis still show a patent epicardial infarct artery. In fact in these patients the lack of ST resolution is caused by the failure of reperfusion at the level of microvasculature rather than at epicardial vessel. Thus, ST resolution represents a powerful predictor of infarct-related artery patency, but it is less accurate for predicting the re-establishment of normal tissue perfusion at microvascular level after fibrinolysis.[9] Therefore, in order to judge the need for adjunctive mechanical reopening of the infarct-related artery after failed fibrinolysis, by the so called "rescue PCI", it is important to integrate clinical and ECG data. It is reasonable to monitor the pattern of ST-segment elevation, cardiac rhythm, and clinical symptoms during the 60–90 minutes after the initiation of fibrinolytic therapy. Non-invasive findings suggesting for a successful reperfusion include relief of symptoms, maintenance or restoration of hemodynamic and electrical stability, and a reduction of at least 50% in the initial ST-segment elevation. In this scenario, the presence of particular arrhythmias, such as not rapid ventricular tachycardia, idioventricular rhythm or not-sustained bradycardia, early after fibrinolytic administration, represents a highly specific marker of reperfusion. Otherwise, persistence of ischemic chest pain, absence of resolution of the qualifying ST-segment elevation, and hemodynamic or electrical instability are generally predictors of failed reperfusion therapy, needing rescue PCI.[10]

There is increasing evidence that the presence of normal epicardial blood flow does not always correlate with microvascular perfusion of the myocardial tissue.[11] The absence of tissue perfusion is the most potent predictor of impaired ventricular function and the risk of death after myocardial infarction.[11] Conversely, resolution of

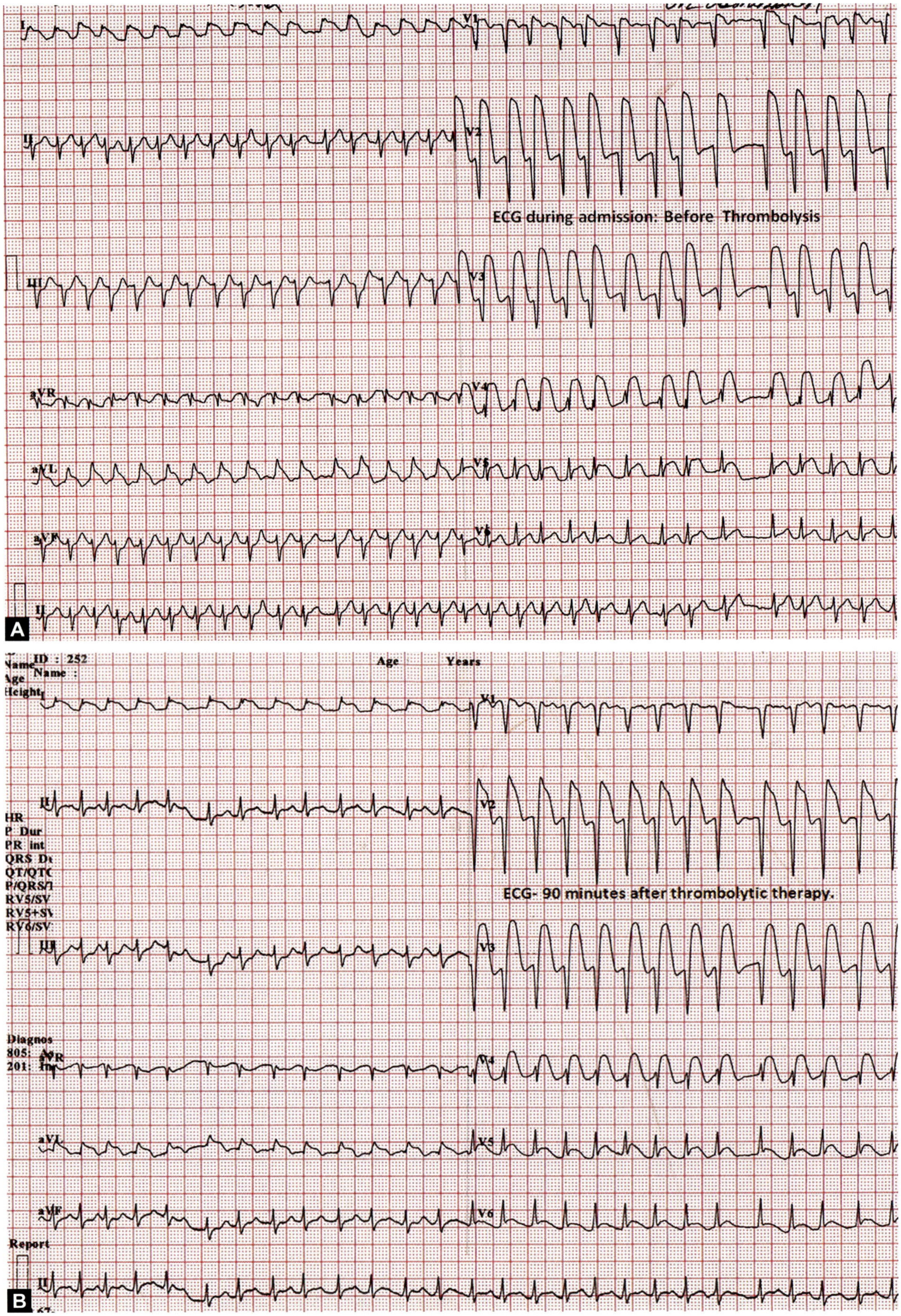

Figs. 9.1A and B: (A) Electrocardiogram during admission (before thrombolysis) shows marked ST-segment elevation in anterior leads (LI, aVL, V1–V5) with fast atrial fibrillation (AF). (B) Electrocardiogram of the same patient (Fig. 9.1A), 90 minutes after initiation of thrombolytic therapy. Note no significant resolution of ST-segment elevation in anterior leads indicating unsuccessful reperfusion therapy.

ST-segment elevation is believed to be an excellent marker of tissue perfusion, and the degree of resolution has proved to be a powerful indicator of short-term (30-day) and long-term (1-year) prognosis.[11]

A reduction in ST-segment elevation by more than 70% in the leads with maximal elevation is associated with the most favorable outcomes (Figs. 9.2A and B).[12-14] Many studies, evaluating the outcomes of PPCI in STEMI, found that persistent ST-segment elevation after coronary flow restoration, is one of the independent determinant of adverse cardiac events.[5,10] Other than resolution of ST-segment elevation, early appearance of T-wave inversion, recovery of reciprocal ST depression and various reperfusion arrhythmias are also regarded as independent predictors of successful reperfusion.

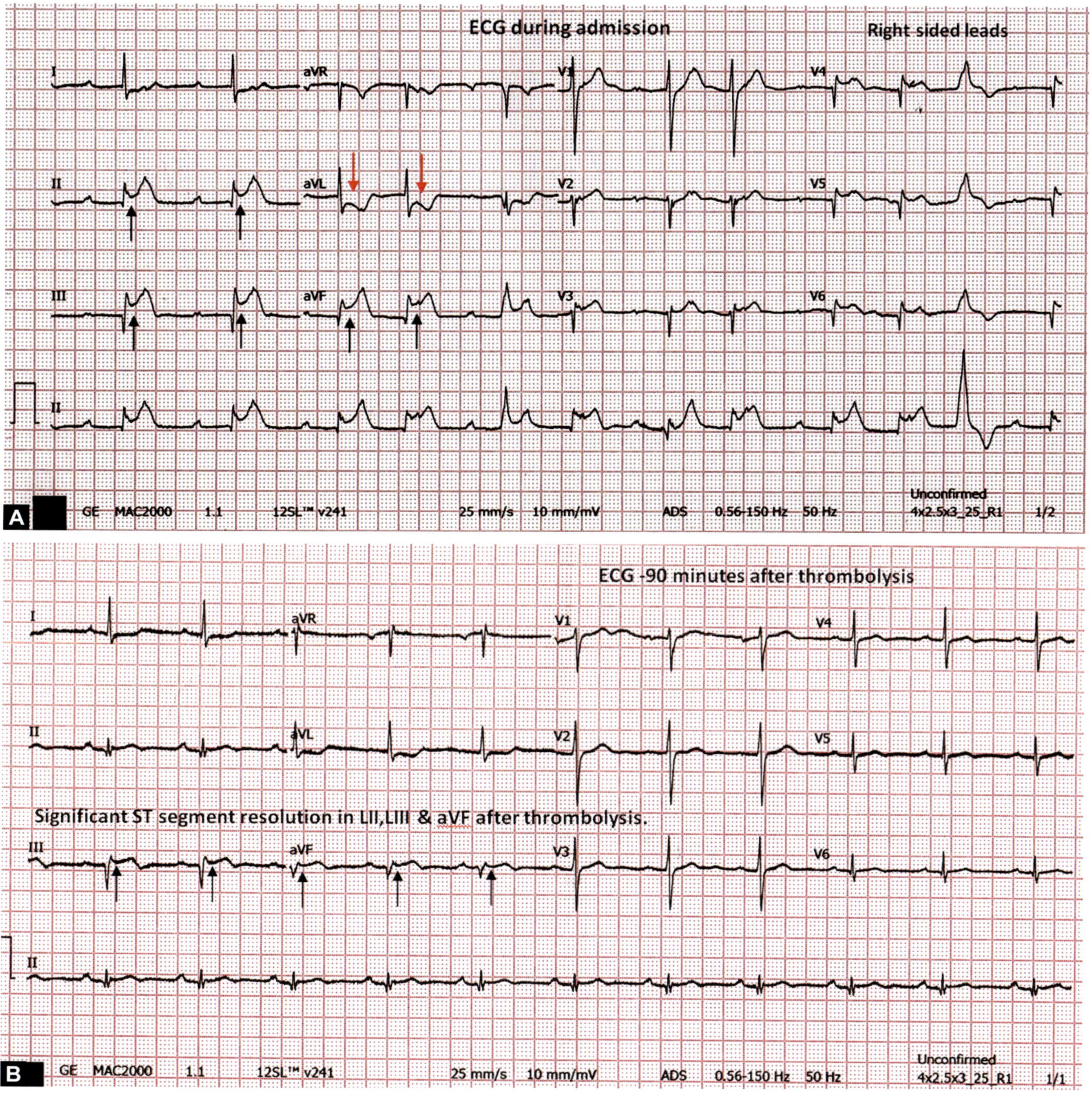

Figs. 9.2A and B: (A) Electrocardiogram of acute inferior STEMI during hospital admission before thrombolysis. Note ST-segment elevation in LII, LIII and aVF (black arrows) with reciprocal ST-segment depression in aVL (*red arrows*). Also note ECG evidence of AV block with significant ST-segment elevation in lead V4R. In this ECG ST elevation in LIII > LII, suggesting possible right coronary artery (RCA) occlusion. (B) Electrocardiogram of the same patient with acute inferior MI (Fig. 9.2A) 90 minutes after thrombolytic therapy shows almost complete resolution of initial ST-segment elevation in inferior leads. Note only mild degree of ST elevation is persisting in LIII and aVF (*arrows*). Also note disappearance of AV block after thrombolysis. (*Source*: Dr APM Sohrabuzzaman, Labaid Cardiac Hospaital).

ELECTROCARDIOGRAM ASSESSMENT OF RESOLUTION OF ST ELEVATION

Resolution of ST-segment elevation can be assessed by three ways:[9]

1. Sum ST-resolution model
2. Single-Lead ST resolution
3. Max ST elevation

Sum ST-segment Resolution

Resolution of the sum of ST-segment elevation (sum STR) after reperfusion therapy either by fibrinolysis or primary percutaneous coronary intervention (PPCI) is used to predict infarct size, left ventricular function, epicardial vessel patency, and mortality. Sum STR is expressed as the percentage from baseline (Figs. 9.3A to D). Measuring ST-segment elevations from all leads related to infarct location, however, is time consuming.[5,15,16]

Single-lead ST-segment Resolution

Single-lead ST-segment resolution (STR) is measured by comparing one ECG lead with the most prominent ST-segment deviation at baseline and at a given time point after reperfusion therapy, irrespective of the ECG lead measure at baseline (Figs. 9.4A to C).This comparison provides percentages of ST-segment deviation recovery independent from any changes in the patient's position or the position of the lead electrodes.[12,17,18]

Max ST-segment Elevation

Max ST-segment elevation (STE) represents the existing maximum ST-segment deviation that is present at a given time of assessment. Max STE is measured as per single-lead STR, but it is not compared with ST-segment deviation on the baseline ECG.

Sum ST resolution (STR) is conventionally categorized as complete (≥70%), partial (<70–30%), and no (≤30%) ST-segment elevation resolution (Box 9.1).[10] Although different time points have been reported across the studies

Box 9.1: ST-segment resolution as a sign of reperfusion.

At 90 minutes, more than 50% reduction in the ST segment elevation is accepted as successful reperfusion.

- *STR > 70%*: Complete resolution may indicate the patency of an epicardial artery as well as restoration of normal myocardial perfusion.
- *STR > 50% but <70%*: May show the patency of an epicardial artery.
- *STR 30–70%*: Partial restoration of myocardial perfusion
- *STR < 30%*: No perfusion.

(STR: ST-segment resolution)

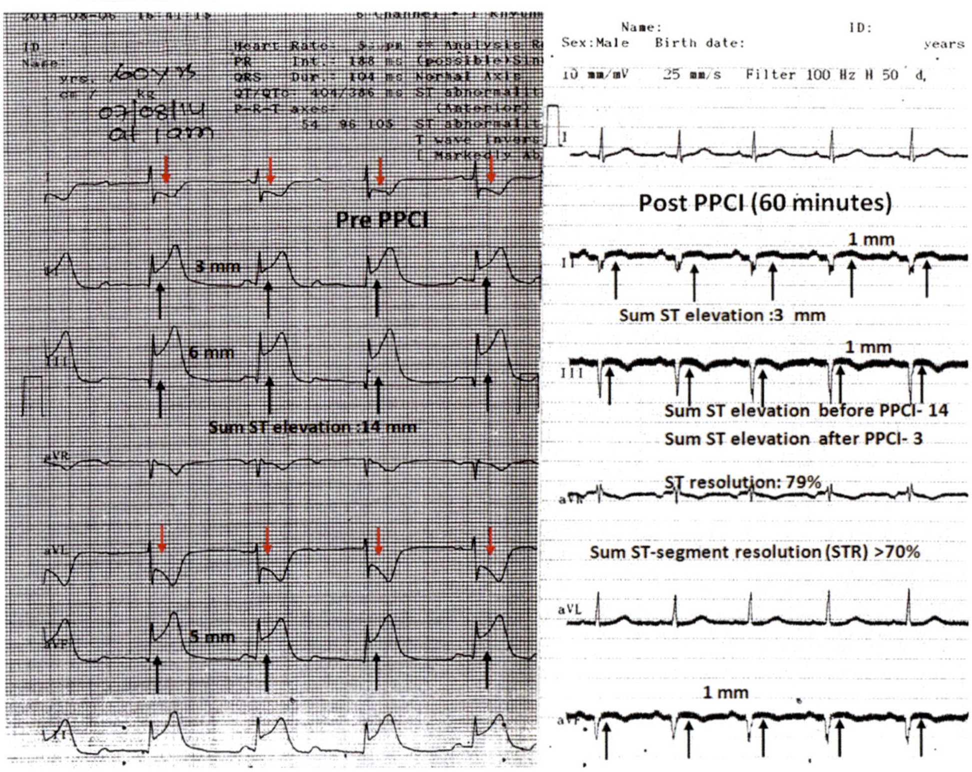

Fig. 9.3A: Two ECGs of inferior STEMI side by side (*left*: before PPCI and right: 60 minutes post PPCI). Note significant ST-segment elevation in inferior leads LII, LIII and aVF (*black arrows*) in pre-PPCI ECG (*left*) with marked reciprocal ST-segment depression in LI and aVL (*red arrows*). Calculated ST-segment elevation in all the three inferior leads (LII-3 mm, LIII-6 mm and aVF-5 mm), so sum of ST elevation = 3 + 6 + 5 = 14. In post-PPCI ECG (after 60 minutes) (*right*) shows remarkable resolution of ST-segment elevation. In the post-PPCI ECG, sum of ST-segment elevation remaining is (LII-1 mm, LIII-1 mm and aVF-1 mm) = 3 mm. So, sum of ST-segment resolution = 79%, which indicates successful reperfusion. Also note the complete disappearance of reciprocal ST-segment depression in leads LI and aVL in post-PPCI ECG. (*Source*: Courtesy by Dr Abduz Zaher, Labaid Cardiac Hospital).

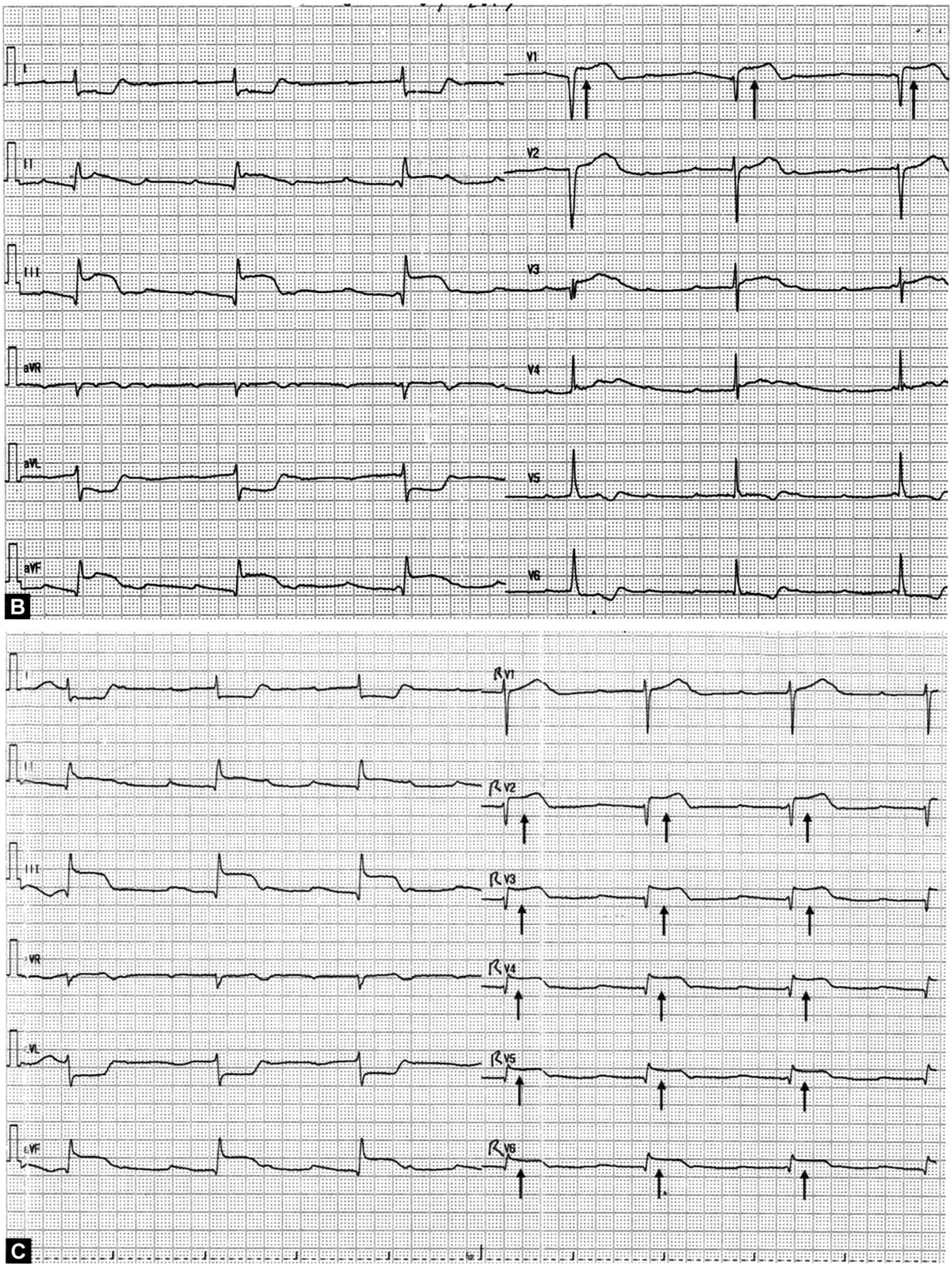

Figs. 9.3B and C: (B) This is the ECG of a patient who presented in the emergency department at late night with history of sudden onset of severe central chest pain of half-an-hour duration. On admission his blood pressure was nonrecordable and this ECG shows evidence of inferior STEMI with complete heart block with rate 35 bpm. Note significant ST-segment elevation in inferior leads LII, LIII and aVF and sum ST-segment elevation in all the three inferior leads, LII + LIII + aVF = 15. Also note ST-segment elevation in lead V1 (*arrows*), suggestive of associated RV infarction. On the standard 12 lead electrocardiogram right ventricular infarction is indicated by signs of inferior infarction, associated with ST-segment elevation in lead V1. With this ECG finding the patient was directly taken to the cath lab for PPCI. (C) Electrocardiogram of the same patient (Fig. 9.3B) taken before PPCI with right-sided leads. This ECG shows marked ST-segment elevation in leads V2R-V6R (*arrows*), which confirms the electrocardiographic diagnosis of concurrent RV infarction. (*Source:* Courtesy by Dr Afzalur Rahman, National Institute of Cardiovascular Diseases, Dhaka).

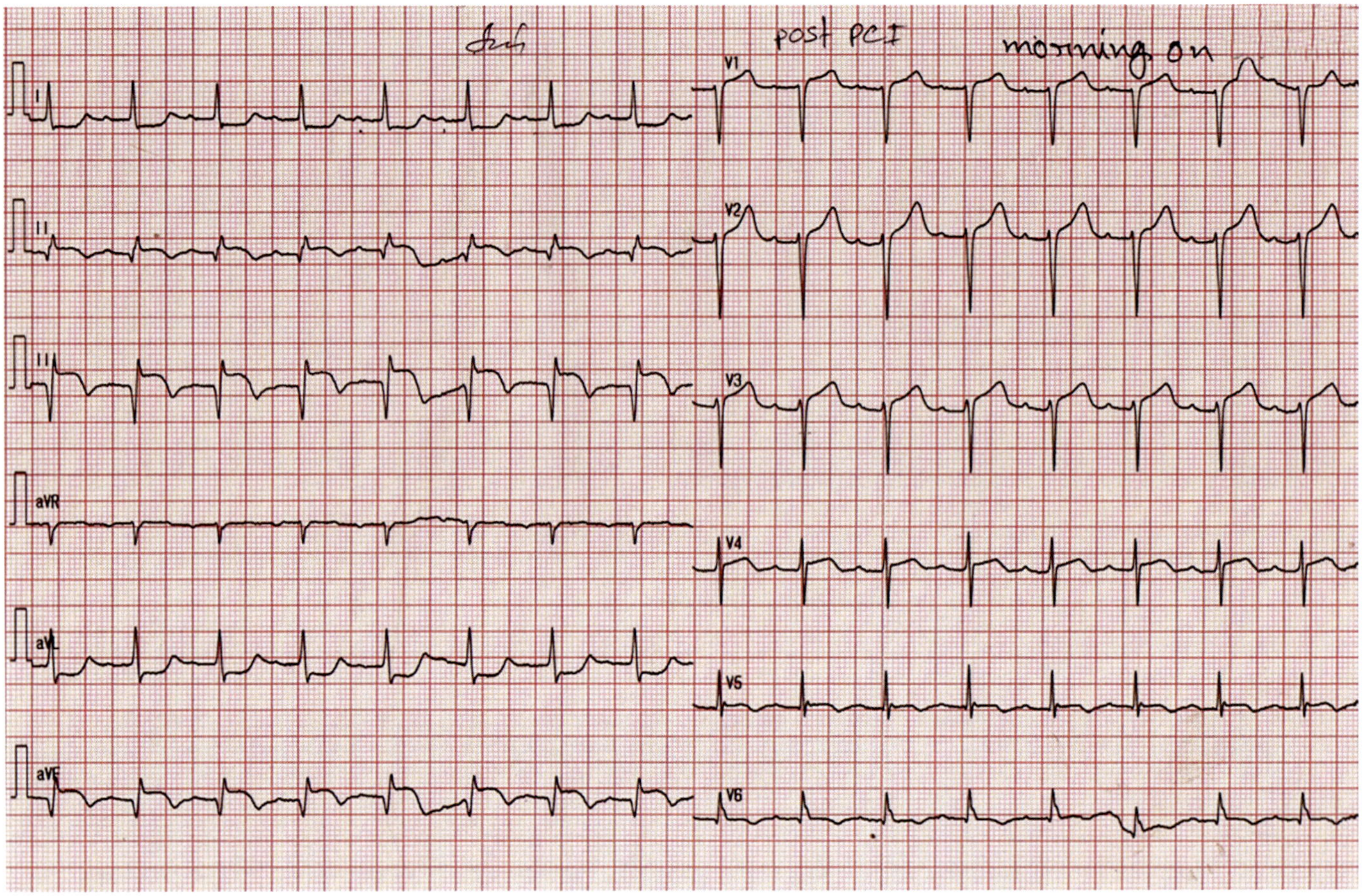

Fig. 9.3D: Electrocardiogram of the same patient (Figs 9.3B and C), taken 90 minutes after PPCI. Coronary angiogram of this patient showed total obstruction of proximal right coronary artery (RCA) and the occluded artery was opened with PCI with stenting. Post-PCI ECG shows marked resolution of ST elevation in inferior leads with disappearance of complete heart block, and now the rhythm is sinus. Post-PCI sum ST-segment elevation in all the three inferior leads, LII + LIII + aVF = 4. Sum of ST elevation before PPCI was 15 and 90 minutes after PPCI is 4. So, sum of ST-segment resolution (STR) is greater than 70%, indicating successful reperfusion. (*Source:* Courtesy by Dr Afzalur Rahman, National Institute of Cardiovascular Diseases, Dhaka).

evaluating the relationship between ST resolution and outcome, such as 30, 60, or even 90 minutes after reperfusion therapy, no significant differences between various time points were found, and the ideal time of measuring ST resolution remains unclear. However, these studies were mostly conducted in patients receiving fibrinolytic therapy, and may not be directly applicable when assessing success of PPCI. In fact, after thrombolysis for STEMI the ECG for measuring ST resolution is usually taken 60–90 minutes after the onset of therapy, in order to detect by means of noninvasive tool the patency of epicardial vessel, rather than the reperfusion at microvascular level.[10]

Primary percutaneous coronary intervention restores epicardial coronary flow in the vast majority of patients with STEMI. However, despite successful primary PCI, a substantial number of patients show signs of suboptimal myocardial reperfusion, manifested by persistent ST-segment elevation and incomplete ST-segment elevation resolution (STR). Absent or incomplete STR after PCI is a strong predictor for impaired left ventricular function and adverse clinical outcomes.[19]

After thrombolysis for STEMI, the ECG for measuring STR is usually taken 60–90 minutes after onset of therapy.[20-22] But, the timing of the ECG after PPCI for determination of STR is highly variable. It ranges from the time of arrival on the coronary care unit (CCU), approximately 30 minutes after PCI, to another 30 minutes or even several hours later.[19,23] Earlier studies showed that STR at 30 minutes after PPCI correlated better with other markers of myocardial perfusion than STR at 60–90 minutes.[24,25]

APPEARANCE OF EARLY T-WAVE INVERSION

One important electrocardiographic markers of reperfusion include T-wave inversion within 4 hours after reperfusion therapy. T-wave inversion that occurs during the first few hours of reperfusion therapy is a highly specific sign of successful reperfusion.[26] T-wave inversion that develops more than 4 hours after the start of reperfusion therapy is consistent with the normal electrocardiographic evolution

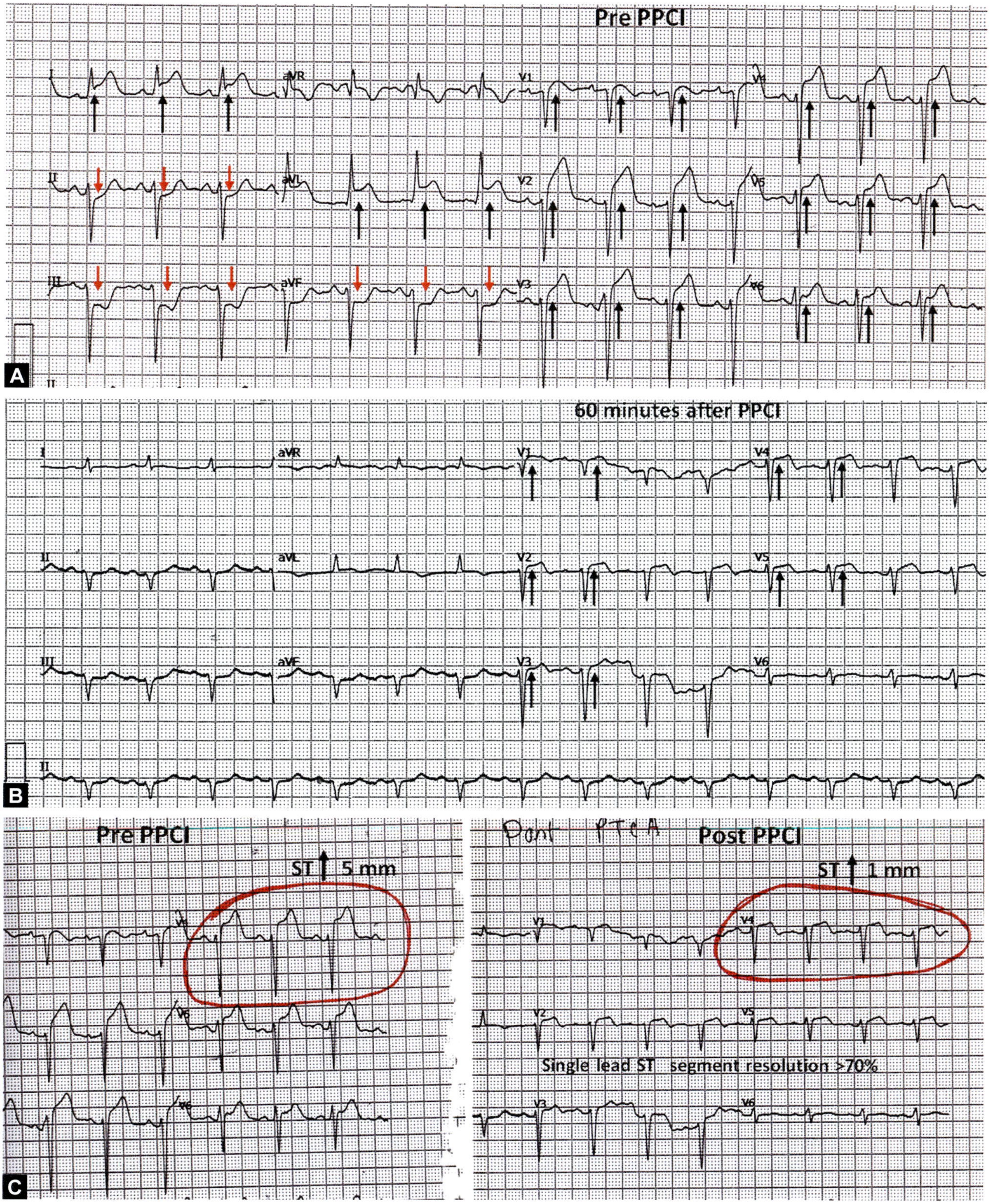

Figs. 9.4A to C: (A) Electrocardiogram (before PPCI) is suggestive of extensive anterior STEMI showing ST elevation in LI, aVL, V1-V6 (*black arrows*) with reciprocal ST-segment depression in leads LII, LIII and aVF (*red arrows*). (B) Electrocardiogram (60 minutes after PPCI) of the same patient (Fig. 9.4A) showing remarkable ST-segment resolution in anterior leads. Only 1–2 mm ST elevation is still persisting in leads V1-V5 (*arrows*). Note complete normalization of ST-segment elevation in leads LI, aVL and V6. Also note complete disappearance of reciprocal ST depression within 60 minutes post-PPCI in leads LII, LIII and aVF. (C) Electrocardiogram showing single lead ST-segment resolution (STR) in same patient (Fig. 9.4A) pre- and post-PPCI. Note maximum ST-segment elevation pre-PPCI was recorded in lead V4 (5 mm) and 60 minutes after PPCI, in the same lead only around 1 mm ST elevation is persisting, indicating successful reperfusion therapy (single lead STR in V4 > 70%). (*Source*: Courtesy by Dr Mahbubor Rahman, Labaid Cardiac Hospital). (PPCI: primary percutaneous coronary intervention).

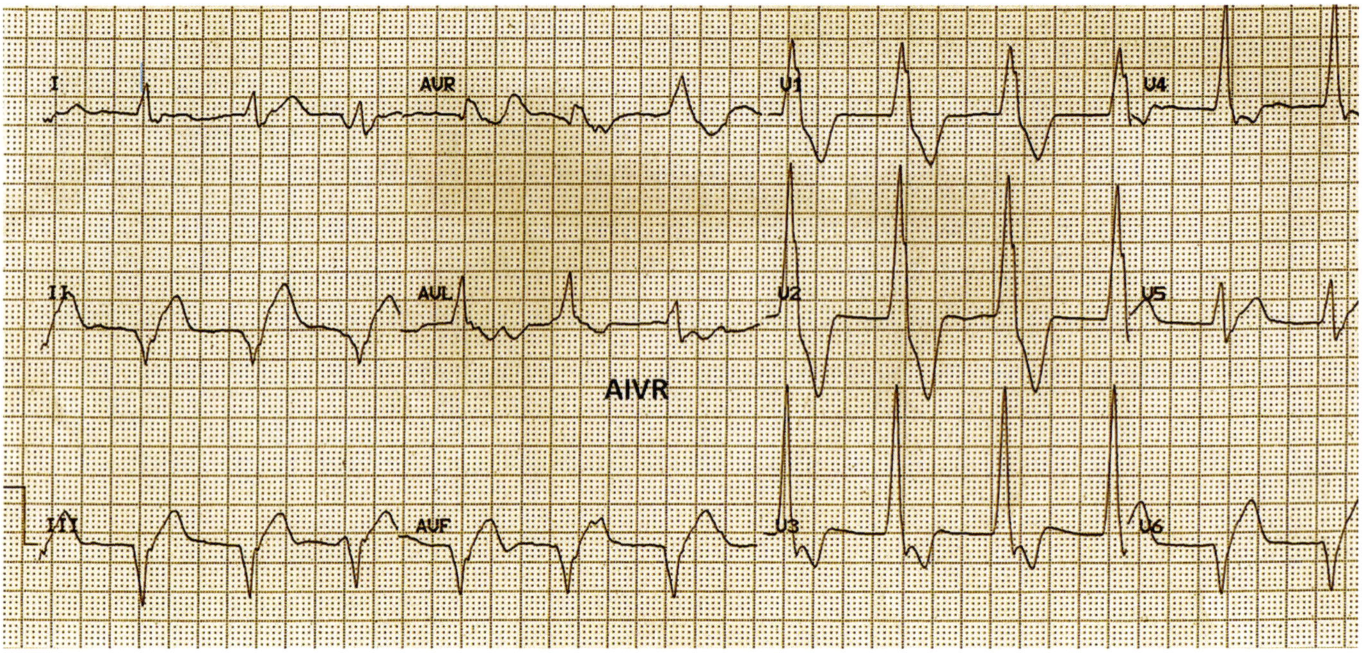

Fig. 9.5: ECG is suggestive of accelerated idioventricular rhythm (AIVR), an arrhythmia regarded as a sign of success of reperfusion therapy.

of myocardial infarction and does not indicate that reperfusion has occurred.[11]

Pseudonormalization of T waves is an ECG sign of re-occlusion. Thus, where reperfusion of the IRA leads to T-wave inversion, if inverted T waves become suddenly upright, this is diagnostic of re-occlusion of the IRA.

ARRHYTHMIAS FOLLOWING ST ELEVATION MYOCARDIAL INFARCTION

Arrhythmias following STEMI may be of two types.

1. Ischemic arrhythmias
2. Reperfusion arrhythmias

Rhythm disorders associated with coronary occlusion are defined as *ischemic arrhythmias*, whereas arrhythmias occurring as the result of increased myocardial perfusion are called *reperfusion arrhythmias.*

ACCELERATED IDIOVENTRICULAR RHYTHM

An accelerated idioventricular rhythm (AIVR) (defined as a heart rate of 40-100 beats/min initiated by a late, coupled, ventricular premature depolarization) is a highly specific marker of reperfusion.[11] This rhythm is benign and should not be suppressed with medication. Accelerated idioventricular rhythm may be a marker of early reperfusion and continuing arterial patency (Fig. 9.5). The presence of AIVR combined with normalization of ST-segment elevation usually indicates successful reperfusion in patients treated with thrombolytics.[27,28]

In the past AIVR was regarded as the most sensitive and specific arrhythmia in cases of successful reperfusion but this view has been changed nowadays.[28] In contrast, Bonnemeier et al. and Terkelsen et al. mentioned that although AIVR does not meet criteria for reperfusion, it may be an indicator of more extensive myocardial damage and delayed microvascular reperfusion in patients who were treated by PPCI.[29,30]

OTHER REPERFUSION ARRHYTHMIAS

Isolated premature ventricular complex (PVC) and non sustained ventricular tachycardia (VT) may also be seen with reperfusion (Fig. 9.6). Polymorphic ventricular tachycardia and ventricular fibrillation may be seen with reperfusion but are rare and should raise the suspicion of ongoing arterial occlusion. In acute myocardial infarction, VT and ventricular fibrillation (VF) may occur due to either complete occlusion or reperfusion (Box 9.2). Engelen et al. demonstrated that at least 97% of patients developed one

Box 9.2: Most frequently observed reperfusion arrhythmias.

The most frequently observed rhythm disorders those are defined as reperfusion arrhythmias are:

- Frequent premature ventricular complex (PVC)
- Accelerated idioventricular rhythm (AIVR)
- Sustained or nonsustained ventricular tachycardia (VT)
- Atrial fibrillation (AF)
- Ventricular fibrillation (VF).

These arrhythmias are thought to be indicators of successful reperfusion. But it is not always true. Sometimes it is very difficult to differentiate reperfusion arrhythmias from ischemic arrhythmias.

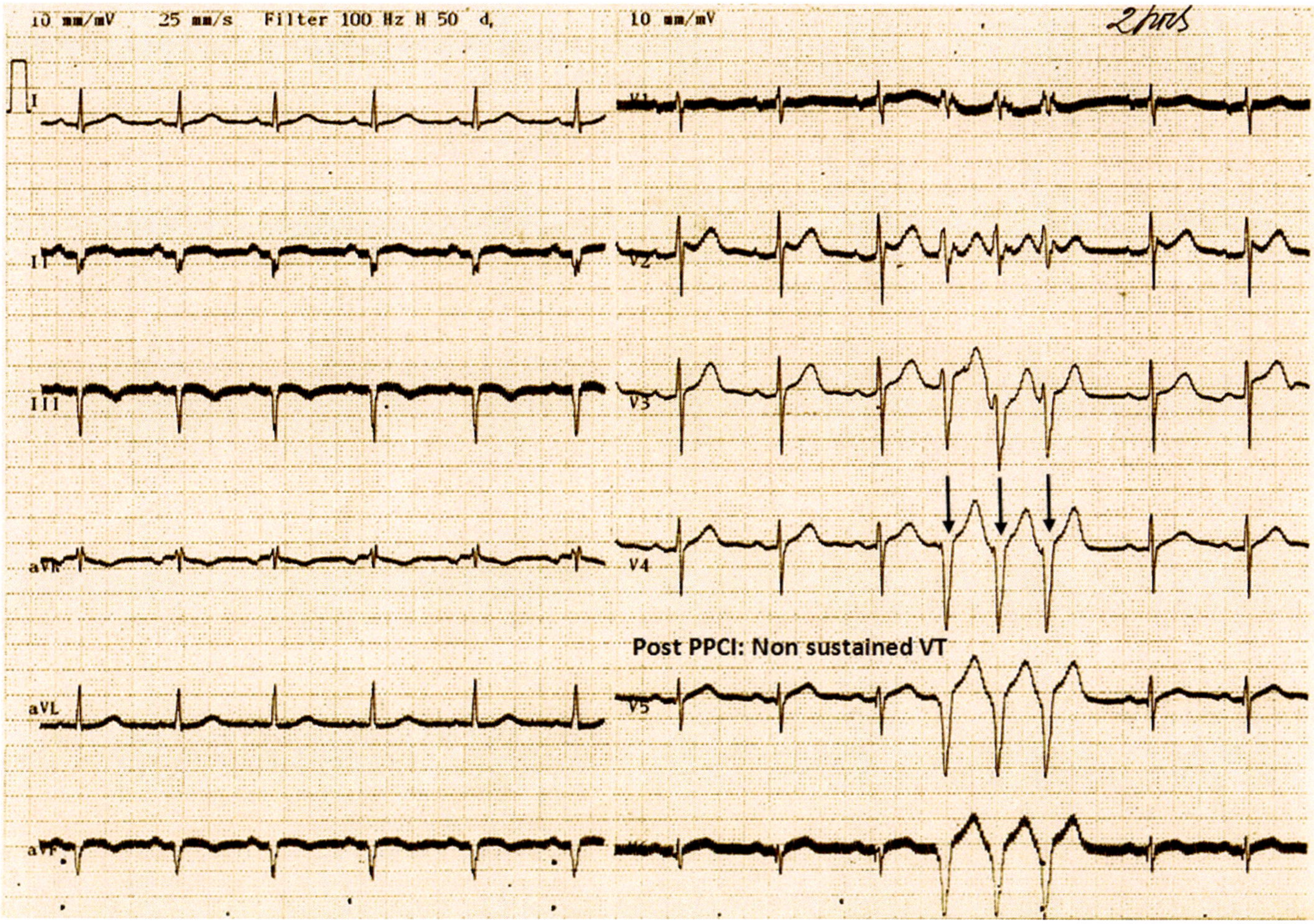

Fig. 9.6: Electrocardiogram taken 2 hours after PPCI for inferior STEMI. This ECG shows nonsustained VT (*arrows*), a possible sign of successful reperfusion. (*Source*: Courtesy by Dr Abduz Zaher, Labaid Cardiac Hospital). (PPCI: primary percutaneous coronary intervention)

ventricular reperfusion arrhythmia in a study group of 62 patients with acute anterior myocardial infarction who underwent PPCI. Non sustained VT, AIVR, and frequent PVC were the most frequent arrhythmias and ventricular arrhythmias correlated with reduced and worsening left ventricular functions after the acute phase of myocardial infarction among the group of patients treated via primary PCI and concluded that reperfusion arrhythmias are noninvasive indicators of myocardial cell damage, rather than a sign of successful reperfusion.[31]

RESOLUTION OF ST-SEGMENT DEPRESSION

Contemporary studies have affirmed the prognostic utility of ST-segment elevation resolution following primary PCI. Less attention has been given towards the evolution of concomitant reciprocal ST-segment depression in patients with STEMI. Despite uncertainty as to its mechanism, concomitant reciprocal ST-segment depression has been associated with poorer clinical outcomes.[32] It is believed that the extent of ST-segment deviation (elevation plus depression) defines the territory at risk and its overall resolution is prognostically relevant.[33,34] Patients with persistent ST-segment depression despite resolution of ST-segment elevation sustained higher in-hospital mortality (13%) compared with those in whom ST-segment depression resolved simultaneously with ST-segment elevation (1%), and to those without baseline ST-segment depression (0%).[32] When concomitant ST depression is present in patients with STEMI undergoing primary PCI, less than 50% resolution of ST depression was associated with worse 90 day clinical outcomes even after accounting for the baseline risk profile, infarct location, PCI procedural outcome, and resolution of ST elevation.[32]

SUMMARY

Assessment of the degree of ST-segment deviation resolution and the presence or absence of reperfusion arrhythmias on a 12-lead ECG, early after reperfusion therapy either by thrombolysis or primary PCI provides strong, remarkably robust, and unambiguous information regarding the success of reperfusion therapy and culprit vessel patency in patients presenting with STEMI.

ECG Criteria of Successful Reperfusion

1. More than 50% resolution of ST-segment elevation at 60–90 minutes following reperfusion therapy is a marker of successful reperfusion.
2. T-wave inversion that occurs during the first 4 hours of reperfusion therapy is a highly specific sign of successful reperfusion.
3. Accelerated idioventricular rhythm (AIVR) may be an ECG marker of successful reperfusion and patency of the culprit vessel.
4. Frequent PVC, nonsustained or sustained VT, and even VF may be the ECG markers of successful reperfusion but polymorphic VT and VF are rare and should raise the suspicion of ongoing arterial occlusion.
5. Resolution of reciprocal ST-segment depression after reperfusion therapy is also considered as a marker of successful reperfusion.

Calculation of ST-Segment Change

Sum of ST-Segment Elevation (sum STE): Sum STE is manually calculated as the sum of ST-segment elevation in all leads using previously validated algorithms as the sum of elevation in LI, aVL V1-6 for anterior infarction and as the sum of elevation in leads II, III, aVF, V5 and V6 for non-anterior infarction.

ST-Segment Resolution (STR): STR is defined as the percent reduction in the sum STE obtained on admission and each time point following reperfusion therapy, thrombolysis or primary PCI. Complete STR is considered for a reduction of greater than or equal to 70%.

Complete (≥70%) resolution of ST elevation is associated with better outcome and preservation of left ventricular function than partial (30% to 70%) or no (<30%) ST-segment resolution. More than or equal to 50% resolution of ST-segment elevation (STR) is a reliable indicator of patency of the IRA, only complete (≥70%) ST elevation resolution is an indicator of restoration of myocardial tissue perfusion.

The presence of AIVR combined with normalization of ST-segments is possibly the best predictor of successful reperfusion in patients treated with reperfusion therapies.

Resolution of ST-segment elevation is a powerful predictor of infarct-related artery patency in STEMI. Absent or incomplete ST-segment elevation resolution is also an important predictor of increased risk of death and congestive heart failure in patients with STEMI treated with thrombolytic therapy. The current theory holds that ST-segment resolution or recovery after reperfusion therapy signifies effective microvascular perfusion, myocardial tissue perfusion, and myocardial salvage.

Reperfusion arrhythmia frequency is not significantly different between patients treated by PPCI and thrombolytics, although PPCI is known to provide better arterial patency. Accelerated idioventricular rhythm, which is so far known as a reperfusion arrhythmia, may indicate myocardial damage and ongoing ischemia rather than vascular patency (successful reperfusion). So the value of AIVR or any other ventricular arrhythmia after reperfusion therapy should be judged cautiously.

REFERENCES

1. O'Gara PT, Kushner KG, Ascheim DD, et al. 2013 ACCF/AHA guideline for the management of ST-elevation myocardial infarction. A report of the American College of Cardiology Foundation/American Heart Association Task Force on Practice Guidelines. Circulation. 2013;127:e362-e425.
2. Antman EM, Anbe DT, Armstrong PW, et al. ACC/AHA guidelines for the management of patients with ST-elevation myocardial infarction–executive summary: a report of the American College of Cardiology/American Heart Association Task Force on Practice Guidelines (Writing Committee to Revise the 1999 Guidelines for the Management of Patients With Acute Myocardial Infarction). Circulation. 2004;110:588-636.
3. Van de Werf F, Bax J, Betriu A, et al. The task force on the management of ST-segment elevation myocardial infarction of the European Society of Cardiology. Management of acute myocardial infarction in patients presenting with persistent ST-segment elevation. Eur Heart J. 2008;29:2909-45.
4. Angeja BG, Gunda M, Murphy SA, et al. LIMIT AMI Study Group. TIMI myocardial perfusion grade and ST segment resolution: association with infarct size as assessed by single photon emission computed tomography imaging. Circulation. 2002;105:282-5.
5. de Lemos JA, Braunwald E. ST segment resolution as a tool for assessing the efficacy of reperfusion therapy. J Am Coll Cardiol. 2001;38:1283-94.
6. Buller CE, Fu Y, Mahaffey KW, et al. ST-segment recovery and outcome after primary PCI for ST elevation myocardial infarction: insights from the APEX AMI Trial. Circulation. 2008;118:1335-46.
7. McLaughlin MG, Stone GW, Aymong E, et al. Prognostic utility of comparative methods for assessment of ST-segment resolution after primary angioplasty for acute myocardial infarction: the Controlled Abciximab and Device Investigation to Lower Late Angioplasty Complications (CADILLAC) trial. J Am Coll Cardiol. 2004;44:1215-23.
8. Prasad A, Stone GW, Aymong E, et al. Impact of ST-segment resolution after primary angioplasty on outcomes after myocardial infarction in elderly patients: an analysis from the CADILLAC trial. Am Heart J. 2004;147:669-75.
9. Schröder R. Prognostic impact of early ST-segment resolution in acute ST-elevation myocardial infarction. Circulation. 2004;110:e506-e510.
10. Napodano M and Paganelli C. ECG in acute myocardial infarction in the reperfusion era. In: Richard Millis RM (Ed). Advances in Electrocardiograms—Clinical Applications. Croatia: InTech; 2012.
11. Zimetbaum PJ, Josephson ME. Use of the electrocardiogram in acute myocardial infarction. N Engl J Med. 2003;348: 933-40.
12. Schroder K, Wegscheider K, Zeymer U, et al. Extent of ST-segment deviation in a single electrocardiogram lead 90 min after thrombolysis as a predictor of medium-term mortality in acute myocardial infarction. Lancet. 2001;358:1479-86.

13. Poli A, Fetiveau R, Vandoni P, et al. Integrated analysis of myocardial blush ST-segment elevation recovery after successful primary angioplasty: real-time grading of microvascular reperfusion and prediction of early and late recovery of left ventricular function. Circulation. 2002;106:313-8.
14. Anderson RD, White HD, Ohman EM, et al. Predicting outcome after thrombolysis in acute myocardial infarction according to ST-segment resolution at 90 minutes: a substudy of the GUSTO-III trial. Global Use of Strategies To Open occluded coronary arteries. Am Heart J. 2002;144: 81-8.
15. van't Hof AW, Liem A, de Boer MJ, et al. Clinical value of 12-lead electrocardiogram after successful reperfusion therapy for acute myocardial infarction. Zwolle Myocardial Infarction Study Group. Lancet. 1997;350:615-9.
16. Zeymer U, Schröder R, Machnig T, et al. Primary percutaneous transluminal coronary angioplasty accelerates early myocardial reperfusion compared to thrombolytic therapy in patients with AMI. Am Heart J. 2003;146:686-91.
17. Schröder K, Wegscheider K, Zeymer U, et al. Extent of ST-segment deviation in the single ECG lead of maximum deviation present 90 or 180 minutes after start of thrombolytic therapy best predicts outcome in acute myocardial infarction. Z Kardiol. 2001;90:557-67.
18. Schröder K, Wegscheider K, Zeymer U, et al. Prediction of long-term outcome by the extent of existing ST-segment deviation in a single electrocardiographic lead shortly after thrombolysis in acute myocardial infarction. Am J Cardiol. 2003;91:454-7.
19. van der Zwaan HB, Stoel MG, von Birgelen C. Early versus late ST-segment resolution and clinical outcomes after percutaneous coronary intervention for acute myocardial infarction. Neth Heart J. 2010;18(9):416-22.
20. Gibson CM, Karha J, Giugliano RP, et al. Association of the timing of ST-segment resolution with TIMI myocardial perfusion grade in acute myocardial infarction. Am Heart J. 2004;147:847-52.
21. Johanson P, Jernberg T, Gunnarsson G, et al. Prognostic value of ST-segment resolution-when and what to measure. Eur Heart J. 2003;24:337-45.
22. Schroder R, Dissmann R, Bruggemann T, et al. Extent of early ST segment elevation resolution: a simple but strong predictor of outcome in patients with acute myocardial infarction. J Am Coll Cardiol. 1994;24:384-91.
23. Brodie BR, Stuckey TD, Hansen C, et al. Relation between electrocardiographic ST-segment resolution and early and late outcomes after primary percutaneous coronary intervention for acute myocardial infarction. Am J Cardiol. 2005;95:343-8.
24. Terkelsen CJ, Norgaard BL, Lassen JF, et al. Potential significance of spontaneous and interventional ST-changes in patients transferred for primary percutaneous coronary intervention: observations from the ST-MONitoring in Acute Myocardial Infarction study (The MONAMI study). Eur Heart J. 2006;27:267-75.
25. Watanabe J, Nakamura S, Sugiura T, et al. Early identification of impaired myocardial reperfusion with serial assessment of ST-segments after percutaneous transluminal coronary angioplasty during acute myocardial infarction. Am J Cardiol. 2001;88:956-9.
26. Wehrens X, Doevendans P, Ophuis TJ, et al. A comparison of electrocardiographic changes during reperfusion of acute myocardial infarction by thrombolysis or percutaneous transluminal coronary angioplasty. Am Heart J. 2000;139:430-6.
27. Chiladakis JA, Vlachos N, Patsouras N, et al. Usefulness of reperfusion ventricular arrhythmias in non-invasive prediction of early reperfusion and sustained coronary artery patency in acute myocardial infarction. J Thromb Thrombolys. 2001;12(3):231-6.
28. Tatli E, Alicik G, Buturak A, et al. Arrhythmias following revascularization procedures in the course of acute myocardial infarction: are they indicators of reperfusion or ongoing ischemia? Scientific World J. 2013; 2013:7
29. Bonnemeier H, Ortak J, Wiegand UKH, et al. Accelerated idioventricular rhythm in the post-thrombolytic era: incidence, prognostic implications, and modulating mechanisms after direct percutaneous coronary intervention. Ann Noninvas Electro. 2005;10(2):179-87.
30. Terkelsen CJ, Sorensen JT, Kaltoft AK, et al. Prevalence and significance of accelerated idioventricular rhythm in patients with ST-elevation myocardial infarction treated with primary percutaneous coronary intervention. Am J Cardiol. 2009;104(12):1641-6.
31. Engelen DJ, Gressin V, Krucoff MW, et al. Usefulness of frequent arrhythmias after epicardial recanalization in anterior wall acute myocardial infarction as a marker of cellular injury leading to poor recovery of left ventricular function. Am J Cardiol. 2003;92(10):1143-9.
32. Tjandrawidjaja MC, Fu Y, Westerhout CM, et al. Resolution of ST-segment depression: a new prognostic marker in ST-segment elevation myocardial infarction. Eur Heart J. 2010;31:573-81.
33. Toma M, Fu Y, Wagner G, et al. Risk stratification in ST-elevation myocardial infarction is enhanced by combining baseline ST deviation and subsequent ST-segment resolution. Heart. 2008;94:e6.
34. De Luca G, Maas AC, Suryapranata H, et al. Prognostic significance of residual cumulative ST-segment deviation after mechanical reperfusion in patients with ST-segment elevation myocardial infarction. Am Heart J. 2005;150:1248-54.

Chapter 10

Ectopic and Escape Beats

INTRODUCTION

The terms ectopic beat, extrasystole or premature contraction are, for practical purposes, synonymous. They refer to an impulse originating from atria, atrioventricular (AV) junction or ventricles, which arise prematurely in the cardiac cycle. Ectopic beats are by definition premature. Thus the interval between the ectopic beat and the preceding beat (i.e. the coupling interval) is shorter than the cycle length of the dominant rhythm (Fig. 10.1).[1]

Ectopic beats are classified by their origin. They are classified into three groups:

1. Premature atrial complex (PAC)
2. Premature junctional complex (PJC)
3. Premature ventricular complex (PVC).

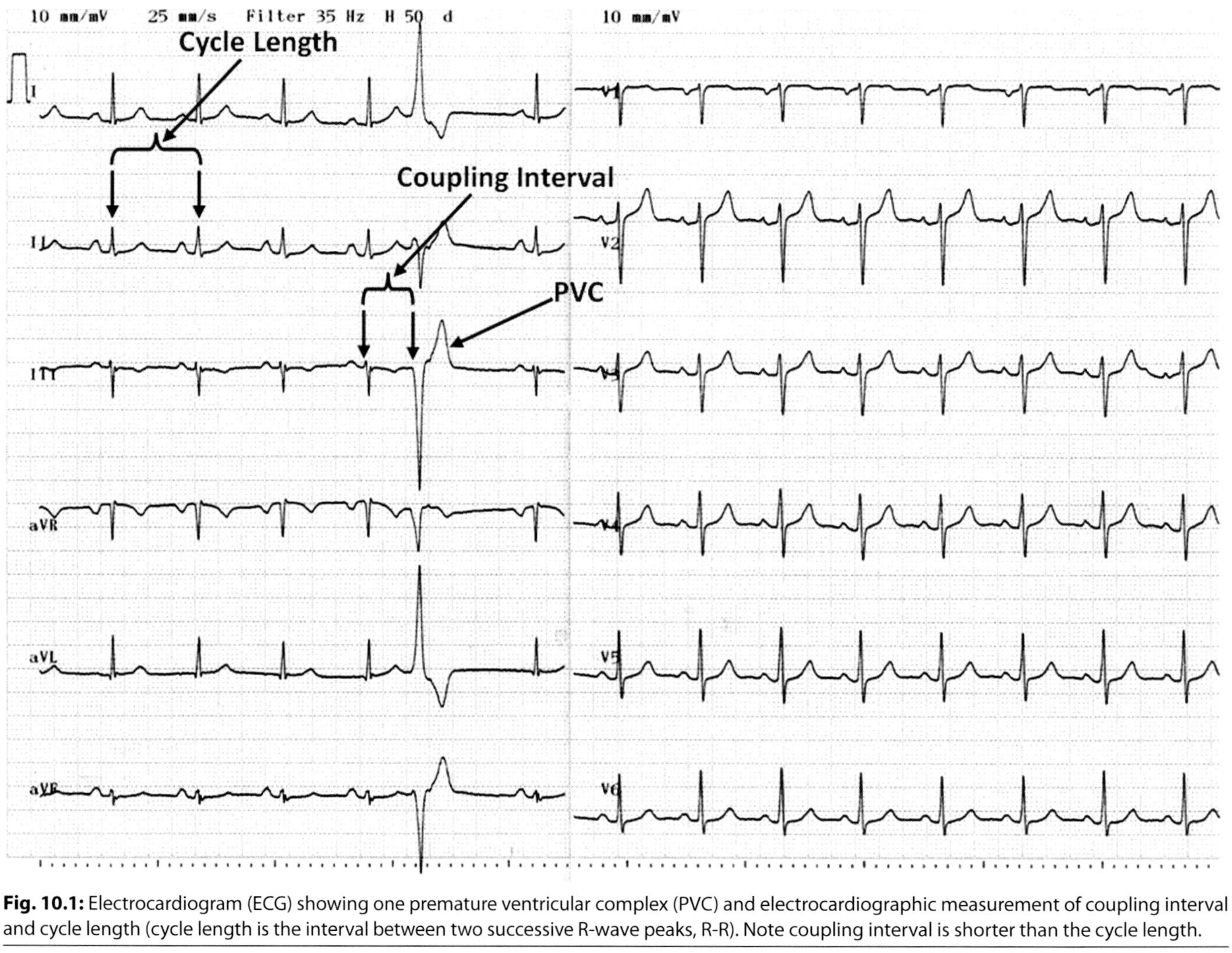

Fig. 10.1: Electrocardiogram (ECG) showing one premature ventricular complex (PVC) and electrocardiographic measurement of coupling interval and cycle length (cycle length is the interval between two successive R-wave peaks, R-R). Note coupling interval is shorter than the cycle length.

PREMATURE ATRIAL COMPLEX

Premature atrial complex (PAC), also known as atrial premature complex (APC) or atrial premature beat (APB) occurs when a focus in the atrium [not the sinoatrial (SA) node], generates an action potential before the next scheduled SA node action potential. These arise from ectopic pacemaking tissue within the atria. There is an abnormal P-wave, usually followed by a normal QRS complex.

There are four main characteristics of PACs: They are *premature*. That is they occur earlier than you would expect if you measure the previous P to P intervals. They are *ectopic*, meaning originating outside of the SA node. Thus the P-wave morphology would be different than the normal sinus P-wave (Figs. 10.2A and 2B). They are narrow complexes. Since they come from the atrium, they will eventually travel through the AV node and use the normal conduction system to spread to the ventricles. There is a compensatory pause

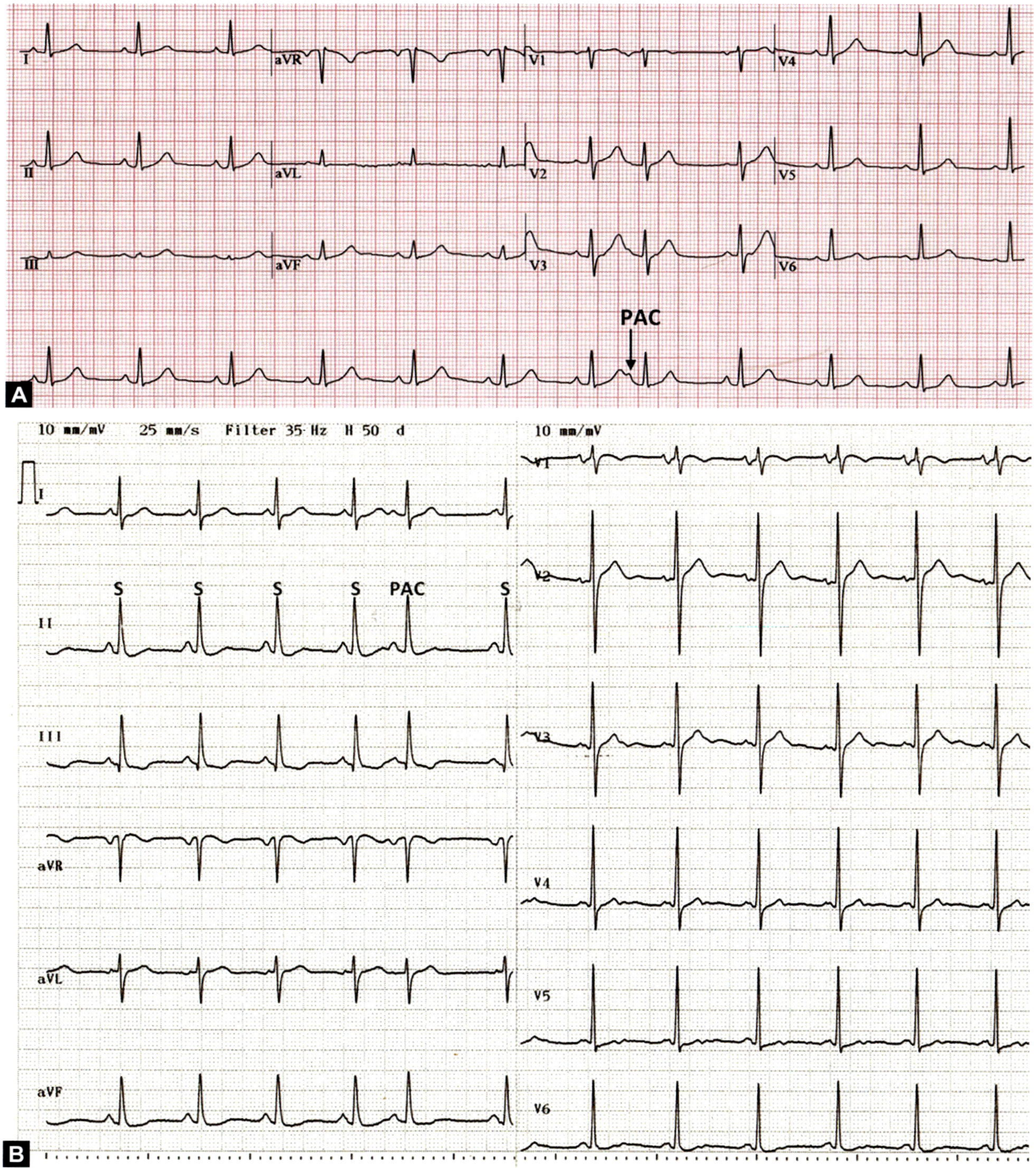

Figs. 10.2A and B: (A) Electrocardiogram shows single premature atrial complex (PAC) (arrow). Note morphology of the P in PAC is different from normal sinus P-wave. (B) ECG shows a single PAC. Note QRS complex is of normal morphology.

after the PAC and it is usually incomplete. A compensatory pause is described as being "complete" when the interval between two sinus beats flanking an ectopic beat is equal to two sinus cycles (Fig. 10.3) and "incomplete" when it is shorter (Fig. 10.4). The extra atrial action potential causes the SA node to become refractory to generating its next scheduled beat. Thus, it must "skip a beat". If a premature atrial contraction occurs when the AV node has not yet recovered from the refractory period, the PAC will fail to conduct to the ventricles and there will not be a QRS complex afterward. In this situation the electrocardiogram (ECG) will show a premature, ectopic P-wave occurring and then no QRS complex afterward. PAC may be unifocal or multifocal. Unifocal, arising from a single ectopic focus and each PAC is identical. Multifocal, arising from two or more ectopic foci and multiple P-wave morphologies are reflected.

Premature atrial complex may be due to multiple causes as follows:[2]

- Anxiety and stress
- Tobacco/alcohol
- Sympathomimetics
- Beta-agonists
- Excess caffeine
- Hypokalemia
- Hypomagnesemia
- Digoxin toxicity
- Coronary artery disease (CAD).

Premature atrial complexes may be asymptomatic or cause symptoms such as a sensation of "skipping" or palpitations. PACs are often single and isolated, but may be frequent and may occur in a bigeminal or trigeminal pattern. In atrial bigeminy, the PAC follows every normal sinus beat (Fig. 10.5) and in atrial trigeminy, there are two normal beats followed by a PAC.

Although PACs have a wide array of manifestations, they are not life-threatening by themselves. The great majority of PACs are completely benign and require little if any treatment at all. In rare cases, PACs may be a sign of underlying cardiac disease. In predisposed individuals, PACs may initiate supraventricular and less commonly, ventricular arrhythmias.[2,3] Atrial fibrillation (AF) is the most common arrhythmia induced by PACs, particularly

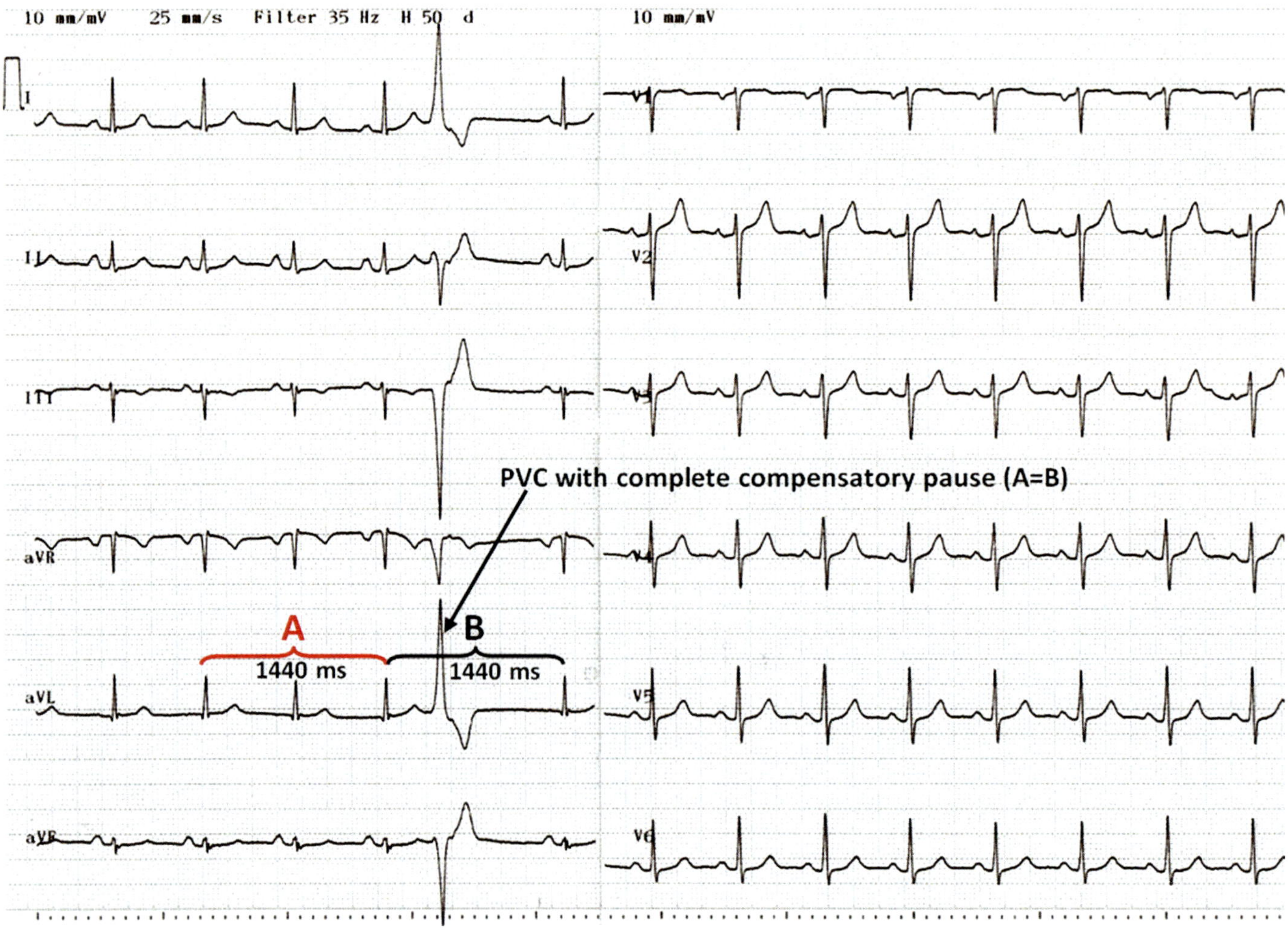

Fig. 10.3: Electrocardiogram showing PVC with complete compensatory pause. Note the distance between two impulses straddling a sinus impulse (distance A, 1440 ms) is equal to the distance between two sinus impulses straddling a PVC (distance B, 1440 ms).

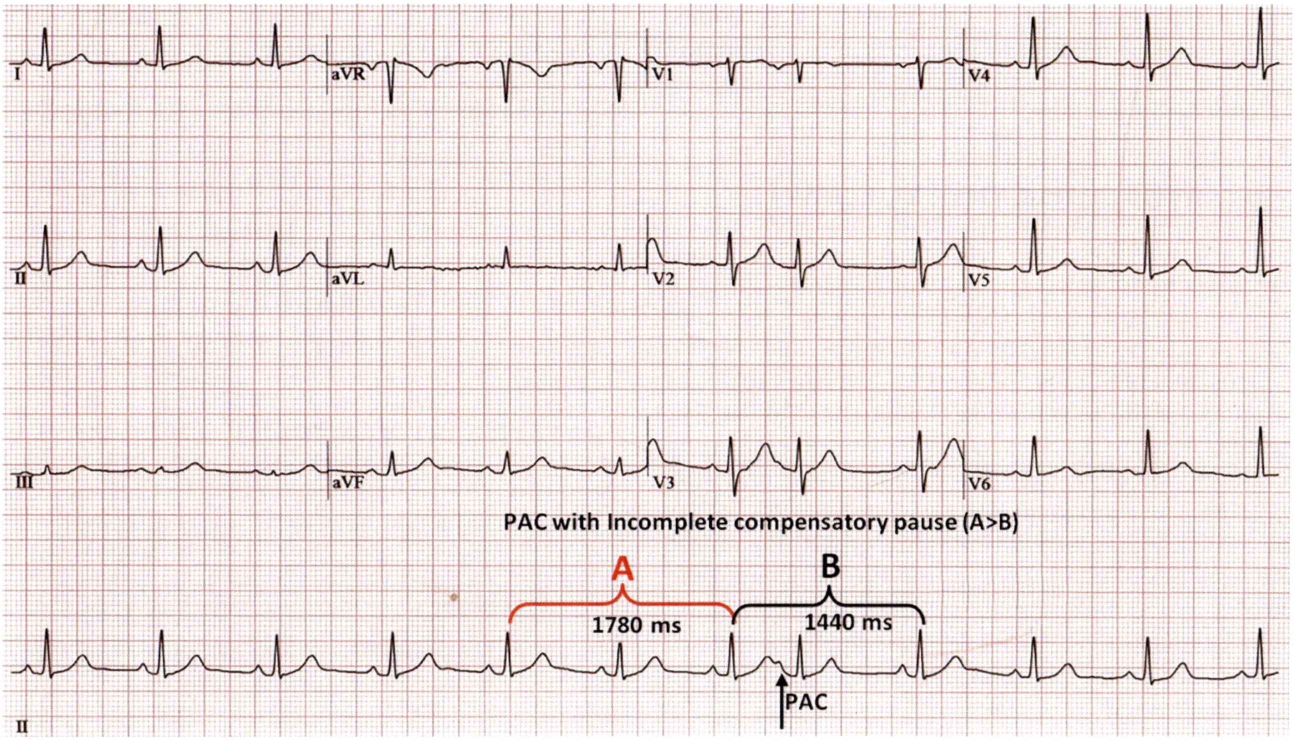

Fig. 10.4: Electrocardiogram showing PAC with incomplete compensatory pause. Note the distance between two impulses straddling a sinus impulse (distance A, 1780 ms) is higher than the distance between two sinus impulses straddling a PAC (distance B, 1440 ms).

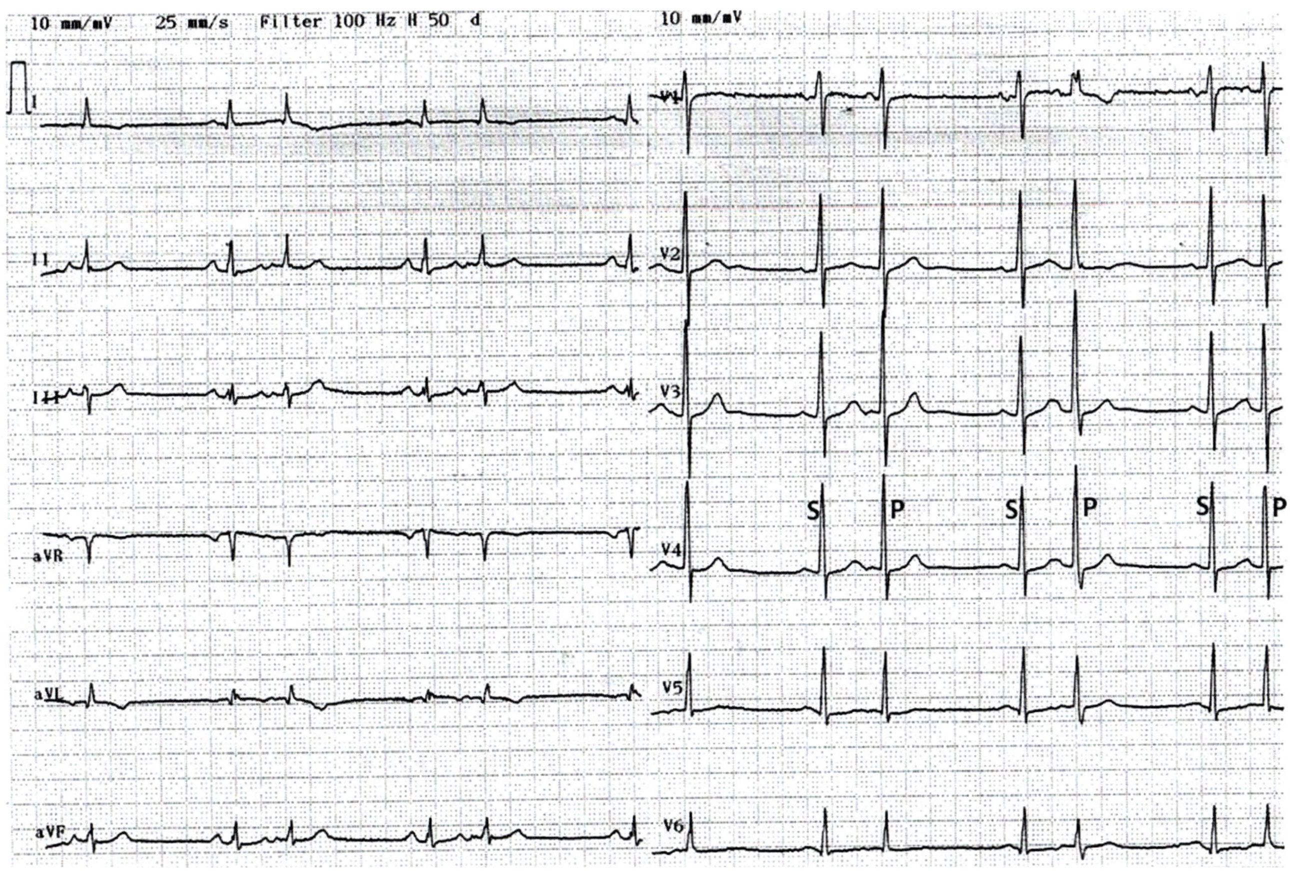

Fig. 10.5: Electrocardiogram shows atrial bigeminy. PAC (P) follows every normal sinus beat (S). Note normal QRS configuration, so premature beats are not PVCs.

those originate around the pulmonary vein.[4] The presence and frequency of PACs have been shown to predict the development of AF after cardiac surgery and the recurrence of AF after cardioversion.[5,6]

PREMATURE JUNCTIONAL COMPLEX

Premature junctional complex (PJC) is also termed as AV junctional ectopic beats or nodal beats. PJCs are recognized by a premature QRS complex which is similar in appearance to that occurring in sinus rhythm. The PJC focus, located in the AV junction, captures the atria (retrograde) and the ventricles (antegrade). So the PJC focus may activate the atria as well as ventricles, leading to a retrograde P-wave (i.e. negative in LII, LIII, and aVF) (Fig. 10.6). The retrograde P waves may precede, follow or be buried within the QRS complex, depending on the relative speeds of conduction of the PJC impulse to the ventricles and to the atria.[1] PJC beats are not as common as atrial or ventricular ectopics. PJCs are similar to PAC's in clinical implications, but occur less frequently. Treatment is rarely necessary.

Premature junctional complexes are distinguished from PACs by the P-wave. PAC has a fairly normal looking P-wave, upright and round. PJCs, however, do not originate in the atria, therefore, the atrial depolarization moves up toward the base of the heart, rather than downward toward the apex. P-waves from PJCs will be inverted (Fig. 10.7) and often, the P-wave will occur along with the QRS complex, and will therefore be hidden from view (Fig. 10.8).

Junctional rhythms are arbitrarily classified by their rate:

1. Junctional escape rhythm: 40-60 beats/min (Figs. 10.9A and B)
2. Accelerated junctional rhythm: 60–100 beats/min (Fig. 10.10)
3. Junctional tachycardia: Greater than 100 beats/min (Fig. 10.11).

These premature beats can be seen occasionally in healthy subjects and more commonly in some pathological conditions, typically in the case of cardiac drug toxicity, electrolyte imbalance, postmitral valve surgery, and cold water immersion.

PREMATURE VENTRICULAR COMPLEX

Premature ventricular complexes (PVCs), also called ventricular premature complex (VPC), ventricular premature beat (VPB), or ventricular extrasystole (VES) are common with an estimated prevalence of 1–4% in the general population. In a normal healthy population, PVCs have been detected in 1% of subjects on standard 12-lead electrocardiography and between 40% and 75% of subjects on 24- to 48-hour Holter monitoring. Their prevalence is generally age-dependent, ranging from <1% in children less than 11 years to 69% in subjects >75 years. Commonly thought to be a benign entity but may be associated with sudden death.[7] A population study showed that PVCs were recorded on standard 12-lead ECGs in 0.8% of subjects in a healthy military population, with a prevalence of 0.5% in those under the age of 20 years and 2.2% in those over 50 years of age. In the Framingham Heart Study, the prevalence of patients having greater than

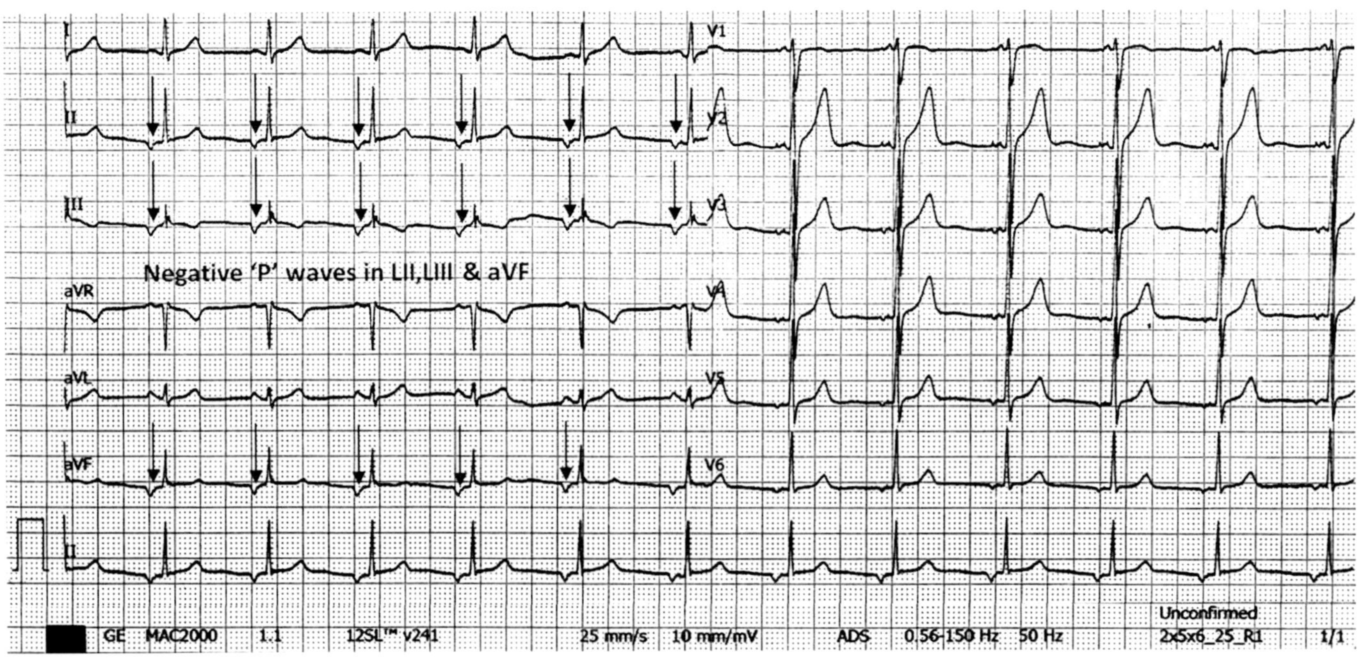

Fig. 10.6: Electrocardiogram is suggestive of junctional or nodal rhythm. Note negative "P" waves in LII, LIII, and aVF (*arrows*).

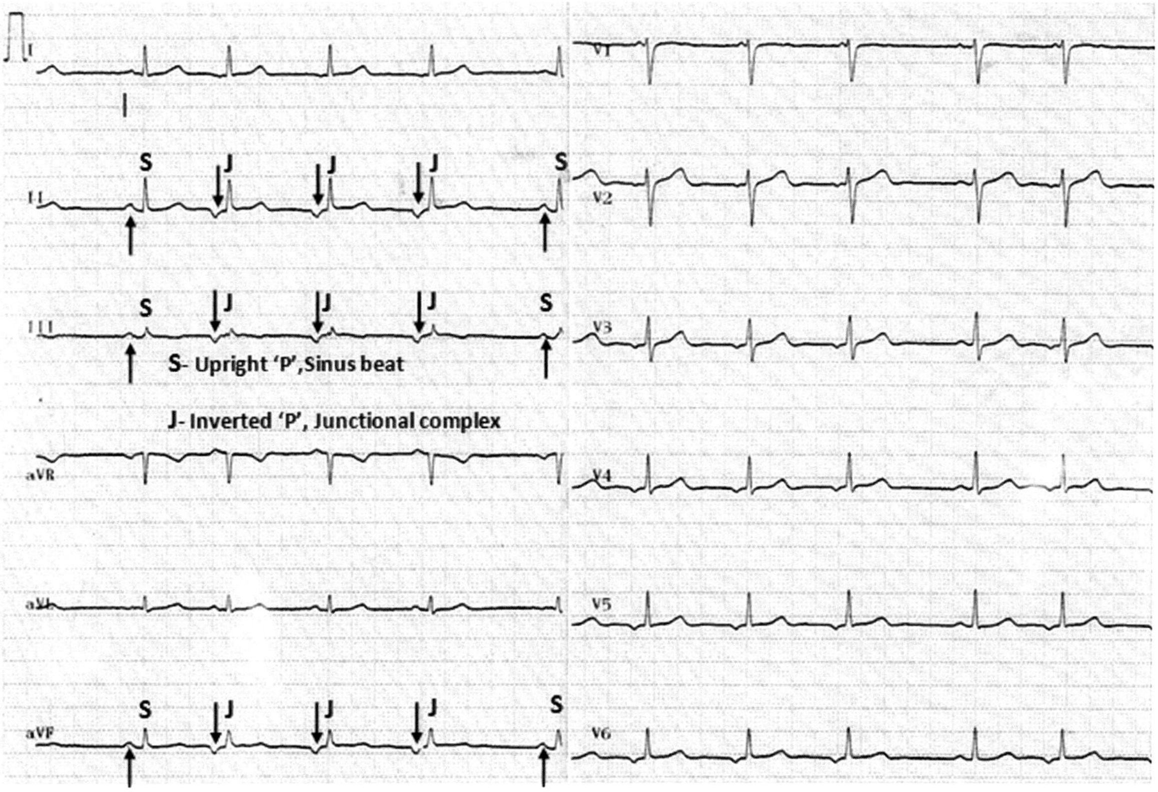

Fig. 10.7: Electrocardiogram shows both sinus beat and junctional complex. In sinus beat "P" upright in LII, LIII, and aVF (*upfacing arrows*) and negative in same leads in junctional beat (*downfacing arrows*).

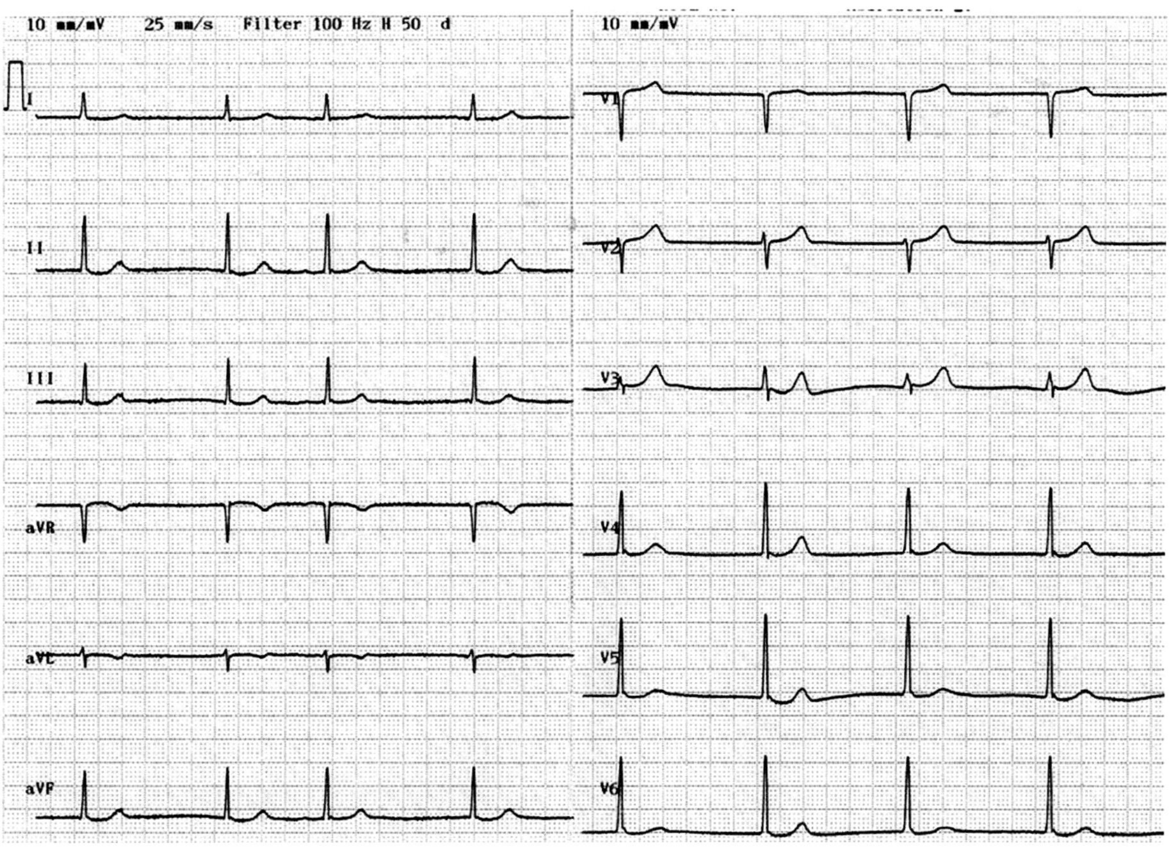

Fig. 10.8: Electrocardiogram of junctional rhythm. Note no "P" wave preceding QRS complex. "P" waves are possibly buried inside the QRS complexes.

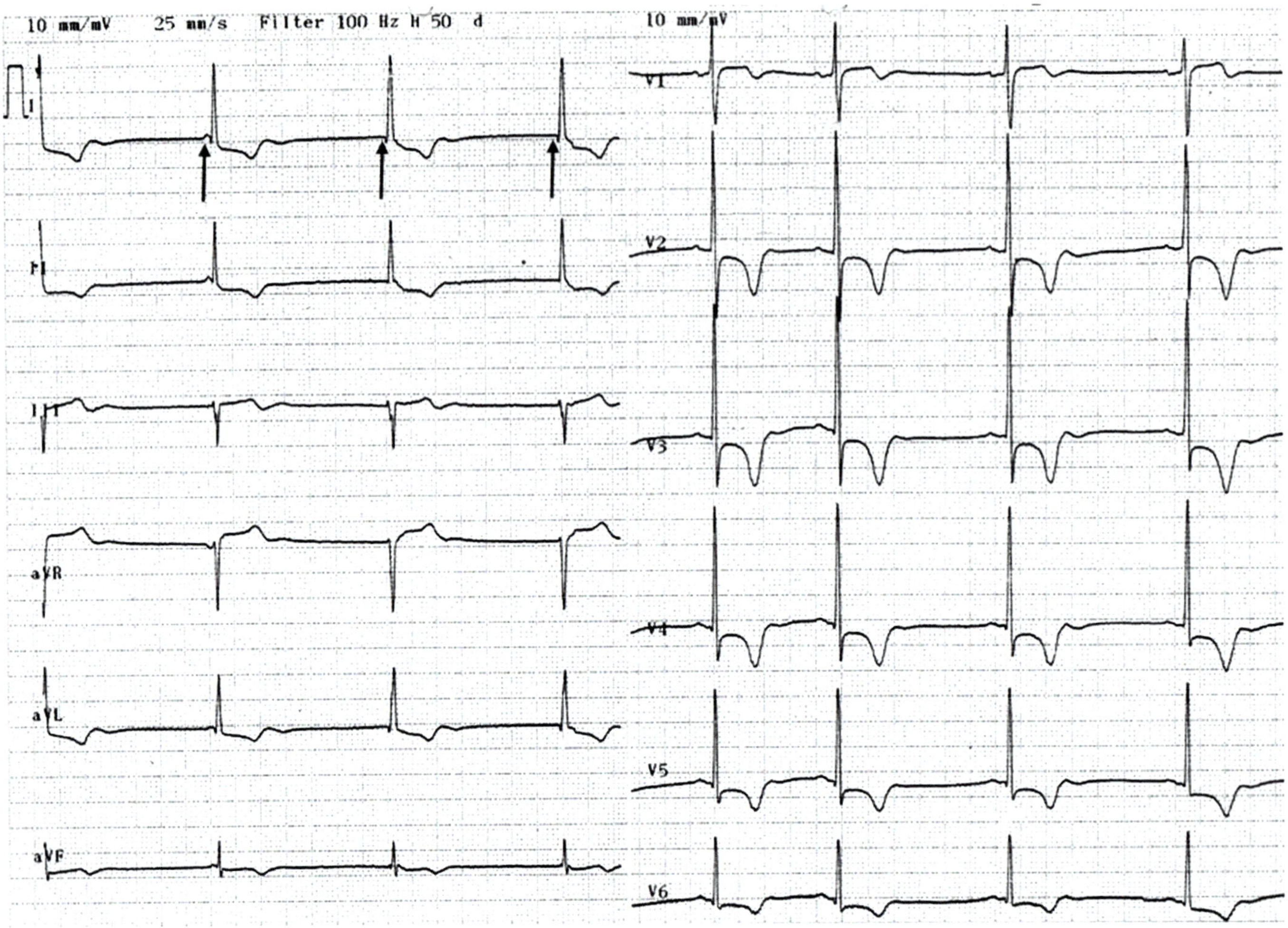

Fig. 10.9A: Intermittent Junctional escape rhythm (heart rate 48 bpm). Note most of the QRS complexes of left side of the ECG panel are not preceded by "P" wave. In this ECG either "P" waves are absent or PR interval is very short (*arrows*).

or equal to 1 PVC/h in a 1-hour ambulatory ECG monitoring was 33% in men and 32% in women without CAD. Among patients with established CAD, the prevalence was 58% in men and 49% in women.[8,9] Patients without structural heart disease and low-to-modest PVC burdens do not always require treatment. PVCs at higher burdens (typically more than 15–20% of heart beats) or strung together in runs of ventricular tachycardia (VT) pose a higher risk of tachycardia-related cardiomyopathy and heart failure, even if asymptomatic.[10,11] PVCs result in a premature QRS complex which is broad greater than 0.12 seconds (greater than 120 ms), bizarre in shape and in contrast to atrial ectopic beats, will not be preceded by an ectopic P-wave.

Electrocardiogram Criteria for Diagnosis of Premature Ventricular Complex (Fig. 10.12)

There are several main characteristics of premature ventricular complexes (PVCs):

- They are premature.
- They are ectopic, meaning originating outside of the SA node. Thus the QRS morphology would be different than the normal QRS morphology when the action potential travels through the normal conduction system.
- They are wide complexes. Since they come from the ventricles and do not use the normal ventricular conduction system, the action potential needs to travel from myocyte to myocyte instead which is much slower, thus the QRS complex is wide. Unlike a premature atrial contraction, which is usually narrow-complexed since it uses the normal ventricular conduction system (unless a baseline right or left bundle branch block is present).
- Discordant ST segment and T-wave changes are present. Discordance describes a pattern of repolarization abnormality (typically seen with left bundle branch block, paced rhythms, and VT) in which the ST segment and T-wave are directed opposite to the main vector of the QRS complex.
- There is a full compensatory pause after the PVC. The extra action potential causes the SA node to become refractory to generating its next scheduled beat.

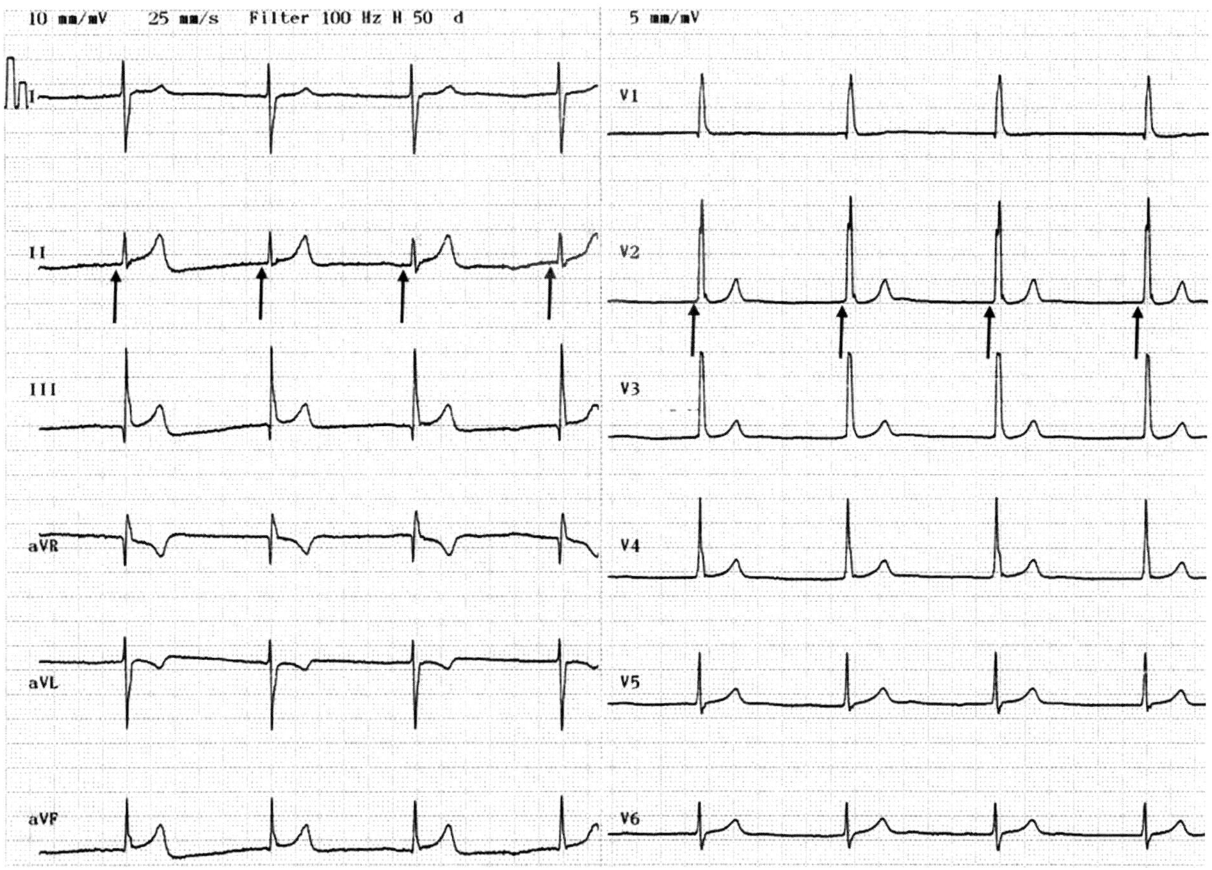

Fig. 10.9B: Junctional escape rhythm (heart rate 50 bpm). Note absence of "P" waves preceding QRS complexes (*arrows*).

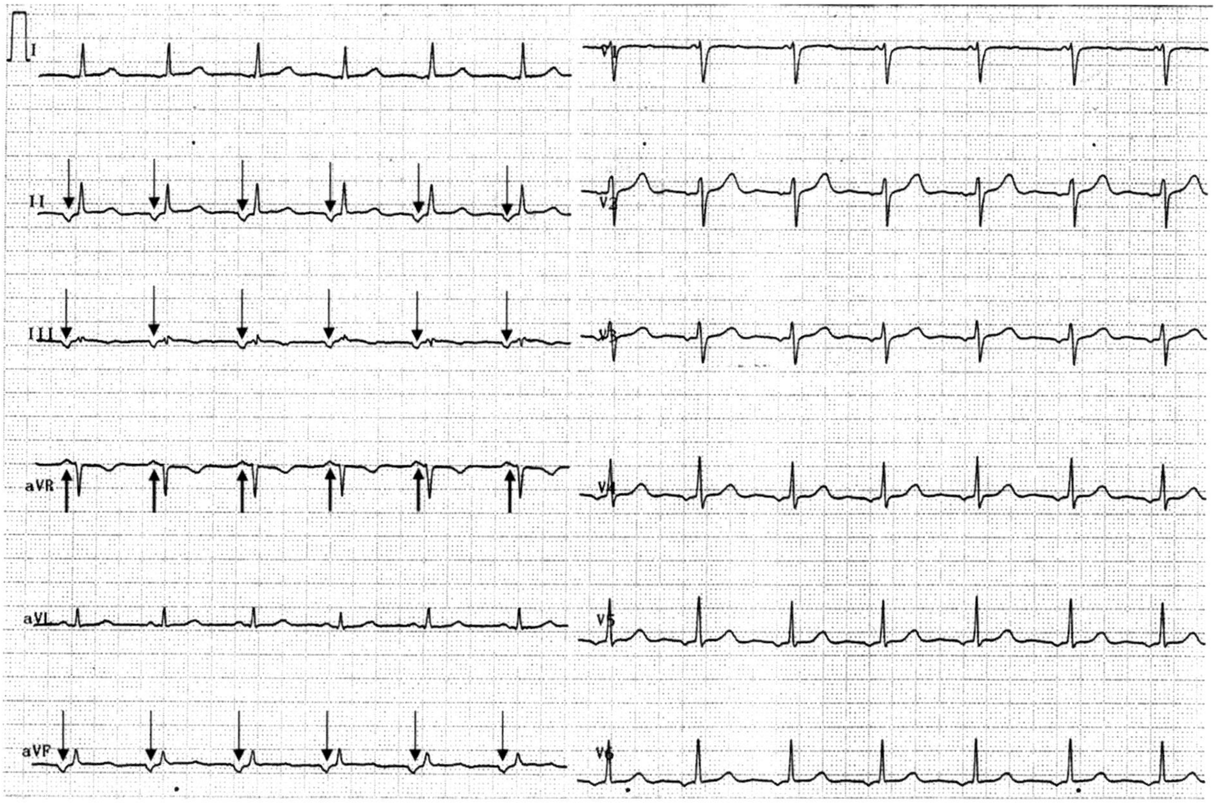

Fig. 10.10: Accelerated junctional rhythm (76 bpm). Note negative "P" waves in LII, LIII, and aVF (*downfacing arrows*) and positive "P" waves in lead aVR (*upfacing arrows*).

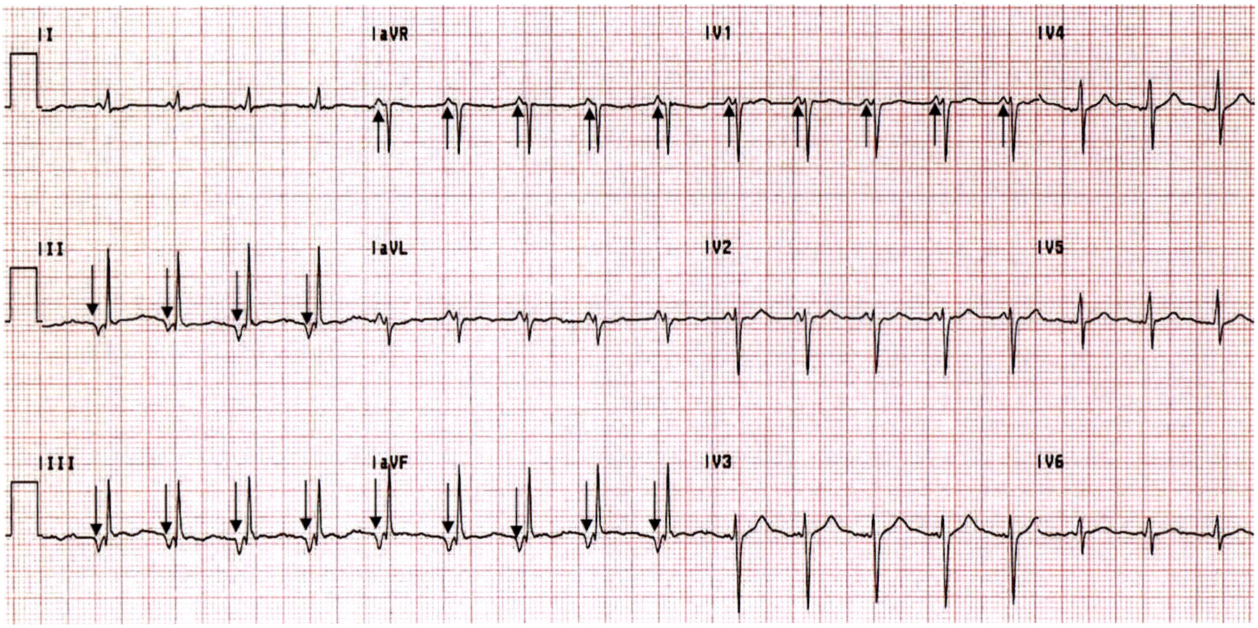

Fig. 10.11: Junctional tachycardia (112 bpm). ECG shows narrow complex tachycardia at 112 bpm, retrograde (inverted) P waves in II, III, and aVF and upright "P" in V1 and aVR. Presence of short PR interval less than 0.12 seconds (less than 120 ms) indicates a junctional rhythm rather than atrial focus.

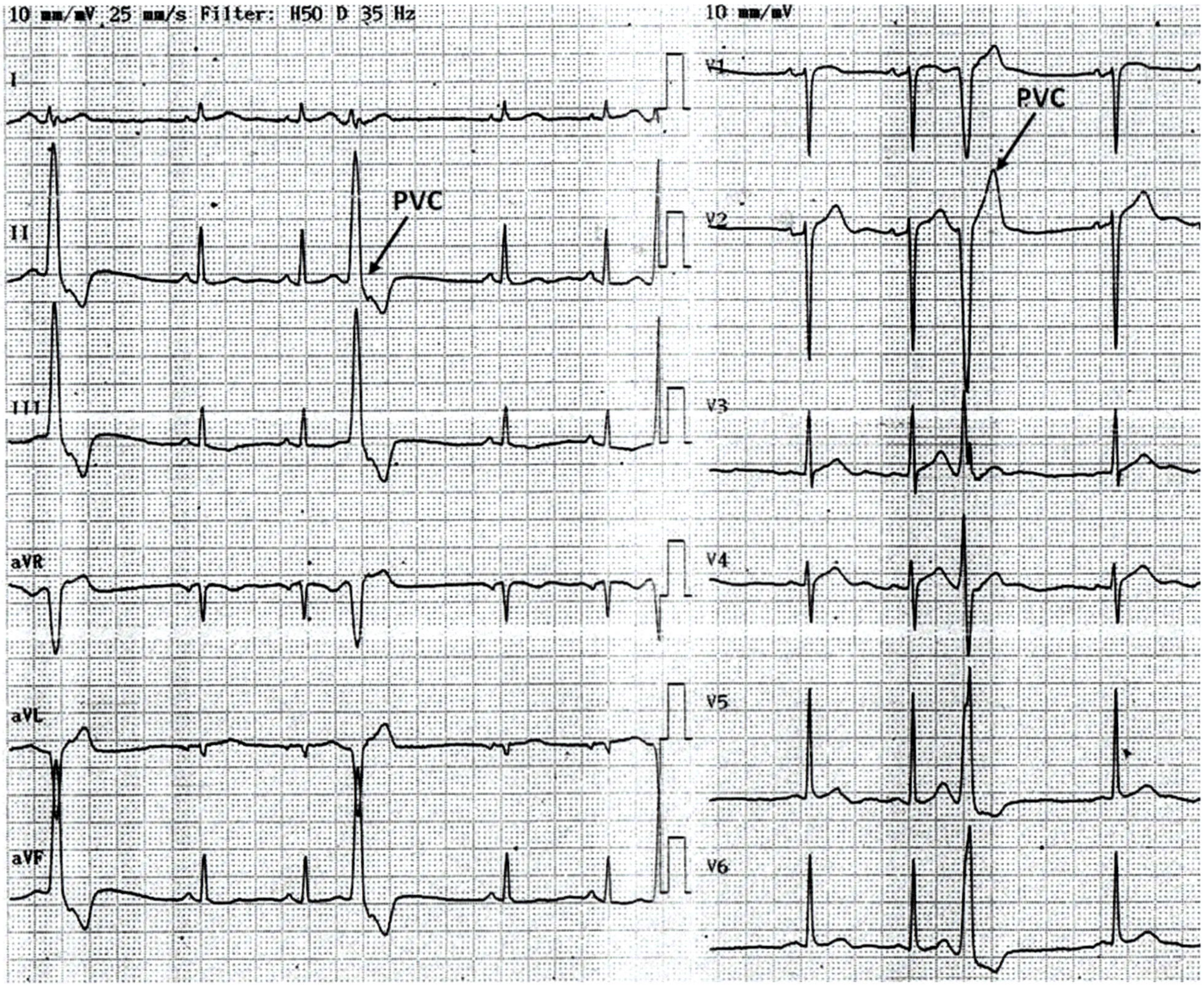

Fig. 10.12: Electrocardiogram shows typical PVCs (*arrows*). PVCs are premature, ectopic and are of wide complexes. Also note discordance of ST segment and T waves (*ST segment and T waves are directed opposite to the main vector of the QRS complex*).

- The QRS complex of a PVC is widened, often notched, and with a QRS duration usually greater than 0.12 seconds (>120 ms). It will have a morphology that resembles a right or left bundle branch block depending upon the location of origin. It is assumed that the PVC originates in the left ventricle when it has a positive deflection or tall R-wave in V1 (right bundle branch block configuration), while a negative complex with a deep S-wave in V1 (resembling a left bundle branch block morphology) originates in the right ventricle (Box 10.1). Other findings on the ECG include marked repolarization abnormalities, manifested as ST segment and T-wave abnormalities.

There can be many sinus node responses to a PVC. Most commonly, a full compensatory pause follows the PVC; thus, the PP interval between the QRS complexes before and after the premature beat is twice the PP interval between two successive sinus beats.

Causes of Premature Ventricular Contraction

- *Cardiac causes include*:
  - Acute myocardial infarction (AMI)
  - Valvular heart disease
  - Mitral valve prolapse (MVP)
  - Cardiomyopathy (e.g. ischemic, dilated, hypertrophic, and infiltrative)
  - Myocarditis.
- *Noncardiac causes include*:
  - Electrolyte disturbances (hypokalemia, hypomagnesemia, or hypercalcemia)
  - Medications (e.g. digoxin, tricyclic antidepressants, aminophylline, amitriptyline, pseudoephedrine, and fluoxetine)
  - Other drugs (e.g. cocaine, amphetamines, caffeine, and alcohol)
  - Anesthetics
  - Surgery
  - Infection
  - Stress.

Three common mechanisms exist for PVCs,

1. Automaticity,
2. Reentry, and
3. Triggered activity.

Automaticity is the development of a new site of depolarization in nonnodal ventricular tissue, which can lead to a PVC. Increased automaticity could be due to electrolyte abnormalities or ischemic myocardium. Reentry typically occurs when slow-conducting tissue (e.g. infarcted myocardium) is present adjacent to normal tissue. The slow-conducting tissue could be due to scarred myocardium, as in the case of a healed myocardial infarction. Triggered activity can induce PVC. After depolarizations triggered by a preceding impulse can lead to premature activation if the threshold is reached, and this can cause a PVC.

Because PVCs arise within an ectopic focus within the ventricular muscle, the QRS complex is wide, bizarre, and unrelated to a preceding P-wave. There is usually a constant relationship (timing) between the preceding sinus beat and a subsequent ventricular beat, because the preceding beat influences the ectopic focus. The ventricular beat is not usually conducted back into the atria. The atrial impulse that occurred, or was about to occur when the PVCs take place is usually blocked, but the subsequent atrial beat will occur on time, and be conducted normally. Rarely, the ventricular beat may be conducted retrogradely and captures the atrium, resulting in a P-wave after the QRS, with an abnormal morphology as conduction through the atrium is retrograde.

Because the intrinsic rate of an ectopic focus often tends to be slow, extrasystoles will tend to arise more commonly with slower rates. In addition, if the rate is varying, extrasystoles will tend to "squeeze in" during long RR intervals. Some have called this the "rule of bigeminy."

Premature Ventricular Contractions are classified on the basis of their origin:

Unifocal PVCs: Unifocal PVCs originate from the same focus. They all have the same shape, or morphology (morphologies of QRS complexes to be compared in the same lead, not in different leads) (Fig. 10.13).

Multifocal PVCs: Multifocal PVCs have different sites of origin, which means their coupling intervals (coupling interval is the distance between the PVC and the preceding QRS complex) are usually different (Fig. 10.14).

Multiformed PVCs: Multiformed PVCs usually have the same coupling intervals (because they originate in the same ectopic site but their conduction through the ventricles differ). Multiformed PVCs are common in digitalis intoxication (Fig. 10.15).

Premature ventricular contractions are also classified by their frequency:

- *Bigeminy*: If each normal contraction is followed by a single PVC, this is termed as bigeminy (Fig. 10.16).
- *Trigeminy*: If two normal contractions are followed by a single PVC, it is called trigeminy (Fig. 10.17).
- *Quadrigeminy*: If three normal contractions are followed by a single PVC, it is called quadrigeminy. In quadrigeminy every fourth beat is a PVC (Fig. 10.18).
- *Couplet*: Two PVCs in a row is called a couplet (Fig. 10.19).
- *Triplet*: Three consecutive PVCs (Fig. 10.20).

Box 10.1: Morphology of premature ventricular complexes.

- *Left ventricular (LV) origin*: Right bundle branch block (RBBB) pattern
- *Right ventricular (RV) origin*: Left bundle branch block (LBBB) pattern
- *Interventricular septum (IVS) origin*: LBBB pattern

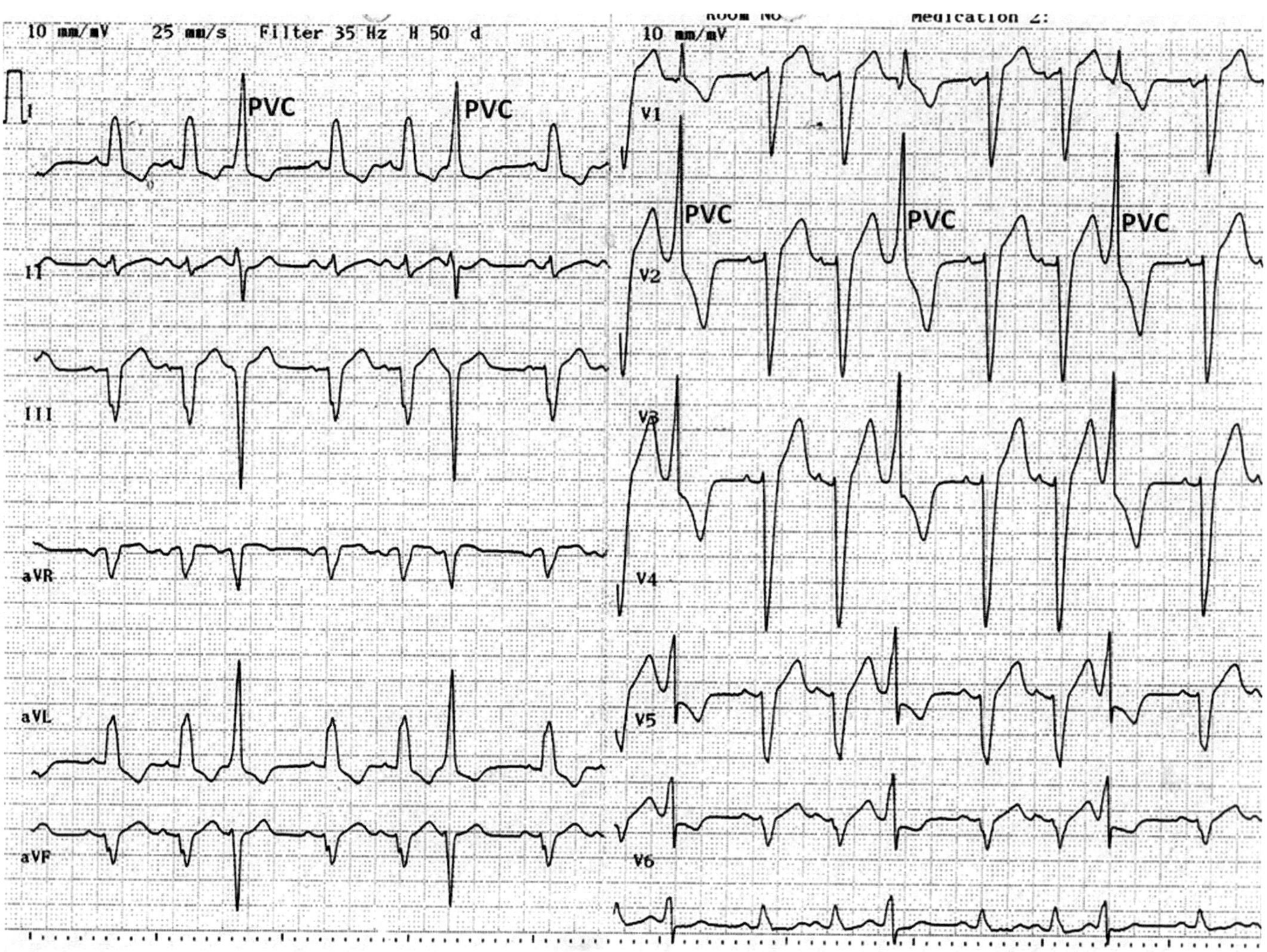

Fig. 10.13: Electrocardiogram strip shows unifocal PVCs. They all have the same shape, or morphology (morphologies of QRS complexes to be compared in the same lead, not in different leads).

- *Salvos*: More than three ectopic beats in succession is called a salvo. If the duration is less than 30 seconds, then this is also called "self-terminating VT" (Fig. 10.21).

R-ON-T PHENOMENON

The appearance of a PVC on the preceding T-wave is called R-on-T phenomenon. PVCs manifesting the R-on-T phenomenon have short coupling interval, usually measuring less than or equal to 0.40 seconds (400 ms). As the coupling interval is short, the PVCs occur on the downslope of the T-wave of the previous complex (Fig. 10.22). The "R-on-T" phenomenon was first described by Smirk in 1949. He observed that abnormal electrocardiogram morphology preceded the start of ventricular fibrillation (VF). Smirk described this morphology as an R-wave superimposed on T waves, representing a ventricular depolarization of an ectopic beat on the preceding T-wave. He believed that these early beats were precursors for VF and sudden death.[12,13] Beats those occur very early in the cardiac cycle will be superimposed on the T-wave of the preceding beat and described as "R-on-T" (Fig. 10.23). When it occurs during the vulnerable period of ventricular repolarization, it may induce VT or VF and sudden death. Anderson et al. have suggested that almost one-third of all sustained monomorphic VTs start with R-on-T PVCs.[14,15] Most episodes of VF and many episodes of VT are initiated by "R-on-T phenomenon," though by no means do all of the "R-on-T phenomenon" ectopic beats precipitate these life-threatening arrhythmias.

INTERPOLATED BEAT

Usually there is a pause after each PVC. When there is no pause and the PVC is thus sandwiched between two normal beats, the PVC is said to be "interpolated" (Figs. 10.24A and B). Interpolated ventricular ectopic beats are recognized as wide bizarre QRS complexes, not preceded by a P-wave. These are called interpolated ectopic beats because they are not disturbing the basic sinus rhythm. This usually occurs

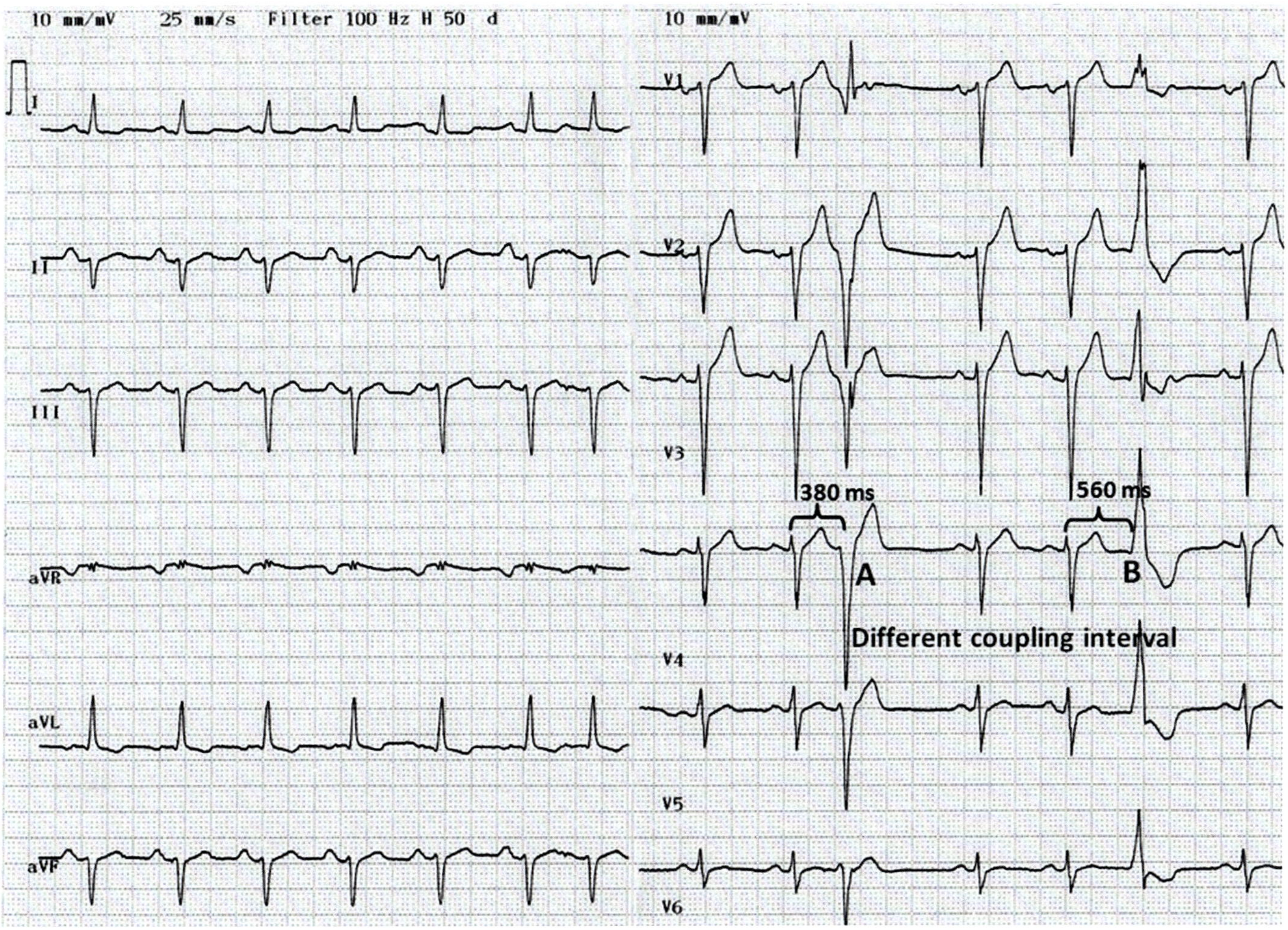

Fig. 10.14: Electrocardiogram shows multifocal PVCs. The PVCs are not of same morphology. They are multifocal as their coupling intervals (coupling interval is the distance between the PVC and the preceding QRS complex) are different. Coupling interval of PVC "A" is 380 ms and "B" is 560 ms.

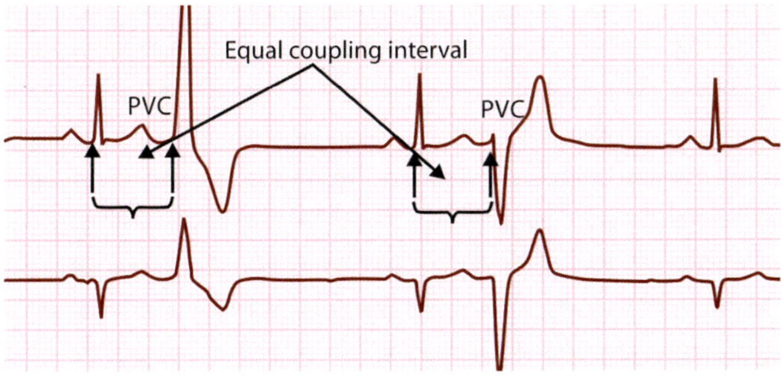

Fig. 10.15: Electrocardiogram shows multiformed PVCs. The morphology of the PVCs are different but their coupling intervals are equal (*arrows*). They originate in the same ectopic site but their conduction through the ventricles differ.

when the sinus rhythm is slower. Interpolation also implies that the ventricular ectopic beat is not getting conducted up to the sinus node to reset it; nor it is blocking the antegrade conduction of the subsequent sinus beat at the AV node. If it does so, varying degrees of AV block can occur for the subsequent sinus beat. Sometimes it will manifest just as prolongation of PR interval, while at the other extreme it might totally be nonconducted. In that case the ectopic beat will no longer be "interpolated" and there will be a compensatory pause visible. In interpolated ectopic beats, there is no pause at all (Fig. 10.25).

PARASYSTOLE

Parasystole usually is considered a rare phenomenon, but its prevalence depends on how it is sought and by whom. Routine electrocardiograms have yielded a prevalence of 0.13%, while the prevalence among patients, who may have more than 1 electrocardiogram to review, is greater (0.3%). When Holter monitoring is used for the search, the prevalence is much higher. The parasystolic focus is more often in the ventricles (>50%) than in the atria (20%) or AV junction (20%). Parasystolic rhythms per se appear to carry no significant risk.[16]

Unifocal ventricular ectopic beats have a constant coupling interval. Ventricular parasystole, which is uncommon, is an exception to this rule. In this arrhythmia

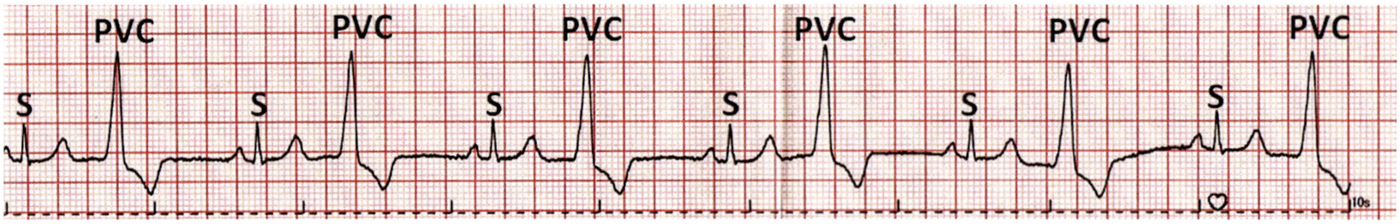

Fig. 10.16: Electrocardiogram is suggestive of ventricular bigeminy, each normal sinus conducted complex (S) is followed by a single PVC.

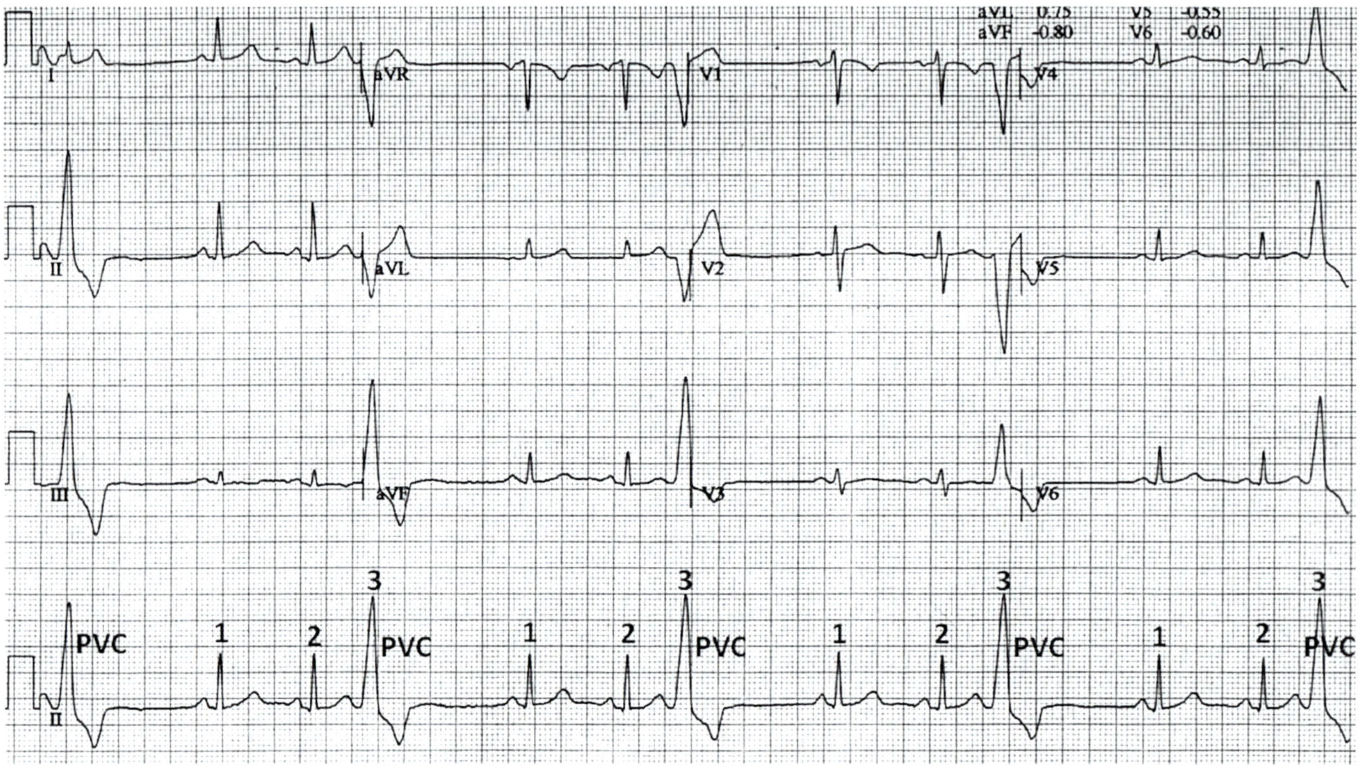

Fig. 10.17: Electrocardiogram is suggestive of sinus rhythm with frequent PVCs in a pattern of ventricular trigeminy. Note every third beat is a PVC.

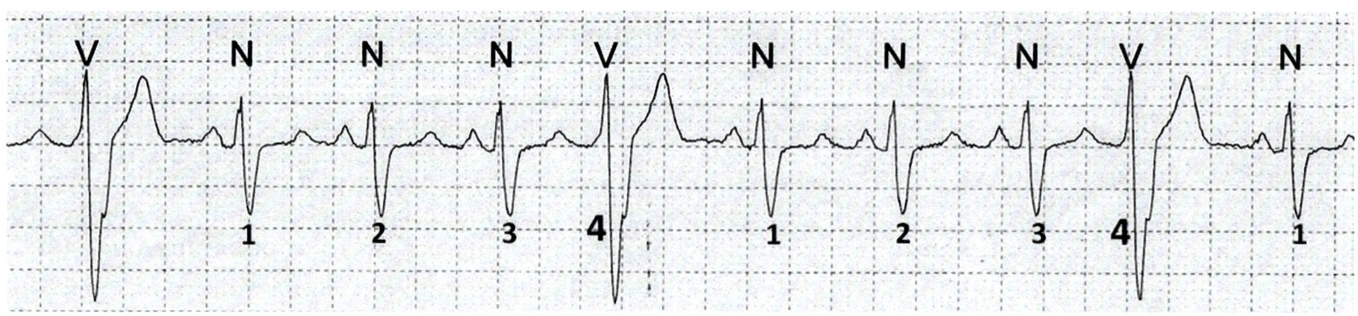

Fig. 10.18: Sinus rhythm with frequent PVCs in a pattern of quadrigeminy—every fourth beat is a PVC. Sinus conducted beat (N) and PVC (V).

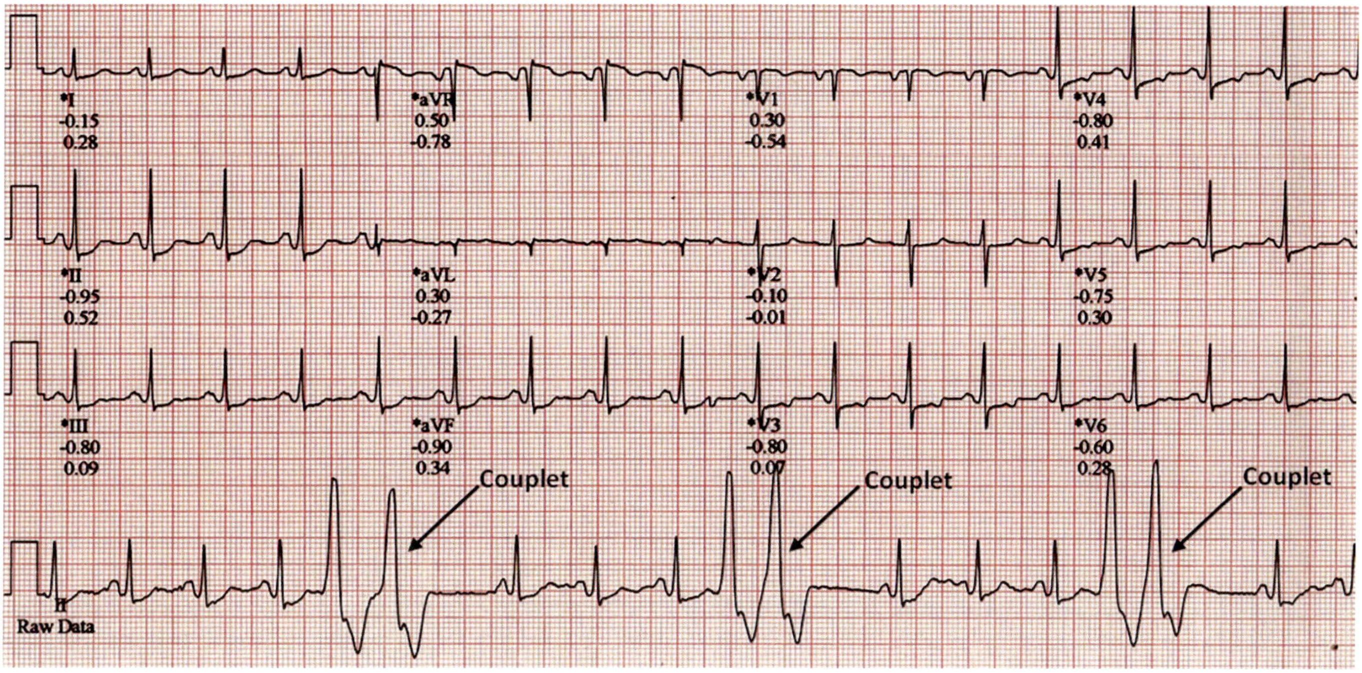

Fig. 10.19: Sinus rhythm with frequent couplets, two consecutive PVCs (*arrows*).

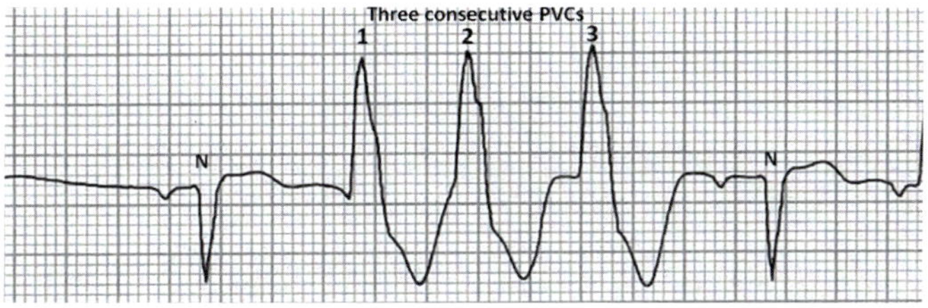

Fig. 10.20: Electrocardiogram strip showing ventricular triplet—three consecutive PVCs in a row (N-normal sinus beat).

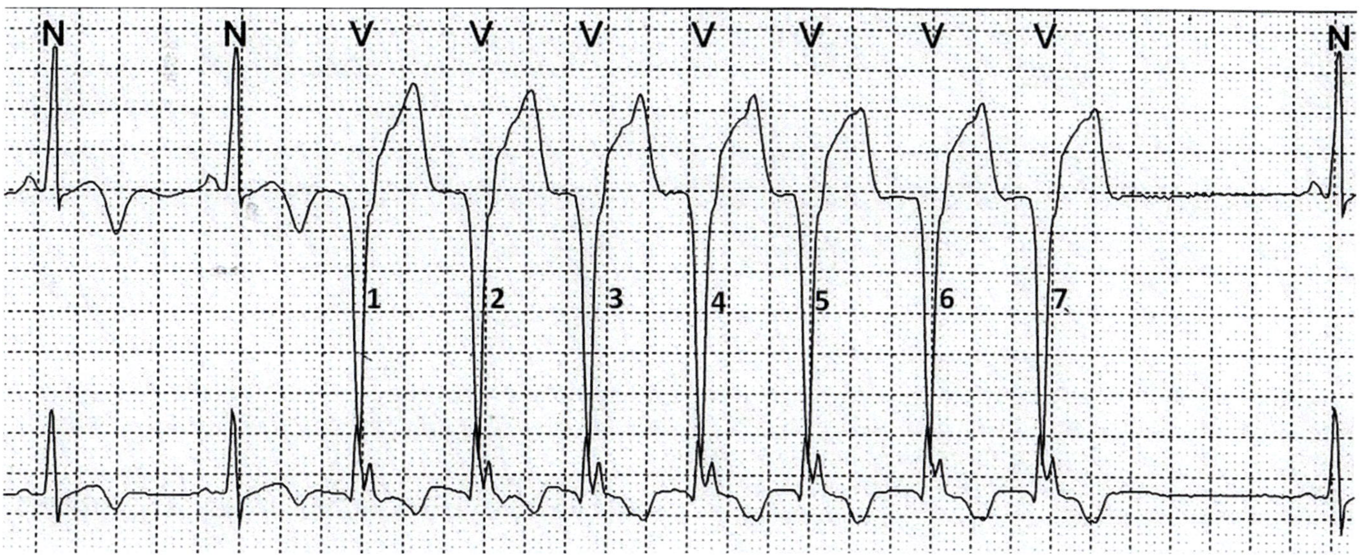

Fig. 10.21: Electrocardiogram strip shows PVCs in salvo—seven PVCs in a row (N-normal sinus beat, V-PVC).

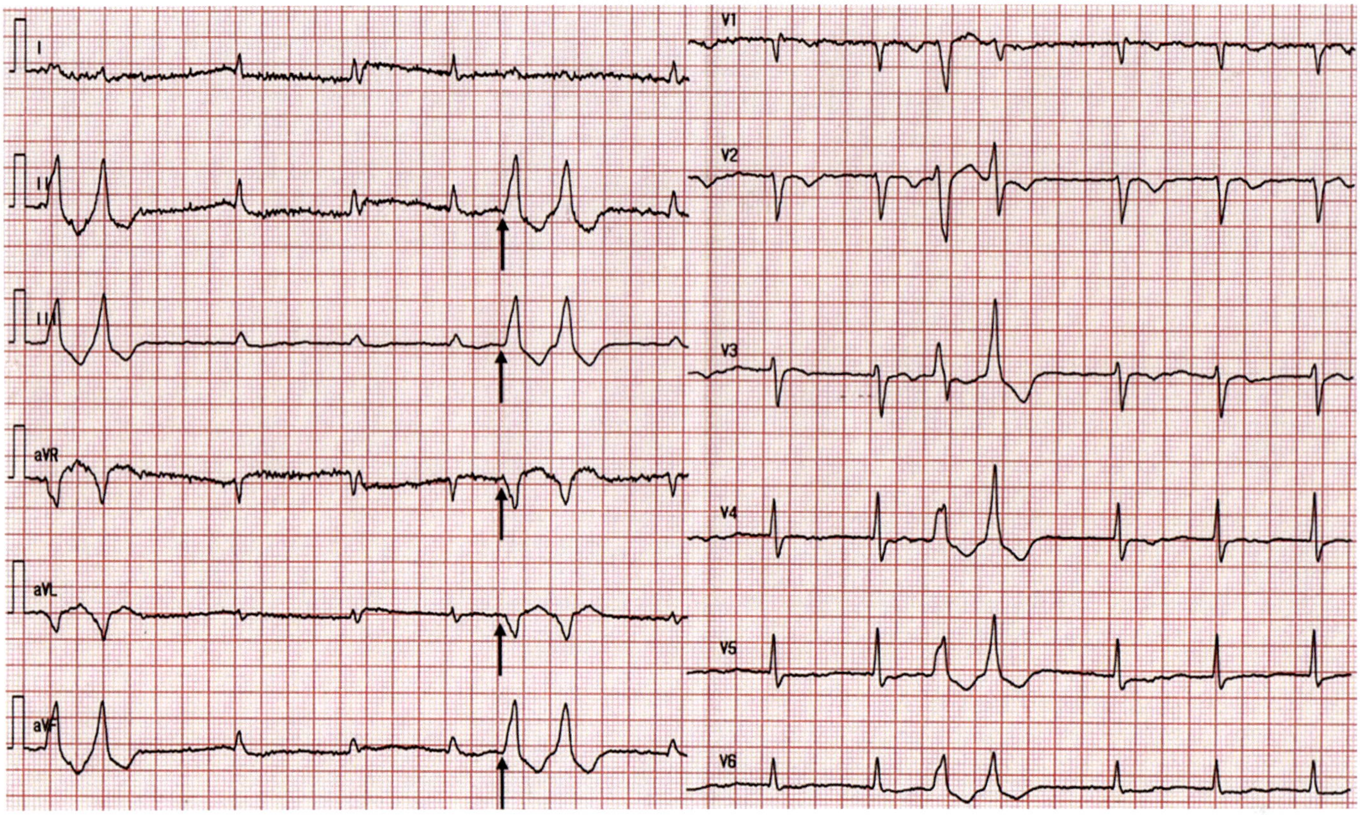

Fig. 10.22: Electrocardiogram illustrating R on T phenomenon. PVCs in the patterns of couplets occur on the downslope of the T-wave of the previous complex (*arrows*).

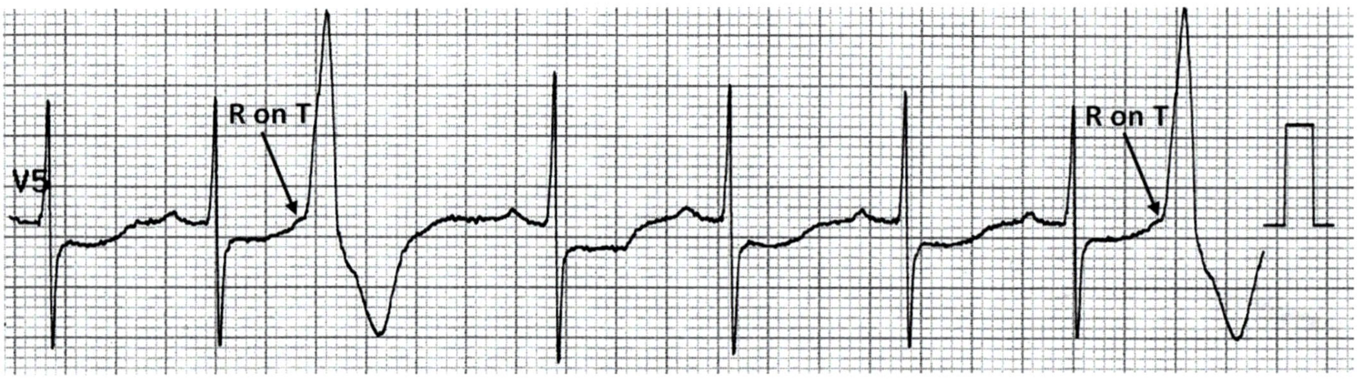

Fig. 10.23: Electrocardiogram showing PVCs manifesting the typical R on T phenomenon. The PVCs occur on the peak of the T-wave of the previous complex (*arrows*).

a ventricular ectopic focus discharges regularly and undisturbed by the dominant rhythm (Fig. 10.26). Rhythm is governed by two pacemakers, one in the SA node and another in the ventricle and ECG sometimes mimic ventricular bigeminy. Ventricular parasystole is characterized by a variable coupling interval and interectopic intervals which are multiples of a common factor.[1] PVCs have uniform morphology unless fusion beats occur. During parasystole the ventricles may by chance be simultaneously activated by both ectopic and normal pacemaker, resulting in formation of a fusion beat (QRS complexes those are in appearance of a fusion between normal and ectopic beats) (Fig. 10.27).

DIFFERENTIATION BETWEEN ABERRANT VENTRICULAR CONDUCTION AND PREMATURE VENTRICULAR COMPLEX

Aberrant ventricular conduction is sometimes confused with PVC and their differentiation is always problematic.

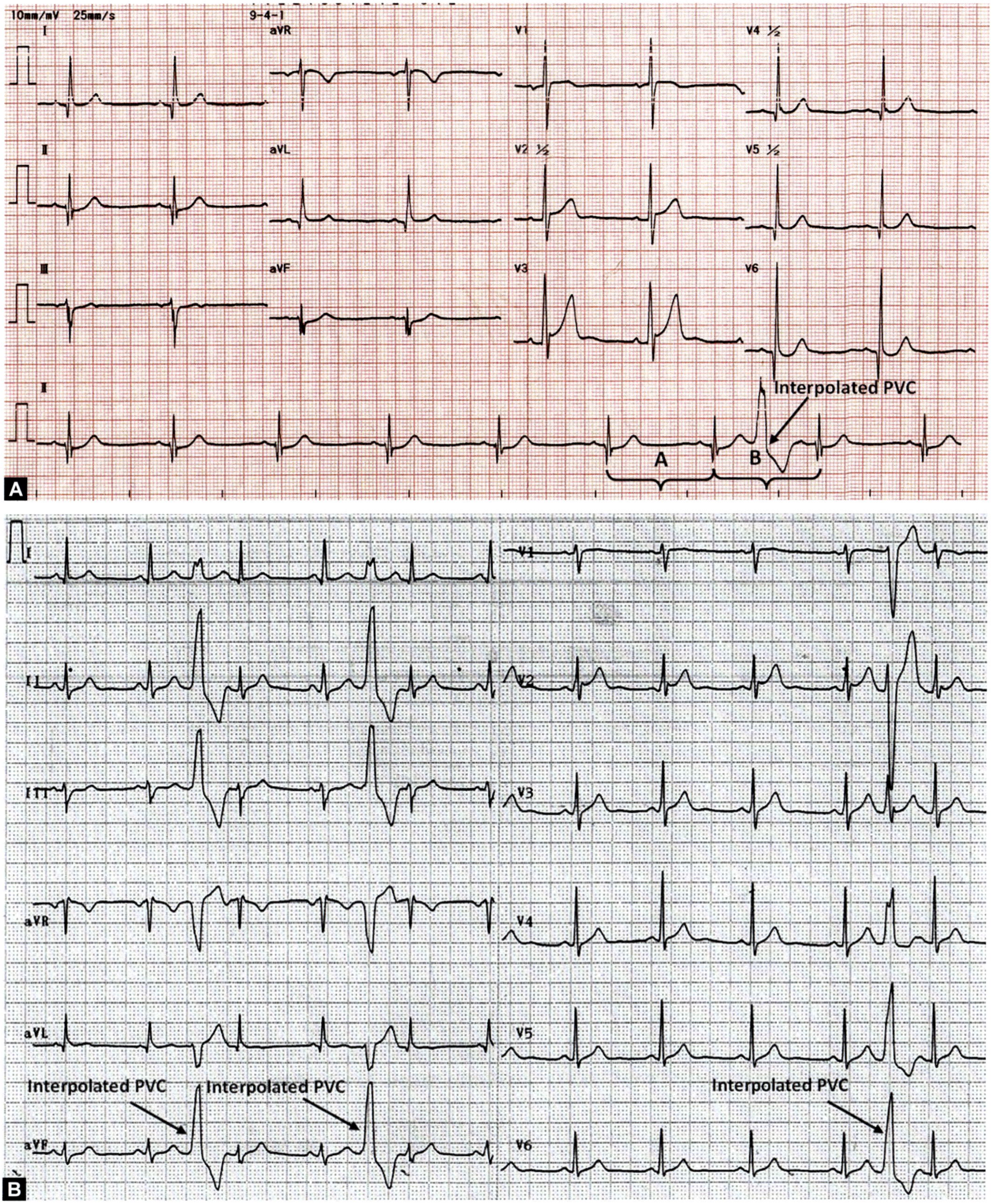

Figs. 10.24A and B: (A) Electrocardiogram shows a single interpolated PVC (*arrow*).The PVC is sandwiched between two normal beats, so the PVC is said to be "interpolated." Note the distance "A" is equal to the distance "B." Interpolated PVC is recognized by its (1) wide bizarre QRS complex, (2) not preceded by a P-wave, and (3) no compensatory pause. (B) ECG shows multiple interpolated PVCs (*arrows*). The PVCs are sandwiched between two normal beats, so no compensatory pause.

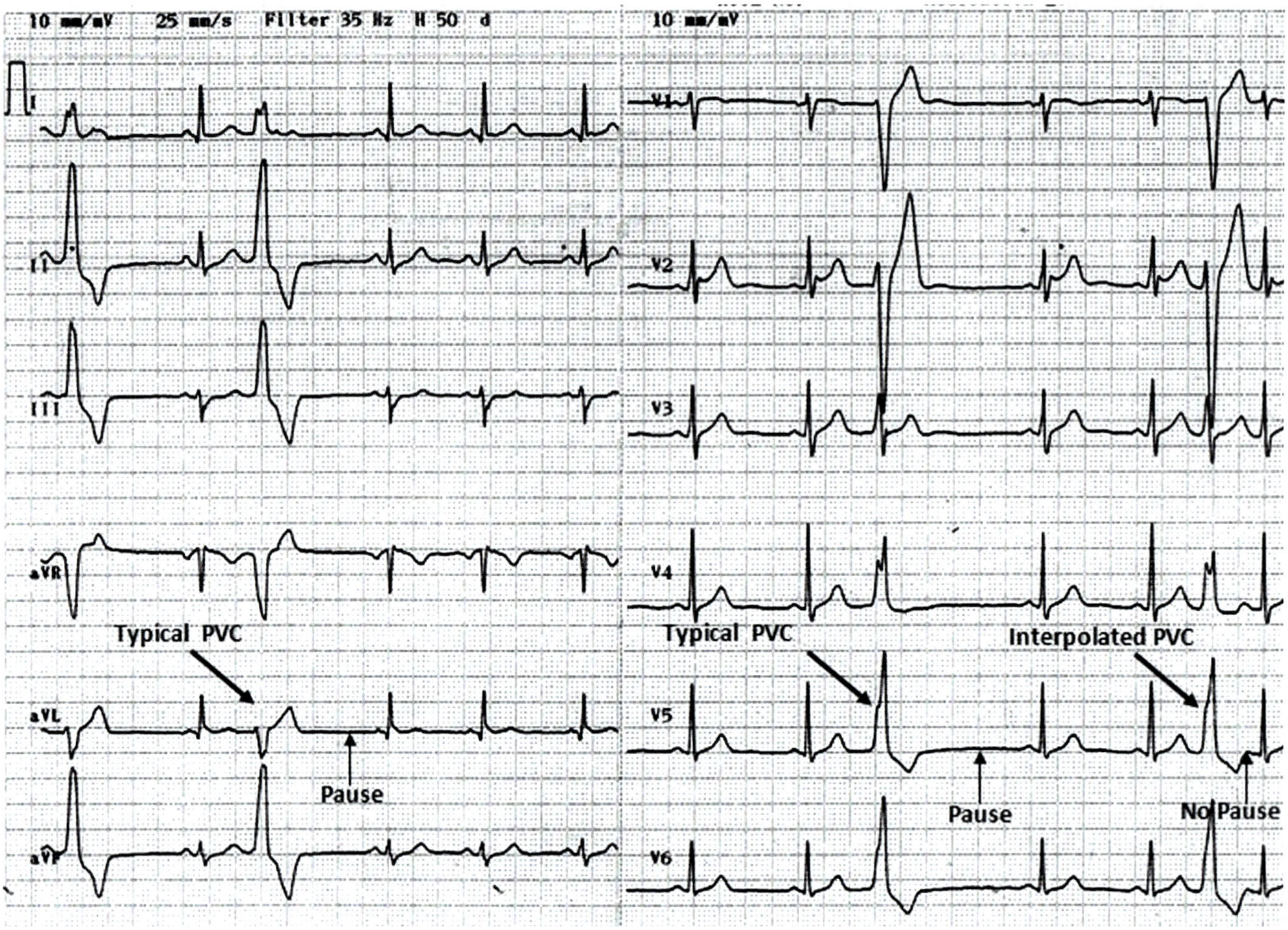

Fig. 10.25: Electrocardiogram shows "typical PVCs" and an "interpolated PVC" in the same strip (*thick arrows*). Typical PVCs are followed by a complete compensatory pause but interpolated PVC is not followed by compensatory pause (*thin arrows*) and thus sandwiched between two normal beats.

Aberrant ventricular conduction is defined as the intermittent abnormal intraventricular conduction of a supraventricular impulse. The phenomenon comes about because of unequal refractoriness of the bundle branches and critical prematurity of a supraventricular impulse. With such critical prematurity, the supraventricular impulse encounters one bundle branch (or fascicle) which is responsive, and the other which is refractory, and is consequently conducted with a bundle branch block or fascicular block pattern.

Preceding ectopic P-wave usually hidden in the ST-T wave of the previous beat favors aberrant ventricular conduction. The compensatory pause can differentiate a PVC from aberrancy. PVC is usually followed by a complete compensatory pause. A complete pause favors PVC and an incomplete pause favors aberrant ventricular conduction.

Morphology of QRS complex in lead V1 gives a clue whether the complex is a PVC or ventricular aberrant conduction. Since aberrancy is almost always in the form of a bundle branch block morphology, V1 is the best lead for differentiating right bundle branch block (RBBB) from left bundle branch block (LBBB); RBBB creates a positive deflection, and LBBB, a negative deflection and can differentiate between these conditions.

If the QRS in V1 is Mostly Positive

Right bundle branch block pattern of rsR' or rSR' QRS morphologies to suggest RBBB aberrancy greater than 90% of the time and monophasic R waves or R waves with a notch or slur on the downstroke of the R waves suggest ventricular ectopy greater than 90% of the time.

If the QRS in V1 is Mostly Negative

Rapid downstroke of the S-wave with or without a preceding "thin" r-wave suggests LBBB aberrancy but a notch/slurring on downstroke of S-wave always suggests PVC.

Premature ventricular complexes are a common cause of palpitations. Related symptoms include difficulty in breathing, chest pain, fatigue, and dizziness. PVCs are also commonly detected incidentally on electrocardiography

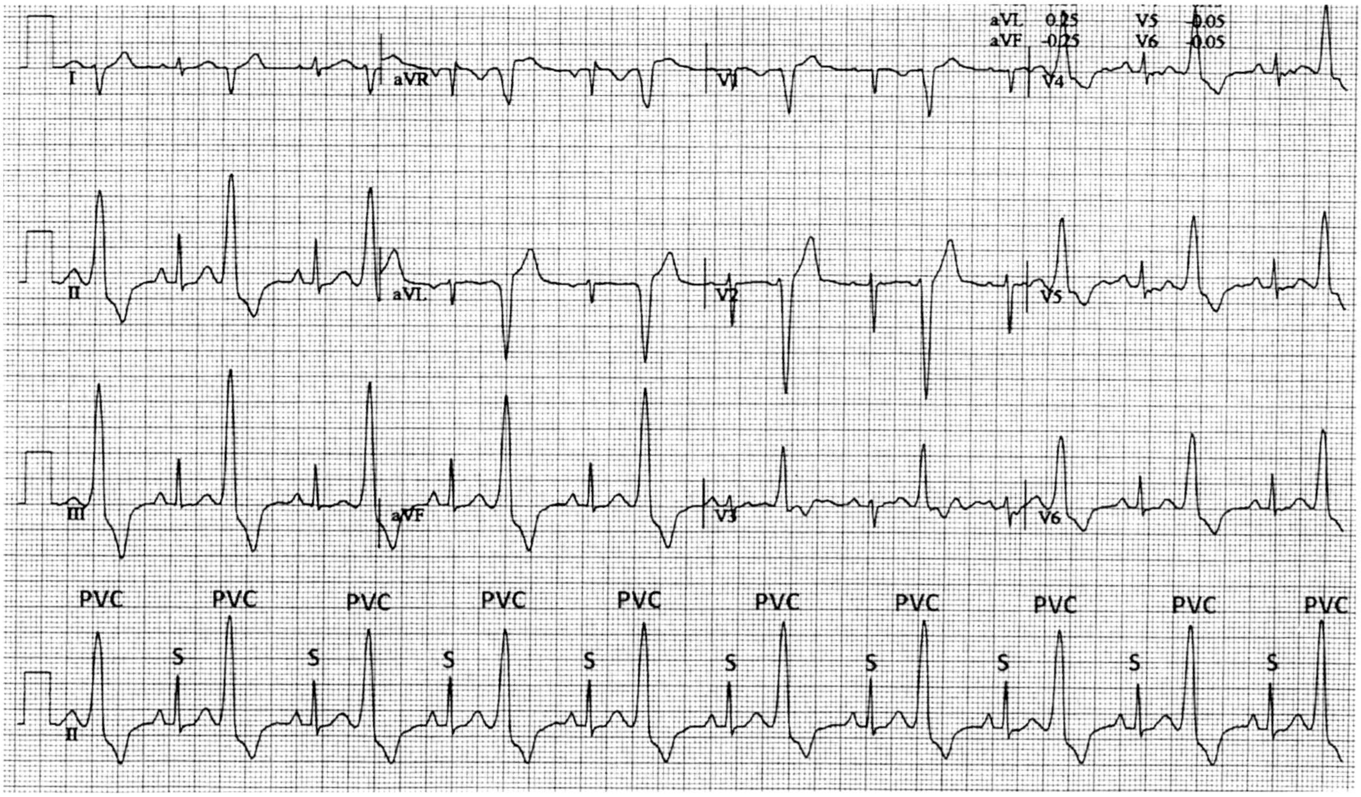

Fig. 10.26: Electrocardiogram showing ventricular parasystole in which the ventricular ectopic focus discharges regularly and undisturbed by the dominant sinus rhythm. Rhythm is governed by two pacemakers, one in the sinoatrial (SA) node (S) and another in the ventricle (PVC) and ECG mimics ventricular bigeminy pattern but ventricular parasystole is characterized by a variable coupling interval.

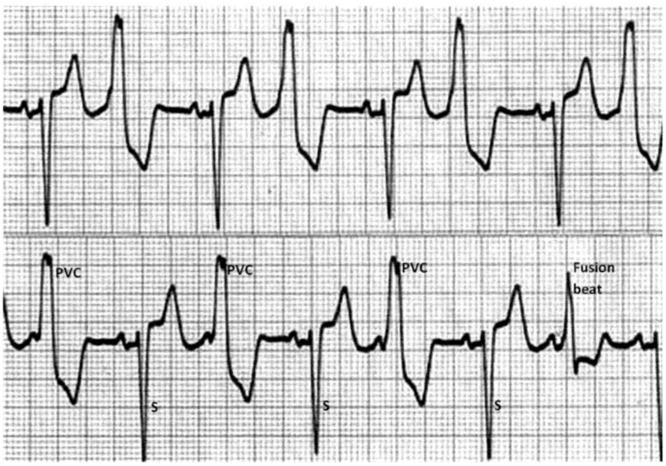

Fig. 10.27: Electrocardiogram showing ventricular parasystole with nonfixed coupled PVCs and PVCs have uniform morphology with one fusion beat.

and are usually benign and do not need any active treatment. But when the PVCs occur near the peak of the T-wave of the preceding beat (R-on-T) or in salvos, these beats predispose the patient to VT or VF. R-on-T pattern is often seen in patients with AMI or long QT intervals.

Lown grading system can be taken into consideration in detecting subjects with high risk (Table 10.1).

There are six grades of PVCs: The first three grades are mostly benign and do not need to be treated if the patient is hemodynamically stable and not symptomatic. Grades 3–5 need cardiac assessment and may require treatment; as if they are left untreated they can potentially develop into fatal rhythms such as VT or VF. A 24-hour ECG should be conducted so as to grade the severity of the patient's PVCs. The higher the grade the higher the risk of VT or VF.

In general, multimorphic PVCs connote a poorer prognosis than uniform morphologic PVCs. In post-MI patients, frequent PVCs (greater than 10/h) were associated with increased mortality in the prethrombolytic era, but the association in patients receiving thrombolysis is weak. Most studies on PVC prognosis in "normal hearts" did not use advanced tests to rule out structural heart disease. Among these patients, PVCs are associated with a worse cardiovascular outcome if patients are older and have higher cardiovascular risk.[17] In two studies, a frequent PVC (defined as the presence of seven or more PVCs per minute during any given stage, ventricular bigeminy, ventricular trigeminy, ventricular couplets, ventricular triplets, sustained or nonsustained VT, ventricular flutter, torsades de pointes, or VF) during exercise was an independent predictor of death.[18,19] However, in another study, frequent PVCs only during exercise did not independently predict an

Table 10.1: Lown grading system of premature ventricular complex (PVC).

Grade	Feature
Grade 0	No PVC
Grade 1	Occasional PVCs (<30/h)
Grade 2	Frequent PVCs (>30/h) e.g. bigeminy
Grade 3	Multifocal
Grade 4	Repetitive (couplets, triplets, and salvos)
Grade 5	R-on-T phenomenon

increased risk; instead frequent PVCs during recovery was a stronger predictor of death.[20] Frequent PVCs, especially when they occur in a bigeminal pattern, can precipitate tachycardia-induced cardiomyopathy that can be reversed by elimination of the PVCs through catheter ablation.[18-22]

ESCAPE BEATS

When the dominant pacemaker fails to discharge, escape beats may arise from subsidiary pacemaker tissue (Fig. 10.28). In contrast to ectopic beats, escape beats are always late, i.e. the coupling interval is greater than the cycle length of the dominant rhythm. Differentiation between escape and ectopic beats are important because the escape beats suggest impaired pacemaker function and an ectopic beat may be entirely benign. Escape beat themselves require no treatment and if treatment is necessary, it is to accelerate the basic rhythm.[1]

The SA-node is able to remain as the dominant pacemaker through automaticity and overdrive suppression. However, when the SA-node fails to depolarize, surrounding cells with automaticity are able to spontaneously depolarize, taking over as the pacemaker for the heart. These secondary pacemaker cells each have an intrinsic rate, allowing us to predict which cells are pacing the heart. When not overdrive-suppressed, the atria is able to spontaneously depolarize and pace the heart at a rate of 60–80 beats/min, which is termed as atrial rhythm or atrial escape rhythm. If the atria fail to spontaneously depolarize, then the AV-junction is able to pace the heart at a rate of 40–60 beats/min, termed as junctional escape rhythm. In junctional (AV junctional) beat or rhythm the atrial depolarization current points cephalad and to the right, away from lead II and towards lead aVR. Therefore, the P-wave, if seen, would be negative in lead II and positive in lead aVR. However this P-wave is usually buried by the QRS complex and not visible. On less common occasions when the P-wave is visible, it may be either immediately before or immediately after the QRS complex.

Should the SA node, atria, and AV junction fail to pace the heart, the last hope is the ventricles themselves, which can spontaneously depolarize at a rate of 20–40 beats/min, and is predictably referred to as a ventricular escape rhythm.

Escape beats usually arise from the AV junction, less commonly, they originate from the ventricles. The QRS duration and configuration of junctional escape beats are similar to those during normal sinus rhythm (Fig. 10.29). Ventricular escape beats have a similar configuration to PVC (Fig. 10.30).

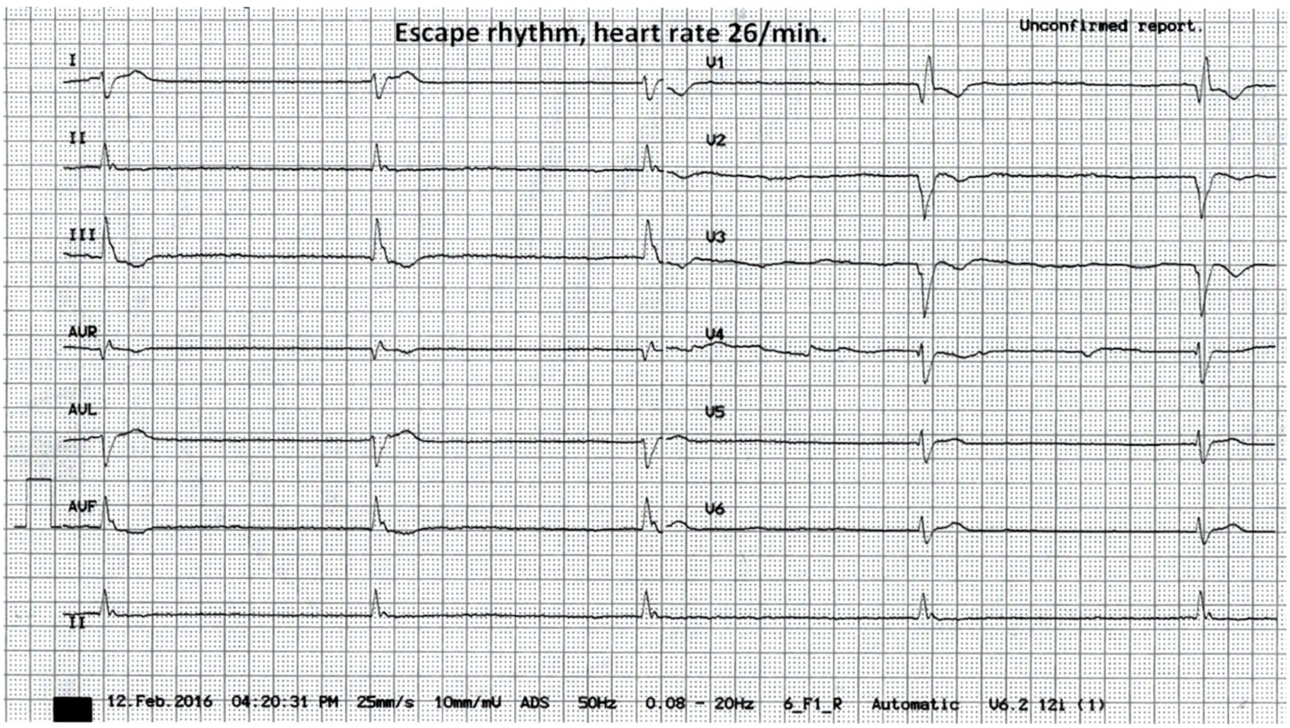

Fig. 10.28: Electrocardiogram is suggestive of escape rhythm with marked bradycardia. Note no P-wave preceding the QRS complexes and QRS complexes appear broad and bizarre suggesting ventricular origin.

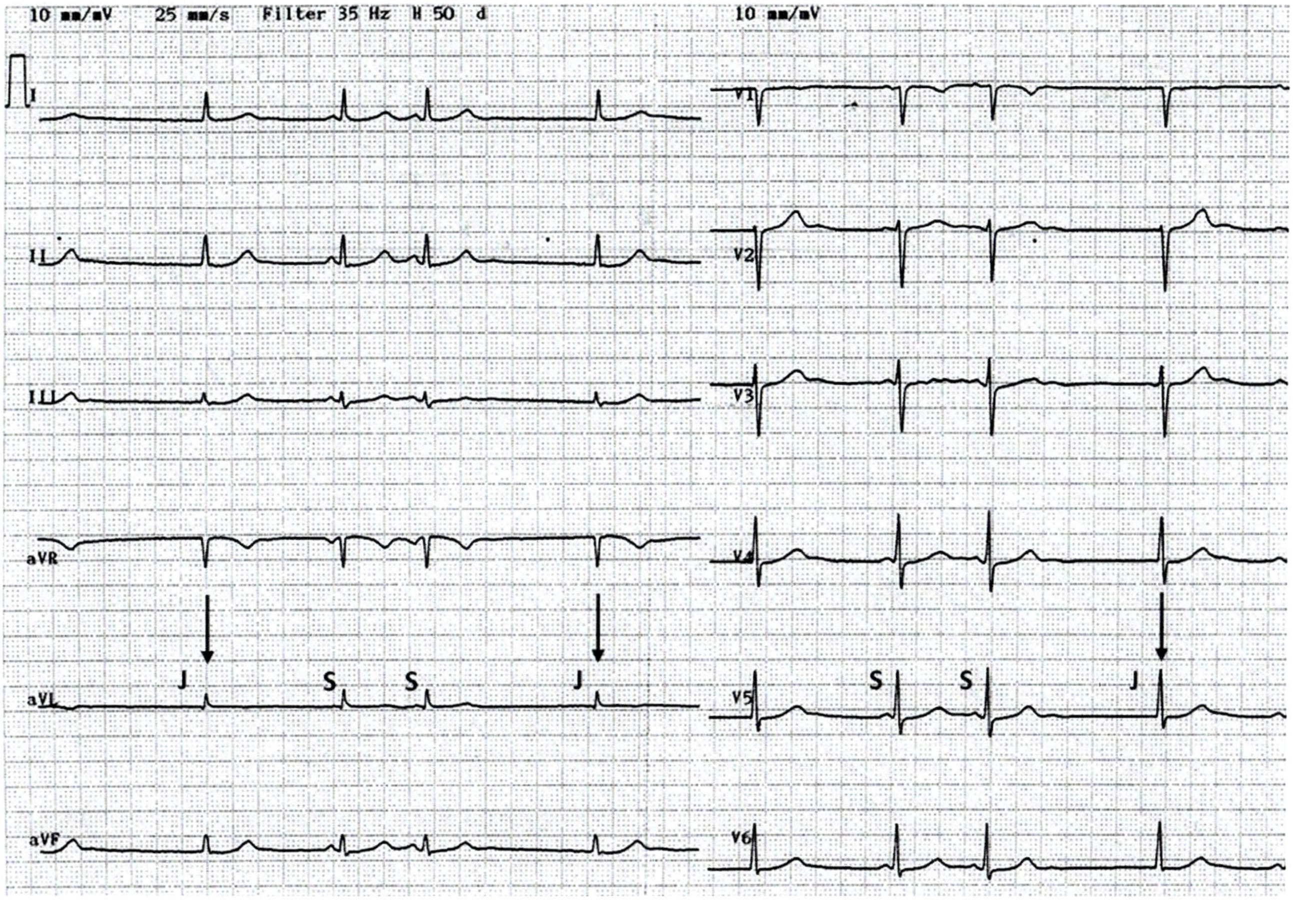

Fig. 10.29: Electrocardiogram showing junctional escape beats (*arrows*). Note there is no P-wave preceding the QRS complexes and QRS duration and configuration of junctional escape beats (J) are similar to those during normal sinus rhythm (S).

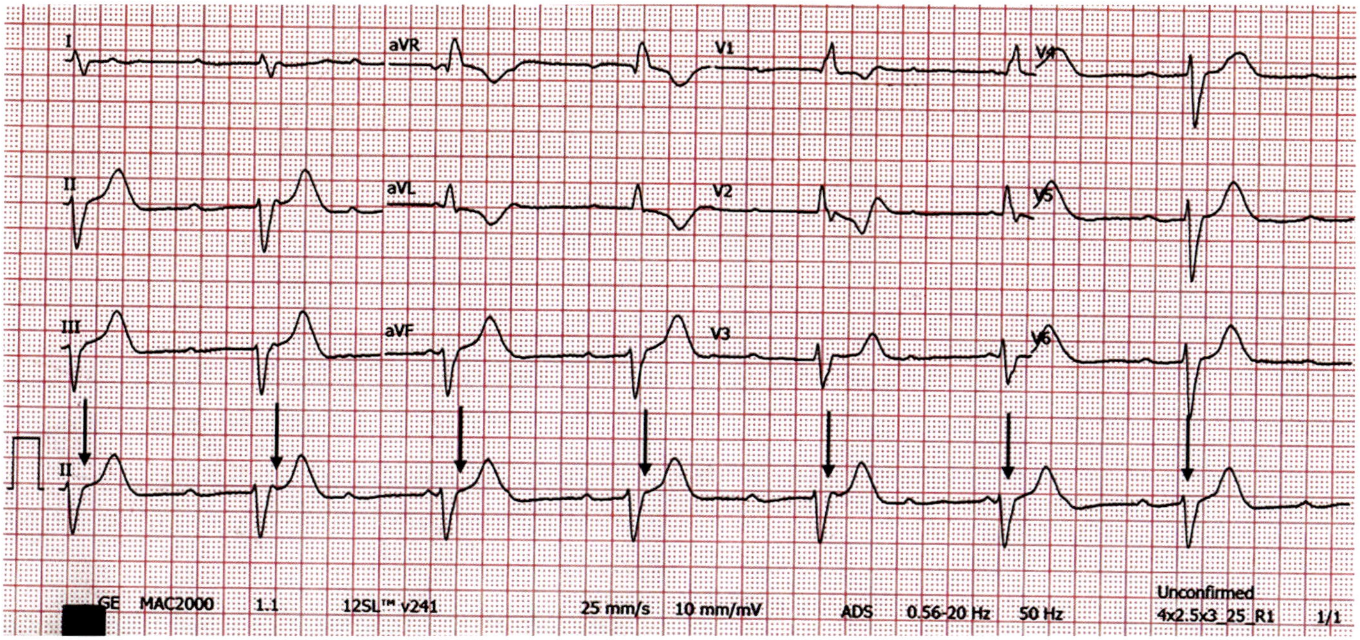

Fig. 10.30: Ventricular escape rhythm during complete heart block at a rate 42 beats/min (*arrows*). Note ventricular escape beats have a similar configuration to PVC.

SUMMARY

Ectopic beats may be of three different types: (1) premature atrial complex (PAC), (2) premature junctional complex (PJC), and (3) premature ventricular complex (PVC) (Box 10.2).

Characteristics of Premature Atrial Complex

- Shape of ectopic P-wave is different from the sinus P-wave.
- RR interval is irregular.
- Narrow QRS complex if conduction in the ventricles is undisturbed. QRS complex is of normal configuration and measures less than 0.12 seconds (120 ms).
- If the PAC occurs so early that the AV node has not fully repolarized from the previous impulse, the AV node will be unable to conduct to the ventricles and the premature P-wave will not be followed by a QRS complex. This is known as a blocked or nonconducted PAC and is the most common cause of a pause during sinus rhythm.
- PR interval may be normal, short, prolonged or absent.
- Premature atrial complex occurs so early that it distorts the T-wave of the previous QRS complex. An abnormal or notched T-wave followed by an early QRS complex should always arouse the suspicion of a PAC.
- Premature atrial complex is followed by an incomplete compensatory pause.

In the majority of cases, PACs occur in normal healthy individuals without any evidence of heart disease. Stress or stimulants such as tea, coffee, or alcohol can increase the frequency of PACs. In the minority of cases, PACs can be associated with CAD, hypertension or valvular heart disease.

The great majority of PACs is completely benign and requires little if any treatment at all. In rare cases, PACs may be a sign of underlying cardiac disease. Important causes of PACs include: anxiety and stress, tobacco/alcohol, beta-agonists (salbutamol, albuterol, salmeterol, terbutaline, etc.), excess caffeine, electrolyte imbalance, digoxin toxicity, and rarely due to CAD.

Electrocardiogram Characteristics of Premature Junctional Complex

- P-wave usually inverted due to retrograde depolarization. P-wave may occur before or after the QRS complex or be buried under the QRS complex.
- *PR interval*: If the P-wave precedes the QRS complex, the PR interval is shortened to less than the normal 0.12 seconds. If P-wave occurs during or after the QRS complex, it cannot be measured.
- *QRS complex*: Because the ventricles are usually depolarized normally, the QRS complex usually has a normal duration of less than 0.12 seconds (120 ms) and a normal appearance. The QRS complex in a PJC is commonly followed by an incomplete compensatory pause.
- *T-wave*: Usually normal configuration.
- Important causes of PJCs include cardiac drug toxicity, electrolyte imbalance, and postmitral valve surgery.

Electrocardiogram Characteristics of Premature Ventricular Complex

- The QRS complex is wide and often premature with increased amplitude and of a bizarre shape.
- The QRS width is 0.12 seconds (120 ms) or wider.
- The T-wave is of opposite polarity to QRS complex.
- There is no related P-wave (unless there is retrograde conduction back through the AV node, which causes the P-wave to occur in or after the QRS complex).
- Usually the PVC is followed by a full compensated pause.

When the pause surrounding the ectopic beat is equal to double the preceding RR interval, this is called "full compensatory pause" (usually seen in PVC). If the pause surrounding the ectopic is less than the double the preceding RR interval then it is called "incomplete compensatory pause" (usually seen in PAC).

Premature ventricular complexes may be unifocal (all look the same), multifocal or multiformed (QRS complexes are of different morphology). Multifocal PVCs have different

Box 10.2: Electrocardiogram criteria of premature atrial complex (PAC), premature junctional complex (PJC), and premature ventricular complex (PVC).

ECG criteria of PAC, PJC and PVC

Premature atrial complex
- They are premature and ectopic, originating outside of the sinoatrial (SA) node. Thus the P-wave morphology would be different than the normal sinus P-wave.
- They are narrow complexes.
- There is an incomplete compensatory pause after the PAC.

Premature junctional complex
- Narrow QRS complex, either
  - Without a preceding P wave or
  - Preceded by an abnormal P-wave with a short PR interval of less than 120 ms or
  - "Retrograde" P waves inverted in leads II, III, and aVF.
- The QRS morphology is very similar to the sinus complexes.
- Followed by an incomplete compensatory pause.

Premature ventricular complex
- Broad QRS complex greater than or equal to 0.12 seconds (≥ 120 ms) with abnormal morphology.
- QRS complex is usually not preceded by P-wave.
- Usually followed by a complete compensatory pause.
- Discordant ST segment and T-wave changes.

Box 10.3: Patterns of premature ventricular complex.

Bigeminy: Every other beat is a PVC.

Trigeminy: Every third beat is a PVC.

Quadrigeminy: Every fourth beat is a PVC.

Couplet: Two consecutive PVCs.

Triplet: Three consecutive PVCs

Salvo: More PVCs in a row.

sites of origin, which means their coupling intervals are usually different but multiformed PVCs usually have the same coupling intervals, because they originate in the same ectopic site but their conduction through the ventricles differ. If PVC recurs every other beat, it is called bigeminy, every third beat is trigeminy, and every fourth beat is quadrigeminy (Box 10.3).

R-On-T Phenomenon

The appearance of a PVC on the preceding T-wave is called R-on-T phenomenon. PVCs manifesting the R-on-T phenomenon have short coupling interval, usually measuring less than or equal to 0.40 seconds (400 ms). As the coupling interval is short, the PVCs occur on the downslope of the T-wave of the previous complex, which corresponds to the vulnerable period of the ventricles and this may potentially trigger VT/VF.

Interpolated Premature Ventricular Complex

Not all PVCs are followed by a pause. If a PVC occurs early enough (especially if the heart rate is slow), it may appear sandwiched in between two normal beats. This is called an interpolated PVC.

Ventricular Parasystole

Ventricular parasystole is a protected, independent, and regular ectopic ventricular rhythm. Independence of the parasystolic focus from the basic cardiac rhythm is the reason for the occurrence of fusion beats and variable coupling intervals. Ventricular parasytolic rhythm is believed to be automatic. Rhythm is governed by two pacemakers, one in the SA node and another in the ventricle and ECG sometimes mimic ventricular bigeminy.

The usual criteria for the diagnosis of parasystole are:

- Premature ventricular complexes have uniform morphology,
- Varying coupling intervals
- Frequent appearance of fusion beats, and
- Temporary or "continuous" independence of the ectopic rhythm from the basic rhythm.

The origin of each PVC can be discerned from the QRS morphology:

- Premature ventricular complexes arising from the *right* ventricle have a left bundle branch block morphology (dominant S-wave in V1).
- Premature ventricular complexes arising from the *left* ventricle have a right bundle branch block morphology (dominant R-wave in V1).

Important causes of PVCs include AMI, valvular heart disease, MVP, myocarditis, cardiomyopathies, electrolyte disturbances (e.g. hypokalemia), drug induced (e.g. digoxin and tricyclic antidepressants toxicity), alcohol, after surgery and infection.

Differences Between Premature Atrial Complex and Premature Ventricular Complex (Table 10.2)

Pacemaker cells are found at various sites throughout the conducting system, with each site capable of independently sustaining the heart rhythm. When the SA node fails to depolarize, surrounding cells with automaticity are able to spontaneously depolarize, taking over as the pacemaker for the heart. The rate of spontaneous depolarization of pacemaker cells decreases down the conducting system:

- Atrial escape rhythm (60–80 bpm)
- Atrioventricular junctional escape rhythm (40–60 bpm)
- Ventricular escape rhythm (20–40 bpm).

Differences Between Ectopic Beat and Escape Beat (Table 10.3)

Ventricular ectopic beats are frequently seen in clinical practice and are usually benign. Presence of heart disease should be sought and, if absent, indicate good prognosis in patients with PVCs.

Escape beats are always late but ectopic beats are always premature. Escape beat usually arises from the AV junction and less commonly from the ventricles.

Table 10.2: Premature atrial complex (PAC) versus premature ventricular complex (PVC).

PAC	*PVC*
QRS complex is of normal configuration	QRS is wide and bizarre looking
Usually preceded by a premature P-wave	Not Preceded by a P-wave
QRS duration <0.12 secs (120 ms)	QRS will be broad >0.12 secs (120 ms)
QRS complex is followed by an incomplete compensatory pause.	QRS complex is followed by a complete compensatory pause

Table 10.3: Ectopic beat versus escape beat.

Ectopic beat	*Escape beat*
Ectopic beats are always premature	Escape beats are always late
The interval between the ectopic beat and the preceding beat (i.e. coupling interval) is shorter than the cycle length of the dominant rhythm.	The coupling interval is greater than the cycle length of the dominant rhythm.

REFERENCES

1. Bennett DH. Cardiac Arrhythmias, 4th edition. Oxford: Butterworth-Heinemann Ltd.; 1993.
2. Nallasivan M, Appel RA, Welch WJ, et al. Ventricular tachycardia due to bundle branch reentry: induction by spontaneous atrial premature beats. Am Heart J. 1988;116(2 Pt. 1):552-5.
3. Berman ND. Ventricular tachycardia initiated by both normally and aberrantly conducted atrial premature beats. Pacing Clin Electrophysiol. 1980;3:51
4. Haissaguerre M, Jaïs P, Shah DC, et al. Spontaneous initiation of atrial fibrillation by ectopic beats originating in the pulmonary veins. N Engl J Med. 1998;339(10):659-66.
5. Jideus L, Kesek M, Joachimsson PO, et al. The role of premature atrial contractions as the main triggers of postoperative atrial fibrillation. J Electrocardiol. 2006;39(1):48-54.
6. Maounis T, Kyrozi E, Katsaros K, et al. The prognostic significance of atrial arrhythmias recorded early after cardioversion for atrial fibrillation. Pacing Clin Electrophysiol. 2001;24(7):1076-81.
7. Cha YM, Lee GK, Klarich KW, et al. Premature ventricular contraction-induced cardiomyopathy: a treatable condition. Circ Arrhythm Electrophysiol. 2012;5(1):229-36.
8. Morshedi-Meibodi A, Evans JC, Levy D, et al. Clinical correlates and prognostic significance of exercise-induced ventricular premature beats in the community: the Framingham Heart Study. Circulation. 2004;109(20):2417-22.
9. Omar AR, Lee LC, Seow SC, et al. Managing ventricular ectopics: are ventricular ectopic beats just an annoyance? Singapore Med J. 2011;52(10):707-14.
10. Cantillon DJ. Evaluation and management of premature ventricular complexes. Cleve Clin J Med. 2013;80(6):377-87.
11. Niwano S, Wakisaka Y, Niwano H, et al. Prognostic significance of frequent premature ventricular contractions originating from the ventricular outflow tract in patients with normal left ventricular function. Heart. 2009;95(15):1230-7.
12. Engel TR, Meister SG, Frankl WS. The "R-on-T" phenomenon: an update and critical review. Ann Intern Med. 1978;88(2):221-5.
13. Nguyen AN, Sarmast SA, Kowal RC, et al. Cardiac arrest due to torsades de pointes in a patient with complete heart block: the "R-on-T" phenomenon. Proc (Bayl Univ Med Cent). 2010;23(4):361-2
14. Anderson KP, Shusterman V, Aysin B, et al. Distinctive RR dynamics preceding two modes of onset of spontaneous sustained ventricular tachycardia. J Cardiovasc Electrophysiol. 1999;10(7):897-904.
15. Oupadia P, Ramaswamy K. "R-on-T" Phenomenon. N Engl J Med. 1998;338:1812.
16. Glancy DL. Group beating resulting from ventricular parasystole. Proc (Bayl Univ Med Cent). 2003;16(3):352-3.
17. Lee V, Hemingway H, Harb R, et al. The prognostic significance of premature ventricular complexes in adults without clinically apparent heart disease: a meta-analysis and systematic review. Heart. 2012;98:1290-8.
18. Jouven X, Zureik M, Desnos M, et al. Long-term outcome in asymptomatic men with exercise-induced premature ventricular depolarizations. N Engl J Med. 2000;343(12):826-33.
19. O'Neill JO, Young JB, Pothier CE, et al. Severe frequent ventricular ectopy after exercise as a predictor of death in patients with heart failure. J Am Coll Cardiol. 2004;44(4):820-6.
20. Frolkis JP, Pothier CE, Blackstone EH, et al. Frequent ventricular ectopy after exercise as a predictor of death. N Engl J Med. 2003;348:781-90.
21. Adams JC, Srivathsan K, Shen WK. Advances in management of premature ventricular contractions. J Interv Card Electrophysiol. 2012;35(2):137-49.
22. Baman TS, Lange DC, Ilg KJ, et al. Relationship between burden of premature ventricular complexes and left ventricular function. Heart Rhythm. 2010;7(7):865-9.

Chapter 11

Narrow Complex Tachycardia

INTRODUCTION

Tachycardias are broadly categorized based upon the width of the QRS complex on the electrocardiogram (ECG). A narrow QRS complex <0.12 seconds (less than 120 ms) reflects rapid activation of the ventricles via the normal His-Purkinje system, which in turn suggests that the arrhythmia originates above or within the His bundle [i.e. a supraventricular tachycardia (SVT)]. The site of origin may be in the sinus node, the atria, the atrioventricular (AV) node, the His bundle, or some combination of these sites.

Basic ECG criteria for the diagnosis of narrow complex tachycardia are:

- Rate is greater than 100 beats per minute (bpm).
- QRS complex duration is less than 0.12 seconds (<120 ms).

Narrow complex tachycardias usually originate from the atria or AV junction and are therefore supraventricular in origin. They have one thing in common—as because they arise from above the level of the bundle branches, they usually result in narrow ventricular complexes.

The clinical importance of a tachycardia in an individual patient is related to the ventricular rate, the presence of any underlying heart disease, and the integrity of cardiovascular reflexes. As a general rule, the faster the ventricular rate, the more likely the presence of symptoms—for example, chest pain, faintness, and breathlessness. Urgent treatment is needed for severely symptomatic patients with a narrow complex tachycardia. Differentiation between different types of SVT may be difficult, particularly when ventricular rate exceeds 150 bpm. Evaluation of atrial activity on the ECG is crucial in this process. Analysis of the ventricular rate and rhythm may also be helpful, although this rate will depend on the degree of AV block. Increasing AV block by maneuvers such as carotid sinus massage or administration of intravenous adenosine may be of diagnostic value as slowing the ventricular rate allows more accurate visualization of atrial activity. Such maneuvers will not usually stop the tachycardia, however, unless it is due to re-entry involving the AV node.[1] Supraventricular tachycardias may be divided into two distinct groups depending on whether they arise from the atria or the AV junction. Electrocardiographic analysis should include measurement of the ventricular rate, assessment of the ventricular rhythm, identification of P, F, or f waves, measurement of the atrial rate, and establishment of the relation of P waves to the ventricular complexes.[1]

Narrow complex tachycardias are broadly divided into two groups:[2]

1. *Regular*
   a. Sinus tachycardia (ST)
   b. Sinus node reentrant tachycardia (SNRT)
   c. Atrial flutter
   d. Atrioventricular nodal reentrant tachycardia (AVNRT)
   e. Atrioventricular reentrant tachycardia (AVRT).
2. *Irregular*
   a. Atrial fibrillation
   b. Atrial flutter with variable block
   c. Multifocal atrial tachycardia (MAT).

The differentiation of narrow complex tachycardias is a commonly encountered diagnostic dilemma. Some narrow complex tachycardias (e.g. ST) are secondary to the presenting complaint (e.g. fever, anxiety, and pain) and will respond to appropriate treatment of the inciting pathologic insult. Alternatively, other narrow complex tachycardias (e.g. atrial fibrillation and AV nodal reentrant tachycardia) may indeed be the cause of the chief complaint (e.g. palpitations and lightheadedness from poor perfusion) and must be positively identified and primarily managed. An appreciation of the similarities and differences among these narrow complex tachycardias is necessary for appropriate recognition.

SINUS TACHYCARDIA

Physiologic sinus tachycardia (ST) refers to a narrow complex tachycardia that originates from the SA node and is due to increased automaticity, rather than a reentrant mechanism. The atrial rate is greater than 100 bpm and is largely regular with slight variations over time. The P-wave morphology is identical to that seen in sinus rhythm and appears positive in leads I, II, III, and augmented vector foot (aVF) and biphasic or negative in lead V1[3] (Fig. 11.1). The onset of ST is gradual, exhibiting a "warm up" period, and is not initiated by atrial or ventricular premature beats.[4-9] Perhaps the most telling feature of ST is that it occurs in the setting of underlying physiologic stress or pharmacologic influence, namely fever, infection, anxiety, stimulant drug use, or hypotension, among many others.[4-6] When frequent premature atrial contractions (PACs) accompany ST, it may be difficult to differentiate from MAT.[3]

SINUS NODE REENTRANT TACHYCARDIA

Sinus node reentrant tachycardia is due to a reentrant mechanism within or adjacent to the sinus nodal tissue.[6] This rhythm is indistinguishable from ST on a simple 12-lead ECG as the P-wave position, axis, and morphology are essentially identical to those of the ST.[3,5] The rate is usually 100–150 bpm, and the rhythm is regular.[6] In contrast to ST, the onset of SNRT is abrupt and often initiated by a premature atrial impulse.[4,9-11] Termination is similarly abrupt and may be terminated with vagal maneuvers or adenosine administration.[3] This rhythm is often an incidental finding seen on Holter monitoring, is typically nonsustained, and rarely causes clinically significant symptomatology, may terminate with vagal maneuvers.[3]

MULTIFOCAL ATRIAL TACHYCARDIA

Multifocal atrial tachycardia (heart rate is greater than 100 bpm) occurs because of multiple atrial premature beats in an atrium caused by hypoxia, increased atrial pressure, and, perhaps most important, theophylline. Multifocal atrial tachycardia is gradual in onset because the underlying rhythm is generally ST, and the heart rates with MAT are only slightly faster than these baseline rates. The rhythm is irregular, and on ECG, P waves with abnormal morphologic characteristics (three abnormal P waves necessary for the diagnosis) precede each QRS complex (Fig. 11.2).[12]

Multifocal atrial tachycardia is an irregular narrow complex tachycardias with a frequency of 0.08–0.36% among hospitalized patients.[13,14] It typically occurs in the elderly in the setting of cardiopulmonary disease and

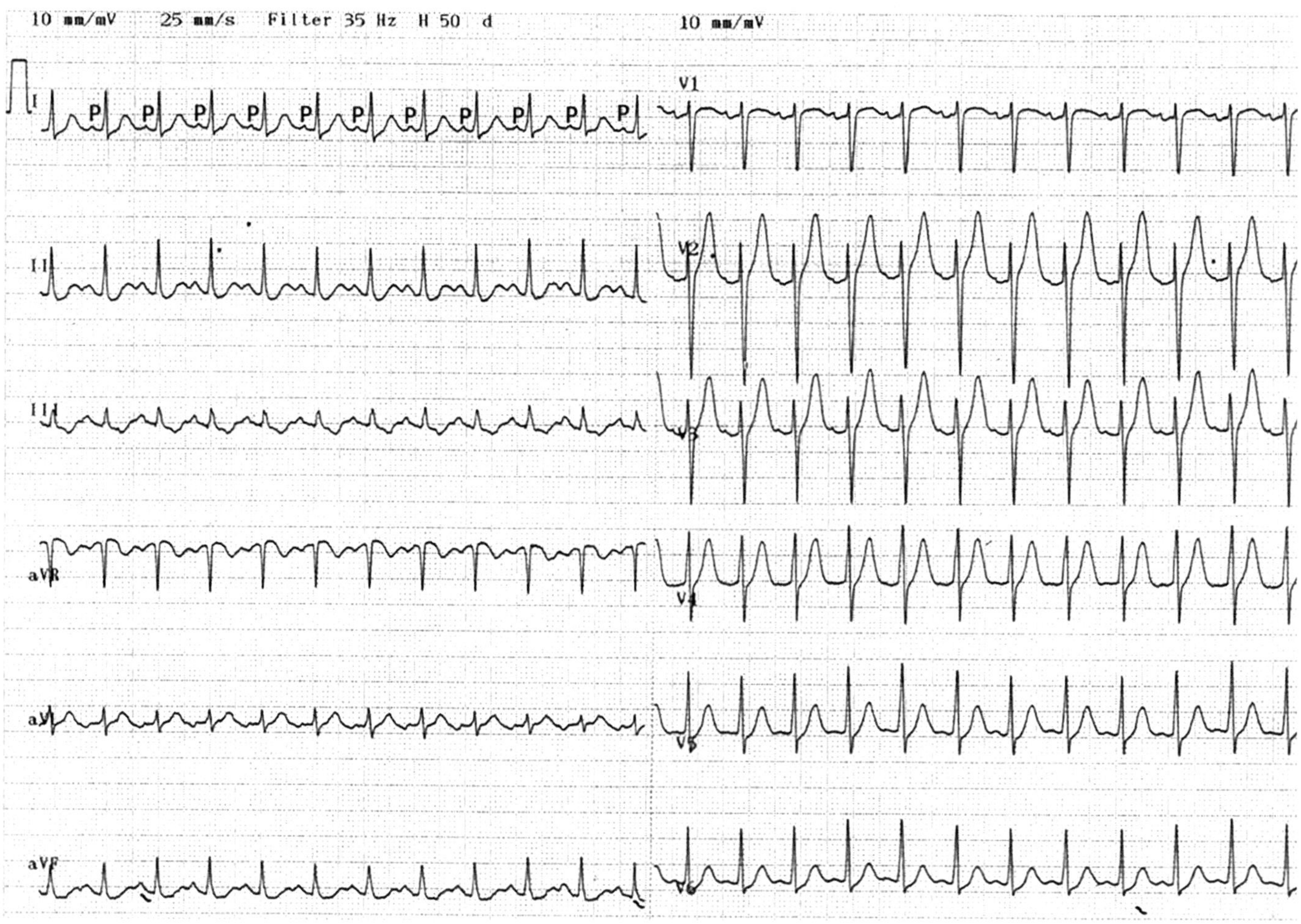

Fig. 11.1: Electrocardiogram (ECG) is suggestive of sinus tachycardia (rate is 148 bpm). The heart rate is regular and P waves precede each and every QRS complex (P).

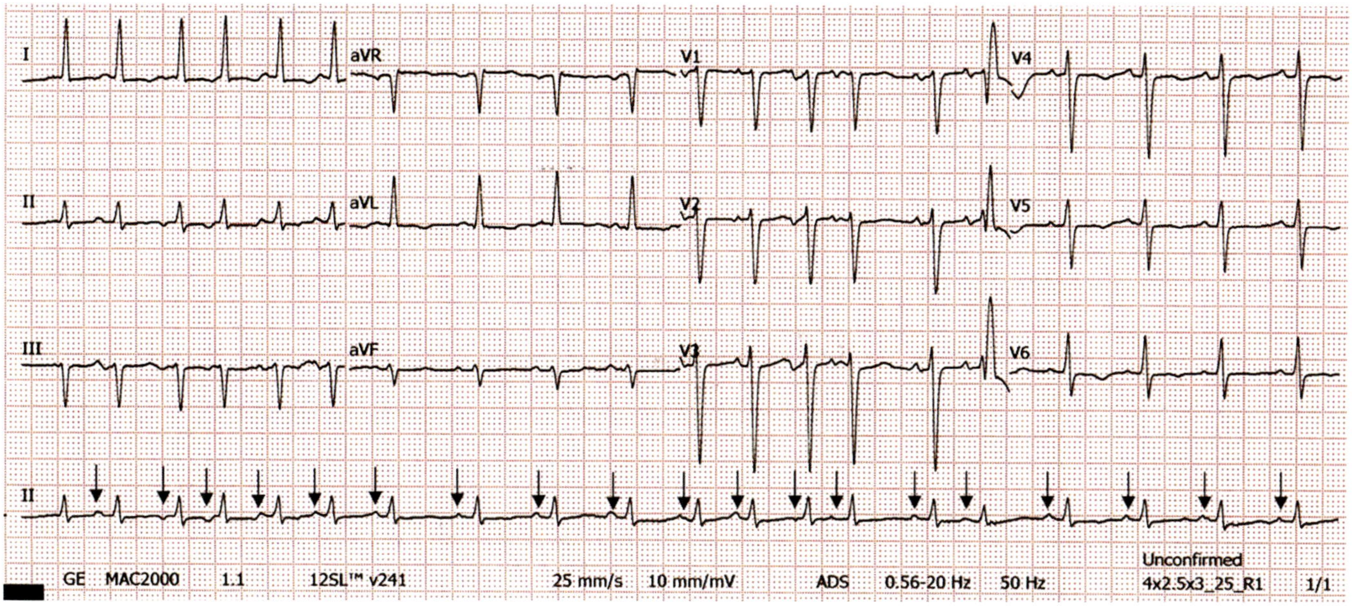

Fig. 11.2: Electrocardiogram shows multifocal atrial tachycardia (MAT), heart rate is greater than 100 bpm, irregularly irregular rhythm with varying PP, PR, and RR intervals and more than three distinct P-wave morphologies in the same lead, some P waves are upright, some are inverted and some are biphasic (arrows) but all the QRS complexes are preceded by P waves, but their morphologies are different.

is most commonly associated with chronic obstructive pulmonary disease (COPD). Associations also exist with pulmonary embolism, hypoxemia, and hypokalemia.[14] Triggered activity and enhanced automaticity have been proposed as likely mechanisms; however, consensus is lacking, and the precise mechanism remains elusive.[15,16]

ATRIAL FIBRILLATION

Atrial fibrillation (AF) is a supraventricular tachyarrhythmia characterized by uncoordinated atrial activation with consequent deterioration of mechanical function (Fig. 11.3). AF is the most common sustained cardiac rhythm disturbance, increasing in prevalence with age. AF is often associated with structural heart disease although a substantial proportion of patients with AF have no detectable heart disease.[17] This is the most common sustained arrhythmia encountered in clinical practice. Approximately 0.4% of persons in the general population have permanent or intermittent AF, and the prevalence of the arrhythmia increases to 6% in persons older than 80 years.[18] Atrial fibrillation can result in serious complications, including congestive heart failure, myocardial infarction, and thromboembolism. Considerable evidence has accumulated that AF occurring in a background of rheumatic heart disease, is decidedly associated with increased risk of stroke. In the Framingham Heart Study, patients with rheumatic heart disease and AF had a 17-fold increased risk of stroke compared with age-matched controls, and the attributable risk was five times greater than in those with nonrheumatic AF.[19]

Most common causes of AF include coronary artery disease, hypertension, mitral stenosis, thyrotoxicosis, and lone AF.

Mechanisms of Atrial Fibrillation

- *Focal activation*: In focal activation, AF originates from an area of focal activity. This activity may be triggered, due to increased automaticity, or from micro reentry and is often located in the pulmonary veins.
- *Multiple wavelet formation*: Multiple wavelet formation in which multiple small wandering wavelets are formed. The fibrillation is maintained by reentry circuits formed by some of the wavelets. This process is potentiated in the presence of a dilated LA.

Atrial fibrillation is often described as "Fast AF," if the ventricular rate is greater than 100 bpm (Fig. 11.4) and "Slow AF," if ventricular rate is less than 60 bpm (Fig. 11.5).

Causes of Atrial Fibrillation

Cardiac

- Coronary artery disease
- Mitral stenosis
- Hypertensive heart disease
- Congestive heart failure
- Multiple valvular heart disease
- Pericarditis
- Dilated cardiomyopathy
- Hypertrophic cardiomyopathy
- Postcardiac surgery.

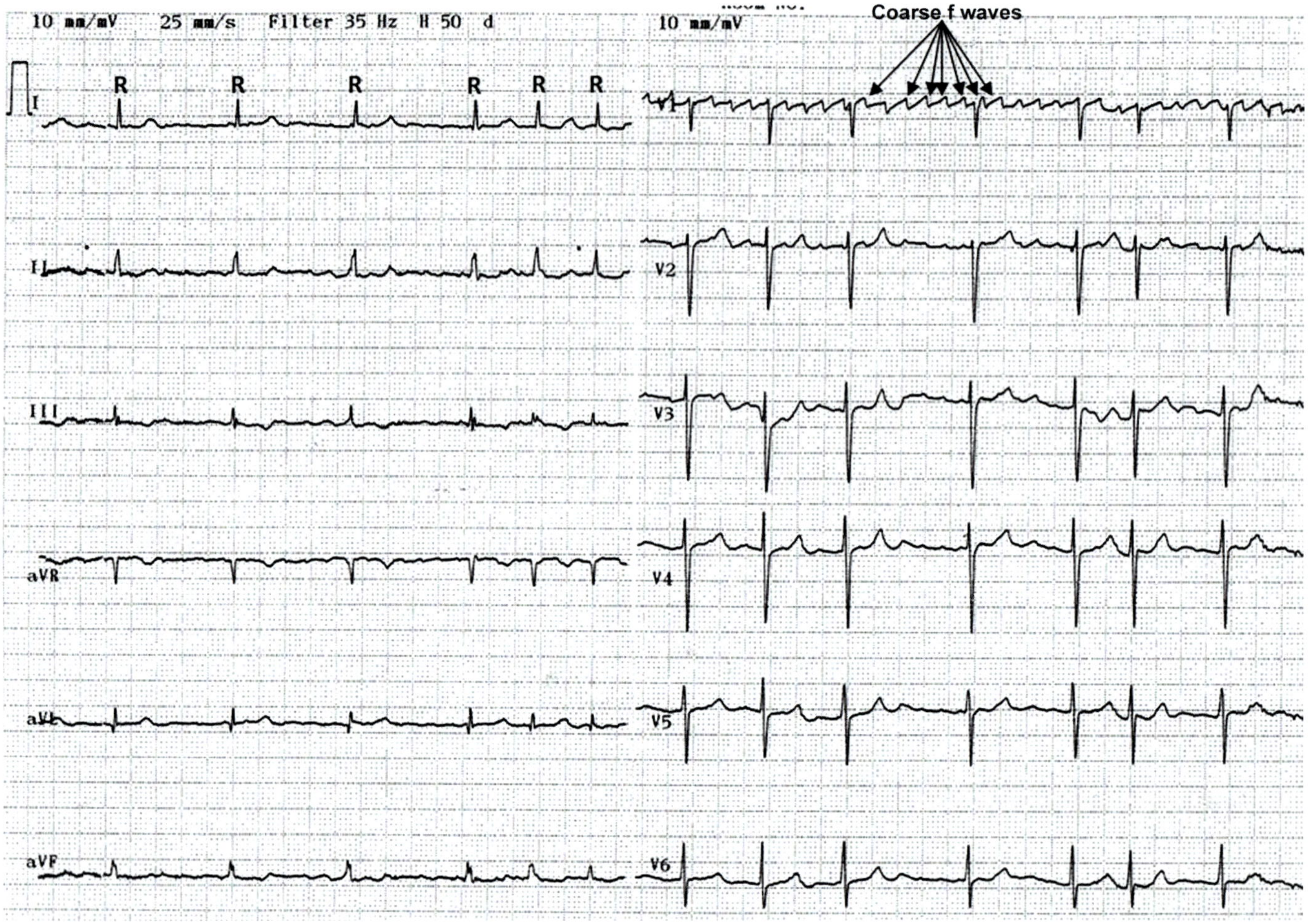

Fig. 11.3: Electrocardiogram is suggestive of typical atrial fibrillation (AF) [P waves are absent, the RR intervals are not equal resulting in an irregular rhythm and note fibrillation (f) waves instead of P waves (*arrows*)]. The "f" waves result in an oscillating irregular baseline.

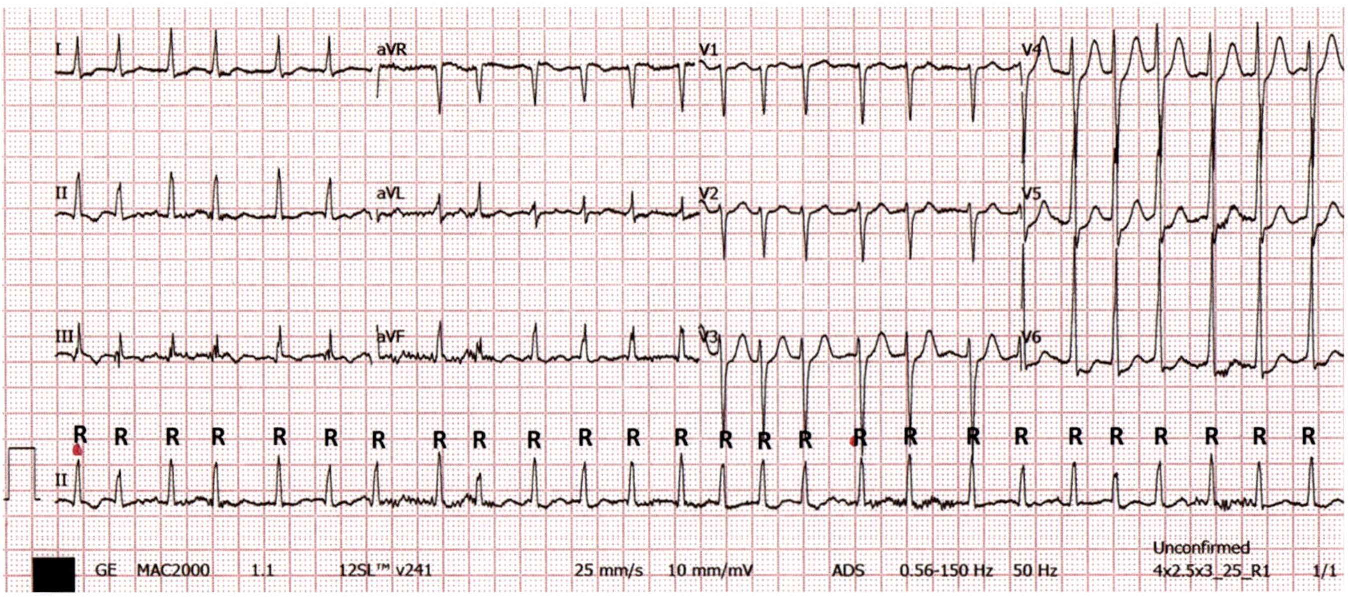

Fig. 11.4: Electrocardiogram of fast AF (rate is 156 bpm).

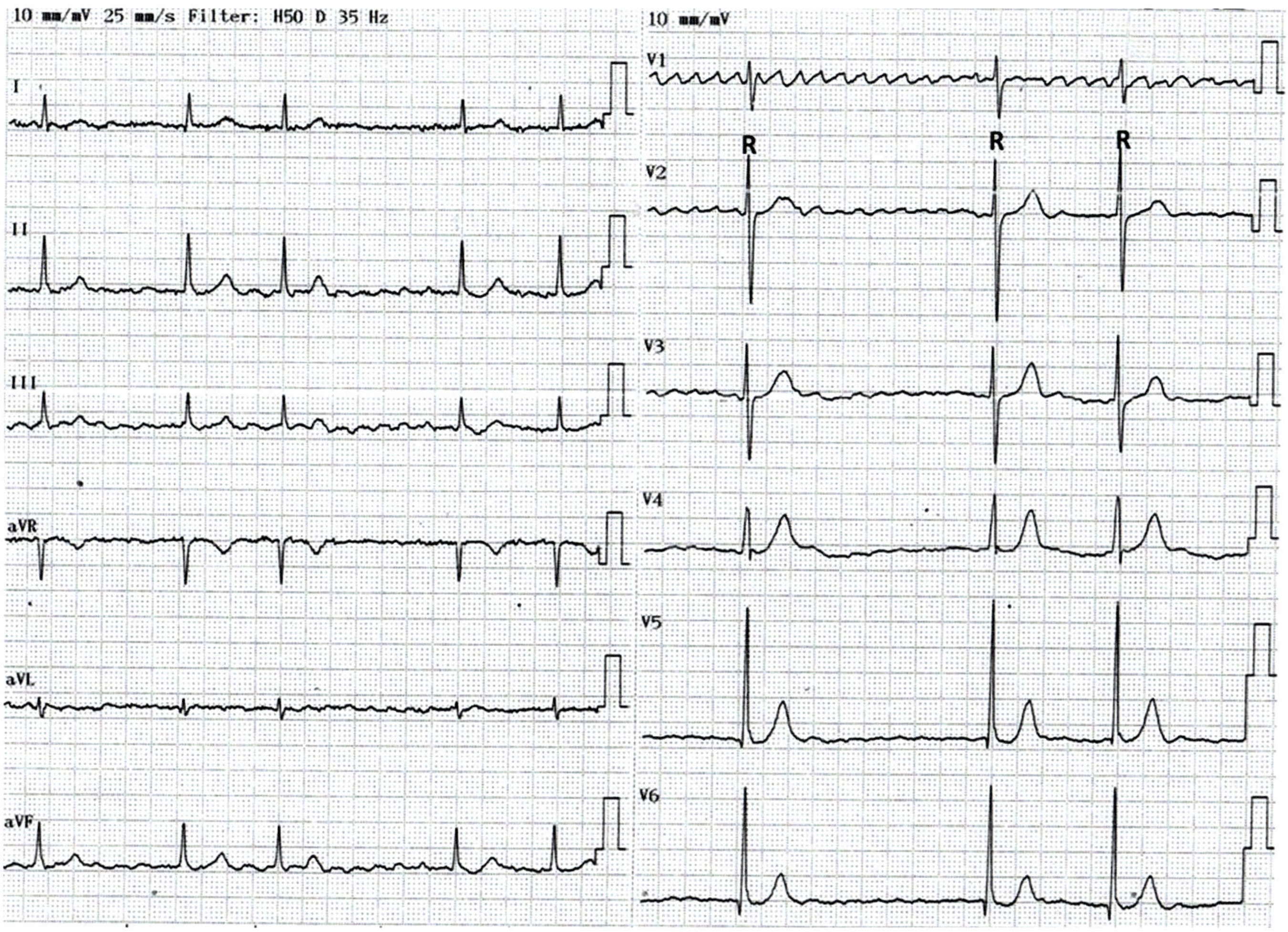

Fig. 11.5: Electrocardiogram of slow AF (rate is 46 bpm).

Noncardiac

- Thyrotoxicosis
- Electrolyte imbalance, e.g. hypokalemia and hypomagnesemia
- Pneumonia
- Lung cancer
- Sarcoidosis
- Excessive alcohol consumption ("binge drinking" or "holiday heart syndrome")
- Lone AF.

Classification of Atrial Fibrillation Based on the Temporal Pattern of the Arrhythmia[20]

1. Paroxysmal
   a. Spontaneous termination in less than 7 days and most often less than 48 hours.
   b. Usually recurrent.
2. Persistent
   a. Not self-terminating
   b. Lasting greater than 7 days or prior cardioversion
   c. Usually recurrent.

   Long-standing persistent AF sustains >1 year.
3. Permanent
   a. Duration is greater than 1 year in which rhythm control interventions are not pursued or are unsuccessful.
   b. Not terminated
   c. Terminated but relapsed
   d. No cardioversion attempt
   e. Established AF.

The ECG is the mainstay for diagnosis of AF. An irregularly irregular rhythm, inconsistent R-R interval, and absence of P waves are the main ECG features of AF. AF waves (f waves), which are small, irregular waves seen as a rapid-cycle baseline fluctuation (Figs. 11.6A and B), indicate rapid atrial activity (usually between 450 bpm and 600 bpm) and are the hallmark of the arrhythmia, although they may not always be visible on a surface ECG. AF should also be distinguished from atrial tachycardia with variable AV block, which usually presents with an atrial rate of 120–200 bpm. In this condition, the atrial rate is regular (unlike the irregular disorganized f waves of AF), but conduction to the ventricles is irregular. The resultant irregularly irregular ventricular rhythm may be difficult to

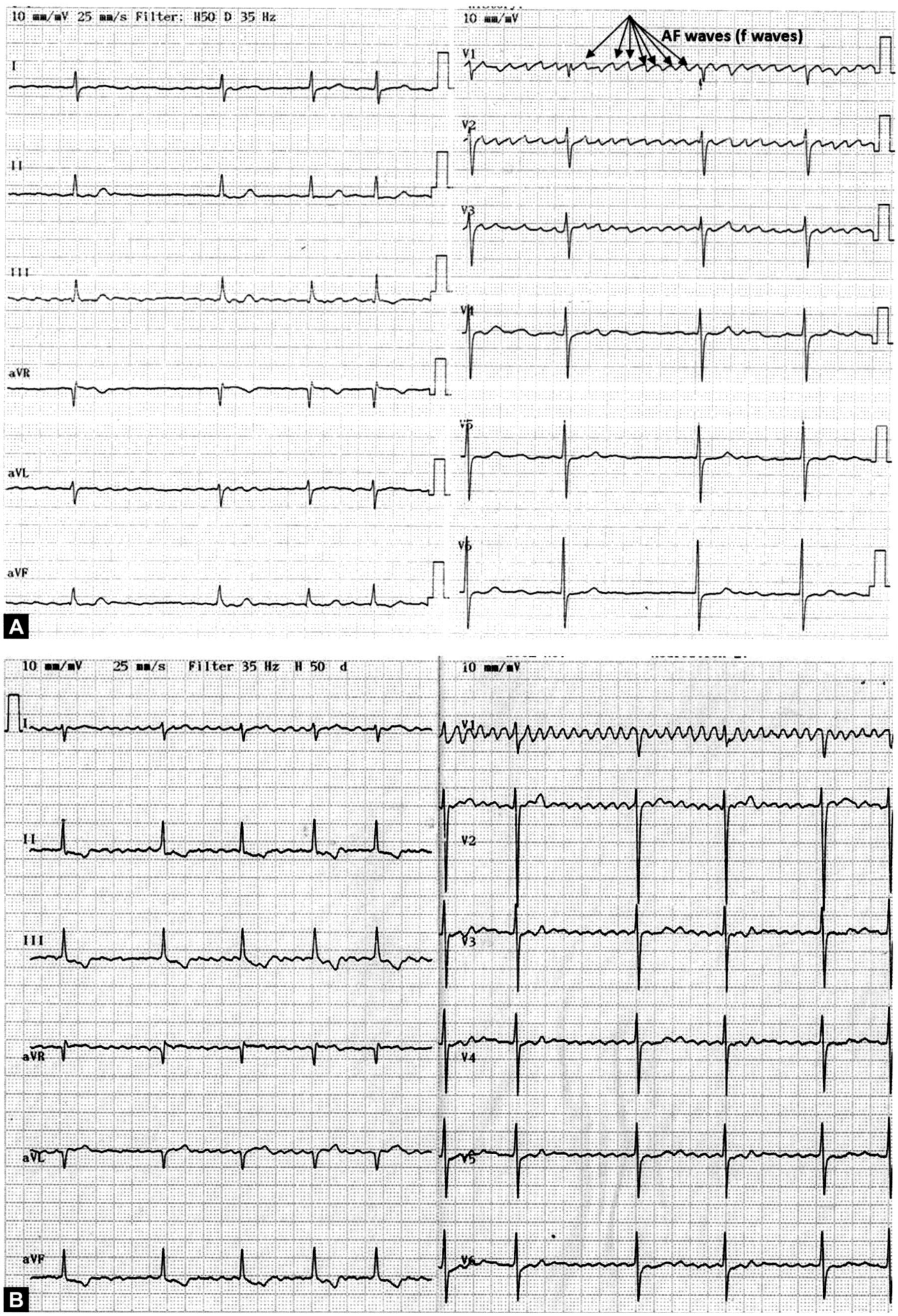

Figs. 11.6A and B: (A) Electrocardiogram showing AF waves (f waves). "f" are small, irregular waves (arrows) seen as a rapid-cycle baseline fluctuation, indicate rapid atrial activity and are the hallmark of the arrhythmia, although they may not always be visible on a surface ECG. (B) ECG suggestive of coarse AF with typical f waves in lead V1. Sometimes it may be difficult to distinguish coarse AF from atrial flutter. But AF has less organized activity in the atria and thus provides less uniform "f" waves and AF has an higher atrial rate (450–600 bpm versus 250–350 bpm for atrial flutter).

differentiate from AF. However, for emergency practice it is useful to consider any irregularly irregular tachycardia with no clear P waves seen as AF unless proven otherwise.[2]

The basic ECG criteria to diagnose AF are:

- Absence of P wave
- Irregularly irregular rhythm with variable RR interval
- Presence of "f" wave.

The baseline may be isoelectric or may exhibit fibrillatory waves (f wave) of varying morphology.[3,20] The amplitude of the fibrillatory waves may suggest the pathogenesis of the underlying pathology. Fine fibrillatory waves (≤0.5 mm amplitude) are associated with ischemic heart disease, while coarse waves (>0.5 mm) signify left atrial enlargement.[3,21,22] In some leads, "f" waves may not be apparent whereas in other leads, especially in lead V1, the waves may appear so coarse that atrial flutter is suspected. In the absence of P waves, even if "f" waves are not seen, a totally irregular ventricular rhythm is diagnostic of AF (Fig. 11.7). If, however, there is complete AV block, ventricular response will, of course, be slow and regular (Fig. 11.8). QRS complexes during AF are of normal duration unless there is established bundle branch block, Wolff–Parkinson–White syndrome or aberrant intraventricular conduction (Figs. 11.9A and B).

Lone Atrial Fibrillation

A subset of patients with AF is less than 60 years and routine evaluation, including physical examination, laboratory tests including thyroid function, echocardiography, and exercise stress testing, does not reveal any abnormalities. These patients are considered to suffer from "lone" AF, i.e. AF without an underlying (cardiovascular) disorder.[23] There is increasing evidence that, from a pathophysiological point of view, the underlying mechanism of lone AF is different than that of AF in the setting of underlying disease. The latter is "substrate related," i.e. due to diseased and dilated atria with stretch and fibrosis. In contrast, lone AF is probably more related to electrophysiological phenomena (triggers) in structurally normal atria. This explains why patients with real lone AF have a normal life expectancy when compared with individuals without arrhythmia, a low risk for stroke, and why paroxysmal lone AF does not often progress to persistent or permanent AF. In contrast, AF in the setting of underlying cardiac pathology usually progresses from paroxysmal to persistent and permanent AF together with the progression of the underlying cardiac substrate and is associated with an increased incidence of stroke. It is usually suggested that a diagnosis of lone AF should be restricted to patients less than 60 years of age.[18,23]

Ashman phenomenon, also known as Ashman beats, describes a particular type of wide QRS complex, often seen isolated that is typically seen in AF. It is more often misinterpreted as a premature ventricular complex (PVC). Typical Ashman aberrancy occurs when a long RR interval is followed by a short RR interval (Fig. 11.10). This wide QRS complex typically has a right bundle branch block (RBBB) morphology (Fig. 11.11) and represents an aberrantly conducted complex that originates above the AV node, rather than a complex that originates in either the right or left ventricle. So, Ashman beats are aberrantly conducted complex, not PVCs.

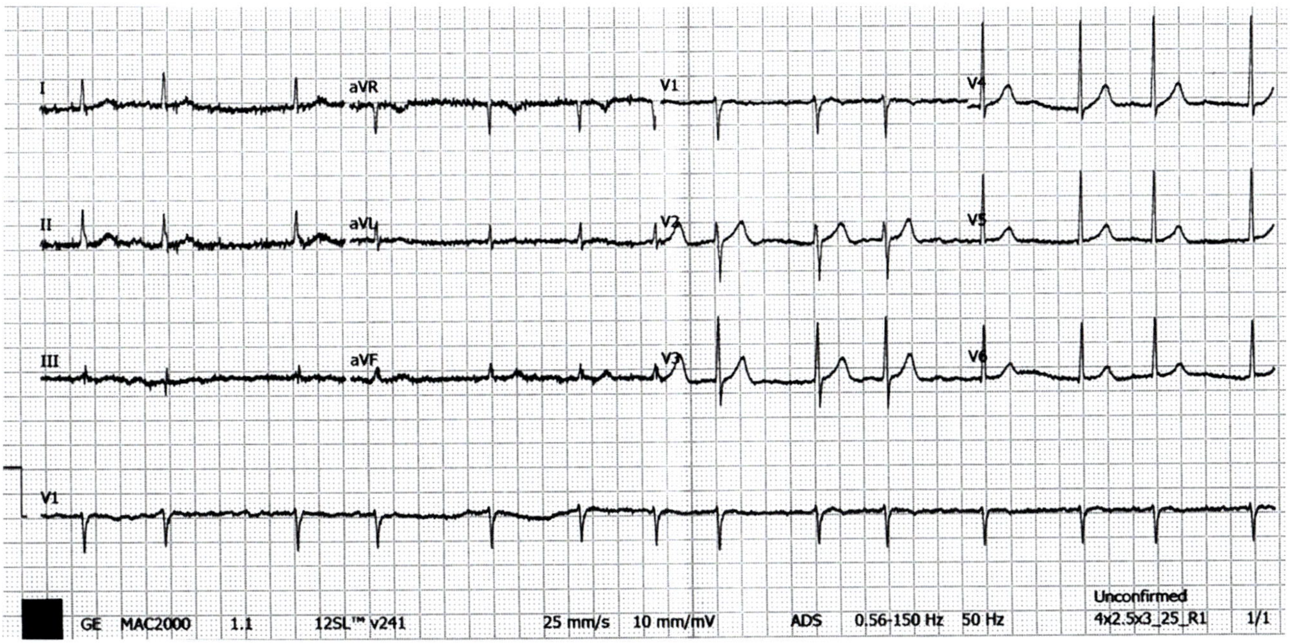

Fig. 11.7: Electrocardiogram strip showing AF (heart rate is 82 bpm) without any discernible "f" (fibrillatory) waves. In the absence of P waves, even if "f" waves are not seen, a totally irregular ventricular rhythm is diagnostic of AF.

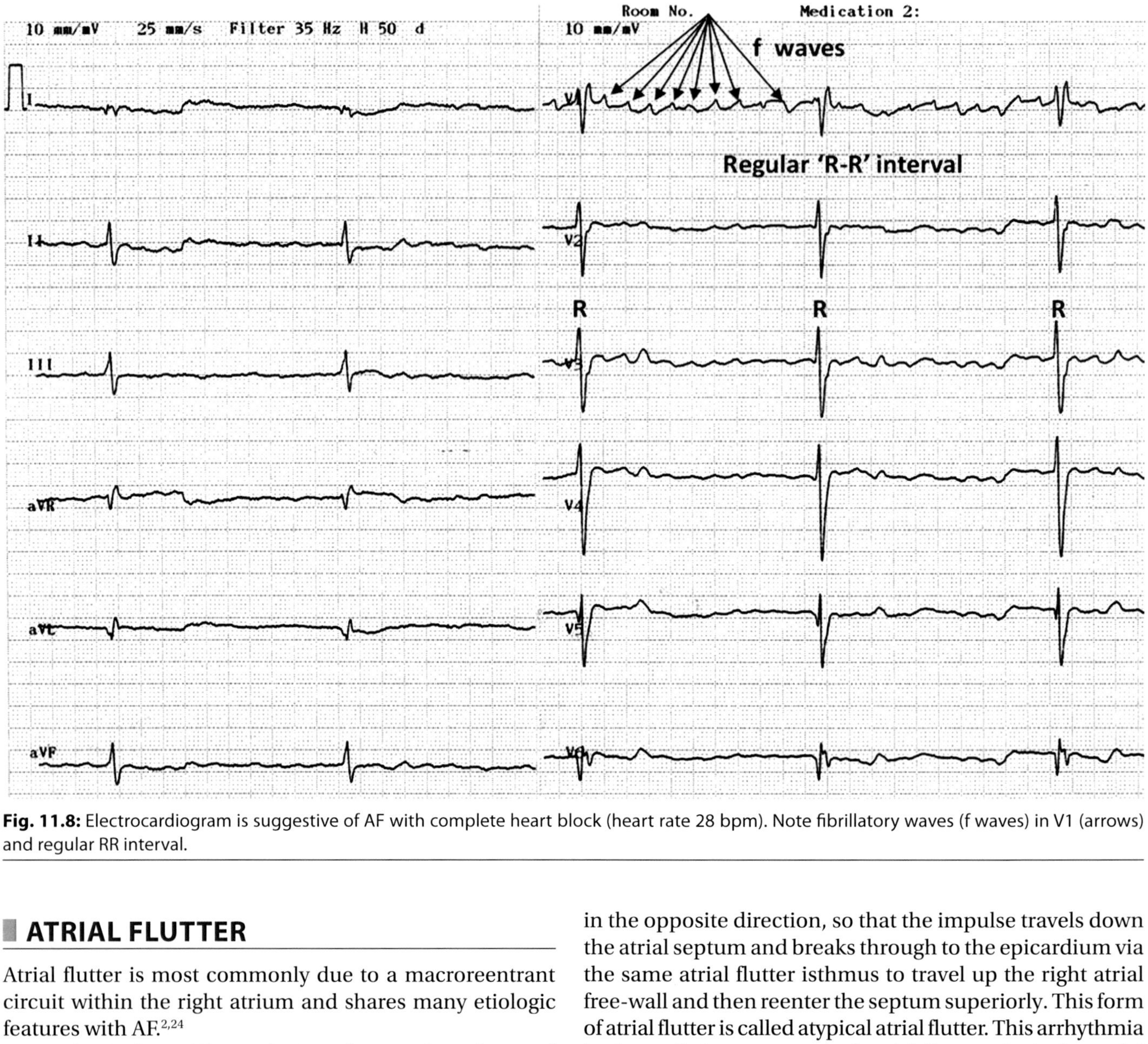

Fig. 11.8: Electrocardiogram is suggestive of AF with complete heart block (heart rate 28 bpm). Note fibrillatory waves (f waves) in V1 (arrows) and regular RR interval.

ATRIAL FLUTTER

Atrial flutter is most commonly due to a macroreentrant circuit within the right atrium and shares many etiologic features with AF.[2,24]

In classical atrial flutter the impulse travels up the atrial septum, with epicardial breakthrough superiorly in the right atrium where the impulse then travels inferiorly down the right atrial free-wall to reenter the atrial septum. In atrial flutter the atria discharges at a rate between 250 bpm and 350 bpm. In most cases, the atrial rate is close to 300 bpm. Atrial flutter may be paroxysmal or sustained. It is usually initiated by an atrial ectopic. It may degenerate into AF. Indeed, it may often be confused with "coarse" AF.[3]

Atrial flutter is of two types:

1. Typical atrial flutter (Type 1 flutter)
2. Atypical atrial flutter (Type 2 flutter).

Typical atrial flutter is also known as common atrial flutter and counterclockwise atrial flutter. A 12-lead ECG during typical atrial flutter shows characteristic negative "sawtooth" atrial flutter waves (F waves) in leads II, III, and aVF and upright flutter waves in V1 (Fig. 11.12).[24,25] It is also recognized that impulses can travel in this reentrant circuit in the opposite direction, so that the impulse travels down the atrial septum and breaks through to the epicardium via the same atrial flutter isthmus to travel up the right atrial free-wall and then reenter the septum superiorly. This form of atrial flutter is called atypical atrial flutter. This arrhythmia is also called reverse typical atrial flutter, clockwise atrial flutter, uncommon atrial flutter, and rare atrial flutter.[2] A 12-lead ECG during reverse typical atrial flutter reflects characteristic positive flutter waves in leads II, III, and aVF (Fig. 11.13). Other atrial flutter circuits have been described originating in both the left and right atrium, often in patients with atrial scar related to prior surgical procedures. These are characterized by regular flutter waves with a rate typically between 250 bpm and 350 bpm and a morphology determined by the flutter circuit. Atrial flutter generally presents as narrow complex tachycardia with a sawtooth baseline. Flutter with 2:1 A:V conduction is common, and so atrial flutter should be considered for any arrhythmia with narrow complexes at the rate of greater than 150 bpm (Figs. 11.14A and B). Atrial flutter can appear as 2:1, 3:1, and 4:1 or as variable A:V conduction (Figs. 11.15 and 16). Although atrial flutter can present with nearly any ventricular rate, 1:1 A:V conduction with ventricular rates of up to and above 300

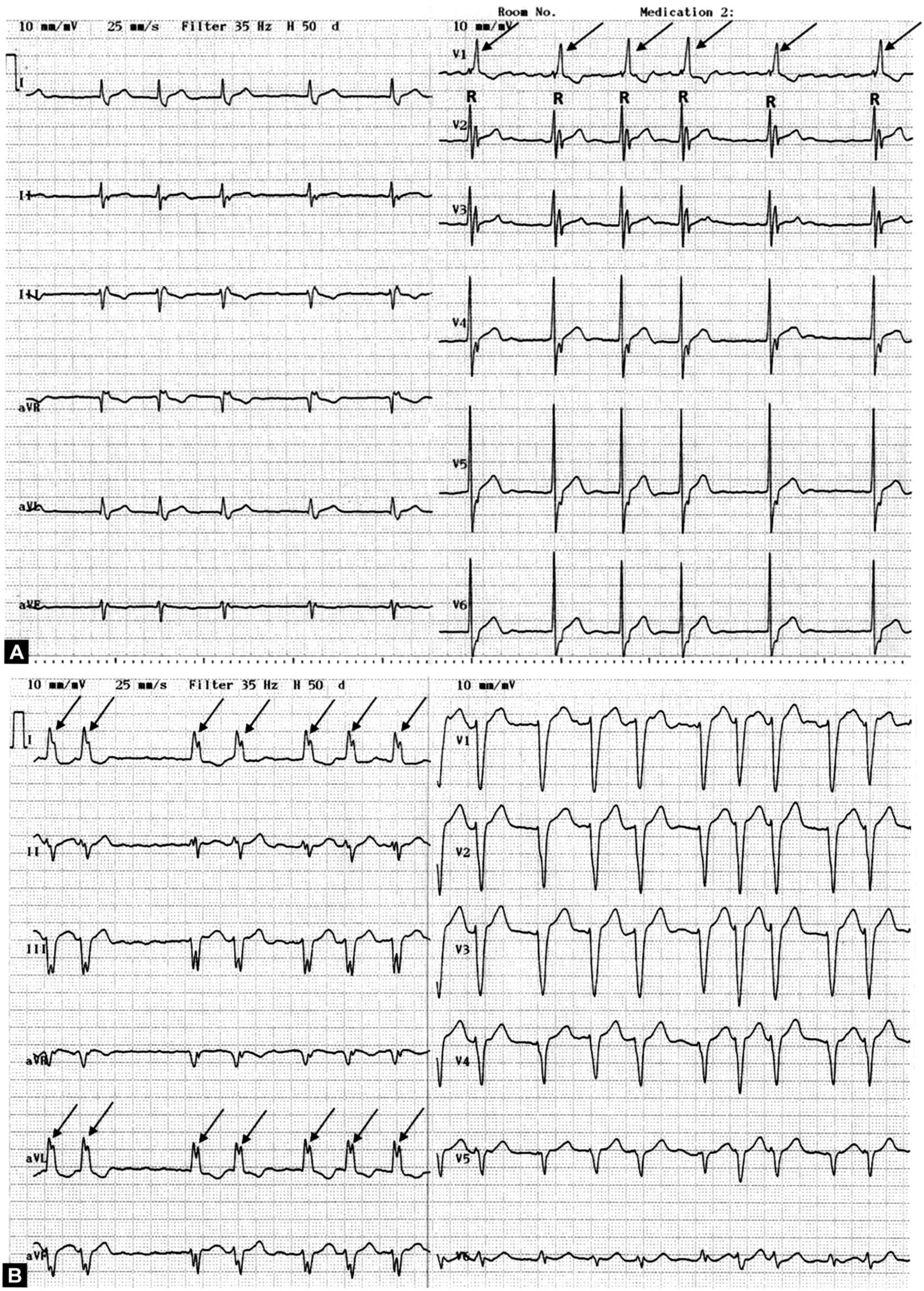

Figs. 11.9A and B: (A) Atrial fibrillation with complete right bundle branch block (RBBB). Note rsR pattern (arrows) in lead V1 and irregular RR interval. QRS complexes during AF are usually of normal duration but in this ECG, QRS duration is prolonged (120 ms) due to preexisting RBBB. (B) Atrial fibrillation with complete left bundle branch block (LBBB). Note "M" pattern QRS complexes in LI and aVL (arrows) with irregular RR interval. QRS complexes during AF are usually of normal duration but in this ECG, QRS duration is prolonged (140 ms) due to preexisting LBBB.

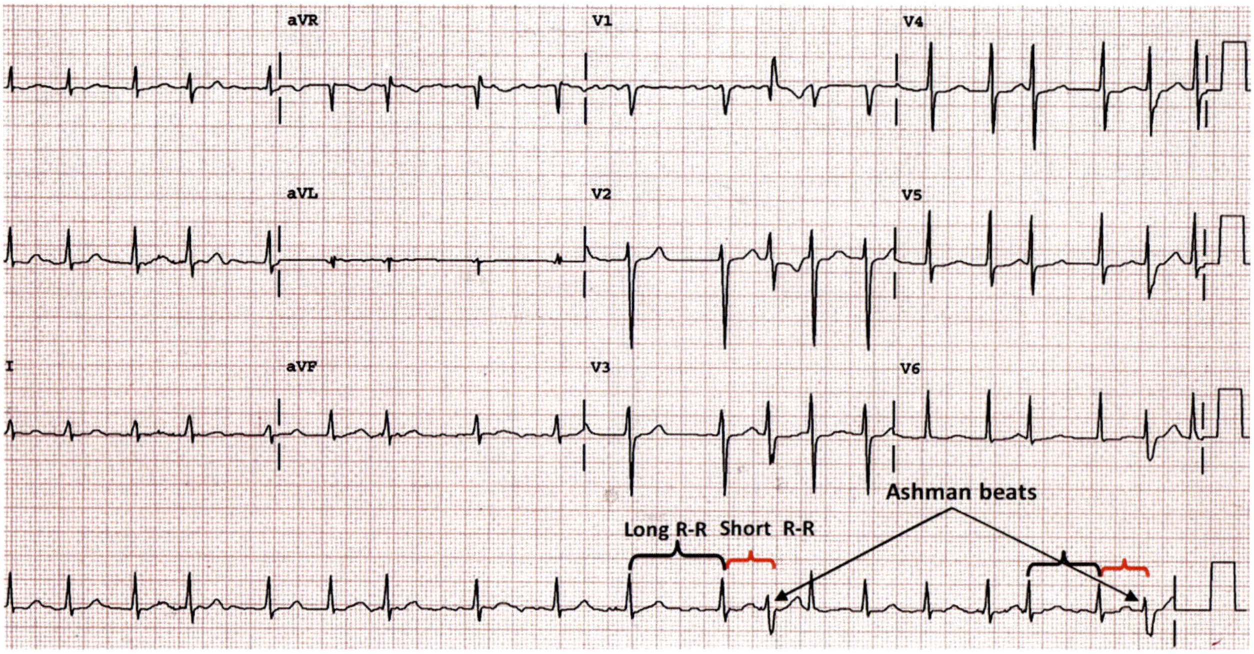

Fig. 11.10: Electrocardiogram shows two Ashman beats (arrows). Typical Ashman aberrancy occurs when a long RR interval (black bracket) is followed by a short RR interval (red bracket). QRS complexes of Ashman beats look like premature ventricular complexes (PVCs) but Ashman beats are aberrantly conducted complex not PVCs.

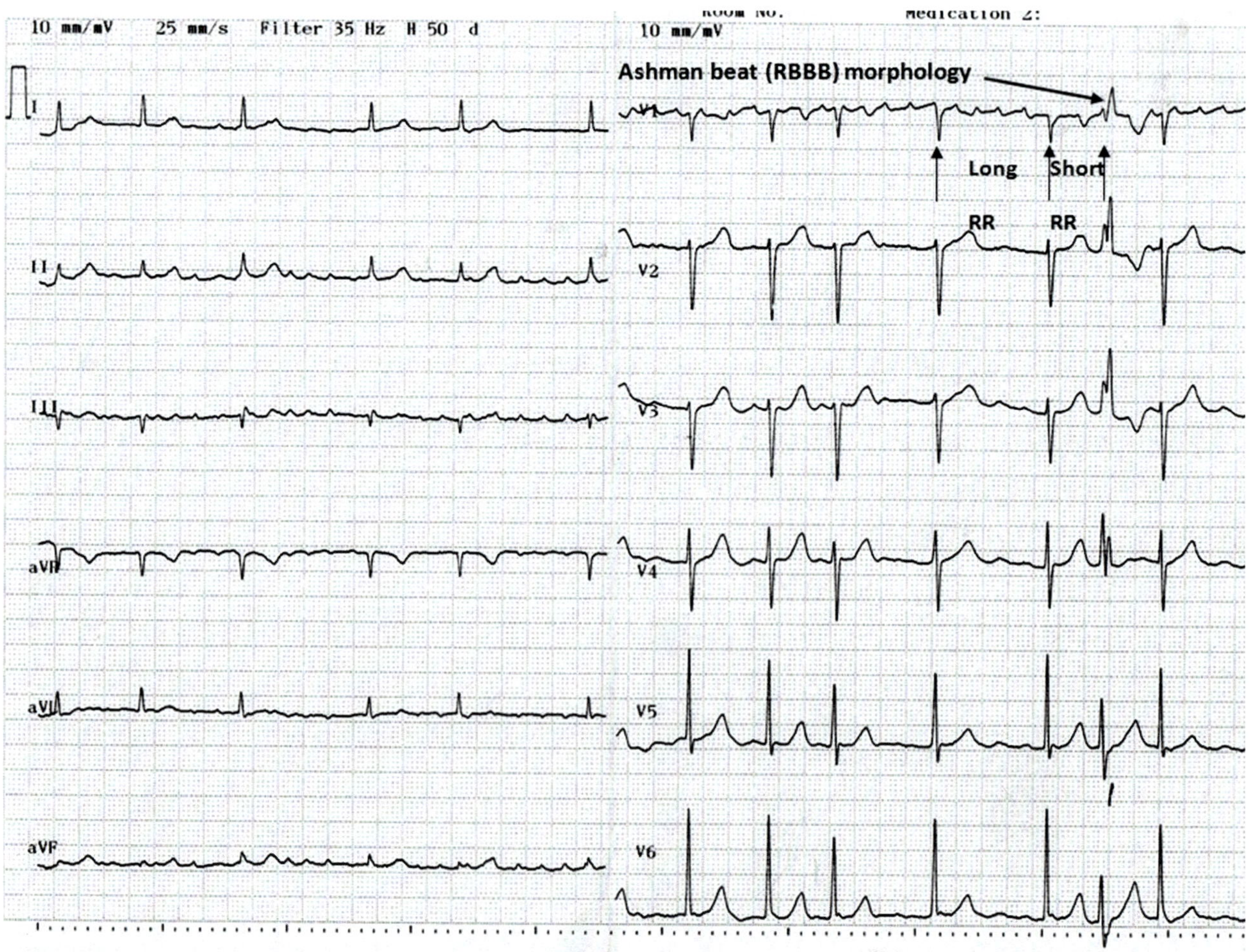

Fig. 11.11: Electrocardiogram shows AF with one Ashman beat (arrow) of RBBB morphology. Ashman phenomenon (Ashman beat) occurs when a premature supraventricular beat occurs before the right bundle branch has recovered from its refractory period. This results in the premature beat displaying a RBBB pattern.

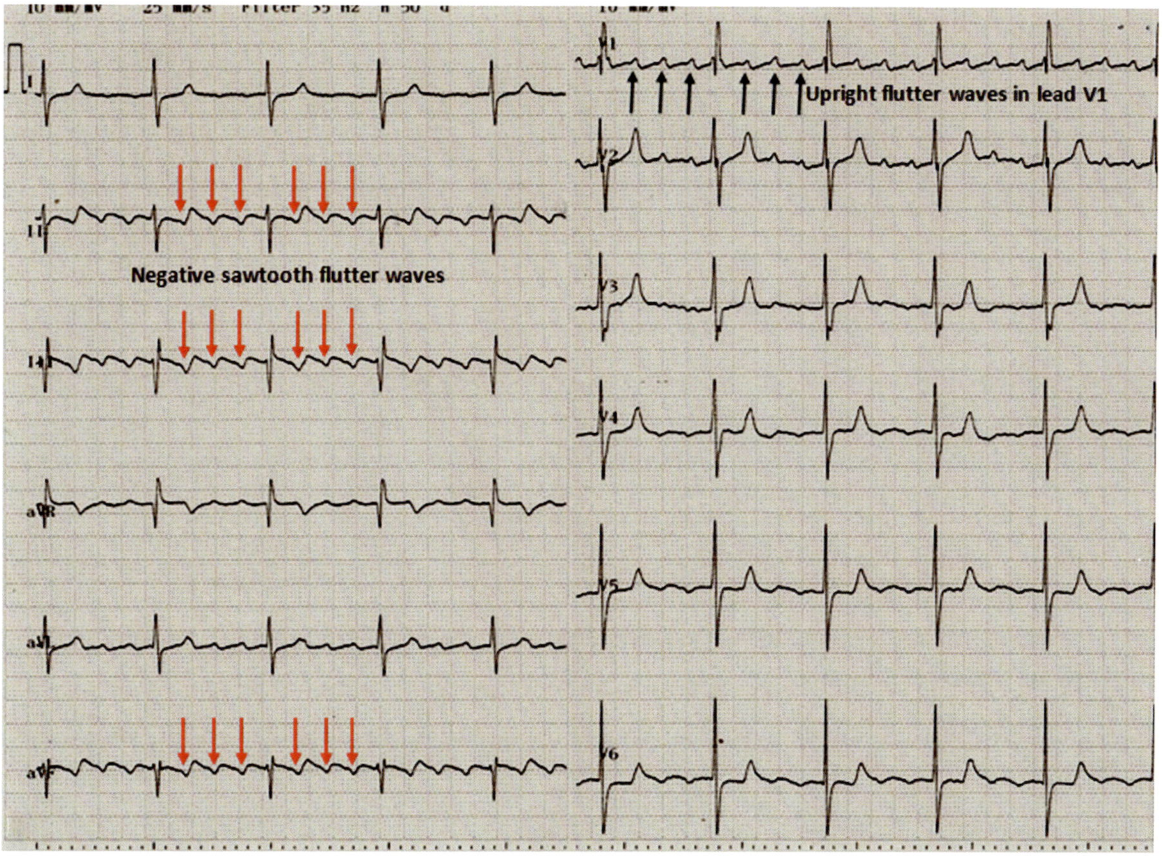

Fig. 11.12: 12-lead ECG showing typical atrial flutter with negative 'sawtooth' atrial flutter waves in leads II, III, and aVF (red arrow) and upright flutter waves in V1 (black arrows).

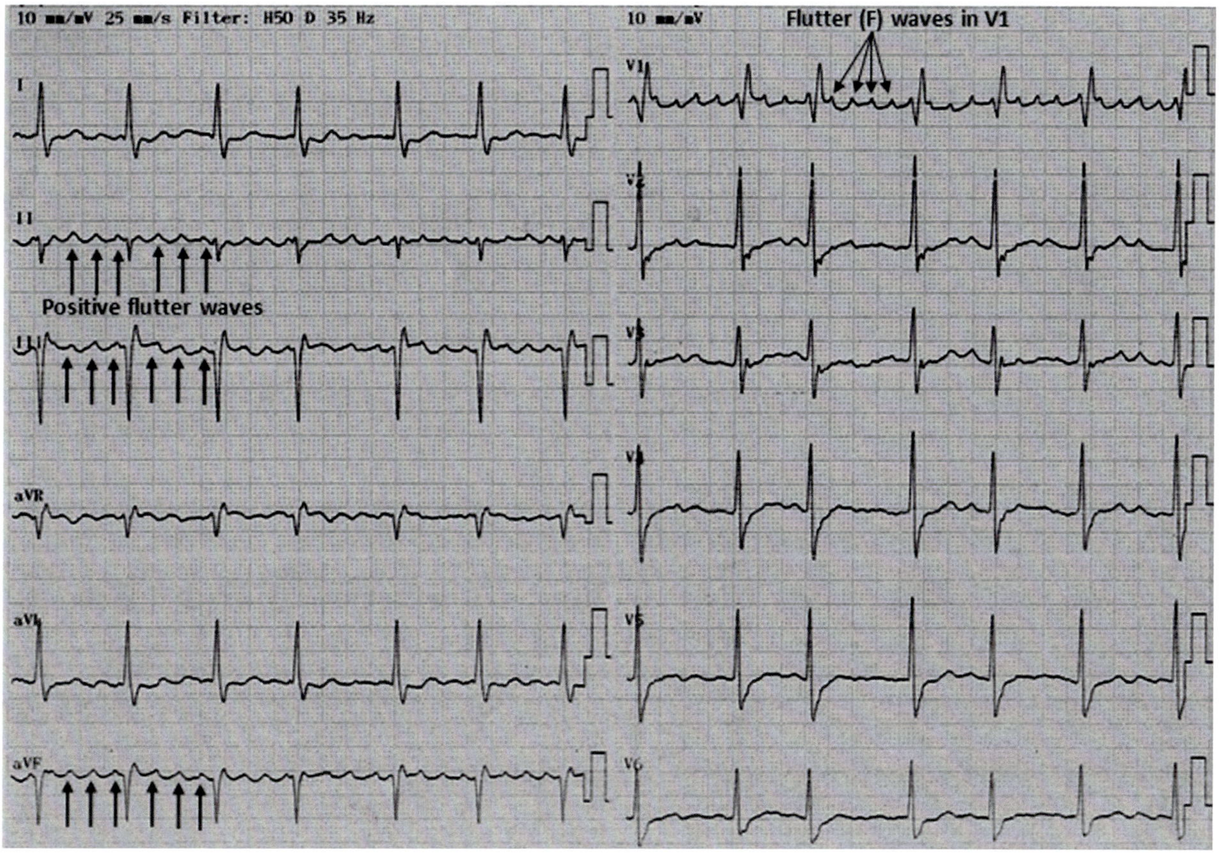

Fig. 11.13: Electrocardiogram showing atypical atrial flutter with positive flutter waves in leads II, III, and aVF (arrows). Also note flutter waves (F waves) in VI.

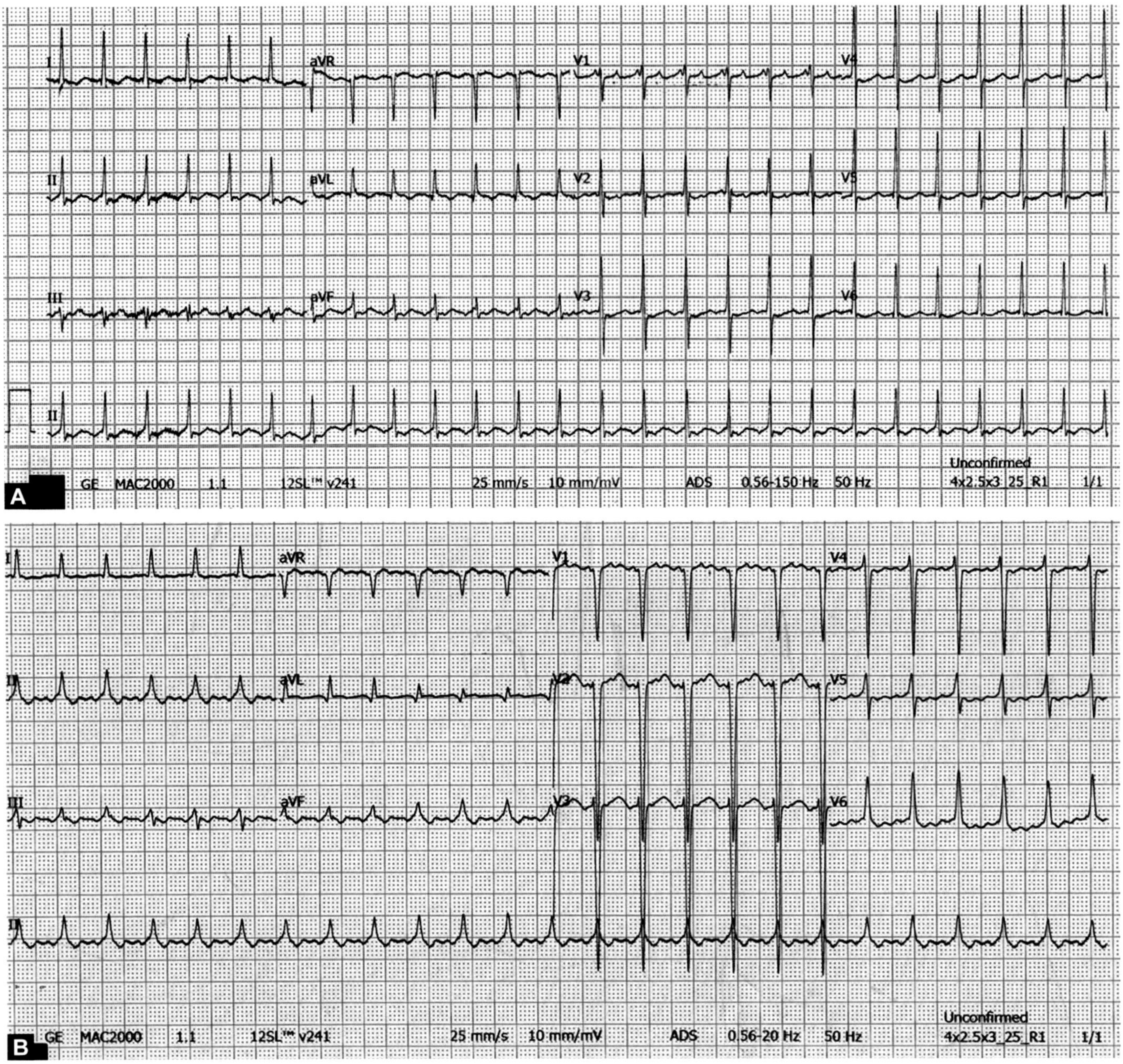

Figs. 11.14A and B: (A) Electrocardiogram showing atrial flutter with 2:1 A:V conduction (rate is 154 bpm). Atrial flutter should be considered for any arrhythmia with narrow complexes at the rate of greater than 150 beats per minute. (B) ECG showing atrial flutter with 2:1 A:V conduction (rate is 150 bpm).

bpm is occasionally encountered (either with a narrow QRS or with aberrant conduction producing a wide QRS).[25,26]

PAROXYSMAL SUPRAVENTRICULAR TACHYCARDIA

Paroxysmal supraventricular tachycardia (PSVT) is a common group of arrhythmias that present with narrow complex tachycardia. PSVT in the absence of structural heart disease can present at any age but most commonly first presents between ages 12 and 30. Most patients with PSVT due to atrioventricular nodal reentrant tachycardia (AVNRT) or atrioventricular reentrant tachycardia (AVRT) do not have associated structural heart disease, although exceptions (e.g. Ebstein's anomaly and pre-excitation syndromes) do exist. Atrial tachycardias (AT) are another cause of PSVT and are often associated with structural heart disease. A 12-lead ECG during tachycardia is helpful for defining the mechanism of PSVT. Patients with panic disorder report symptoms similar to those of PSVT, and an ECG during palpitation shows mostly ST thus aiding in diagnosis.

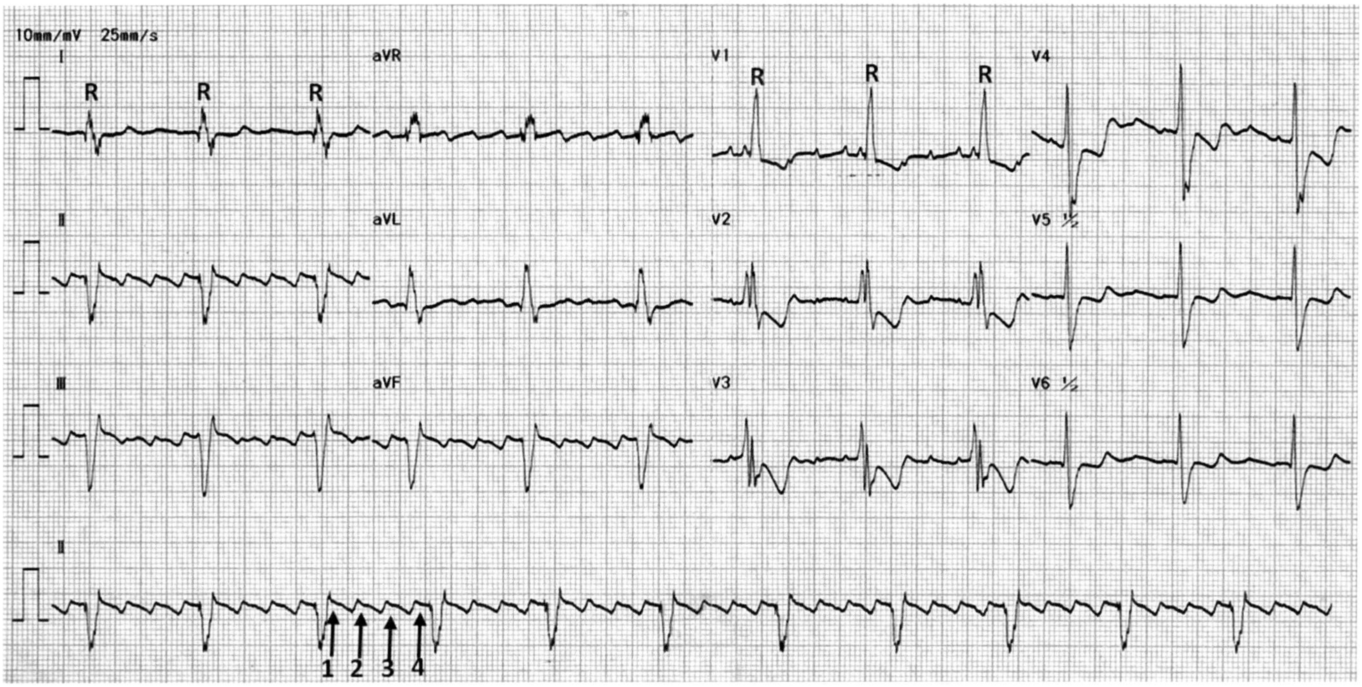

Fig. 11.15: Atrial flutter with 4:1 atrioventricular (AV) conduction. Note regular RR interval and positive flutter waves in V1 resembling P waves.

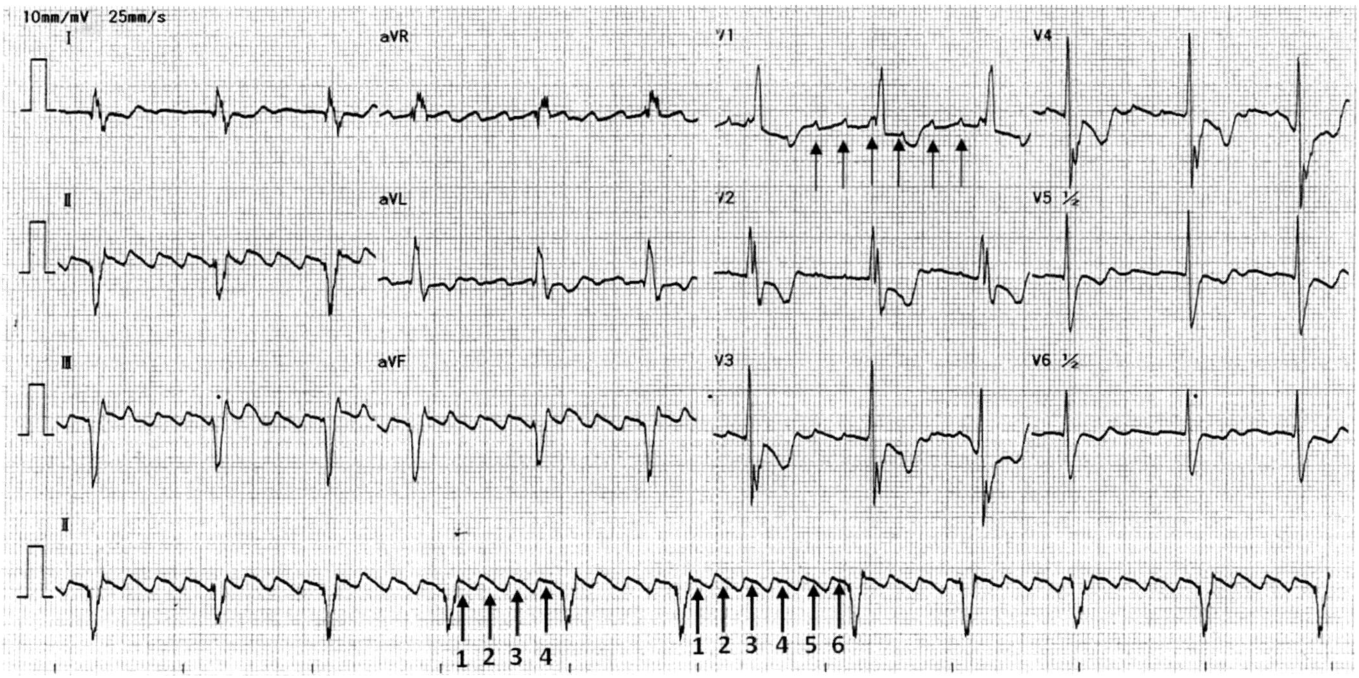

Fig. 11.16: Atrial flutter with variable AV conduction (arrows), AV block varies from 4:1 to 6:1. Note irregular RR interval and positive flutter waves in V1 resembling P waves (arrows).

ATRIOVENTRICULAR NODAL RE-ENTRANT TACHYCARDIA

The three most common SVTs—AVNRT, AVRT or AV reciprocating tachycardia, and atrial tachycardia—are often considered to be a triumvirate because they share many characteristics, including rapid onset, heart rates of 140–280 bpm, and regularity of the ventricular response. Atrioventricular nodal reentrant tachycardia and AV reciprocating tachycardia are caused by the presence of abnormal electrical circuits, whereas atrial tachycardia can be focal or caused by very small abnormal circuits. These

SVTs occur in approximately 1 person per 500 population. Atrioventricular nodal reentrant tachycardia is most common among persons older than 20 years of age (mean age of onset 32 years), whereas AV reciprocating tachycardia occurs more frequently in the pediatric population. Atrial tachycardia is the least common of the three.[12]

Atrioventricular nodal reentrant tachycardia is typically paroxysmal and may occur spontaneously in patients or upon provocation with exertion, coffee, tea, or alcohol. It is more common in women than men (~75% of cases occurring in women) and may occur in young and healthy patients as well as those suffering from chronic heart disease. Patients will typically complain of the sudden onset of rapid, regular palpitations. The patient may experience a brief fall in blood pressure causing presyncope or occasionally syncope. If the patient has underlying coronary artery disease the patient may experience chest pain similar to angina (tight band around the chest radiating to left arm or left side of the jaw). The patient may complain of shortness of breath, anxiety, and occasionally polyuria due to elevated atrial pressure releasing atrial natriuretic peptide. The tachycardia typically ranges between 140 bpm and 280 bpm and is regular in nature. It may cease spontaneously (and abruptly) or continue indefinitely until medical treatment is sought. The condition is generally well-tolerated and is rarely life threatening in patients with preexisting heart disease.[27]

The pathogenesis of AVNRT depends on so called "dual AV nodal pathway," which indicates that the AV node has two distinct tracts capable of conducting impulses, one of which conducts slowly but has a short refractory period, and the other of which conducts rapidly but has a relatively longer refractory period. During sinus rhythm, impulses are typically carried by the "fast" (also known as "beta") pathway, and the "slow" (also known as "alpha") pathway is unused (Fig. 11.17).[3]

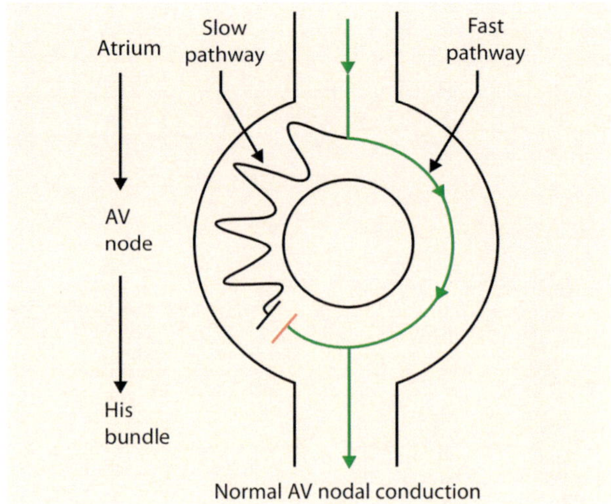

Fig. 11.17: Normal AV nodal conduction during sinus rhythm. During sinus rhythm, impulses are typically carried by the "fast" pathway, and the "slow" pathway is unused.

Types of Atrioventricular Nodal Reentrant Tachycardia[27,28]

1. *Slow-fast AVNRT (common AVNRT)*: Accounts for 80–90% of AVNRT
2. *Fast-slow AVNRT (uncommon AVNRT)*: Accounts for 10% of AVNRT
3. *Slow-slow AVNRT (atypical AVNRT)*: Accounts for 1–5% of AVNRT.

Common AVNRT is initiated when a premature atrial impulse finds the fast pathway refractory and instead uses the slow pathway to conduct to the His-Purkinje system. By the time the impulse reaches the ventricles, the fast pathway has repolarized, and the impulse is carried by this tract in a retrograde fashion. This pattern continues in order to produce "common" AVNRT (also known as typical AVNRT or slow-fast AVNRT) (Fig. 11.18). A premature ventricular impulse may also initiate this rhythm, if the impulse is blocked in the retrograde direction by the slow pathway and follows the fast pathway. The impulse then proceeds via the slow pathway in the antegrade direction and back up the fast pathway for retrograde transmission.[3] In most cases of common AVNRT, the P waves are absent during tachyarrhythmia (Fig. 11.19). P waves are often hidden—being embedded in the QRS complexes. Pseudo r' wave may be seen in V1 and pseudo S waves may be seen in leads II, III, or aVF.

In uncommon AVNRT, the fast pathway may have a shorter refractory period than the slow pathway, allowing for reversal of the circuit.[3,29-32] "Uncommon" AVNRT (also known as fast-slow AVNRT) occurs when antegrade conduction follows the fast pathway and retrograde conduction is carried by the slow pathway. It is generally initiated by a premature ventricular impulse.[30] In ECG of uncommon AVNRT, the retrograde P wave may appear after the corresponding QRS. Then P waves are visible between the QRS and T waves (Fig. 11.20). During slow-slow AVNRT (atypical AVNRT) in ECG, P wave is seen in mid-diastole, effectively appearing before the QRS complex, confusing as a P wave appearing before the QRS complex in the face of a tachycardia might honestly be read as a ST. The distinction between "fast-slow" and "slow-slow" forms is not unanimously defined, and probably of no practical significance. It is suggested that AVNRT should be classified as typical or atypical according to the His-atrial interval.[33]

ECG Characteristics of Atrioventricular Nodal Reentrant Tachycardia

During tachycardia rate is in the range of 140–280 bpm (commonly 170–200 bpm). It usually presents as a narrow complex tachycardia with no visible P waves. It starts abruptly due to a premature atrial complex (PAC) and ends abruptly. The PAC that initiates the tachycardia generally is conducted with a prolonged PR interval. In

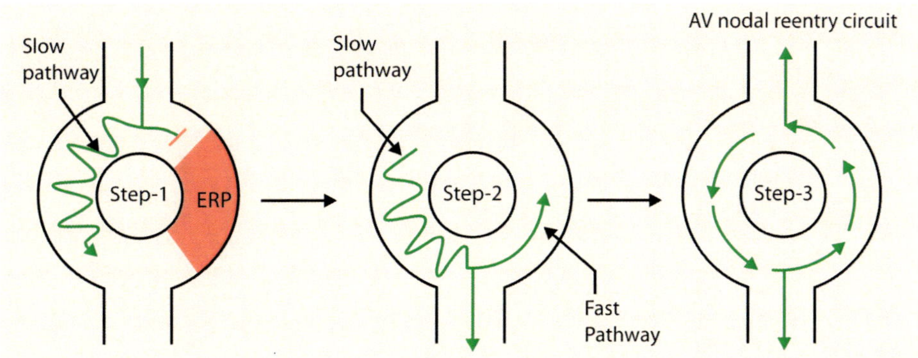

Fig. 11.18: Mechanism of reentry in "slow-fast" or common atrioventricular nodal reentrant tachycardia (AVNRT). Step 1: A premature atrial contraction (PAC) arrives while the fast pathway is still refractory, the electrical impulse will be directed solely down the slow pathway. Step 2: By the time the premature impulse reaches the end of the slow pathway, the fast pathway is no longer refractory, hence the impulse is permitted to recycle retrogradely up the fast pathway. Step 3: This creates a circus movement whereby the impulse continually cycles around the two pathways. (ERP: effective refractory period)

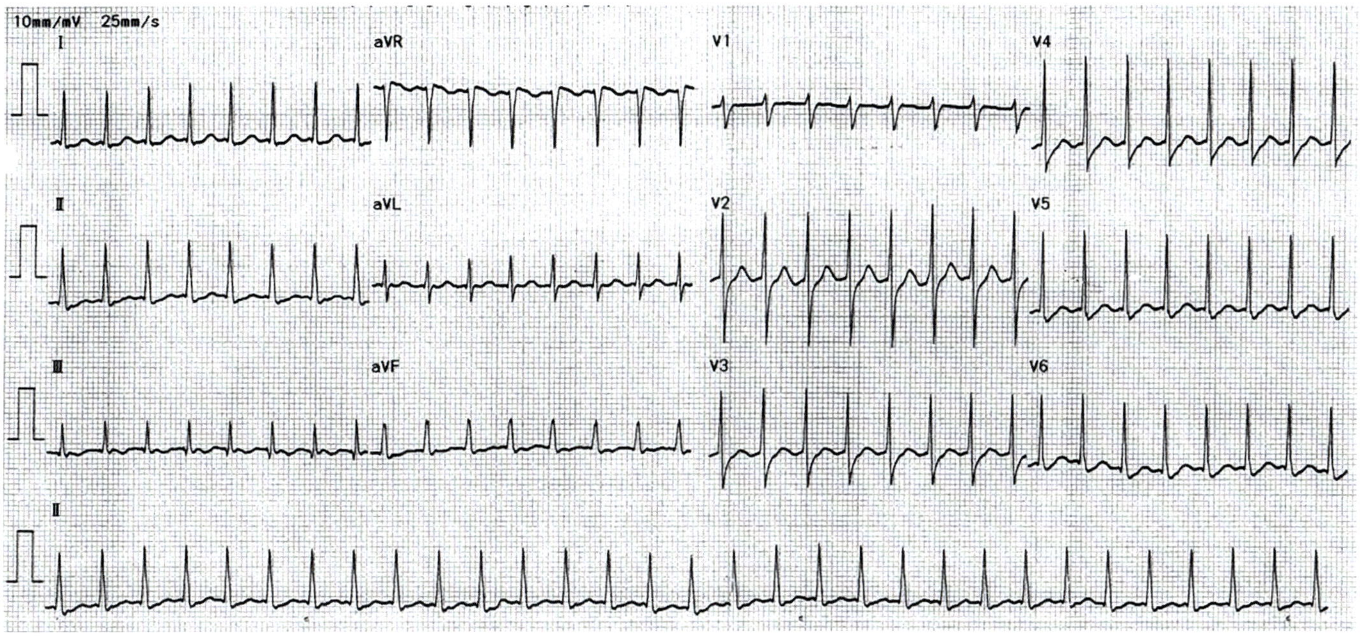

Fig. 11.19: Electrocardiogram is suggestive of common atrioventricular nodal reentrant tachycardia (AVNRT) at rate of 184 bpm. It is narrow complex tachycardia with no visible P wave, possibly a slow–fast (common or typical) AVNRT.

typical, slow pathway-antegrade, fast pathway-retrograde (slow–fast AVNRT), the P wave is either not seen or is visible in the terminal portion of the QRS (especially in lead V1). Practically during common AVNRT, P waves are generally not seen as they are buried in the QRS complex and do not manifest in surface ECG. However, if the tachycardia occurs through the fast–slow pathway (uncommon AVNRT), then P waves may be visible after the QRS complex due to slow conduction over the retrograde pathway. It must be remembered that both the fast and slow pathways are within the AV node.

ATRIOVENTRICULAR REENTRANT TACHYCARDIA

Atrioventricular reentrant tachycardias (AVRT) also known as atrioventricular reciprocating tachycardias occur as a result of an anatomically distinct AV connection. This accessory conduction pathway allows the atrial impulse to bypass the AV node and activate the ventricles prematurely (ventricular preexcitation). The presence of the accessory pathway (AP) allows a reentry circuit to form and paroxysmal AVRT to occur. Atrioventricular reentrant tachycardia

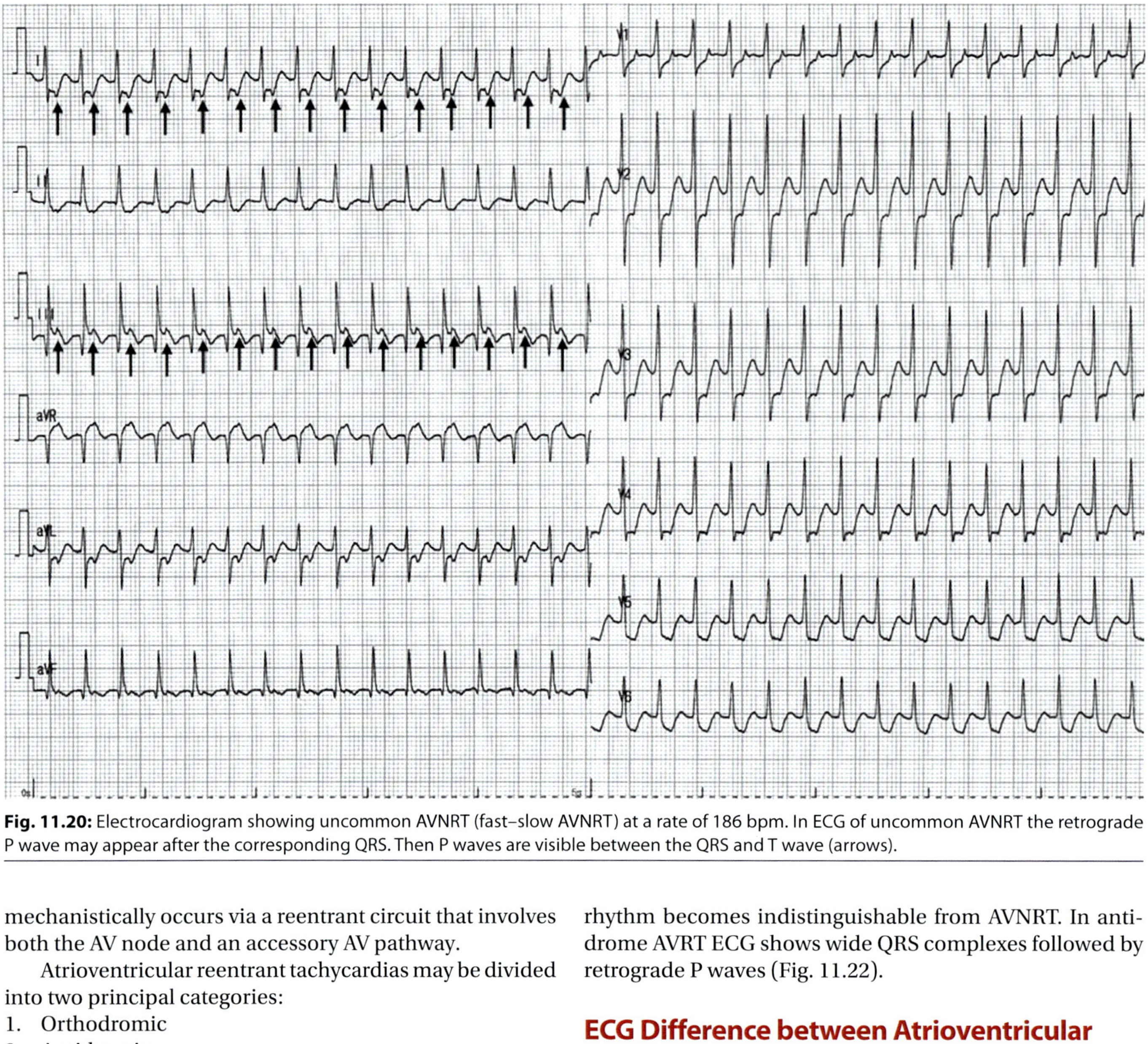

Fig. 11.20: Electrocardiogram showing uncommon AVNRT (fast–slow AVNRT) at a rate of 186 bpm. In ECG of uncommon AVNRT the retrograde P wave may appear after the corresponding QRS. Then P waves are visible between the QRS and T wave (arrows).

mechanistically occurs via a reentrant circuit that involves both the AV node and an accessory AV pathway.

Atrioventricular reentrant tachycardias may be divided into two principal categories:

1. Orthodromic
2. Antidromic.

Orthodromic AVRT indicates that antegrade conduction occurs through the AV node with retrograde conduction via the AP, resulting in a narrow QRS complex tachycardia (Figs. 11.21A and B). Conversely, antidromic AVRT occurs with antegrade conduction down the AP and retrograde conduction through the AV node, producing a wide QRS complex tachycardia (Fig. 11.22). Onset of AVRT is abrupt and is typically initiated by a premature atrial or ventricular impulse.[8-11,33] Rates typically range from 140 bpm to 280 bpm.[3] ST-segment elevation is seen in lead aVR, due to retrograde atrial activation; this finding can be helpful in differentiating AVRT from AVNRT.[34] During tachycardia ECG features of orthodrome AVRT includes a narrow QRS complex, may be preceded by a P wave. P waves may be buried in QRS complex or retrograde (Figs. 11.21A and B). Sometimes there are no discernible P waves and then the rhythm becomes indistinguishable from AVNRT. In antidrome AVRT ECG shows wide QRS complexes followed by retrograde P waves (Fig. 11.22).

ECG Difference between Atrioventricular Nodal Reentrant Tachycardia and Atrioventricular Reentrant Tachycardia[2,3,34-41]

1. A visible P wave is classically uncommon in AVNRT. In typical, slow pathway-antegrade, fast pathway-retrograde AVNRT, the P wave is either not seen or is visible in the terminal portion of the QRS (especially in lead V1). In typical AVNRT, the P wave and QRS are usually simultaneous so cannot see the P wave on surface ECG. Absence of visible P wave is rather uncommon during AVRT.
2. The finding of a pseudo "s" (lead II) or pseudo "r'" (lead V1) during tachycardia are the most frequent ECG features observed during AVNRT. Such patterns are not noted during AVRT.
3. The presence of ST-segment elevation in lead aVR is suggestive of AVRT. No such phenomenon is seen in AVNRT.

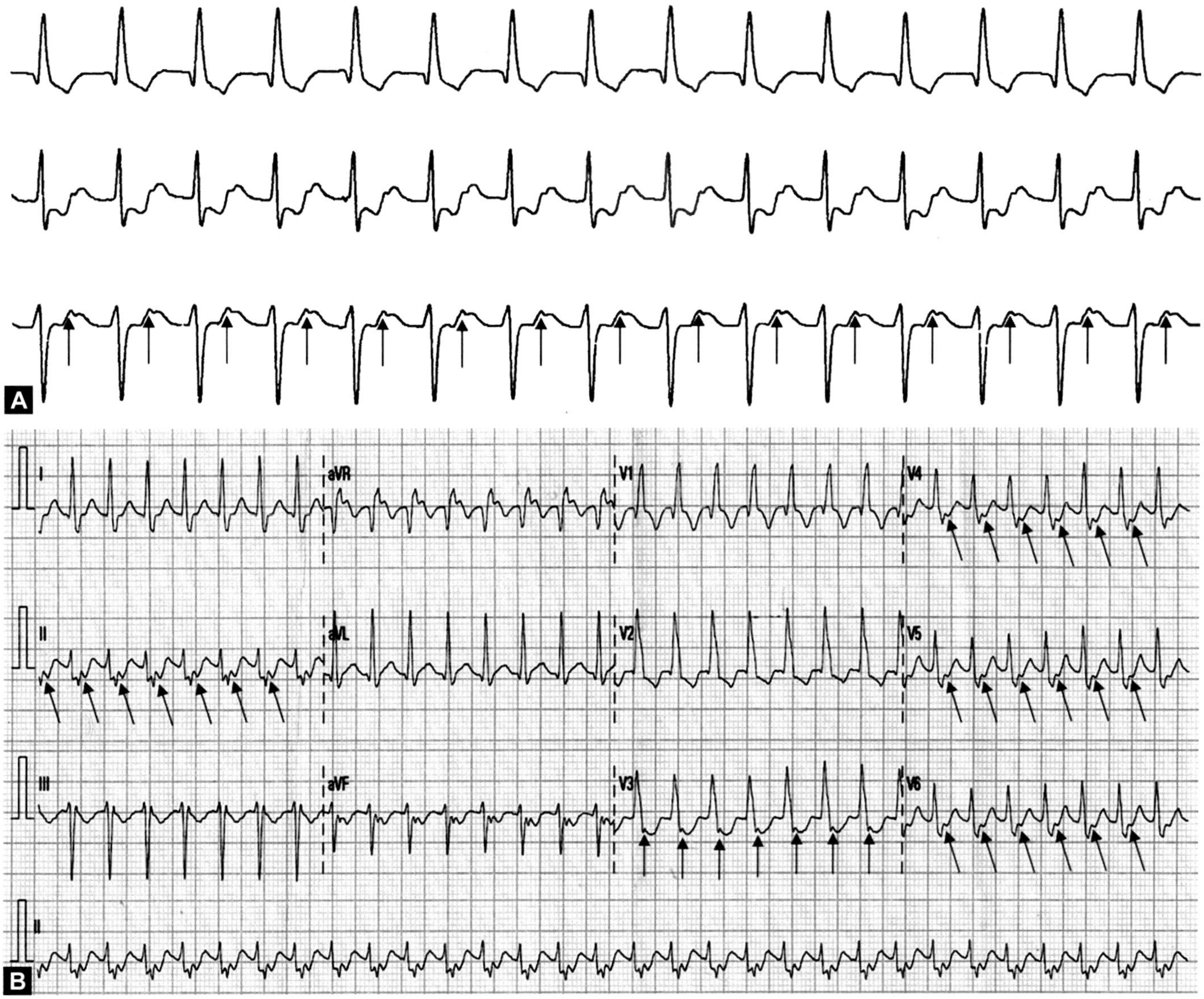

Figs. 11.21A and B: (A) Atrioventricular reentrant tachycardia (AVRT). This is a narrow complex tachycardia (orthodromic AVRT) and there is a P wave after each QRS complex (*arrows*) which is superimposed on the T wave and T appears bifid. (B) ECG is suggestive of AVRT with regular, narrow complex tachycardia at 185 bpm with discernible retrograde P waves in multiple leads most prominent in LII, V3–V6 (arrows). Classically on surface ECG of narrow complex tachycardia, visibility of P waves favor AVRT.

4. During tachycardia, the presence of a notch in lead aVL is suggestive of AVNRT which is usually absent in case of AVRT.
5. QRS alternans suggests AVRT. QRS alternans are rare in AVNRT.
6. The presence of a delta wave during sinus rhythm is highly suggestive of AVRT. This wave is not reflected on surface ECG in AVNRT.
7. The absence of ST-segment depression during SVT in the left precordial leads (V4–V6) is highly suggestive of AVNRT. Whereas ST-segment depression and QRS alternans display the highest predictive ability favoring the diagnosis of AVRT.

ATRIAL TACHYCARDIA

Atrial tachycardia (rate >100 bpm) is the least common form of PSVT in normal individuals but predominates in patients with significant atrial scarring, especially from prior atrial surgery. Atrial tachycardia (AT) may occur in hypertension, congestive heart failure, valvular heart disease, and simply aging of the heart. Brief atrial tachycardia is seen on ambulatory ECG monitoring in the elderly and is frequently asymptomatic.[2] Atrial tachycardias may be caused by enhanced or triggered automaticity or by a micro-reentrant circuit. Because the AV node and ventricle are not required participants in the arrhythmia, AV block commonly occurs.

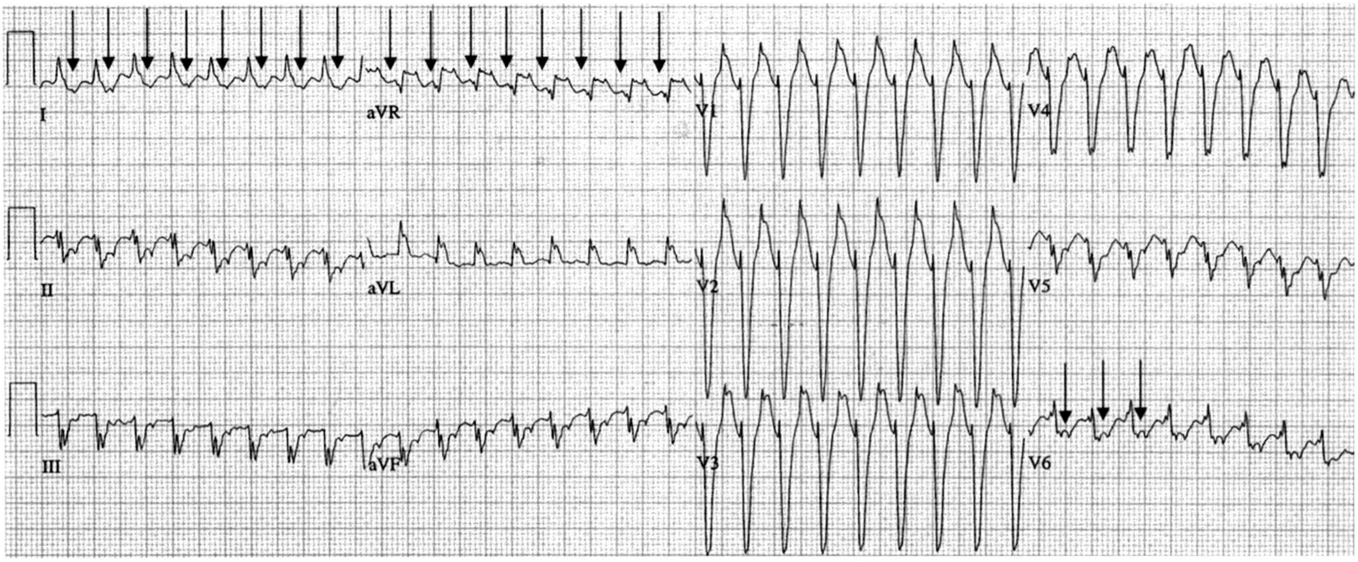

Fig. 11.22: Atrioventricular reentrant tachycardia. This is a wide complex tachycardia (QRS 140 ms), at rate of 205 bpm with evidence of retrograde P wave distorting the ST-segment in multiple leads best seen in LI, aVR, and V6 (arrows) suggestive of antidromic AVRT.

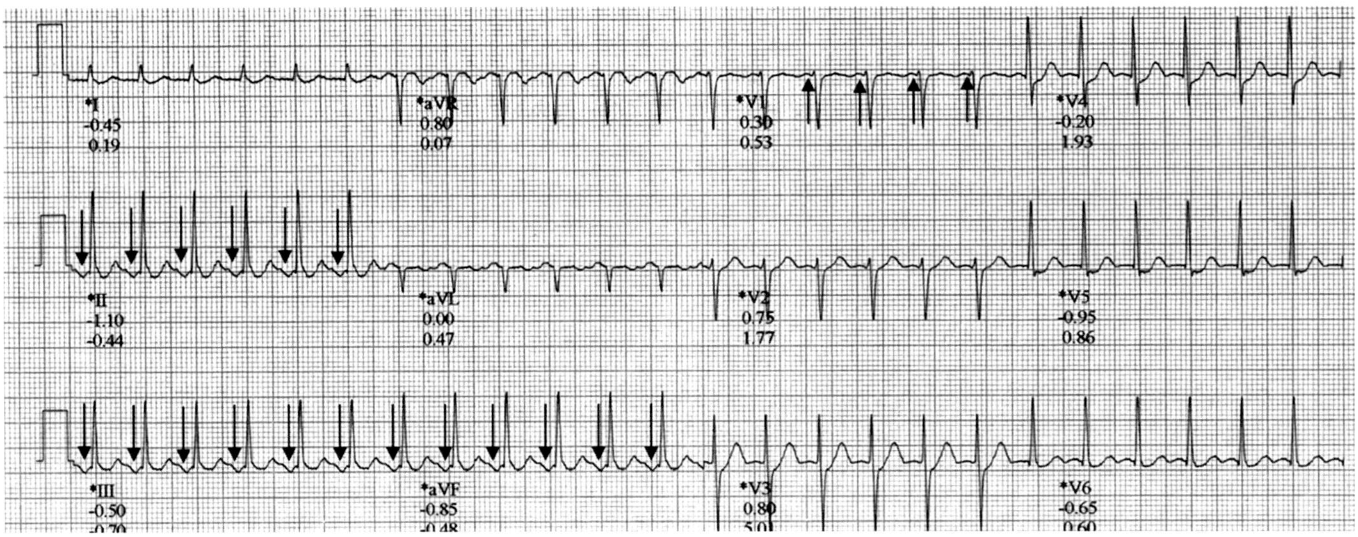

Fig. 11.23: Atrial tachycardia at rate of 148 bpm. Each QRS complex is preceded by an abnormal P wave, upright in V1 (arrows), inverted in the inferior leads II, III, and aVF (arrows).

The PR or apparent RP' intervals depend on AV conduction properties. P-wave morphology depends on the site of origin in the atrium. If the site of origin is within or involves the sinus node region, sinus node reentrant or inappropriate ST is identified.

There are two unique characteristics of atrial tachycardias: (1) they may occur in repetitive short bursts, and (2) they are frequently characterized by a warm-up phenomenon in which the atrial rate increases slightly over the first 5–10 seconds before stabilizing. Surface ECGs show a P wave preceding each QRS complex but P-wave morphology is abnormal when compared with sinus P wave due to ectopic origin (Fig. 11.23). Due to rapid heart rates, the P wave may be obscured by the T wave.[12] Frequently there is AV block evident in cases of atrial tachycardia and thus more P waves are seen than QRS complexes, thus simplifying diagnosis. When atrial tachycardia occurs with a 2:1 conduction block, digoxin toxicity should be considered.

SUMMARY

Electrocardiogram criteria for the diagnosis of narrow complex tachycardia are:

- Rate is greater than 100 bpm
- QRS complex duration is less than 0.12 seconds (<120 ms).

Narrow complex tachycardias usually originate from the atria or AV junction and are therefore supraventricular in origin.

Sinus Tachycardia

It is the most common form of narrow complex tachycardia (rate >100 bpm) and is not a pathologic arrhythmia. Sinus tachycardia (ST) is gradual in onset and recession. The heart rate is regular and classically does not exceed 220 bpm minus the patient's age. In ST, P waves precede the QRS complex.

Sinus Node Reentrant Tachycardia

Due to a reentry circuit, either in or near the sinus node with abrupt onset and offset. P waves are similar or identical to sinus P waves (i.e. high right atrium to low right atrium activation sequence), so resembles ST; but starts and ends abruptly. Heart rate usually is 100–150 bpm, and ECG usually demonstrates a normal sinus P-wave morphology.

Electrocardiogram criteria of SNRT:

- Surface ECG indistinguishable from ST.
- Heart rate usually is 100–150 bpm.

Multifocal Atrial Tachycardia

Specific ECG criteria of MAT include:

- Rate greater than 100 bpm
- Three or more distinct nonsinus P-wave morphologies (in the same lead)
- An isoelectric baseline (i.e. no flutter or fibrillation waves)
- Irregularity of the PP, PR, and RR intervals.

Multifocal atrial tachycardia is most commonly associated with COPD.

Atrial Fibrillation

Atrial fibrillation is the most common pathologic SVT. Risk factors for AF include older age, male sex, hypertension, coronary artery disease, thyrotoxicosis, mitral stenosis, and cardiomyopathies (Box 11.1).

Electrocardiogram features of AF include:

1. P waves are absent.
2. The RR intervals are not equal resulting in an irregular rhythm.
3. There are fibrillation (f) waves instead of P waves. The "f" waves result in an oscillating irregular baseline.

Classification of Atrial Fibrillation

Classification is dependent on the presentation and duration of AF (Box 11.2) as below:

1. *First episode*: Initial detection of AF regardless of symptoms or duration.
2. *Recurrent AF*: More than two episodes of AF
3. *Paroxysmal AF*: Self-terminating episode, duration is less than 7 days
4. *Persistent AF:* Not self-terminating, duration is greater than 7 days
5. *Long-standing persistent AF*: Duration is greater than 1 year.
6. *Permanent AF*: Duration is greater than 1 year in which rhythm control interventions are not pursued or are unsuccessful.

Atrial fibrillation may be of two types according to ventricular response:

1. *Fast AF*: Atrial fibrillation is often described as having "rapid ventricular response" once the ventricular rate is greater than 100 bpm.
2. *Slow AF*: When in AF ventricular rate is less than 60 bpm, it is termed as slow AF.

Lone atrial fibrillation: No detectable cause.

- Absence of clinical or echocardiographic findings of other cardiovascular disease (including hypertension), related pulmonary disease, or cardiac abnormalities such as enlargement of the left atrium.
- Age under 60 years.

Nonvalvular AF: Absence of rheumatic mitral valve disease, a prosthetic heart valve, or mitral valve repair.

Box 11.1: Common causes of atrial fibrillation.

1. Coronary artery disease
2. Mitral stenosis
3. Hypertensive heart disease
4. Congestive heart failure
5. Thyrotoxicosis
6. Lone AF

Box 11.2: Classification of AF according to duration.

Paroxysmal AF: Less than 7 days
Persistent AF: Greater than 7 days
Permanent: AF: Greater than 1 year

Atrial Flutter

Atrial flutter has similar etiology to atrial fibrillation but flutter is less common than AF. During atrial flutter, the atria discharge regularly at a rate of approximately 300 bpm. Flutter waves (F waves) are of "sawtooth" appearance which is usually best seen in leads LII, LIII, and aVF. Atrial flutter is recognized on an ECG by presence of characteristic flutter waves at a regular rate. Individual flutter waves may be symmetrical, resembling P waves, or may be asymmetrical with a "sawtooth" shape.

Electrocardiogram features of atrial flutter include:

1. ECG shows sawtooth flutter waves, best seen in leads II, III, and aVF, with atrial rates of 250–350. A 12-lead ECG is gold standard for diagnosis.
2. The ventricular response may be regular or irregular.
3. Variable AV conduction can also be seen (commonly present with 2:1 or 3:1 AV conduction).

Atrioventricular Nodal Reentrant Tachycardia and Atrioventricular Reentrant Tachycardia

The most common SVT is AVNRT (60%), followed by AVRT (30%) and AT (10%). AVNRT is more common in women (75%) and mean age of onset 32 years. AVRT is more common in men and children. Atrial tachycardia is more common with older age and structural heart disease.

Atrioventricular Nodal Reentrant Tachycardia

Atrioventricular nodal reentrant tachycardia (AVNRT) is typically found in patients with no structural heart disease. It may produce symptoms like palpitations, polyuria, etc. It can also produce angina, syncope, heart failure or even shock. AVNRT is a common arrhythmia which occurs in patients with two functionally distinct conduction pathways through the AV node, typically fast and slow pathways (Box 11.3). The slow pathway usually has a shorter refractory period than the fast pathway. Both the fast and slow pathways are necessary to maintain AVNRT. The common form of AVNRT is typically initiated when an atrial premature beat blocks in the fast pathway, conducts down the slow pathway, and returns retrograde via the fast pathway to depolarize the atrium, thus creating a reentrant circuit in the AV node.

In AVNRT, the ECG will typically show a tachycardia of 140–280 bpm with normal and regular QRS complexes. ECG features include:

1. No visible P waves (hidden within the QRS complex)
2. Rhythm is regular
3. QRS complex is usually of normal morphology during common AVNRT.

Atrioventricular Reentrant Tachycardia

Atrioventricular reentrant tachycardia (AVRT) is less common than AVNRT and the patients usually younger. AVRT uses two distinct pathways, the normal AV conduction system and an AV accessory pathway (AP). Keeping this in mind there will be two ways the conduction will travel. The first most common variety occurs when the impulses travel down the AV node to the ventricle and up the AP. This is called orthodromic AV reentry tachycardia. The second type occurs when the AP is used in the antegrade direction to the ventricle and retrograde conduction occurs up the AV node. This is called antidromic AV reentry tachycardia. Both can be initiated by atrial or ventricular premature beats. Electrocardiogram features of both are:

1. *Orthodromic AVRT*: The heart rate is regular and ranges between 140 bpm and 280 bpm. The P-wave is visible and inscribed within the ST-T wave segment. The QRS is narrow.
2. *Antidromic AVRT*: The heart rate is regular and ranges between140 bpm and 280 bpm. It is characterized by a preexcited wide QRS complex. Sometimes the P wave may be more difficult to see because of the wide QRS and ST and T wave.

Orthodromic AVRT usually presents with narrow complex tachycardia whereas antidromic AVRT always produces wide complex tachycardia.

Electrocardiogram difference between AVNRT and AVRT is shown in Table 11.1.

Box 11.3: Atrioventricular nodal reentrant tachycardia.

AV conduction: Normal sinus rhythm:

During sinus rhythm, electrical impulses travel down both pathways simultaneously. The impulse transmitted down the fast pathway enters the distal end of the slow pathway and the two impulses cancel each other out. During sinus rhythm, impulses are typically carried by the "fast" pathway, and the "slow" pathway is unused.

Mechanism of re-entry in "slow–fast" or common AVNRT:

Step 1: If a premature atrial contraction (PAC) arrives while the fast pathway is still refractory, the electrical impulse will be directed solely down the slow pathway.

Step 2: By the time the premature impulse reaches the end of the slow pathway, the fast pathway is no longer refractory, hence, the impulse is permitted to recycle retrogradely up the fast pathway.

Step 3: This creates a circus movement whereby the impulse continually cycles around the two pathways, activating the bundle of His antegradely and the atria retrogradely. The short cycle length is responsible for the rapid heart rate.

Table 11.1: Difference between atrioventricular nodal reentrant tachycardia **(AVNRT)** and atrioventricular reentrant tachycardia **(AVRT)** in electrocardiogram.

Atrioventricular nodal reentrant tachycardia	*Atrioventricular reentrant tachycardia*
P-wave is usually not visible on the surface ECG in AVNRT	P waves may be visible on the surface ECG
QRS alternans are rare in AVNRT and usually not seen	The finding of QRS alternans during tachycardia is suggestive of AVRT
The finding of a pseudo "s" (lead II) or pseudo "r'" (lead V1) during tachycardia goes in favor of AVNRT	Such patterns are not noted during AVRT
ST elevation in aVR: No such phenomenon is seen in AVNRT	The presence of ST segment elevation in lead aVR is suggestive of AVRT
Delta wave is not reflected on surface ECG in AVNRT	The presence of a delta wave during sinus rhythm is highly suggestive of AVRT

Atrial Tachycardia

Atrial tachycardia has a more or less regular heart rate greater than 100 bpm, with narrow QRS complexes but P waves that do not originate from the sinus node but from another site in the atria. The P waves usually have a different configuration and their nonsinus origin can easily be recognized if the P waves are negative in I and/or aVF.

REFERENCES

1. Goodacre S, Irons R. Atrial arrhythmias. BMJ. 2002;324:594-1002.
2. Ray IB. Narrow Complex Tachycardia: Recognition and Management in the Emergency Room. J Assoc Physicians India. 2004;52:816-24.
3. Borloz MP, Mark DG, Pines JM, et al. ECG differential diagnosis of narrow QRS complex tachycardia in the emergency department: a review of common rhythms and distinguishing features. Emergencias. 2010;22:369-80.
4. Kazzi AA, Wong H. Other supraventricular tachydysrhythmias. In: Chan TC, Brady WJ, Harrigan RA, Ornato JP, Rosen P (Eds). ECG in Emergency Medicine and Acute Care, 1st edition. Philadelphia, PA: Elsevier; 2005. pp. 104-11.
5. Carnell J, Singh A. An evidence-based approach to supraventricular tachydysrhythmias. Emerg Med Pract. 2008;10:1-26.
6. Wathen MS, Klein GJ, Yee R, et al. Classification and terminology of supraventricular tachycardia. Diagnosis and management of the atrial tachycardias. Cardiol Clin. 1993;11:109-20.
7. Chan TC. P wave. In: Chan TC, Brady WJ, Harrigan RA, Ornato JP, Rosen P (Eds). ECG in Emergency Medicine and Acute Care, 1st edition. Philadelphia, PA: Elsevier; 2005. pp. 48-52.
8. Xie B, Thakur RK, Shah CP, et al. Clinical differentiation of narrow QRS complex tachycardias. Emerg Med Clin North Am. 1998;16(2):295-330.
9. Josephson ME, Wellens HJ. Differential diagnosis of supraventricular tachycardia. Cardiol Clin. 1990;8(3):411-42.
10. Ganz LI, Friedman PL. Supraventricular tachycardia. N Engl J Med. 1995;332(3):162-73.
11. Wu D. Supraventricular tachycardias. JAMA. 1983;249(24):3357-60.
12. Link MS. Evaluation and initial treatment of supraventricular tachycardia. N Engl J Med. 2012;367(15):1438-48.
13. Scher DL, Arsura EL. Multifocal atrial tachycardia: mechanisms, clinical correlates, and treatment. Am Heart J. 1989;118(3):574-80.
14. McCord J, Borzak S. Multifocal atrial tachycardia. Chest. 1998;113(1):203-9.
15. Kumar UN, Rao RK, Scheinman MM. The 12-lead electrocardiogram in supraventricular tachycardia. Cardiol Clin. 2006;24(3):427-37.
16. Schwartz M, Rodman D, Lowenstein SR. Recognition and treatment of multifocal atrial tachycardia: a critical review. J Emerg Med. 1994;12(3):353-60.
17. Wann S, Curtis AB, Ellenbogen KA, et al. 2011 ACCF/AHA/HRS focused update on the management of patients with atrial fibrillation (updating the 2006 guideline): a report of the American College of Cardiology Foundation/American Heart Association Task Force on Practice Guidelines. Circulation. 2011;123(1):104-23.
18. Fuster V, Ryden LE, Cannom DS, et al. ACC/AHA/ESC 2006 guidelines for the management of patients with atrial fibrillation: a report of the American College of Cardiology/American Heart Association Task Force on Practice Guidelines and the European Society of Cardiology Committee for Practice Guidelines (Writing Committee to Revise the 2001 Guidelines for the Management of Patients With Atrial Fibrillation): developed in collaboration with the European Heart Rhythm Association and the Heart Rhythm Society. Circulation. 2006;114(7):e257-354.
19. Wolf PA, Abott RD, Kannel WB. Atrial fibrillation as an independent risk factor for stroke: the Framingham Study. Stroke. 1991;22(8):983-8.
20. Levy S, Camm AJ, Saksena S, et al. International consensus on nomenclature and classification of atrial fibrillation. Europace. 2003;5(2):119-22.
21. Stahmer SA, Cowan R. Tachydysrhythmias. Emerg Med Clin North Am. 2006;24(1):11-40.
22. Sager PT, Bhandari AK. Narrow complex tachycardia. Differential diagnosis and management. Cardiol Clin. 1991;9:619-40.
23. Frost L. Lone atrial fibrillation: good, bad, or ugly? Circulation. 2007;115:3040-1.
24. Garcia-Cosio F, Fuentes AP, Angulo AN. Clinical approach to atrial tachycardia and atrial flutter from an understanding of the mechanisms. Electrophysiology based on anatomy. Rev Esp Cardiol. 2012;65(4):363-75.
25. Weinberg KM, Denes P, Kadish AH, et al. Development and validation of diagnostic criteria for atrial flutter on the surface electrocardiogram. Ann Noninvasive Electrocardiol. 2008;13(2):145-54.
26. Kawabata M, Hirao K, Higuchi K, et al. Clinical and electrophysiological characteristics of patients having atrial flutter with 1:1 atrioventricular conduction. Europace. 2008;10:284-8.
27. Goyal R, Zivin A, Souza J, et al. Comparison of the ages of tachycardia onset in patients with atrioventricular nodal reentrant tachycardia and accessory pathway-mediated tachycardia. Am Heart J. 1996;132(4):765-7.
28. Katritsis DG, Camm AJ. Atrioventricular nodal reentrant tachycardia. Circulation. 2010;122(8):831-40.
29. Wu D, Denes P, Amat-Y-Leon F, et al. Clinical, electrocardiographic and electrophysiologic observations in patients with paroxysmal supraventricular tachycardia. Am J Cardiol. 1978;41(6):1045-51.
30. Brugada P, Bär FW, Vanagt EJ, et al. Observations in patients showing A-V junctional echoes with a shorter P-R than R-P interval. Am J Cardiol. 1981;48(4):611-22.
31. Rodriguez LM, de Chillou C, Schläpfer J, et al. Age at onset and gender of patients with different types of supraventricular tachycardias. Am J Cardiol. 1992;70(13):1213-5.
32. Akhtar M, Jazayeri MR, Sra J, et al. Atrioventricular nodal reentry. Clinical, electrophysiological, and therapeutic considerations. Circulation. 1993;88(1):282-95.
33. Katritsis DG, Josephson ME. Classification of electrophysiological types of atrioventricular nodal re-entrant tachycardia: a reappraisal. Europace. 2013;15(9):1231-40.

34. Gorgels AP, Engelen DJ, Wellens HJ. Lead aVR, a mostly ignored but very valuable lead in clinical electrocardiography. J Am Coll Cardiol. 2001;38(5):1355-6.
35. Maury P, Zimmermann M, Metzger J. Distinction between atrioventricular reciprocating tachycardia and atrioventricular node re-entrant tachycardia in the adult population based on P wave location; should we reconsider the value of some ECG criteria according to gender and age? Europace 2003;5(1):57-64.
36. Toro DD, Hadid C, Lopez C, et al. Utility of the aVL lead in the electrocardiographic diagnosis of atrioventricular node re-entrant tachycardia. Europace. 2009;11(7):944-8.
37. Ferguson JD, DiMarco JP. Contemporary management of paroxysmal supraventricular tachycardia. Circulation. 2003;107(8):1096-9.
38. Wellens HJ, Conover MB. The ECG in Emergency Decision Making, 2nd edition. Philadelphia: Saunders; 2006.
39. Obel OA, Camm AJ. Supraventricular tachycardia: ECG diagnosis and anatomy. Eur Heart J. 1997;18(Suppl C): C2-11.
40. Letsas KP, Weber R, Siklody CH, et al. Electrocardiographic differentiation of common type atrioventricular nodal reentrant tachycardia from atrioventricular reciprocating tachycardia via a concealed accessory pathway. Acta Cardiol. 2010;65(2):171-6.
41. Kossaify A, Zeeny M. Electrocardiographic and electrophysiologic insights into atrioventricular nodal re-entry tachycardia: diagnostic update. Clin Med Insights Cardiol. 2012;6:111-7.

Chapter 12

Broad Complex Tachycardia

INTRODUCTION

When confronted with a tachycardia having a broad QRS complex, it is important to be able to differentiate between a supraventricular tachycardia (SVT) and a ventricular tachycardia (VT). Medication given for the treatment of an SVT may be harmful to a patient with a VT. A reasonable hemodynamic condition during a tachycardia may erroneously lead to the wrong diagnosis of an SVT. Familiarity with the ECG signs allowing the diagnosis of a VT is therefore essential. ECG not only tells us how to distinguish VT from other tachycardias with a broad QRS complex, but also to suspect its etiology and its site of origin in the ventricle. Both aspects are important in decision making about the prognostic significance of VT and correct treatment.[1] In the emergency setting, most broad complex tachycardias have a ventricular origin. However, an arrhythmia arising from the atria or the atrioventricular (AV) junction will produce a broad complex, if associated with ventricular preexcitation or bundle branch block (BBB). The causes of VT and SVT are generally quite different, with widely differing prognoses. Most importantly, the treatment of a broad complex tachycardia depends on the origin of the tachycardia.[2]

Broad complex tachycardia is defined as:

- Heart rate is >100 beats/min.
- Duration of QRS is >0.12 seconds (>120 ms).

The basic difference between VT and SVT is QRS duration. If QRS duration is less than 0.12 seconds (<120 ms) then it is possibly SVT and if duration is greater than 0.12 seconds (>120 ms) then it is probably VT (Fig. 12.1).

CAUSES OF BROAD COMPLEX TACHYCARDIA

- Ventricular tachycardia
- Supraventricular tachycardia with aberrant conduction due to BBB
- Supraventricular tachycardia with aberrant conduction due to the Wolff-Parkinson-White syndrome (WPW syndrome)
- Pacemaker mediated tachycardia
- Metabolic derangements (e.g. hyperkalemia)
- Drug-induced tachycardia (e.g. tricyclic antidepressants).

VENTRICULAR TACHYCARDIA

Ventricular tachycardia is defined as three or more ventricular extrasystoles in succession at a rate of more than 100 bpm (according to some authorities VT rate should be >120 bpm) and VT may be of right bundle branch block (RBBB) and left bundle branch block (LBBB) morphology (Figs. 12.2A to D). But typical features of RBBB or LBBB morphology are absent. The tachycardia may be self-terminating but is described as "sustained VT", if it lasts longer than 30 seconds. If it sustains less than 30 seconds it is termed as "nonsustained VT" (Figs. 12.3A and B).

Electrocardiogram Criteria of Ventricular Tachycardia

- Three or more ventricular extrasystoles in succession
- Broad QRS complexes (>120 ms)
- Rapid heart rate (>100 bpm).

Accelerated idioventricular rhythm (AIVR) is ventricular rhythm with a rate of between 40 beats/min and 100 beats/min. AIVR is distinguished from other ventricular rhythms with rates less than 40 (ventricular escape) and those faster than 100 (VT). It is also referred as "slow VT."[1-3]

Ventricular tachycardia is a syndrome with diverse etiologies. There have been many classifications of VT depending on the site of origin, etiology and the morphology of the ECG complexes produced. But from ECG, VT can be categorized depending on the morphology of the QRS complex.

Ventricular tachycardia may be of following types:[3]

- Monomorphic VT
- Polymorphic VT with long QT
- Polymorphic VT with normal QT
- Fascicular tachycardia
- Right ventricular outflow tract (RVOT) tachycardia.

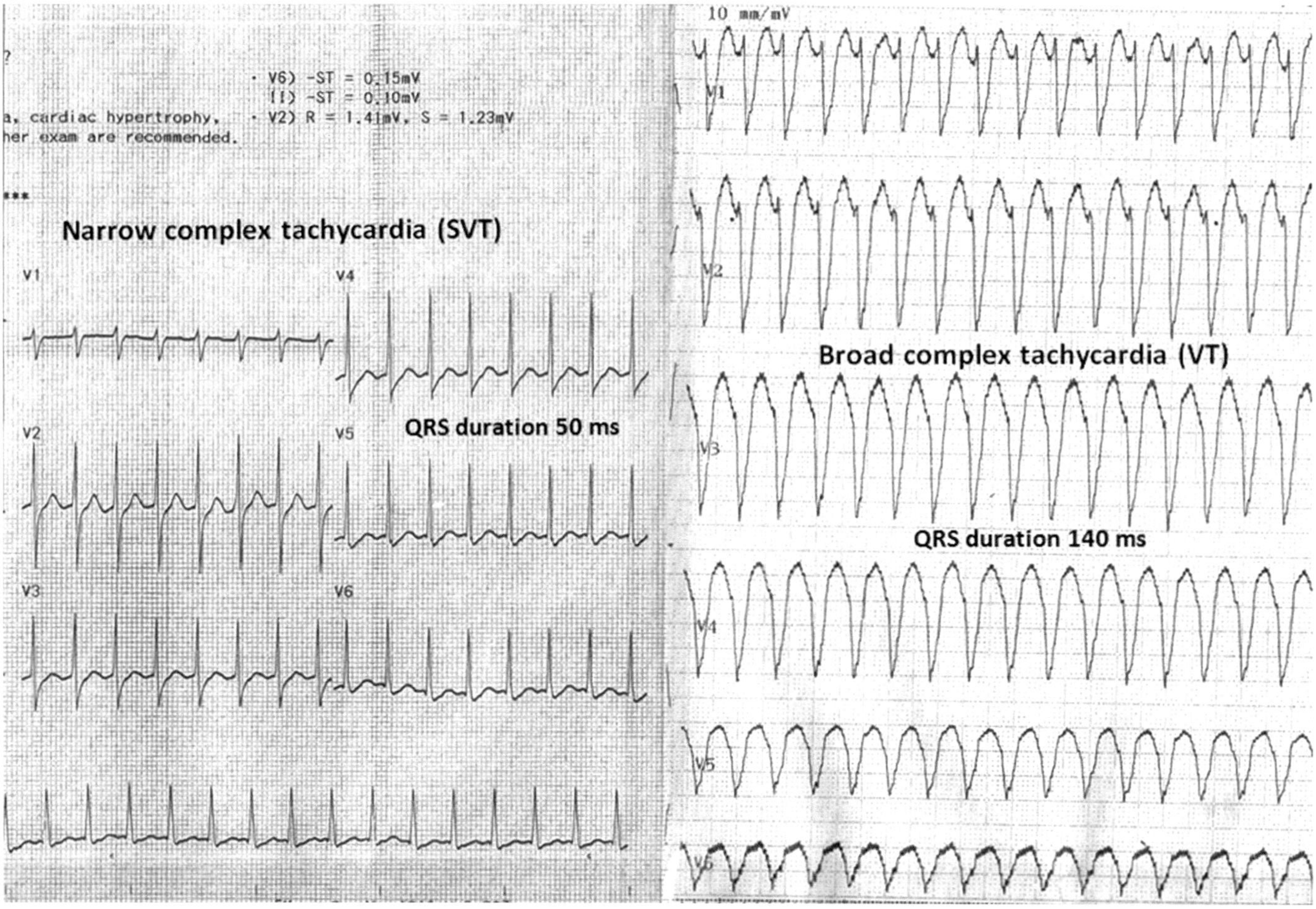

Fig. 12.1: Electrocardiogram shows narrow complex tachycardia (QRS duration is 50 ms and rate is 188 bpm) (left) and broad complex tachycardia (QRS duration is 140 ms and rate is 200 bpm) (right).

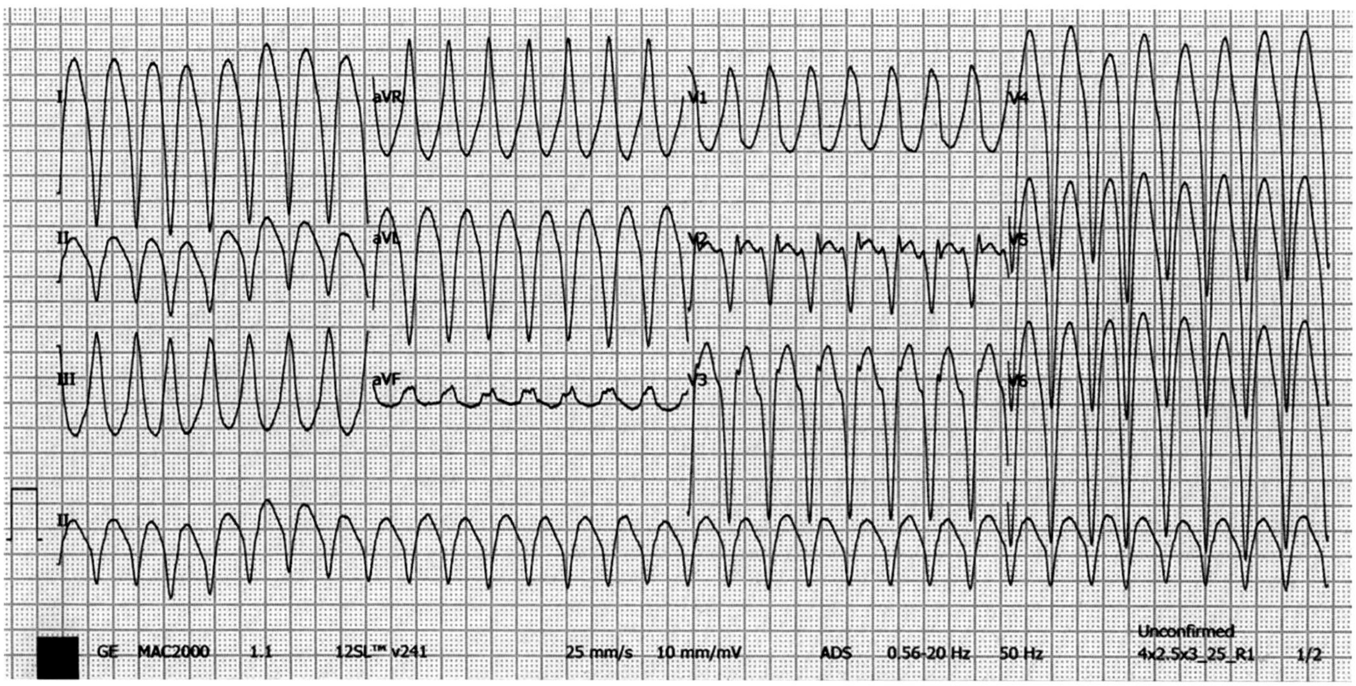

Fig. 12.2A: Broad complex tachycardia suggestive of ventricular tachycardia (rate is 192 bpm and QRS duration is 216 ms with extreme axis deviation).

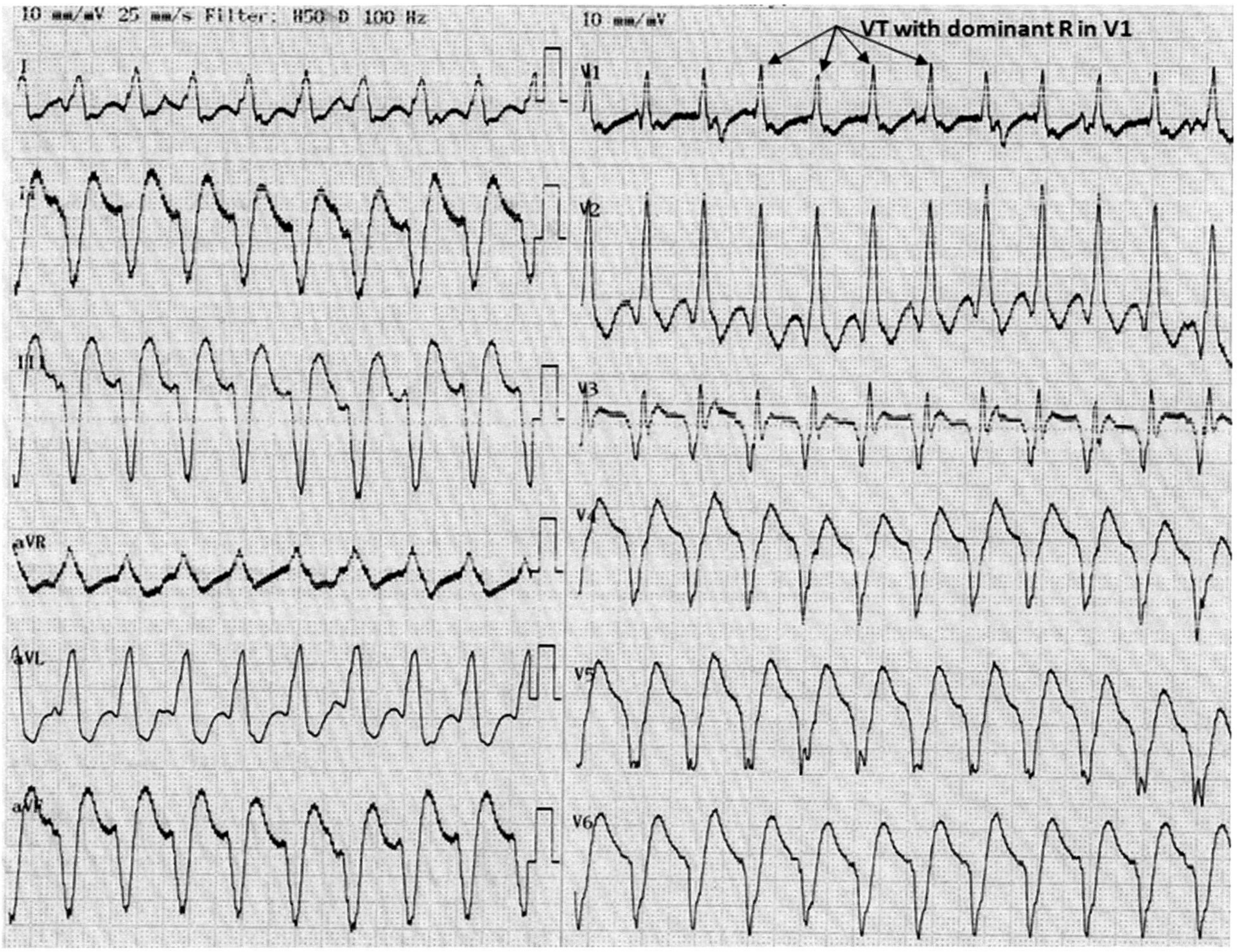

Fig. 12.2B: Broad complex tachycardia with right bundle branch block pattern showing dominant R wave (*arrows*) in V1 (ventricular tachycardia with right bundle branch block-like morphology).

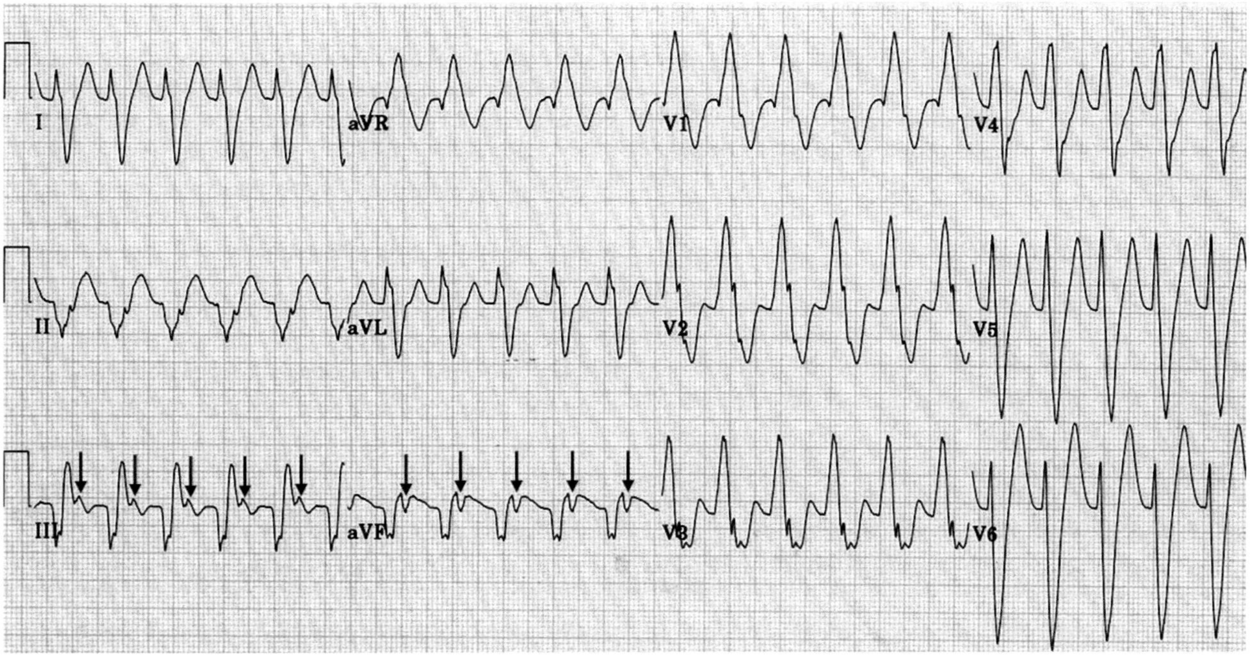

Fig. 12.2C: This electrocardiogram illustrates broad complex tachycardia (QRS is 160 ms) at a rate of 140 bpm with right bundle branch block pattern showing dominant R wave in V1 (ventricular tachycardia with right bundle branch block-like morphology). Note retrograde P waves in LIII and aVF (*arrows*) with 1:1 retrograde activation of atria. This type of 1:1 retrograde activation of the atria may occur in up to one-fourth of cases of VT.

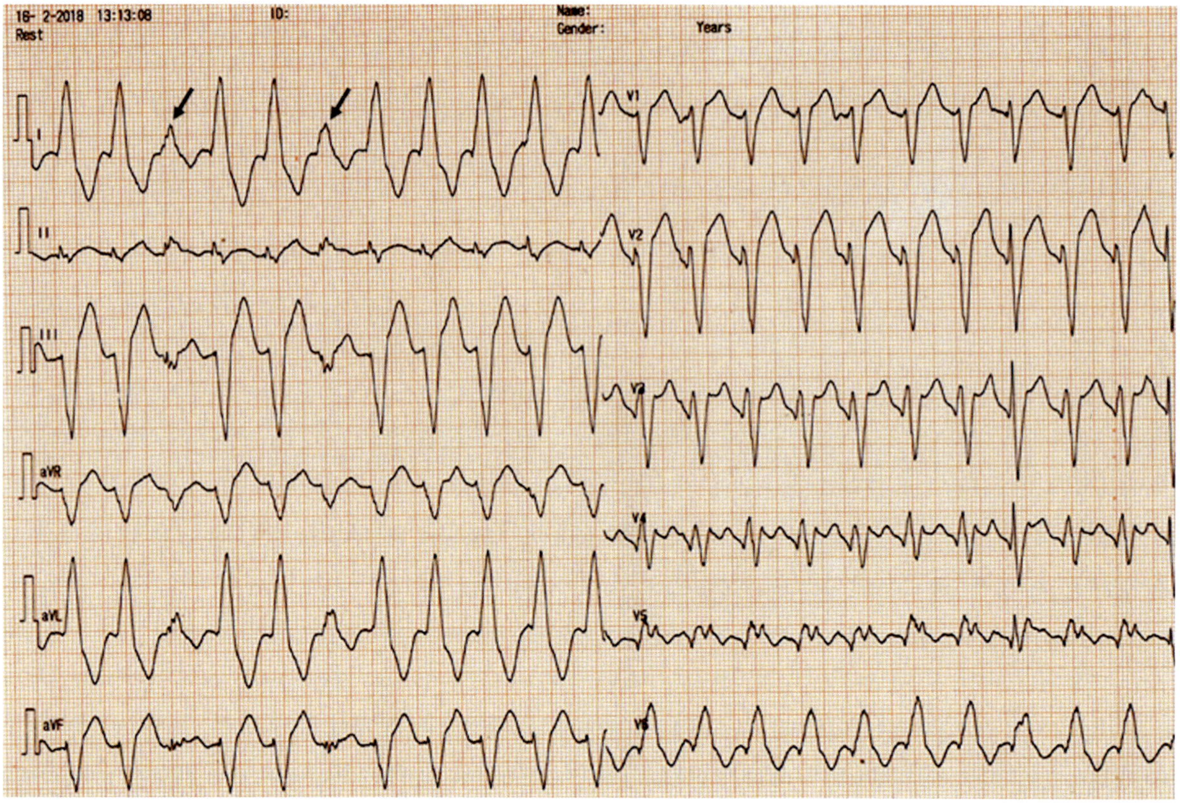

Fig. 12.2D: Broad complex tachycardia (rate 132 bpm) with LBBB pattern, showing dominant S wave in V1 (VT with LBBB-like morphology). Also note two fusion beats (arrows).

(*Courtesy:* Dr Abul Khayer, Labaid Cardiac Hospital)

Monomorphic VT, fascicular tachycardia, and RVOT tachycardia are usually regular but polymorphic VT (e.g. torsades de pointes tachycardia) is usually irregular.

Monomorphic Ventricular Tachycardia

Monomorphic VT means that the appearance of all the beats matches each other in each lead of a surface ECG. There is no beat-to-beat variation in the QRS morphology in the same lead (Figs. 12.4A and B). Monomorphic VT is most frequently due to scar-related reentry, typically in the setting of coronary artery disease, prior myocardial infarction (MI), and left ventricular dysfunction.

Less frequently encountered (10% of sustained VT) is idiopathic VT. This typically occurs in the setting of a structurally normal heart, and often responds to beta-blocker or nondihydropyridine calcium channel blocker therapy. VT arising from the right or left ventricular outflow tract is especially common in this setting; clues to its diagnosis include VT in the setting of a structurally normal heart and tall R waves in the inferior leads. Other monomorphic VTs (bundle branch reentry and right ventricular dysplasia associated VT) should be treated acutely similarly to scar-related VT.

The structural changes in the ventricles of patients with cardiac disease can create the substrate for ventricular arrhythmias. The most common substrate for VT is ventricular scarring related to ischemic heart disease, which is present in approximately 60% of patients.[4] However, patients with dilated cardiomyopathies, arrhythmogenic right ventricular cardiomyopathy (ARVC), prior cardiac surgery (particularly for correction of congenital anomalies or valve surgery), sarcoidosis, or hypertrophic cardiomyopathy can also have ventricular scarring and VT.[5] Ventricular scars consist of dense fibrosis, with surviving myocardial bundles traversing the scar and creating channels. These channels often have interstitial fibrosis, which can create separations between the muscle bundles and, therefore, circuitous patterns of activation through the bundles. In addition, cell-to-cell coupling between the myocytes is reduced.[6,7] This combination creates slow conduction through the channels. Large ventricular scars seem to predispose the patient to the development of VT by supporting a greater number of channels than do smaller scars. Patients with structural heart disease and VT tend to have numerous channels, as evidenced by multiple inducible morphologies of scar-related VT.[8-10] These channels can be identified with substrate mapping in patients with postinfarction cardiomyopathy and VT.[11]

Bundle branch reentry is a unique form of reentrant monomorphic VT that occurs predominantly in patients with dilated cardiomyopathy. This condition comprises a macroreentrant circuit that involves the Purkinje system. The most common form of bundle branch reentry features

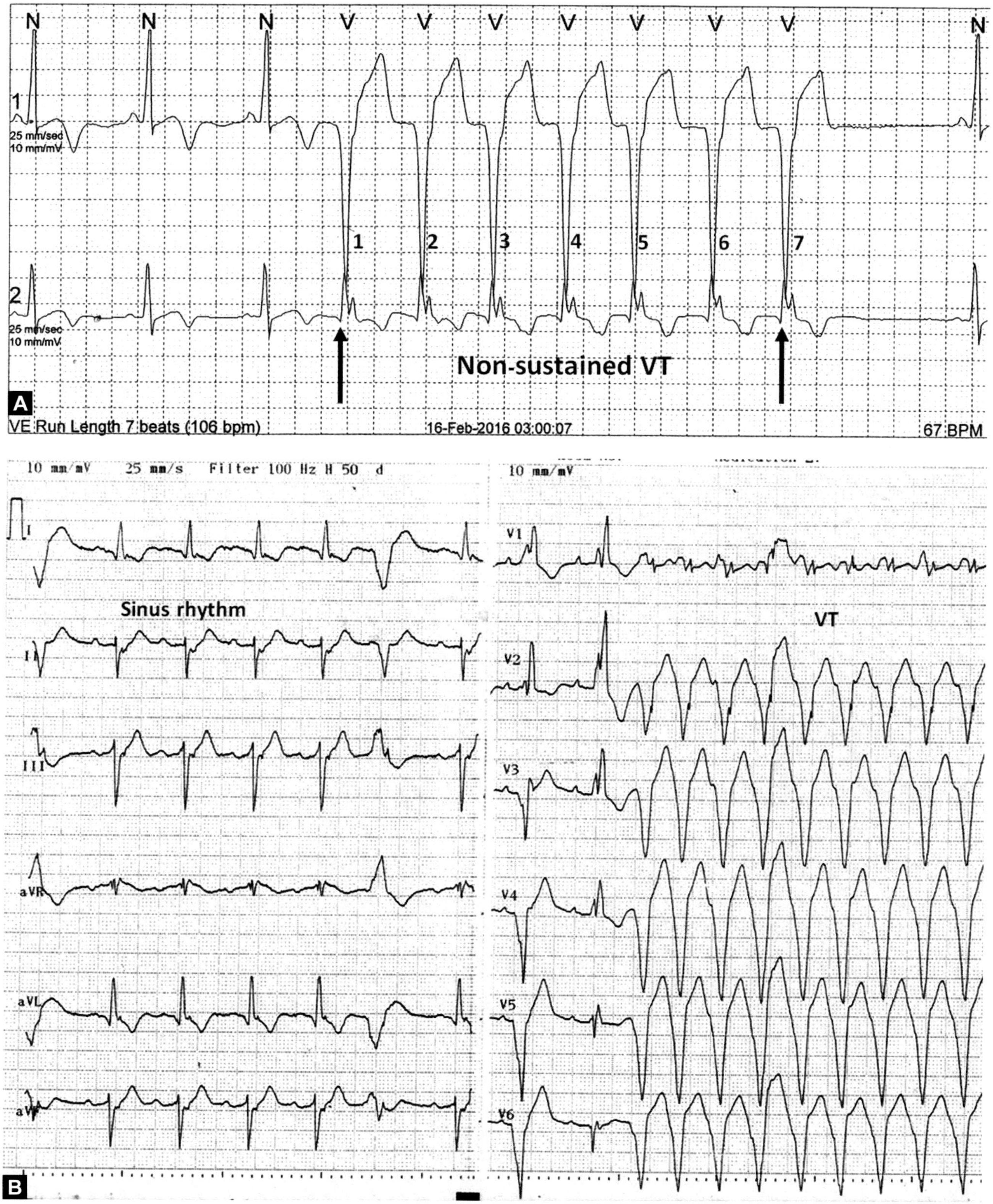

Figs. 12.3A and B: (A) This Holter monitoring electrocardiogram strip shows nonsustained VT. Note first three beats and last beat are sinus conducted (N) and middle seven beats (V) are suggestive of nonsustained ventricular tachycardia (*arrows*). (B) Nonsustained ventricular tachycardia in a patient admitted with acute coronary syndrome. Patient was having recurrent bouts of nonsustained ventricular tachycardia during his stay in coronary care unit and developed ventricular tachycardia during taking routine bedside 12-lead electrocardiogram. [*Courtesy:* Dr APM Sohrabuzzaman (A), Dr Habibur Rahman (B), Labaid Cardiac Hospital].

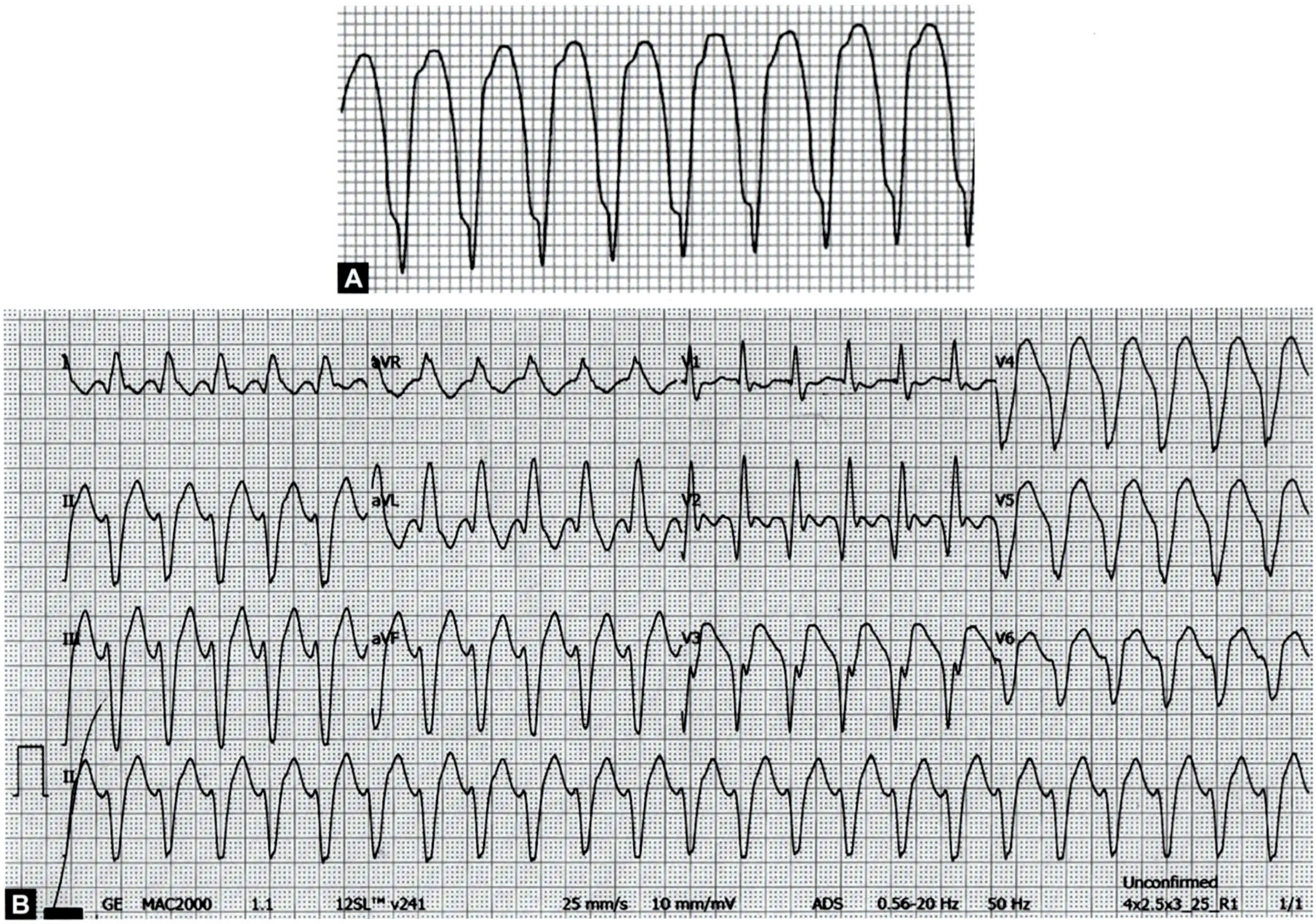

Figs. 12.4A and B: (A) Classic monomorphic ventricular tachycardia with uniform QRS complexes. (B) Electrocardiogram is suggestive of monomorphic ventricular tachycardia, the rate is 190 bpm (broad complex tachycardia with no beat-to-beat variations in the QRS morphology in the same lead). [*Courtesy:* Dr Arun Kumar Sharma (B), Labaid Cardiac Hospital]

the right bundle as the antegrade limb and the left bundle as the retrograde limb, leading to an LBBB morphology during VT. Rarely, the circuit can occur in the opposite direction, giving rise to an RBBB pattern. Commonly, these patients have evidence of conduction system disease. Importantly, this form of VT responds poorly to pharmacological therapy, but can be eliminated by catheter ablation of the right bundle.[5,12]

Polymorphic Ventricular Tachycardia

Polymorphic VT is a form of VT in which there are multiple ventricular foci with the resultant QRS complexes varying in amplitude, axis, and duration (Figs. 12.5A and B). The most common cause of polymorphic VT is myocardial ischemia.

Polymorphic Ventricular Tachycardia with Normal QT

Polymorphic VT with a normal QT interval is most frequently caused by acute ischemia or myocardial infarction (MI). It is usually initiated during sinus tachycardia, with a premature ventricular beat with a short coupling interval. It is usually poorly tolerated and tends to degenerate into VF quickly. Rarely, polymorphic VT with a normal QT interval is caused by ARVC, idiopathic polymorphic VT ("short-coupled variant of torsades de pointes") or familial catecholaminergic polymorphic VT.[3]

Polymorphic VT with normal QT

- Has the same ECG characteristics as torsades de pointes but in sinus rhythm (SR) the QT interval is normal.
- The ECG trace is also similar to that of atrial fibrillation (AF) with preexcitation.
- It is much less common than torsades de pointes.
- It can occur in acute MI and may deteriorate into ventricular fibrillation (VF).

Polymorphic Ventricular Tachycardia with Long QT (Torsades de Pointes)

Torsades de pointes is a type of ventricular arrhythmia that is classically accompanied by certain characteristics including QT prolongation (Figs. 12.6A and B). The initiation of the

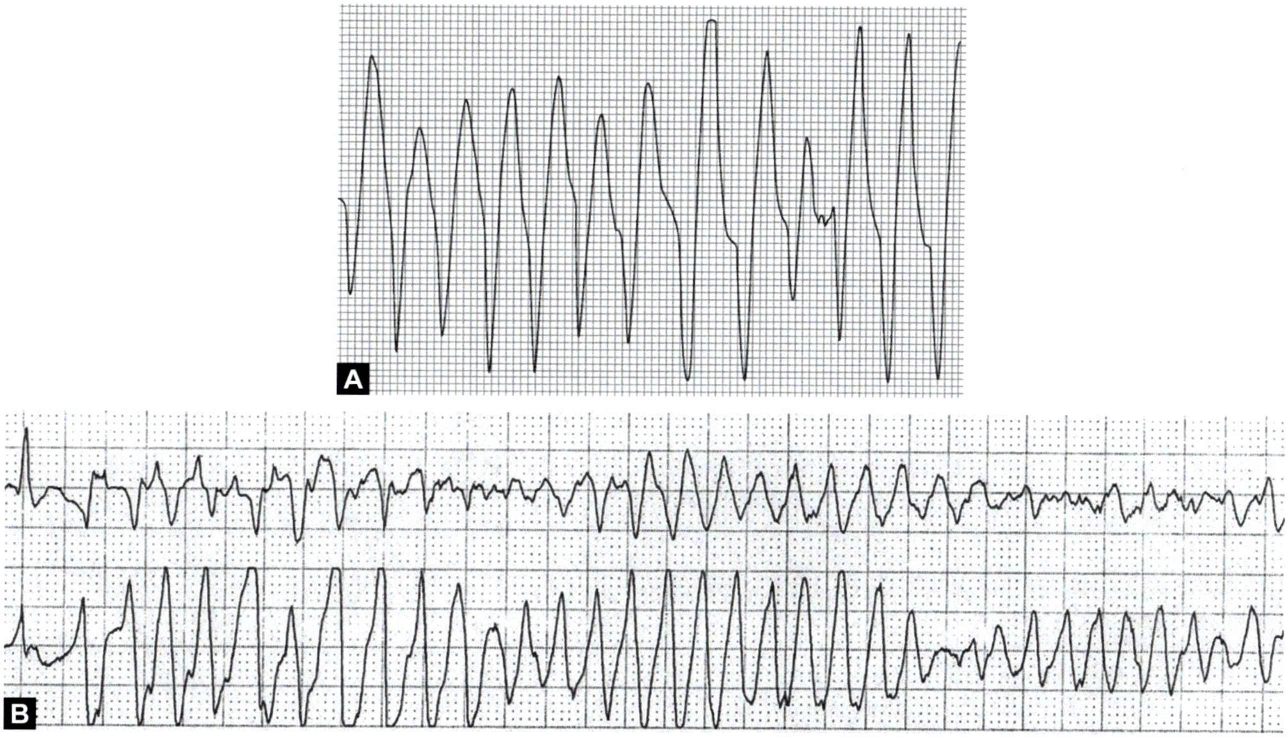

Figs. 12.5A and B: (A) Polymorphic ventricular tachycardia showing broad complex tachycardia with multiple QRS morphologies. (B) Polymorphic ventricular tachycardia showing QRS complexes varying in amplitude and duration.

tachycardia is pause-dependent, with late coupled PVC (long-short initiating sequence). On the resting ECG long QTc and abnormally shaped T waves are characteristic (Fig. 12.6B). QT prolonging drugs, bradycardia, hypokalemia, and hypomagnesemia are usually the precipitating factors.[3] Torsades de pointes means (twisting of points). In this type of polymorphic VT the cardiac axis rotates over a sequence of 5–20 beats, changing from one direction to another and back again. The QRS amplitude varies similarly, such that the complexes appear to twist around the baseline. In SR, the QT interval is prolonged and prominent U waves may be seen. Torsades de pointes is not usually sustained, but it will recur unless the underlying cause is corrected. Occasionally it may be prolonged or may degenerate into VF. It is associated with conditions that prolong the QT interval. Transient prolongation of the QT interval is often seen in the acute phase of MI, and this may lead to torsades de pointes. Ability to recognize torsades de pointes is important because its management is different from the management of other VTs.[2]

CAUSES OF TORSADES DE POINTES

Coronary artery disease: Acute ST elevation MI, non-ST elevation MI, and unstable angina.

Drugs

Antiarrhythmic drugs:

- Class Ia (disopyramide, procainamide, and quinidine)
- Class III (amiodarone, bretylium, and sotalol).

Antibacterials: Erythromycin, fluoroquinolones, and trimethoprim.

Other drugs: Terfenadine, cisapride, tricyclic antidepressants, haloperidol, lithium, phenothiazines, chloroquine, and thioridazine.

Electrolyte disturbances: Hypokalemia and hypomagnesemia.

Congenital syndromes: Jervell and Lange-Nielsen syndrome and Romano-Ward syndrome.

Other causes: Myxedema and bradycardia due to sick sinus syndrome or complete heart block, and subarachnoid hemorrhage.

VENTRICULAR FLUTTER

Ventricular flutter is an arrhythmia, more specifically a tachycardia affecting the ventricles with a rate over 250–350 beats/min. It is characterized on the ECG by a sinusoidal waveform without clear definition of the QRS and T waves. It has been considered as a possible transition stage between VT and fibrillation, and is a critically unstable arrhythmia that can result in sudden cardiac death (SCD). It can occur in infancy, youth and also in adult.[13,14] It can be induced by programmed electrical stimulation.[15,16]

Electrocardiogram Criteria of Ventricular Flutter (Fig. 12.7)

- Extreme form of VT with loss of organized electrical activity

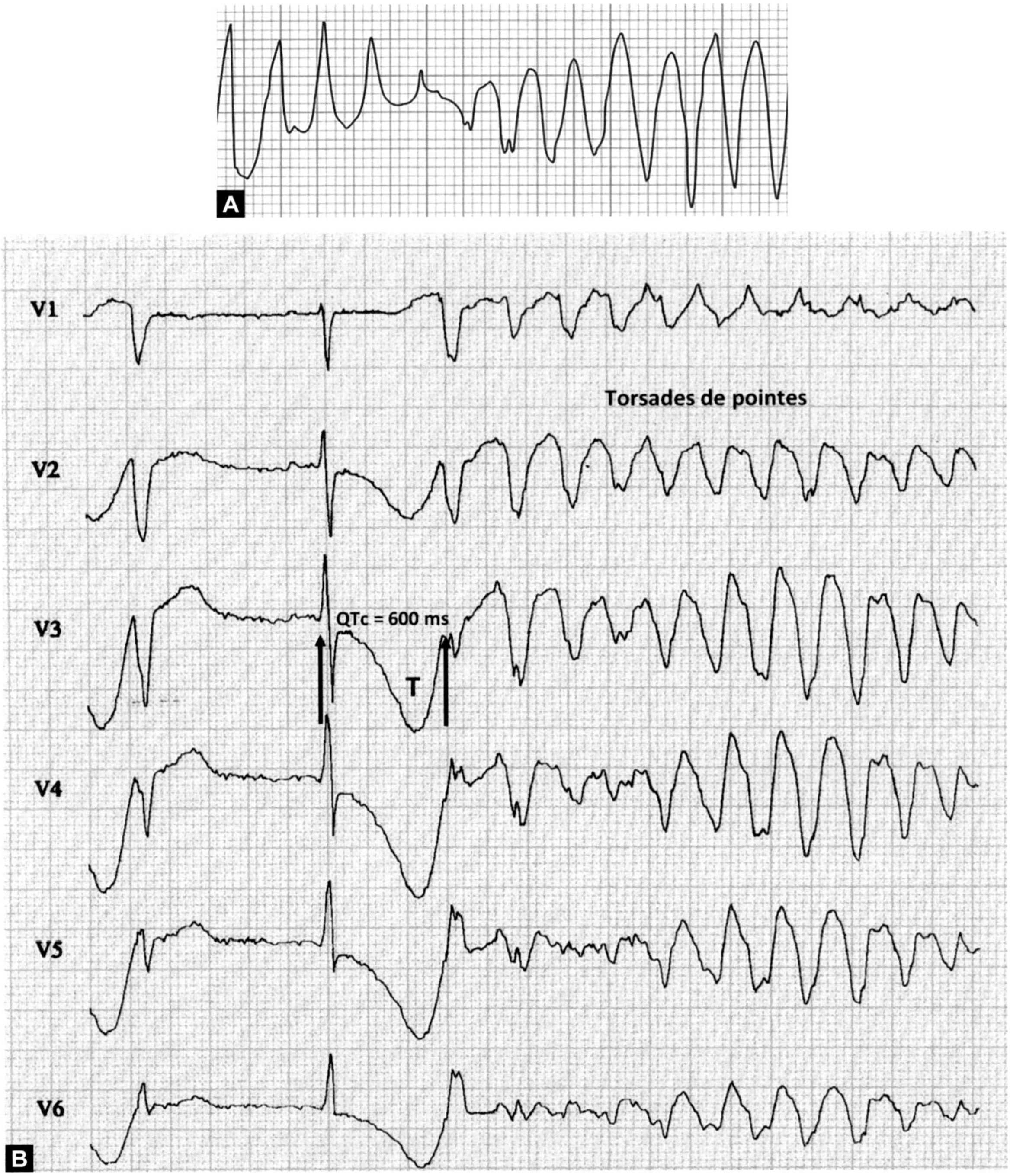

Figs. 12.6A and B: (A) Electrocardiogram is suggestive of torsades de pointes showing gradual change in the amplitude and twisting of the QRS complexes around the isoelectric line. (B) Electrocardiogram tracing is suggestive of torsades de pointes ventricular tachycardia in the presence of marked QT prolongation. QTc preceding torsades de pointes ventricular tachycardia is 600 ms (*arrows*).

- Continuous sine wave
- No identifiable P waves, QRS complexes, or T waves
- Rate usually is greater than 250 beats/min
- The ECG looks identical when viewed upside down.

Ventricular flutter is associated with rapid and profound hemodynamic compromise and it is usually short lived due to progression to VF.

VENTRICULAR FIBRILLATION

Ventricular fibrillation is a condition in which there is uncoordinated contraction of the cardiac muscle of the ventricles in the heart, making them quiver rather than contract properly. This rapid and irregular electrical activity renders the ventricles unable to contract in a synchronized manner, resulting in immediate loss of cardiac output. VF is the most commonly identified arrhythmia in cardiac arrest patients particularly in patients with coronary artery disease. VF is a medical emergency that requires prompt Advanced Life Support interventions. If this arrhythmia continues for more than a few seconds, it will likely degenerate further into asystole (ECG becomes flatline). This condition results in cardiogenic shock and cessation of effective blood circulation. As a consequence, SCD will result in a matter of minutes.

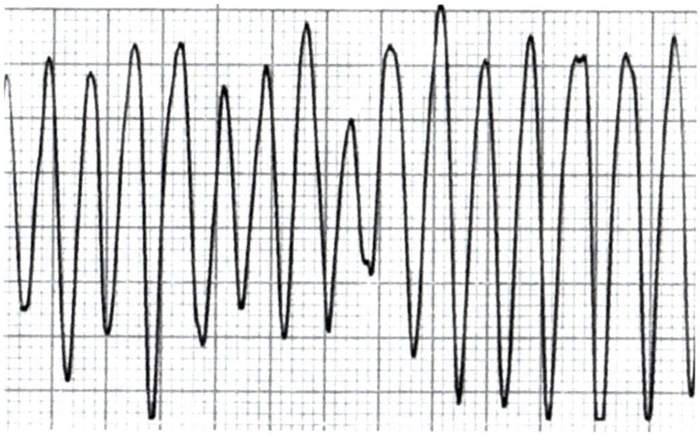

Fig. 12.7: Electrocardiogram is suggestive of ventricular flutter showing a sinusoidal waveform without any clear definition of the QRS complex and T waves.

Electrocardiogram Criteria of Ventricular Fibrillation (Fig. 12.8)

- Electrocardiogram shows chaotic irregular deflections of varying amplitude.
- No identifiable P waves, QRS complexes, or T waves on surface ECG.
- Rate usually varies from 150 bpm to 500 bpm but difficult to count.
- Amplitude decreases with duration and coarse VF turns into fine VF.

FASCICULAR VENTRICULAR TACHYCARDIA

Idiopathic fascicular VT is an important cardiac arrhythmia with specific electrocardiographic features and therapeutic options. It is characterized by relatively narrow QRS complex and RBBB pattern (Fig. 12.9). The QRS axis depends on which fascicle is involved in the reentry. Left axis deviation is noted with left posterior fascicular tachycardia (Fig. 12.10) and right axis deviation with left anterior fascicular

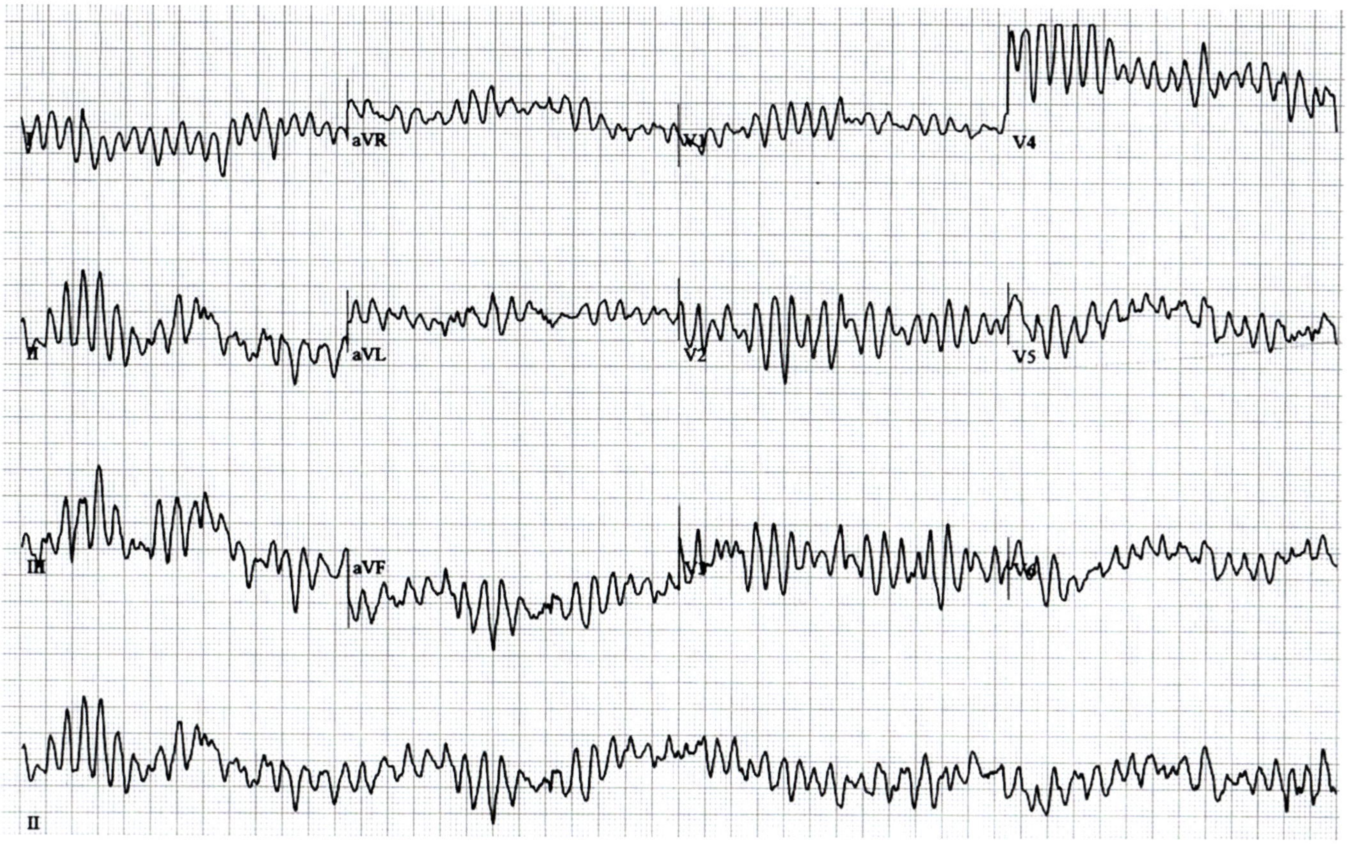

Fig. 12.8: Electrocardiogram of ventricular fibrillation showing chaotic irregular deflections of varying amplitude without any identifiable P waves, QRS complexes, or T waves. The patient developed VT/VF during stress test.

(*Courtesy:* Dr. SM Mustafa Zaman, Bangabandhu Sheikh Mujib Medical University)

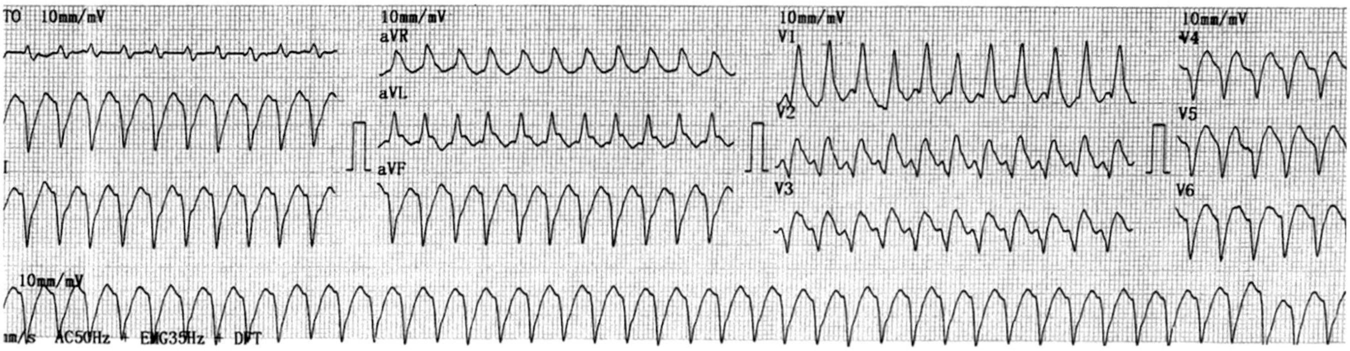

Fig. 12.9: Fascicular ventricular tachycardia is characterized by relatively narrow QRS complex (QRS is 130 ms) and right bundle branch block pattern.

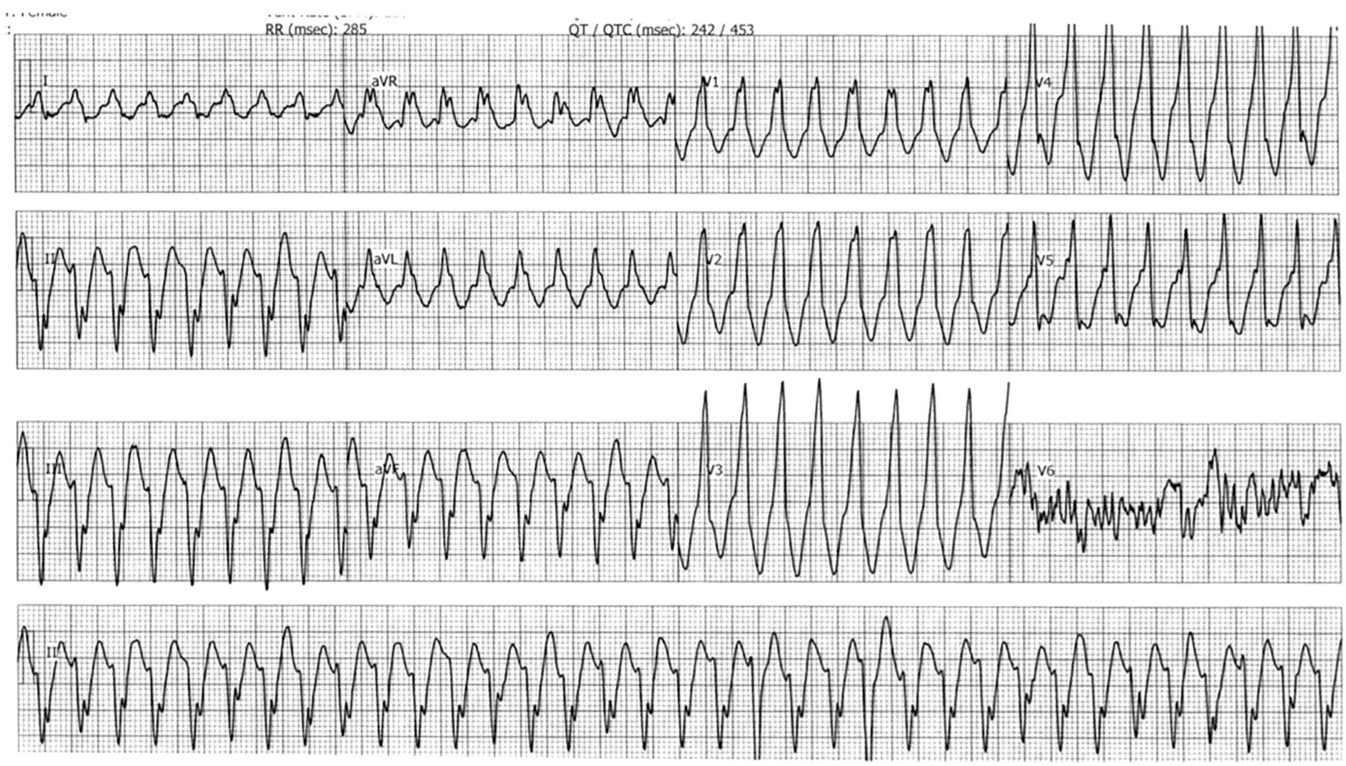

Fig. 12.10: Fascicular ventricular tachycardia (left posterior fascicular tachycardia) with left axis deviation.

tachycardia (Fig. 12.11). A left septal fascicular tachycardia with normal axis has also been described. Fascicular tachycardia is usually seen in individuals without structural heart disease [17]

Fascicular VT usually originates from the region of the posterior fascicle (or occasionally the anterior fascicle) of the left bundle branch and is partly propagated by the His-Purkinje network. It, therefore, produces QRS complexes of relatively short duration (0.11–0.14 seconds). Consequently, this arrhythmia is commonly misdiagnosed as SVT. The QRS complexes have an RBBB pattern, often with a small Q wave rather than primary R wave in lead V1 and a deep S wave in lead V6. When the tachycardia originates from the posterior fascicle, the frontal plane axis of the QRS complex is deviated to the left; when it originates from the anterior fascicle, right axis deviation is seen.[2] Response to verapamil is an important feature of fascicular tachycardia.[17]

RIGHT VENTRICULAR OUTFLOW TRACT TACHYCARDIA

The most common form of idiopathic VT originates from the ventricular outflow tract. Approximately, 90% arise from the RVOT, whereas the remainders are from the left.[18] Right ventricular outflow tract VT is a form of monomorphic VT originating from the outflow tract of the right ventricle or occasionally from the tricuspid annulus. It is usually seen

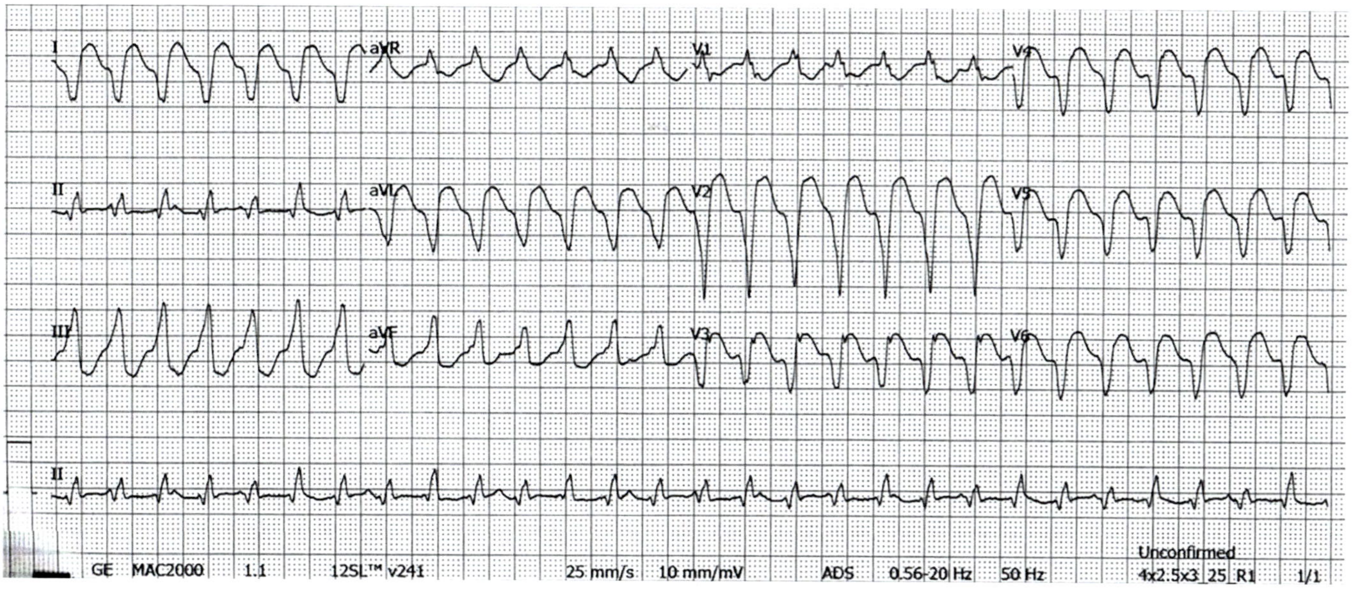

Fig. 12.11: Fascicular ventricular tachycardia (left anterior fascicular tachycardia) with right axis deviation (rate is 170 bpm and QRS duration is 130 ms).

in patients without underlying structural heart disease, although may also occur in the context of ARVC.

Two clinical manifestations of this tachycardia have been described—exercise (stress) induced VT and repetitive monomorphic VT (which occurs at rest).[19] Pioneering studies have shown that some of these arrhythmias are caused by inherited channelopathies—for example, long QT syndrome, Brugada syndrome, and catecholaminergic VT.[20,21] The mechanisms underlying some other forms of idiopathic VT, such as verapamil sensitive fascicular tachycardia and idiopathic VF, remain unclear, although it is known that they originate from Purkinje fibers.[18,22]

The electrocardiogram typically shows right axis deviation, with an LBBB pattern (Fig. 12.12). The tachycardia may be brief and self-terminating or sustained, and it may be provoked by catecholamine release, sudden changes in heart rate, and exercise.[2] Unlike any other form of VT, this tachycardia terminates in response to adenosine, beta-blockers, calcium channel blockers, and valsalva maneuvers.[23,24] Occasionally, the arrhythmia stops with adenosine treatment and so may be misdiagnosed as SVT.[2]

BIDIRECTIONAL VENTRICULAR TACHYCARDIA

Bidirectional VT is a rare ventricular dysrhythmia characterized by a beat-to-beat alternation of the frontal QRS axis (Fig. 12.13). The QRS axis may shift 180° from left to right with each alternate beat or there may be alternating LBBB and RBBB pattern. This rhythm is most commonly associated with severe digoxin toxicity. It may be the presenting rhythm in patients with familial catecholaminergic polymorphic VT. This type of VT has also been reported with herbal aconite poisoning.

Accelerated Idioventricular Rhythm

Monomorphic VT with a rate less than 100 bpm is termed as accelerated idioventricular rhythm or slow VT (Fig. 12.14). It is usually noticed during acute MI and treatment is not necessary for this rhythm. AIVR is considered to be the most common reperfusion arrhythmia associated with successful reperfusion. ST-segment resolution (STR) greater than 70% along with AIVR possibly indicates successful reperfusion after thrombolysis/primary percutaneous coronary intervention (PPCI).

BROAD COMPLEX TACHYCARDIAS OF SUPRAVENTRICULAR ORIGIN

In the presence of aberrant conduction or ventricular preexcitation, any SVT may present as a broad complex tachycardia and mimic VT. There are three main diagnostic possibilities of all broad complex tachycardia:

- VT
- SVT with aberrant conduction due to bundle branch block
- SVT with aberrant conduction due to the Wolff-Parkinson-White syndrome.

The most important distinction is whether the rhythm is ventricular (VT) or supraventricular (SVT with aberrancy), as this will significantly influence the management of the patient. But, the electrocardiographic differentiation of VT

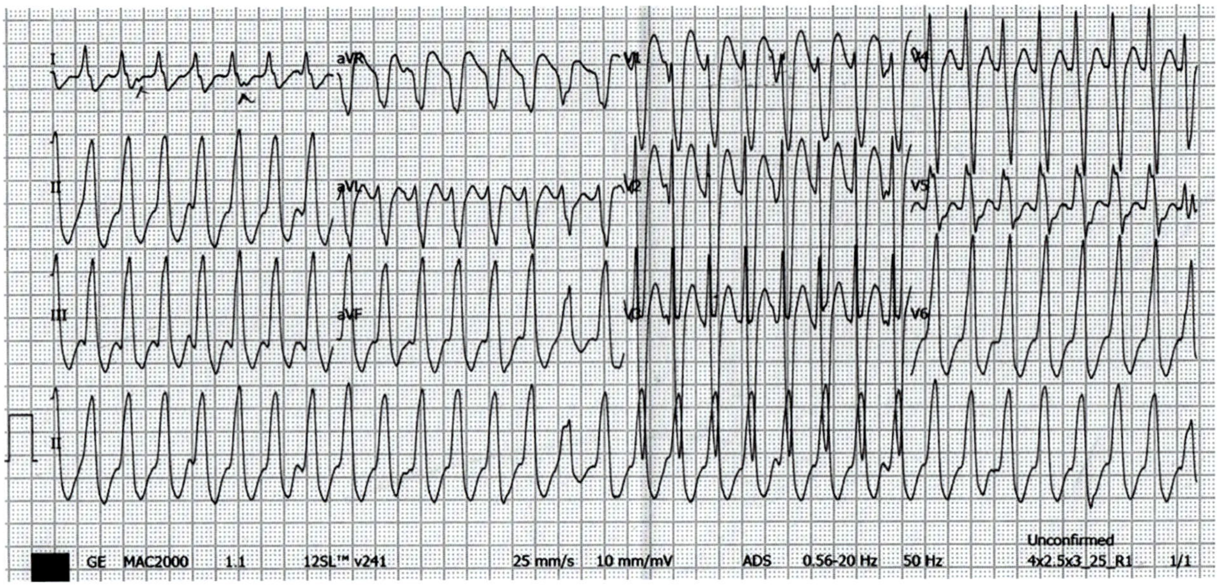

Fig. 12.12: Right ventricular outflow tract–ventricular tachycardia—Electrocardiogram shows ventricular tachycardia originating from the right ventricular outflow tract. The ventricular tachycardia is directed inferiorly, as is apparent by the positive complexes in LII, LIII, and aVF and by the negative complexes in leads aVR and aVL. Lead V1 is negative, consistent with a right ventricular outflow tract focus.

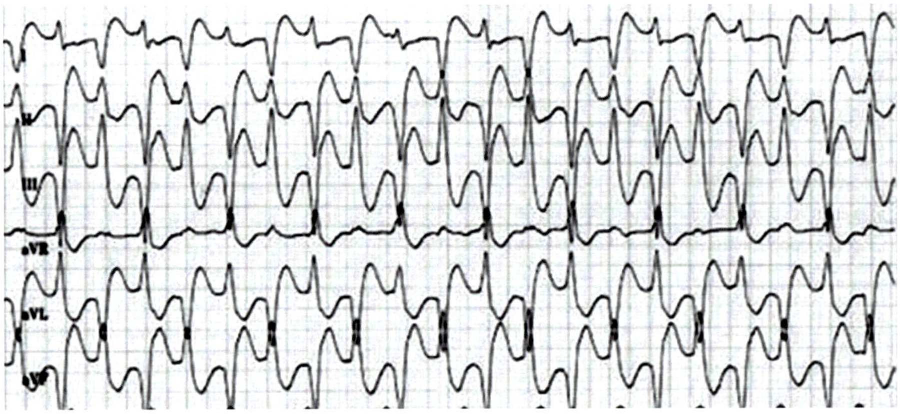

Fig. 12.13: Bidirectional ventricular tachycardia recorded in limb leads. The QRS axis shift from left to right with each alternate beat.

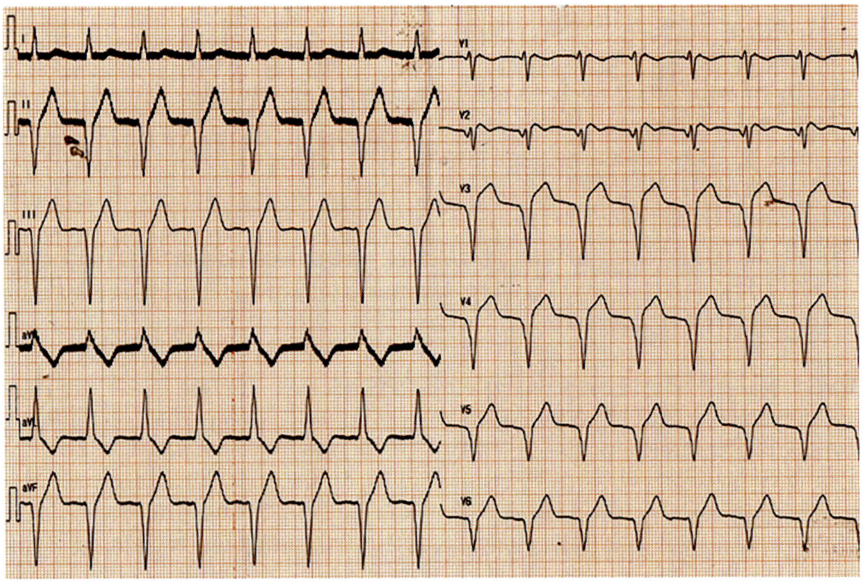

Fig. 12.14: ECG is consistent with accelerated idioventricular rhythm (AIVR). ECG shows slow monomophic VT (rate 88 bpm) suggestive of AIVR. This patient developed AIVR immediately after primary percutaneous coronary intervention (PPCI).

(*Courtesy:* Dr Mahbubor Rahman, Labaid Cardiac Hospital)

from SVT with aberrancy is not easy and not always possible also.

Supraventricular Tachycardia with Aberrant Conduction

Supraventricular tachycardia with aberrant conduction is defined as conduction through the AV node with delay or block, resulting in a broader QRS complex. Aberrant conduction usually manifests as LBBB or RBBB, both of which have characteristic features. The BBB may predate the tachycardia, or it may be a rate-related functional block, occurring when atrial impulses arrive too rapidly for a bundle branch to conduct normally.

If the tachycardia is known with certainty to be supraventricular in origin, it can be treated as a narrow QRS complex tachycardia.[25] In some cases, it can prove challenging to differentiate VT from SVT with aberrancy. It must be remembered in this context that 80% of broad complex tachycardias are VTs and a minority are actually SVTs. However, it is important to remember that at the bedside, if it is difficult to differentiate between the two; all such rhythms must be taken as VT and treated as such. Far more costly mistakes are made at the bedside by incorrectly diagnosing VT as SVT than conversely by incorrectly diagnosing SVT as VT. An arrhythmia that has been definitively diagnosed as SVT with aberrancy can be treated according to the typical care for that SVT; any broad complex tachycardia that does not have definitive features of SVT should be treated as VT until proven otherwise.[3]

Supraventricular Tachycardia with Accessory Pathway

Accessory pathways are anomalous extranodal connections which connect the epicardial surface of the atrium and ventricle along the AV groove. Accessory pathways which are capable only of retrograde conduction are concealed whereas those capable of antegrade conduction are manifested, demonstrating preexcitation on a standard ECG. AVRT can present with a wide QRS complex, preexcited tachycardia as a result of manifest anterograde accessory pathway conduction. These patients may have WPW syndrome that can be diagnosed by the resting sinus ECG, based on the delta wave and short PR interval. It is also possible to have a normal ECG during sinus rhythm (SR), if the accessory pathway conduction is slow compared to the AV nodal conduction.

The term "WPW syndrome" is reserved for patients who have both preexcitation (wide QRS in SR due to presence of delta wave) and symptomatic tachyarrhythmias. It is important to remember that even amongst patients with the WPW syndrome, when they present with tachyarrhythmia; orthodromic AVRT with a narrow complex tachycardia is the most common form, occurring in 90% of these patients. AVRT is subclassified into orthodromic and antidromic AVRT. During orthodromic AVRT, the reentrant impulse utilizes the AV node and specialized conduction system for conduction from the atrium to the ventricle, and utilizes the accessory pathway for conduction from the ventricle to the atrium. During antidromic AVRT, the reentrant impulse travels in the reverse direction with conduction from the atrium to the ventricle occurring via the accessory pathway, so patient presents with broad complex tachycardia. AF is a potentially life-threatening arrhythmia in patients with the WPW syndrome as it can result in a very rapid ventricular response, and rarely VF. Patients with WPW syndrome have a delta wave seen in an SR ECG. A broad complex tachycardia is generally seen when these patients present with antidromic conduction over the accessory pathway. Patients with WPW syndrome and AF can present with a broad complex irregular ECG mimicking polymorphic VT. If no previous ECG is present and it is difficult to be certain they should be treated as if they have VT.

BROAD COMPLEX TACHYCARDIAS: VENTRICULAR TACHYCARDIA VERSUS SUPRAVENTRICULAR TACHYCARDIA WITH ABERRANCY

Broad QRS complex tachycardia still presents a diagnostic challenge when confronted with a 12-lead ECG. The ECG differential diagnosis includes VT versus SVT with aberrant conduction, preexisting BBB, intraventricular conduction disturbances, or preexcitation. VT is the most important differential diagnosis because of its least favorable prognostic value. An accurate diagnosis with an immediate treatment is usually required. Delay or misdiagnosing VT with an inappropriate intravenous administration of drugs used for the treatment of SVT, such as verapamil and adenosine, can cause severe hemodynamic deterioration and may provoke VF and cardiac arrest.[26-31] VT is the most common cause of regular broad complex tachycardia, accounting for up to 80% of all cases. The history of prior MI, congestive heart failure, and recent angina pectoris has positive predictive values for VT of 98, 100, and 100%, respectively.[32] The most safe option is to regard a broad complex tachycardia of uncertain origin as VT unless good evidence suggests a supraventricular origin. If a VT is wrongly treated as SVT, the consequences may be extremely serious.

CERTAIN ELECTROCARDIOGRAM FEATURES MAY DIFFERENTIATE VENTRICULAR TACHYCARDIA FROM SUPRAVENTRICULAR TACHYCARDIA WITH ABERRANCY

- Atrioventricular dissociation
- *Concordant patterns*: All the precordial leads have predominantly positive or negative QRS pattern.

- Presence of fusion beats
- Presence of capture beats
- Extreme left axis deviation is more likely to be VT. Axis in "no man's land" (right superior, i.e. between –90° and ±180°) is almost always VT.
- QRS duration greater than 140 ms (RBBB QRS configuration) or greater than 160 ms (LBBB QRS configuration) is suggestive of VT.
- Presence of Q waves indicates presence of old MI and thus VT is the likely diagnosis.
- Notching or slurring of the S wave (Josephson's sign) in V1, V2 suggests VT.

Atrioventricular Dissociation

Atrioventricular dissociation is a condition in which the atria and ventricles do not activate in a synchronous fashion but beat independent of each other (Fig. 12.15). This is one of the most useful criteria for distinguishing VT from SVT with aberrancy. It occurs in 20–50% of VT and almost never in SVT.[33-35] It is often very difficult to ascertain the presence of AV dissociation, particularly in rapid tachycardia. It usually demands long 12-lead ECG recordings and careful ECG analysis. However, retrograde ventriculoatrial (VA) conduction, whether 1 to 1 or 2 to 1, or Wenckebach VA conduction occurs in up to 50% of all VT.[36,37] AV dissociation can also be seen in rare cases of AVNRT and uncommon types of Mahaim tachycardia (nodo-fascicular/ nodo-ventricular), in which the retrograde conduction is absent.[38,39] AV dissociation is generally detectable in a lead where the P wave is most prominent whether anterograde or retrograde. This lead is usually one of the inferior leads considering the lead in which the QRS complex is the most modest, i.e. least interfering with the relatively prominent P wave. QRS variability can indicate AV dissociation. Obviously, care should be taken to record technically excellent ECGs without disturbances of the baseline.[38] The use of the Lewis lead can be helpful in detecting the P waves on the ECG.[40]

The ECG should be scrutinized to find out hidden P waves—these are often superimposed on the QRS complexes and may be difficult to see. If P waves are present at a different rate to the QRS complexes, AV dissociation is present and VT is diagnosed.

CONCORDANT PATTERNS

Concordance exists when all the QRS complexes in the chest leads are either predominantly positive or predominantly negative. The presence of concordance suggests that the tachycardia has a ventricular origin. Positive concordance probably indicates that the origin of the tachycardia lies on the posterior ventricular wall; the wave of depolarization moves toward all the chest leads and produces positive complexes. Similarly, negative concordance is thought to correlate with a tachycardia originating in the anterior ventricular wall.[2] If all precordial leads are predominantly negative, a VT is the likely diagnosis (Fig. 12.16). If all precordial leads are predominantly positive, the differential

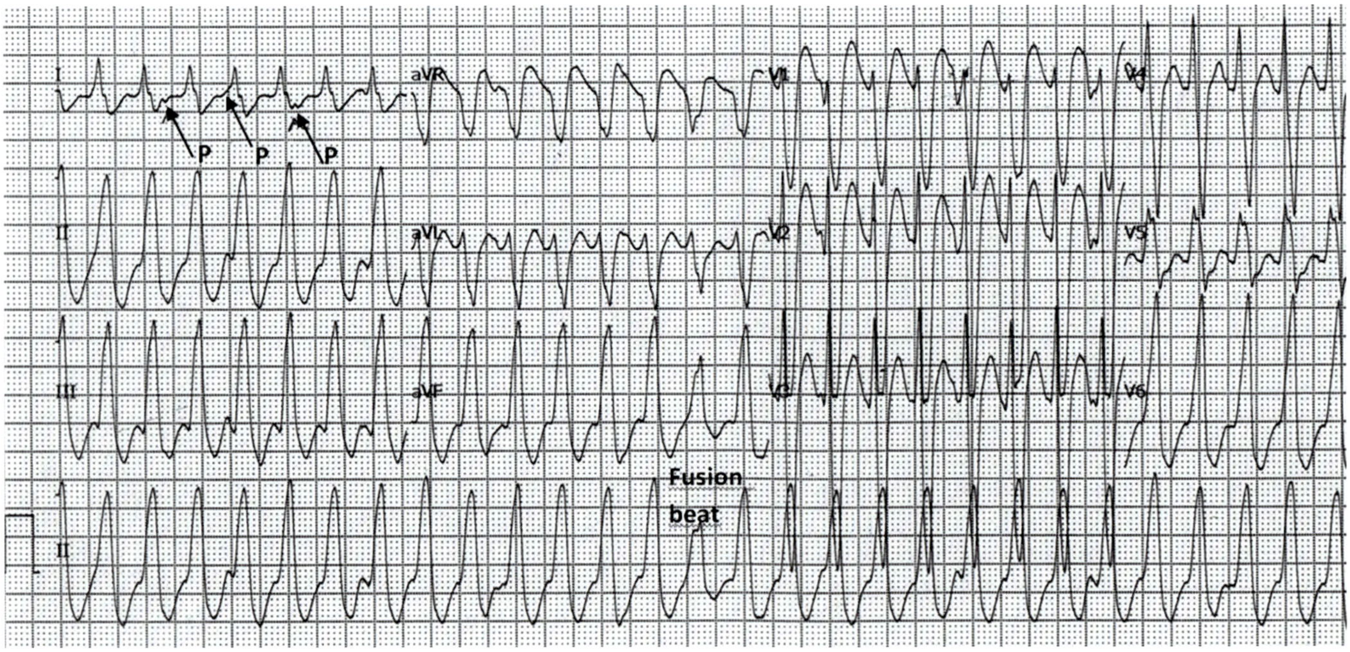

Fig. 12.15: Ventricular tachycardia with atrioventricular dissociation (P and QRS complexes at different rates). Note visible P waves in L1 (*arrows*) and some P waves are superimposed on the QRS complexes and may be difficult to see. Also note a fusion beat.

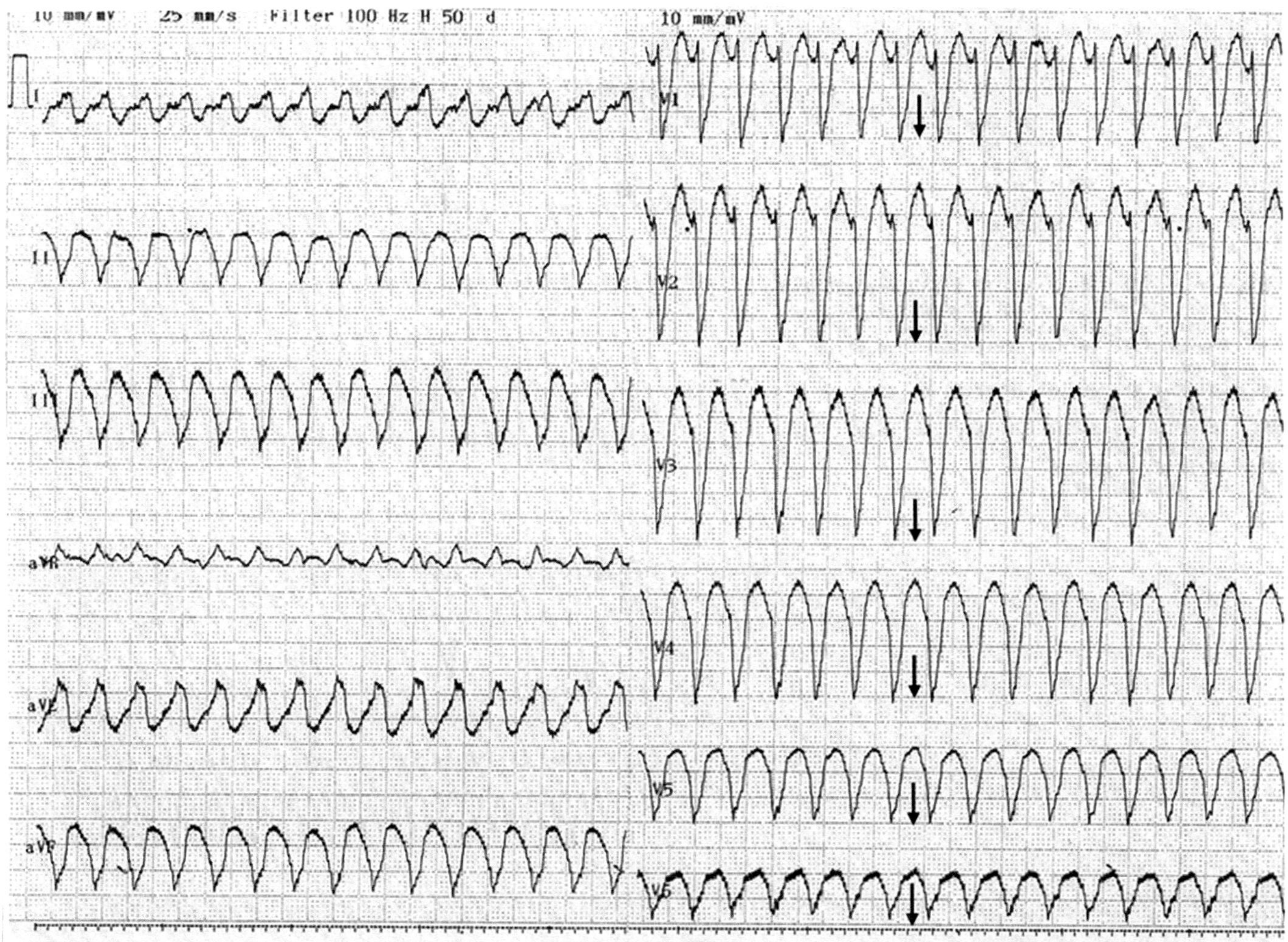

Fig. 12.16: Electrocardiogram shows broad complex tachycardia (rate is 194 bpm) with negative concordance. Note all precordial leads are predominantly negative (*arrows*). If all precordial leads are predominantly negative, a ventricular tachycardia is the likely diagnosis.

diagnosis is an antidromic tachycardia using a left-sided accessory pathway or a VT.

PRESENCE OF FUSION BEATS

A fusion beat occurs when a sinus beat conducts to the ventricles via the AV node and fuses with a beat arising in the ventricles. As the ventricles are depolarized partly by the impulse conducted through the His-Purkinje system and partly by the impulse arising in the ventricle, the resulting QRS complex has an appearance intermediate between a normal beat and a tachycardia beat (Figs. 12.17A and B). Like capture beats, fusion beats are uncommon, and though they support a diagnosis of VT, their absence does not exclude the diagnosis.[2]

CAPTURE BEATS

Occasionally during VT an atrial impulse may cause ventricular depolarization via the normal conduction system. The resulting QRS complex appears normal and narrow (Figs. 12.18A and B). Such a beat shows that even at rapid rates the conduction system is able to conduct normally, thus making a diagnosis of SVT with aberrancy unlikely. Capture beats are uncommon, and though they confirm a diagnosis of VT, their absence does not exclude the diagnosis.[2]

EXTREME LEFT AXIS DEVIATION

A frontal axis of between –90° and ±180° cannot be achieved by any combination of BBB and therefore suggests VT. Thus, predominantly negative QRS complexes in LI, LII, and LIII are useful criteria for identifying a VT. The QRS axis is not only important for the differentiation of the broad QRS tachycardias but also to identify its site of origin and etiology.[1,41]

QRS DURATION

It is of interest that a QRS width of more than 0.14 seconds (140 ms) in RBBB tachycardias and 0.16 seconds (160 ms) during LBBB argues for a VT.[33,36] The site of origin of the VT plays a role in the width of the QRS complex. When the arrhythmia arises in the lateral free wall of the ventricle sequential activation of the ventricles occur resulting in a

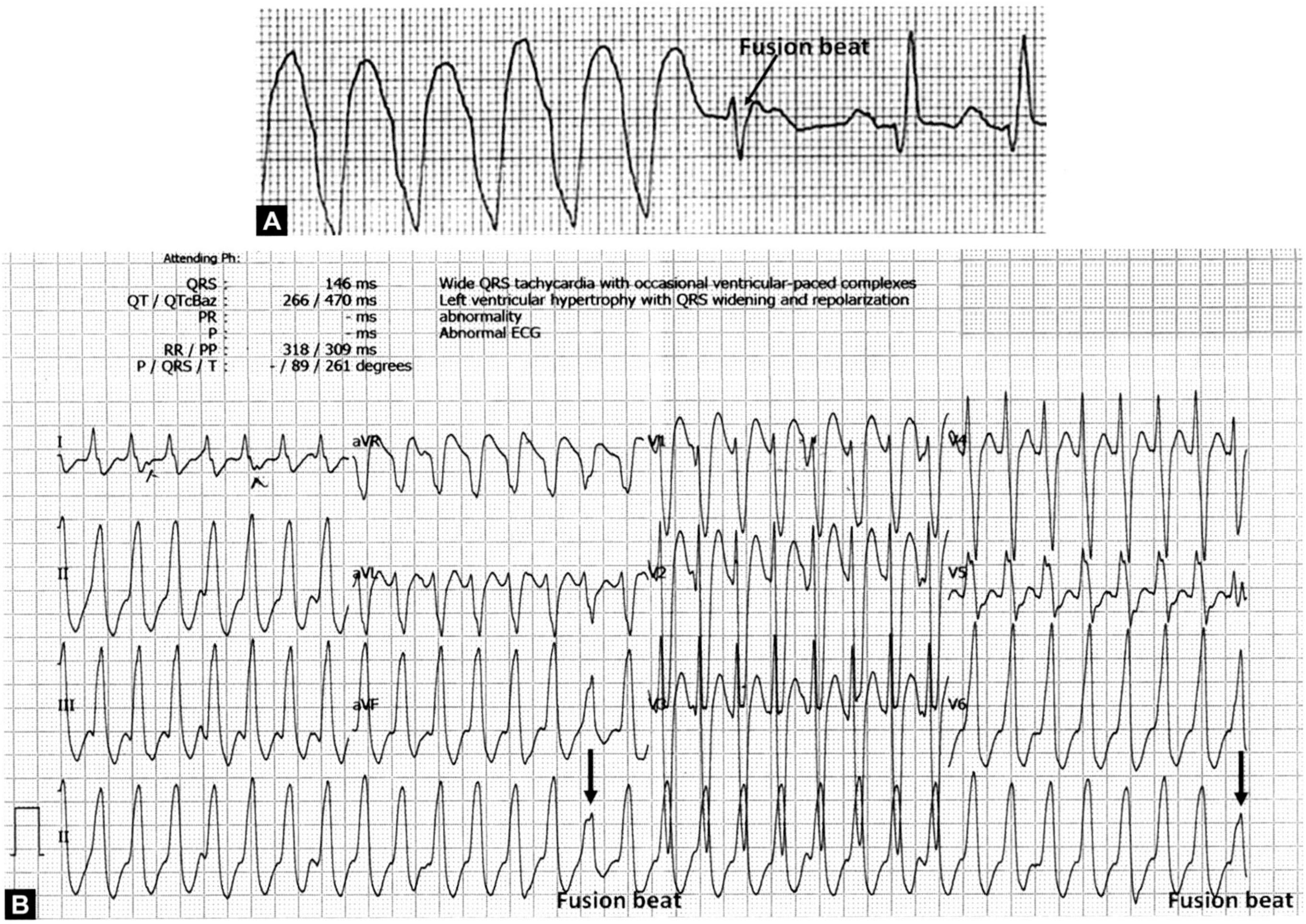

Figs. 12.17A and B: (A) Electrocardiogram showing nonsustained ventricular tachycardia with a fusion beat (*arrow*), the resulting QRS complex has an appearance intermediate between a normal sinus node conducted beat (QRS complexes of right panel) and a tachycardia beat (QRS complexes of left panel). (B) Electrocardiogram showing broad complex tachycardia with two fusion beats (*arrows*) suggestive of ventricular tachycardia. Also note atrioventricular dissociation.

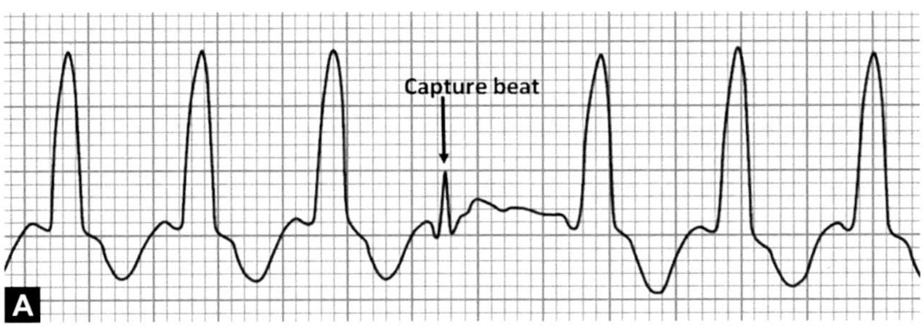

Fig. 12.18A: Electrocardiogram strip shows ventricular tachycardia with one capture beat (*arrow*). Capture beat produces a QRS complex of normal duration in the midst of atrioventricular dissociation. Presence of capture beat is suggestive of ventricular tachycardia.

very wide QRS. The QRS complex will be smaller when the VT has its origin in or close to the interventricular septum. But other factors also play a role in the QRS width during VT, such as scar tissue (after MI), ventricular hypertrophy, and muscular disarray (as in hypertrophic cardiomyopathy). A QRS width below such values may occur in VTs having their origin in or close to the interventricular septum.[1] Of course, QRS width is not helpful in differentiating VT from a tachycardia with AV conduction over an accessory AV pathway because such a pathway inserts into the ventricle leading to eccentric ventricular activation and a wide QRS complex.[1] An SVT can have a QRS width of more than 140 ms (RBBB) or 160 ms (LBBB) under three circumstances: (1) In the presence of preexistent BBB in the elderly with fibrosis in the bundle branch system and ventricular myocardium; (2) when during SVT, AV conduction occurs over an accessory

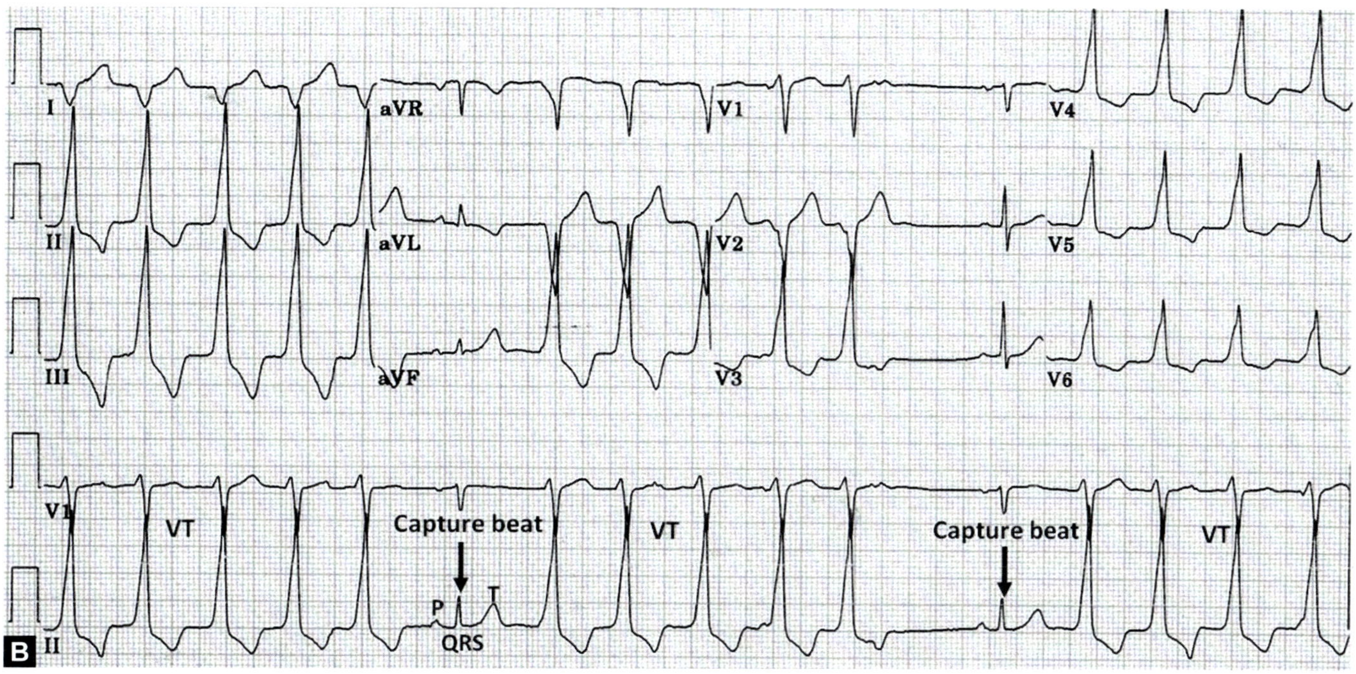

Fig. 12.18B: Electrocardiogram tracing illustrates relatively slow monomorphic ventricular tachycardia with two capture beats (*arrows*). Sinus conducted beats captured the ventricles during pauses of ventricular tachycardia. The QRS complexes of capture beats are of normal duration and configuration and preceded by "P" wave of normal morphology.

AV pathway; (3) when class IC drugs (especially flecainide) are present during SVT.[1]

PRESENCE OF Q WAVES

Presence of Q waves indicates the presence of old MI and thus VT is the likely diagnosis. QR (but not a QS) complex during a broad QRS tachycardia indicates a scar in the myocardium usually caused by MI and hence suggests VT. QR complexes during VT are present in approximately 40% of VTs after MI.[42,43]

JOSEPHSON'S SIGN

This sign is one of the important electrocardiographic criteria for establishing the diagnosis of VT in presence of wide complex LBBB morphology tachycardias. Notching on the downstroke of the S wave in V1 or V2 is known as Josephson's sign and suggests VT (Fig. 12.19).

TACHYCARDIA QRS MORE NARROW THAN SINUS QRS

When during tachycardia, the QRS is more narrow than during sinus rhythm (SR), a VT should be diagnosed. A very wide QRS is present during SR because of sequential activation of first the right and then the left ventricle. During tachycardia, the QRS is more narrow. This can only be explained by a ventricular origin of the arrhythmia close to the interventricular septum, resulting in more simultaneous activation of the right and left ventricle than during SR.[1]

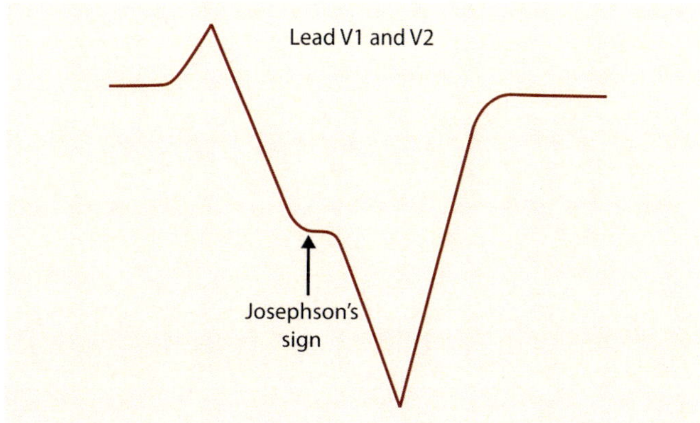

Fig. 12.19: In broad complex tachycardia notching on the downstroke of the S wave in V1 or V2 (*arrow*) is known as Josephson's sign and suggest ventricular tachycardia.

NEWER CRITERIA TO DIFFERENTIATE BETWEEN VENTRICULAR TACHYCARDIA AND SUPRAVENTRICULAR TACHYCARDIA WITH ABERRANCY

Marriott and Sandler noticed that "concordant" precordial patterns, whether entirely upright or entirely inverted, were almost diagnostic for ventricular origin. Positive concordance may also occur during antidromic tachycardia using a left posterior or left lateral accessory pathway. Negative concordance is nearly always VT.[30,44] Marriott also introduced in 1971 the term "*Rabbit ear sign*" for a double-peaked R wave in lead V1. Whereas a "good rabbit" with a taller right peak being typical for RBBB aberrancy, a "bad rabbit" with a taller left peak suggests ventricular origin (Figs. 12.20A to C).[38] In 1978, Wellens et al. used His bundle recording for the first time to determine the site of origin of tachycardia with broad QRS complex and created the so-called "*classical criteria*".[34,37,45] Wellens VT diagnostic criteria include: (1) QRS complex duration of more than 140 ms in RBBB pattern tachycardia and QRS more than 160 ms in LBBB pattern tachycardia; (2) Left axis deviation; (3) AV dissociation; (4) Capture and/or fusion beats; (5) If RBBB morphology tachycardia, then RSR' pattern in V1, mono or biphasic QRS in V1, or monophasic QS in V6 suggests VT. If LBBB pattern tachycardia, then presence of initial R in V1 more than 30 ms, slurring or notching of the downstroke of the S wave in V1, V2, beginning of QRS to nadir of S wave more than 70 ms in V1, V2 and any Q in V6 suggest VT.[34,37]

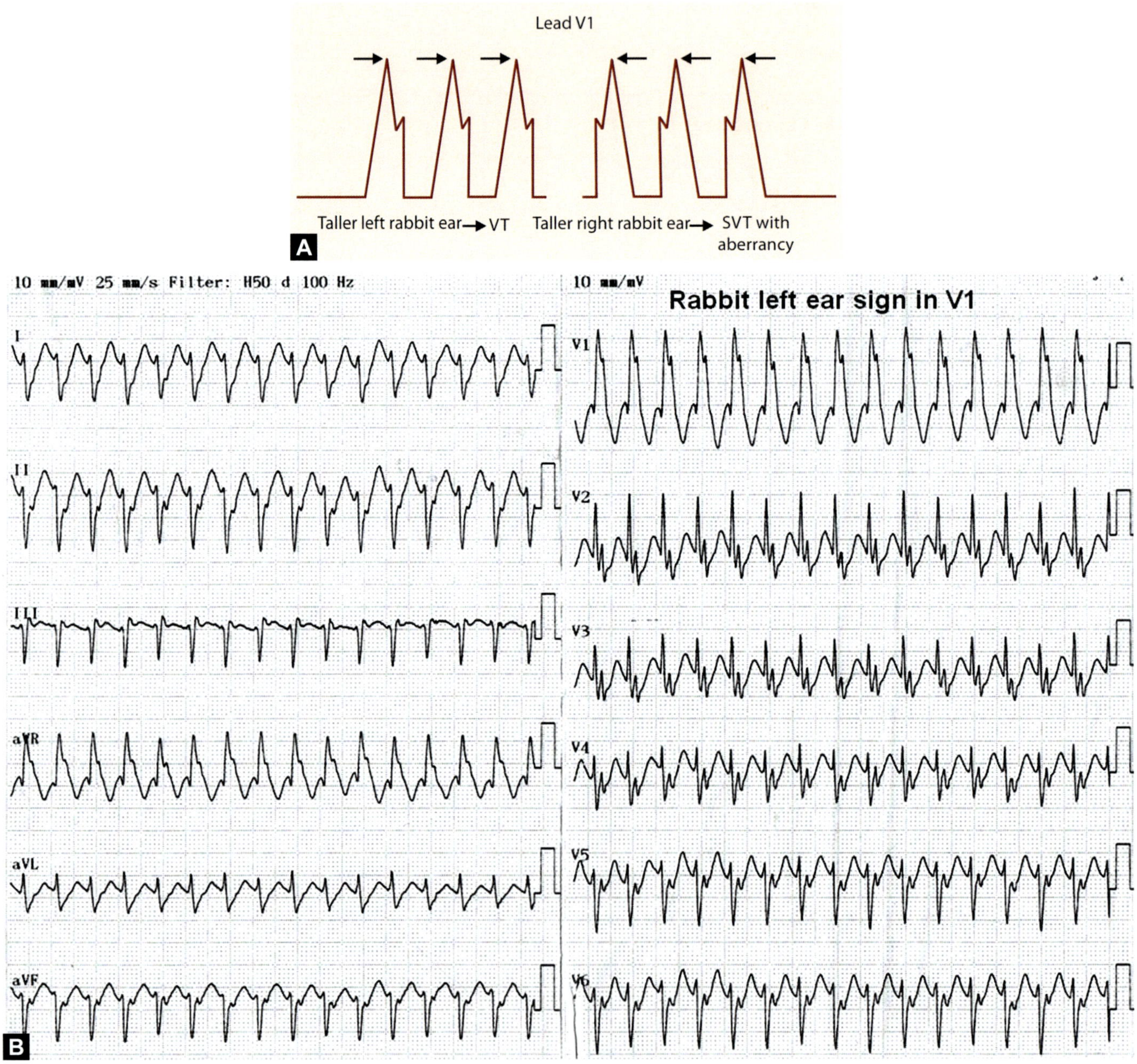

Figs. 12.20A and B: (A) Rabbit ear sign to differentiate between ventricular tachycardia and supraventricular tachycardia with aberrancy. A taller right peak being typical for supraventricular tachycardia with aberrancy (*arrows*) and a taller left peak suggests ventricular tachycardia. (B) Electrocardiogram is consistent with broad complex tachycardia, QRS duration is 140 ms (0.14 seconds) at rate of 200 bpm with a "bad rabbit" (rabbit ear sign) with a taller left peak in V1 suggests ventricular tachycardia (Marriott's sign).
[*Courtesy:* Dr Abduz Zaher, Labaid Cardiac Hospital (B)]

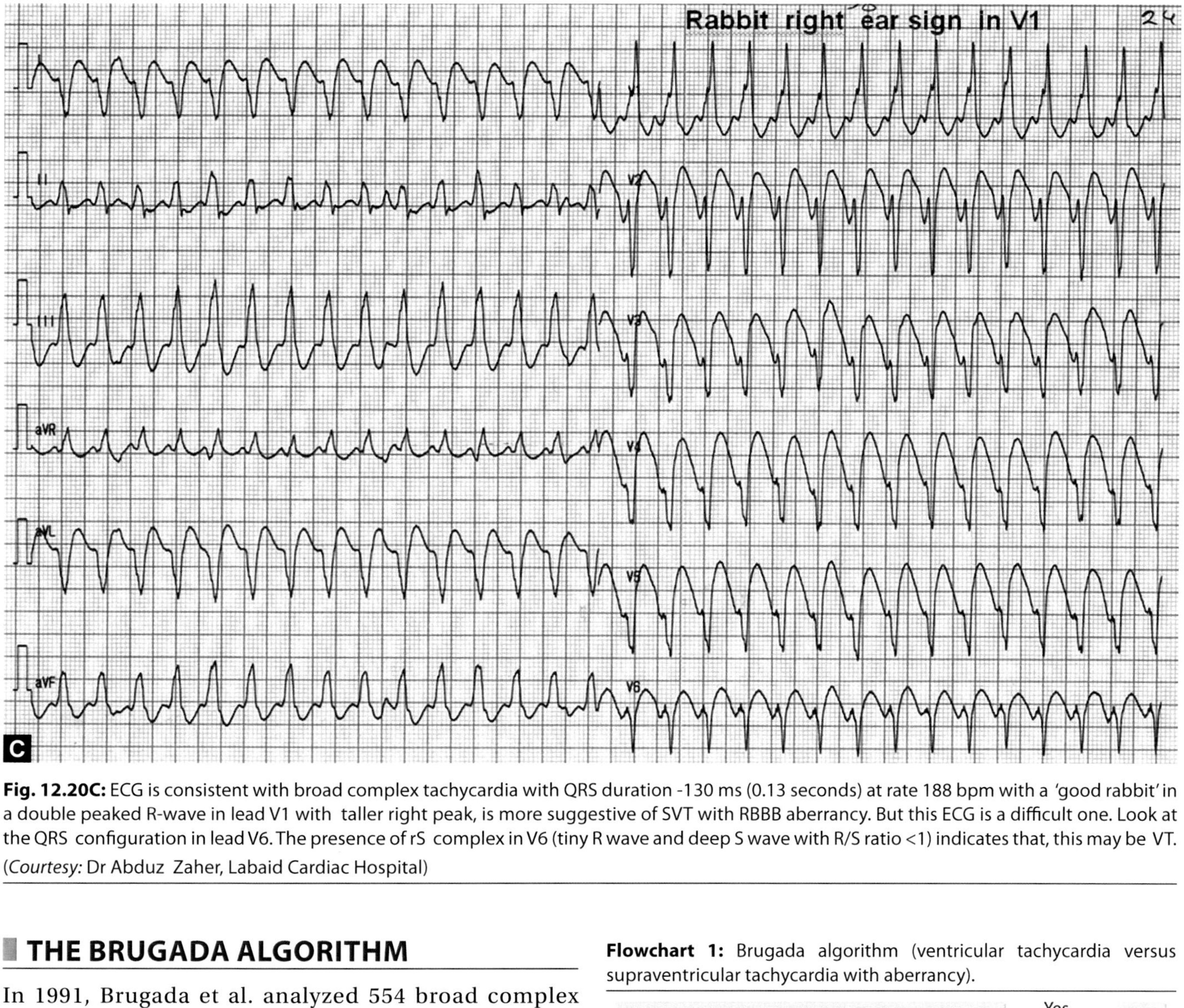

Fig. 12.20C: ECG is consistent with broad complex tachycardia with QRS duration -130 ms (0.13 seconds) at rate 188 bpm with a 'good rabbit' in a double peaked R-wave in lead V1 with taller right peak, is more suggestive of SVT with RBBB aberrancy. But this ECG is a difficult one. Look at the QRS configuration in lead V6. The presence of rS complex in V6 (tiny R wave and deep S wave with R/S ratio <1) indicates that, this may be VT. (*Courtesy:* Dr Abduz Zaher, Labaid Cardiac Hospital)

THE BRUGADA ALGORITHM

In 1991, Brugada et al. analyzed 554 broad complex tachycardia ECGs and produced simple criteria in a stepwise approach irrespective of the QRS complex morphology, whether RBBB- or LBBB-like, with a sensitivity and specificity of 0.987 and 0.965, respectively. The algorithm begins with the identification of an RS complex in any precordial lead.

The Brugada criteria algorithm involves four steps (Flowchart 1):[46]

Step-1: The algorithm begins with the identification of an RS complex in any precordial lead, if failed the diagnosis of VT is made.

Step-2: If an RS complex is present in one or more precordial leads, the next step is to measure the longest RS interval. If an RS interval is longer than 100 ms, the diagnosis of VT is made (Figs. 12.21A and B). If not, the next step of the algorithm is to consider whether AV dissociation is present.

Step-3: If AV dissociation is present, the diagnosis of VT is made.

Step-4: If AV dissociation is absent, the classical morphology criteria for VT are used. If both lead V1 and V6 fulfill the criteria for VT, the diagnosis of VT is made. If not, the diagnosis of SVT with aberrant conduction is made by exclusion of VT.

Flowchart 1: Brugada algorithm (ventricular tachycardia versus supraventricular tachycardia with aberrancy).

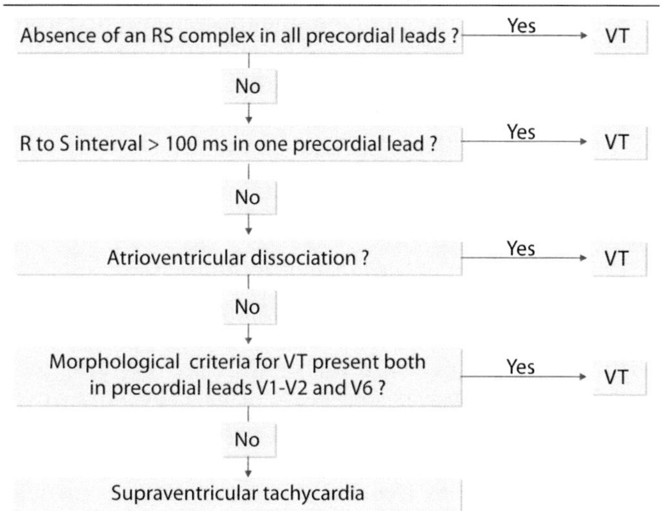

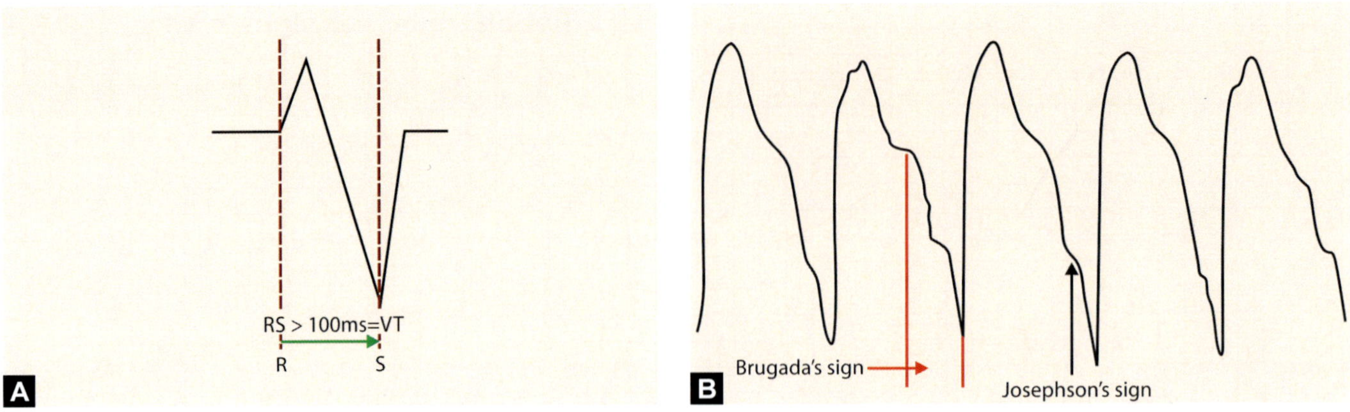

Figs. 12.21A and B: (A) If an RS complex is present in precordial leads and if the RS interval is longer than 100 ms, the diagnosis of ventricular tachycardia is made. (B) Broad complex tachycardia with the presence of Brugada's sign and Josephson's sign are suggestive of ventricular tachycardia (*Brugada's sign*—the distance from the onset of the QRS complex to the nadir of the S wave is greater than 100 ms and Josephson's sign—Notching near the nadir of the S wave).

VERECKEI "THE aVR" ALGORITHM[47,48]

In 2007, a new algorithm analyzed in 287 patients with a high accuracy has been proposed by Vereckei et al. They found that the following criteria were suggestive of VT—(1) the presence of AV dissociation; (2) the presence of an initial R wave in lead aVR, and (3) measuring the voltage during the initial 40 ms (V_i), the terminal 40 ms (V_t), their ratio (V_i/V_t), and that V_i/V_t is less than or equal to 1 was suggestive of VT (Fig. 12.22). In 2008, the same group presented a simplified algorithm using only lead aVR, analyzed in 313 patients with the same accuracy as their first algorithm. Criteria for VT in lead aVR are—(1) the presence of an initial R wave, (2) width of an initial r- or q-wave is greater than 40 ms, (3) notching on the initial downstroke of a predominantly negative QRS complex, and (4) V_i/V_t is less than or equal to 1.

There are some overlaps between the Vereckei and Brugada algorithms, but one of the most useful tips from the Vereckei algorithm is to examine the QRS complex:

- A dominant initial R wave in aVR is indicative of VT.
- A dominant terminal R' wave in aVR (i.e. following a Q/S wave) is more likely SVT with aberrancy.

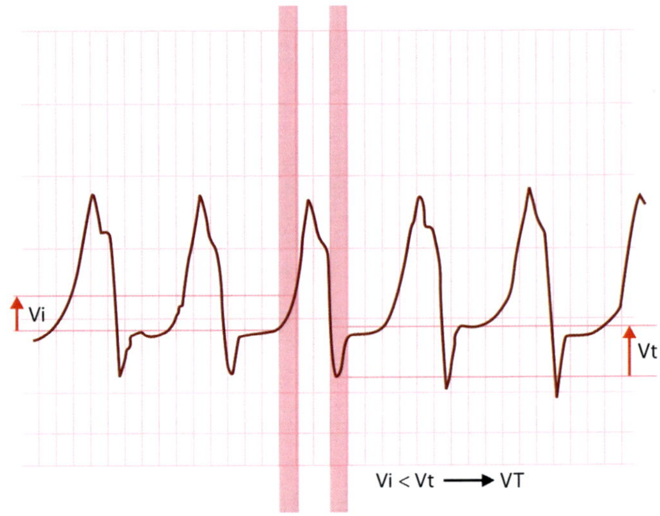

Fig. 12.22: According to Vereckei's algorithm measuring the voltage during the initial 40 ms (*Vi*), the terminal 40 ms (*Vt*) and their ratio (*Vi/Vt*) may be helpful in the electrocardiogram diagnosis of ventricular tachycardia. *Vi* is less than *Vt*, is suggestive of ventricular tachycardia.

GRIFFITH ALGORITHM[49-51]

In 1991, Griffith et al. performed a multivariate analysis in 102 patients to identify which of 15 clinical or 11 ECG variables are independent predictors of VT. They found that (1) the history of previous MI, (2) in lead aVF, a predominant negative deflection was suggestive of VT especially when Q wave was present in RBBB pattern tachycardia. In LBBB pattern tachycardia, a QS or qR waveform in lead aVF is highly suggestive for VT, whereas an Rs complex was specific for SVT, (3) in RBBB pattern tachycardia, a monophasic or biphasic waveform in lead V1 suggested VT, a triphasic RSR', rSR configuration suggested SVT, and (4) change in axis of more than 40° between SR and tachycardia were independent predictors of VT. If none of the above variables was found, the diagnosis was almost certainly SVT. If one criterion was found, the diagnosis was probably SVT. If two criteria were found, then the diagnosis was probably VT. If three or four criteria were found, the diagnosis was almost certainly VT.

THE BAYESIAN APPROACH[52]

Despite numerous attempts at devising algorithms for diagnosing broad complex tachycardia on the basis of the ECG, misdiagnosis is still common. The reason for this may lie with difficulty in implementing existent algorithms in practice, due to imperfect ascertainment of ECG features within them. An attempt was made to approach the problem afresh with the Bayesian inference by the construction of a diagnostic algorithm centered around the likelihood ratio (LR). Previously studied ECG features most effective in discriminating VT from SVT with aberrant conduction, according to their LR values, were selected for inclusion into a Bayesian diagnostic algorithm. A test set of 244 broad complex tachycardia ECGs was assembled and shown to three independent observers who were blinded to the diagnoses made at electrophysiological study. Their diagnostic accuracy by the Bayesian algorithm was compared against that by clinical judgment with the diagnoses from electrophysiologic study as the standard. Clinical judgment correctly diagnosed 35% of SVT with aberrant conduction, 85% of VT, and 47% of fascicular tachycardia. In comparison, by the Bayesian algorithm devised, 52% of SVT with aberrant conduction, 95% of VT, and 97% of fascicular tachycardia were correctly diagnosed.

ULTRA SIMPLE BRUGADA CRITERION: R WAVE PEAK TIME[53]

In 2010, Joseph Brugada et al. published a new criterion to differentiate VT from SVT in broad complex tachycardias—the R wave peak time (RWPT) in lead II. They suggest measuring the duration of onset of the QRS to the first change in polarity (either nadir Q or peak R) in lead II. If the RWPT is greater than or equal to 50 ms, then the likelihood of a VT is very high (Fig. 12.23).

Several ECG algorithms have been developed to differentiate broad QRS-complex tachycardias. Most of them performed very well in the population they were based upon. A review tested five commonly used algorithms in a control population and found that each of them only performed reasonably well in differentiating VT from SVT (accuracy 66–77%).[54] The five criteria tested were:

1. *Brugada algorithm*: This is the most commonly used algorithm. Sensitivity 89% and specificity 59.2%.[46]
2. *RWPT*: The lead II R-wave-peak-time. Sensitivity 60% and specificity 82.7%.[53]
3. *The aVR algorithm*: Sensitivity 87.1% and specificity 48%.[47]
4. *The Bayesian algorithm*: This calculates a score based on 19 morphologic features. Sensitivity 89% and specificity 52%.[52]
5. *The Griffith algorithm*: Sensitivity 94.2% and specificity 39.8%.[51]

"Head-to-head" comparison of several electrocardiographic methods for broad complex tachycardia differentiation suggested that the newer algorithms/criteria were not more accurate than the classic Brugada algorithm.[54] As such, no one algorithm/criterion can be recommended as a preferred method for broad complex tachycardia diagnosis. It may be best that physicians should select the algorithm with which they are most familiar.

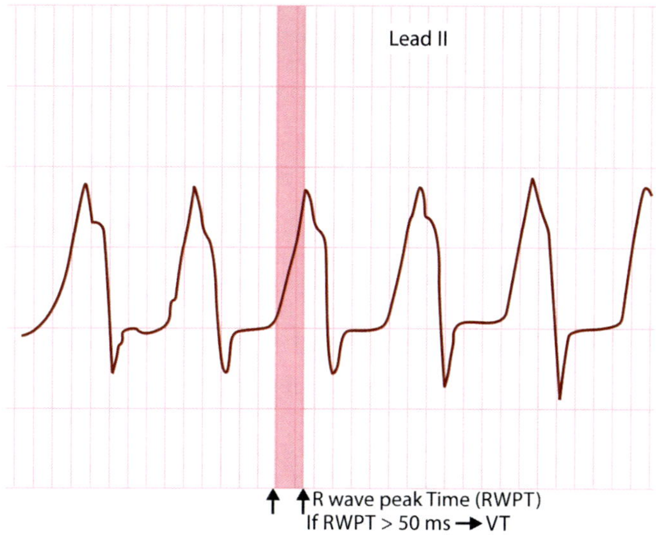

Fig. 12.23: During electrocardiogram evaluation of broad complex tachycardias, ventricular tachycardia may be differentiated from supraventricular tachycardia by measuring the R wave peak time in LII. If the RWPT is greater than or equal to 50 ms, the likelihood of a VT is very high.

SUMMARY

Broad complex tachycardia is defined as

- Heart rate is greater than 100 beats/min
- Duration of QRS is greater than 0.12 seconds (>120 ms).

The differentiation between supraventricular and ventricular origin of the arrhythmia is important to guide therapy. Several algorithms have been developed to aid in this differentiation. It is important to keep in mind that a good estimate of VT versus SVT can be made based on the clinical vignette. Older patient with previous MI with broad complex tachycardia, the most likely diagnosis is VT but in younger patient with known paroxysmal tachycardias and who is hemodynamically to stable, the most likely diagnosis is SVT with aberrancy or BBB. VT is the most common cause of broad complex tachycardia.

Important causes of broad-complex tachycardia include (Box 12.1):

- Ventricular tachycardia
- Supraventricular tachycardia with BBB
- Supraventricular tachycardia with antegrade conduction over an accessory pathway (preexcited tachycardia)
- Congenital heart disease
- Drug toxicities
- Electrolyte imbalances

Ventricular tachycardia refers to a broad QRS complex tachycardia (QRS duration >120 ms) originating in the ventricles at a rate of greater than 100 bpm (Box 12.2). This can be hemodynamically unstable causing severe hypotension and thus can be life-threatening. VF, asystole, and SCD can occur soon after VT, if necessary measures are not taken immediately.

Box 12.1: Three common diagnostic possibilities of broad complex tachycardia.

Broad complex tachycardia—three common diagnostic possibilities:
1. Ventricular tachycardia
2. Supraventricular tachycardia with aberrant conduction due to BBB
3. Supraventricular tachycardia with aberrant conduction due to the WPW syndrome.

Patterns of Ventricular Rhythms

- *Ventricular escape*: Ventricular rhythm with rates less than 40 bpm.
- *Accelerated idioventricular rhythm*: Ventricular rhythm with a rate of between 40 bpm and 100 bpm. AIVR is also referred as "slow VT."
- *Ventricular tachycardia*: Ventricular rhythm with rates faster than 100 bpm.

Mechanism of Ventricular Tachycardia

- Reentry phenomenon
- Enhanced automaticity, which may be spontaneous or triggered.

The tachycardia is usually initiated by an extrasystole and involves two pathways of conduction with differing electrical properties. The reentry circuits that support VT can be "micro" or "macro" in scale and often occur in the zone of ischemia or fibrosis surrounding damaged myocardium. VT may result from direct damage to the myocardium secondary to ischemia or cardiomyopathy, or from the effects of myocarditis or drugs—for example, class 1 antiarrhythmics (such as flecainide, quinidine, and disopyramide). Monomorphic VT usually occurs after MI and is a sign of extensive myocardial damage.

Causes of Ventricular Tachycardia

1. Acute MI or ischemia
2. Post MI
3. Dilated cardiomyopathy
4. Hypertrophic cardiomyopathy
5. Myocarditis
6. Arrhythmogenic right ventricular dysplasia/cardiomyopathy
7. Mitral valve prolapse
8. Rheumatic valvular heart disease
9. Postcardiac surgery
10. Idiopathic.

Ventricular tachycardia can be categorized as follows (Box 12.3):

- *Nonsustained VT*: Three or more ventricular beats with a maximal duration of 30 seconds.
- *Sustained VT*: A VT of more than 30 seconds duration.
- *Monomorphic VT*: All ventricular beats have the same configuration in the same lead. Monomorphic VT is the most common form of sustained VT.

Box 12.2: Definition of ventricular tachycardia.

Ventricular tachycardia is defined as:
- Greater than or equal to three consecutive premature ventricular complexes with
- QRS duration greater than 0.12 seconds (120 ms) and
- Rate greater than 100 bpm.

Box 12.3: Types of ventricular tachycardia.

Types of VT are:
- *Nonsustained*: Three or more consecutive ventricular complexes terminating spontaneously in less than 30 seconds.
- *Sustained*: Duration is greater than 30 seconds or requiring intervention due to hemodynamic compromise.

- *Polymorphic VT*: The ventricular beats have a changing configuration. May be of irregular rhythm, with beat-to-beat variation in QRS complexes.

Polymorphic VT is either *torsades de pointes* (associated with a long QT on the baseline 12-lead ECG) or non-*torsades* (usually associated with ischemia or other organic heart disease).

Torsades de pointes is an uncommon and distinctive form of polymorphic VT characterized by a gradual change in the amplitude and twisting of the QRS complexes around the isoelectric line. Torsades de pointes is associated with a prolonged QT interval, which may be congenital or acquired. By definition torsades de pointes is paroxysmal and nonsustained. This arrhythmia often has a rate above 200 bpm, and usually lasts 5–20 cycles. Interestingly torsades de pointes frequently develops in the setting of bradycardia with preceding prolonged QT interval. This arrhythmia may terminate spontaneously but frequently recurs and may degenerate into VF.

- *Bidirectional VT*: A VT with a QRS complex that alternates from beat to beat with change in axis. Associated with digoxin intoxication and long QT syndrome.

Patterns of Ventricular Tachycardia

Regular

- Monomorphic VT
- Fascicular VT
- Right ventricular outflow tract tachycardia.

Irregular

- Polymorphic VT
- Torsades de pointes tachycardia.

Morphological Criteria for Ventricular Tachycardia

Leads V1-2 may be assessed for characteristic features of VT. There are two sets of morphological criteria depending on the appearance of the QRS complex in V1:

1. If there is a dominant R wave in V1 → VT with RBBB-like morphology.

2. If there is a dominant S wave in V1 → VT with LBBB-like morphology.

Broad Complex Tachycardias due to Supraventricular Tachycardia with Aberrancy

Supraventricular tachycardia with aberrancy may manifest as broad complex tachycardia. Two important causes of SVT manifesting as broad complex tachycardia are:

1. Supraventricular tachycardia with aberrant conduction due to BBB
2. Supraventricular tachycardia with aberrant conduction due to the WPW syndrome.

Unfortunately, the electrocardiographic differentiation of VT from SVT with aberrancy is not always possible (Box 12.4). It must be remembered that 80% of broad complex tachycardias are VTs and a minority are actually SVTs. However, it is important to remember that at the bedside, if it is difficult to differentiate between the two; all such rhythms must be taken as VT and treated as such.

Electrocardiogram Difference between Ventricular Tachycardia and Supraventricular Tachycardia with Aberrant Conduction

- Atrioventricular dissociation with a ventricular rate faster than the atrial rate generally proves the diagnosis of VT but is clearly discernible in only 20–50% of all VTs.
  - Dissociation means that the atria are being driven by one pacemaker (usually the sinus node) while the ventricles are being driven by an ectopic rhythm in the junction or in the ventricles. The two rhythms are independent. This is an important ECG finding in the diagnosis of VT. Usually ECG shows discernible independent P waves marching through the ventricular complexes. But sometimes the dissociated P waves are obvious and sometimes not.
- Fusion beats are pathognomonic of VT. Fusion beats occur when a sinus and ventricular beat coincides to produce a hybrid complex.
- Capture beats occur when the SA node transiently "captures" the ventricles, in the midst of AV dissociation, to produce a QRS complex of normal duration. Presence of capture beat is suggestive of VT.

Box 12.4: Electrocardiogram features suggesting ventricular tachycardia.

A broad QRS tachycardia is VT until proven otherwise. Important ECG features suggesting VT include:

- Evidence of AV dissociation
- Capture or fusion beats
- Very wide QRS complexes (>140 ms)
- QRS concordance (chest leads all positive or negative)
- Extreme left axis deviation.

- *Width of the QRS Complex*: A QRS width of more than 0.14 seconds (140 ms) with RBBB morphology or 0.16 seconds (160 ms) during LBBB pattern of tachycardia favors VT.
- *QRS concordance*: Positive or negative concordance throughout the chest leads, i.e. leads V1-6 show entirely positive (R) or entirely negative (QS) complexes, with no RS complexes seen, is suggestive of VT.
  - A QRS pattern with negative concordance in the precordial leads is diagnostic for VT ("negative concordance" means that the QRS patterns in all of the precordial leads are similar, and with QS complexes). Positive concordance also suggests VT but does not exclude the possibility of antidromic AVRT over a left posterior accessory pathway.
- Extreme left axis deviation is more likely to be VT.
- QR complexes indicate a myocardial scar and are present in approximately 40% of patients with VTs after MI.
- When there are two positive peaks in lead V1, VT is very likely if the left peak is taller and if the right peak is taller, SVT with aberrancy is the probable diagnosis (Box 12.5). This ECG change in lead V1 is called *Rabbit ear sign*.

Box 12.5: Morphological criteria for VT /SVT with aberrancy in leads V1-2 and V6 in broad complex tachycardia.

RBBB Morphology: Dominant R Wave in V1 or V2

Lead V1 morphology consistent with VT:

- Notched downslope of the R wave, the taller left rabbit ear (Marriott's sign positive) >VT
- Monophasic R wave in V1 >VT
- A qR complex (small Q wave, tall R wave) in V1 >VT
- RBBB morphology with 'good rabbit' with a taller right peak >SVT with RBBB aberrancy. But possibility of VT to be excluded by observing the QRS morphology in V6. Look at the QRS complex of V6:
  - QS complex in V6—a completely negative complex with no R wave > suggestive of VT
  - rS complex in V6 with r/S ratio <1—small R wave, deep S wave >VT only if left axis deviation is also present
  - RBBB morphology in V1 with a taller right peak and no QS or rS pattern in V6 >SVT with aberrancy.

LBBB Morphology: Dominant S Wave in V1 or V2

Lead V1 morphology consistent with VT:

With a dominant S wave in V1, the following three features are diagnostic of VT:

- Initial R wave >30 ms duration.
- Notching or slurring of the S wave (Josephson's sign).
- RS interval (time from R wave onset to S wave nadir) >70 ms.

Appearance of QRS complex in V6 in LBBB morphology

With a LBBB-pattern broad complex tachycardia, the presence of Q waves in V6 is indicative of VT. There are two possible patterns:

- QS waves in V6 >VT
- qR pattern in V6 (small Q wave, large R wave) >VT.

Conversely, SVT with LBBB is associated with absent Q waves in V6.

- *Brugada's sign*: If the distance from the onset of the QRS complex to the nadir of the S wave is greater than 100 ms, then VT is the most likely diagnosis.

Ventricular Fibrillation

Ventricular fibrillation is a leading cause of SCD. In VF, irregular electrical activity renders the ventricles unable to contract in a synchronized manner, resulting in immediate loss of cardiac output and the heart is no longer an effective pump. Unless cardiopulmonary resuscitation is rapidly instituted, this rhythm is invariably fatal. Important causes of VF are acute coronary syndromes, electrolyte imbalance, cardiomyopathies (dilated, hypertrophic or restrictive), long QT (acquired/congenital), and Brugada syndrome, etc.
Electrocardiogram criteria of VF are:

- Chaotic irregular electrical deflections of varying amplitude.
- No identifiable P waves, QRS complexes, or T waves on surface ECG
- Amplitude decreases with duration and coarse VF converts into fine VF.
- Heart rate is difficult to measure but on ECG tracing usually varies from 150 bpm to 500 bpm.

REFERENCES

1. Wellens HJJ. Ventricular tachycardia: diagnosis of broad QRS complex tachycardia. Heart. 2001;86(5):579-85.
2. Edhouse J, Morris F. Broad complex tachycardia—Part I. BMJ. 2002;324(7339):666-722.
3. Ray IB. Wide complex tachycardia: recognition and management in the emergency room. JAPI. 2004;52:882-7.
4. Sacher F, Tedrow UB, Field ME, et al. Ventricular tachycardia ablation: evolution of patients and procedures over 8 years. Circ Arrhythm Electrophysiol. 2008;1(3):153-61.
5. Roberts-Thomson KC, Lau DH, Sanders P. The diagnosis and management of ventricular arrhythmias. Nat Rev Cardiol. 2011;8(6):311-21.
6. de Bakker JM, van Capeiie FJ, Janse MJ, et al. Slow conduction in the infarcted human heart. 'Zigzag' course of activation. Circulation. 1993;88(3):915-26.
7. Peters NS, Coromilas J, Severs NJ, et al. Disturbed connexin43 gap junction distribution correlates with the location of reentrant circuits in the epicardial border zone of healing canine infarcts that cause ventricular tachycardia. Circulation. 1997;95(4):988-96.
8. Haqqani HM, Kalman JM, Roberts-Thomson KC, et al. Fundamental differences in electrophysiologic and electroanatomic substrate between ischemic cardiomyopathy patients with and without clinical ventricular tachycardia. J Am Coll Cardiol. 2009;54(2):166-73.
9. Calkins H, Epstein A, Packer D, et al. Catheter ablation of ventricular tachycardia in patients with structural heart disease using cooled radiofrequency energy: results of a prospective multicenter study. Cooled RF Multi Center investigators Group. J Am Coll Cardiol. 2000;35(7):1905-14.
10. Stevenson WG, Wilber DJ, Natale A, et al. Irrigated radiofrequency catheter ablation guided by electroanatomic mapping for recurrent ventricular tachycardia after myocardial infarction: the multicenter thermocool ventricular tachycardia ablation trial. Circulation. 2008;118(25): 2773-82.
11. Mountantonakis SE, Park RE, Frankel DS, et al. Relationship between Voltage Map "Channels" and the Location of Critical Isthmus Sites in Patients With Post-Infarction Cardiomyopathy and Ventricular Tachycardia. J Am Coll Cardiol. 2013;61(20):2088-95.
12. Cohen TJ, Chien WW, Lurie KG, et al. Radiofrequency catheter ablation for treatment of bundle branch reentrant ventricular tachycardia: results and long-term follow-up. J Am Coll Cardiol. 1991;18(7):1767-73.
13. Thies KC, Boos K, Müller-Deile K, et al. Ventricular flutter in a neonate--severe electrolyte imbalance caused by urinary tract infection in the presence of urinary tract malformation. J Emerg Med. 2000;18(1):47-50.
14. Hayashi M, Murata M, Satoh M, et al. Sudden nocturnal death in young males from ventricular flutter. Jpn Heart J. 1985;26(4):585-91.
15. Gurevitz O, Viskin S, Glikson M, et al. Long-term prognosis of inducible ventricular flutter: not an innocent finding. Am Heart J. 2004:147(4):649-54.
16. Viskin S, Ish-Shalom M, Koifman E, et al. Ventricular flutter induced during electrophysiologic studies in patients with old myocardial infarction: clinical and electrophysiologic predictors, and prognostic significance. J Cardiovasc Electrophysiol. 2003;14(9):913-9.
17. Francis J, Venugopal K, Gupta AK. Idiopathic fascicular ventricular tachycardia. Indian Pacing Electrophysiol J. 2004;4(3):98-103.
18. Lerman BB, Stein KM, Markowitz SM, et al. Ventricular tachycardia in patients with structurally normal hearts. In: Zipes DP, Jaife J (Eds). Cardiac electrophysiology: from cell to bedside, 4th edition. Philadelphia: WB Saunders; 2004, p. 668.
19. Farzaneh-Far A, Lerman BB. Idiopathic ventricular outflow tract tachycardia. Heart. 2005;91(2):136-8.
20. Glassner IW, Kass RS, Clancy CE. Mechanism of genetic arrhythmias: from DNA to ECG. Prog Cardiovasc Dis. 2003;46(3):259-70.
21. Priori SG, Napolitano C, Memmi M, et al. Clinical and molecular characterization of patients with catecholaminergic polymorphic ventricular tachycardia. Circulation. 2002;106(1):69-74.
22. Haissaguerre M, Shah DC, Jais P, et al. Role of Purkinje conducting system in triggering of idiopathic ventricular fibrillation. Lancet. 2002;359(9307):677-8.
23. Lerman BB, Belardinelli L, West GA, et al. Adenosine-sensitive ventricular tachycardia: evidence suggesting cyclic AMP-mediated triggered activity. Circulation. 1986;74(2):270-80.
24. Lerman BB, Stein K, Engelstein ED, et al. Mechanism of repetitive monomorphic ventricular tachycardia. Circulation. 1995;92(3):421-9.
25. Ferguson JD, DiMarco JP. Contemporary management of paroxysmal supraventricular tachycardia. Circulation. 2003;107(8):1096-9.
26. Stewart RB, Bardy GH, Greene HL. Wide complex tachycardia: misdiagnosis and outcome after emergent therapy. Ann Intern Med. 1986;104(6):766-71.
27. Dancy M, Camm AJ, Ward D. Misdiagnosis of chronic recurrent ventricular tachycardia. Lancet. 1985;2(8450):320-3.

28. Biaggioni I, Killian TJ, Mosqueda-Garcia R, et al. Adenosine increases sympathetic nerve traffic in humans. Circulation. 1991;83(5):1668-75.
29. Buxton AE, Marchlinski FE, Doherty JU, et al. Hazards of intravenous verapamil for sustained ventricular tachycardia. Am J Cardiol. 1987;59(12):1107-10.
30. ECC Committee, Subcommittees and Task Forces of the American Heart Association, 2005. American Heart Association Guidelines for Cardiopulmonary Resuscitation and Emergency Cardiovascular Care. Circulation. 2005;112:203-9.
31. Pelleg A, Pennock RS, Kutalek SP. Proarrhythmic effects of adenosine: one decade of clinical data. Am J Ther. 2002;9(2):141-7.
32. Baerman JM, Morady F, DiCarlo LA Jr, et al. Differentiation of ventricular tachycardia from supraventricular tachycardia with aberration: value of the clinical history. Ann Emerg Med. 1987;16(1):40-3.
33. Akhtar M, Shenasa M, Jazayeri M, et al. Wide QRS complex tachycardia. Reappraisal of a common clinical problem. Ann Intern Med. 1988;109(11):905-12.
34. Wellen HJJ, Bar FW, Lie KI. The value of the electrocardiogram in the differential diagnosis of a tachycardia with a widened QRS complex. Am J Med. 1978;64(1):27-33.
35. Kremers MS, Black WH, Wells PJ, et al. Effect of preexisting bundle branch block on the electrocardiographic diagnosis of ventricular tachycardia. Am J Cardiol. 1988;62(17):1208-12.
36. Wellens HJJ, Brugada P. Diagnosis of ventricular tachycardia from the twelve lead electrocardiogram. Cardiol Clin. 1987;5(3):511-25.
37. Wellens HJJ, Bar F, Brugada P, et al. The differentiation between ventricular tachycardia and supraventricular tachycardia with aberrant conduction: the value of the 12 lead electrocardiogram. In: Wellens HJJ, Kulbertus HE (Eds). What's New in Electrocardiography? The Hague: Martinus Nijhoff; 1981. pp. 184-99.
38. Alzand BSN, Crijns HJGM. Diagnostic criteria of broad QRS complex tachycardia: decades of evolution. Europace. 2011;13(4):465-72.
39. Marriott HJ. Differential diagnosis of supraventricular and ventricular tachycardia. Cardiology. 1990;77(3):209-20.
40. Bakker AL, Nijkerk G, Groenemeijer BE, et al. The Lewis lead: making recognition of P waves easy during wide QRS complex tachycardia. Circulation. 2009;119(24):e592-3.
41. Kindwall E, Brown J, Josephson ME. Electrocardiographic criteria for ventricular tachycardia in wide complex left bundle branch block morphology tachycardia. Am J Cardiol. 1988;61(15):1279-83.
42. Coumel P, Leclerq JF, Attuel P, et al. The QRS morphology in post-myocardial infarction ventricular tachycardia. A study of 100 tracings compared with 70 cases of idiopathic ventricular tachycardia. Eur Heart J. 1984;5(10):792-805.
43. Topol E, Wellens HJJ. The electrocardiographic diagnosis of arrhythmias. In: Topol E (Ed). Textbook of cardiovascular medicine. Philadelphia, PA: Lippincott-Raven; 1998. pp. 1591-609.
44. Marriott HJ, Sandler IA. Criteria, old and new, for differentiating between ectopic ventricular beat and aberrant ventricular conduction in the presence of atrial fibrillation. Prog Cardiovasc Dis. 1966;9(1):18-28.
45. Volders PG, Timmermans C, Rodriguez LM, et al. Wide QRS complex tachycardia with negative precordial concordance: always a ventricular origin? J Cardiovasc Electrophysiol. 2003;14(1):109-11.
46. Brugada P, Brugada J, Mont L, et al. A new approach to the differential diagnosis of a regular tachycardia with a wide QRS complex. Circulation. 1991;83(5):1649-59.
47. Vereckei A, Duray G, Szenasi G, et al. Application of a new algorithm in the differential diagnosis of wide QRS complex tachycardia. Eur Heart J. 2007;28(5):589-600.
48. Vereckei A, Duray G, Szenasi G, et al. New algorithm using only lead aVR for differential diagnosis of wide QRS complex tachycardia. Heart Rhythm. 2008;5(1):89-98.
49. Griffith M, de Belder MA, Linker NJ, et al. Multivariate analysis to simplify the differential diagnosis of broad complex tachycardia. Br Heart J. 1991;66(2):166.
50. Griffith M, de Belder MA, Linker NJ, et al. Difficulties in the use of electrocardiographic criteria for the differential diagnosis of left bundle branch block pattern tachycardia in patients with a structurally normal heart. Eur Heart J. 1992;13(4):478-83.
51. Griffith MJ, Garatt CJ, Mounsey P. Ventricular tachycardia as default diagnosis in broad complex tachycardia. Lancet. 1994;343(8894):386-8.
52. Lau EW, Pathamanathan RK, Ng GA, et al. The Bayesian approach improves the electrocardiographic diagnosis of broad complex tachycardia. Pacing Clin Electrophysiol. 2000;23(10 Pt 1):1519-26.
53. Pava LF, Perafan P, Badiel M, et al. R-wave peak time at Lead II: a new criterion for differentiating between wide complex QRS tachycardias. Heart Rhythm. 2010;7(7):922-6.
54. Jastrzebski M, Kukla P, Czarnecka D, et al. Comparison of five electrocardiographic methods for differentiation of wide QRS-complex tachycardias. Europace. 2012;14(8):1165-71.

Chapter 13

Bundle-Branch Block

INTRODUCTION

The electrical activity of heart begins in the sinoatrial node, which is situated on the upper right atrium. The impulse travels next through the left and right atria and summates at the atrioventricular (AV) node through the internodal fibers (Fig. 13.1). From the AV node, the electrical impulse travels down the bundle of His and divides into the right and left bundle branches. The right bundle branch contains one fascicle. The left bundle branch subdivides into two fascicles: (1) The left anterior fascicle and (2) the left posterior fascicle. The thicker left posterior fascicle bifurcates, with one fascicle being in the septal aspect. Ultimately, the fascicles divide into millions of Purkinje fibers which in turn interdigitize with individual cardiac myocytes, allowing for rapid, coordinated, and synchronous physiologic depolarization of the ventricles.

The term intraventricular conduction disturbance refers to abnormalities in the intraventricular propagation of supraventricular impulses that give rise to changes in the shape and/or duration of the QRS complex. These changes in intraventricular conduction may be fixed and present at all heart rates, or they may be intermittent and be tachycardia or bradycardia dependent. They may be caused by structural abnormalities in the His-Purkinje conduction system or ventricular myocardium that result from necrosis, fibrosis, calcification, infiltrative lesions, or impaired vascular supply.[1]

When a bundle branch or fascicle becomes affected due to underlying degenerative or coronary artery disease, it may cease to conduct electrical impulses appropriately. This results in altered pathways for ventricular depolarization. Since the electrical impulse can no longer use the preferred pathway across the bundle branch, it may move instead through muscle fibers in a way that both slows the electrical movement and changes the directional propagation of the impulses. As a result, there is a loss of ventricular synchrony and ventricular depolarization is prolonged.

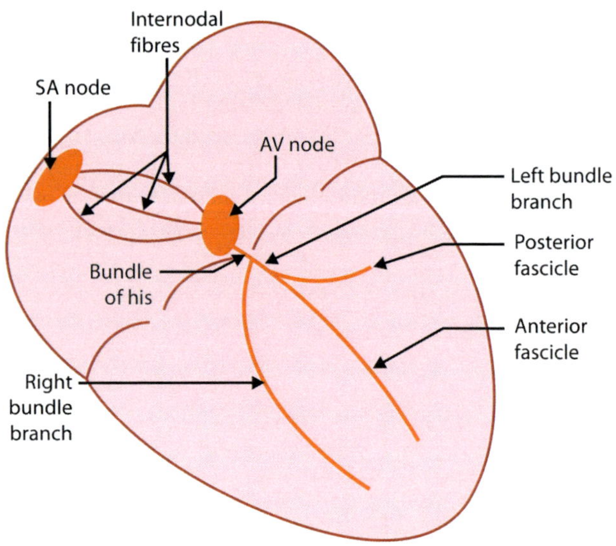

Fig. 13.1: Diagram showing conductive system of heart.

BUNDLE-BRANCH BLOCK: BASIC PRINCIPLES

Normally both right and left ventricles are depolarized simultaneously. Bundle branch block (BBB) is caused by a conduction defect in the right or in the left bundle branch. The blocked bundle branch delays the conduction of the depolarization wave to the ventricle that it supplies. So, in BBB, the unblocked bundle conducts impulse normally but impulse transmission in the blocked bundle proceeds slowly through the surrounding muscle to stimulate the bundle branch below the level of block. After this delay, depolarization impulse proceeds normally below the block. For this delayed conduction in BBB, both the ventricles cannot be depolarized simultaneously. In fact in BBB, one ventricle is depolarized slightly later than the other. So, two fused wave forms are reflected in the QRS complexes of patients with BBB. First part of the QRS complex is due to normal conduction in the unblocked ventricle and second part is due to delayed conduction in the blocked ventricle. So, "joined QRS" complexes appear on ECG

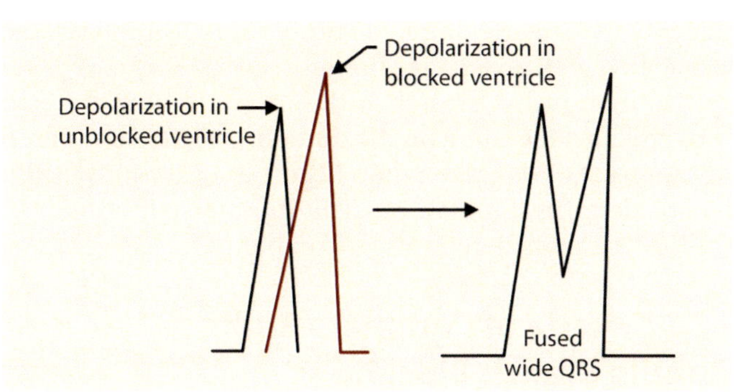

Fig. 13.2: Diagram showing "fused QRS" complex in bundle branch block (BBB). In BBB, the unblocked ventricle depolarizes normally but blocked ventricle depolarizes slightly later and both the waves fuse together producing a joined QRS (large arrow), which appears widened on electrocardiogram (ECG) paper.

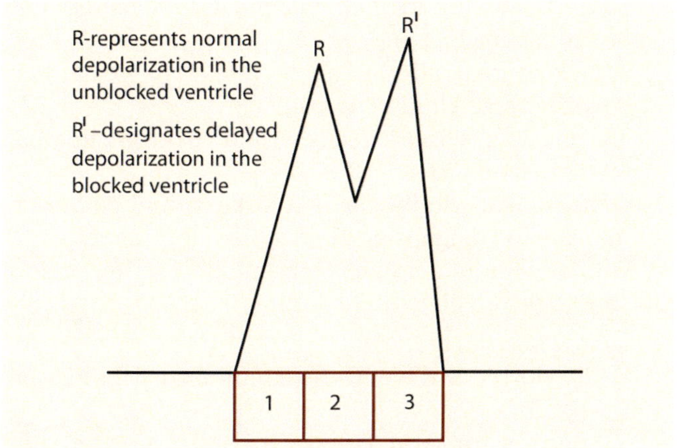

Fig. 13.3: In BBB, QRS becomes widened and duration is usually greater than 120 ms (0.12 seconds) which is more than three small squares on the ECG paper (1, 2, and 3 designates three small squares on the ECG paper). "R" indicates normal impulse conduction in the unblocked ventricle and R' represents delayed conduction in the blocked ventricle.

(Fig. 13.2). Due to fusion of two depolarization waves, in BBB the QRS duration is widened, usually greater than 0.12 seconds (120 ms), which is greater than three small squares on ECG paper (Fig. 13.3). Two "R" waves appear on ECG tracing, "R" designates normal conduction in the unblocked ventricle and R' indicates the delayed conduction through the blocked ventricle. In left bundle branch block (LBBB), the depolarization of the left ventricle is delayed and in right bundle branch block (RBBB) the depolarization of the right ventricle is delayed. In LBBB, left ventricular (LV) depolarization is delayed but right ventricular (RV) depolarization occurs normally. So "R" indicates normal RV depolarization and "R'" represents delayed LV depolarization. In RBBB, LV depolarizes normally, so "R" represents normal LV depolarization and "R'" represents delayed RV depolarization (Fig. 13.4).

TYPES OF BUNDLE-BRANCH BLOCKS

Depending on the anatomical location of the defect which leads to a BBB, the blocks are further classified into:

- Right bundle branch block
- Left bundle branch block

The LBBB can be further subclassified into:

- *Left anterior hemiblock (LAHB)*: In this case only the anterior half of the left bundle branch (fascicle) is involved.
- *Left posterior hemiblock (LPHB)*: Only the posterior part of the left bundle branch is involved.

Other classifications of BBBs are:

Bifascicular block: This is a combination of RBBB and either LAHB or LPHB.

Trifascicular block: This is a combination of RBBB with either LAHB or LPHB together with a first degree AV block.

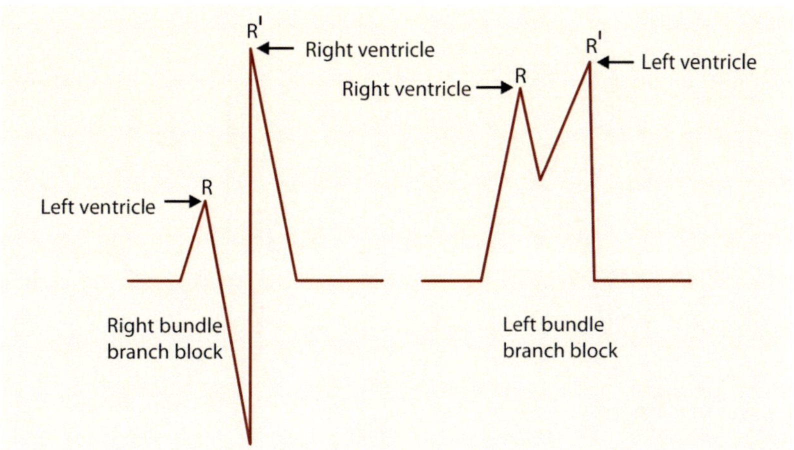

Fig. 13.4: Diagram showing pattern of depolarization in BBB. In right bundle branch block (RBBB), right ventricular depolarization is delayed and in left bundle branch block (LBBB), left ventricular depolarization is delayed, so two depolarization waves (R and R') fuse together to produce a wide QRS complex on ECG (arrows).

RIGHT BUNDLE BRANCH BLOCK

When conduction in the right bundle branch is blocked, depolarization of the right ventricle is delayed. The left ventricle depolarizes in the normal way and thus the early part of the QRS complex appears normal. The wave of depolarization then spreads to the right ventricle through nonspecialized conducting tissue, with slow depolarization of the right ventricle in a left to right direction. As LV depolarization is complete, the forces of RV depolarization are unopposed. Thus the later part of the QRS complex is abnormal; the right precordial leads have a prominent and late R-wave, and the left precordial and limb leads have a terminal S-wave. These terminal deflections are wide and slurred (Figs. 13.5A and B). Presence of RSR' pattern in V1–V3, broad QRS >120 ms (0.12 seconds), along with slurred S-wave in the lateral leads (I, aVL, and V5–6) are suggestive of RBBB (Figs. 13.6A and B). Abnormal ventricular depolarization is associated with secondary repolarization changes, giving rise to changes in the ST-T waves in the right chest leads (Fig. 13.7).[2]

Right bundle branch block is generally considered as a benign finding that does not imply increased risk when found in asymptomatic healthy individuals.[3-5] The prevalence of RBBB is known to increase with age, to be higher in men, diabetics, and in patients with hypertension.[4,6-8] The prevalence of RBBB is approximately twice as high in men as in women and was highly age-dependent ranging from 0.6% in women below the age of 40 to 14.3% in men above the age of 80.[3,9,10] The higher prevalence of RBBB in men compared with women was not caused by differences in risk factor distribution and remains largely unexplained.[11] RBBB may also indicate affection of the right side of the heart through cor pulmonale, myocardial ischemia/infarction, pulmonary embolism, myocarditis, or congenital heart disease. Among patients with heart failure, the presence of RBBB has been associated with an adverse prognosis.[12,13]

Right bundle branch block may be complete or incomplete depending on the duration of QRS complex. If duration of QRS is greater than 120 ms (0.12 seconds) RBBB is considered as complete but if the duration is less than 120 ms RBBB is considered to be incomplete.

ECG Criteria of Complete Right Bundle Branch Block[1]

1. QRS duration is greater than or equal to 120 ms in adults, greater than 100 ms in children ages 4–16 years, and greater than 90 ms in children less than 4 years of age.
2. rsR', Rsr', or rSR' in leads V1 or V2. The R' or r' deflection is usually wider than the initial R-wave. In a minority of patients, a wide and often notched R-wave pattern may be seen in lead V1 and/or V2.
3. S-wave of greater duration than R-wave or greater than 40 ms in leads I and V6 in adults.
4. Normal R peak time in leads V5 and V6 but greater than 50 ms in lead V1.

   Of the above criteria, the first three should be present to make the diagnosis. When a pure dominant R-wave with or without a notch is present in V1, criterion four should be satisfied.

Associated features of RBBB

1. Wide, slurred S-wave in the lateral leads (I, aVL, and V5–6).
2. ST depression and T-wave inversion in the right precordial leads (V1–3).

Sometimes rather than an RSR' pattern in V1, there may be a monophasic R-wave (Fig. 13.8) or a qR complex (Fig. 13.9).

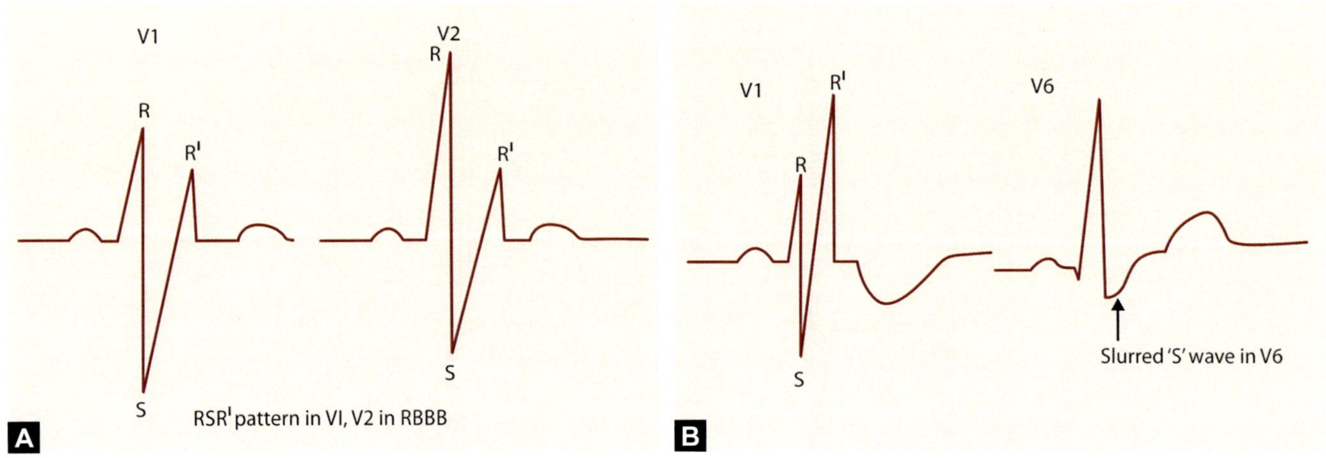

Figs. 13.5A and B: (A) Diagram showing RSR' pattern wide QRS complex in right precordial leads V1 and V2, which is suggestive of RBBB. (B) Diagram showing RSR' pattern wide QRS complex in V1 along with slurred and wide S wave in lead V6, which are suggestive of RBBB. RSR' pattern QRS in V1–V3 along with wide and slurred S wave in the lateral leads (I, aVL, and V5–6) are typical ECG features of RBBB.

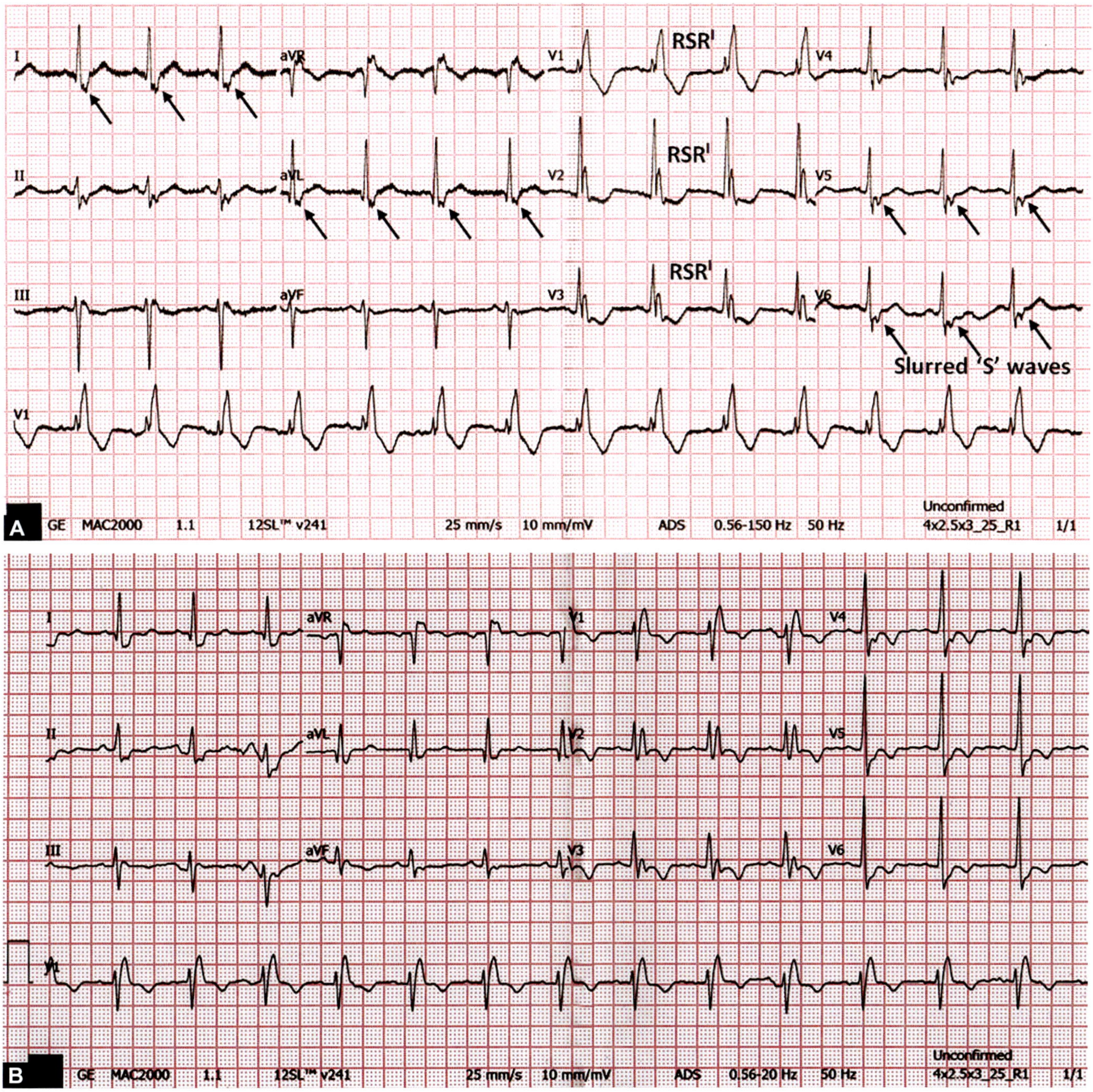

Figs. 13.6A and B: (A) Electrocardiogram showing typical features of complete RBBB. RSR' pattern wide QRS complex (QRS is 146 ms) in V1–V3 along with slurred and wide S-waves in lateral leads LI, aVL, and V5–V6 (arrows). (B) Electrocardiogram showing typical features of complete RBBB. Note RSR' pattern wide QRS complex (QRS is 166 ms) in V1–V3 along with slurred and wide S waves in lateral leads LI, aVL, and V5–V6.

Incomplete Right Bundle Branch Block

Whereas complete RBBB patterns are relatively rare in electrocardiograms in the general population, incomplete RBBB (IRBBB), with a near normal duration of the QRS complex, is a common finding. Most persons with IRBBB have no clinical evidence of structural heart disease and IRBBB is seen relatively frequently in healthy young athletes.[14] Incomplete RBBB is thus regarded as a benign condition but IRBBB has a considerably higher likelihood of developing complete RBBB at follow-up.[14,15] This ECG pattern is also commonly seen in patients with ASD.

ECG Criteria of Incomplete Right Bundle Branch Block[1]

Incomplete RBBB is defined by RSR' pattern in V1-V3 along with QRS duration between 110 ms and 120 ms in

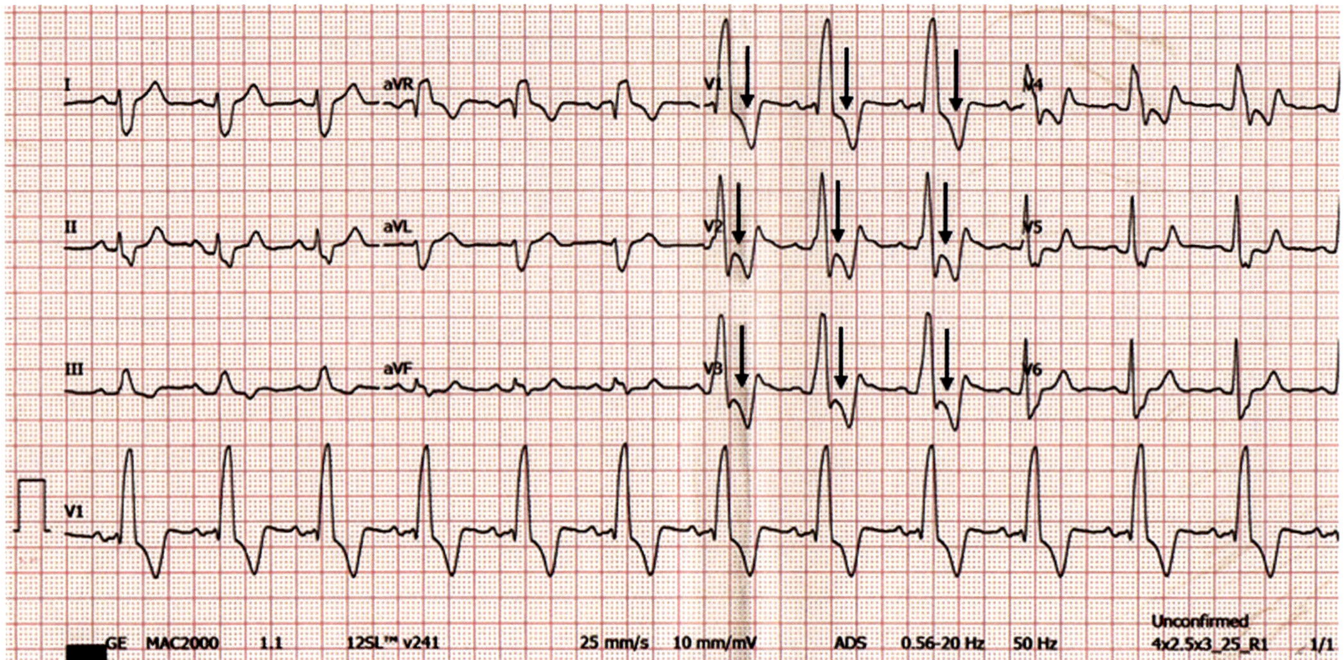

Fig. 13.7: Electrocardiogram showing typical features of complete RBBB with rSR' pattern wide QRS complex (QRS is 170 ms) in V1–V3 along with slurred and wide S waves in lateral leads LI, aVL, and V5–V6. Note marked ST-segment depression and T-wave inversions in right precordial leads V1–V3 (arrows).

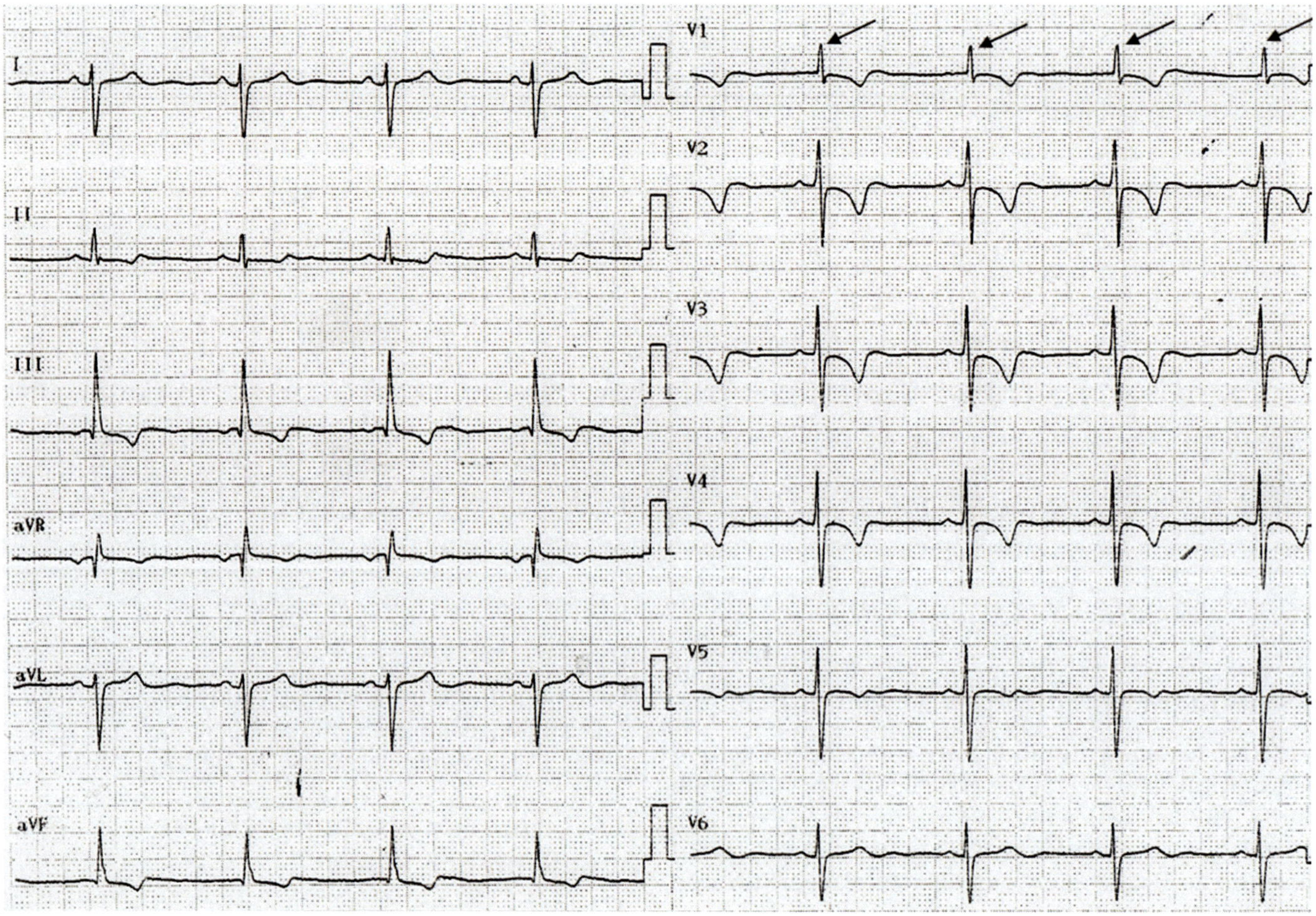

Fig. 13.8: Electrocardiogram is suggestive of incomplete RBBB with monophasic R-wave in V1. Note deep S waves in lateral leads along with secondary ST-segment depression and T-wave inversions in leads V1–V4 but QRS is not widened. This pattern of ECG may be confused with normal variant ECG, commonly seen in children of no clinical significance.

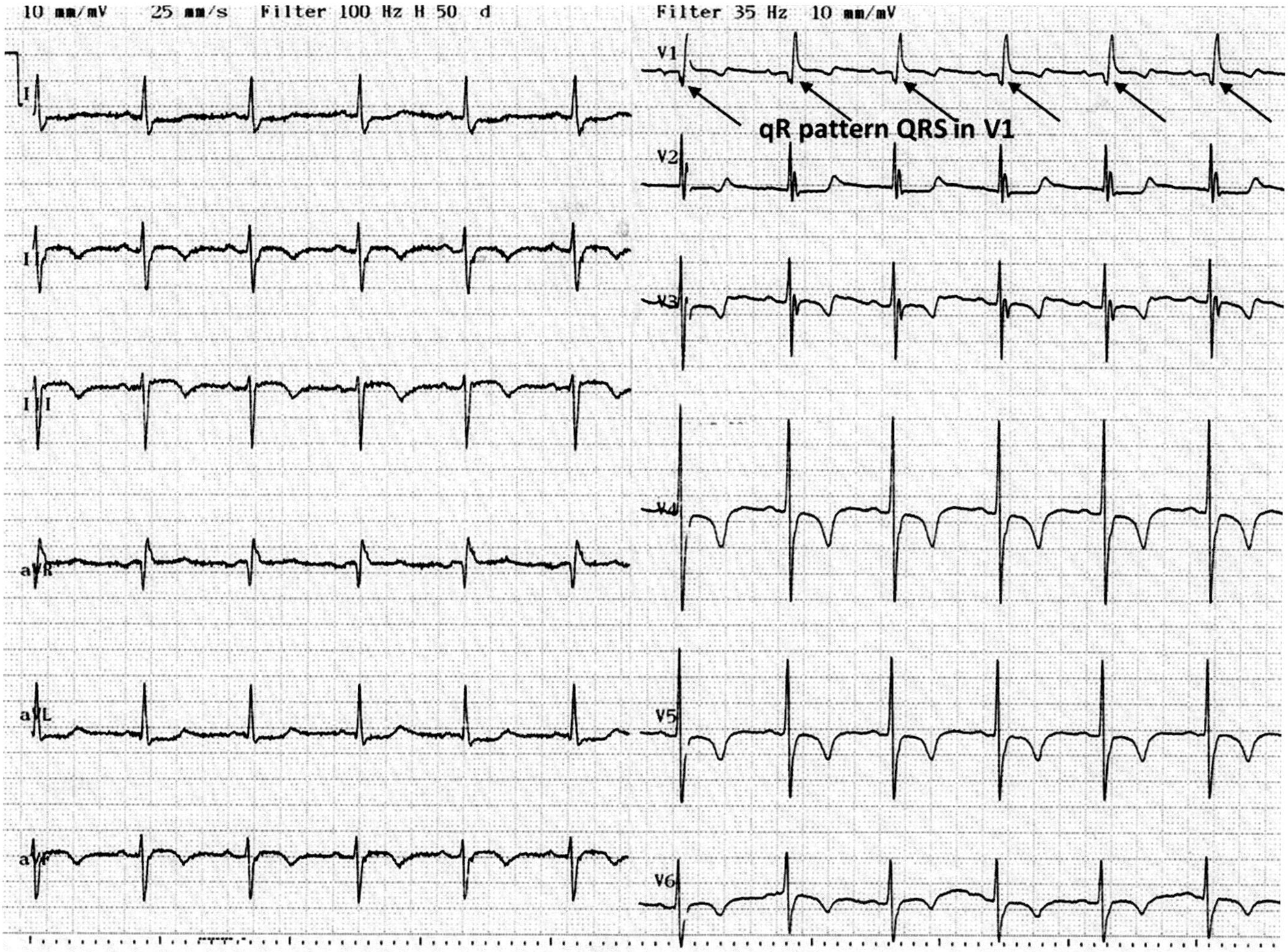

Fig. 13.9: Electrocardiogram is suggestive of RBBB with qR pattern QRS (*arrows*) in V1 (QRS is 120 ms). Note slurred and deep S waves in lateral leads along with secondary ST-segment depression and T inversions in chest leads.

adults, between 90 ms and 100 ms in children between 8 years and 16 years of age, and between 86 ms and 90 ms in children less than 8 years of age. Other criteria are the same as for complete RBBB (Figs. 13.10A and B).

LEFT BUNDLE BRANCH BLOCK

In LBBB, activation of the left ventricle is delayed, which causes the left ventricle to contract later than the right ventricle. The intraventricular conduction system of the left ventricle is composed of fibers of the bundle of His that become the main left bundle branch and then divide into anterior and posterior fascicles, further branching to become the distal conduction system. In contrast to the right bundle branch, which is a discrete structure that can be acutely injured with a small focal insult, the left bundle branch is a large and diffuse structure that typically requires a large insult to lead to acute injury.[16]

Left bundle branch block may be the result of an aging and/or fibrotic conduction system, chronic ischemic heart disease, acute coronary syndrome (ACS), left ventricular hypertrophy (most commonly from long-standing hypertension), adverse ventricular remodeling from congestive heart failure, or valvular heart disease.[17] Patients with a suspected ACS in the setting of LBBB, present an important diagnostic and therapeutic challenge to the clinician. Not only is the ECG diagnosis of acute myocardial infarction (AMI) difficult due to "masking" of characteristic ECG changes by altered ventricular depolarization, but these patients may be at higher risk for arrhythmia, congestive heart failure, and death compared with patients without LBBB.[18-20] When a new LBBB is caused by AMI, the site of infarction is usually anterior or anteroseptal, with the infarction involving a large myocardial territory.[21] Inferior or posterior infarctions may uncommonly result in a new LBBB from involvement of the more proximal portion of the conduction system supplied by the AV nodal artery. However, the majority of LBBB in AMI are not a result of focal infarctions since either a discrete lesion just distal to the bundle of His or extensive myocardial damage involving a large portion of the distal conduction system including both fascicles would be required to cause LBBB.[17,21]

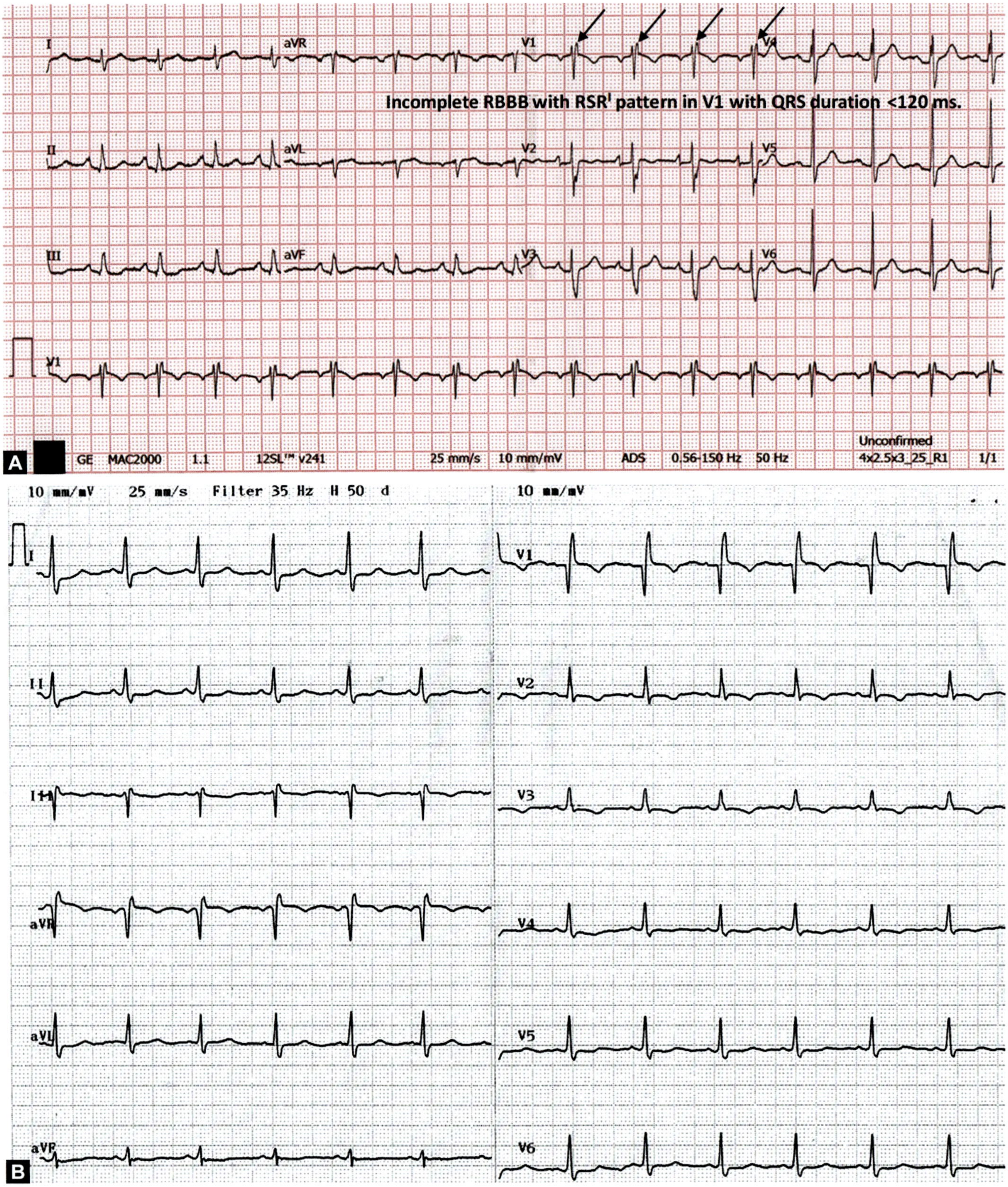

Figs. 13.10A and B: (A) Electrocardiogram illustrates the features of incomplete RBBB with RSR' pattern QRS in V1 (arrows) but QRS duration is less than 120 ms. Also note the slurred and deep S waves in lateral leads. (B) Electrocardiogram illustrates the features of incomplete RBBB with QR pattern QRS in V1 and the QRS duration is 116 ms. Note the slurred S waves in lateral leads.

Normally the septum is activated from left to right, producing small Q waves in the lateral leads. In LBBB, the normal direction of septal depolarization is reversed (becomes right to left), as the impulse spreads first to the RV via the right bundle branch and then to the LV via the septum. This sequence of activation increases the QRS duration to greater than 120 ms and eliminates the normal septal Q waves in the lateral leads. The overall direction of depolarization (from right to left) produces tall R waves in the lateral leads (I, aVL, and V5–V6) and deep S waves in the right precordial leads (V1–V3). The QRS complex in V1 may be either: rS complex (small R-wave, deep S-wave) or QS complex (deep Q/S-wave with no preceding R-wave) (Fig. 13.11). As the ventricles are activated sequentially (right, then left) rather than simultaneously, this produces a broad or notched ("M"-shaped) R-wave in the lateral leads (Fig. 13.12).

ECG Criteria of Left Bundle Branch Block[1]

Complete Left Bundle Branch Block (Fig. 13.13)

- QRS duration greater than or equal to 120 ms (0.12 seconds) in adults, greater than 100 ms in children 4–16 years of age, and greater than 90 ms in children less than 4 years of age.
- Broad, notched or slurred R-wave (M pattern) in leads I, aVL, V5, and V6 and an occasional RS pattern in

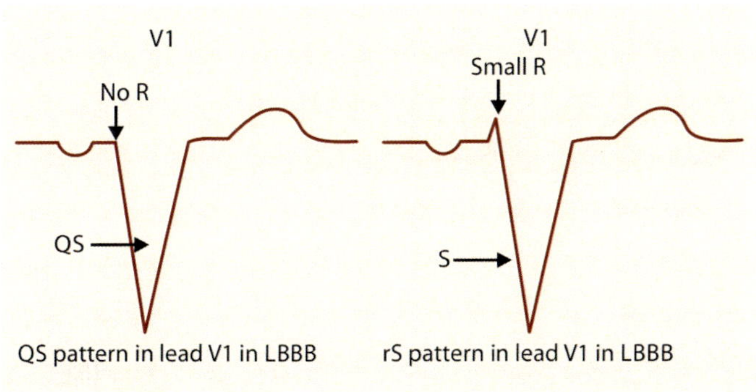

Fig. 13.11: Diagram shows typical QRS complex morphology in lead V1 in LBBB on ECG. The QRS complex in V1 may be either: rS complex (small R wave, deep S wave) (right panel) or QS complex (deep Q/S wave with no preceding R wave) (left panel).

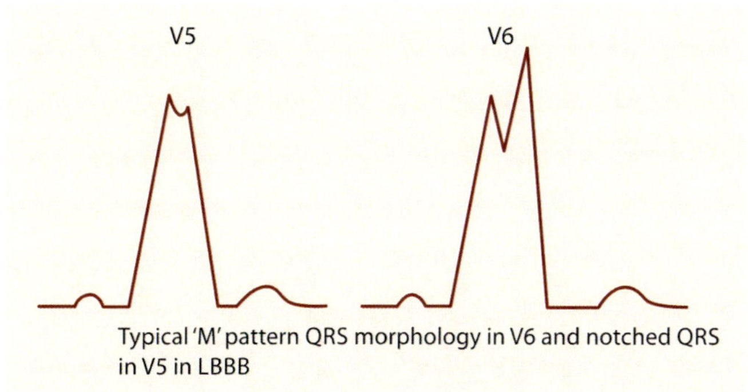

Fig. 13.12: Diagram showing typical "M" pattern morphology of QRS complex in leads V5 and V6 in LBBB. As the ventricles are activated sequentially (right, then left) rather than simultaneously, this produces a broad or notched ("M"-shaped) R wave in the lateral leads.

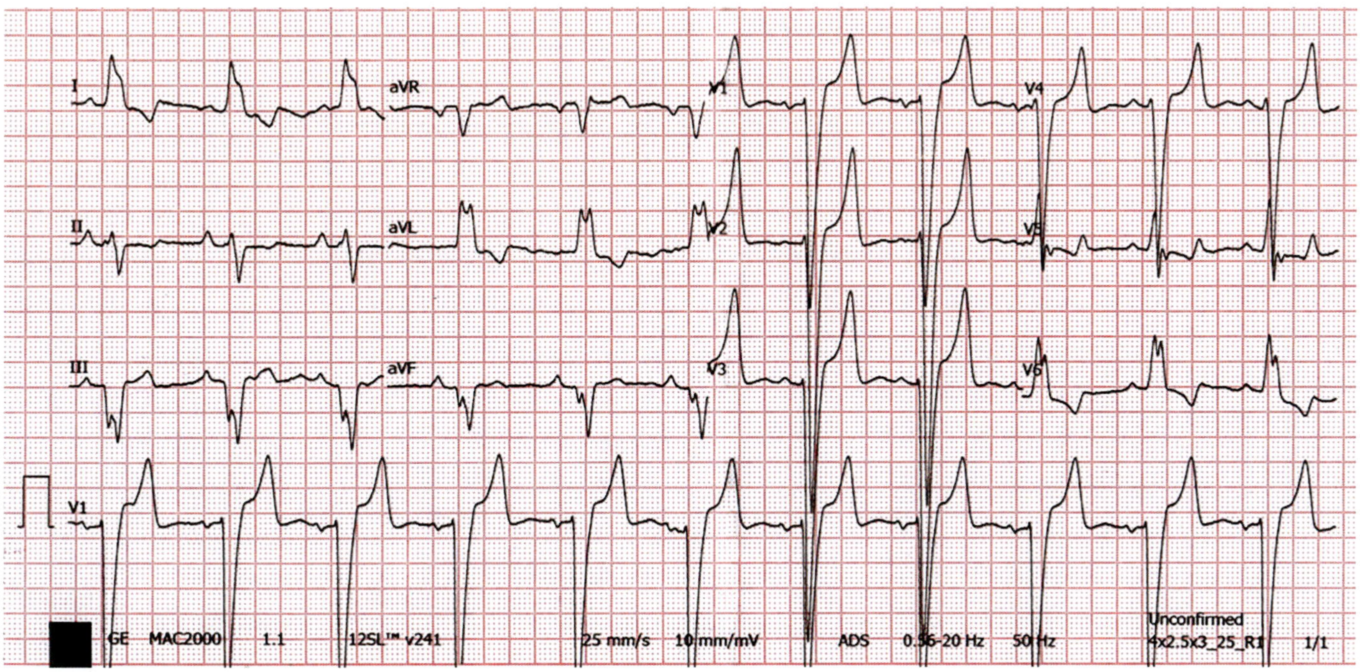

Fig. 13.13: Electrocardiogram showing typical ECG features of complete LBBB. Note (1) broad biphasic (M pattern) QRS complex (QRS is 170 ms) in aVL and V6, and notched QRS in L1; (2) rS morphology with poor R-wave progression in chest leads; (3) left axis deviation (dominant R wave in LI and aVL with negative QRS complex in LII, LIII, and aVF); (4) absent normal septal Q waves in leads I, aVL, V5, and V6; (5) ST and T waves are opposite in direction to QRS.

V5 and V6 attributed to displaced transition of QRS complex along with dominant S-wave in V1 with QS or rS configuration of QRS complex (Figs. 13.14A to C).

- Absent normal septal Q waves in leads I, V5, and V6, but in the lead aVL, a narrow Q-wave may be present in the absence of myocardial pathology.
- R peak time greater than 60 ms in leads V5 and V6 but normal in leads V1, V2, and V3, when small initial R waves can be discerned in the above leads.
- ST and T waves usually opposite in direction to QRS (Fig. 13.15).
- The appearance of LBBB may change the mean QRS axis in the frontal plane to the right, to the left, or to a superior, in some cases in a rate-dependent manner.

Incomplete Left Bundle Branch Block[1] (Fig. 13.16)

- QRS duration between 110 ms and 119 ms in adults, between 90 ms and 100 ms in children 8–16 years of age, and between 80 ms and 90 ms in children less than 8 years of age.

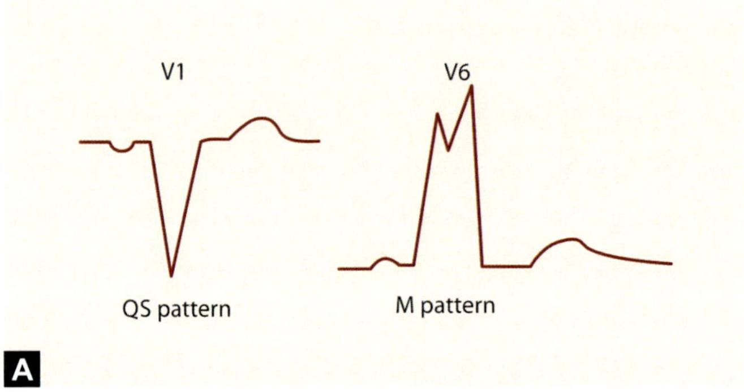

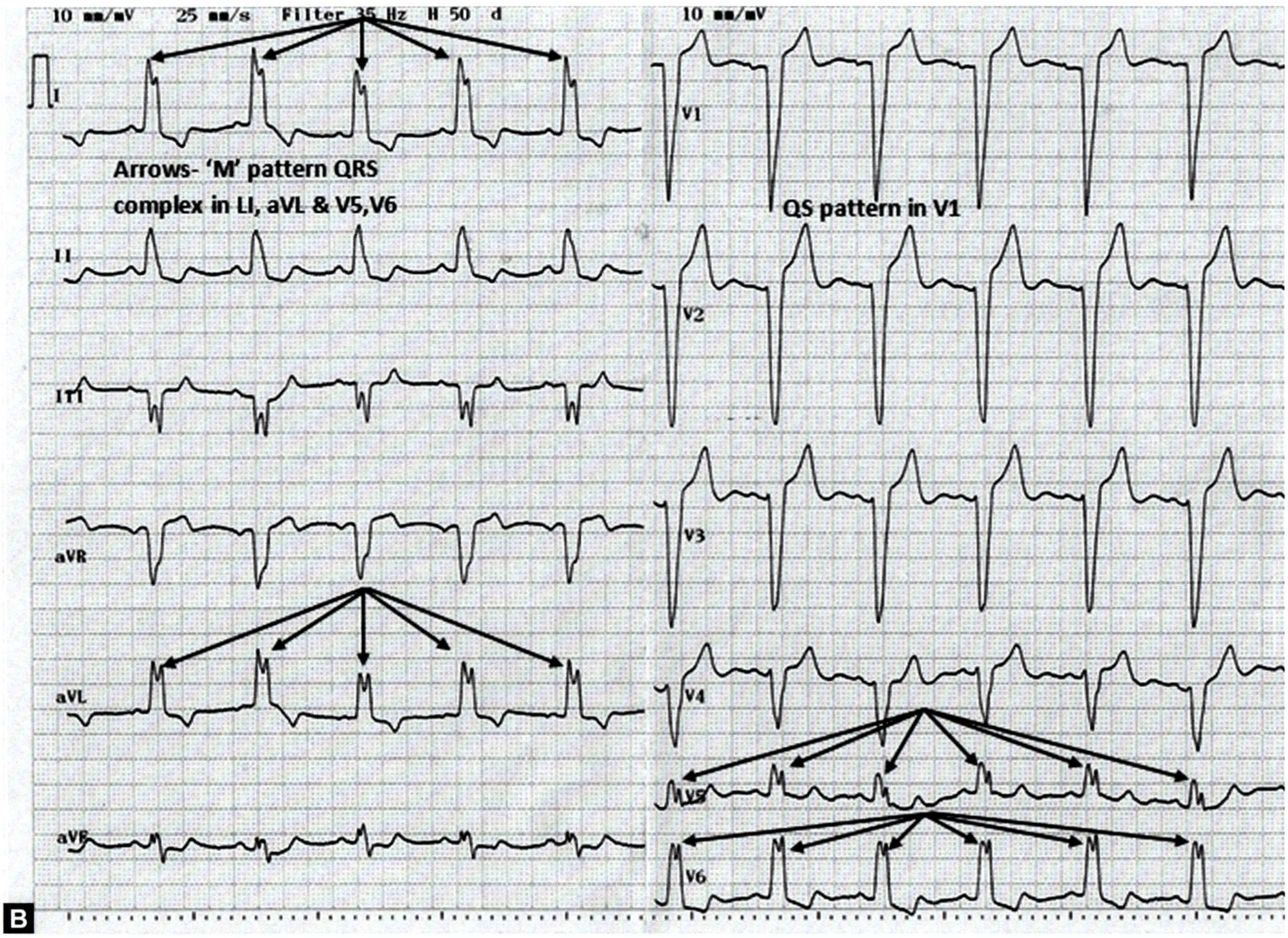

Figs. 13.14A and B: (A) Diagram showing typical QS pattern of QRS morphology in V1 and M pattern QRS complex in V6 in LBBB. (B) Electrocardiogram illustrates the typical QS pattern of QRS morphology in V1 and M pattern morphology in LI, aVL, V5, and V6 (*arrows*). QRS duration in this ECG is around 150 ms.

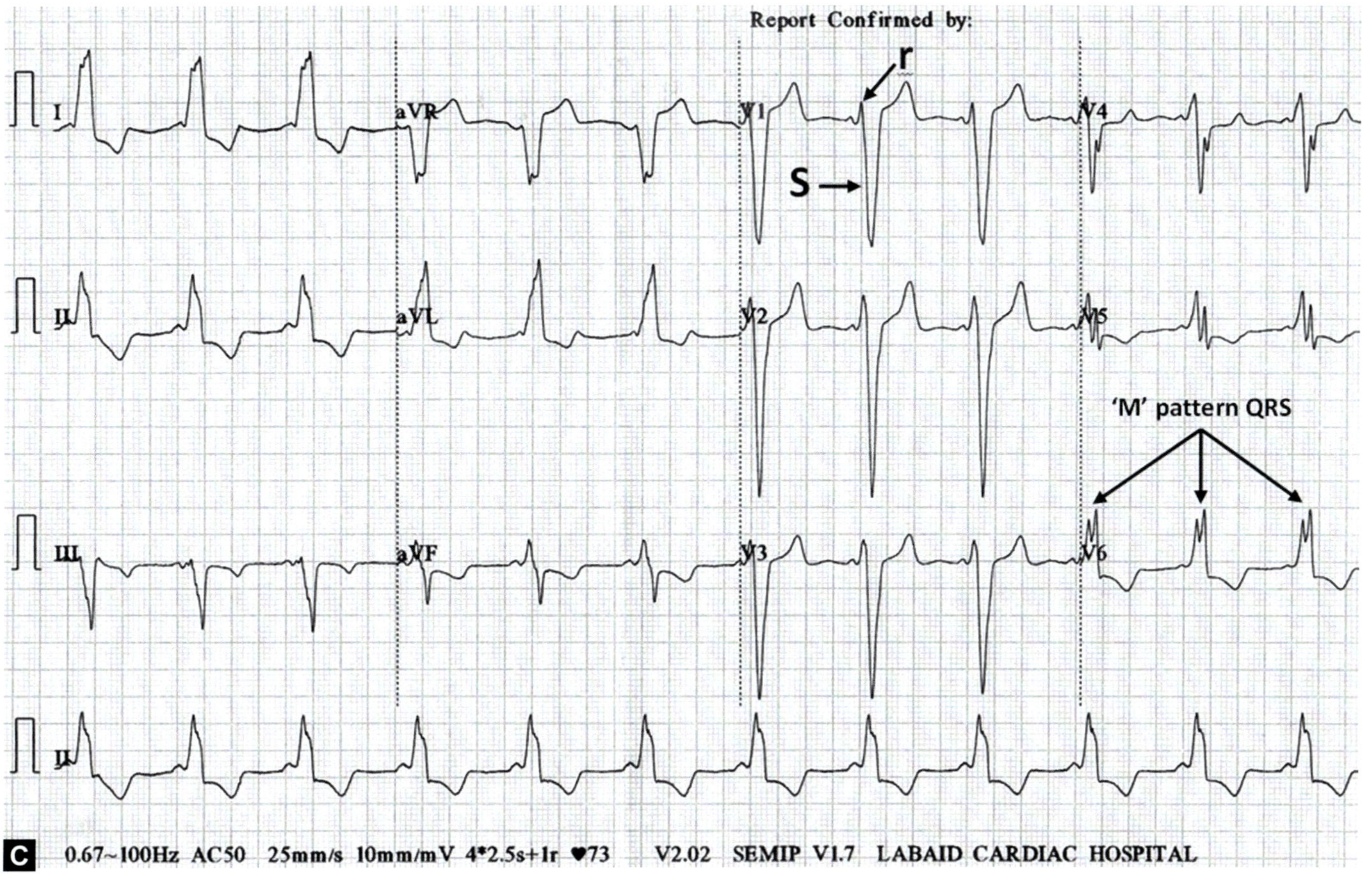

Fig. 13.14C: Electrocardiogram showing LBBB (QRS duration is 160 ms) with rS complex in V1 and M pattern morphology in V5 and V6 with notched and broad QRS in LI and aVL.

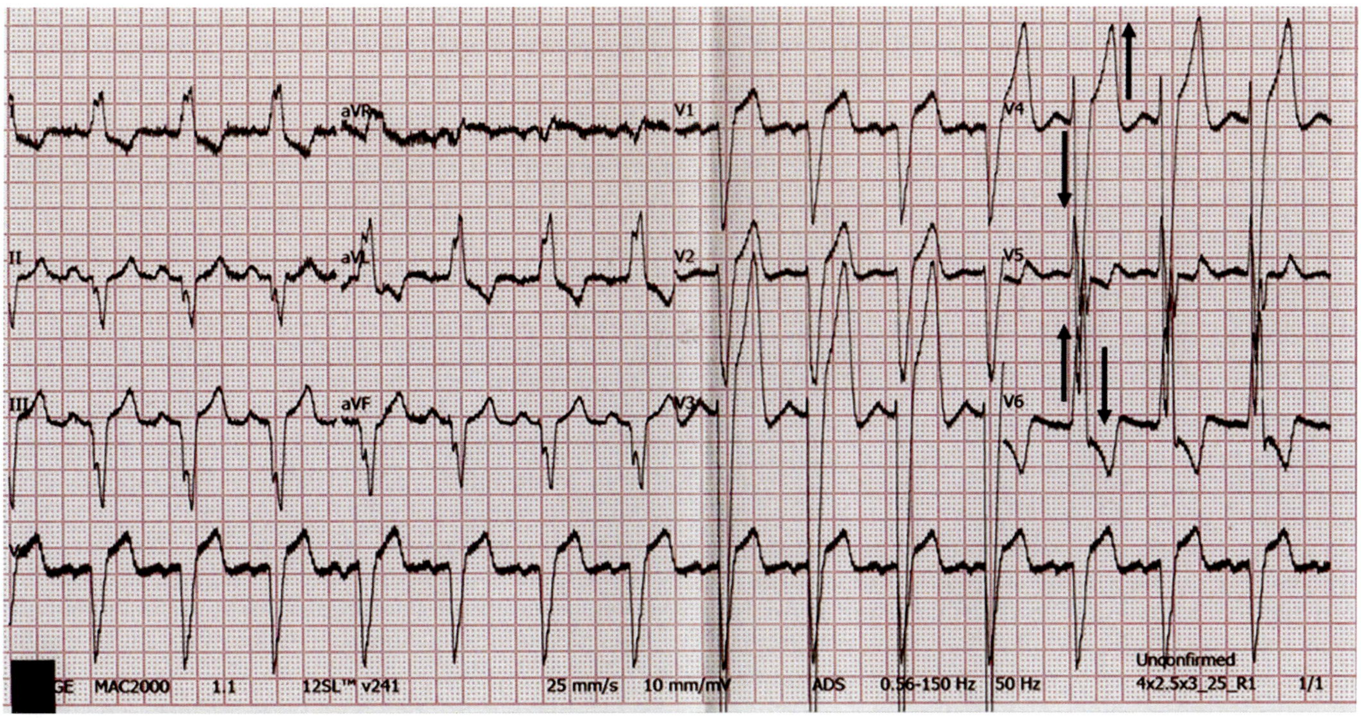

Fig. 13.15: Electrocardiogram showing ST and T waves changes in LBBB. In LBBB, ST segments and T waves always go in the opposite direction (discordance) to the main vector of the QRS complex (arrows).

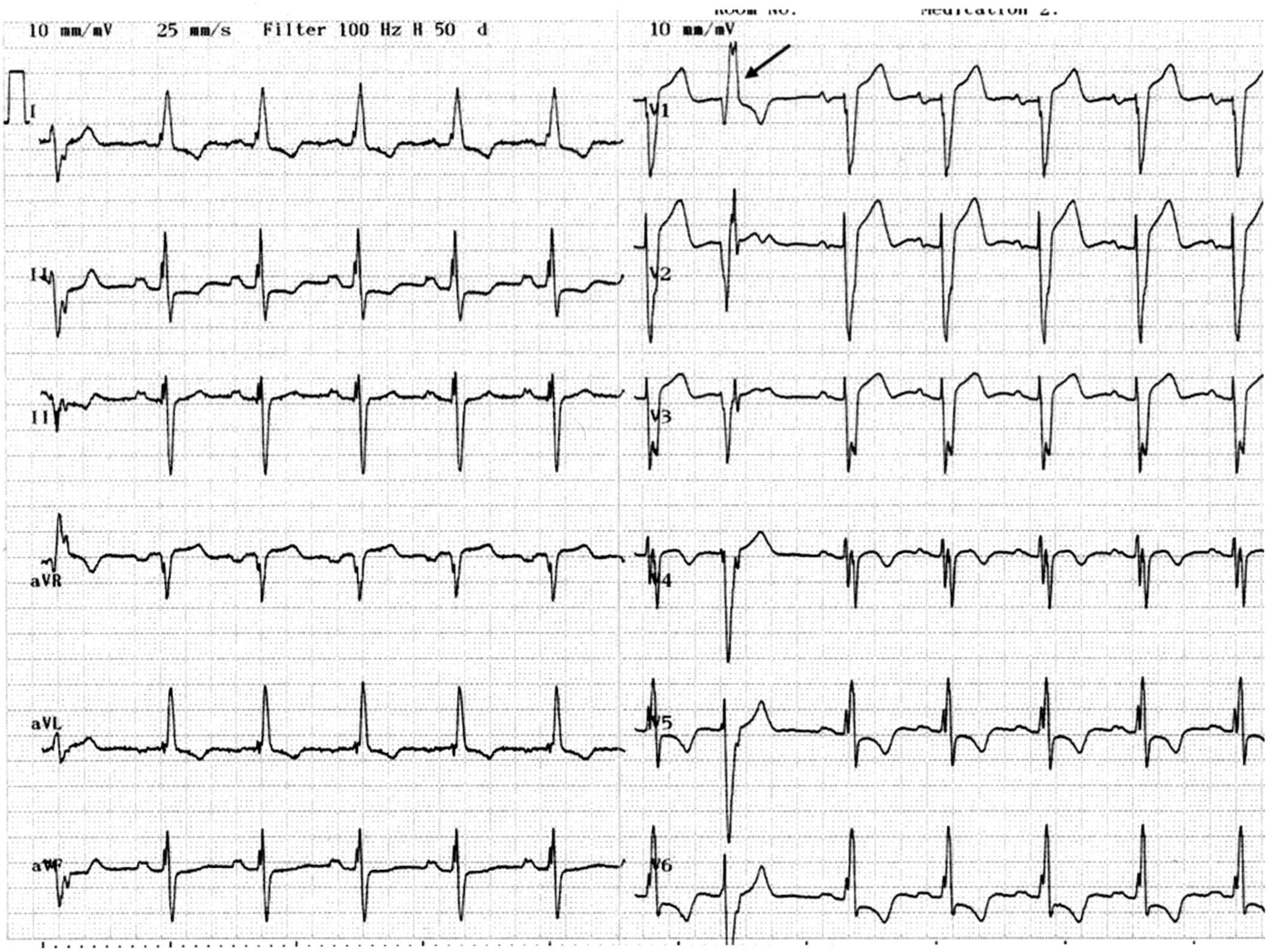

Fig. 13.16: Electrocardiogram illustrates the features of incomplete LBBB, slurred and notched QRS complex (QRS duration is 110 ms) in leads L1, aVL, V5, and V6 but QRS duration is less than 120 ms, rS pattern in V1 and absent normal septal Q waves in leads I, aVL, V5, and V6. Note one premature ventricular complex (PVC) in chest leads (arrow).

- Poor R-wave progression in the right precordial leads
- Absence of normal septal Q-wave in leads I, V5, and V6
- R peak time greater than 60 ms in leads V4, V5, and V6.

The morphology of QRS complex in lateral leads (L1, aVL, V5, and V6) in presence of LBBB may be of "M-shaped" (Fig. 13.17), notched (Fig. 13.18), monophasic (Fig. 13.19), or RS complex (Fig. 13.20). The diagnosis of left ventricular hypertrophy is possible in cases of LBBB by using the criteria of QRS amplitude in the left precordial leads. On the other hand, the diagnosis of myocardial infarction is more difficult, the criteria being very specific but having sensitivity less than 50%.[22]

Long term follow-up study showed that individuals with left, but not right, BBB had a markedly increased risk of dying from coronary disease and that two-thirds of these deaths occurred outside hospital, indicating probable fatal arrhythmia. One in six of the men with LBBB progressed to high-degree AV block or to requiring a pacemaker. Individual with RBBB also progress to high-degree AV block and/or to requiring a pacemaker to a greater extent than men without BBB, but otherwise did not have an increased risk of cardiovascular disease or death.[23,24]

HEMIBLOCK CONCEPT

Normal activation of the left ventricle proceeds down the left bundle branch, which consist of three fascicles, the left anterior fascicle, the left posterior fascicle, and the septal fascicle. The posterior fascicle supplies the posterior and inferoposterior walls of the LV, the anterior fascicle supplies the upper and anterior parts of the LV and the septal fascicle supplies the septal wall with innervation.

Though anatomically left bundle branch divides into three fascicles, but the third fascicle (septal fascicle) is not very important from clinical point of view. So depending on the anatomical location of the defect the LBBB can be further subclassified into:

- *Left anterior hemiblock (left anterior fascicular block, LAFB)*: In this case, only the anterior half of the left bundle branch (fascicle) is involved.

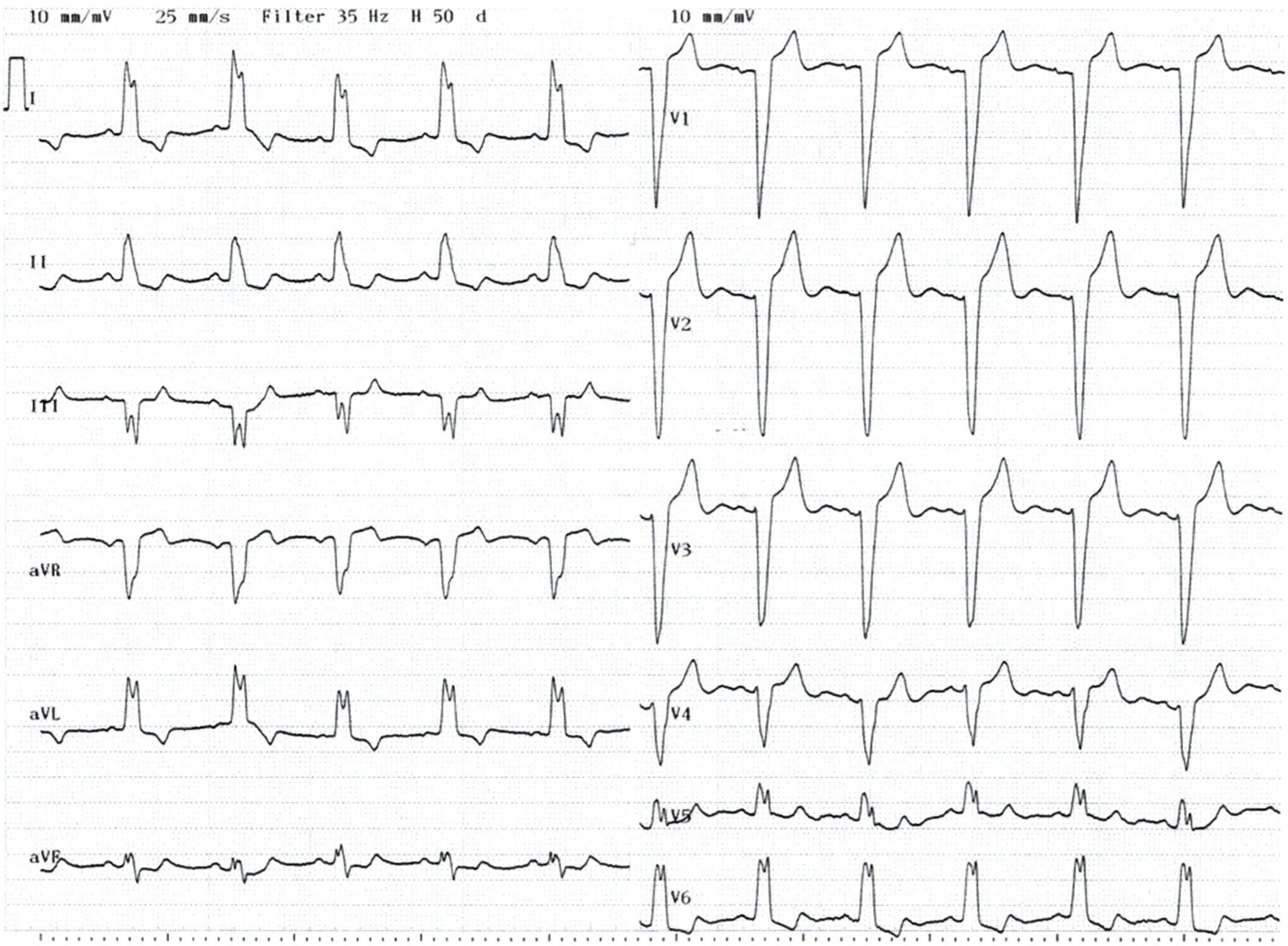

Fig. 13.17: Electrocardiogram showing typical features of complete LBBB with "M" pattern QRS complexes in LI, aVL, V5, and V6.

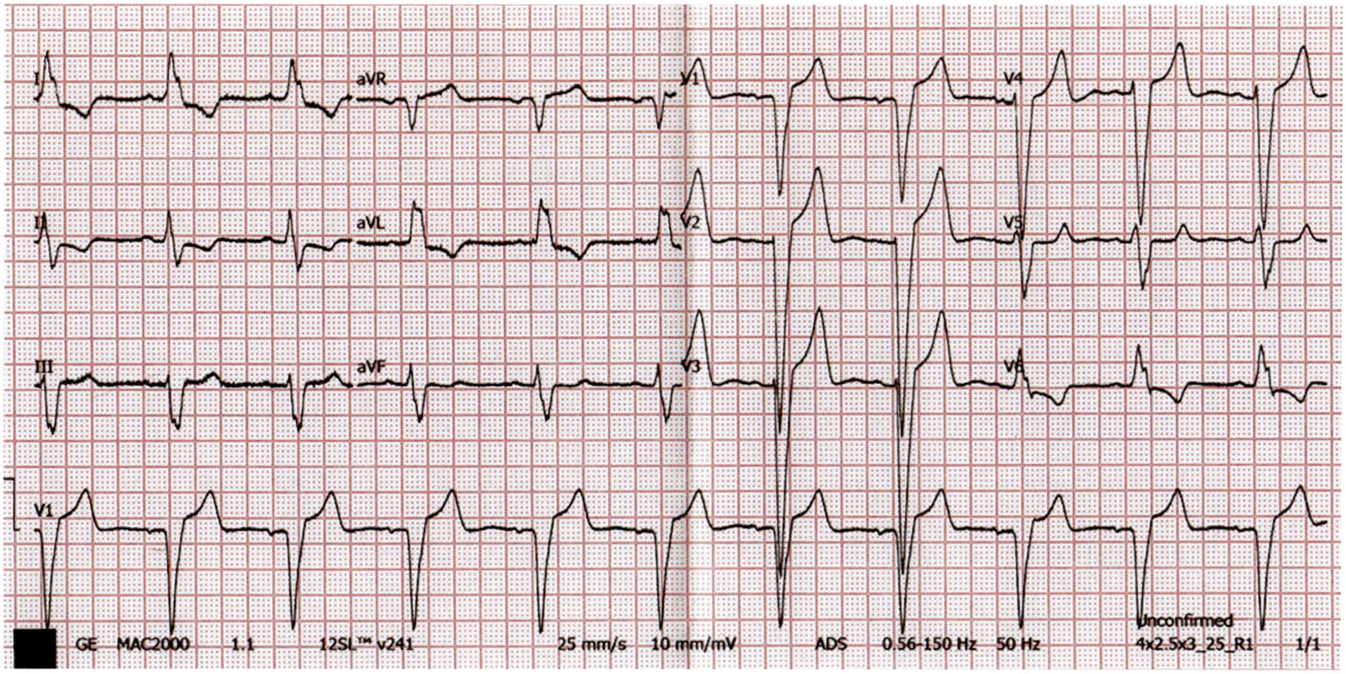

Fig. 13.18: Electrocardiogram showing features of complete LBBB with "notched" QRS complexes in LI, aVL, V5, and V6.

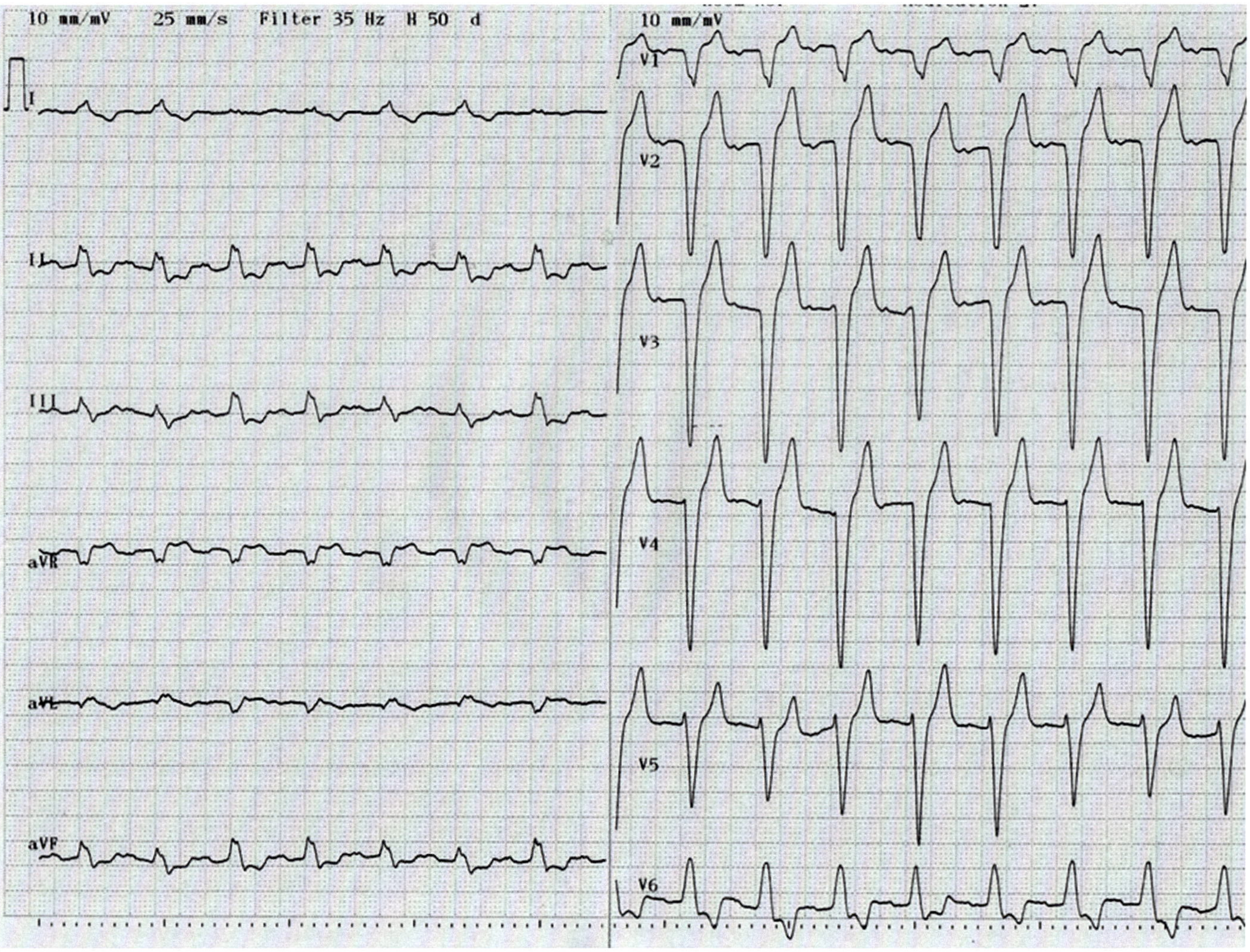

Fig. 13.19: Electrocardiogram showing features of LBBB with monophasic QRS complex in V6.

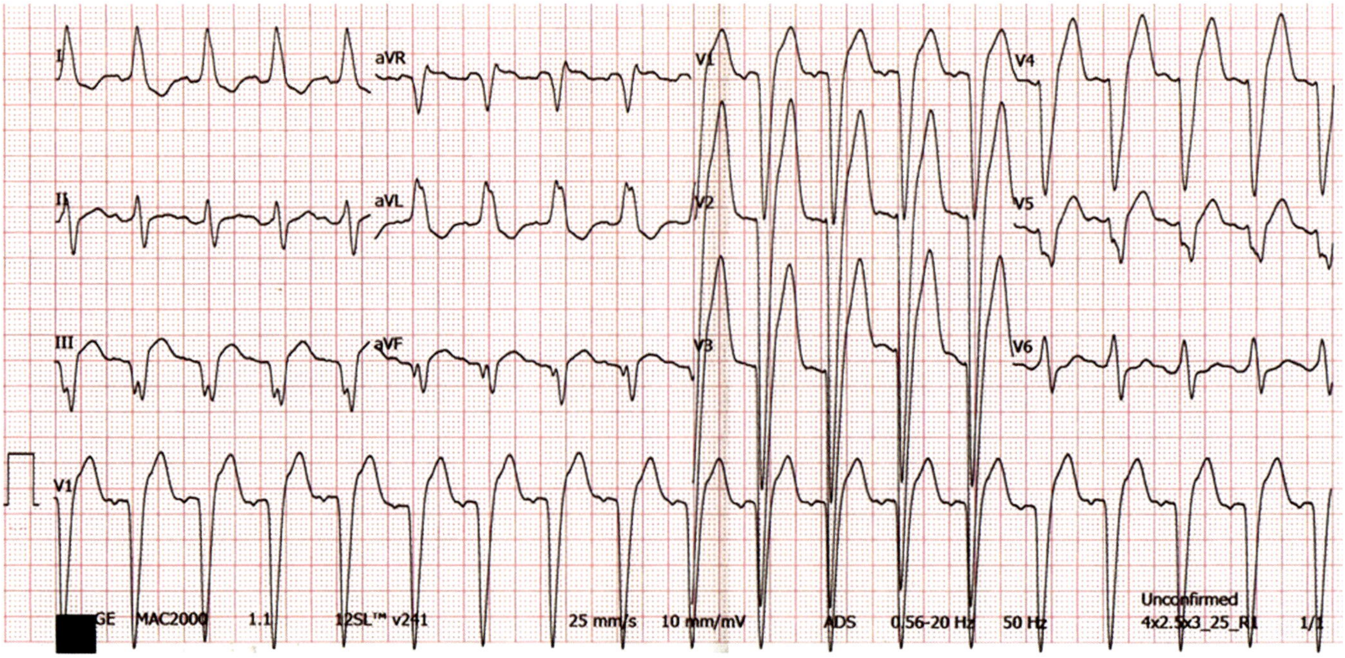

Fig. 13.20: Electrocardiogram showing features of LBBB with RS pattern QRS complex in V6.

- *Left posterior hemiblock (left posterior fascicular block, LPFB)*: Only the posterior part of the left bundle branch is involved.

One of the most important problems related to hemiblocks is that they may simulate or conceal the electrocardiographic signs of myocardial infarction or myocardial ischemia and may mask or simulate ventricular hypertrophy. One of the most common causes of hemiblocks is coronary artery disease, and there is a particularly frequent association between anteroseptal myocardial infarction and left anterior hemiblock. The second most important cause is arterial hypertension, followed by cardiomyopathies and Lev and Lenegre diseases. The hemiblocks may also occur in aortic valve disease and congenital heart diseases. Left anterior hemiblock is more common in men and increases in frequency with advancing age. Isolated left anterior hemiblock is a relatively frequent finding in subjects devoid of evidence of structural heart disease. Conversely, isolated left posterior hemiblock is a very rare finding.

Left Anterior Hemiblock (LAHB)

In LAHB, also called LAFB impulses are conducted to the left ventricle via the left posterior fascicle, which inserts into the infero-septal wall of the left ventricle along its endocardial surface (Fig. 13.21). On reaching the left ventricle, the initial electrical vector is therefore directed downward and rightward (as excitation spreads outward from endocardium to epicardium), producing small R waves in the inferior leads (II, III, and aVF) and small Q waves in the left-sided leads (I and aVL) (Fig. 13.22). The major wave of depolarization then spreads in an upward and leftward direction, producing large positive voltages (tall R waves) in the left-sided leads and large negative voltages (deep S waves) in the inferior leads (Fig. 13.23). This process takes about 20 ms longer than simultaneous conduction via both fascicles, resulting in a slight widening of the QRS. The impulse reaches the left-sided leads later than normal, resulting in an increased R-wave peak time (the time from onset of the QRS to the peak of the R-wave) in aVL. The ECG criteria of LAHB include: (1) Frontal plane axis between –45° and –90°; (2) Small Q waves with tall R waves (qR complexes) in leads I and aVL and small R waves with deep S waves (rS complexes) in leads II, III, and aVF; (3) R-peak time in lead aVL of 45 ms or more, and (4) QRS duration less than 120 ms (Fig. 13.24).[1]

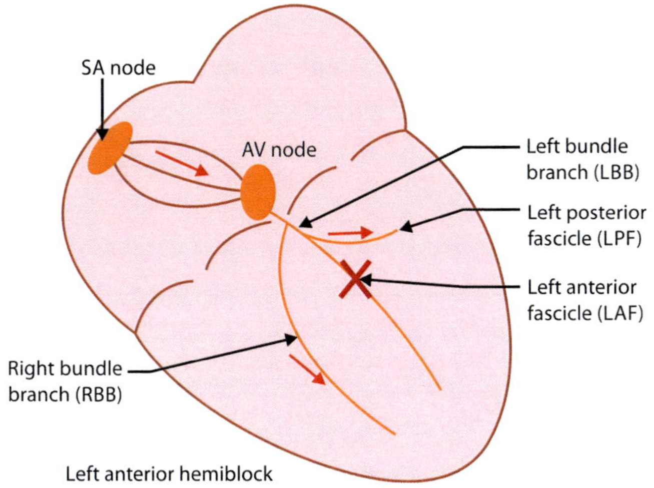

Fig. 13.21: Diagram showing impulse conduction in left anterior hemiblock. From left bundle impulse conducts through left posterior fascicle as left anterior fascicle is blocked. Conduction in right bundle is normal.

Left anterior hemiblock may be seen in 4% cases of acute MI. It is the most common type of intraventricular conduction defect seen in acute anterior myocardial infarction, and the left anterior descending artery is usually the culprit vessel. LAHB is difficult to diagnose when a prior inferior wall myocardial infarction is evident on the ECG. Inferior MI can also cause extreme left-axis deviation, but will manifest with Q waves in the inferior leads II, III, and aVF. By contrast, QRS complexes in the inferior leads should begin with R waves in LAHB.

Left Posterior Hemiblock (LPHB)

In LPHB, also called LPFB impulses are conducted to the left ventricle via the left anterior fascicle, which inserts into the upper, lateral wall of the left ventricle along its endocardial surface (Fig. 13.25). On reaching the ventricle, the initial electrical vector is therefore directed upward and leftward (as excitation spreads outward from endocardium to epicardium), causing small R waves in the lateral leads (I and aVL) and small Q waves in the inferior leads (II, III, and aVF) (Fig. 13.26). The major wave of depolarization then spreads along the free LV wall in a downward and rightward direction, producing large positive voltages (tall R waves) in the inferior leads and large negative voltages (deep S waves) in the lateral leads (Fig. 13.27). This process takes up to 20 ms longer than simultaneous conduction via both fascicles, resulting in a slight widening of the QRS. The impulse reaches the inferior leads later than normal, resulting in an increased R-wave peak time (the time from onset of the QRS to the peak of the R-wave) in aVF. The ECG criteria of LPHB include: (1) Frontal plane axis between greater than +90° and 180° in adults. Owing to the more rightward axis in children up to 16 years of age, this criterion should only be applied to them when a distinct rightward change in axis is documented; (2) rS pattern in leads I and aVL; (3) qR pattern in leads II, III, and aVF and; (4) QRS duration is less than 120 ms (Figs. 13.28A and B).[1]

Left Septal Hemiblock

Left septal hemiblock (LSHB) also known as left septal fascicular block (LSFB) is not a well-defined ECG entity.

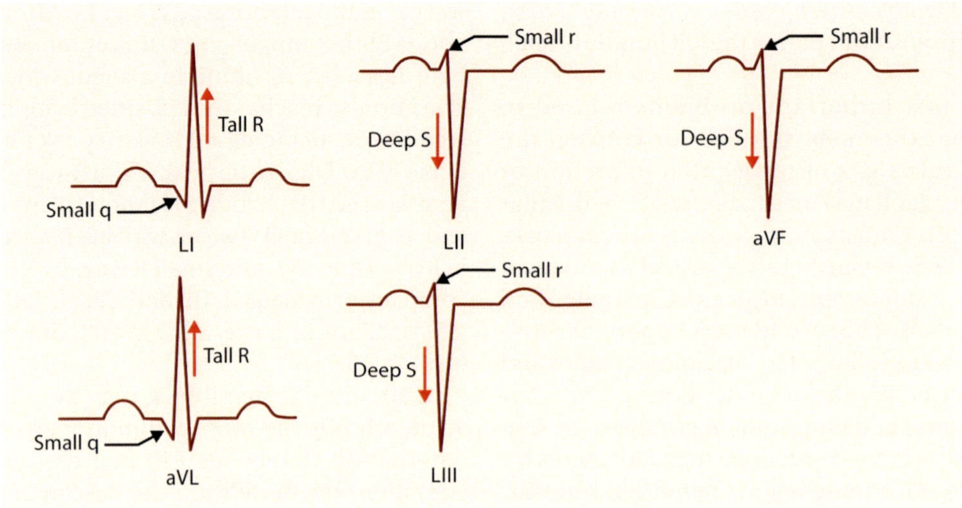

Fig. 13.22: Diagram showing typical ECG criteria of left anterior hemiblock. Note small Q waves with tall R waves (qR complexes) in leads I and aVL and small R waves with deep S waves (rS complexes) in leads II, III, and aVF with left axis deviation.

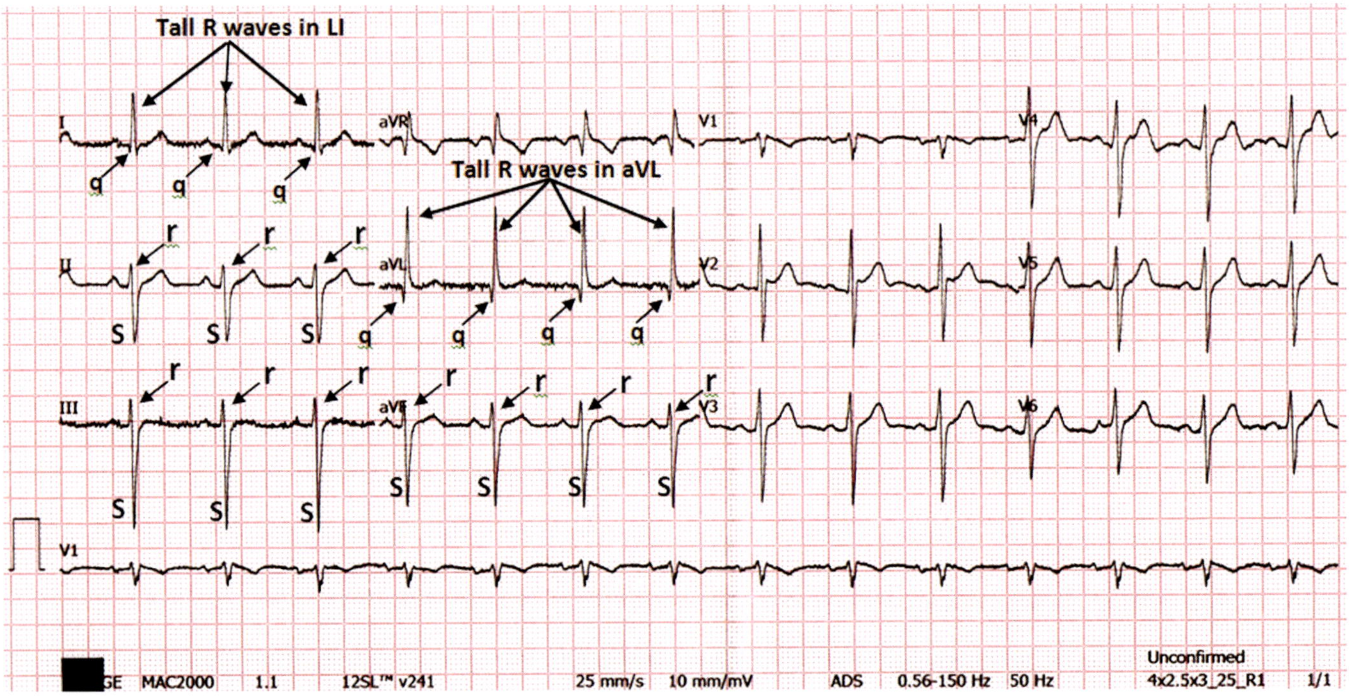

Fig. 13.23: Electrocardiogram illustrates the typical features of left anterior hemiblock. Note small Q waves with tall R waves (qR complexes) in leads I and aVL and small R waves with deep S waves (rS complexes) in leads II, III, and aVF with left axis deviation. Also note the normal QRS duration.

Anatomic studies have shown that the left bundle branch divides into three fascicles in most humans. Changes in the 12-lead ECG due to conduction abnormalities of the left anterior fascicle and left posterior fascicle are well documented. But there are no standard criteria for detecting conduction defects involving the third left fascicle, the septal or median fascicle, and the very existence of such defects is still a matter of controversy. Most of the published data opined that LSFB is a polymorphic conduction defect. Various criteria for LSHB (LSFB) have been proposed based on case reports. It may present with multiple morphologies, and is frequently combined with other conduction abnormalities which obscure its presence.[25,26]

Proposed ECG criteria for LSHB (LSFB):[25,26]

- Septal Q waves are markedly diminished or lost by shift in initial QRS forces to the left, this means loss of normal septal Q waves from I, V5–V6.
- Loss of initial R waves in right precordial leads accompanied by loss of septal Q waves (which implies posterior as well as leftward orientation of initial QRS forces).

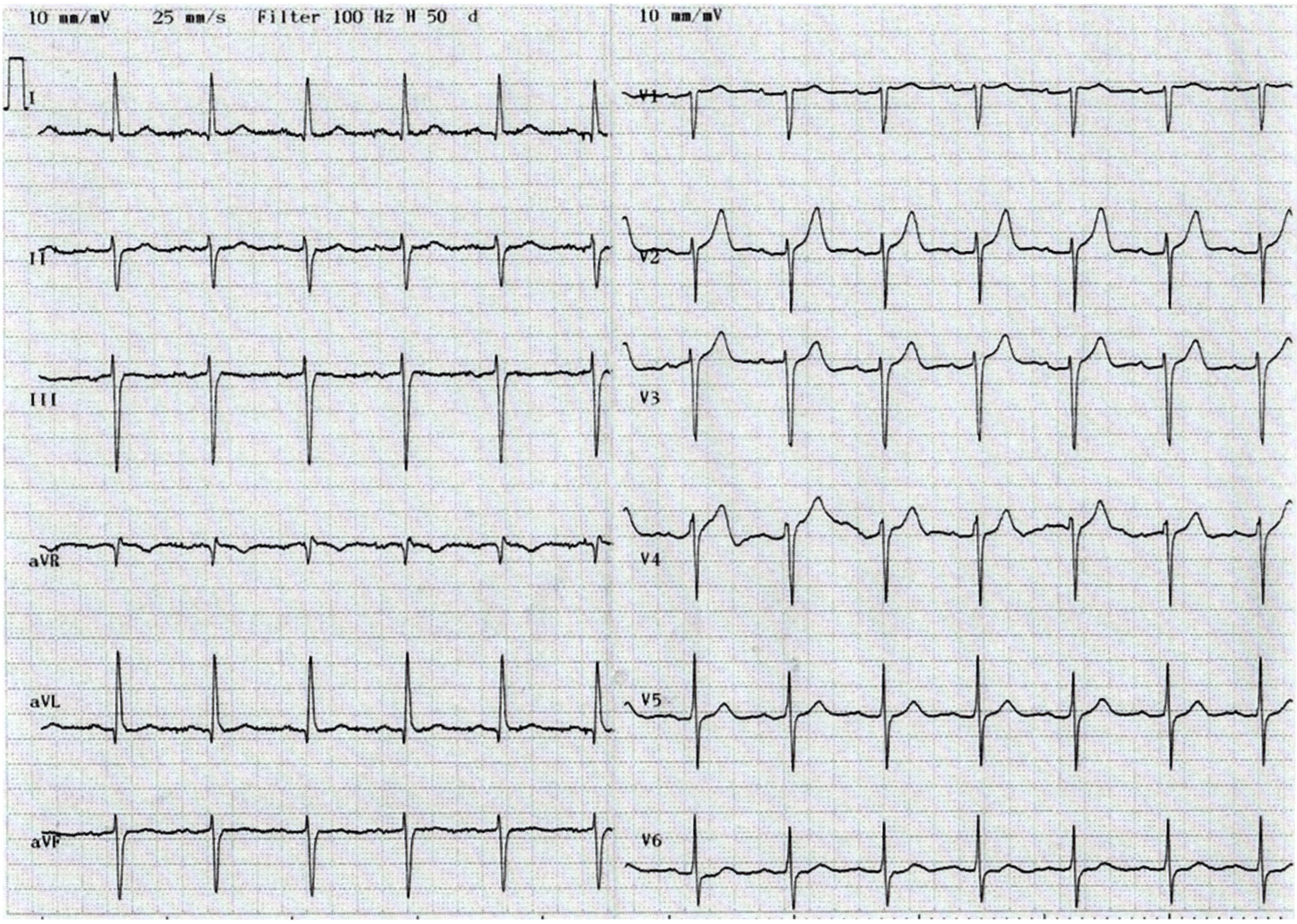

Fig. 13.24: Electrocardiogram showing typical features of left anterior hemiblock. Note small Q waves with tall R waves (qR complexes) in leads I and aVL and small R waves with deep S waves (rS complexes) in leads II, III, and aVF with left axis deviation. Note also the normal QRS duration.

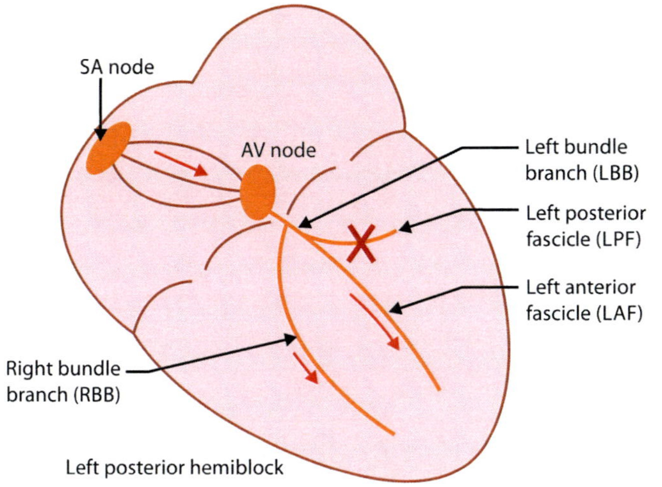

Fig. 13.25: Diagram showing impulse conduction in left posterior hemiblock. From left bundle impulse conducts through left anterior fascicle as left posterior fascicle is blocked. Conduction in right bundle is normal.

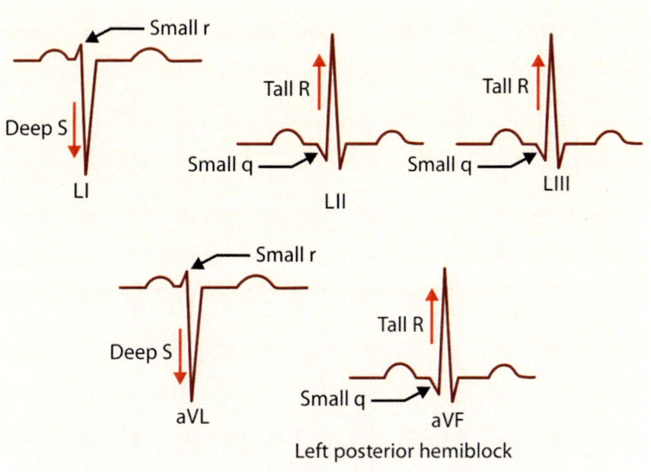

Fig. 13.26: Diagram showing ECG features of typical left posterior hemiblock. Note small Q waves with tall R waves (qR complexes) in leads II, III, and aVF and small R waves with deep S waves (rS complexes) in leads I and aVL along with right axis deviation.

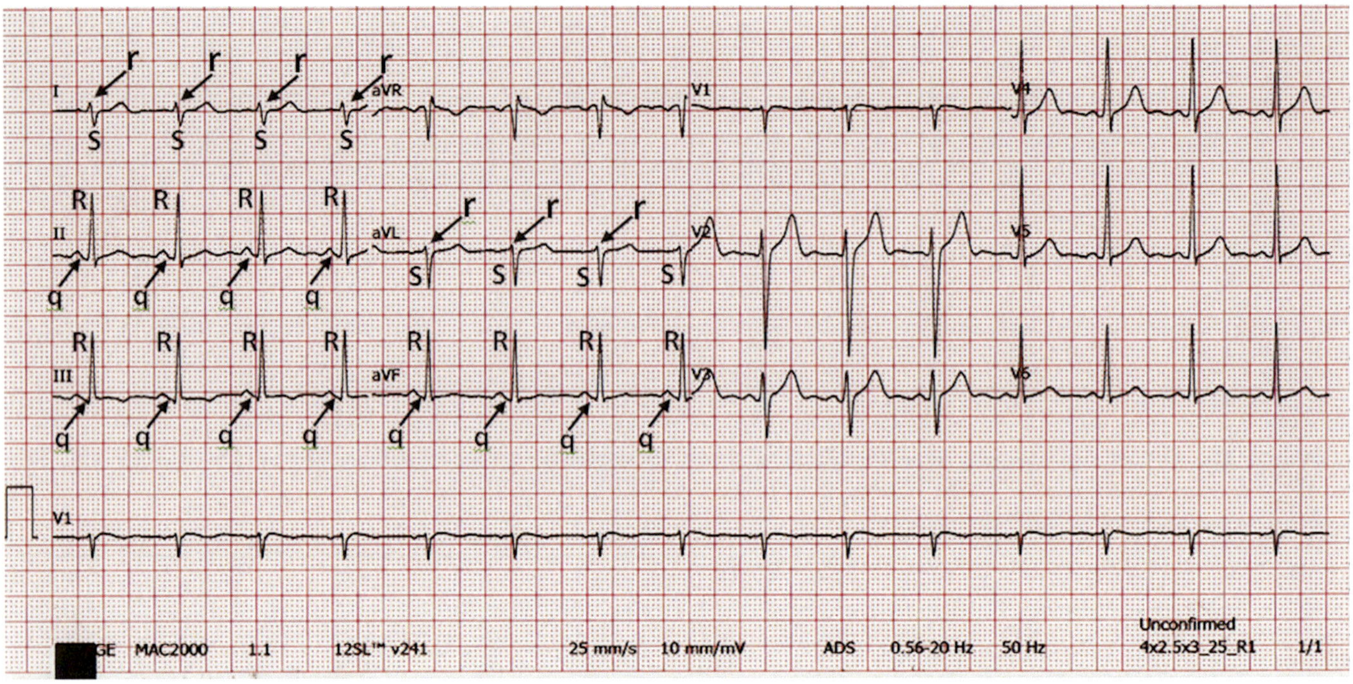

Fig. 13.27: Electrocardiogram illustrates the typical electrocardiographic features of left posterior hemiblock. Note small Q waves with tall R waves (qR complexes) in leads II, III and aVF and small R waves with deep S waves (rS complexes) in leads I and aVL along with right axis deviation. Also note normal QRS duration.

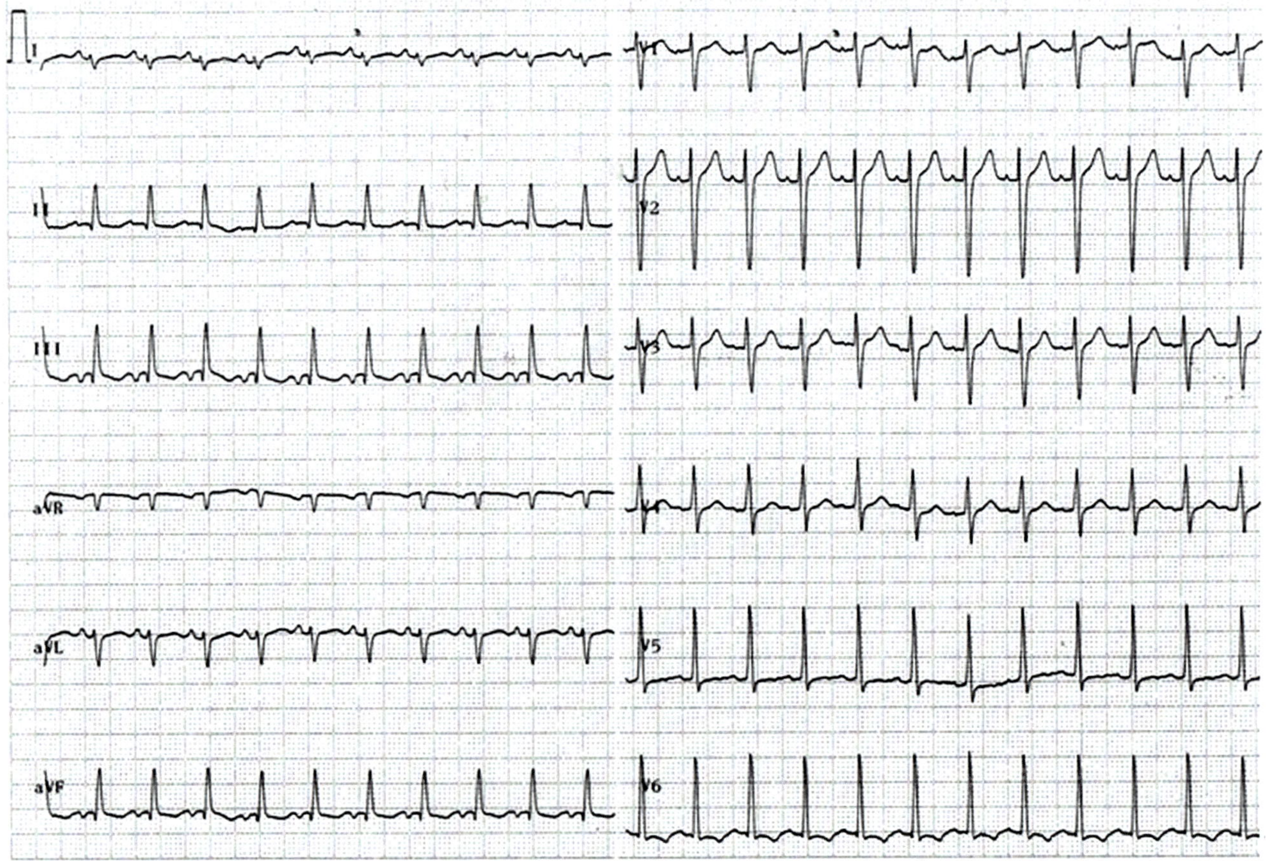

Fig. 13.28A: Electrocardiogram showing features of left posterior hemiblock with marked sinus tachycardia (136 bpm). Note small Q waves with tall R waves (qR complexes) in leads II, III, and aVF and small R waves with deep S waves (rS complexes) in leads I and aVL along with right axis deviation. Also note normal QRS duration (QRS duration is 80 ms).

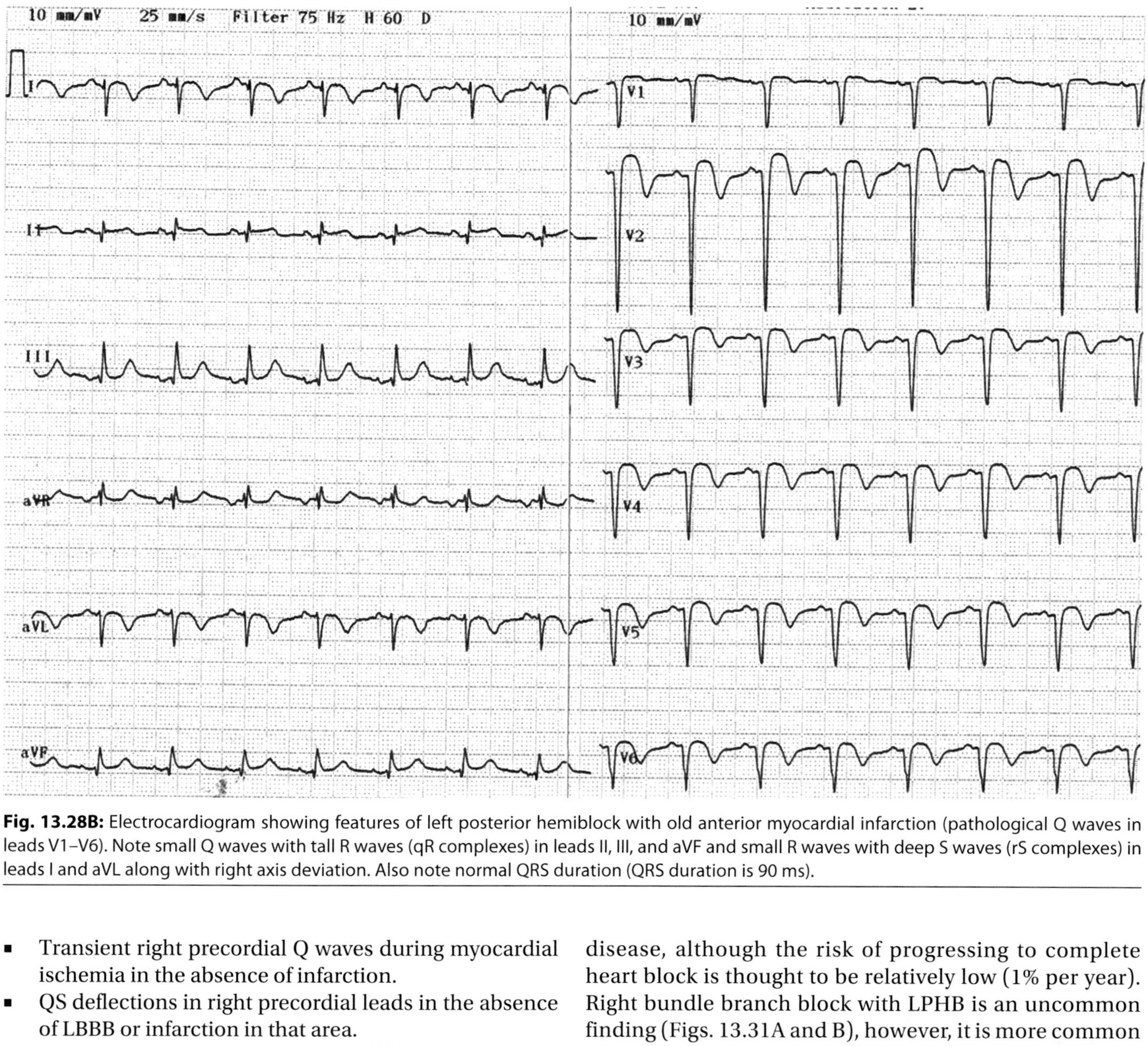

Fig. 13.28B: Electrocardiogram showing features of left posterior hemiblock with old anterior myocardial infarction (pathological Q waves in leads V1–V6). Note small Q waves with tall R waves (qR complexes) in leads II, III, and aVF and small R waves with deep S waves (rS complexes) in leads I and aVL along with right axis deviation. Also note normal QRS duration (QRS duration is 90 ms).

- Transient right precordial Q waves during myocardial ischemia in the absence of infarction.
- QS deflections in right precordial leads in the absence of LBBB or infarction in that area.
- Atypical cases of incomplete LBBB in which left ventricular activation time remains normal and the sense of initial septal activation may not be strictly right-to-left.

BIFASCICULAR/TRIFASCICULAR BLOCK

Bifascicular block most commonly refers to conduction disturbances below the AV node in which the right bundle branch and one of the two fascicles (anterior or posterior) of the left bundle branch are involved (Figs. 13.29A to C). Some authors, including those of the guidelines on the management of syncope include LBBB in the definition of bifascicular block since LBBB implies block in both fascicles.[27,28] Most common type of bifascicular block is RBBB with LAHB (Figs. 13.30A to C) and most commonly seen in patients with coronary artery disease.[29] Bifascicular block is a sign of extensive conducting system disease, although the risk of progressing to complete heart block is thought to be relatively low (1% per year). Right bundle branch block with LPHB is an uncommon finding (Figs. 13.31A and B), however, it is more common than isolated LPHB and appears to progress to complete heart block more frequently than does the combination of RBBB and LAHB.[29] Important causes of bifascicular block include chronic ischemic heart disease, hypertension, acute ST-elevation anterior myocardial infarction, aortic stenosis, primary degenerative disease of the conducting system (Lenegre's/Lev's disease), congenital heart disease, etc.

The term trifascicular block is also confusing, since involvement of the right bundle branch and both fascicles of the left bundle branch would be manifested as complete heart block. Thus, trifascicular block is most often arbitrarily applied to patients with bifascicular block and prolongation of the PR interval (Figs. 13.32A to C). LBBB with first degree AV block is also considered as a type of trifascicular block by some authors, since the PR interval prolongation could indicate that the conduction in the right bundle is also affected (Fig. 13.33). Rarely it could be due to a coexistent

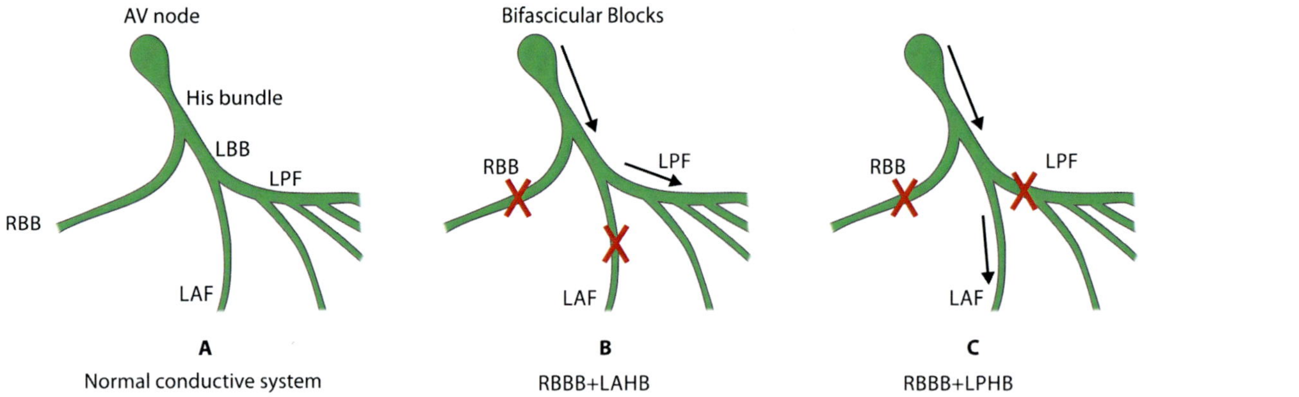

Figs. 13.29A to C: Diagram showing different patterns of bifascicular blocks. (A) Normal ventricular conductive system. (B) Bifascicular block: RBBB + LAHB. (C) Bifascicular block: RBBB + LPHB. (AV node: atrioventricular node; LBB: left bundle branch; RBB: right bundle branch; LAF: left anterior fascicle; LPF: left posterior fascicle)

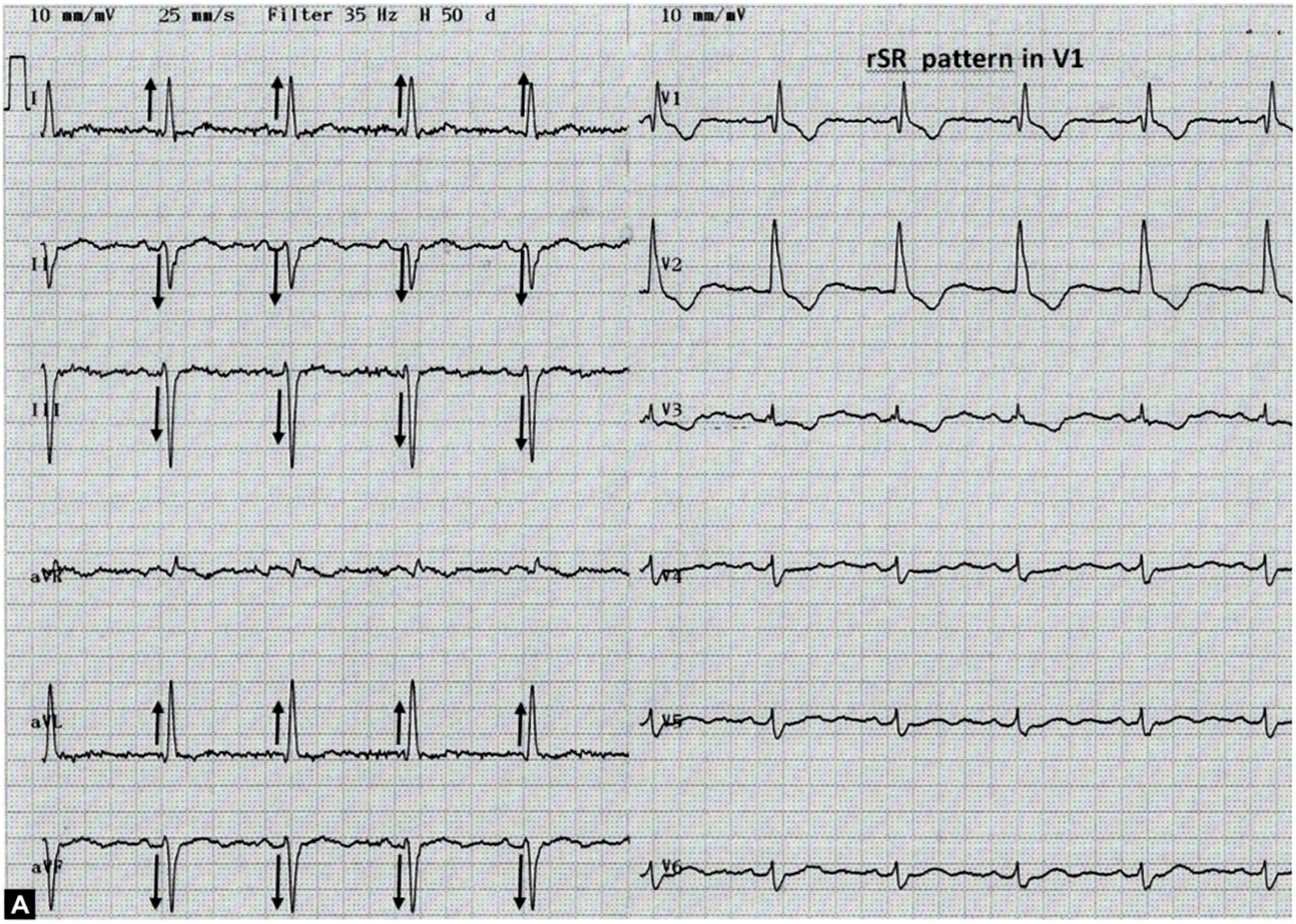

Fig. 13.30A: Electrocardiogram illustrates typical features of bifascicular block (RBBB + LAHB). Note rSR pattern QRS complex in V1 (QRS duration is 142 ms) suggestive of RBBB along with small Q and tall R waves in LI and aVL and small R with deep S waves in LII, LIII, and aVF (arrows) suggestive of LAHB. Note also left axis deviation and normal PR interval.

conduction delay in the AV node, rather than in the infra Hisian conduction system. LBBB with first degree AV block may be considered as a fore runner of complete AV block. RBBB with alternating left anterior and left posterior hemiblock or alternating LBBB and RBBB are also considered as trifascicular block.

Trifascicular block usually include:
1. Right bundle branch block + left anterior hemiblock + first degree heart block.
2. Right bundle branch block + left posterior hemiblock + first degree heart block.
3. Left bundle branch block + first degree heart block.

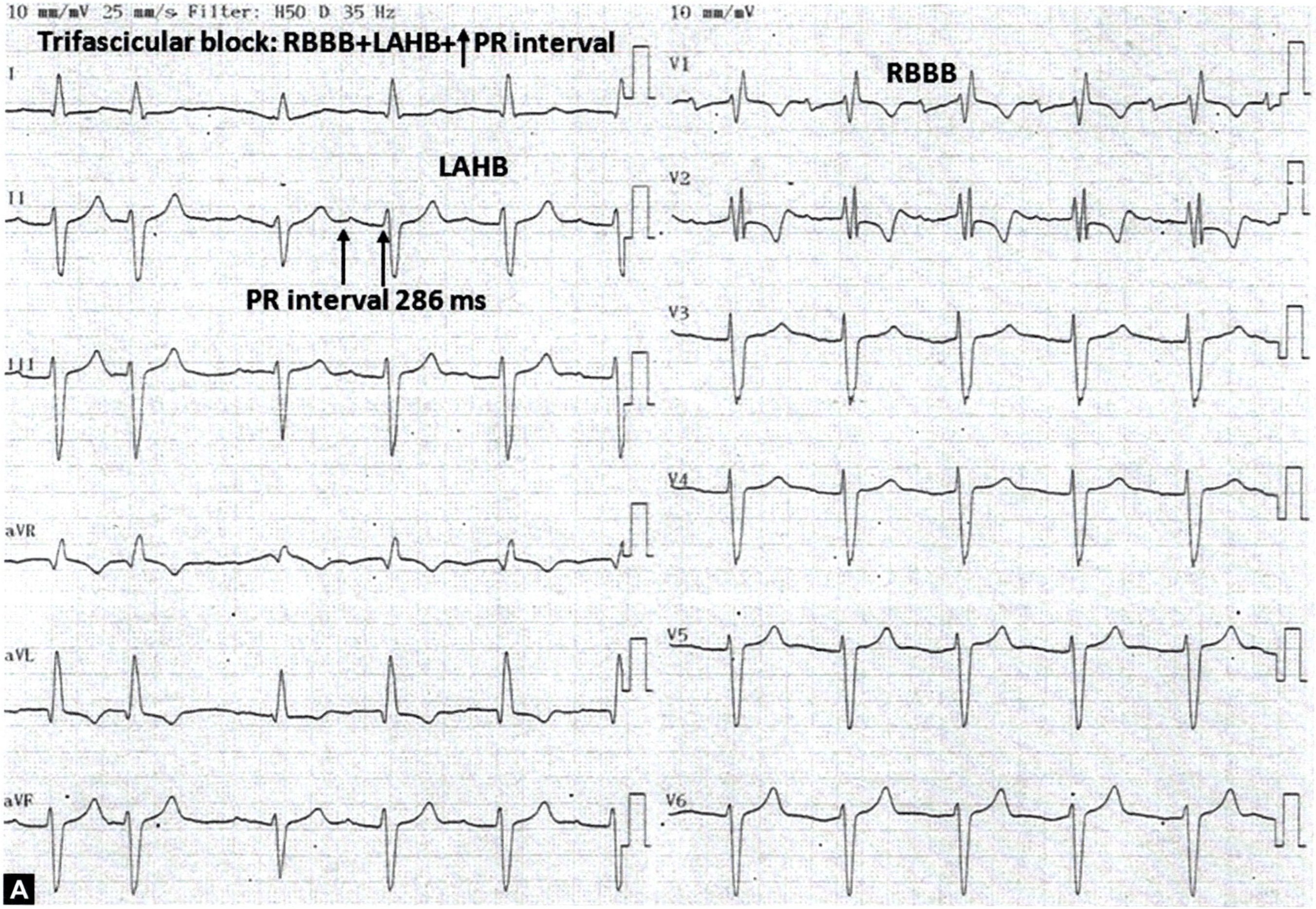

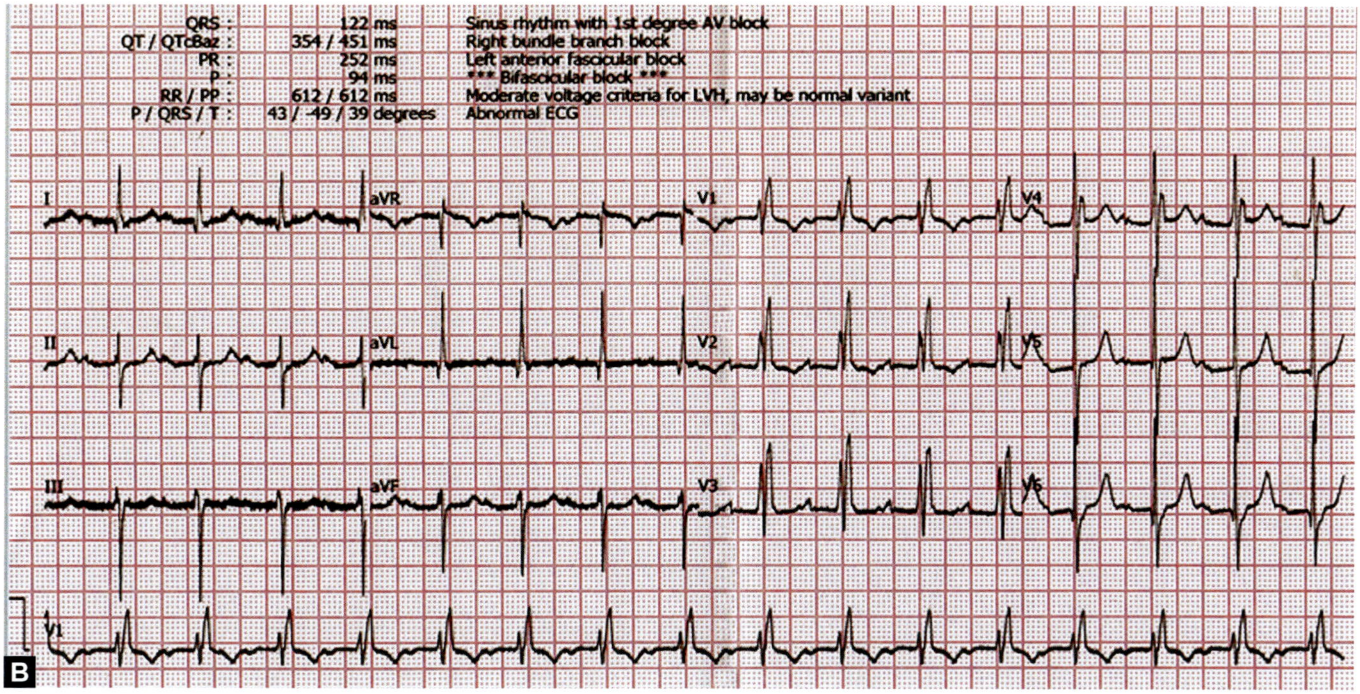

Figs. 13.32A and B: (A) Electrocardiogram illustrates features of trifascicular block. RBBB (rsR pattern QRS in V1 and V2 with duration 150 ms) + LAHB (small Q waves with tall R waves, qR complexes in LI and aVL and small R waves with deep S waves, rS complexes in LII, LIII, and aVF) + first degree heart block (PR interval is 286 ms). Note one ectopic beat in limb leads. (B) Electrocardiogram showing features of trifascicular block. RBBB + LAHB + first degree heart block (PR interval is 252 ms).

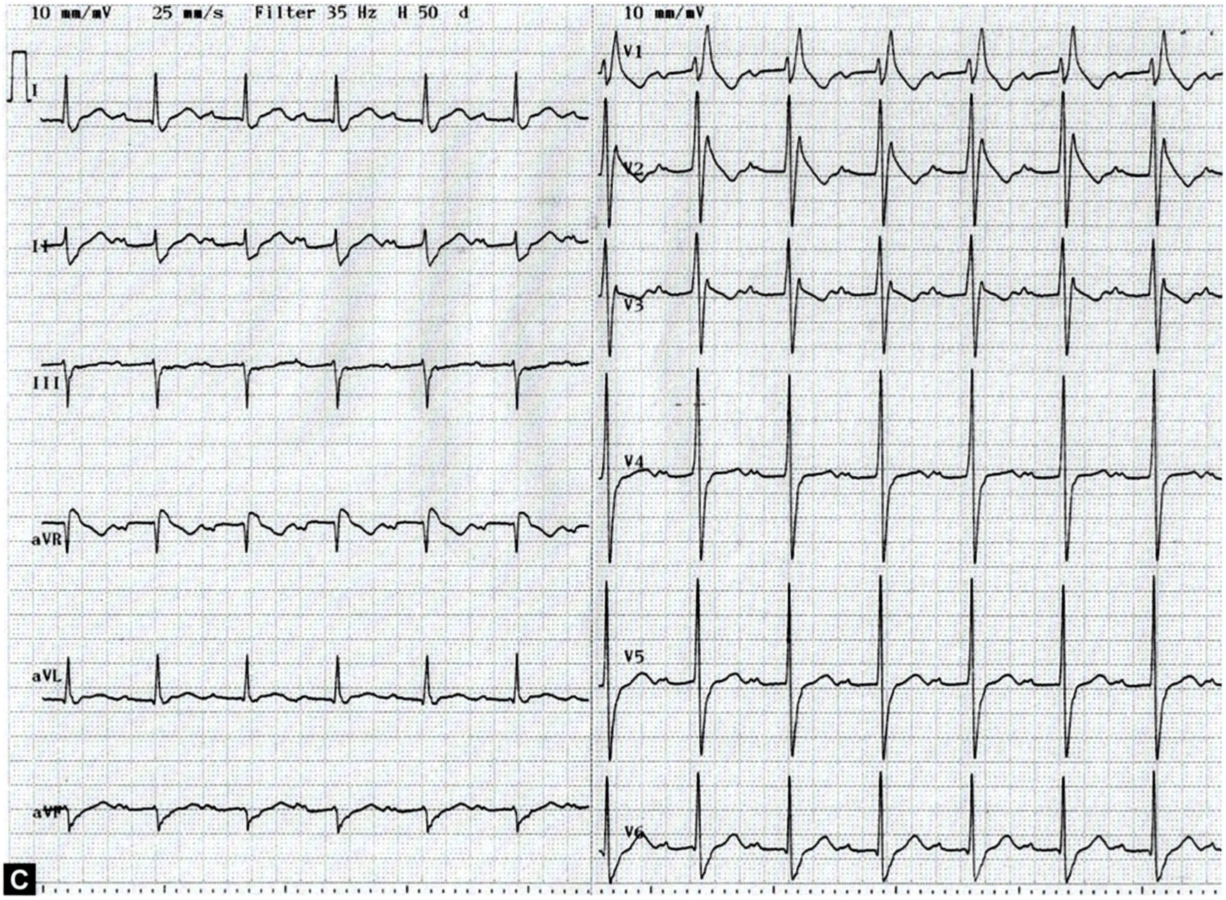

Fig. 13.32C: Electrocardiogram showing features of trifascicular block. RBBB + LAHB + first degree heart block (PR interval is 326 ms).

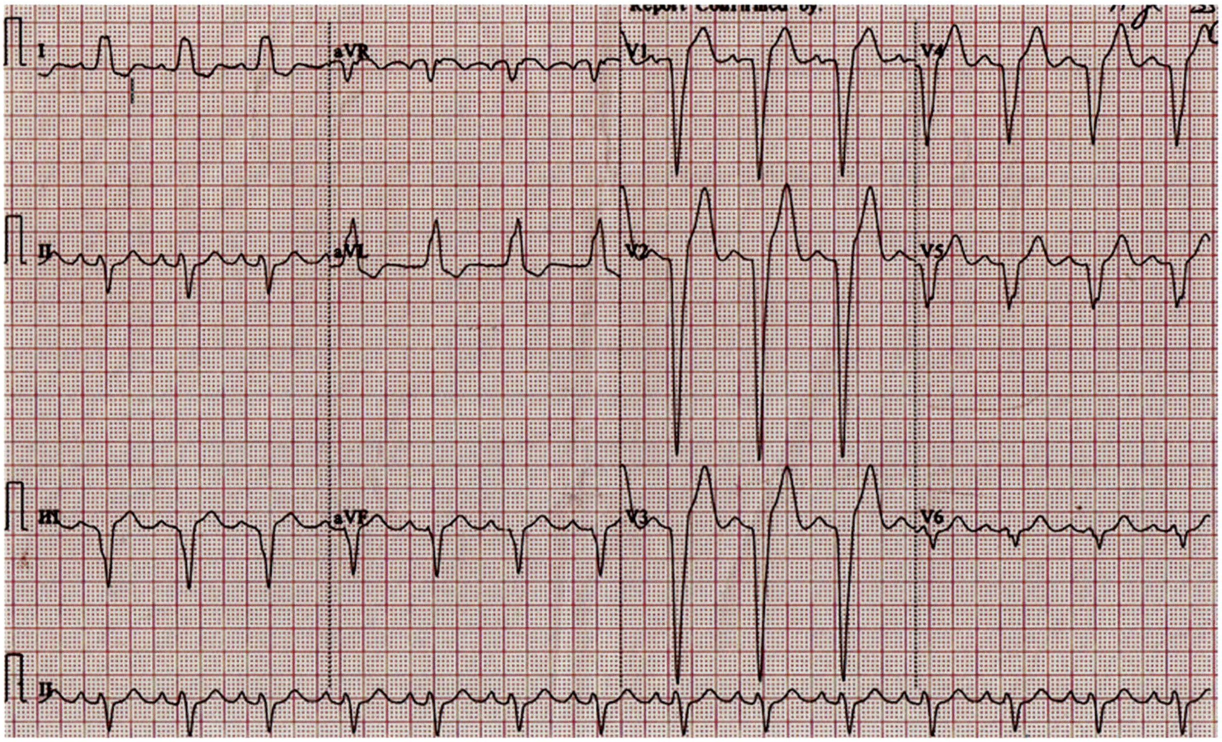

Fig. 13.33: Electrocardiogram showing features of trifascicular block (LBBB + first degree heart block, PR interval is 230 ms). LBBB with first degree AV block is sometimes considered as a type of trifascicular block, since the PR interval prolongation could indicate that the conduction in the right bundle is also affected.

PERI-INFARCTION BLOCK

Conduction defect that is limited to the area surrounding the infarcted myocardium is termed as "peri-infarction block." The ECG criteria of peri-infarction block (Fig. 13.34):[30,31]

- Evidence of myocardial infarction on surface ECG.
- Notching or slurred QRS complexes in the leads those show infarction pattern.
- The terminal portion of the QRS complex is wide. So, QRS duration is mildly prolonged, usually between 110 ms and 120 ms.
- Ventricular activation time may be prolonged in the leads overlying the infarcted area.

In peri-infarction block fibers of the distant Purkinje system surrounding the infarcted area is usually involved. The term "peri-ischemic block" is recommended when a transient increase in QRS duration accompanies the ST-segment deviation seen with acute injury.[1,32,33]

NONSPECIFIC INTRAVENTRICULAR CONDUCTION DISTURBANCE

QRS duration greater than 110 ms in adults, greater than 90 ms in children 8–16 years of age, and greater than 80 ms in children less than 8 years of age without criteria for RBBB or LBBB are considered as intraventricular conduction disturbance (Figs. 13.35A and B). The definition may also be applied to a pattern with RBBB criteria in the precordial leads and LBBB criteria in the limb leads, and vice versa.[1]

SUMMARY

In ECG, if the QRS complex is wider than 0.12 seconds, this is mostly caused by a delay in the conduction tissue of one of the bundle branches, RBBB, LBBB, or intraventricular conduction delay (Box 13.1). A left or right axis rotation can be caused by a LAHB or LPHB.

In RBBB, activation of the right ventricle is delayed as depolarization has to spread across the septum from the left ventricle. The left ventricle is activated normally, meaning that the early part of the QRS complex is unchanged. The delayed RV activation produces a secondary R wave ($R^{\prime}$) in the right precordial leads (V1–3) and a wide, slurred S wave in the lateral leads. Delayed activation of the right ventricle also gives rise to secondary repolarization abnormalities, with ST depression and T-wave inversion in the right precordial leads (V1–V3). In isolated RBBB the cardiac axis is unchanged, as left ventricular activation proceeds normally via the left bundle branch. RBBB may be complete or incomplete. Incomplete RBBB is mostly a normal variant,

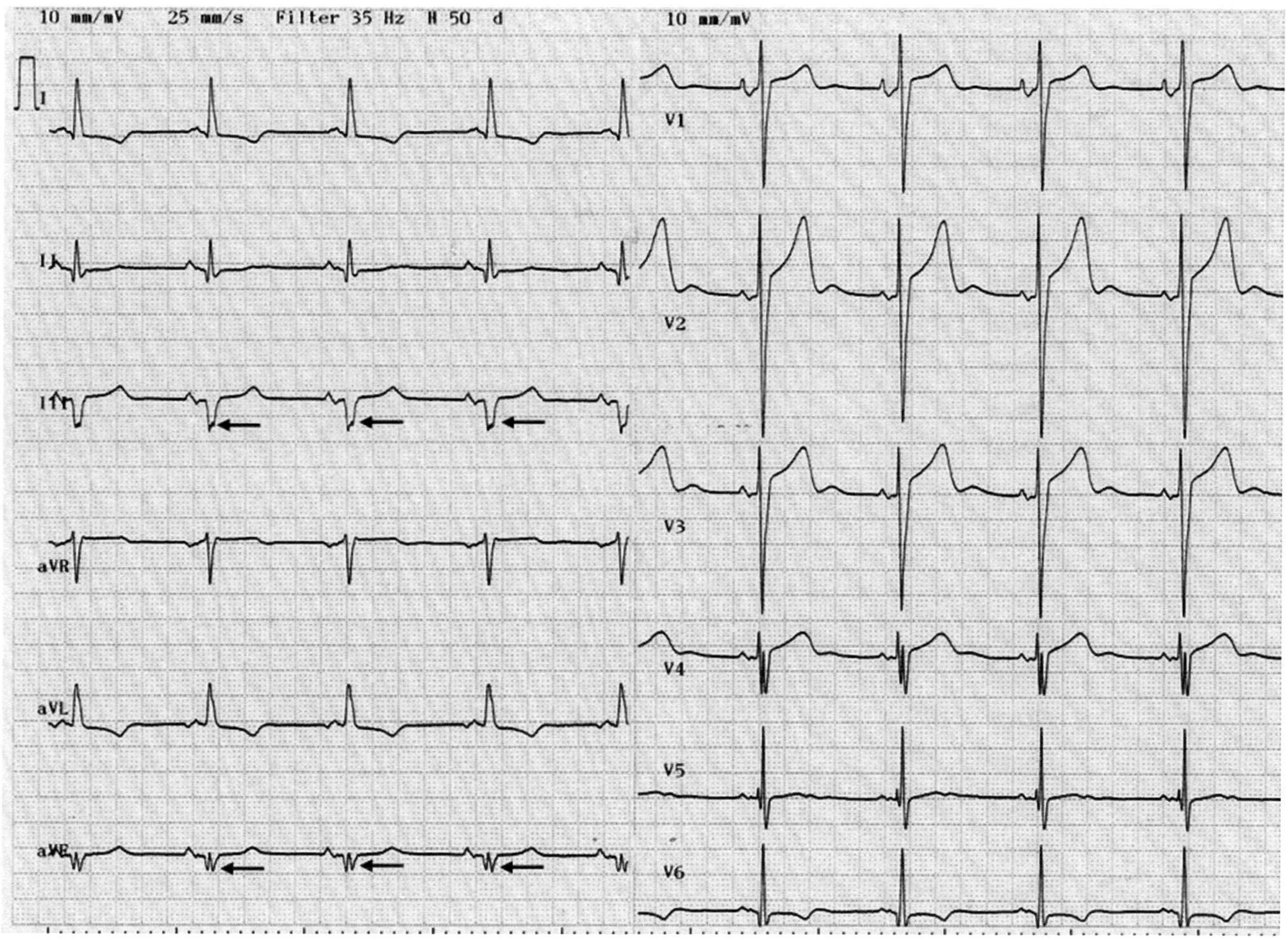

Fig. 13.34: Electrocardiogram shows peri-infarction block in inferior myocardial infarction. Note the presence of wide and slurred QRS complex (arrows) in LIII and aVF.

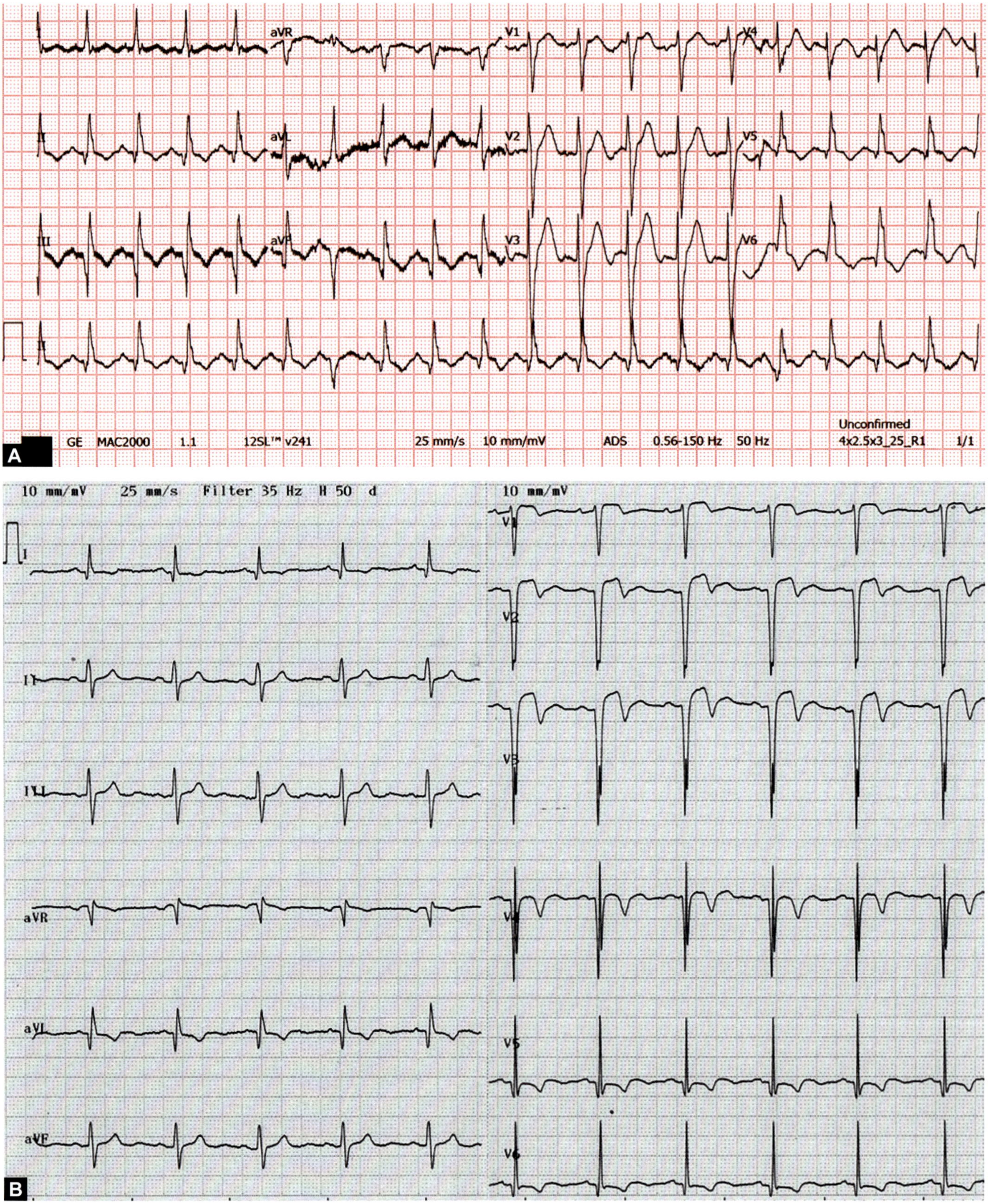

Figs. 13.35A and B: (A) Electrocardiogram showing broad and slurred QRS complexes (QRS duration is 125 ms) in LII, LIII, aVF, aVL, and V4–V6 suggestive of intraventricular conduction defect. Also note pathological Q waves in LII, LIII, and aVF suggestive of old inferior MI. (B) Electrocardiogram showing broad and slurred QRS complexes (QRS duration is 126 ms) in V2–V4 suggestive of intraventricular conduction defect. Note also the features of recent anterior MI.

Box 13.1: Diagnostic criteria of bundle branch block.

Diagnostic criteria of RBBB
- RSR' pattern in V1–3
- Broad QRS >120 ms (0.12 seconds)
- Wide and slurred S wave in the lateral leads (I, aVL, and V5–6)
- Secondary ST depression and T-wave inversion in the right precordial leads (V1–3)

Diagnostic criteria of LBBB
- Broad biphasic (M pattern) or monophasic R wave in lateral leads (I, aVL, and V5–V6).
- Dominant S wave in V1
- QRS duration of greater than 120 ms (0.12 seconds)
- Poor R-wave progression in the chest leads
- ST segments and T waves always go in the opposite direction (discordance) to the main vector of the QRS complex.
- Left axis deviation.

(*In complete BBB QRS duration is greater than 120 ms and in incomplete BBB, QRS duration is less than 120 ms but other ECG features are almost same as complete BBB.*)

commonly seen in children and healthy young athletes of no clinical significance. RBBB is two to three times more common among men than women.

Causes of Right Bundle Branch Block

- Congenital heart disease (e.g. atrial septal defect)
- Right ventricular hypertrophy (RVH)/cor pulmonale
- Ischemic heart disease
- Rheumatic heart disease
- Myocarditis
- Cardiomyopathy
- Pulmonary embolus
- Degenerative disease of the conduction system.

Diagnostic Criteria of Complete Right Bundle Branch Block

- RSR' pattern in V1–V3 (sometimes "M-shaped" QRS complex)
- Wide and slurred S wave in the lateral leads (I, aVL, and V5–V6)
- Broad QRS >120 ms
- Secondary ST depression and T-wave inversion in the right precordial leads (V1–V3).

Diagnostic Criteria of Incomplete Right Bundle Branch Block

- RSR' pattern in V1–V3 or slurred QRS complex in V1–V3.
- QRS duration is less than 120 ms.

Left Bundle Branch Block

In LBBB, the normal direction of septal depolarization is reversed, becomes right to left, as the impulse spreads first to the right ventricle via the right bundle branch and then to the left ventricle via the septum. Normally, the septum is activated from left to right, producing small Q waves in the lateral leads. But the altered sequence of activation extends the QRS duration to greater than 120 ms and eliminates the normal septal Q waves in the lateral leads. The overall direction of depolarization (from right to left) produces tall R waves in the lateral leads (I and V5–6) and deep S waves in the right precordial leads (V1–3), and usually leads to left axis deviation. As the ventricles are activated sequentially (right, then left) rather than simultaneously, this produces a broad or notched ("M"-shaped) R wave in the L1, aVL, and V5–V6.

Causes of Left Bundle Branch Block

- Chronic ischemic heart disease
- ST-elevation myocardial infarction
- Primary degenerative disease (fibrosis) of the conducting system
- Hypertension
- Aortic stenosis
- Dilated cardiomyopathy
- Lenegre's disease
- Hyperkalemia.

Diagnostic Criteria of Complete Left Bundle Branch Block

- Broad and slurred QRS complex in lateral leads (LI, aVL, and V5–V6). QRS morphology in the lateral leads may be of "M"-shaped, notched, monophasic, or RS complex.
- QRS duration of greater than 120 ms
- Dominant S wave in V1 with poor R-wave progression in the chest leads
- Absence of normal septal Q waves in lateral leads.
- Left axis deviation
- Discordance of the ST segments and T waves. ST segment and T waves always go in the opposite direction to the main vector of the QRS complex.
- Prolonged R-wave peak time >60 ms in left precordial leads (V5–V6).

Diagnostic Criteria of Incomplete Left Bundle Branch Block

Incomplete LBBB is diagnosed when typical LBBB morphology is associated with a QRS duration <120 ms.

Right Bundle Branch Block versus Left Bundle Branch Block

Check V1 when QRS is greater than 0.12 seconds. When the "terminal force" of the QRS in V1 is below the baseline (i.e. QS-wave), a LBBB is the most likely diagnosis. When the "terminal force" of the QRS in V1 is above the baseline (i.e.

RSR' wave), it's a RBBB. If the QRS is greater than 110 ms, but the morphological criteria of LBBB or RBBB do not apply, it is called intraventricular conduction delay.

Sometimes, BBB is rate-dependent. The BBB occurs only at higher heart rates and disappears at slower heart rates. RBBB is considered more benign compared to LBBB. Individual with LBBB but not with RBBB had a markedly increased risk of dying from coronary disease.

Hemiblocks

Anatomically left bundle branch divides into three fascicles, left anterior fascicle, left posterior fascicle, and a small septal fascicle. But the third fascicle (septal fascicle) is not very important from clinical point of view.

The fascicles can also be damaged, leading to what is called hemiblock or fascicular to block, usually specified as left anterior hemiblock (LAHB) or left anterior fascicular block (LAFB) and left posterior hemiblock (LPHB) or left posterior fascicular block (LPFB). Left anterior hemiblock is a common ECG finding but isolated left posterior hemiblock is very rare.

Causes of hemiblocks are as follows:

- Coronary artery disease
- Hypertension
- Cardiomyopathies
- Advancing age
- Normal variant without any structural heart disease.
- Lev and Lenegre diseases
- Aortic valvular disease.

ECG Criteria: Left Anterior Hemiblock (LAHB)

- Small Q waves with tall R waves (qR complexes) in leads I and aVL
- Small R waves with deep S waves (rS complexes) in leads II, III, and aVF
- Left axis deviation (usually between –45° and –90°)
- QRS duration is normal or slightly prolonged (80–110 ms)
- Prolonged R-wave peak time in aVL >45 ms.

Clinical Significance of Left Anterior Hemiblock

- It can be seen in approximately 4% of cases of AMI.
- It is the most common type of intraventricular conduction defect seen in acute anterior myocardial infarction.
- It also can be seen with acute inferior wall myocardial infarction.
- It is also associated with hypertensive heart disease, aortic valvular disease, cardiomyopathies, and degenerative fibrotic disease of the cardiac skeleton.

ECG Criteria: Left Posterior Hemiblock (LPHB)

- Small Q waves with tall R waves (qR complexes) in leads II, III, and aVF
- Small R waves with deep S waves (rS complexes) in leads I and aVL
- Right axis deviation (> +90°)
- QRS duration is normal or slightly prolonged (80–110 ms)
- No evidence of RV hypertrophy or any other cause for right axis deviation.

Clinical Significance of Left Posterior Hemiblock

Left posterior hemiblock is much less common than LAHB, as the broad bundle of fibers that comprise the left posterior fascicle are relatively resistant to damage when compared with the slim single tract that makes up the left anterior fascicle. It is extremely rare to see LPHB in isolation. It usually occurs along with RBBB in the context of a bifascicular block. It is not wise to diagnose LPHB until the other more significant causes of right axis deviation, i.e. RVH, lateral MI, pulmonary embolism, etc. are ruled out.

Left Septal Hemiblock

Left septal hemiblock is also known as LSFB is not a well-defined ECG entity. There are no standard criteria for detecting conduction defects involving the third left fascicle, the septal or median fascicle, and the very existence of such defects is still a matter of controversy. But the proposed criteria of ECG diagnosis of LSHB (LSFB) are: (1) Loss of initial R waves in right precordial leads accompanied by loss of septal Q waves (LI, V5, and V6); (2) Transient right precordial Q waves during myocardial ischemia in the absence of infarction; (3) QS complexes in right precordial leads in the absence of LBBB or infarction.

Bifascicular Block

A bifascicular block occurs when both the right bundle branch and either the left anterior or posterior fascicle are blocked. It is a combination of RBBB with either LAHB or LPHB (RBBB + LAHB or RBBB + LPHB pattern). In this situation, conduction to the ventricles is sustained via the single remaining fascicle. The ECG will show typical features of RBBB plus either left or right axis deviation. RBBB + LAHB is the most common of the two patterns. Some authors consider LBBB to be a "bifascicular block," because both fascicles of the left bundle branch are blocked.

Causes of Bifascicular Block

- Coronary artery disease
- Hypertension

- Valvular heart disease
- Advanced age
- Primary degenerative disease of the conducting system (Lenegre's/Lev's disease)
- Congenital heart disease
- Hyperkalemia.

Trifascicular Block

Bifascicular block + first degree AV block is referred as trifascicular block. Trifascicular block include:

- RBBB + LAHB + first degree heart block.
- RBBB + LPHB + first degree heart block.
- LBBB + first degree heart block.

Trifascicular block may progress to complete heart block.

REFERENCES

1. Surawicz B, Childers R, Deal BJ, et al. AHA/ACCF/HRS recommendations for the standardization and interpretation of the electrocardiogram. Part III: intraventricular conduction disturbances: a scientific statement from the American Heart Association Electrocardiography and Arrhythmias Committee, Council on Clinical Cardiology; the American College of Cardiology Foundation; and the Heart Rhythm Society: endorsed by the international society for computerized electrocardiology. Circulation. 2009;119:e235-e240.
2. Costa D, Brady WJ, Edhouse J. Bradycardias and atrioventricular conduction block. BMJ. 2002;324(7336): 535-8.
3. Fahy GJ, Pinski SL, Miller DP, et al. Natural history of isolated bundle branch block. Am J Cardiol. 1996;77(14):1185-90.
4. Eriksson P, Hansson PO, Eriksson H, et al. Bundle-branch block in a general male population: the study of men born 1913. Circulation. 1998;98(22):2494-500.
5. Fleg JL, Das DN, Lakatta EG. Right bundle branch block: long-term prognosis in apparently healthy men. J Am Coll Cardiol. 1983;1(3):887-92.
6. Movahed MR. Diabetes as a risk factor for cardiac conduction defects: a review. Diabetes Obes Metab. 2007;9(3):276-81.
7. Miller WL, Hodge DO, Hammill SC. Association of uncomplicated electrocardiographic conduction blocks with subsequent cardiac morbidity in a community-based population (Olmsted County, Minnesota). Am J Cardiol. 2008;101(1):102-6.
8. Jeong JH, Kim JH, Park YH, et al. Incidence of and risk factors for bundle branch block in adults older than 40 years. Korean J Intern Med. 2004;19(3):171-8.
9. Thrainsdottir IS, Hardarson T, Thorgeirsson G, et al. The epidemiology of right bundle branch block and its association with cardiovascular morbidity—the Reykjavik Study. Eur Heart J. 1993;14(12):1590-6.
10. Schneider JF, Thomas HE, Kreger BE, et al. Newly acquired right bundle-branch block: the Framingham Study. Ann Intern Med. 1980;92(1):37-44.
11. Bussink BE, Holst AG, Jespersen L, et al. Right bundle branch block: prevalence, risk factors, and outcome in the general population: results from the Copenhagen City Heart Study Eur Heart J. 2012;34(2):138-46.
12. Barsheshet A, Goldenberg I, Garty M, et al. Relation of bundle branch block to long-term (four-year) mortality in hospitalized patients with systolic heart failure. Am J Cardiol. 2011;107(4):540-4.
13. Abdel-Qadir HM, Tu JV, Austin PC, et al. Bundle branch block patterns and long-term outcomes in heart failure. Int J Cardiol. 2011;146(2):213-8.
14. Le VV, Wheeler MT, Mandic S, et al. Addition of the electrocardiogram to the preparticipation examination of college athletes. Clin J Sport Med. 2010;20(2):98-105.
15. Liao Y, Emidy LA, Dyer A, et al. Characteristics and prognosis of incomplete right bundle branch block: an epidemiologic study. J Am Coll Cardiol. 1986;7(3):492-9.
16. Godman MJ, Lassers BW, Julian DG. Complete bundle-branch block complicating acute myocardial infarction. N Engl J Med. 1970;282(5):237-40.
17. Neeland IJ, Kontos MC, de Lemos JA. Evolving considerations in the management of patients with left bundle branch block and suspected myocardial infarction. J Am Coll Cardiol. 2012;60(2):96-105.
18. Bansilal S, Aneja A, Mathew V, et al. Long-term cardiovascular outcomes in patients with angina pectoris presenting with bundle branch block. Am J Cardiol. 2011;107(11):1565-70.
19. Go AS, Barron HV, Rundle AC, et al. Bundle-branch block and inhospital mortality in acute myocardial infarction. National Registry of Myocardial Infarction 2 Investigators. Ann Intern Med. 1998;129(9):690-7.
20. Cannon CP, McCabe CH, Stone PH, et al. The electrocardiogram predicts one-year outcome of patients with unstable angina and non-Q wave myocardial infarction: results of the TIMI III Registry ECG Ancillary Study. Thrombolysis in Myocardial Ischemia. J Am Coll Cardiol. 1997;30(1):133-40.
21. Hindman MC, Wagner GS, JaRo M, et al. The clinical significance of bundle branch block complicating acute myocardial infarction. Clinical characteristics, hospital mortality, and one-year follow-up. Circulation. 1978;58(4):679-88.
22. Deharo JC. Left bundle branch block. Electrocardiographic and prognostic aspects. Arch Mal Coeur Vaiss. 2000;93(3):31-7.
23. Eriksson P, Wilhelmsen L, Rosengren A. Bundle-branch block in middle-aged men: risk of complications and death over 28 years. The Primary Prevention Study in Göteborg, Sweden. Eur Heart J. 2005;26(21):2300-6.
24. van Hemel NM. Left is worse than right: the outcome of bundle branch block in middle-aged men. Eur Heart J. 2005;26(21):2222-3.
25. MacAlpin RN. Left septal fascicular block: myth or reality? Indian Pacing Electrophysiol J. 2003;3(3):157-77.
26. Perez Riera AR, Ferreira C, Ferreira Filho C, et al. Electrovectorcardiographic diagnosis of left septal fascicular block: anatomic and clinical considerations. Ann Noninvasive Electrocardiol. 2011;16(2):196-207.
27. Epstein AE, DiMarco JP, Ellenbogen KA, et al. ACC/AHA/HRS 2008 guidelines for device-based therapy of cardiac rhythm abnormalities: a report of the American College of Cardiology/American Heart Association Task Force on Practice Guidelines (Writing committee to revise the ACC/AHA/NASPE 2002 Guideline update for implantation of cardiac pacemakers and antiarrhythmia devices): developed in collaboration with the American Association for Thoracic

Surgery and Society of Thoracic Surgeons. Circulation. 2008;117:e350.
28. Moya A, Sutton R, Ammirati F, et al. Guidelines for the diagnosis and management of syncope (version 2009). The task force for the diagnosis and management of syncope of the European Society of Cardiology (ESC). Eur Heart J. 2009;30(21):2631-71.
29. Harrigan RA, Pollack ML, Chan TC. Electrocardiographic manifestations: bundle branch blocks and fascicular blocks. J Emerg Med. 2003;25(1):67-77.
30. Grant RP. Peri-infarction block. Prog Cardiovasc Dis. 1959;2:237-47.
31. Vassallo JA, Cassidy DM, Marchlinski FE, et al. Abnormalities of endocardial activation pattern in patients with previous healed myocardial infarction and ventricular tachycardia. Am J Cardiol. 1986;58(6):479-84.
32. Wagner NB, Sevilla DC, Krucoff MW, et al. Transient alterations of the QRS complex and ST segment during percutaneous transluminal balloon angioplasty of the left anterior descending coronary artery. Am J Cardiol. 1988;62(16):1038-142.
33. Surawicz B. Reversible QRS changes during acute myocardial ischemia. J Electrocardiol. 1998;31(3):209-20.

Chapter 14

Sick Sinus Syndrome

INTRODUCTION

The sinoatrial (SA) node is a collection of specialized cells located in the sulcus terminalis at the junction of the superior vena cava and the right atrium that depolarize spontaneously. The sinus node is supplied with blood by the sinus node artery, which originates from the proximal right coronary artery in 65% of patients, the circumflex artery in 25%, and both in 10%. Normally, impulses originate in the sinus node and propagate through the right atrium to the atrioventricular (AV) node in the low septal right atrium.[1,2]

The SA node represents the integrated activity of pacemaker cells, sometimes called P cells, in a compact region at the junction of the high right atrium and the superior vena cava. Perinodal cells, sometimes called transitional or T cells, transmit the electrical impulse from the SA node to the right atrium. Each of these cell types has distinct expression profiles of ion channels and gap junctions. Given the architecture of the SA node, SA nodal dysfunction typically results from either abnormalities in impulse generation by the P cells or abnormalities in conduction across the T cells. SA nodal dysfunction is more commonly an acquired condition, but in some patients it can be inherited, with gene mutations having been described in some forms of inherited SA nodal dysfunction.[3] Patients with SA nodal dysfunction may be asymptomatic or highly symptomatic as in cases of sick sinus syndrome.

Sick sinus syndrome (sinus node dysfunction) may be due to intrinsic pathologic characteristics of the sinus node itself, or it may be due to extrinsic causes. Intrinsic disease is characterized by the replacement of nodal tissue with fibrous tissue. Since the sinus node is a complex of cells in the atrial wall, permanent injury by infarction or infection is uncommon. Extrinsic causes of sinus node dysfunction include the use of pharmacologic agents (e.g. β-adrenergic blockers, calcium-channel blockers, digoxin, some antihypertensive agents, and antiarrhythmic drugs), electrolyte imbalance, hypothermia, hypothyroidism, increased intracranial pressure, and excessive vagal tone.[2,4-10]

The possible electrocardiographic features include persistent sinus bradycardia, periods of SA block, sinus arrest, junctional or ventricular escape rhythms, tachycardia-bradycardia syndrome, paroxysmal atrial flutter, and atrial fibrillation (AF). The most common electrocardiographic feature is an inappropriate, persistent, and often severe sinus bradycardia.[11] Sick sinus syndrome, either intrinsic or extrinsic, may have several electrocardiographic presentations. Sinus bradycardia is due to depressed automaticity in the sinus node itself. Sinus pauses or sinus arrest may be due to failure of either impulse formation or conduction out of the nodal region to the surrounding atrium. Abnormal automaticity and conduction in the atrium predispose patients to AF and flutter, and the tachycardia-bradycardia syndrome is also a common manifestation of sick sinus syndrome. The combination of tachycardia and sinus bradycardia in patients with sinus node dysfunction is particularly worrisome.[11]

SINUS BRADYCARDIA

Sinus bradycardia is a common finding in the sick sinus syndrome (Fig. 14.1). The rate may fall as low as 30–35 beats/minute (Fig. 14.2).

SINUS ARREST

In addition to sustained sinus bradycardia, sick sinus syndrome may occur intermittently, ranging from a delayed beat (sinus pause) (Fig. 14.3) to long periods of asystole (sinus arrest-pause >3 seconds) (Figs. 14.4A and B). Sinus arrest occurs when there is transient cessation of impulse formation at the SA node; it manifests as a prolonged pause without P wave activity (Figs. 14.5A to C). The pause is unrelated to the length of the P-P cycle.

ESCAPE RHYTHMS

In sinus arrest, the SA node transiently ceases to generate the electrical impulses that normally stimulate the myocardial tissues to contract and thus the heart to beat. Since the heart contains multiple pacemakers, this interruption of the cardiac cycle generally lasts only a few seconds before another part of the heart begins pacing and restores the cardiac rhythm. If a pacemaker other than the SA node

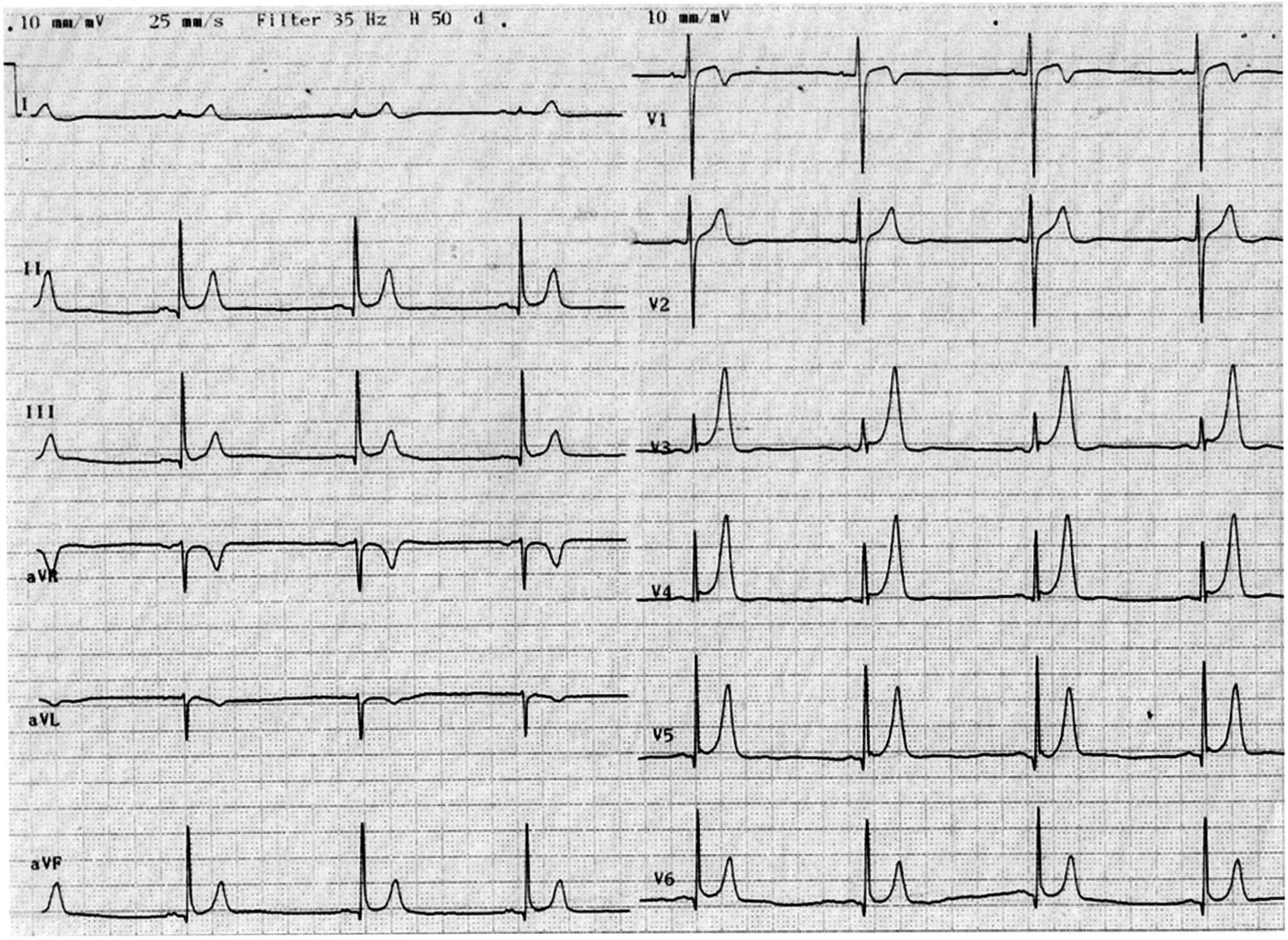

Fig. 14.1: ECG is suggestive of marked sinus bradycardia [heart rate 45 beats per minute (bpm)]. Note all the QRS complexes are preceded by a P wave. Marked sinus bradycardia may be the initial ECG manifestation of sick sinus syndrome.

is pacing the heart, this condition is known as an escape rhythm (Fig. 14.6). Extreme sinus bradycardia interspersed with escape beat during long pause may be the ECG manifestation of sick sinus syndrome (Fig. 14.7). Escape rhythms are the result of spontaneous activity from a subsidiary pacemaker, located in the atria, AV junction, or ventricles. Atrial escape (rate 60–80) originates within atria other than sinus node, so normal P morphology is lost. Junctional escape (rate 40–60) originates near the AV node (Fig. 14.8); a normal P wave is not seen, may be occasionally seen as a retrograde P wave. Ventricular escape (rate 20–40) originates in ventricular conduction system with no P wave and manifests on ECG with wide and abnormal QRS complex (Fig. 14.9). Escape rhythms take over when normal impulse formation or conduction fails and may be associated with any profound bradycardia.

TACHYCARDIA-BRADYCARDIA SYNDROME

Tachycardia-bradycardia syndrome is a variant of sick sinus syndrome in which the arrhythmia alternates between slow and fast heart rates (Figs. 14.10A and B). Sometimes runs of tachycardia interspersed with long sinus pauses are seen (Figs. 14.11A and B). Sometimes sinus beats are followed by paroxysms of junctional tachycardia.

Several tachycardias of supraventricular origin may occur in patients with the sick sinus syndrome. Among them paroxysmal AF and flutter are the most common. Slow AF may be a manifestation of sick sinus syndrome (Fig. 14.12). Atrial tachycardia can also occur. Sinus node automaticity is often depressed by these tachycardias, so sinus bradycardia or arrest follows tachycardia. Conversely, tachycardias often arise as an escape rhythm following bradycardia. Thus, tachycardia often alternates with bradycardia. The combination of tachycardia and sinus bradycardia in patients with sick sinus syndrome is particularly worrisome, since overdrive suppression of sinus automaticity may result in long pauses and syncope when tachycardia terminates. Therapy to control the ventricular rate during tachycardia by blocking AV conduction with β-adrenergic blockers, calcium-channel blockers, or digitalis may not be possible, because it may further depress the sinus node.[2]

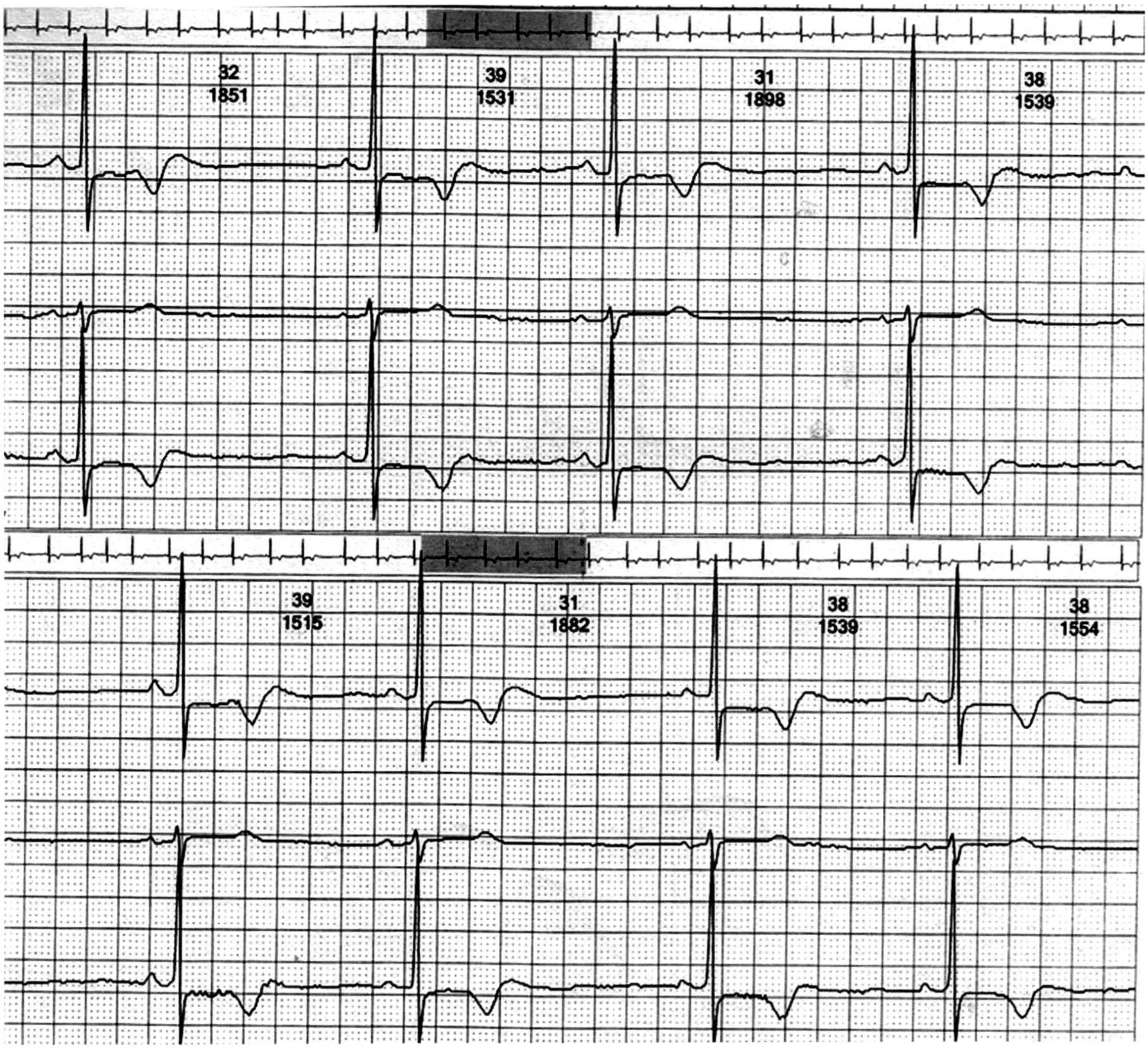

Fig. 14.2: ECG (Holter strip) is suggestive of extreme sinus bradycardia (heart rate 34 bpm), which may be the presentation of sick sinus syndrome.

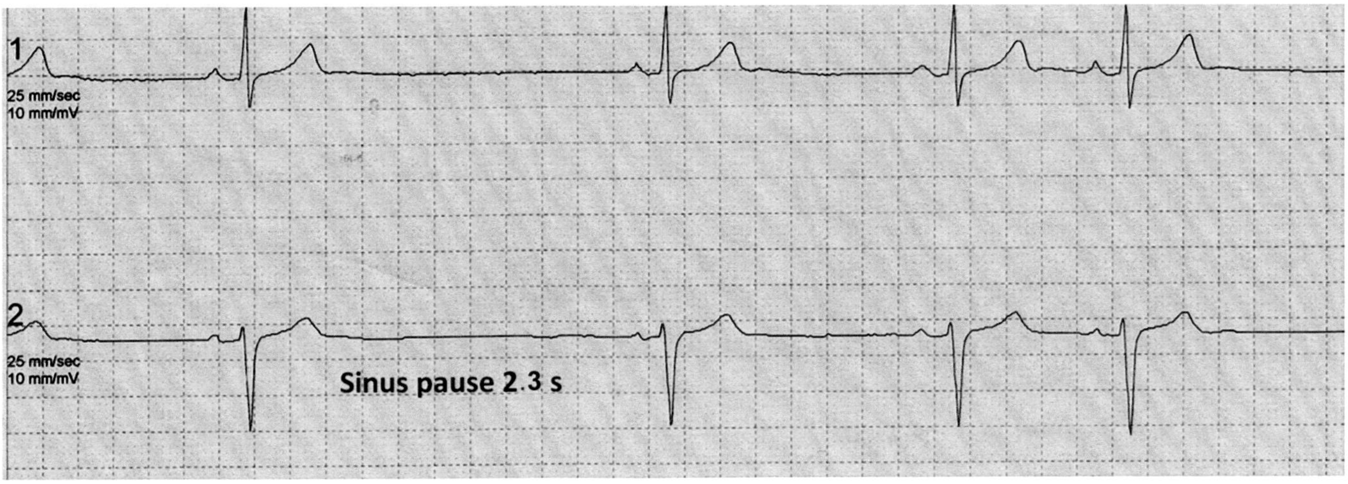

Fig. 14.3: Holter ECG strip showing 2.3 seconds sinus pause.

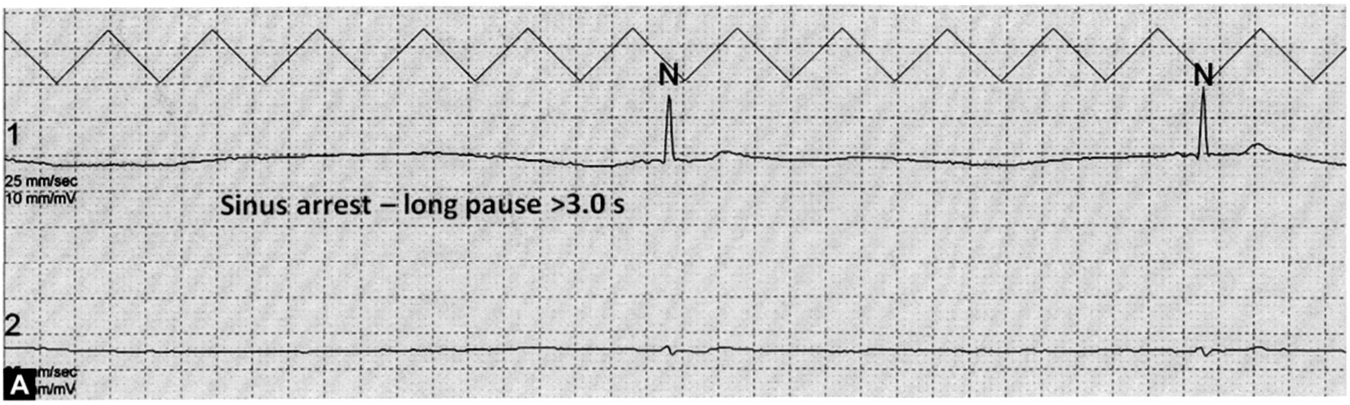

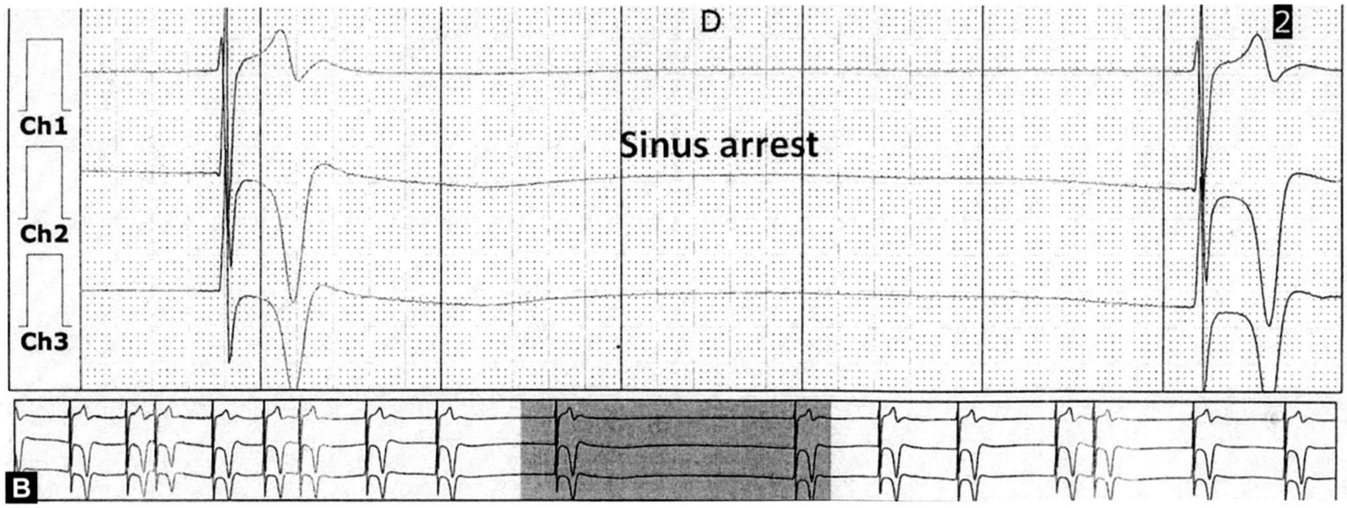

Figs. 14.4A and B: (A) ECG strip illustrates sinus arrest (long pause >3.0 s). Prolonged absence of sinus node activity (absent P waves) greater than 3 seconds is suggestive of sinus arrest; (B) Holter ECG strip illustrates sinus arrest (long pause >3.0 s). Note prolonged absence of P waves suggestive of sinus arrest.

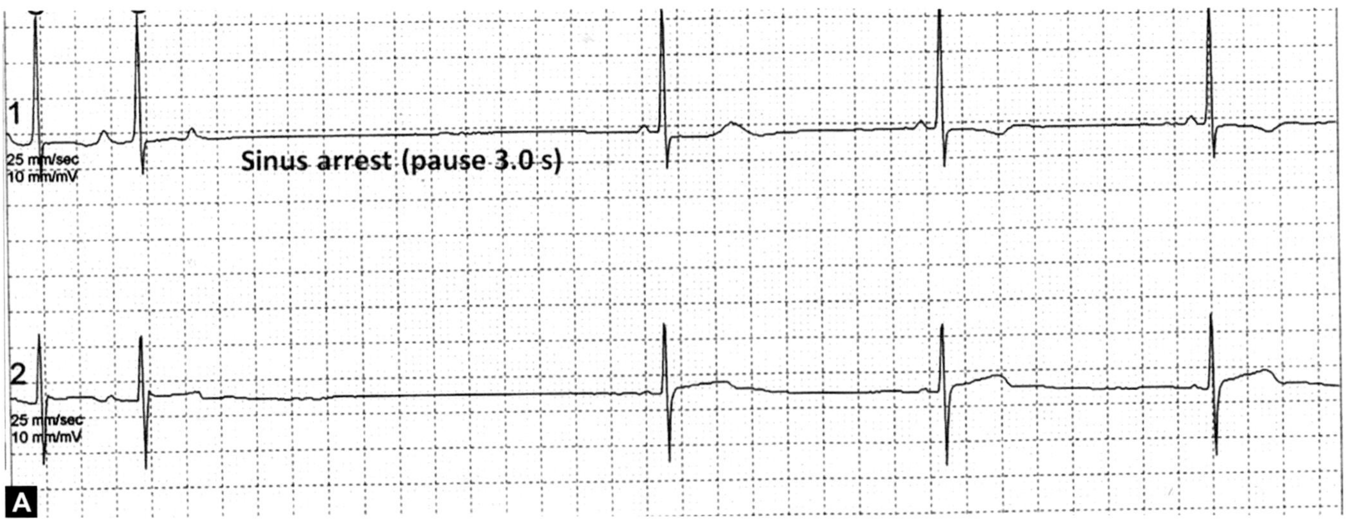

Fig. 14.5A: ECG strip is suggestive of sinus arrest (pause 3.0 s). Note no P wave during the period of prolonged pause.

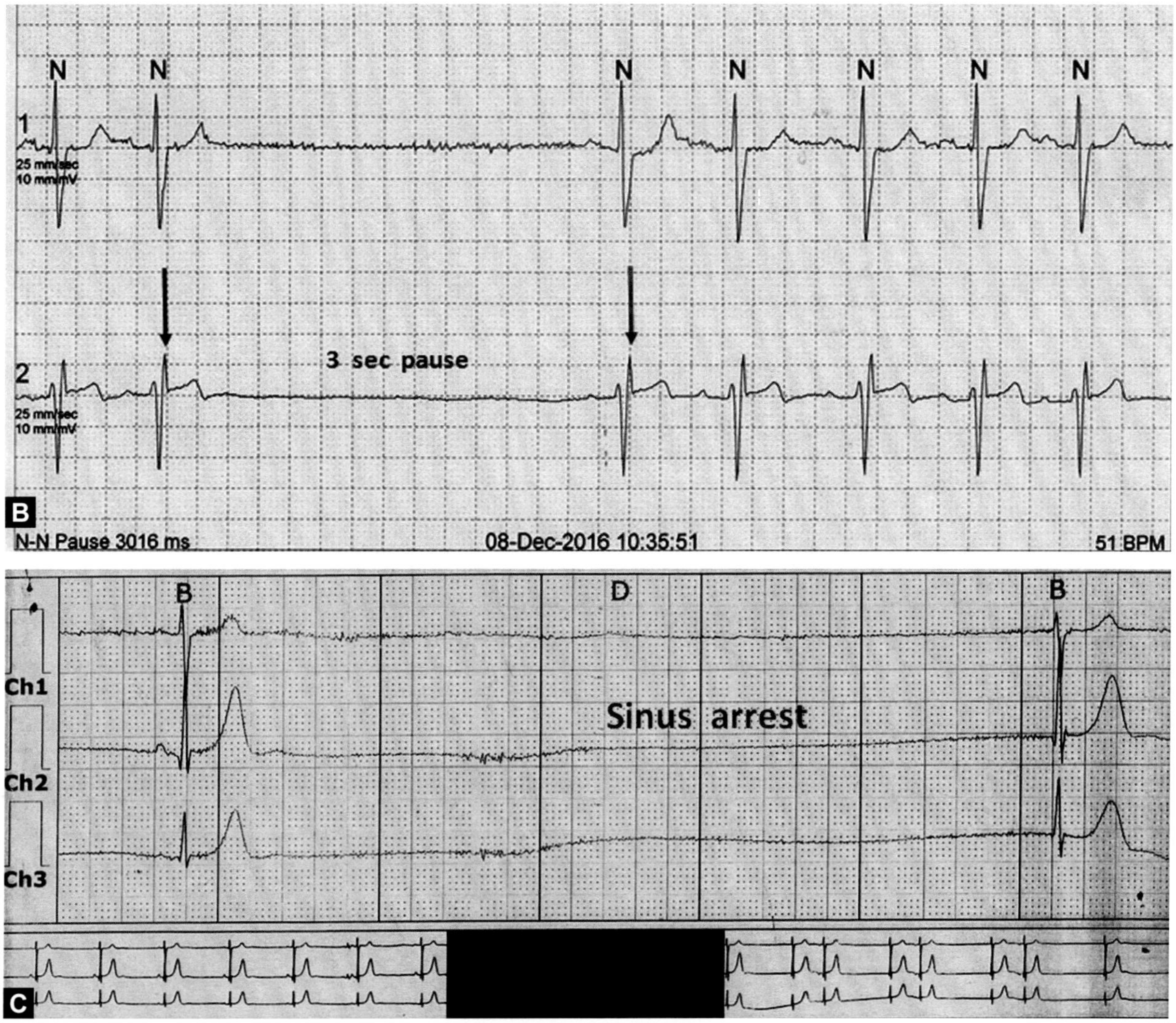

Figs. 14.5B and C: (B) ECG strip showing 3.0 seconds pause. Pause greater than 3.0 seconds is always significant and is an indication of permanent pacemaker implantation; (C) ECG strip illustrates sinus arrest. Note >3.0 s pause without any P wave.

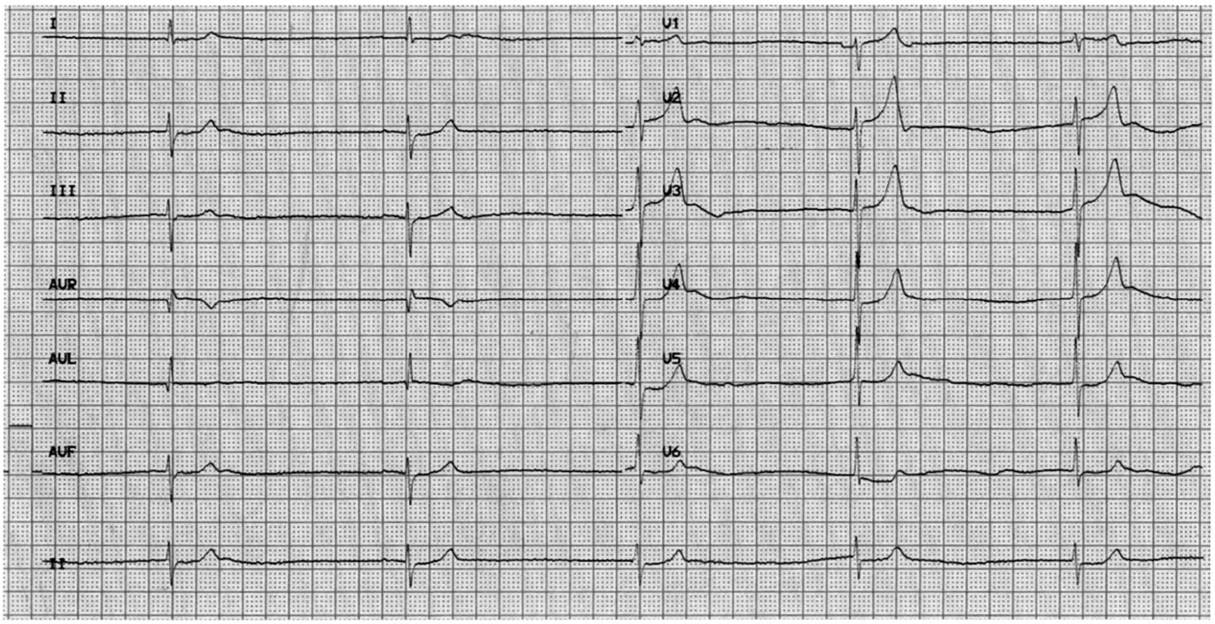

Fig. 14.6: ECG illustrates escape rhythm (rate 30 bpm). Possibly escape rhythm originates in supra-His region, so QRS complexes appear narrow.

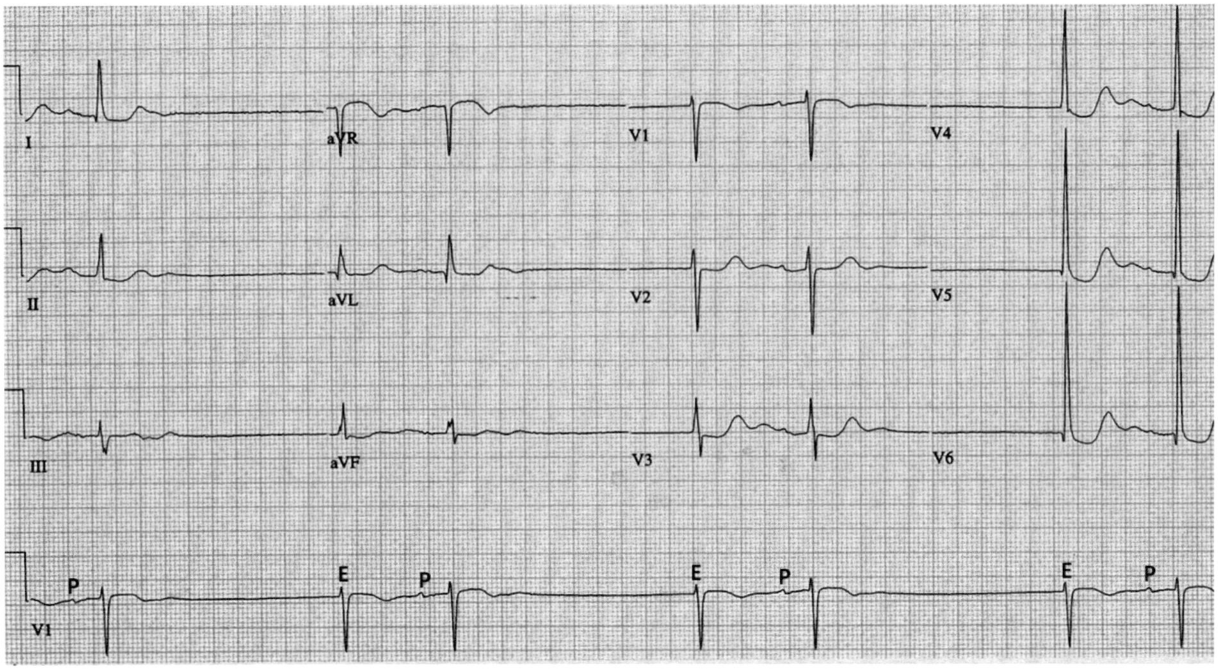

Fig. 14.7: ECG is consistent with extreme sinus bradycardia interspersed with escape beats suggestive of sick sinus syndrome. Note P waves with normal polarity with prolonged PR interval throughout the tracing with severe bradycardia and after long pauses narrow QRS complexes similar in morphology to the conducted beats, representing junctional escape beats (E). These junctional beats appear not to reset the sinus node as the sinus cycle length remains rather constant with only minor variations, giving the appearance of "group beating". Note sinus conducted QRS complexes are preceded by P waves but escape beats (E) are not preceded by any P wave.

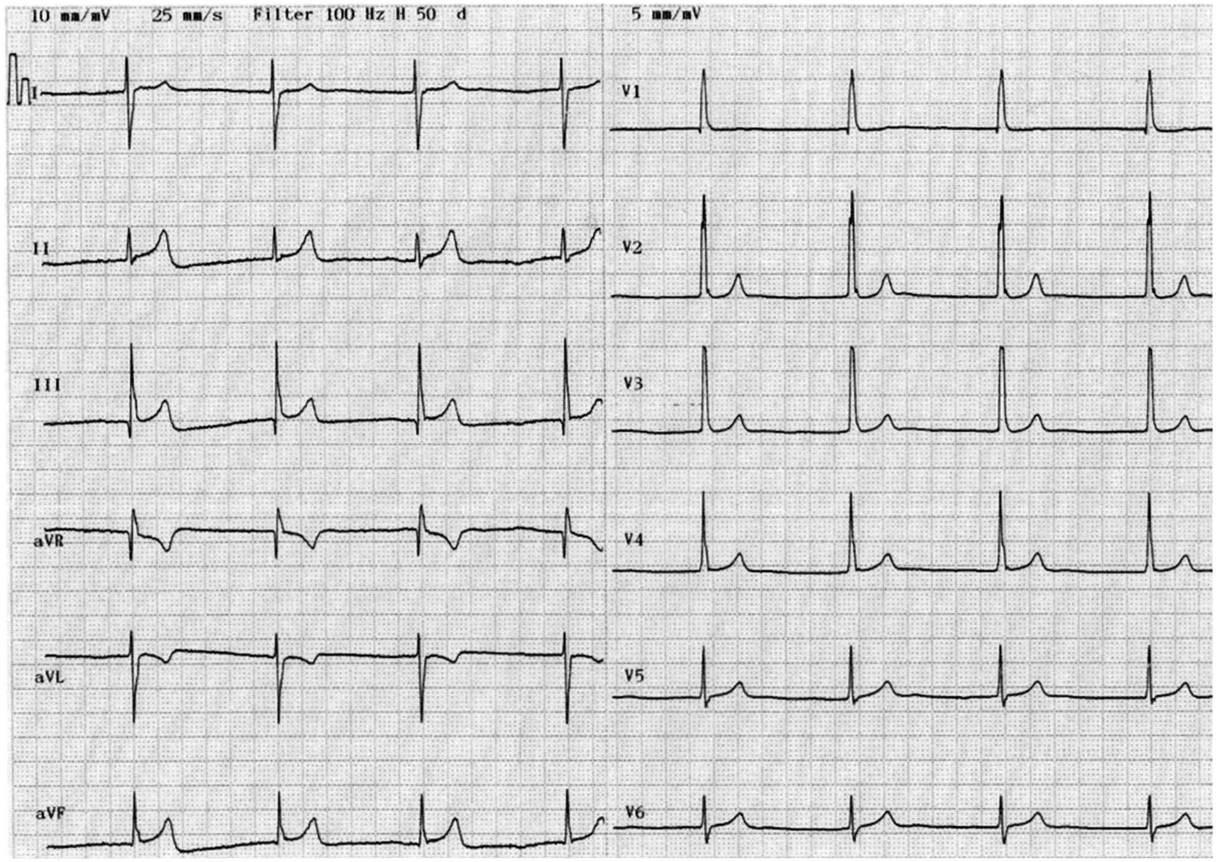

Fig. 14.8: ECG is suggestive of junctional escape rhythm (rate 50 bpm). No P wave manifest on ECG preceding QRS complexes.

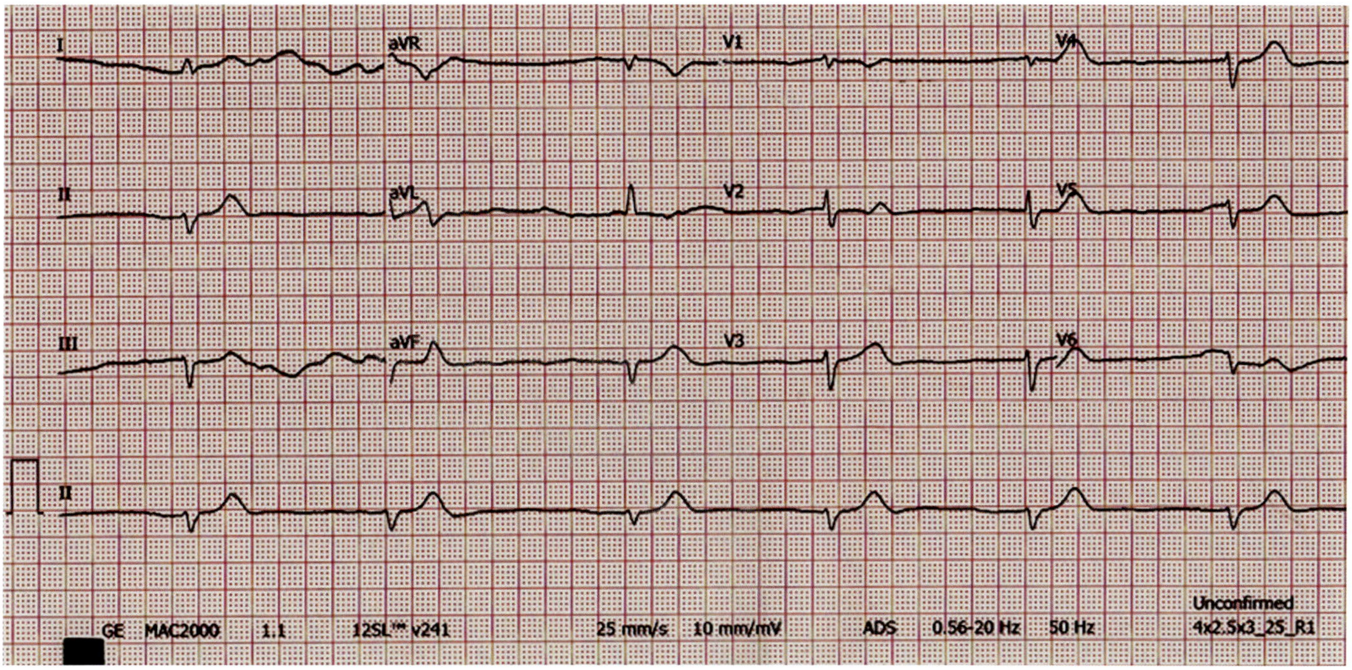

Fig. 14.9: ECG is suggestive of sick sinus syndrome with ventricular escape rhythm (no P waves) with extreme bradycardia (heart rate 38 bpm). Escape rhythm originates in ventricular conduction system with no P wave and manifests on ECG with wide and abnormal QRS complex.

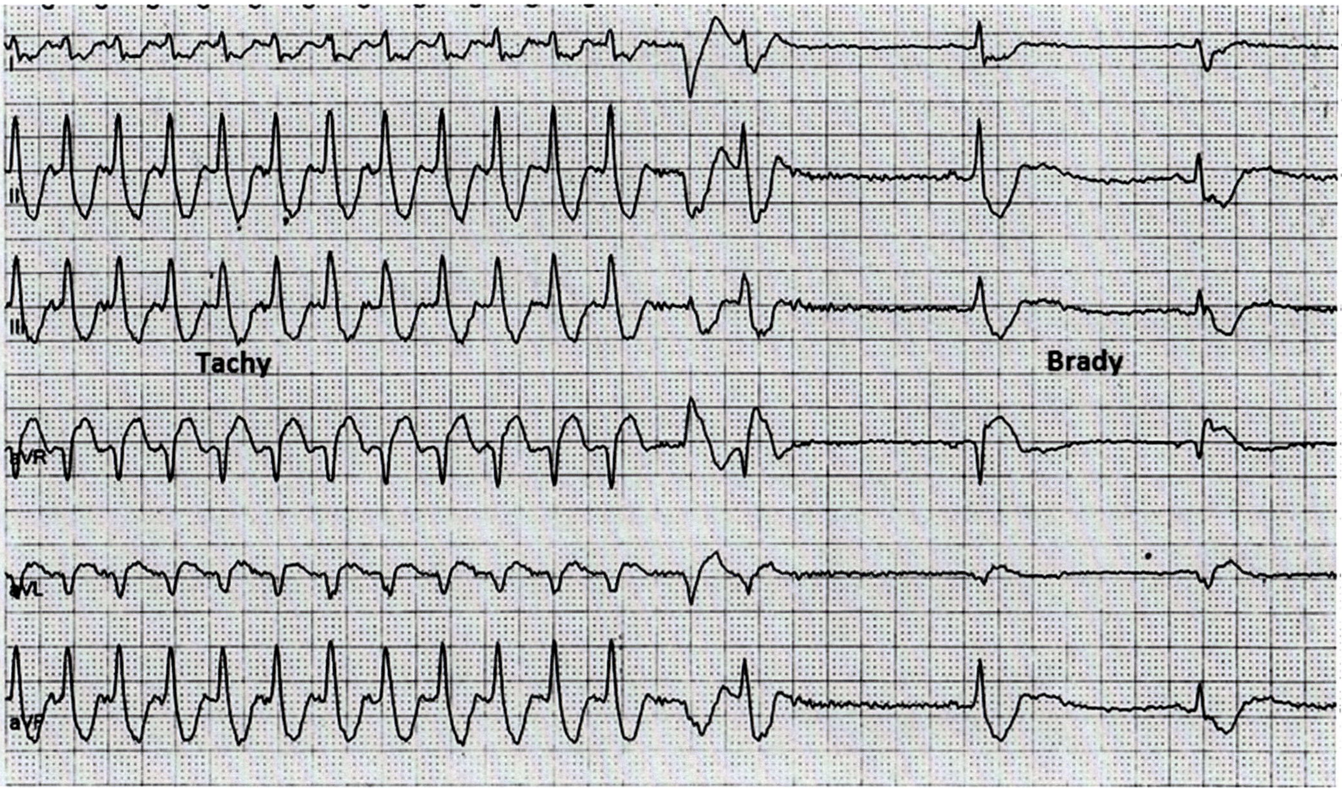

Fig. 14.10A: ECG strip shows tachycardia-bradycardia syndrome. *Note* tachy (left side of the ECG) followed by brady (right side).

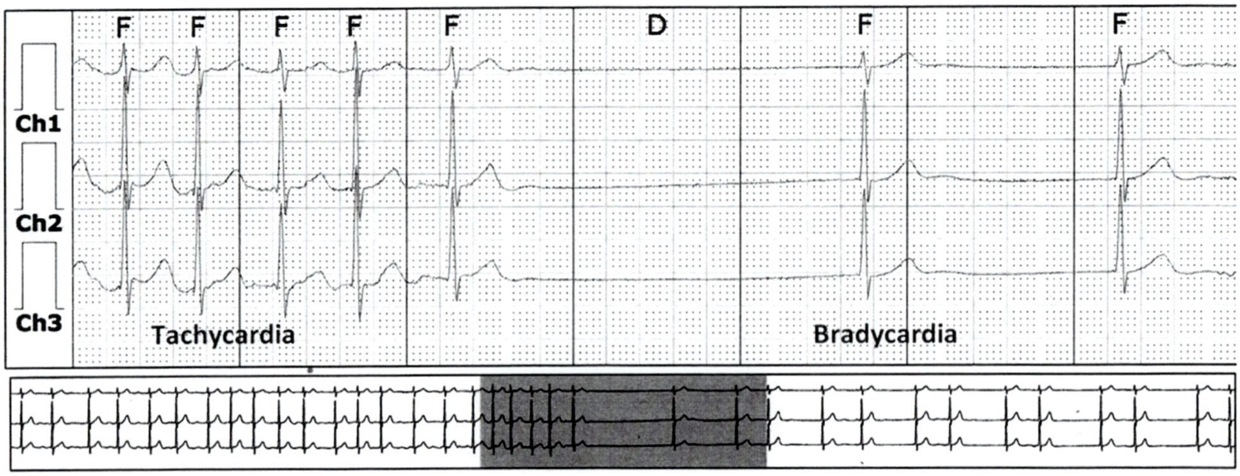

Fig. 14.10B: ECG strip shows tachycardia-bradycardia syndrome. Left side of the Holter monitoring strip shows tachycardia and right side shows severe bradyarrhythmia.

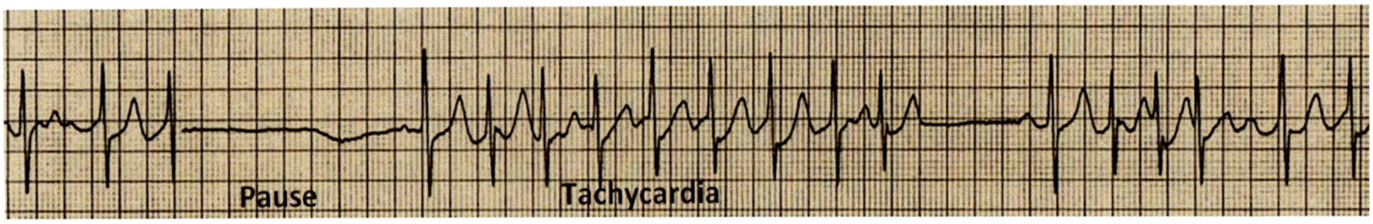

Fig. 14.11A: ECG strip illustrates a variant of tachycardia-bradycardia syndrome. In tachycardia-bradycardia syndrome, sometimes runs of tachycardia interspersed with long sinus pauses are seen.

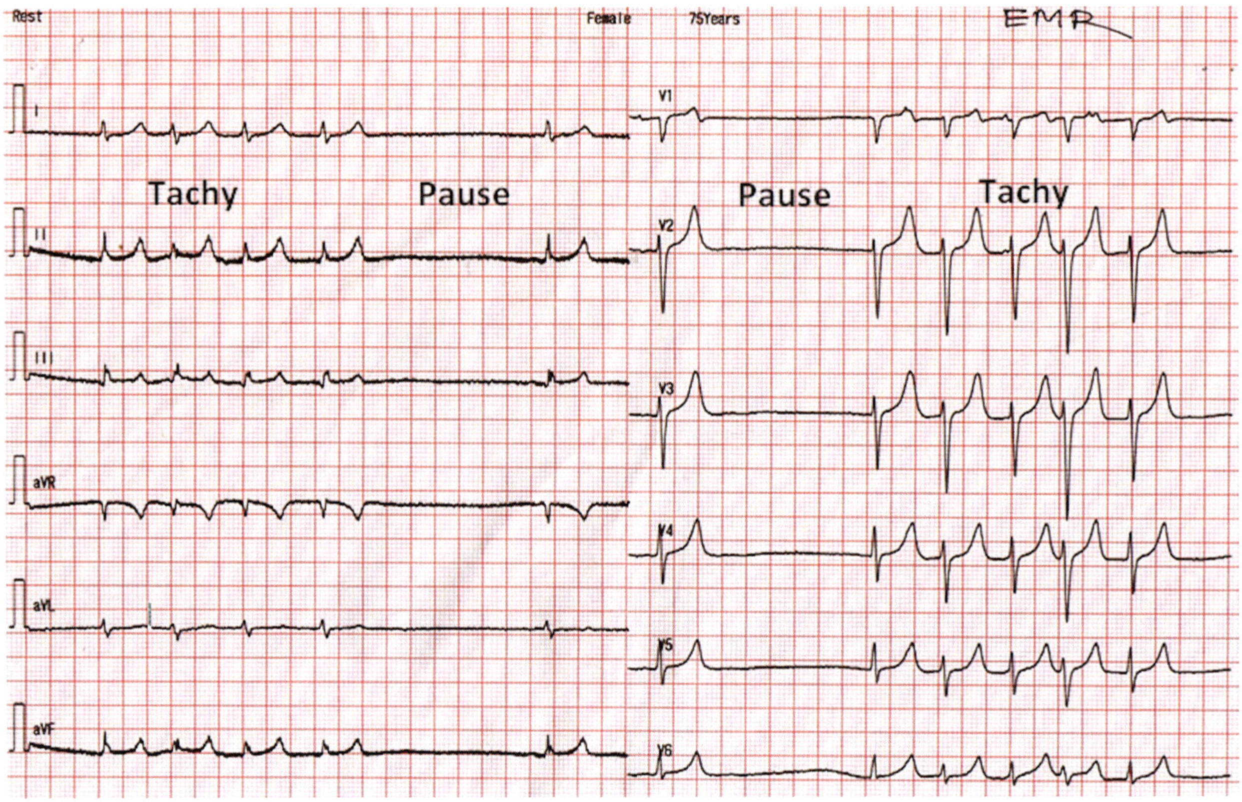

Fig. 14.11B: ECG of a patient with sick sinus syndrome presenting with tachycardia-bradycardia syndrome and this electrocardiogram shows recurrent tachycardia and pause, documented during taking standard bedside 12 lead ECG.

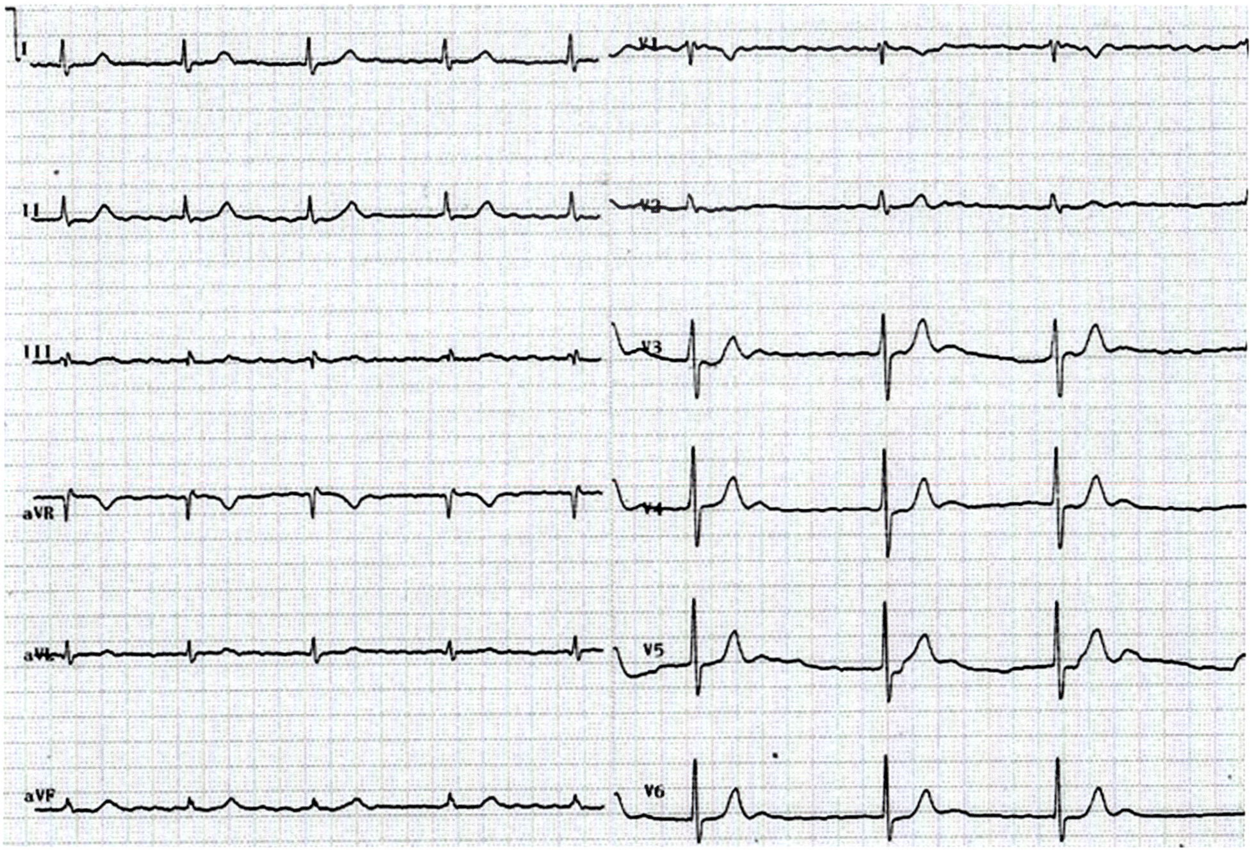

Fig. 14.12: ECG is suggestive of slow atrial fibrillation (AF) (rate 48 bpm). Remember sick sinus syndrome (SSS) may present with slow AF.

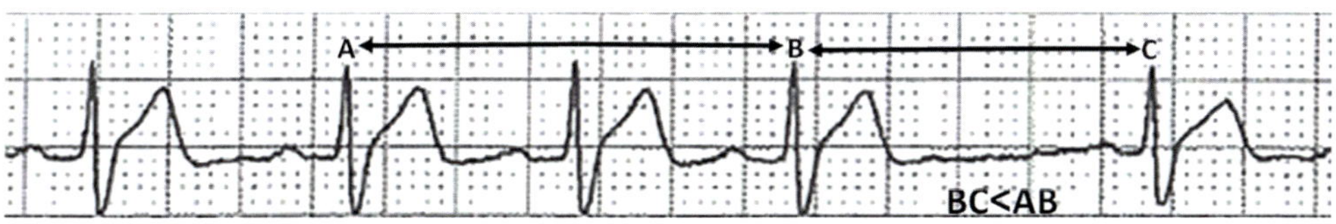

Fig. 14.13: ECG shows second-degree type I sinoatrial (SA) exit block (Wenckebach). Note progressive shortening of the R-R intervals until a P wave is blocked in the SA node (which does not appear on the ECG) and a sinus pause ensues afterward and the sinus pause is shorter than two of the preceding R-R intervals (distance B to C < the distance A to B).

SINOATRIAL EXIT BLOCK

In a sinoatrial exit block (SA exit block), the electrical impulse is delayed or blocked on the way to the atria, thus delaying atrial depolarization. This is different from an AV block which occurs in the AV node and delays ventricular depolarization. SA blocks are categorized into three classes based on the length of the delay: (1) first-degree SA block, (2) second-degree SA block, and (3) third-degree SA block.

First-Degree SA Block

In first-degree SA block, there is a lag between the time that the SA node fires and actual depolarization of the atria. This rhythm is not recognizable on an ECG strip because a strip does not denote when the SA node fires. It can only be detected during an electrophysiology study.

Second-Degree SA Blocks

Second-degree SA block can be recognized on the surface ECG (i.e. intermittent conduction failure between the sinus node and the right atrium). Second-degree SA blocks are divided into two subcategories just like AV blocks: (1) type I block and (2) type II block.

Type I Block or Wenckebach Block

Second-degree type I SA exit block (Wenckebach) manifests with progressive shortening of the R-R or P-P intervals until a P wave is blocked in the SA node, so P wave does not appear on the ECG. A "sinus pause" ensues afterward which would be shorter than two of the preceding R-R intervals (Fig. 14.13).

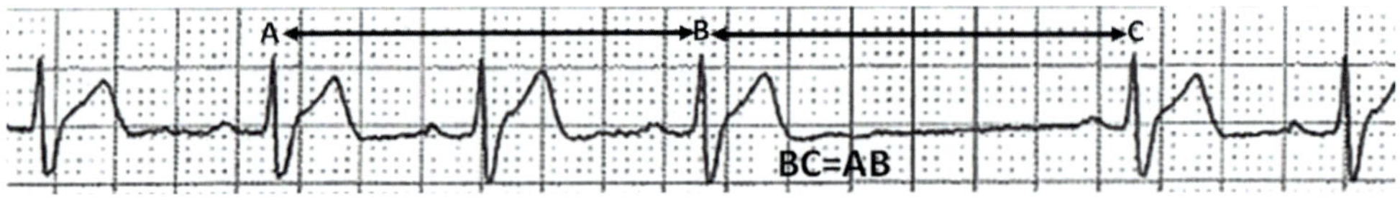

Fig. 14.14A: ECG shows second-degree type II sinoatrial (SA) exit block. Second-degree type II SA exit block occurs when there are consistent R-R and P-P intervals, then a P wave is blocked in the SA node (which is not seen on the ECG). The subsequent sinus pause is an exact interval of the preceding R-R intervals, usually two times (distance BC = AB).

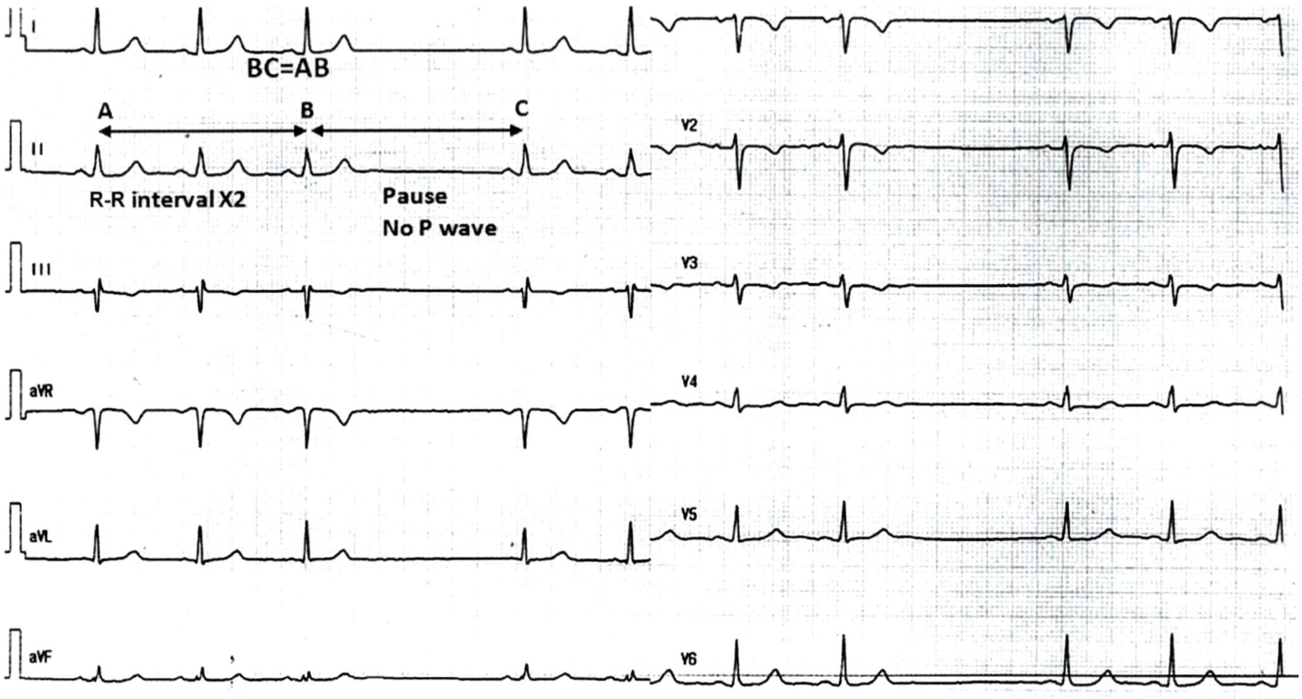

Fig. 14.14B: ECG shows second degree type II sinoatrial exit block. Note consistent R-R & P-P intervals, then a P wave is blocked, which is not seen on the ECG. The pause around the dropped P wave is approximately twice the basic PP interval (PP interval is measured from the onset of one P wave to the onset of the next P wave. In sinus rhythm, PP and RR intervals are the same). In this ECG the distance BC=AB. Intermittent P waves drop out of the rhythm, while subsequent P waves arrive on due time.

Type II SA Block

Second-degree type II SA exit block occurs when there are consistent R-R and P-P intervals, then a P wave is blocked in the SA node (not seen on the ECG). The subsequent "sinus pause" is an exact interval of the preceding R-R intervals (usually two times) (Figs. 14.14A and B).

Third-Degree SA Block

Third-degree SA exit block occurs when no SA nodal action potentials are able to leave the SA node. No P waves are seen on the ECG. A third-degree SA block looks very similar to a sinus arrest. However, a sinus arrest is caused by a failure to form impulses. In third-degree SA exit block when a junctional escape ensues and the rhythm may be confused with a junctional rhythm. If there is no junctional escape rhythm that is present, a long pause can occur resulting in asystole and cardiac arrest.

SUMMARY

Sick Sinus Syndrome

Sick sinus syndrome (sinus node dysfunction) is the result of dysfunction of the SA node, with impairment of its ability to generate and conduct impulses. Important causes of sick sinus syndrome are idiopathic fibrosis, ischemia, high vagal tone, myocarditis, digoxin toxicity, etc. It is a common cause of syncope, dizzy spell and palpitation.

Sick sinus syndrome may be due to intrinsic or extrinsic causes:

Intrinsic causes:

- Idiopathic degenerative fibrosis (the most common cause)
- Coronary artery disease
- Cardiomyopathies
- Congenital abnormalities.

Extrinsic causes:
- Drugs, e.g. digoxin, beta-blockers, calcium channel blockers
- Autonomic dysfunction
- Hypothyroidism
- Hypothermia
- Hyperkalemia
- Infiltrative diseases, e.g. sarcoidosis, hemochromatosis
- Increased intracranial pressure.

Sick sinus syndrome may be manifested on ECG as:
1. Sinus bradycardia
2. Sinus arrest (pause >3 seconds)
3. Escape rhythm
4. Tachycardia-bradycardia syndrome
5. Atrial fibrillation with slow ventricular rate
6. Sinoatrial block.

Marked sinus bradycardia is a common ECG finding in patients with sick sinus syndrome.

Tachycardia-bradycardia syndrome is common in sick sinus syndrome, characterized by bursts of atrial tachycardia interspersed with periods of bradycardia. In this syndrome, tachycardia alternates with bradycardia.

Sinoatrial Exit Block

Sinoatrial exit block occurs when the action potential initiated by the SA node is inhibited or completely blocked before it is able to leave the SA node and reach the atrium, thus no P wave will appear on the ECG.

Three subtypes of SA block can be distinguished:
1. *First-degree SA block*: This rhythm is not recognizable on an ECG and it can only be detected during an electrophysiology study.
2. *Second-degree SA block*: There are two patterns in this type of sinus node dysfunction. Second-degree type I SA exit block (Wenckebach) demonstrates progressive shortening of the R-R or P-P intervals until a P wave is blocked. Second-degree type II SA exit block occurs when there are consistent R-R and P-P intervals, then a P wave is blocked in the SA node, which is not seen on the ECG.
3. *Third-degree SA exit block*: A third-degree SA block looks very similar to a sinus arrest, absence of P waves (can only be diagnosed with an sinus node electrode, during electrophysiological evaluation).

REFERENCES

1. Bouman LN, Jongsma HJ. Structure and function of the sino-atrial node: a review. Eur Heart J. 1986;7:94-104.
2. Mangrum JM, DiMarco JP. The evaluation and management of bradycardia. N Engl J Med. 2000;342:703-9.
3. Park DS, Fishman GI. The cardiac conduction system. Circulation. 2011;123:904-15.
4. Adan V, Crown LA. Diagnosis and treatment of sick sinus syndrome. Am Fam Physician. 2003;67(8):1725-32.
5. Wahls SA. Sick sinus syndrome. Am Fam Physician. 1985;31:117-24.
6. Bower PJ. Sick sinus syndrome. Arch Intern Med. 1978;138:133-7.
7. Lamas GA, Lee K, Sweeney M, et al. The mode selection trial (MOST) in sinus node dysfunction: design, rationale, and baseline characteristics of the first 1000 patients. Am Heart J. 2000;140:541-51.
8. Tierney LM, McPhee SJ, Papadakis MA. Heart conduction disturbances: sick sinus syndrome. In: Papadakis MA, Tierney LM, McPhee SJ (Eds). Current Medical Diagnosis and Treatment, 39th edition. New York, NY: Lange Medical Books/McGraw-Hill; 2000. p. 412.
9. Rodriguez RD, Schocken DD. Update on sick sinus syndrome, a cardiac disorder of aging. Geriatrics. 1990;45:26-30, 33-6.
10. Fuster V, Alexander RW, O'Rourke RA. Hurst's the Heart, 10th edition. New York, NY: McGraw-Hill Medical Publishing Division; 2001.
11. Da Costa D, Brady WJ, Edhouse J. Bradycardias and atrioventricular conduction block. BMJ. 2002;324:535-8.

Chapter 15

Atrioventricular Block

INTRODUCTION

The atrioventricular (AV) node receives its blood supply from the AV nodal artery. This artery arises from the right coronary artery in 80% of patients, the circumflex coronary artery in 10%, and both in the remainder. Impulses are conducted through the AV node to the bundle of His, which courses through the membranous septum, then separates into two major divisions—(1) the right and (2) left bundle branches.[1]

Atrioventricular block occurs when atrial depolarization fails to reach the ventricles or when atrial depolarization is conducted with a delay. Three degrees of AV block are recognized:

1. First-degree AV block
2. Second-degree AV block
3. Third-degree AV block [complete heart block (CHB)].

FIRST-DEGREE ATRIOVENTRICULAR BLOCK

First-degree AV block is manifested in electrocardiogram (ECG) as prolonged PR interval. The PR interval measures the time from the onset of atrial depolarization to the onset of ventricular depolarization.[2,3] This interval sums the time taken for the sequential conduction of electrical impulses from the sinoatrial (SA) node through the atrium, AV node, His bundle, and early fascicular system until the initiation of septal depolarization. Consequently, there are numerous potential causes of PR prolongation including intra-atrial conduction defects, increased vagal tone leading to increased AV nodal delay, conduction disease in the AV node, conduction disease in the His bundle, and the presence of antiarrhythmic medications.[2]

Electrocardiographically first-degree heart block is defined as prolongation of the PR interval to more than 200 ms (0.20 seconds) (Fig. 15.1).[4] The PR interval of the surface ECG is measured from the onset of atrial depolarization (P wave) to the beginning of ventricular depolarization (QRS complex). Normally, this interval should be between 120 ms and 200 ms (0.12–0.20 seconds) in the adult population. First-degree AV block is considered "marked" when the PR interval exceeds 300 ms (0.30 seconds) (Fig. 15.2).[5]

Though conduction is slowed, there are no missed beats. In first-degree AV block, every atrial impulse is transmitted to the ventricles, resulting in a regular ventricular rate. The prevalence of first-degree AV block among young adults ranges from 0.65% to 1.6%. Higher prevalence (8.7%) is reported in studies of trained athletes. The prevalence of first-degree AV block increases with advancing age; first-degree AV block is reported in 5% of men older than 60 years.[6]

A number of specific conditions are associated with first-degree heart block:[7-10]

- *Normal variant:* Healthy individual, athletic training, and well-trained athletes can demonstrate first-degree (and occasionally higher degree) AV block owing to an increase in vagal tone.
- *Coronary artery disease:* First-degree AV block occurs in fewer than 15% of patients with acute ST elevation myocardial infarction (MI) admitted to coronary care units. AV block is more common in the setting of inferior MI (Figs. 15.3A and 3B).
- *Infectious diseases:* Rheumatic fever, infective endocarditis, diphtheria, Chagas disease, Lyme disease, etc. may be associated with first-degree AV block. Extension of the infection to the adjacent myocardium in native or prosthetic valve infective endocarditis (i.e. ring abscess) can cause AV block. Acute myocarditis caused by diphtheria, rheumatic fever, or Chagas disease can result in AV block.
- *Drug-induced first-degree heart block:* Drugs those most commonly cause first-degree AV block include: beta blockers, calcium channel blockers, amiodarone, digoxin or other cardiac glycosides, quinidine, procainamide, disopyramide, flecainide, encainide, propafenone, etc. Although first-degree AV block is not an absolute contraindication for administration of drugs such as calcium channel blockers, beta blockers, digoxin, and amiodarone, extreme caution should be exercised in the use of these medications in patients with first-degree AV block. Exposure to these drugs increase the risk of developing higher degree AV block.

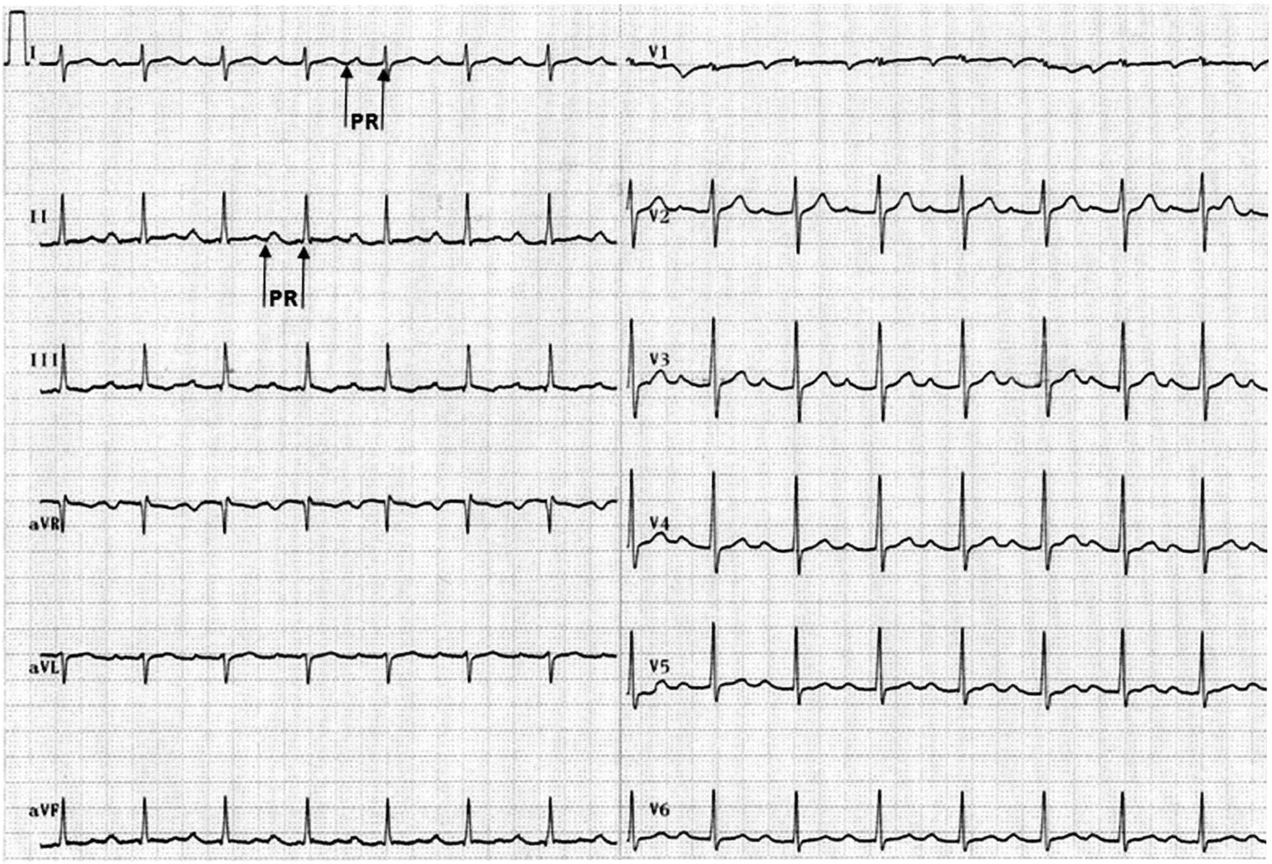

Fig. 15.1: Electrocardiogram (ECG) is consistent with first-degree atrioventricular (AV) block with PR interval 280 ms (*arrows*).

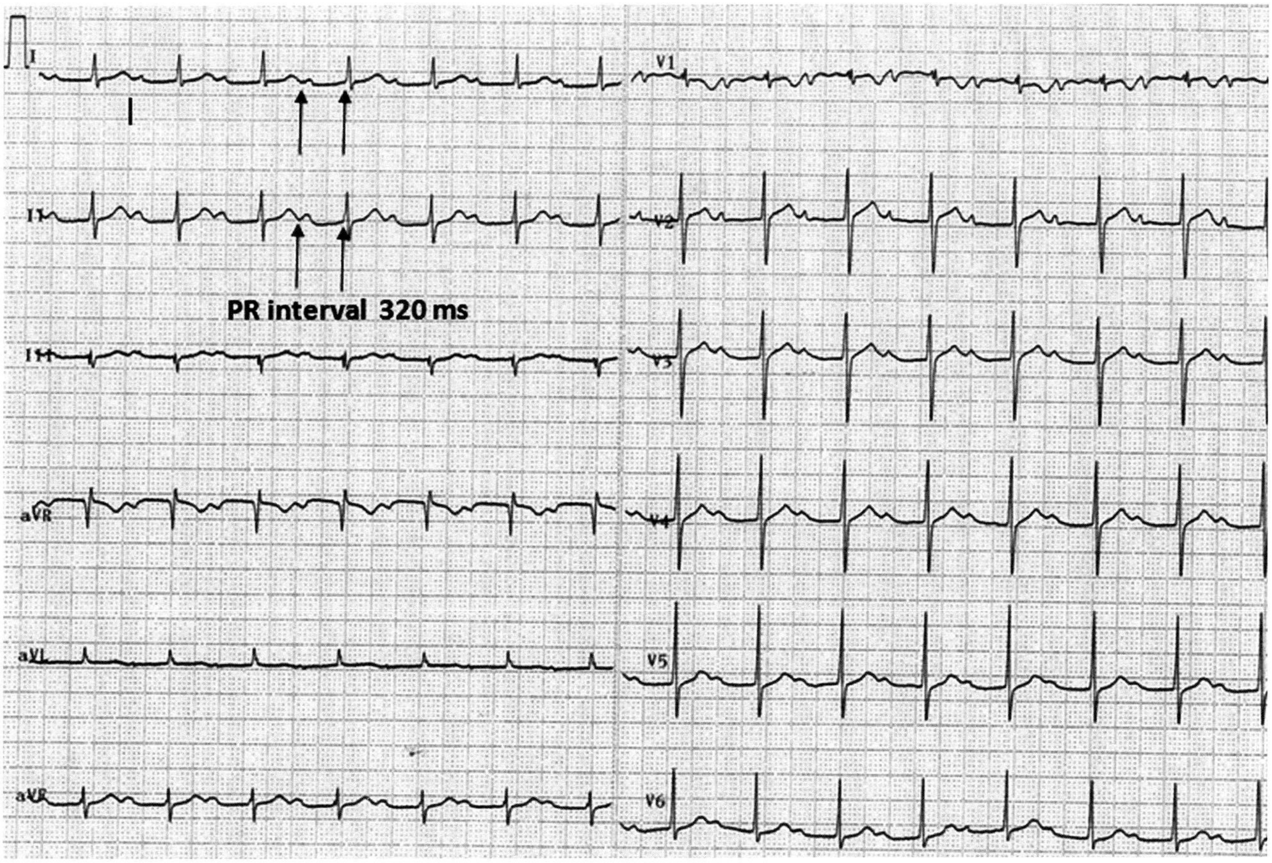

Fig. 15.2: Electrocardiogram (ECG) is consistent with marked first-degree heart block with PR interval 320 ms (*arrows*).

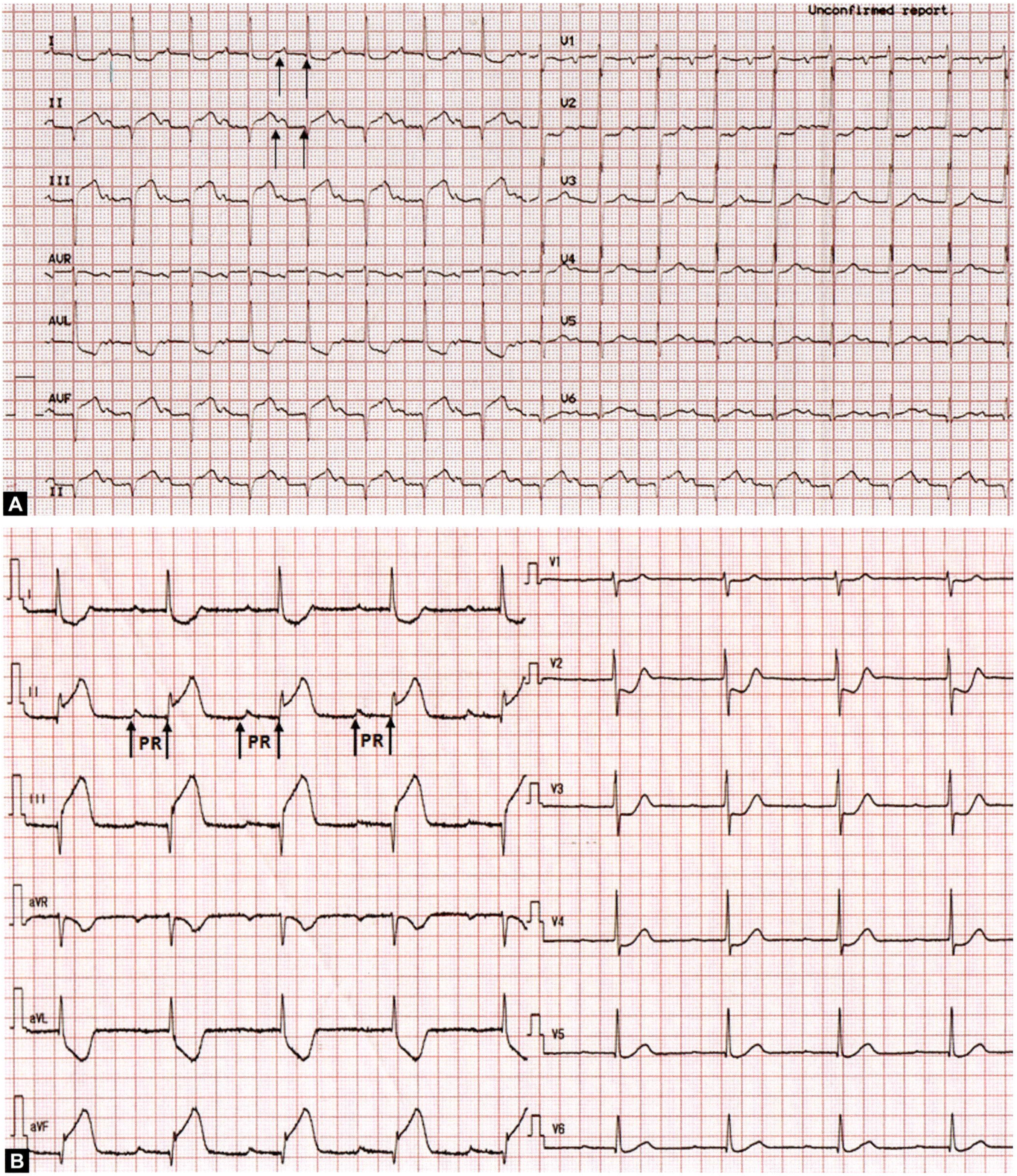

Figs. 15.3A and B: (A) Electrocardiogram (ECG) shows first-degree heart block, PR interval 260 ms (*arrows*) in the presence of acute inferior myocardial infarction (MI). *Note* ST segment elevation in LII, LIII and aVF with reciprocal ST segment depression in LI and aVL suggestive of acute inferior MI; and (B) ECG is consistent with marked first-degree heart block, PR interval 320 ms (*arrows*) in the presence of acute inferior MI. *Note:* ST segment elevation in LII, LIII and aVF with reciprocal ST segment depression in LI, aVL and V2–V4 suggestive of acute inferior MI.

- *Degenerative diseases of conduction system:* Idiopathic sclerosis and fibrosis may produce first-degree heart block. Lev's disease (or Lenegre-Lev syndrome) is associated with first-degree heart block. Lev's disease is due to progressive degenerative fibrosis and calcification of the neighboring cardiac structures, or "sclerosis of the left side of cardiac skeleton" (including the mitral annulus, central fibrous body, membranous septum, base of the aorta, and crest of the ventricular septum).
- *Electrolyte disturbances* (e.g. hypokalemia, hypomagnesemia) may produce ECG evidence of first-degree heart block.
- *Mitral or aortic valve annulus calcification:* The main penetrating bundle of His is located near the base of the anterior leaflet of the mitral valve and the noncoronary cusp of the aortic valve. Heavy calcium deposits in patients with aortic or mitral annular calcification are associated with increased risk of AV block.
- *Collagen vascular diseases:* Rheumatoid arthritis, systemic lupus erythematosus (SLE), and scleroderma all may be associated with first-degree AV block. Rheumatoid nodules may occur in the central fibrous body and result in AV block. Fibrosis of the AV node or the adjacent myocardium in patients with SLE or scleroderma can cause first-degree AV block.
- *Postprocedure first-degree heart block:* First-degree AV block occurs in about 10% of patients who undergo adenosine stress testing and is usually hemodynamically insignificant. Marked first-degree AV block may occur after catheter ablation of the tachyarrhythmias which is usually transient. First-degree AV block (reversible or permanent) has been reported in about 2% of patients who undergo closure of an atrial septal defect (ASD) using the Amplatzer septal occluder.[10] First-degree AV block can occur following cardiac surgery. Transient first-degree AV block may result from right heart catheterization.

Electrocardiogram Criteria of First-degree Heart Block

A first-degree AV block is indicated on the ECG by a prolonged PR interval. The P wave indicates atrial depolarization (initiated by firing of the SA node). The atrial depolarization eventually spreads to the AV node where there is a slight delay before the electrical impulse is conducted to the ventricles. If the AV nodal conduction (dromotropy) is decreased, it will take longer for the impulse to reach the ventricles, so there will be a greater distance between the P wave and the QRS complex. Thus the PR interval will be prolonged.

The PR interval is normally 120–200 ms (0.12–0.20 seconds). A PR interval consistently longer than 0.20 seconds (greater than five small boxes) indicates a first-degree AV block. In first-degree heart block there is a 1:1 ratio between P waves and QRS complexes, unlike second- and third-degree AV nodal block.

First-degree AV block is usually considered as a benign ECG finding and is mostly seen in healthy individuals with no prognostic significance.[2,11,12] However, a growing body of literature has emerged that challenges our established conceptions of apparently "benign" ECG findings such as right bundle branch block, repolarization abnormalities, first-degree AV block, and T-wave morphology.[2,13-18] Framingham study reported that first-degree AV block is associated with an increased risk for atrial fibrillation, pacemaker implantation, and all-cause mortality among community-dwelling adults.[19] First-degree AV block is also associated with heart failure and cardiovascular (CV) mortality in persons with stable coronary artery disease.[2]

SECOND-DEGREE ATRIOVENTRICULAR BLOCK

Second-degree AV block is manifested in ECG with intermittent failure of conduction between the atria and ventricles. Some P waves are not followed by a QRS complex.

There are two types of second-degree AV block:

1. Mobitz type I block (Wenckebach phenomenon)
2. Mobitz type II block (Hay phenomenon).

Both types are named after Woldemar Mobitz. Type I is also named for Dutch anatomist Karel Frederik Wenckebach, and type II is also named for British cardiologist John Hay.[20-23] Woldemar Mobitz, an early 20th century Russian born German internist, analyzed arrhythmias by graphing the relationship of changing atrial rates and premature beats to AV conduction. Through an astute mathematical approach, he was able to classify second-degree AV block into two types, subsequently referred to as Mobitz type I (Wenckebach phenomenon) and Mobitz type II (Hay phenomenon). Type I AV block was most often due to digitalis and was reversible. There were no associated pathological findings. Type II AV block frequently progressed to complete AV block and was associated with seizures, death, and pathological findings.[20]

Mobitz Type I Second-degree Atrioventricular Block (Wenckebach Phenomenon)

Mobitz type I second-degree AV block (Wenckebach phenomenon) is diagnosed when the ECG shows a stable

PP interval and a progressive increase in the PR interval until a P wave fails to conduct (Figs. 15.4A to D). After the blocked P wave, the next PR interval returns to the initial value.[1] Mobitz type I second-degree AV block may be due to coronary artery disease (e.g. acute inferior MI), myocarditis, drug induced: beta-blockers, calcium channel blockers, digoxin, amiodarone, and sometimes may be due to increased vagal tone (e.g. athletes) (Figs. 15.5A to F). Mobitz I is usually a benign rhythm, causing minimal hemodynamic disturbance and with low risk of progression to third-degree heart block. Asymptomatic patients do not require treatment. Symptomatic patients usually respond to atropine. Permanent pacing is rarely required.

Electrocardiogram Criteria: Mobitz I Atrioventricular Block (Wenckebach Phenomenon)

(1) Progressive prolongation of the PR interval followed by a drop beat (a nonconducted P wave); (2) The P-P interval remains relatively constant; (3) The RR interval progressively shortens with each beat of the cycle; (4) The PR interval is longest immediately before the dropped beat; and (5) The PR interval is shortest immediately after the dropped beat.

Mobitz Type II Second-degree Atrioventricular Block (Hay Phenomenon)

Mobitz type II block (Hay phenomenon) was originally described by John Hay in 1906.[23] Type II AV block is defined as the occurrence of a single nonconducted P wave associated with constant PR intervals before and after a single blocked impulse as long as the sinus rate or the P-P interval is constant and there are at least two consecutively conducted P waves (i.e. 3:2 AV block) to determine the behavior of the PR interval.[24] In Mobitz type II block, the PR interval can be normal or prolonged, and the QRS complex can be narrow or wide. Typically, the PR interval is normal and the QRS complex is wide (Figs. 15.6A to C). While Mobitz I is usually due to a functional suppression of AV conduction (e.g. due to drugs, reversible ischemia), Mobitz II is more likely to be due to structural damage to the conducting system (e.g. infarction, fibrosis, and necrosis). Unlike Mobitz I, which is produced by progressive fatigue of the AV nodal cells, Mobitz II is an "all or nothing" phenomenon whereby the His-Purkinje cells suddenly and unexpectedly fail to conduct a supraventricular impulse. Important causes of Mobitz type II block include anterior MI (due to septal infarction with necrosis of the bundle branches), idiopathic fibrosis of the conducting system, drugs: beta blockers, calcium channel blockers, amiodarone, electrolyte imbalance, e.g. hyperkalemia and after cardiac surgery (e.g. mitral valve repair). Rarely it may be due to inflammatory conditions like rheumatic fever, myocarditis, autoimmune diseases, e.g. SLE, systemic sclerosis, and infiltrative myocardial diseases like amyloidosis, hemochromatosis, and sarcoidosis.

Electrocardiogram Criteria: Mobitz II Atrioventricular Block

(1) Intermittent drop beat (nonconducted P waves) without any progressive prolongation of the PR interval; (2) The P waves "march through" at a constant rate and the PR interval in the conducted beats remains constant; and (3) QRS morphology may be wide or may be of normal narrow complex configuration.

Site of Block

A type I AV block with a narrow QRS complex is almost always due to a lesion in the AV node because a type I block in the His bundle is rare. In a type I block with a wide QRS complex (>0.12 seconds), except for acute MI, the block is AV nodal in 30–40% of cases and is in the His-Purkinje system in 60–70% of cases.[25-27] Type I infranodal block indicates diffuse disease of the His-Purkinje system, and its prognosis is believed to be the same as for type II block.[24] The diagnosis of type I infranodal block requires invasive His bundle recordings, and the increments in AV conduction occur in the HV interval.

According to the strict definition, a type II AV block occurs in the His-Purkinje system and rarely above the site of recording of the His bundle potential in the proximal His bundle or nodo-Hisian junction. Type II block has not yet been convincingly demonstrated in the body of the AV node.[24] About 70% of cases of type II block are associated with bundle branch block (Fig. 15.7), and 30% are associated with a narrow QRS complex (Fig. 15.8) and are therefore within the His bundle.[24]

2:1 Atrioventricular Block

Second-degree AV block in the form of a 2:1 AV block or involving two or more consecutively blocked P waves is usually characterized as advanced second-degree AV block.[28,29] A 2:1 AV block can be in the AV node or the His-Purkinje system. In a 2:1 AV block, there is only one conducted P wave for each P wave blocked; thus, only one PR interval is available for examination before the block (Figs. 15.9A to C). So it is difficult to classify a 2:1 AV block as type I or type II.[24] In 2:1 block, a narrow QRS complex and associated periods of Wenckebach block, or simultaneous sinus slowing (*vagotonic block*), suggest that atrioventricular nodal block is present, whereas a wide QRS complex suggests the presence of infranodal block.[1] 2:1 AV block with an initial lengthened PR interval with no wide QRS pattern is suggestive of 2:1 AV block, Wenckebach type (Figs. 15.10A and B), and a widened QRS complex with normal PR interval is suggestive of 2:1 Mobitz type II pattern block (Figs. 15.11A and B) (Table 15.1).

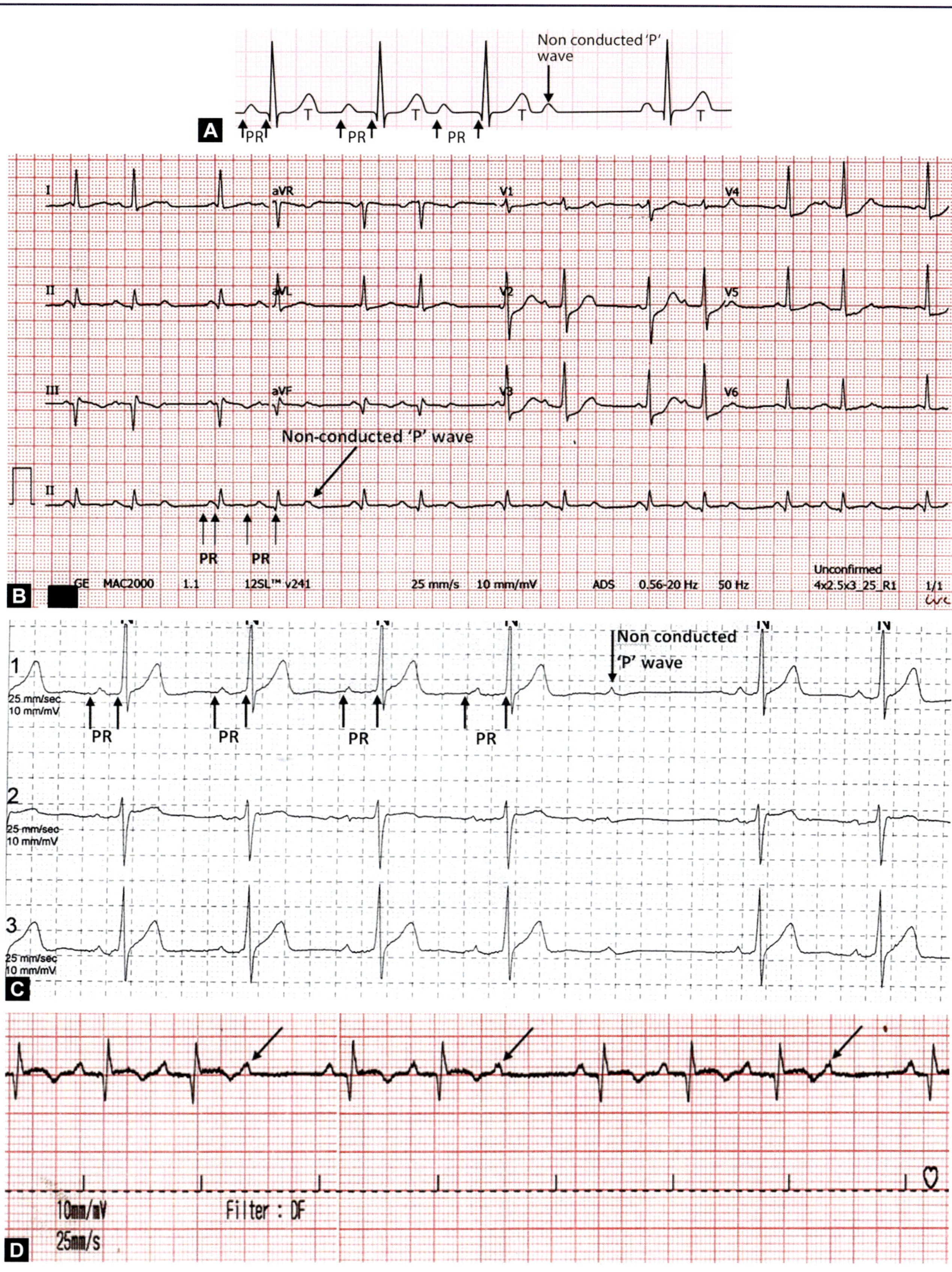

Figs. 15.4A to D: (A) ECG tracing shows Mobitz type I second-degree AV block (Wenckebach phenomenon). *Note:* Progressive increase in the PR interval (*small arrows*) followed by a nonconducted P wave (*large arrow*); (B) ECG is consistent with Wenckebach phenomenon (Mobitz type I block) showing gradual prolongation of PR interval (*paired arrows*) followed by nonconducted "P" wave (*long arrow*). *Note:* Also Q waves in LII, LIII and aVF and tall R waves in leads V1 and V2, suggestive of recent inferior and posterior MI; (C) Holter ECG tracing showing typical Wenckebach phenomenon (Mobitz type I block) with gradual prolongation of PR interval (*paired arrows*) followed by nonconducted "P" wave (*long arrow*); and (D) This ECG rhythm strip shows typical Wenckebach phenomenon (Mobitz type I block) with gradual prolongation of PR interval followed by nonconducted "P" wave (*arrows*). (AV: atrioventricular; ECG: electrocardiogram; MI: myocardial infarction)

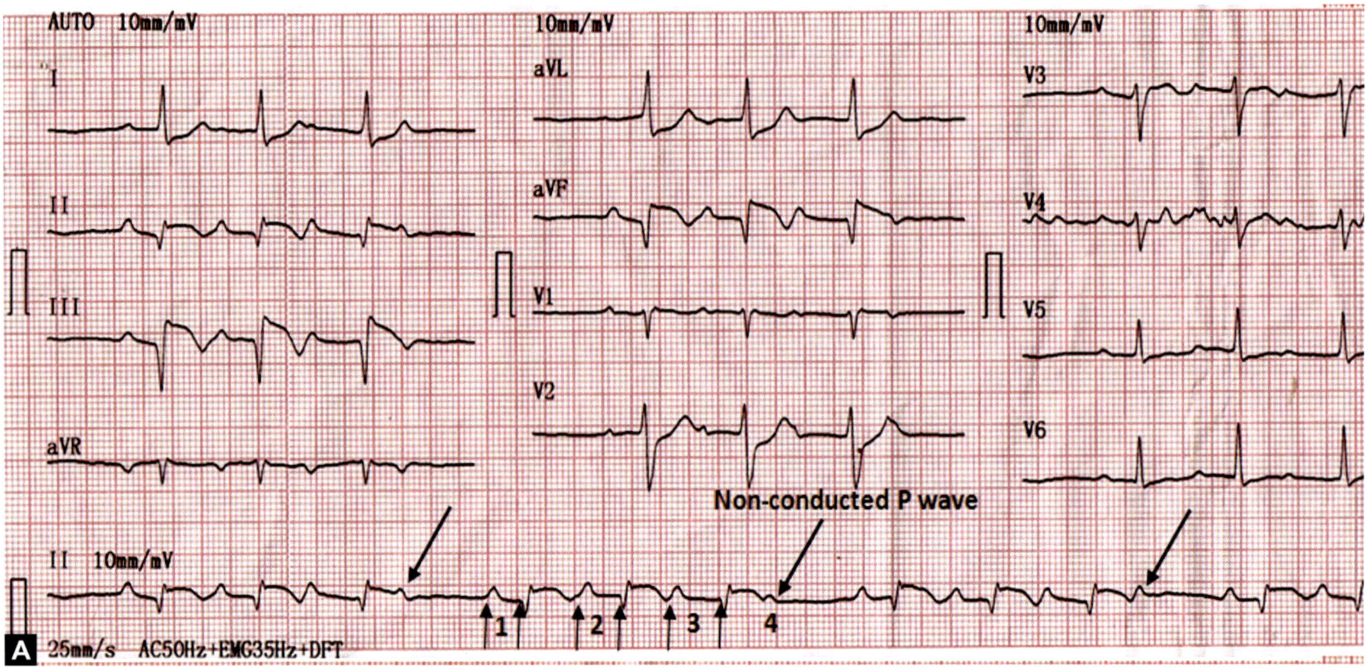

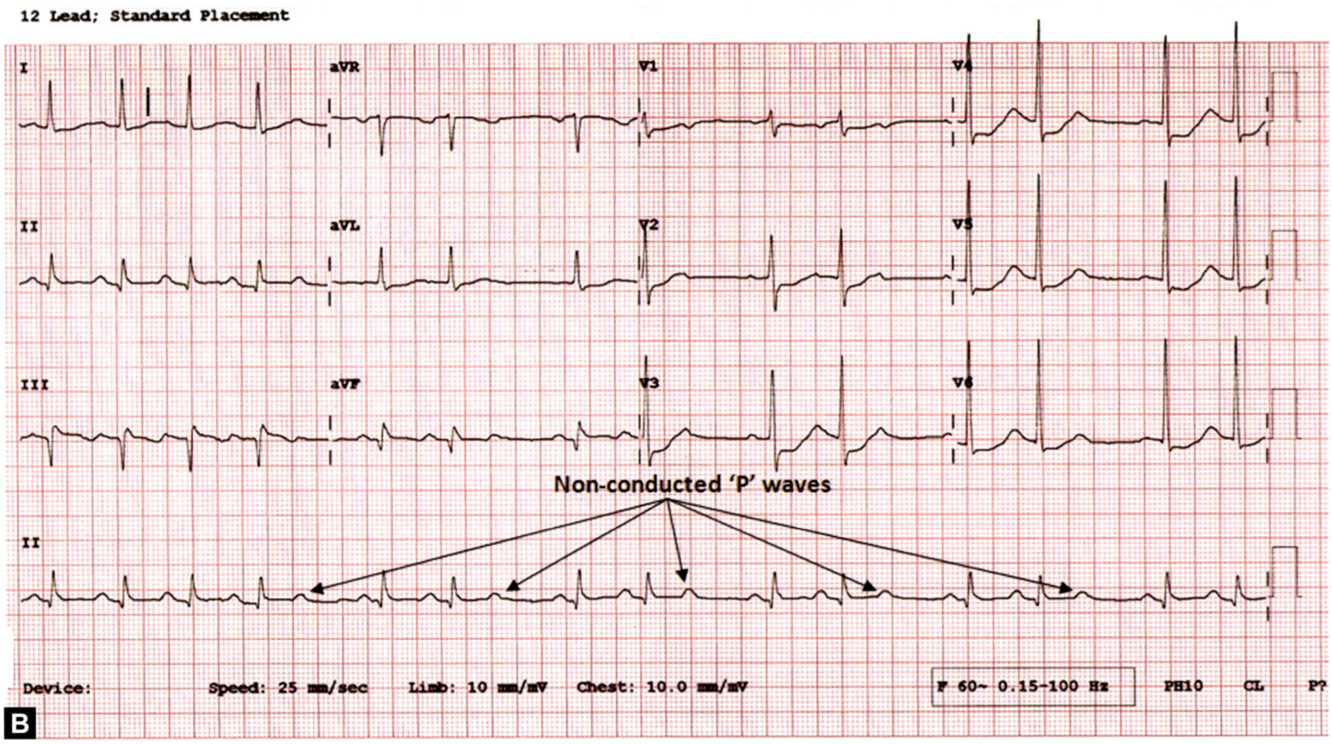

Figs. 15.5A and B: (A) This ECG illustrates typical Wenckebach phenomenon (Mobitz type I block) in a patient with acute inferior myocardial infarction (ST segment elevation and pathological Q waves in LII,LIII and aVF with reciprocal ST depression in LI and aVL) with progressive prolongation of PR interval followed by drop beat. Note every 4th "P" wave is non-conducted (large arrows).The Wenckebach pattern here is repeating in cycles of 4 P waves to 3 QRS complexes (4:3 conduction ratio); (B) ECG is consistent with Wenckebach phenomenon (Mobitz type I block) in a patient with recent inferior and posterior myocardial infarction. *Note:* Nonconducted "P" waves (*arrows*).

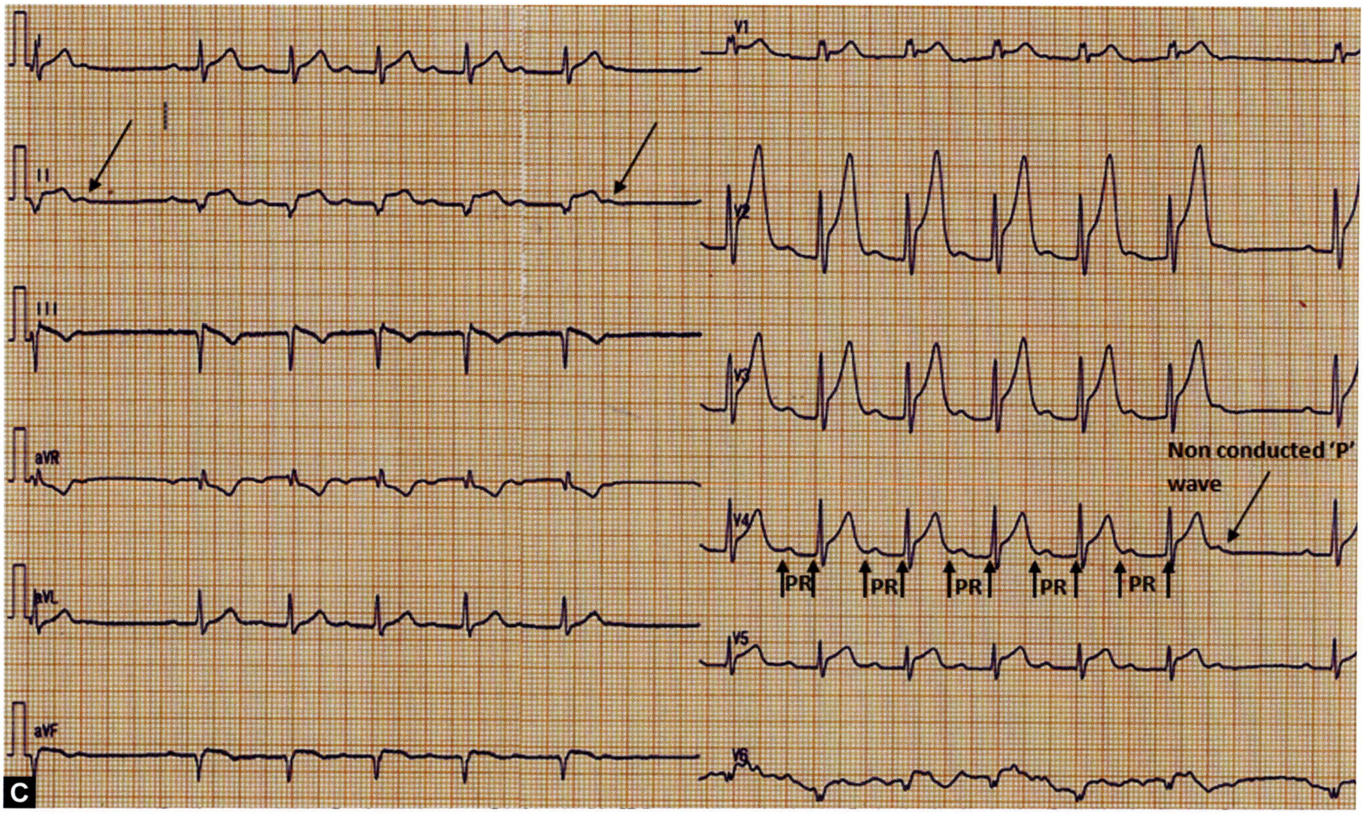

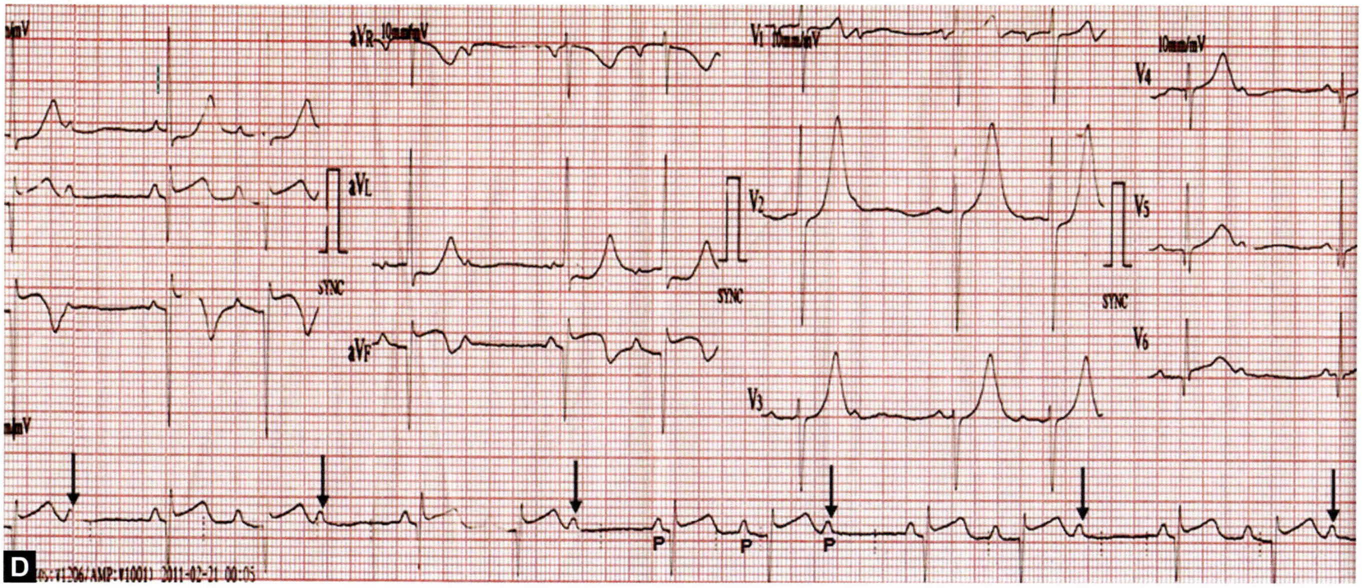

Figs. 15.5C and D: (C) ECG is consistent with Wenckebach phenomenon (Mobitz type I block) in a patient with recent inferior myocardial infarction with ST segment elevation and Q waves in LII, LIII and aVF. *Note:* Gradual prolongation of PR interval (*paired arrows*) with intermittent nonconducted "P" waves (*large arrows*). Also note tall R and upright T waves in right precordial leads suggestive of concurrent posterior MI. (*Courtesy:* Dr Mahbubor Rahman, Labaid Cardiac Hospital); (D) ECG is consistent with Wenckebach phenomenon (Mobitz type I block) in a patient with inferior myocardial infarction (ST segment elevation and pathological Q waves in LII, LIII, and aVF). *Note:* Gradual prolongation of PR interval with intermittent nonconducted "P" waves (*arrows*). The Wenckebach pattern here is repeating in cycles of three P waves to two QRS complexes (3:2 conduction ratio) (*Courtesy:* Dr Atiquzzaman Sohel, Labaid Cardiac Hospital)

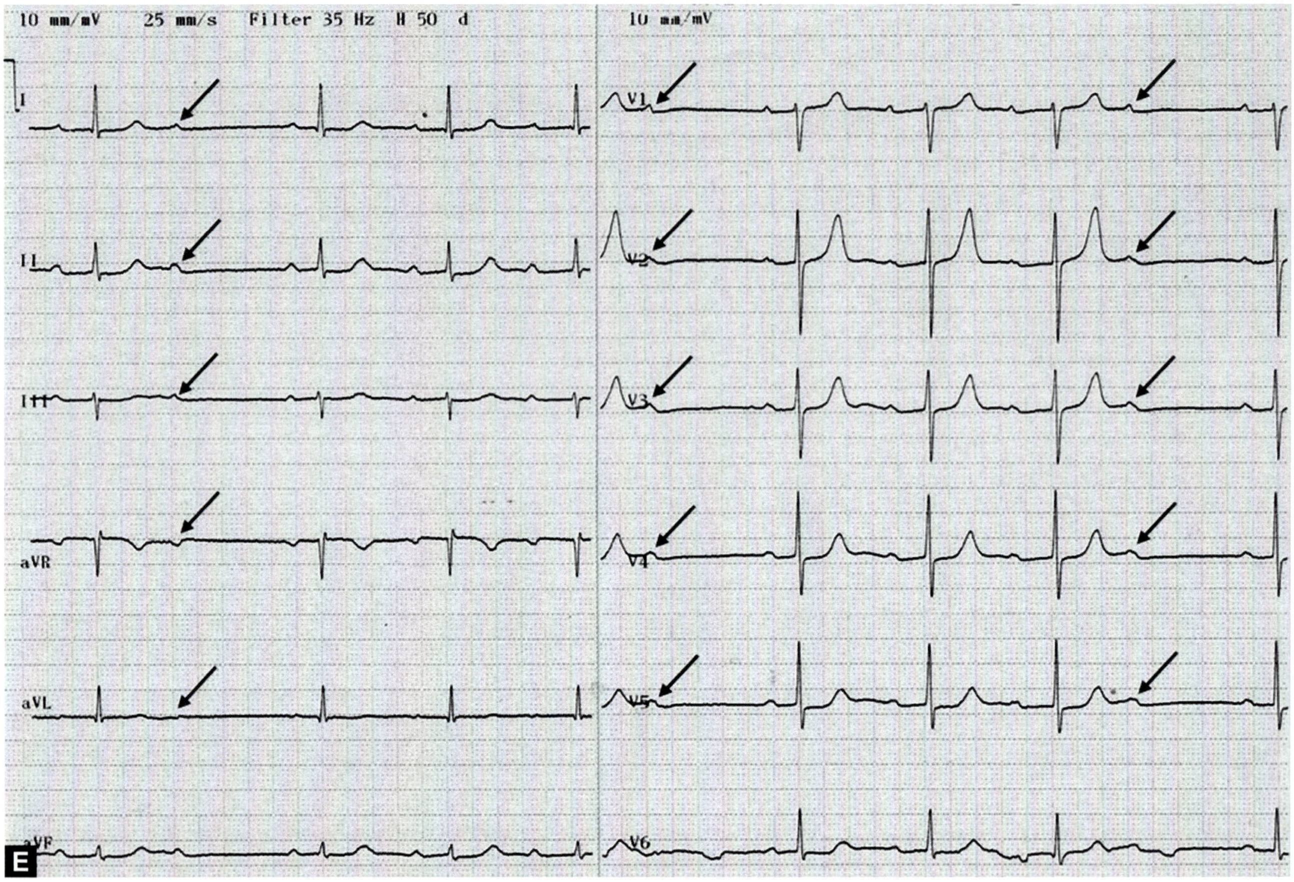

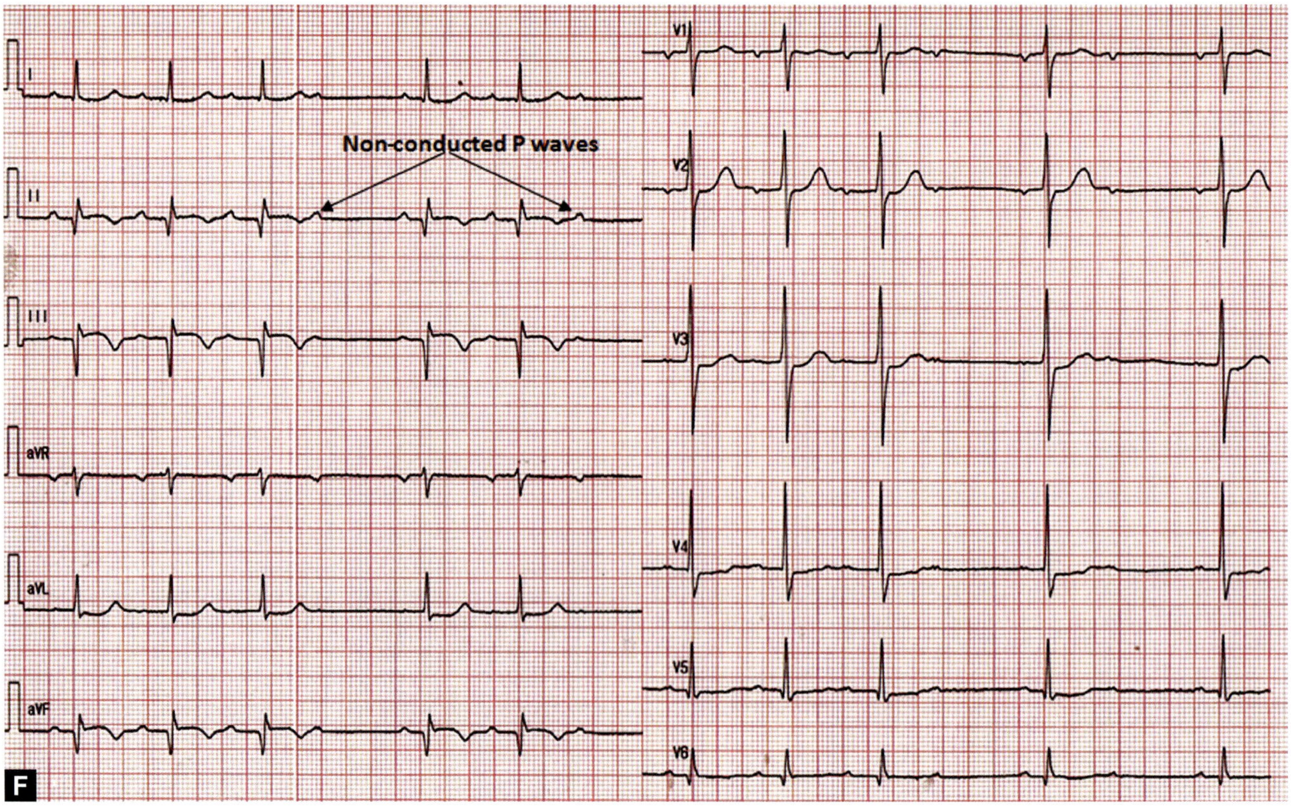

Figs. 15.5E and F: (E) ECG is consistent with Wenckebach phenomenon (Mobitz type I block). *Note:* Gradual prolongation of PR interval with intermittent nonconducted "P" waves (*arrows*) (*Courtesy:* Dr Abul Khayer, Labaid Cardiac Hospital); and (F) ECG is consistent with Wenckebach phenomenon (Mobitz type I block) in a patient with recent inferior myocardial infarction. *Note:* Gradual prolongation of PR interval followed by nonconducted "P" waves (*arrows*). *Note:* Also some ST segment elevation along with pathological Q waves with biphasic T waves in leads LII, LIII, and aVF. (*Courtesy:* Dr Shiblee Sadik Pathan, Labaid Cardiac Hospital)

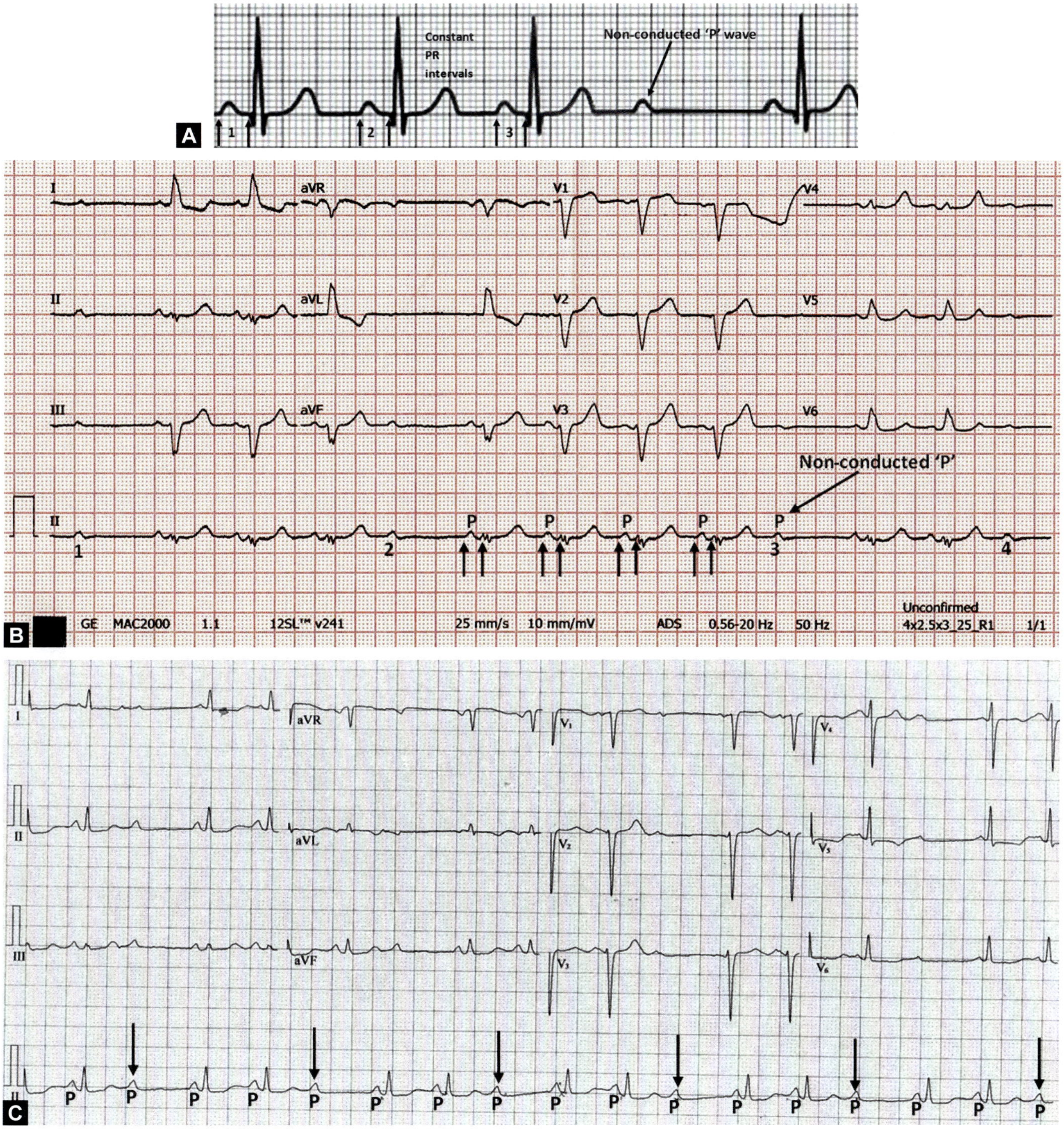

Figs. 15.6A to C: (A) Mobitz type II AV block associated with constant PR intervals (*paired arrows*) followed by single nonconducted P wave (*large arrow*); (B) ECG shows Mobitz type II AV block with intermittent nonconducted P waves without any progressive prolongation of the PR interval, rather PR interval in the conducted beats remains constant (*paired arrows*). *Note:* Four nonconducted "P" waves (marked 1, 2, 3, and 4) in this rhythm strip; and (C) ECG illustrates 3:2 Mobitz type II AV block with intermittent nonconducted P waves without any progressive prolongation of the PR interval. *Note:* Every third "P" is nonconducted (*arrows*). (AV: atrioventricular; ECG: electrocardiogram)

Courtesy: Dr APM Sohrabuzzaman, Labaid Cardiac Hospital

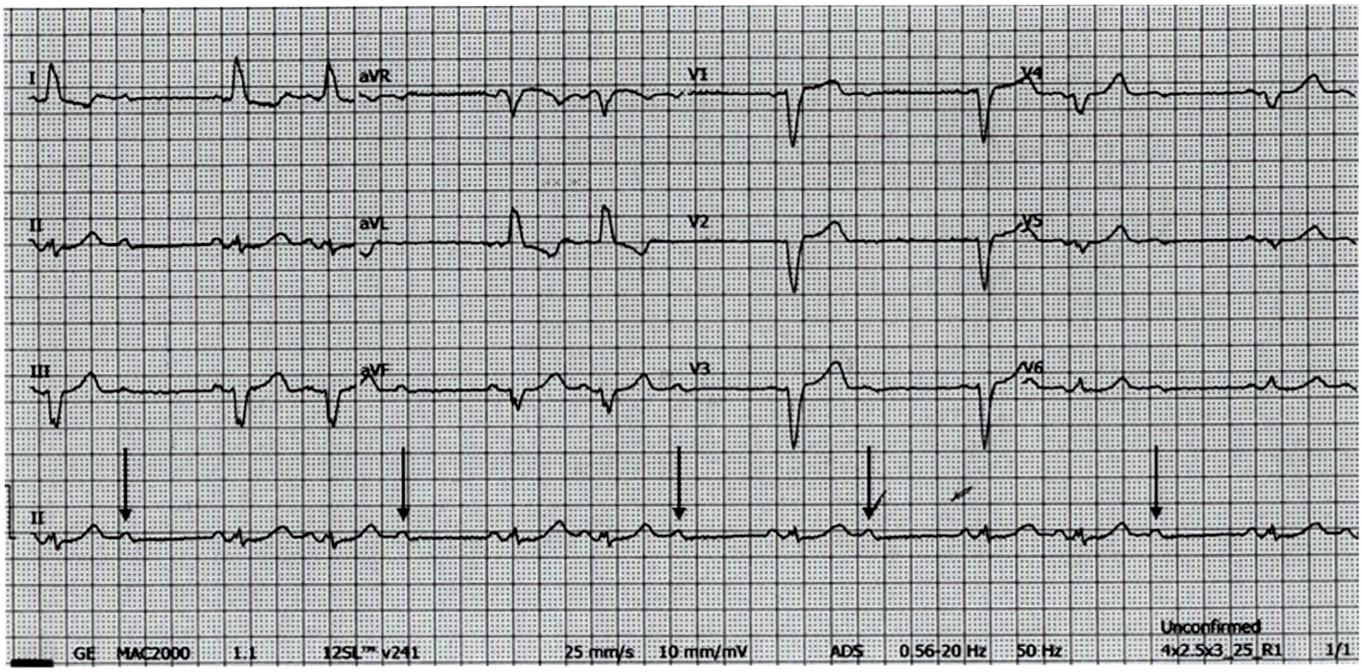

Fig. 15.7: ECG shows Mobitz type II AV block with LBBB pattern (QRS duration 128 ms). ECG illustrates intermittent nonconducted P waves (*arrows*). (AV: atrioventricular; ECG: electrocardiogram; LBBB: left bundle branch block)

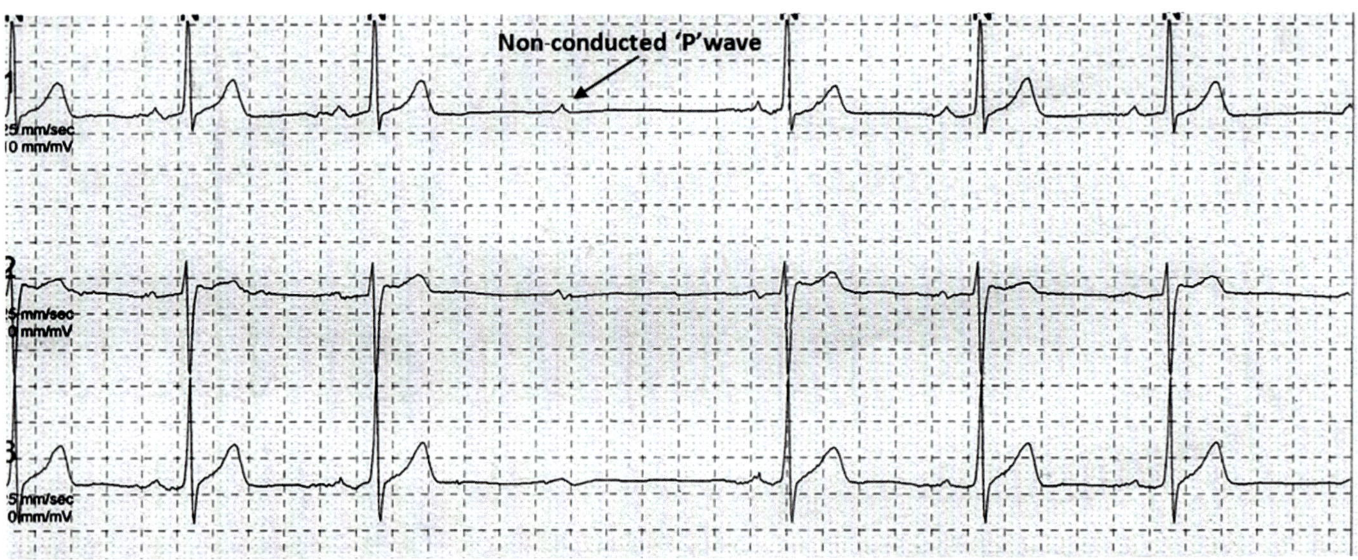

Fig. 15.8: ECG shows Mobitz type II AV block with narrow QRS complex with one nonconducted "P" wave (*arrow*). *Note:* PR intervals are almost constant. (AV: atrioventricular; ECG: electrocardiogram)

Table 15.1: 2:1 Atrioventricular block—2:1 Mobitz type I (Wenckebach) or 2:1 Mobitz type II.

2:1 Atrioventricular (AV) block	*2:1 Mobitz type I*	*2:1 Mobitz type II*
Site of block	AV node	Below AV node, in the bundle of His, or the bundle branches
PR interval	An initial lengthened PR interval is usually present	Often has a normal PR interval
QRS duration	No wide QRS pattern	A widened QRS complex is usually present
Effect of vagal maneuver	Vagal maneuvers increase the parasympathetic inhibition of the AV node and may convert 2:1 Wenckebach block to 3:2 or 4:3 Wenckebach	Vagal maneuvers either eliminate the block, thus producing 1:1 AV conduction or these maneuvers have no effect

Vagally-mediated Atrioventricular Block and Atrioventricular Block in Athletes

A vagal surge can cause simultaneous sinus slowing and AV nodal block, an often benign condition that can superficially resemble type II AV block. It is associated with a narrow QRS complex and results of electrophysiologic investigations are usually normal. A vagally-induced AV block can occur in otherwise normal patients, in those with cough or hiccups, and during swallowing or micturition when vagal discharge is enhanced. A vagally-mediated AV block is characteristically paroxysmal and is often associated with clearly visible sinus slowing on an ECG. Vagal AV block differs from neurally-mediated malignant vasovagal syncope in which head-up tilt testing causes sinus arrest and rarely predominant AV block.[24]

Atrioventricular block in athletes is typically type I second-degree AV block and probably an expression of hypervagotonia related to physical training and it resolves after physical deconditioning.[30,31] This form of AV block may be associated with sinus bradycardia because the relative effects of sympathetic and parasympathetic systems on the AV and sinus node may differ.[24] An AV block in athletes responds to exercise or atropine. Rarely type II second-degree AV block can occur in young athletes.[24]

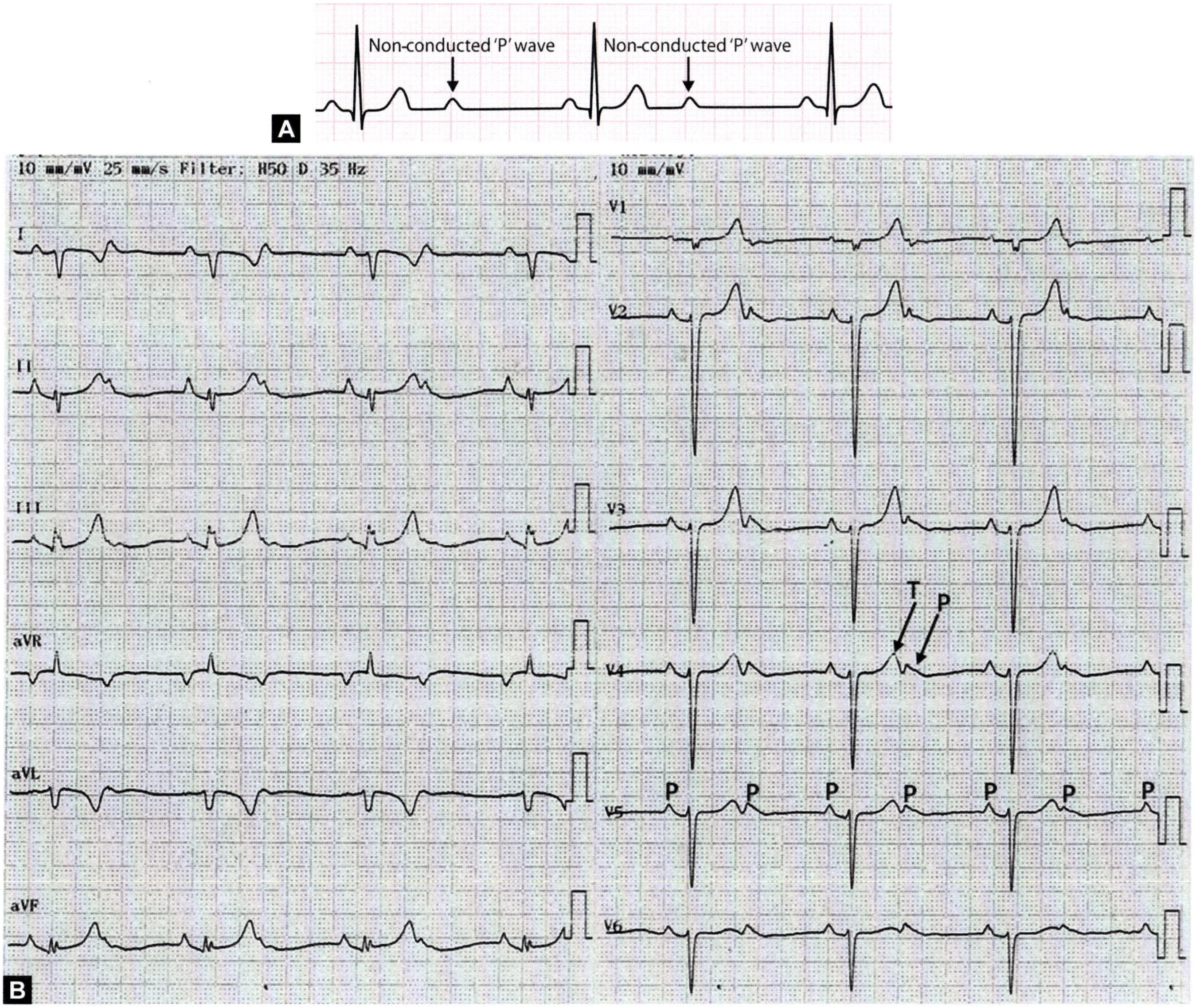

Figs. 15.9A and B: (A) ECG shows 2:1 AV block, every alternate "P" waves are nonconducted (*arrows*). *Note:* PR intervals are constant in all the conducted beats; (B) ECG shows 2:1 AV block, every alternate "P" waves are nonconducted with marked bradycardia (heart rate 43 bpm). *Note:* PR intervals are constant in all the conducted beats. Also note the "P" and "T" waves are fused together and appears biphasic (*arrows*);

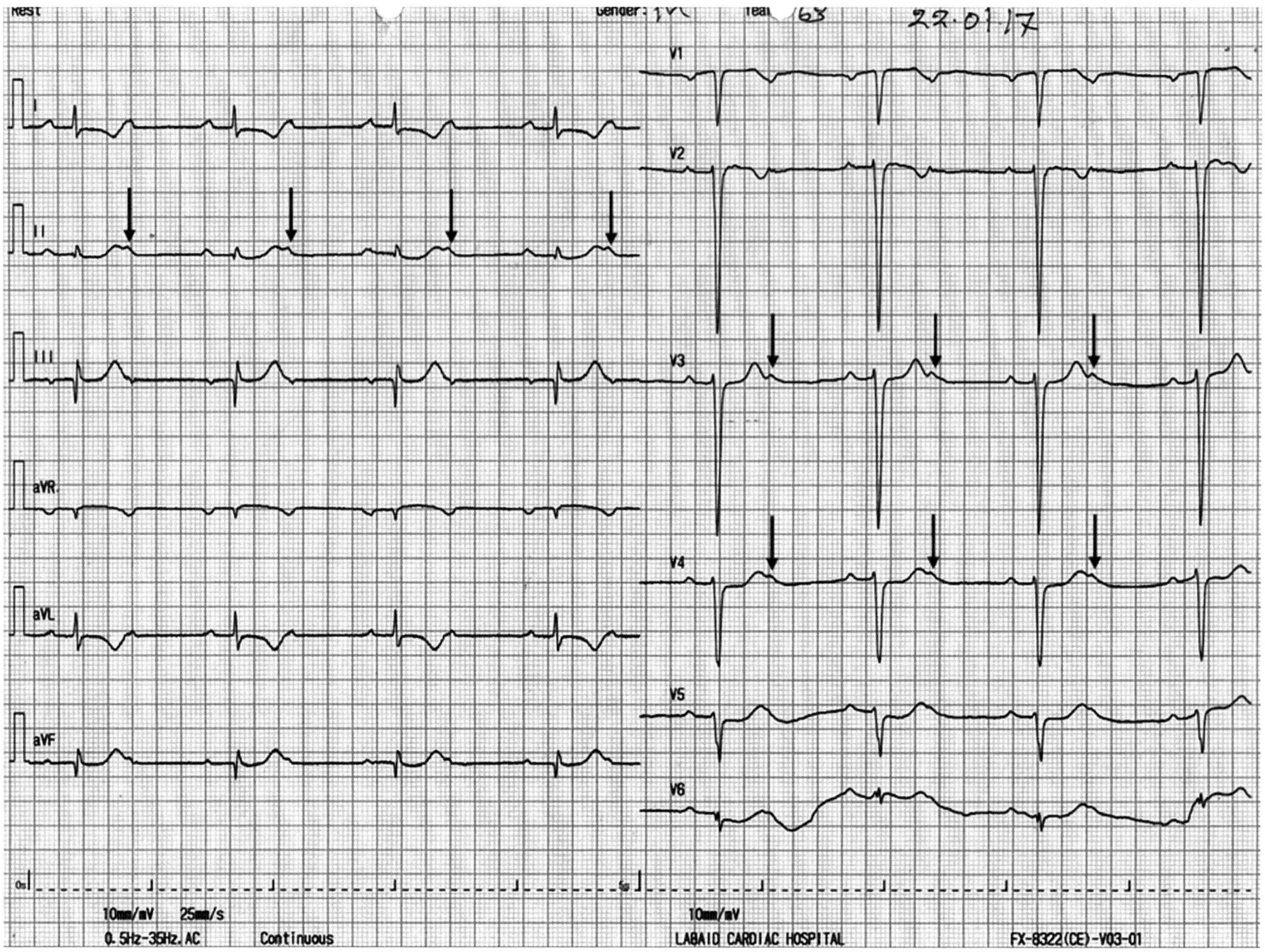

Fig. 15.9C: ECG shows 2:1 AV block, every alternate "P" waves are nonconducted (*arrows*) with marked bradycardia (heart rate 45 bpm). *Note:* PR intervals are constant in all the conducted beats. Also note the "P" and "T" waves are fused together and appears biphasic in most of the leads. (AV: atrioventricular; ECG: electrocardiogram)

THIRD-DEGREE ATRIOVENTRICULAR BLOCK (COMPLETE HEART BLOCK)

Third-degree AV block, also referred to as third-degree heart block or complete heart block (CHB), is a disorder of the cardiac conduction system where there is no conduction through the AV node. Therefore, complete dissociation of the atrial and ventricular activity exists. The ventricular escape mechanism can occur anywhere from the AV node to the bundle-branch Purkinje system.[32,33] It is important to realize that not all patients with AV dissociation have CHB. For example, patients with ventricular tachycardia (VT) have AV dissociation, but not CHB; in VT, AV dissociation is due to the ventricular rate being faster than the intrinsic sinus rate. On ECG, CHB is represented by QRS complexes being conducted at their own rate and totally independent of the P waves. Worldwide prevalence of third-degree AV block is around 0.04%.[34]

Because the impulse is blocked, an accessory pacemaker in the lower chambers will typically activate the ventricles. This is known as an escape rhythm. Since this accessory pacemaker also activates independently of the impulse generated at the SA node, two independent rhythms can be noted on the ECG. ECG features of CHB include (Fig. 15.12):

- The P waves with a regular P to P interval represent the first rhythm.
- The QRS complexes with a regular R to R interval represent the second rhythm.
- The PR interval will be variable.

In third-degree AV block the conduction block may be at the level of the AV node, the bundle of His, or the bundle-branch Purkinje system. In most cases (approximately 60%), the block occurs below the His bundle. Block within the AV node accounts for approximately 20% of all cases, whereas block within the His bundle accounts for slightly fewer than 20% of all cases.[33] The configuration and duration of the escape QRS complex depends on the site of the block and the site of the escape rhythm pacemaker. Pacemakers above the His bundle produce a narrow QRS complex escape rhythm (Fig. 15.13), whereas those at

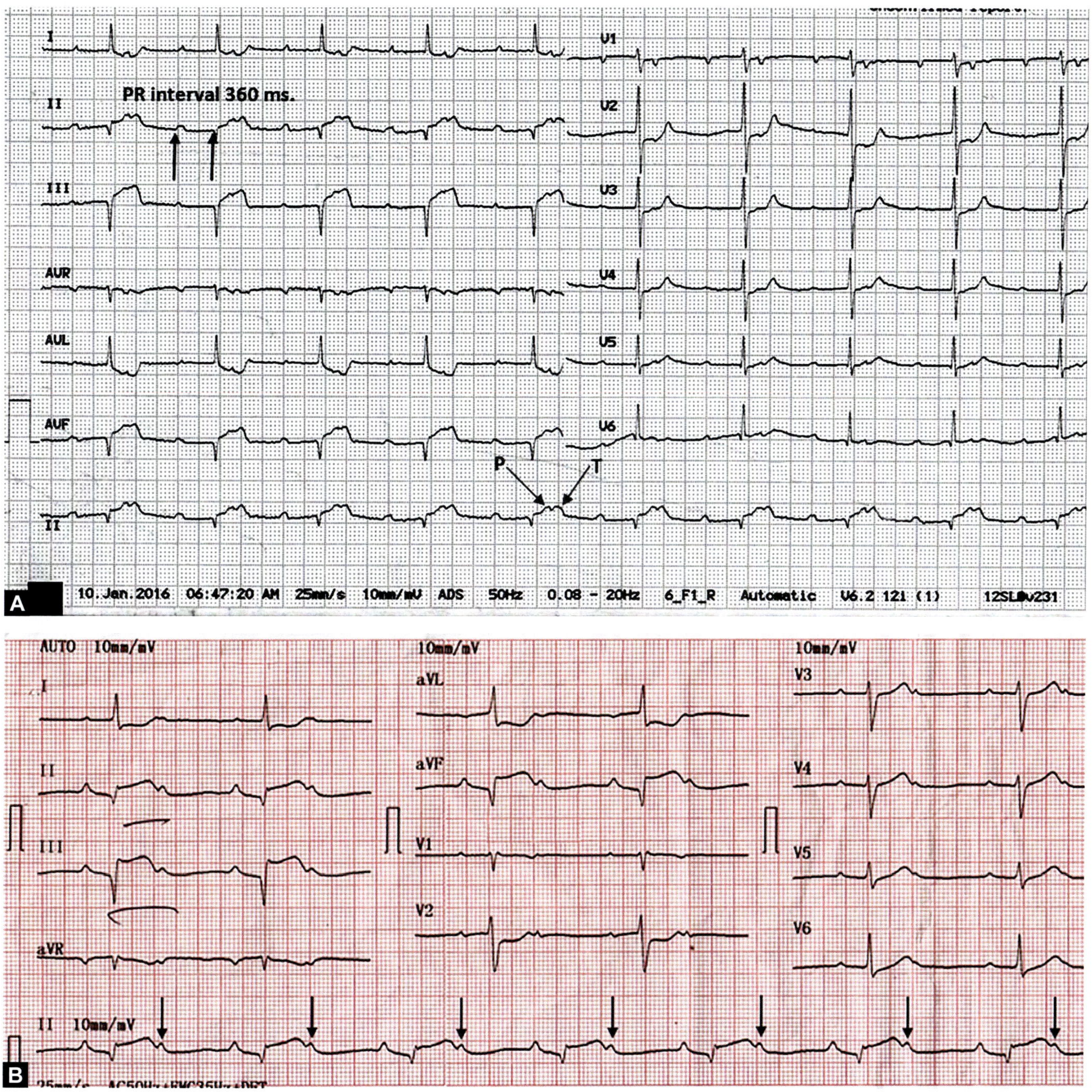

Figs. 15.10A and B: (A) ECG illustrates 2:1 AV block (Wenckebach pattern). *Note:* Lengthened PR interval (PR interval 360 ms) with narrow QRS pattern. Also note "T" waves and nonconducted "P" waves are fused together giving biphasic configuration. ECG also shows features of acute inferior myocardial infarction (ST segment elevation in leads LII, LIII, and aVF along with reciprocal ST depression in anterior leads); and (B) ECG illustrates 2:1 AV block (Wenckebach pattern) with alternate non-conducted P waves (*arrows*). Note lengthened PR interval (PR interval—280 ms) with narrow QRS complex. ECG also shows features of acute inferior myocardial infarction (ST segment elevation with pathological Q waves in leads LII,LIII and aVF) and reciprocal ST segment depression in L1 and aVL.

or below the His bundle produce a wide QRS complex (Fig. 15.14).

When the block is at the level of the AV node, the escape rhythm generally arises from a junctional pacemaker with a rate of 45–60 beats/min. Patients with a junctional pacemaker frequently are hemodynamically stable, and their heart rate increases in response to exercise and atropine. When the block is below the AV node, the escape rhythm arises from the His bundle or the bundle-branch Purkinje system at rates slower than 45 beats/min (usually 30–40 beats/min). These patients generally are hemodynamically unstable, and their heart rate is unresponsive to exercise and atropine.

Many conditions can cause third-degree heart block, but the most common cause is coronary artery disease and progressive degeneration of the electrical conduction system of the heart. This may be preceded by first-degree

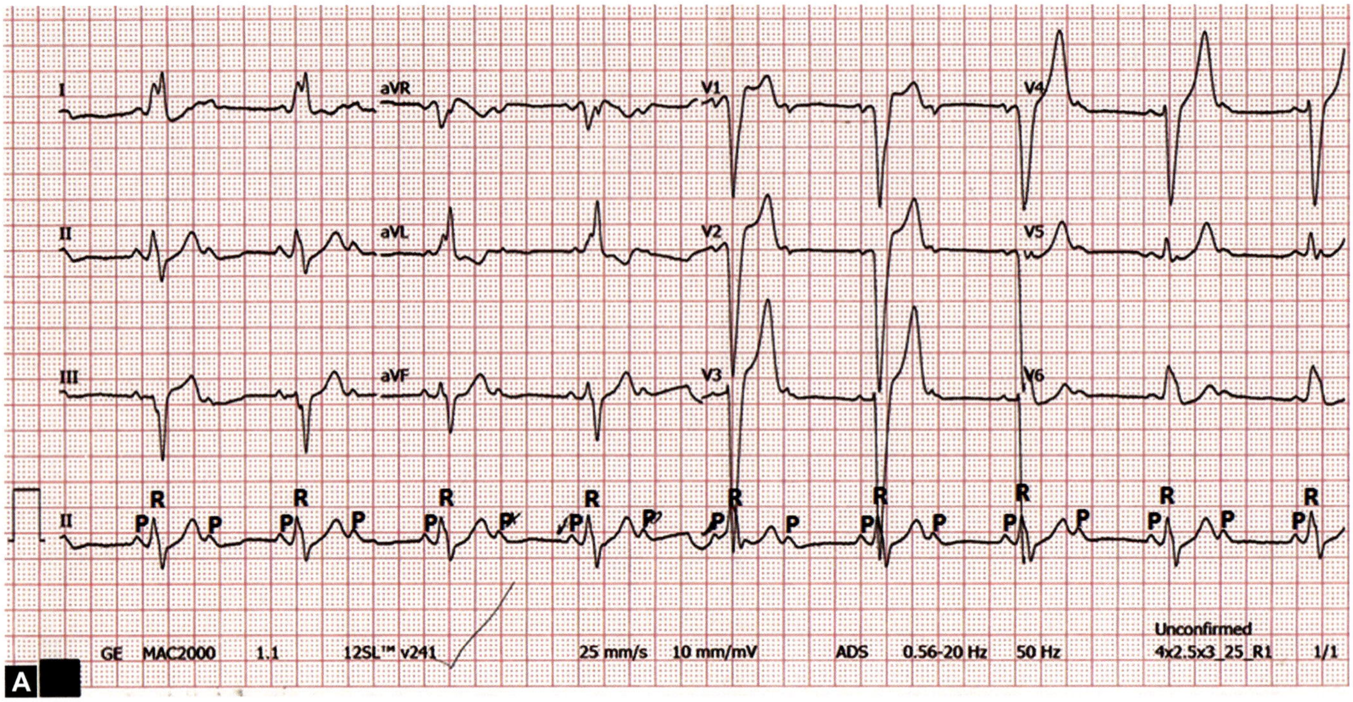

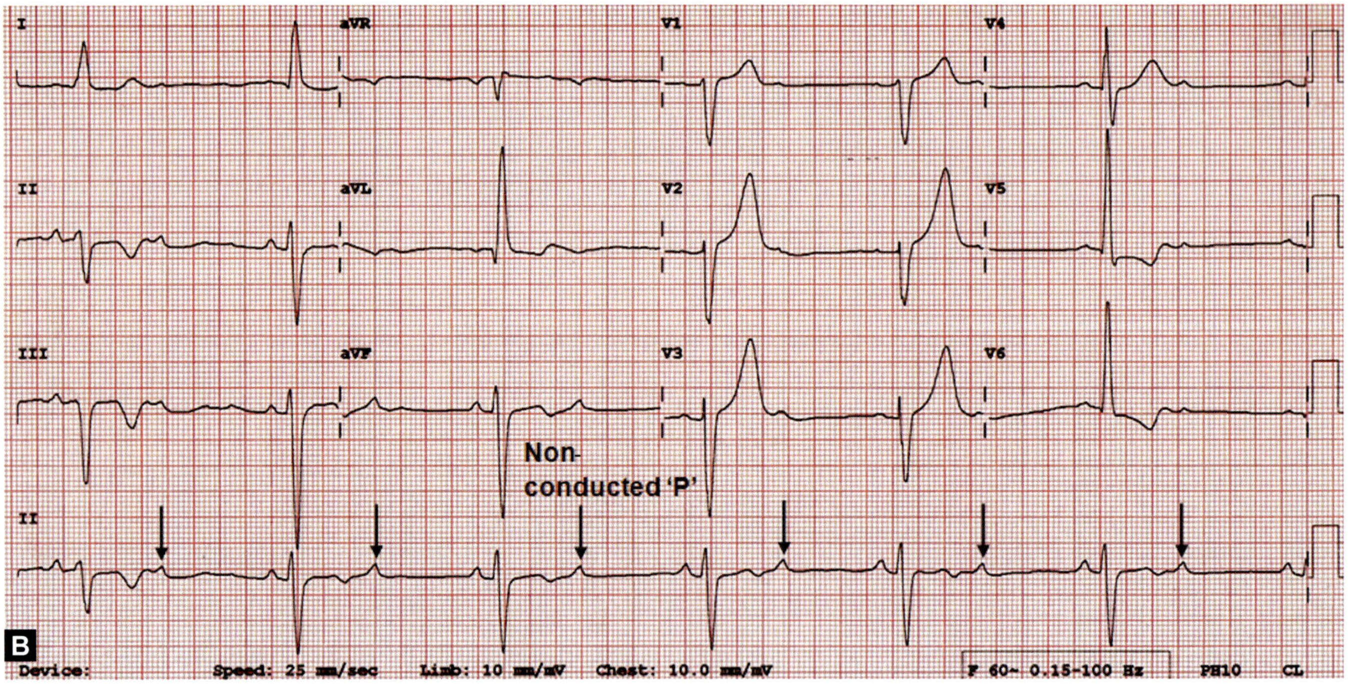

Figs. 15.11A and B: (A) ECG illustrates 2:1 AV block (Mobitz type II pattern). *Note:* Normal and constant PR interval (PR interval 128 ms) with wide QRS pattern (QRS 150 ms); and (B) ECG illustrates 2:1 AV block (Mobitz type II pattern) with heart rate 38 bpm. PR intervals are constant (PR interval 180 ms) in the complexes with conducted "P" waves and QRS complexes are broad (QRS duration 148 ms). Note also the nonconducted "P" waves (arrows). (AV: atrioventricular; ECG: electrocardiogram)

AV block, second-degree AV block, bundle branch block, or bifascicular block. In addition, acute MI may present with third-degree AV block.

An inferior wall MI may cause damage to the AV node, causing third-degree heart block. In this case, the damage is usually transitory. Studies have shown that third-degree heart block in the setting of an inferior wall MI typically resolves within 2 weeks. The escape rhythm typically originates in the AV junction, producing a narrow complex escape rhythm (Figs. 15.15A to C). An anterior wall MI may damage the distal conduction system of the heart, causing third-degree heart block.[35] This is typically extensive, permanent damage to the conduction system, sometimes necessitating a permanent pacemaker to be placed. The escape rhythm typically originates in the ventricles, producing a wide complex escape rhythm (Figs. 15.16A to C). CHB complicating acute anterior wall MI may disappear after successful reperfusion therapy (Figs. 15.17A and B).

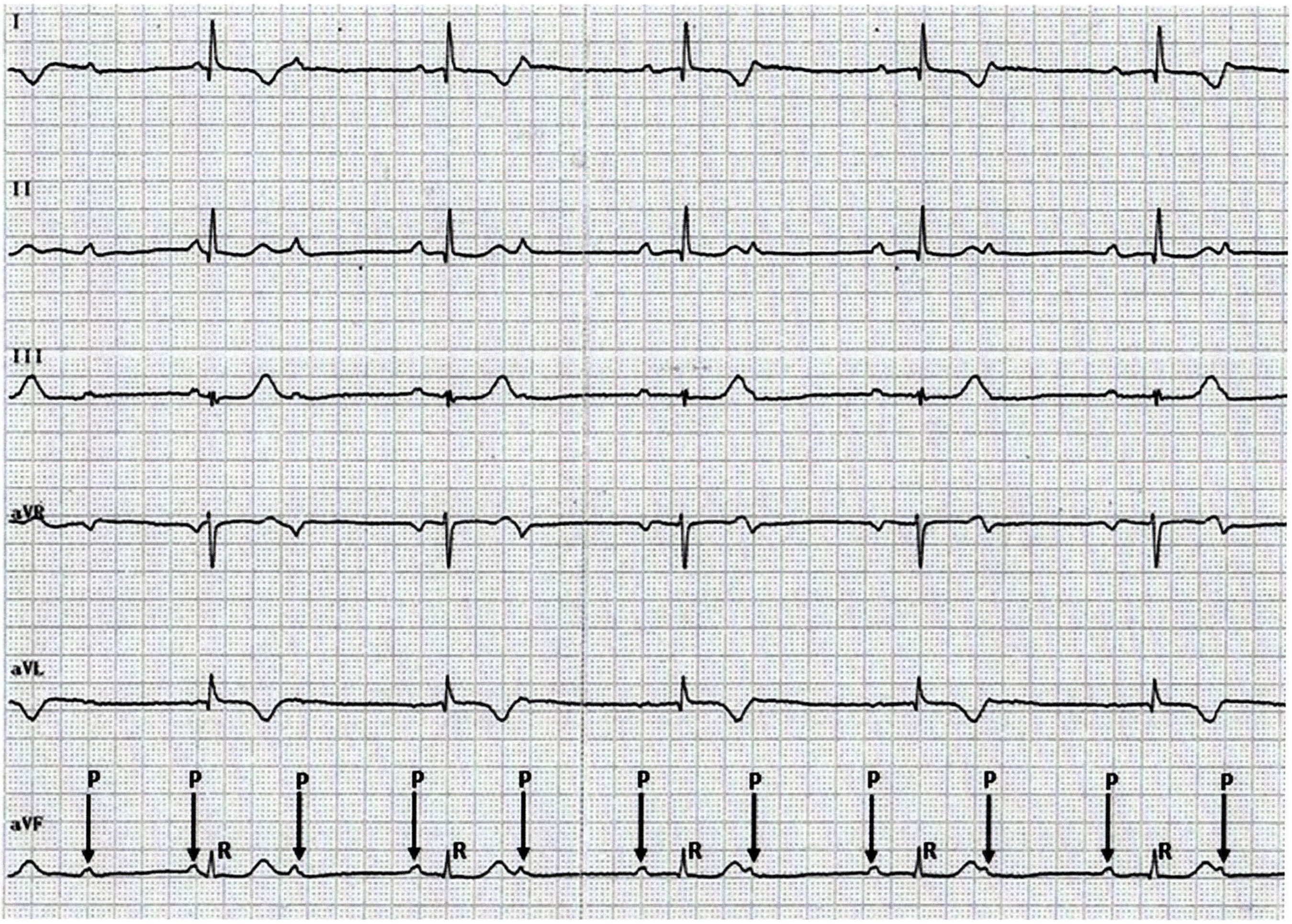

Fig. 15.12: Electrocardiogram (ECG) shows typical features of complete heart block (third-degree heart block) with heart rate 35 bpm. *Note:* P to P intervals are regular, QRS complexes with a regular R to R interval but PR intervals are variable.

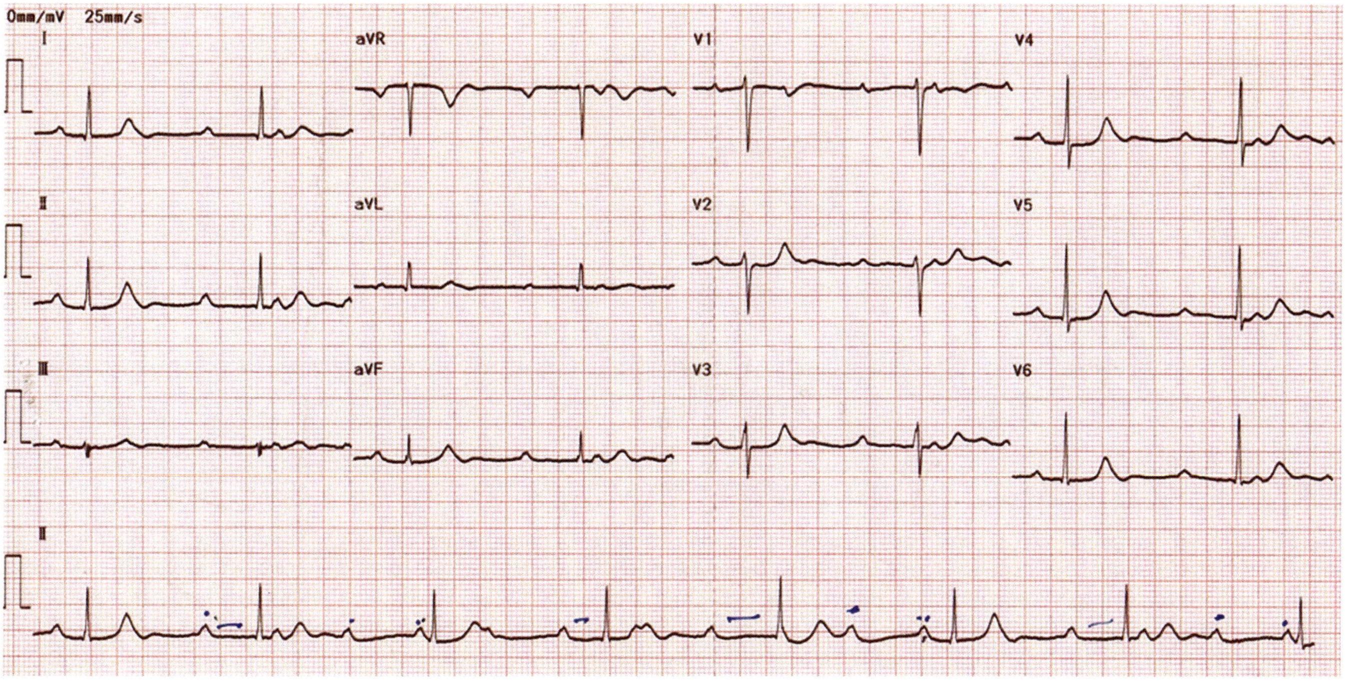

Fig. 15.13: ECG is suggestive of supra-His complete heart block with features of AV dissociation. *Note:* Normal narrow QRS complex with escape rhythm (rate 44 bpm). The configuration and duration of the escape QRS complex depends on the site of the block. Pacemakers above the His bundle produce a narrow QRS complex escape rhythm. (AV: atrioventricular; ECG: electrocardiogram)

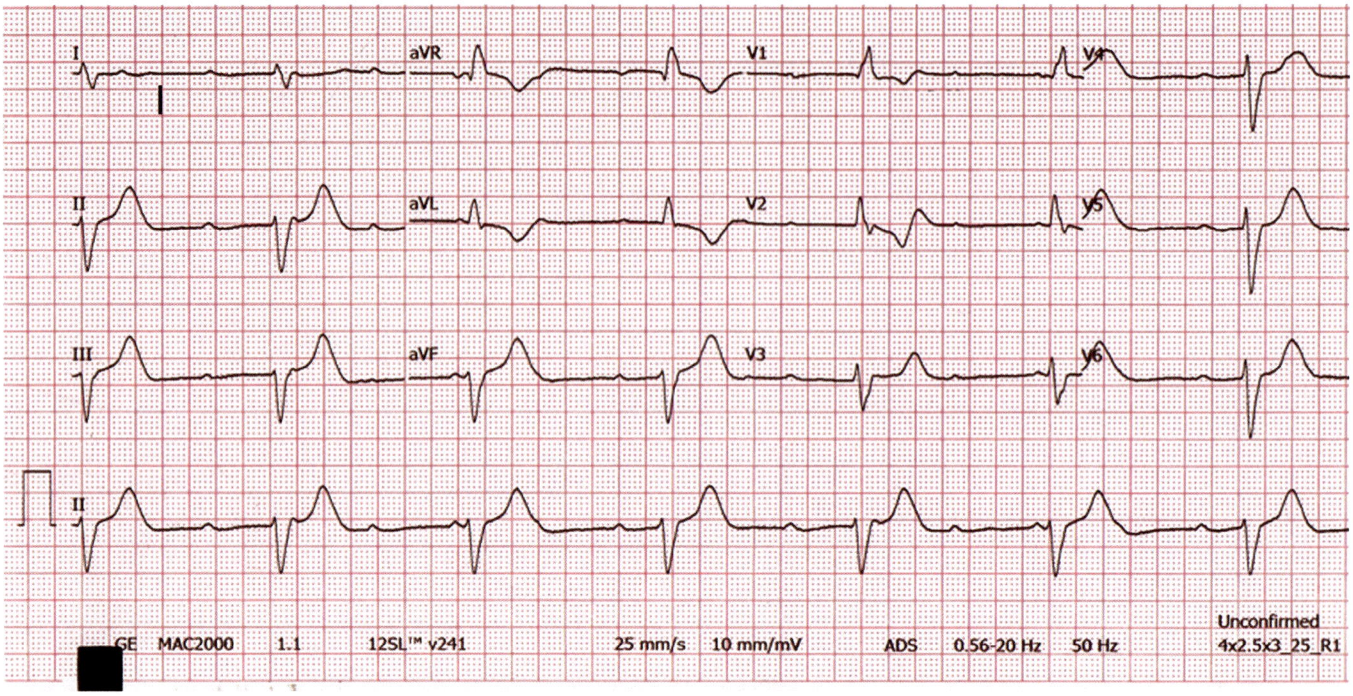

Fig. 15.14: ECG is suggestive of infra-His complete heart block with features of AV dissociation. *Note:* Wide QRS complex (QRS 136 ms) escape rhythm (rate 44 bpm). (AV: atrioventricular; ECG: electrocardiogram)

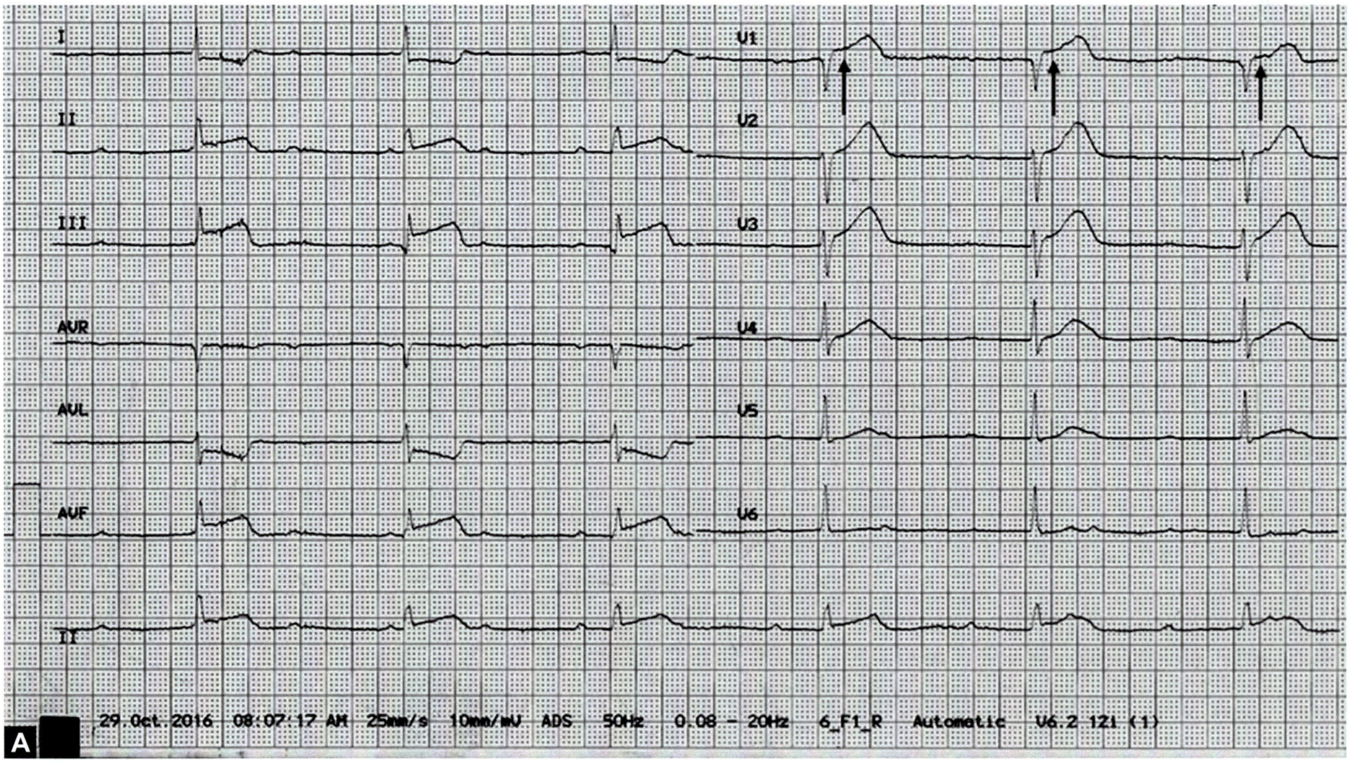

Fig. 15.15A: Electrocardiogram (ECG) shows complete heart block (CHB) in the setting of acute inferior MI (ST segment elevation in LII, LIII, and aVF) with reciprocal ST depression in LI and aVL. *Note:* Normal narrow QRS complex with escape rhythm (rate 36 bpm). Also note some ST segment elevation in lead V1 (*arrows*), which indicates associated right ventricular (RV) infarction in the setting of acute inferior MI. On the standard 12-lead ECG RV infarction is indicated by signs of inferior infarction, associated with ST segment elevation in lead V1. It is unusual for ST segment elevation in lead V1 to occur as an isolated phenomenon

Courtesy: Dr. Mahbubor Rahman, Labaid Cardiac Hospital

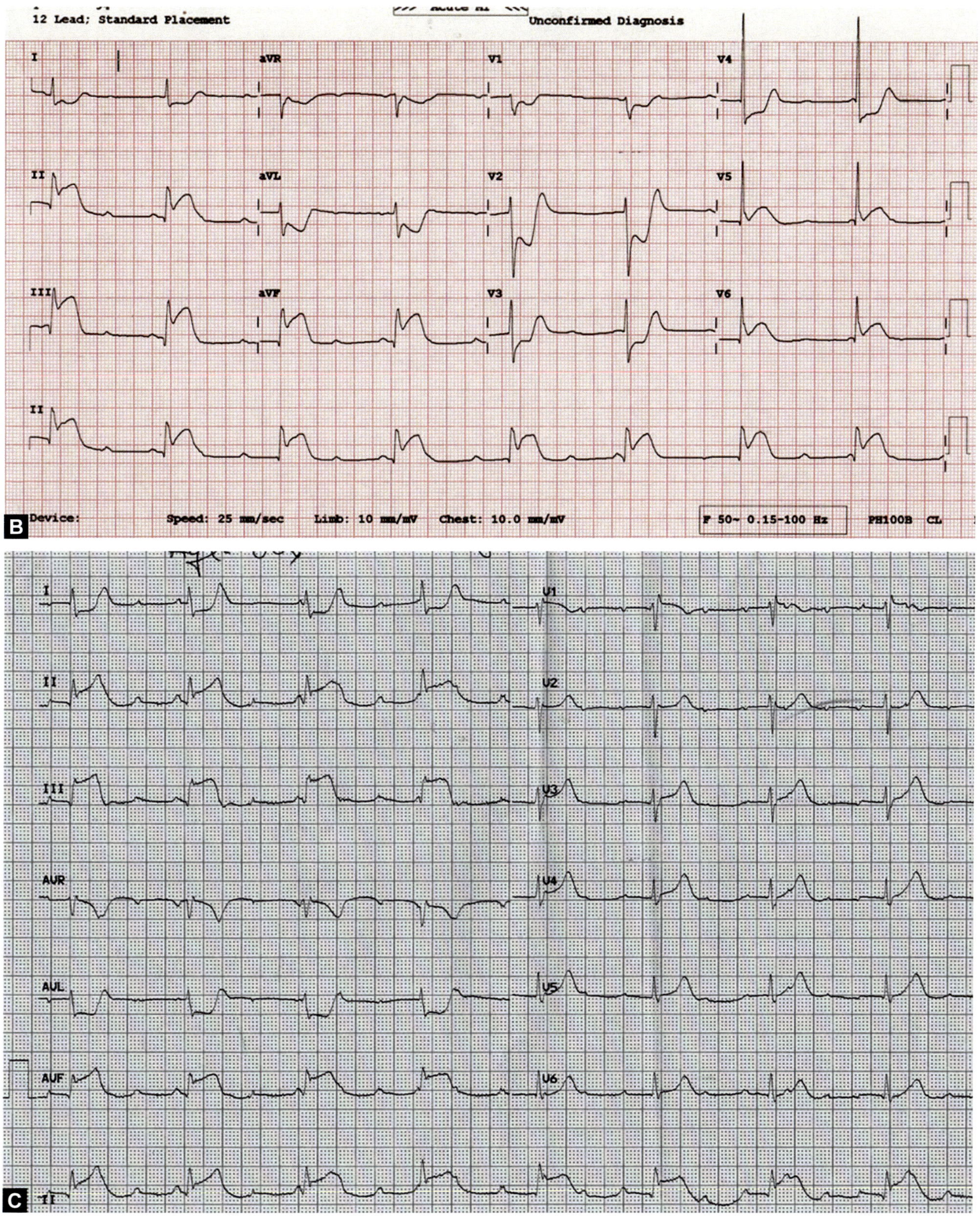

Figs. 15.15B and C: (B) ECG shows CHB in the setting of acute inferior and lateral MI (ST segment elevation in inferior leads, LII, LIII, aVF and V5–V6 with reciprocal ST depression in anterior leads LI, aVL, and V1–V4). The escape rhythm originated in the AV junction, producing a narrow complex escape rhythm (escape rate 48 bpm). Also note marked degree ST segment depression in lead V2, which suggests possible concurrent posterior wall infarction; and (C) ECG shows CHB in the setting of acute inferior MI (ST segment elevation in inferior leads with reciprocal ST depression in LI and aVL). The escape rhythm originated in the AV junction, producing a narrow complex escape rhythm (escape rate 48 bpm). Also note partial right bundle branch block. (AV: atrioventricular; MI: myocardial infarction)

Courtesy: Dr. Mahbubor Rahman, Labaid Cardiac Hospital

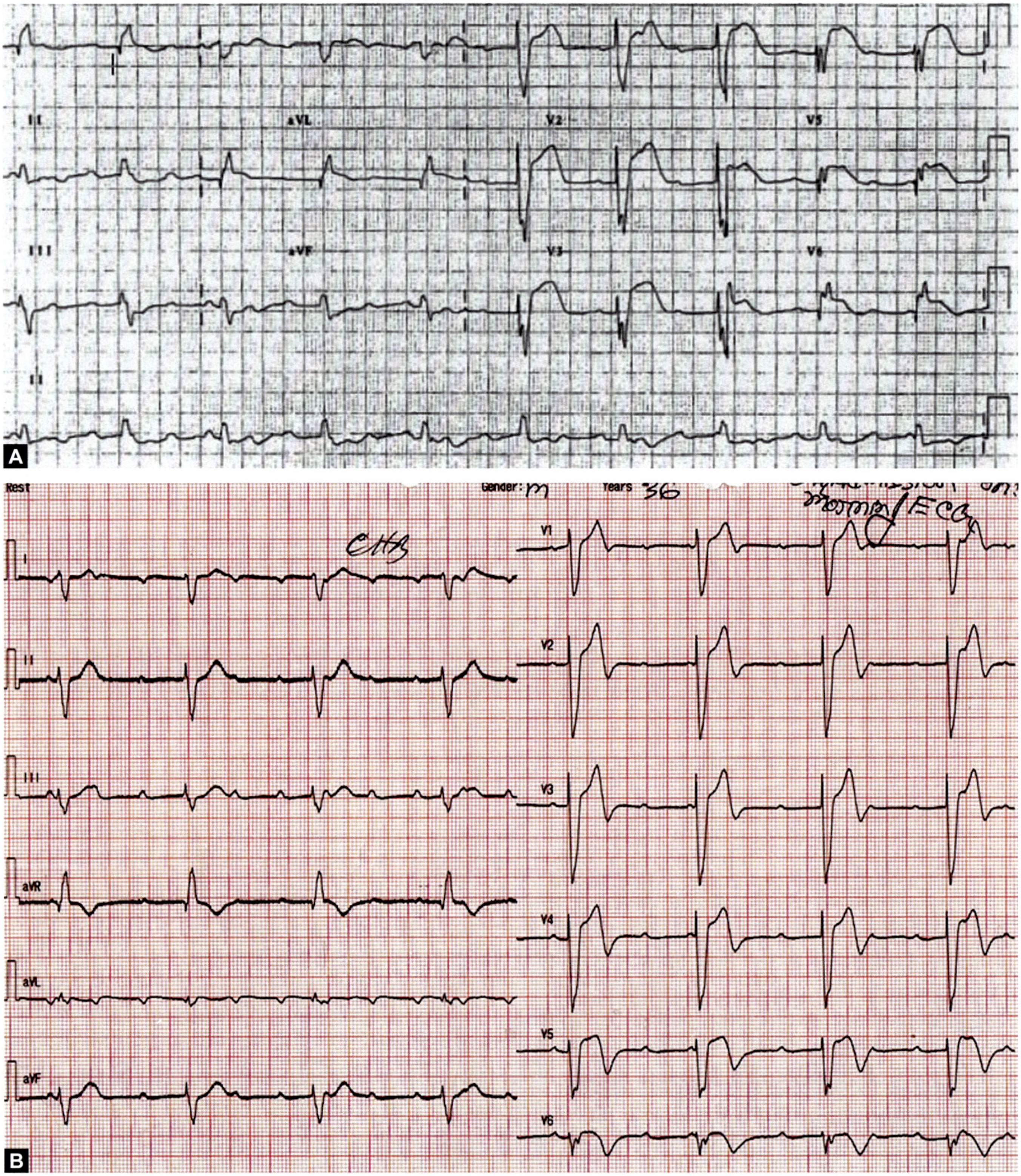

Figs. 15.16A and B: (A) ECG shows complete heart block (CHB) in the setting of acute anterior MI (ST segment elevation in LI, aVL, and V1–V6 with wide QRS complex). The escape rhythm possibly originated in the distal conduction system producing a broad QRS complex escape rhythm (escape rate 58 bpm). An anterior wall myocardial infarction may damage the distal conduction system of the heart, causing third-degree heart block. The escape rhythm typically originates in the ventricles, producing a wide complex escape rhythm; (B) ECG shows CHB in the setting of acute anterior MI with heart rate 48 bpm. *Note:* ST segment elevation with biphasic T waves in leads V1–V6. This patient underwent primary percutaneous coronary intervention (PPCI) for ostioproximal occlusion of left anterior descending coronary artery (*Courtesy:* Dr A K Miah, Labaid Cardiac Hospital)

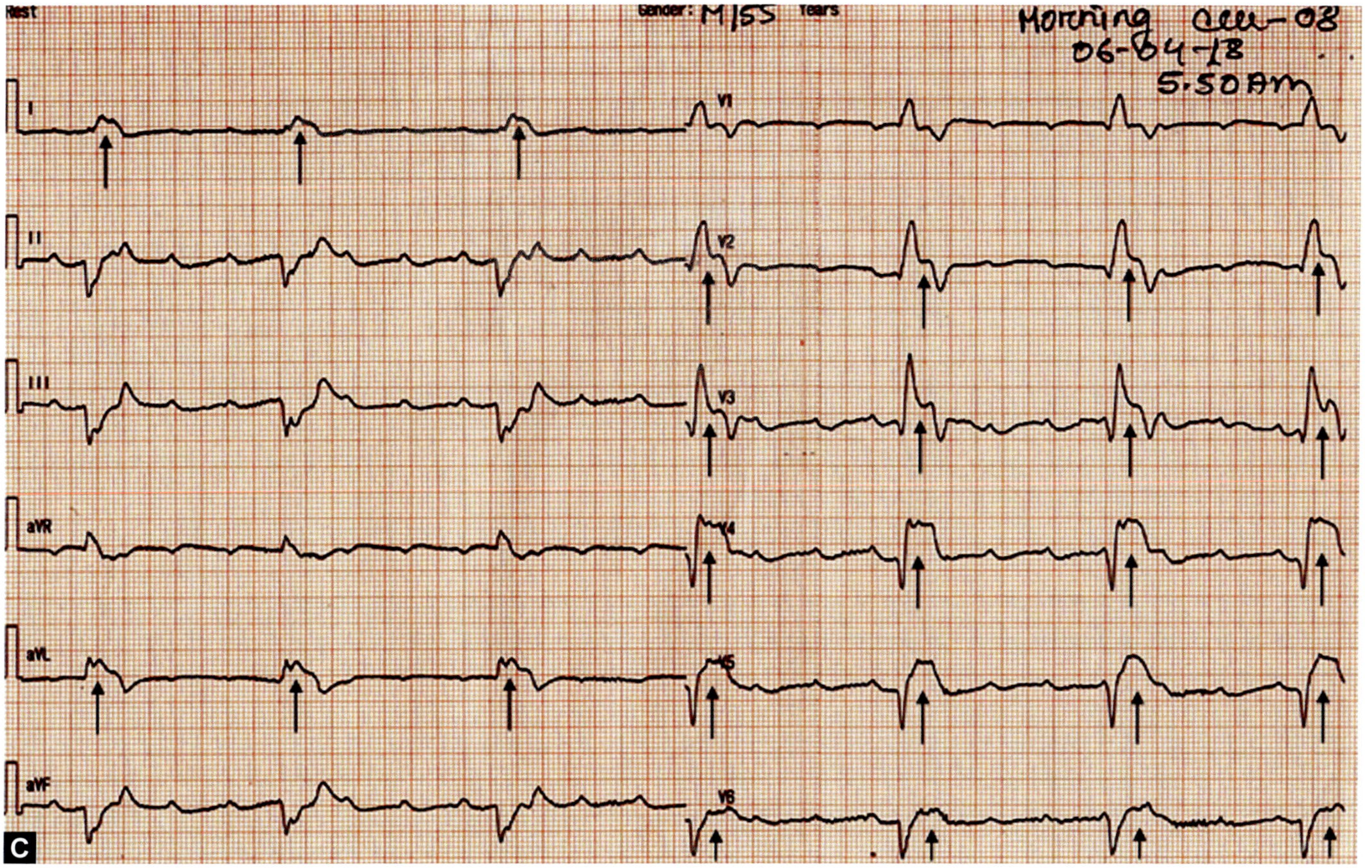

Fig. 15.16C: ECG shows CHB in the setting of acute anterior MI. Note: ST segment elevation in LI, aVL and V2-V6 (arrows) with wide QRS complex (QRS duration 150 ms) with escape rate 37 bpm. (ECG: electrocardiogram; MI: myocardial infarction)

Courtesy: Dr Abul Khayer, Labaid Cardiac Hospital

Third-degree heart block may also be congenital and has been linked to the presence of lupus in the mother. It is thought that maternal antibodies may cross the placenta and attack the heart tissue during gestation.[36] The cause of congenital third-degree heart block in many patients is unknown. Studies suggest that the prevalence of congenital third-degree heart block is between 1 in 15,000 and 1 in 22,000 live births. Lyme disease can also result in third-degree heart block.

If congenital CHB occurs alone, then it is relatively benign, as the block to conduction is at the level of the AV node. The ventricular pacemaker is proximal to the bifurcation of the bundle of His, and therefore the QRS complexes are narrow, and the ventricular conduction system intact (Fig. 15.18). The rate is relatively high and can vary from 40 beats/min to 80 beats/min, and may increase with exercise, atropine, or sympathomimetics.[37,38]

SUMMARY

Heart block can occur anywhere in the specialized conduction system beginning with the SA connections, the AV junction, the bundle branches and their fascicles, and ending in the distal ventricular Purkinje fibers. AV block may manifest as slowed conduction, intermittent conduction defect, or complete conduction failure. AV block is of three types (Box 15.1):

1. First-degree AV block
2. Second-degree AV block
3. Third-degree AV block (CHB).

First-degree heart block is manifested in ECG as prolonged PR interval more than 200 ms (>0.20 seconds). In the presence of marked first-degree AV block (PR interval > 300 ms), P waves may be buried in the preceding T wave. It is usually detected incidentally and often considered as normal variant. Common causes of first-degree heart block include: increased vagal tone, athletic training, inferior MI, rheumatic fever, diphtheria, myocarditis, and AV nodal blocking drugs (e.g. beta blockers, calcium channel blockers, digoxin, amiodarone, etc.). First-degree heart block does not cause hemodynamic disturbance and no specific treatment is required. Though first-degree heart block is usually considered as a benign condition but recent reports opined that this condition may be associated with

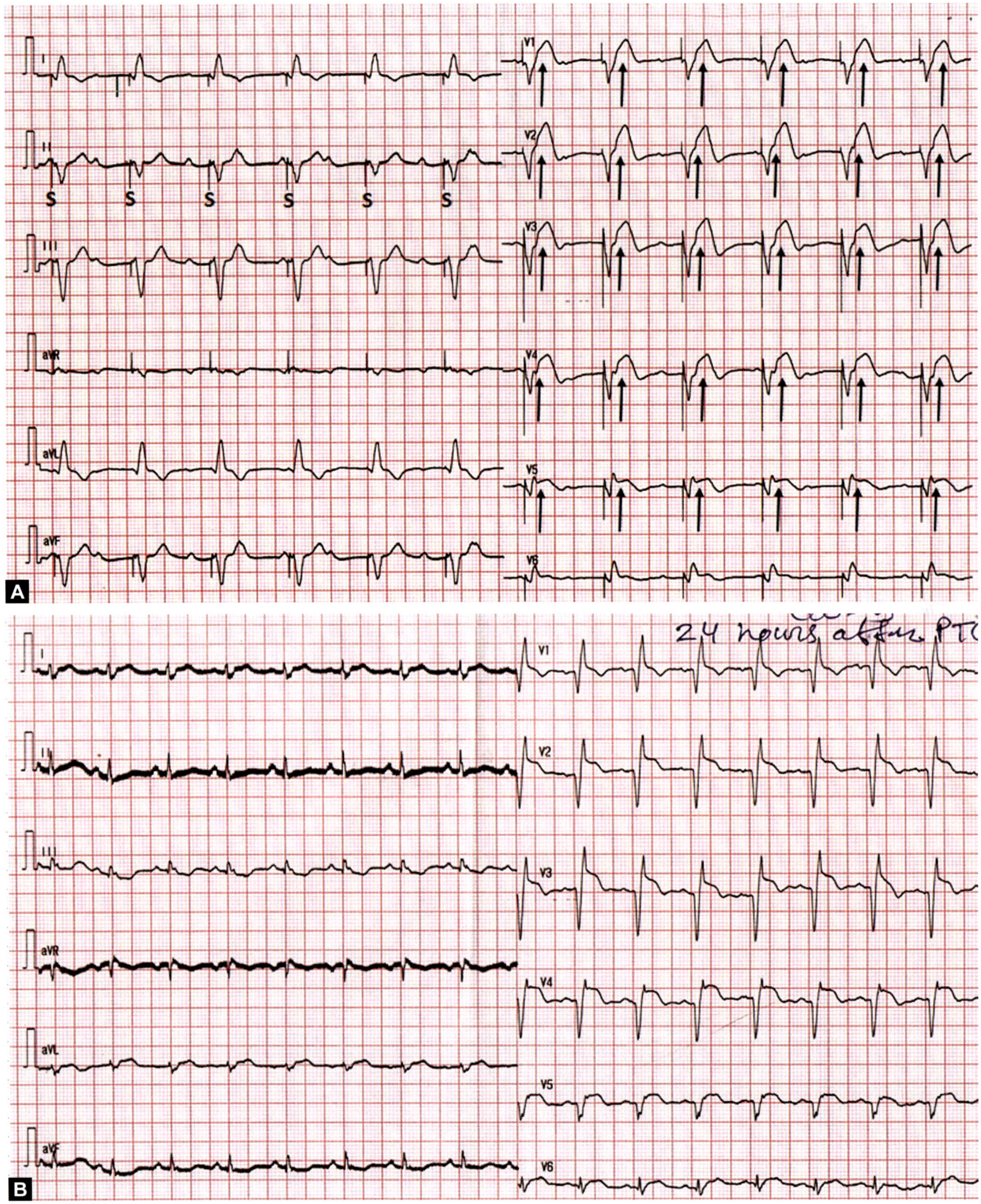

Figs. 15.17A and B: (A) ECG of a patient who presented with anterior STEMI (marked ST segment elevation in leads V1-V5) (*arrows*) with complete heart block. Temporary pacemaker was inserted immediately after admission (note pacing spikes 'S') and patient underwent primary percutaneous coronary intervention (PPCI); and (B) ECG of the same patient shown in Figure 15.17A, 24 hours after primary percutaneous coronary intervention to left anterior descending artery. *Note:* Disappearance of complete heart block and the patient is now in sinus rhythm. Also note appearance of Q waves in leads V1–V6 with RBBB pattern and some ST segment elevations are still persisting in anterior leads. (ECG: electrocardiogram; MI: myocardial infarction; RBBB: right bundle branch block)

Courtesy: Dr Arun Kumar Sharma, Labaid Cardiac Hospital

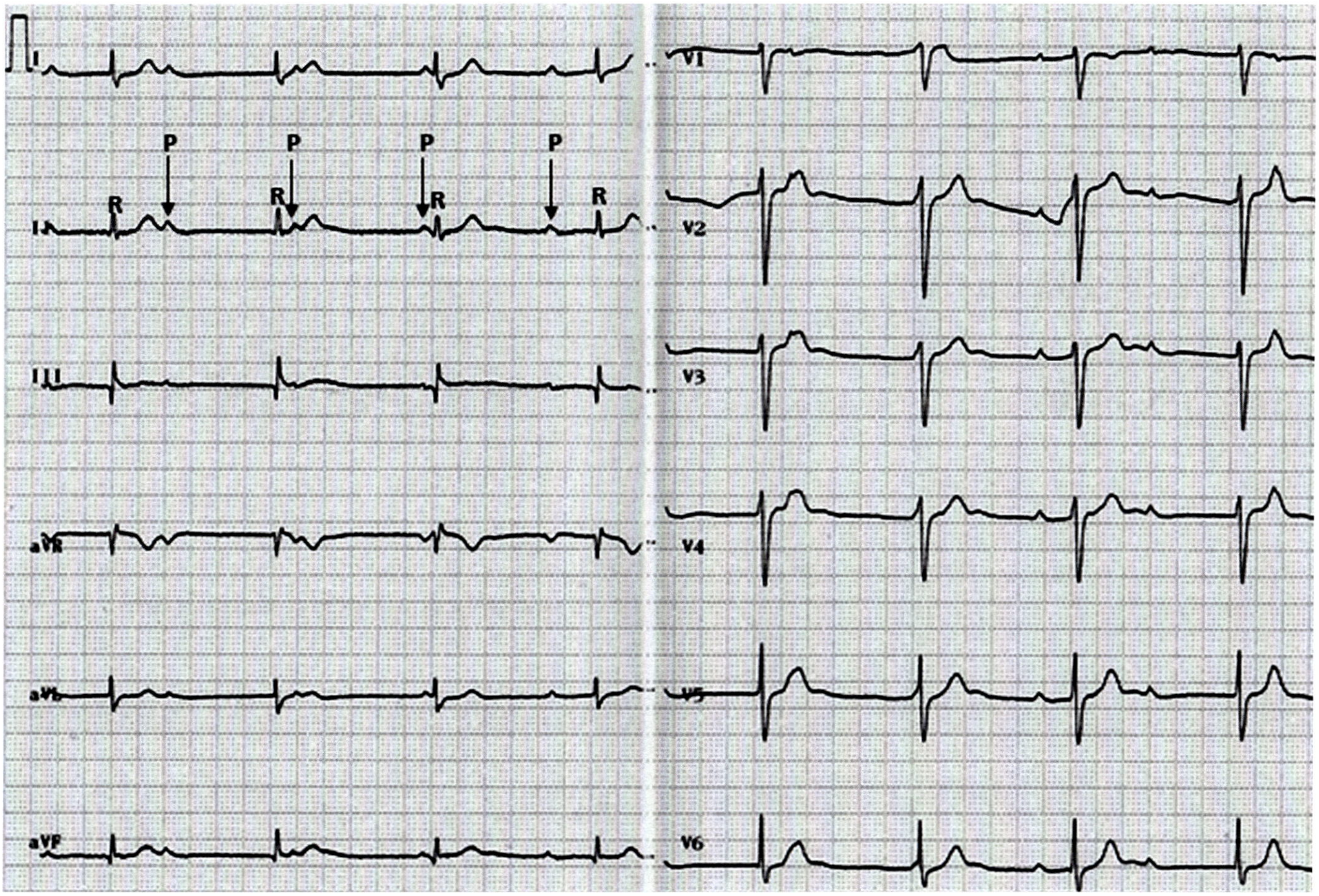

Fig. 15.18: Congenital complete heart block (CHB) in a 15-years old girl. Narrow complex CHB with heart rate 50 bpm. *Note:* Atrioventricular (AV) dissociation.

Box 15.1: ECG criteria of different types of AV block.

First degree heart block:

PR interval > 200 ms (>0.20 seconds) = (>5 small squares).

Second-degree heart block, Mobitz I (Wenckebach phenomenon):

Progressive prolongation of the PR interval followed by a drop beat (a nonconducted P wave).

Second-degree heart block, Mobitz II:

Intermittent drop beat (nonconducted P waves) without any progressive prolongation of the PR interval and the PR interval in the conducted beats remain constant.

Third-degree heart block (complete heart block):

- Usually the heart rate varies from 30–40 beats/minute
- P-P intervals are regular
- R-R intervals are regular but
- PR intervals are not regular (variable).

(AV: atrioventricular; ECG: electrocardiogram)

increased risk for atrial fibrillation, heart failure, and CV mortality.

Mobitz Type I Second-degree Atrioventricular Block (Wenckebach Phenomenon)

Mobitz type I second-degree AV block (Wenckebach phenomenon) is manifested on ECG with the followings:

- Progressive prolongation of the PR interval followed by a drop beat (culminating in a nonconducted P wave).
- The R-R interval progressively shortens with each beat of the cycle.
- The P-P interval remains relatively constant.

Causes of Mobitz Type I (Wenckebach Phenomenon) AV Block

The common causes of Mobitz type I second-degree AV block include:

- Acute inferior MI
- Increased vagal tone
- Myocarditis

- Drug induced, e.g. beta blockers, calcium channel blockers, digoxin, amiodarone, etc.

In Mobitz type I AV block the PR interval is longest immediately before the dropped beat and the PR interval is shortest immediately after the dropped beat. Mobitz I is usually due to reversible conduction block at the level of the AV node. Malfunctioning AV node cells tend to progressively fatigue until they fail to conduct an impulse. This is different to cells of the His-Purkinje system which tend to fail suddenly and unexpectedly (i.e. producing a Mobitz II block).

Mobitz Type II Second-degree Atrioventricular Block (Hay Phenomenon)

Mobitz II is usually due to failure of conduction at the level of the His-Purkinje system (i.e. below the AV node). While Mobitz I is usually due to a functional suppression of AV conduction (e.g. due to drugs, reversible ischemia), Mobitz II is more likely to be due to structural damage to the conducting system (e.g. infarction, fibrosis, and necrosis). In around 70% of cases, the conduction block is located distal to the Bundle of His, producing broad QRS complexes and in the remaining 30% of cases, the conduction block is located within the His Bundle itself, producing narrow QRS complexes.

The common causes of Mobitz type II AV block are:

- Anterior MI
- Idiopathic fibrosis of the conducting system
- Postcardiac surgery
- Inflammatory conditions (rheumatic fever, myocarditis, and Lyme disease)
- Autoimmune diseases, e.g. SLE
- Infiltrative myocardial diseases (amyloidosis, hemochromatosis, and sarcoidosis)
- Hyperkalemia
- *Drugs:* Beta blockers, calcium channel blockers, and amiodarone.

Electrocardiogram Criteria of Mobitz Type II Atrioventricular Block

- Intermittent nonconducted P waves without progressive prolongation of the PR interval.
- The PR interval in the conducted beats remain constant.
- The P waves "march through" at a constant rate.
- Mobitz type II AV block is usually associated with broad QRS complex.

Mobitz I AV block (Wenckebach phenomenon) is usually due to reversible conduction block at the level of the AV node but Mobitz II is usually due to failure of conduction at the level of the His-Purkinje system (i.e. below the AV node). Mobitz II AV block is much more likely than Mobitz type I second-degree AV block to be associated with hemodynamic compromise, severe bradycardia, and progression to CHB.

2:1 Atrioventricular Block

A 2:1 AV block can be in the AV node (Mobitz type I or Wenckebach phenomenon) or in the His-Purkinje system (2:1 Mobitz type II AV block). In a 2:1 AV block, there is only one conducted P wave for each P wave blocked; thus, only one PR interval is available for examination before the block. So it is difficult to classify a 2:1 AV block as type I or type II. If initial PR interval is lengthened with normal QRS complex, the possible diagnosis is 2:1 Wenckebach block (Mobitz type I) but normal PR interval with broad QRS complex is suggestive of 2:1 Mobitz type II block. Differentiation of 2:1 Wenckebach from 2:1 Mobitz type II block is important because Wenckebach is often considered innocuous but 2:1 Mobitz type II block is considered pathological.

Third-degree Atrioventricular Block (Complete Heart Block)

Third-degree AV block (also referred to as CHB) is the complete dissociation of the atria and the ventricles. Third-degree AV block exists when more P waves than QRS complexes exist and no relationship (no conduction) exists between them. The escape rhythm may arise within the AV node (resulting in a narrow QRS complex), or lower in the conduction system (producing a wide QRS complex). The ventricular rate (pulse) varies from 30–40 beats/minute. But when the block is at the level of the AV node, the escape rhythm generally arises from a junctional pacemaker with a rate of 45–60 beats/min. Characteristically in third-degree AV block, the atrial rate is faster than the ventricular rate (60–100 beats/minute).

In CHB, there is complete absence of AV conduction—none of the supraventricular impulses are conducted to the ventricles. The cardiac rhythm is maintained by a junctional or ventricular escape rhythm. Alternatively, the patient may suffer ventricular standstill leading to syncope (if self-terminating) or sudden cardiac death (if prolonged). Typically the patient will have severe bradycardia with independent atrial and ventricular rates, i.e. AV dissociation. Important causes of third-degree heart block include acute MI, idiopathic degeneration of the conducting system, Lev's disease, and AV-nodal blocking drugs (e.g. calcium channel blockers, beta blockers, and digoxin).

Sometimes third-degree heart block may be congenital. In most of the cases of congenital CHB the QRS complexes are narrow, as the ventricular pacemaker is proximal to the bifurcation of the bundle of His. In congenital CHB the rate is relatively high and can vary from 40 beats/min to 80 beats/min, and may increase with exercise, atropine, or sympathomimetics.

Characteristics those can be seen on an ECG include:

- P waves with a regular P to P interval.
- QRS complexes with a regular R to R interval.
- The PR interval will appear variable because there is no relationship between the P waves and the QRS complexes.

P-P intervals are regular, R-R intervals are regular but PR intervals are not regular—these three are considered as the hallmark criteria for the diagnosis of CHB.

Patients with third-degree heart block are at high risk of ventricular standstill and sudden cardiac death and usually require insertion of a permanent pacemaker.

REFERENCES

1. Mangrum JM, DiMarco JP. The evaluation and management of bradycardia. N Engl J Med. 2000;342(10):703-9.
2. Crisel RK, Farzaneh-Far R, Na B, et al. First-degree atrioventricular block is associated with heart failure and death in persons with stable coronary artery disease: data from the Heart and Soul Study. Eur Heart J. 2011;32(15): 1875-80.
3. Libby P, Braunwald E. Braunwald's Heart Disease: A Textbook of Cardiovascular Medicine, 8th edition. Philadelphia: Saunders/Elsevier; 2008.
4. John AD, Fleisher LA. Electrocardiography: the ECG. Anesthesiol Clin. 2006;24(4):697-715.
5. Barold SS, Ilercil A, Leonelli F, et al. First-degree atrioventricular block. Clinical manifestations, indications for pacing, pacemaker management & consequences during cardiac resynchronization. J Interv Card Electrophysiol. 2006;17(2):139-52.
6. Upshaw CB. Comparison of the prevalence of first-degree atrioventricular block in African-American and in Caucasian patients: an electrocardiographic study III. J Natl Med Assoc. 2004;96(6):756-60.
7. Berger PB, Ruocco NA, Ryan TJ, et al. Incidence and prognostic implications of heart block complicating inferior myocardial infarction treated with thrombolytic therapy: results from TIMI II. J Am Coll Cardiol. 1992;20(3):533-40.
8. Sonesson SE, Salomonsson S, Jacobsson LA, et al. Signs of first-degree heart block occur in one-third of fetuses of pregnant women with anti-SSA/Ro 52-kd antibodies. Arthritis Rheum. 2004;50(4):1253-61.
9. Alkoutami GS, Reeves WC, Movahed A. The safety of adenosine pharmacologic stress testing in patients with first-degree atrioventricular block in the presence and absence of atrioventricular blocking medications. J Nucl Cardiol. 1999;6(5):495-7.
10. Suda K, Raboisson MJ, Piette E, et al. Reversible atrioventricular block associated with closure of atrial septal defects using the Amplatzer device. J Am Coll Cardiol. 2004;43(9):1677-82.
11. Johnson RL, Averill KH, Lamb LE. Electrocardiographic findings in 67,375 asymptomatic subjects. VII. Atrioventricular block. Am J Cardiol. 1960;6:153-77.
12. Mymin D, Mathewson FA, Tate RB, et al. The natural history of primary first-degree atrioventricular heart block. N Engl J Med. 1986;315(19):1183-7.
13. Haïssaguerre M, Derval N, Sacher F, et al. Sudden cardiac arrest associated with early repolarization. N Engl J Med. 2008;358(19):2016-23.
14. Garg A, Finneran W, Feld GK. Familial sudden cardiac death associated with a terminal QRS abnormality on surface 12-lead electrocardiogram in the index case. J Cardiovasc Electrophysiol. 1998;9(6):642-7.
15. Porthan K, Viitasalo M, Jula A, et al. Predictive value of electrocardiographic QT interval and T-wave morphology parameters for all-cause and cardiovascular mortality in a general population sample. Heart Rhythm. 2009;6(8):1202-8, 1208.e1.
16. Gussak I, Antzelevitch C. Early repolarization syndrome: clinical characteristics and possible cellular and ionic mechanisms. J Electrocardiol. 2000;33(4):299-309.
17. Miller WL, Hodge DO, Hammill SC. Association of uncomplicated electrocardiographic conduction blocks with subsequent cardiac morbidity in a community-based population (Olmsted County, Minnesota). Am J Cardiol. 2008;101(1):102-6.
18. Takagi M, Aihara N, Takaki H, et al. Clinical characteristics of patients with spontaneous or inducible ventricular fibrillation without apparent heart disease presenting with J wave and ST segment elevation in inferior leads. J Cardiovasc Electrophysiol. 2000;11(8):844-8.
19. Cheng S, Keyes MJ, Larson MG, et al. Long-term outcomes in individuals with prolonged PR interval or first-degree atrioventricular block. JAMA. 2009;301(24):2571-7.
20. Silverman ME, Upshaw CB, Lange HW. Woldemar Mobitz and His 1924 classification of second-degree atrioventricular block. Circulation. 2004;110(9):1162-7.
21. Mobitz W. Über die unvollständige Störung der Erregungsüberleitung zwischen Vorhof und Kammer des menschlichen Herzens [On the partial block of impulse conduction between atrium and ventricle of human hearts]. Z Gesamte Exp Med. 1924;41:180-237.
22. Wenckebach KF. Zur Analyse des unregelmassigne Pulses: II. On the analysis of irregular pulses: II. Z Klin Med. 1899;37:475-88.
23. Hay J. Bradycardia and cardiac arrhythmia produced by depression of certain of the functions of the heart. Lancet. 1906;167(4299):139-43.
24. Barold SS, Hayes DL. Second-degree atrioventricular block: a reappraisal. Mayo Clin Proc. 2001;76(1):44-57.
25. Puech P, Wainwright RJ. Clinical electrophysiology of atrioventricular block. Cardiol Clin. 1983;1(2):209-24.
26. Narula QS. Cardiac Arrhythmias: Electrophysiology, Diagnosis and Management. Baltimore: Williams & Wilkins; 1979. pp. 85-113.
27. Narula QS. Clinical concepts of spontaneous and induced atrioventricular block. In: Mandel WJ (Ed). Cardiac Arrhythmias, 3rd edition. Philadelphia: Lippincott; 1995. pp. 441-59.
28. WHO/ISC Task Force. Definition of terms related to cardiac rhythm. Am Heart J. 1978;95:796-806.
29. Surawicz B, Uhley H, Borun R, et al. The quest for optimal electrocardiography. Tast Force I: standardization of terminology and interpretation. Am J Cardiol. 1978;41(1):130-45.
30. Zaman L, Moleiro F, Rozanski JJ, et al. Multiple electrophysiologic manifestations and clinical implications of vagally mediated AV block. Am Heart J. 1983;106(1 Pt 1):92-9.

31. Barold SS. Cardiac pacing in special and complex situations. Indications and modes of stimulation. Cardiol Clin. 1992;10(4):573-91.
32. Narula OS, Scherlag BJ, Javier RP, et al. Analysis of the A-V conduction defect in complete heart block utilizing His bundle electrograms. Circulation. 1970;41(3):437-48.
33. Rosen KM, Dhingra RC, Loeb HS, et al. Chronic heart block in adults. Clinical and electrophysiological observations. Arch Intern Med. 1973;131(5):663-72.
34. Kojic EM, Hardarson T, Sigfusson N, et al. The prevalence and prognosis of third-degree atrioventricular conduction block: the Reykjavik study. J Intern Med. 1999;246(1):81-6.
35. Ho KW, Koh TH, Wong P, et al. Complete atrioventricular block complicating acute anterior myocardial infarction can be reversed with acute coronary angioplasty. Ann Acad Med Singapore. 2010;39(3):254-7.
36. Costedoat-Chalumeau N, Georgin-Lavialle S, Amoura Z, et al. Anti-SSA/Ro and anti-SSB/La antibody-mediated congenital heart block. Lupus. 2005;14(9):660-4.
37. Reid JM, Coleman EN, Doig W. Complete congenital heart block. Report of 35 cases. Br Heart J. 1982;48(3):236-9.
38. Kumar AU, Sripriya R, Parthasarathy S, et al. Congenital complete heart block and spinal anaesthesia for caesarean section. Indian J Anaesth. 2012;56(1):72-4.

Chapter 16

Electrocardiographic Diagnosis of Cardiac Channelopathies

INTRODUCTION

Cardiac channelopathies are a group of clinical syndromes that affect the cardiovascular electrical system and several mutation-associated cardiac diseases, affecting sodium (Na^+), potassium (K^+), or calcium (Ca^{2+}) ion currents, have been described affecting either the generation of the action potential or calcium homeostasis.[1-4] Cardiac channelopathies may be clinically identified only by the presence of some characteristic electrocardiographic abnormalities.[1] These are not always present in genetic carriers, because the diseases often have a low penetrance.[5-7]

As a result of channelopathy, the electrical properties of the patient's heart are altered, changing the surface electrocardiogram (ECG) and/or predisposing them to life-threatening, proarrhythmic events. These syndromes include:

1. Brugada syndrome (BrS)
2. Long QT syndrome (LQTS)
3. Short QT syndrome (SQTS)
4. Catecholaminergic polymorphic ventricular tachycardia (CPVT).

BRUGADA SYNDROME

Brugada syndrome is a hereditary disease responsible for ventricular fibrillation (VF) and sudden cardiac death (SCD) in the young. The disease is characterized by the presence of right ventricular conduction abnormalities and coved-type ST-segment elevation in the anterior precordial leads (V1-V3) (Fig. 16.1).

First described in 1992 by the Brugada brothers, the disease has since had an exponential rise in the numbers of cases reported, to such an extent that this syndrome is regarded as the second leading cause of sudden death in males less than 40 (after trauma).[8-10] Its incidence seems to be particularly high in Southeast Asia where it had been previously described as sudden unexplained nocturnal death syndrome (SUNDS), indeed it was known colloquially in the Philippines as *bangungut* (to rise and moan in sleep), in Japan as *pokkuri* (sudden and unexpectedly ceased phenomena), and in Thailand as *Lai Tai* (death during sleep). The mean age of sudden death is 41, with the age at diagnosis ranging from 2 days to 84 years.[8-12]

A diagnostic triad characterizes BrS. It consists of (1) complete or incomplete right bundle branch block (RBBB) pattern ECG, (2) ST-segment elevation in leads V1-V3, and (3) SCD. Approximately 50% of patients with BrS noted to have familial occurrence, this suggests a genetic component of the disease. Commonly mutations in gene SCN5A, an encoder for human cardiac sodium channel on chromosome 3p21, cause BrS.[13] The disease exhibits an autosomal dominant pattern of transmission with variable penetrance.[14-16]

When an ECG shows (or is suspicious for) a Brugada pattern (BrP), i.e. the association of a positive terminal deflection and ST-segment elevation in the right precordial leads, the cardiologist often faces several problems. Three important questions are raised by this ECG pattern:

1. Is this really a Brugada ECG pattern?
2. How can be determined whether this patient is at risk for sudden death?

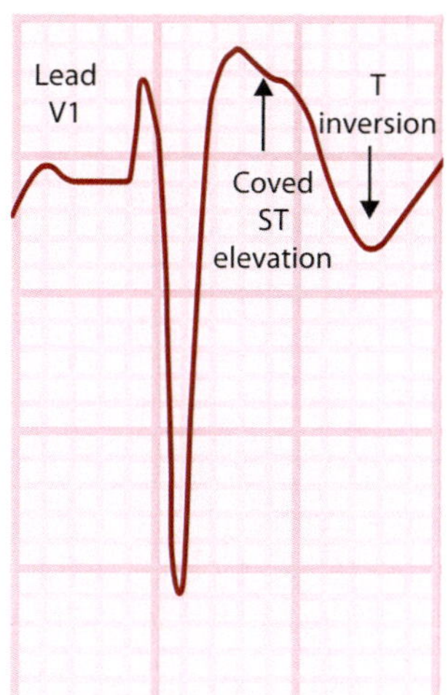

Fig. 16.1: Coved ST-segment elevation greater than 2 mm in lead V1 followed by a negative T wave is the most important ECG abnormality in the type 1 Brugada syndrome . This has been referred to as Brugada sign.

3. Should this patient receive an implantable cardioverter-defibrillator (ICD)?

The term "Brugada syndrome" should be restricted to patients who have diagnostic ECG changes, as well as a history of symptoms. Asymptomatic subjects, in contrast, should be categorized as having a "Brugada ECG pattern" rather than the syndrome.[17] The diagnostic ECG of "BrS" is characterized by a J wave (a terminal positive wave) whose amplitude is greater than or equal to 2 mm, and a "coved"-type ST-segment elevation located in the right precordial leads (Fig. 16.2). These signs are usually present in leads V1 and/or V2 (lead V3 is more rarely involved, and is never the only affected one), but occasionally also can be observed in some of the limb leads (Fig. 16.3).[17]

Types of Brugada Pattern Electrocardiograms

Electrocardiogram abnormalities constitute the hallmark of BrS. They include repolarization and depolarization abnormalities in the absence of identifiable structural cardiac abnormalities or other conditions or agents known to lead to ST-segment elevation in the right precordial leads (V1-V3). Three types of repolarization patterns are recognized.[18]

1. *Type 1*: This pattern is characterized by a prominent coved ST-segment elevation displaying J wave amplitude or ST-segment elevation greater than or equal to 2 mm or 0.2 mV at its peak followed by a negative T wave, with little or no isoelectric separation (Figs. 16.4 and 16.5).
2. *Type 2*: This pattern also has a high take-off ST-segment elevation, but in this case, J wave amplitude (≥2 mm) gives rise to a gradually descending ST-segment elevation (remaining ≥1 mm above the baseline), followed by a positive or biphasic T wave that results in a saddleback configuration (Figs. 16.6 and 16.7).
3. *Type 3*: This pattern reveals right precordial ST-segment elevation of less than 1 mm of saddleback type, coved type, or both (Fig. 16.8).

Type 1 ECG is suggestive of BrS, and type 2 and type 3 ECGs are considered as BrP (Figs. 16.9A to C and 16.10A to C). In BrS, the ST-segment changes may be dynamic. Different patterns may be observed sequentially in the same patient or following the introduction of specific drugs. Intravenous administration of certain drugs may modify the ECG pattern.

Electrocardiographic Criteria for the Diagnosis of Brugada Syndrome

ST-segment and T-wave abnormalities in leads V1-V3 have been shown in Table 16.1.

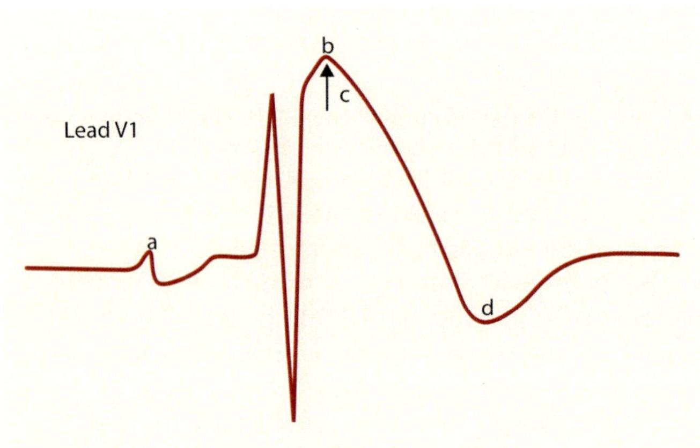

Fig. 16.2: Patterns of different waves in the lead V1 in Brugada syndrome: (a) Biphasic broad P wave, (b) J point elevation (arrow), (c) Coved-type ST-segment elevation, and (d) Inverted T wave.

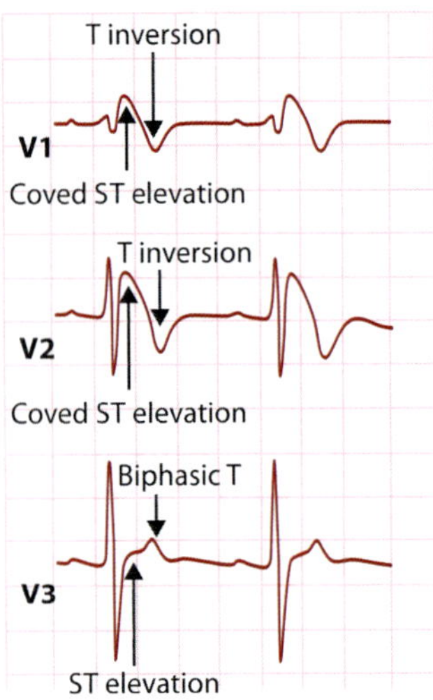

Fig. 16.3: ECG of Brugada syndrome displaying right bundle branch block pattern with coved ST-segment elevation in leads V1-V2 with J point elevation with terminal negative T wave in V1-V2 and biphasic T wave in lead V3.

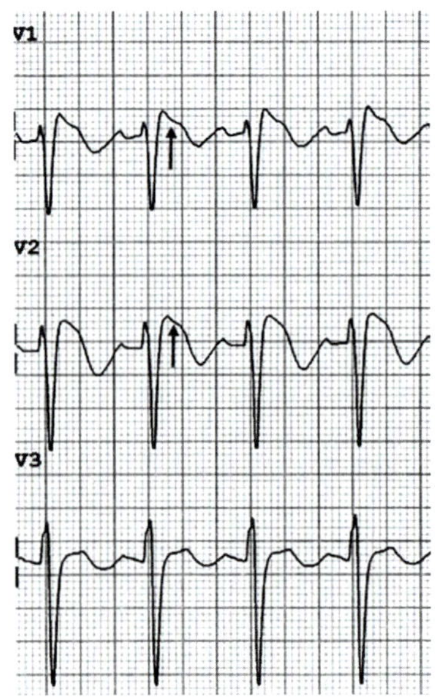

Fig. 16.4: ECG of type 1 Brugada syndrome showing J point elevation with coved ST-segment elevation greater than 2 mm in leads V1-V2 (arrows) followed by negative T waves. Also note some ST-segment elevation followed by biphasic T wave in V3.

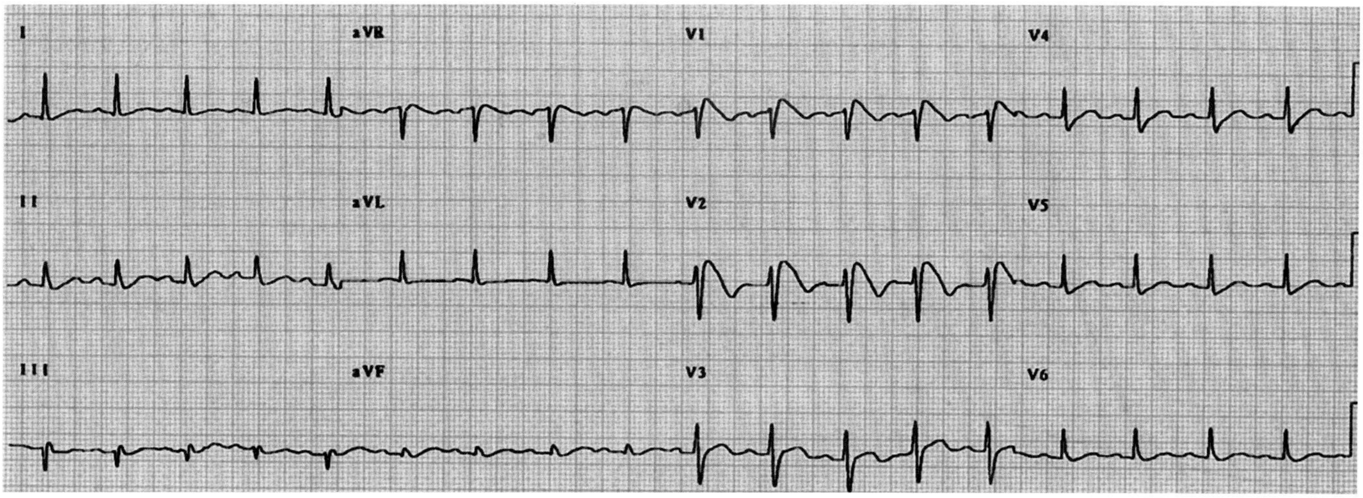

Fig. 16.5: ECG of type 1 Brugada syndrome showing J point elevation with coved ST-segment elevation greater than 2 mm in leads V1-V2 followed by a negative T wave in leads V1-V2 . Also note less than 1 mm ST-segment elevation followed by biphasic T wave in V3.

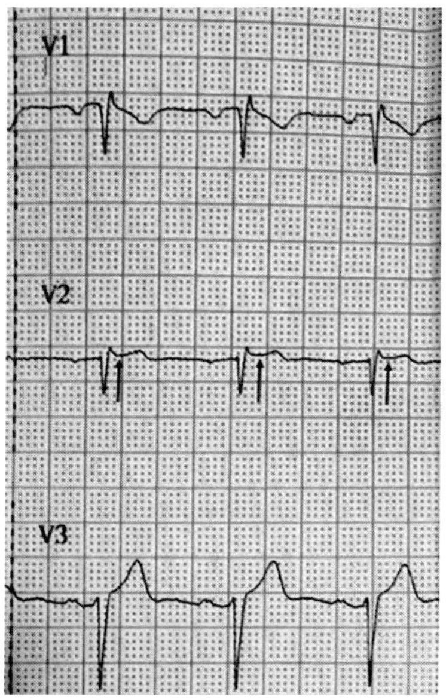

Fig. 16.6: Type 2 Brugada ECG showing greater than 1 mm ST elevation with T-wave inversion in V1 and greater than 1 mm saddleback-shaped ST elevation (arrows) with biphasic T waves in lead V2 typical of type 2 pattern. Also note less than 1 mm ST-segment elevation followed by upright T wave in V3. (*Source:* Courtesy of Dr Shiblee Sadik Pathan)

Drug Challenge to Help the Electrocardiographic Diagnosis

Several studies have already informed about the dynamic character of the ECG in BrS. Class I antiarrhythmic drugs (AADs) are able to reproduce the diagnostic pattern when administered to those patients in whom the ECG spontaneously normalized. Drug challenge for diagnosis of BrS is indicated in cases in which the disease is suspected, but in which the basal ECG is normal (e.g. familial screening) or suspicious, but not diagnostic of type 2 or 3 BrS. Flecainide, ajmaline, procainamide, disopyramide, propafenone, and pilsicainide have been used to unmask Brugada ECG. Drug challenge is only considered positive when a conversion to the diagnostic type 1 occurs.[19-21]

Electrocardiographic features obtained with alternative placement of the right precordial leads in a superior intercostal space in individuals with high clinical suspicion (aborted SCD victims, family members of patients with BrS) may also disclose the presence of the arrhythmic substrate. In selected cases, one may even consider rightward displacement.[22]

Syncope or SCD may be the first symptom in patients with BrS. About 80% of patients with documented VF have a history of syncope. Rapid polymorphic ventricular tachycardia (VT) is a common arrhythmia in patients with BrS. Ventricular tachycardia (VT) usually starts with a short coupling interval. Self-terminating episodes typically lead to repeated episodes of syncope.[19] It has been suggested that there is a higher than normal incidence of supraventricular tachyarrhythmias, including atrial and atrioventricular reentrant tachycardia in the Brugada population.[23] But monomorphic VT is rarely observed.[24,25] Clinical reports indicate that sudden death in patients with BrS most commonly occurs during sleep, in particular during the early morning hours.[26,27] Family history is of paramount importance and is often positive for SCD at a young age.[18]

The basic ECG diagnostic criteria of the BrS is ST-segment elevation in the right precordial leads (V1-V3). But the list of the causes of ST-segment elevation in leads V1-V3 is long. Clinical diagnostic evaluation should be directed toward excluding each of these causes. Discrimination between BrS and arrhythmogenic right ventricular cardiomyopathy (ARVC) may be particularly difficult because ARVC may at times mimic BrS and structural abnormalities may only be found at time of autopsy. Before the diagnosis of BrS is made, a serious attempt should be taken to exclude ARVC. Drug challenge with sodium channel blockers may be useful in discriminating between these two diseases.[18] BrS should also be distinguished from early repolarization pattern (with an eventual elevated J wave amplitude in the left precordial leads) and from normal degrees of right

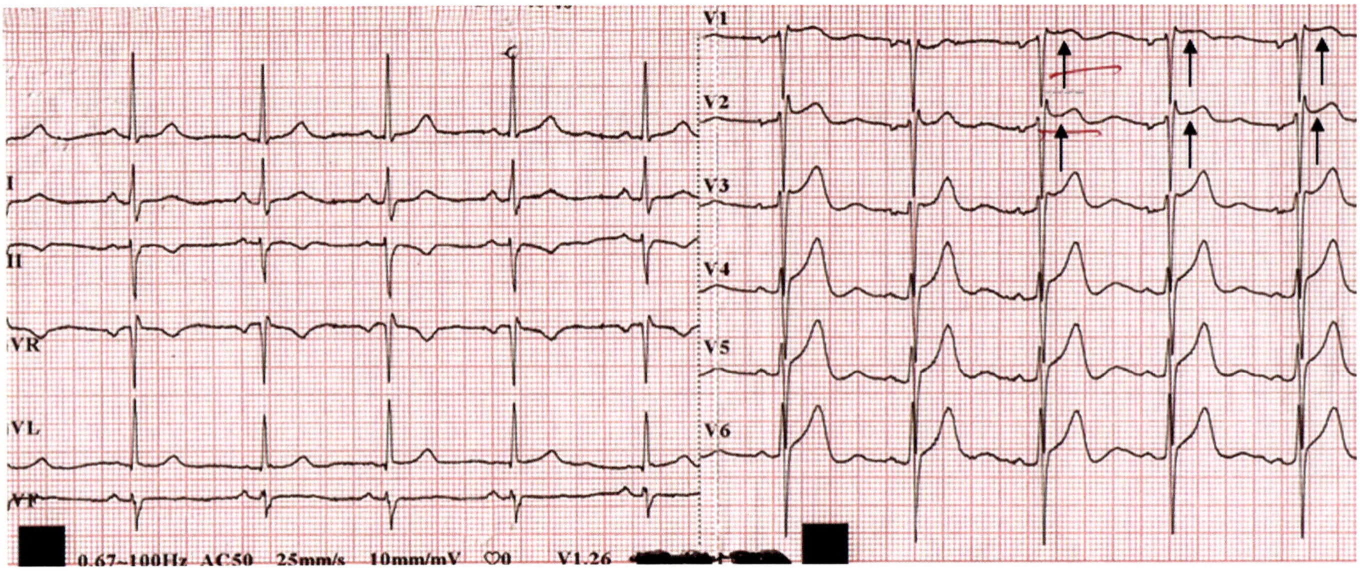

Fig. 16.7: Type 2 Brugada ECG showing greater than 1 mm saddleback-shaped ST elevation (arrows) with biphasic T waves in lead V1 and V2 typical of type 2 pattern. Also note some ST-segment elevation followed by upright T wave in V3. (*Source:* Courtesy of Dr Nur Mohammad)

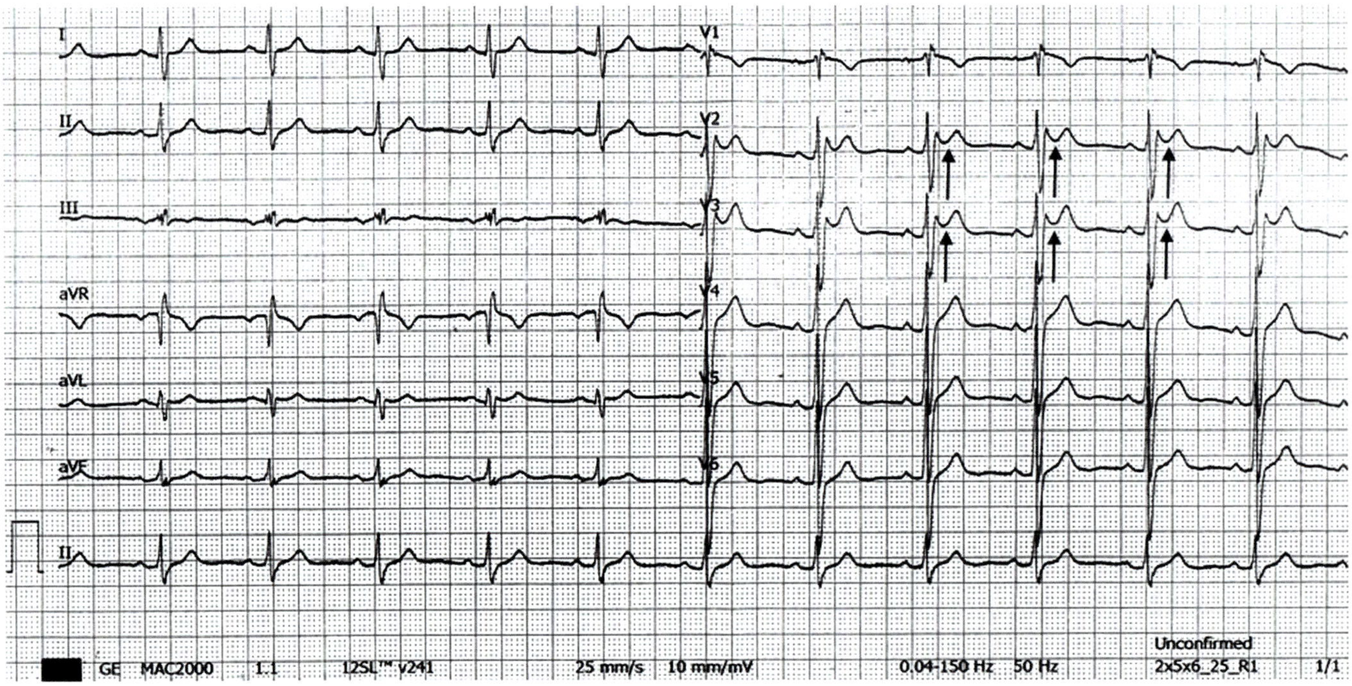

Fig. 16.8: Type 3 Brugada ECG showing less than 1 mm of coved ST-segment elevation in lead V1 followed by T-wave inversion along with saddleback-shaped ST elevation (arrows) in leads V2 and V3 followed by upright T waves. This ECG mimics partial right bundle branch block.

precordial ST elevation in men, which may mimic a type 2 or 3 Brugada ECG pattern. If any difficulty arises to confirm the diagnosis, a drug challenge might provide the clue for a proper diagnosis.[18]

Electrocardiogram Differentiation: Brugada Syndrome/Pattern versus Right Bundle Branch Block

The distinction between Brugada ECG and complete RBBB is straightforward because, in complete RBBB, the ST-segment is not elevated in the right precordial leads, the terminal wave (r' or R') is synchronous with the broad S wave observed in leads I and V6, and the QRS is wider (≥120 ms). In BrS, however, usually no wide S wave is present in the left precordial leads (V5, V6) because the terminal forces of the ventricular complex in V1-V2 can be recorded only by electrodes placed in proximity of the site where the abnormal electrical activity occurs (the outflow tract of the right ventricle) and not from further away leads. Therefore, the QRS in left precordial leads is usually less than 120 milliseconds. In BrS, the r' wave is broad, rounded and

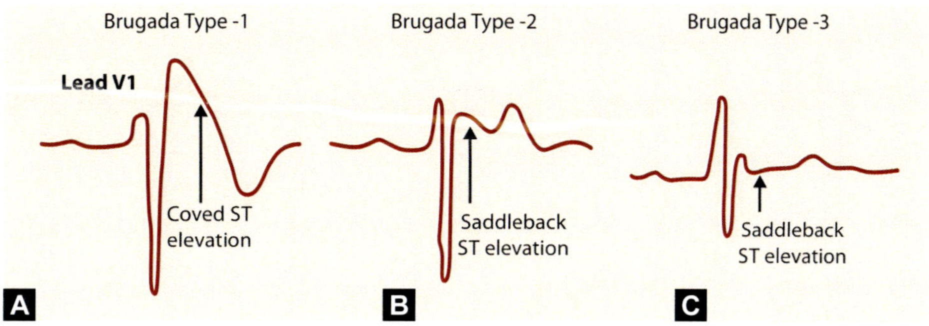

Figs. 16.9A to C: Different patterns of ST-segment elevation in lead V1 in different types of Brugada ECGs. (A) Coved pattern ST-segment elevation in lead V1 in type 1 Brugada syndrome (arrow); (B) Saddleback-shaped ST elevation around 2 mm (arrow) in type 2 Brugada ECG or Brugada pattern; (C) Saddleback-shaped ST elevation around less than 1 mm (arrow) in type 3 Brugada ECG or Brugada pattern.

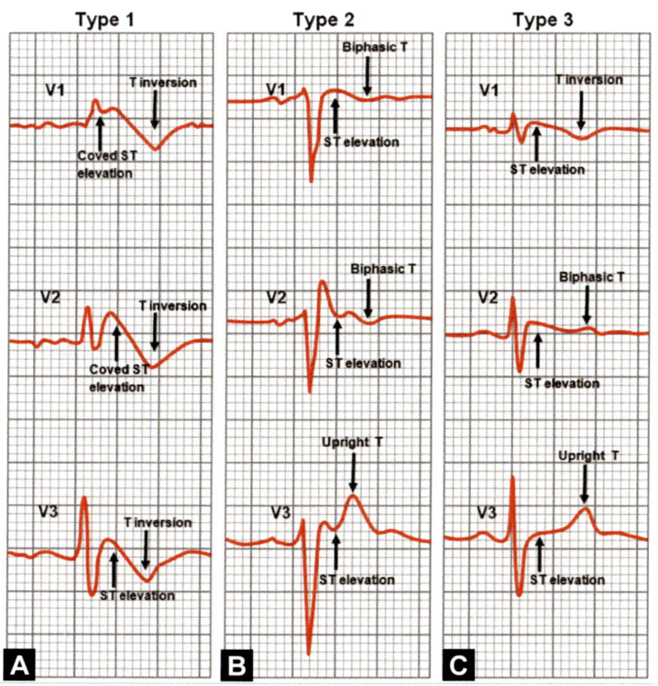

Figs. 16.10A to C: ECGs displaying three different types of Brugada syndrome. (A) Type 1 showing J point elevation with prominent coved ST-segment elevation followed by a negative T wave in leads V1-V3; (B) Type 2 Brugada pattern shows saddleback ST-segment elevation with biphasic T wave in leads V1 and V2 and upright T in lead V3; (C) Type 3 Brugada pattern displays around 1 mm ST elevation in right precordial leads with negative T wave in lead V1, biphasic T in V2 and upright T in lead V3.

Table 16.1: ST-segment and T-wave abnormalities in leads V1-V3 in Brugada ECGs.

ECG change	*Type 1*	*Type 2*	*Type 3*
ST elevation	≥2 mm	≥1 mm	<1 mm
ST-T configuration	Coved type	Saddleback	Saddleback or coved
T wave	Negative	Positive or biphasic	Positive
Terminal portion of ST-segment	Gradually descending	Elevated ≥1 mm	Elevated <1 mm

Note: 1 mm = 0.1 mV. The terminal portion of the ST-segment refers to the latter half of the ST-segment.

generally of low voltage, with a slow descent. In contrast, that of RBBB is pointed.

Type 2 BrP and incomplete RBBB raise more problems: whenever a small positive terminal QRS deflection (r') is present in V1-V2, it is possible to distinguish the r' wave of incomplete RBBB from the terminal positive r' wave of type 2 BrP on the basis of the following: (1) the positive terminal r' wave is peaked in RBBB, whereas, in BrP, type 2 is rounded, wide, and usually of relatively low voltage; (2) in incomplete RBBB, the QRS complex duration in leads V1-V2 is identical to that observed in lead V6. In type 2 BrP, in contrast, the QRS duration is longer in the right precordial leads than in V6 because the terminal deflection observed in V1 (the r' wave) cannot be recorded by the V6 electrode. In other words, in BrP, the QRS complex end is earlier in V6 than in V1-V2.[16-20]

There are a couple of new measurements which may also help to quantify the difference in the r' wave morphology of BrS and incomplete RBBB.

Two angles were measured manually: (1) alpha (α)—the angle between a vertical line and the downslope of the r' wave and (2) beta (β)—the angle between the upslope of the S wave and the downslope of the r' wave (Fig. 16.11).[8,16]

- The α angle (α >50°, sensitivity 71% and specificity 79%) and β angle (β >58°, sensitivity 79%, specificity 83%) are greater in BrS than in incomplete RBBB.
- The duration of the base of the triangle of the r'-wave at 5 mm of the high take-off greater than or equal to 4 mm is a good criterion for BrS and is much shorter in healthy athletes with incomplete RBBB (Fig. 16.12).

For further confirmation drug challenge can be done. AADs particularly sodium channel blockers have been used effectively to unmask BrS. To differentiate between type 2 or type 3 BrP and incomplete RBBB, AAD challenge is helpful.[16,20] Before AAD, two angles are measured from ECG leads V1 and/or V2 showing incomplete RBBB (?BrP): The baseline angle values, alone or combined with QRS duration, are usually compared between patients with negative and positive results on AAD. Change in type 2 and type 3 BrPs into type 1 pattern after drug challenge or change in the α and β angles

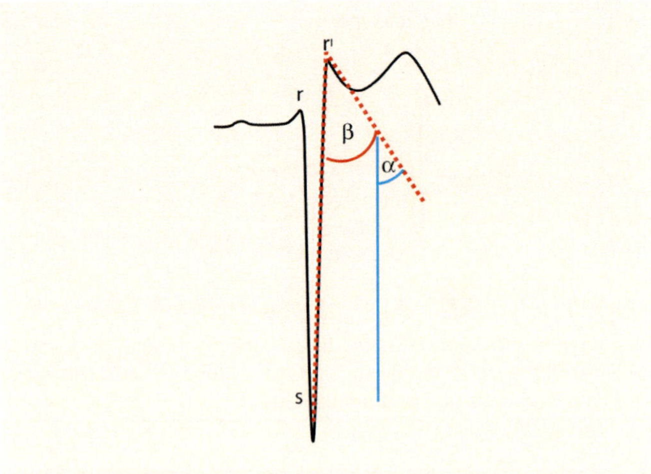

Fig. 16.11: Measuring alpha (α) and beta (β) angles from the r' wave morphology of right precordial leads can differentiate BrS and incomplete RBBB: α—the angle between a vertical line and the downslope of the r' wave, and β—the angle between the upslope of the S wave and the downslope of the r' wave.

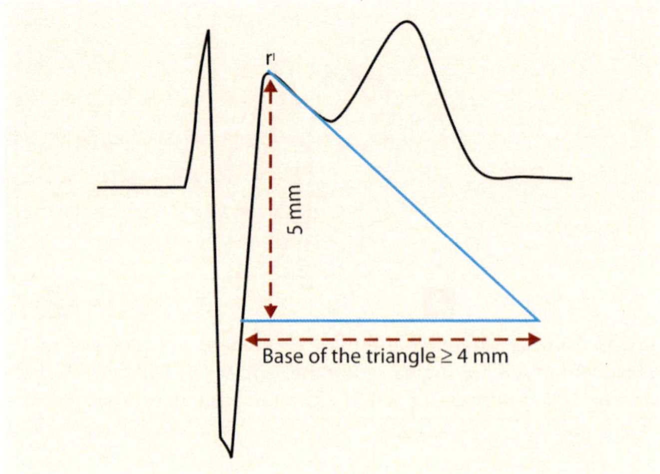

Fig. 16.12: Measuring the base of the triangle, of the r' wave at 5 mm of the high take-off is useful to distinguish between Brugada syndrome (BrS) ECG and incomplete RBBB. The base of the triangle greater than or equal to 4 mm is a good criterion for BrS and is much shorter in healthy athletes with incomplete RBBB.

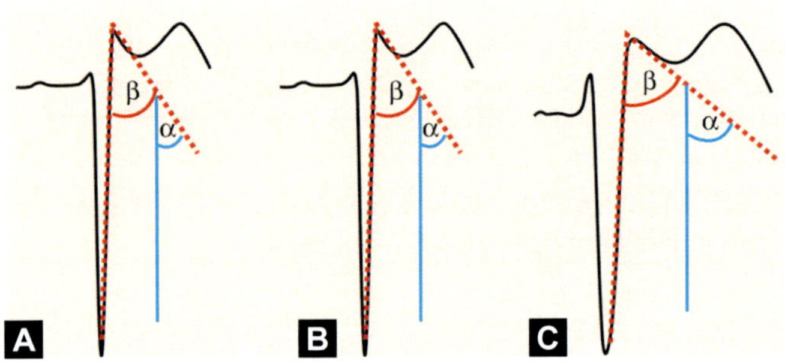

Figs. 16.13A to C: Antiarrhythmic drug (AAD) challenge can differentiate between type 2 or type 3 Brugada pattern and incomplete RBBB. Before AAD challenge, two angles (α and β) are measured from ECG leads V1 and/or V2 showing incomplete RBBB (?BrP). The baseline angles are compared with the angles after drug challenge. Change in type 2 and type 3 Brugada patterns into type 1 pattern after drug challenge or change in the α and β angles of ECG after drug challenge are considered as positive test and suggestive of BrS rather than incomplete RBBB. Widening of angles is also suggestive of Brugada syndrome. (A) Baseline ECG with α and β angles; (B) Negative test, no change in α and β angles after AAD challenge, suggestive of incomplete RBBB; (C) Positive test, widening of both α and β angles after drug challenge, suggestive of BrS.

Box 16.1: Clinical criteria for the diagnosis of Brugada syndrome.

- Brugada syndrome (BrS) is definitely diagnosed when the patient presents with (1) a type 1 ECG (either spontaneously or elicited by drug challenge) and (2) at least one of the below mentioned clinical criteria
- There are three kinds of clinical criteria for the disease:

1. *Data from the family history*:
   a. SCD in a family member younger than 45 years.
   b. ECG type 1 in family members
2. *Arrhythmia-related symptoms*:
   a. Syncope.
   b. Seizures.
   c. Nocturnal agonal respiration
3. *Documented ventricular arrhythmias*:
   a. Polymorphic ventricular tachycardia (PVT)
   b. Ventricular fibrillation (VF)

- *Once we have observed a type 1 ECG in more than one precordial leads, and exclude other conditions that may account for it, we should search for clinical data that support the diagnosis of BrS*

of ECG after drug challenge are considered as positive test and suggestive of BrS rather than incomplete RBBB. Widening of angles is suggestive of BrS (Figs. 16.13A to C).[16,18,20,21]

Several pharmacological approaches have been proposed in the prevention of SCD in BrS, but none has found clinical applicability so far.[28] The presence of a spontaneous type 1 ECG (i.e. no need for drug challenge to make the diagnosis) together with history of syncope consistently identifies subjects who warrant an ICD.

Clinical criteria for the diagnosis of BrS have been shown in Box 16.1.

LONG QT SYNDROME

Long QT syndrome (LQTS) is defined as an arrhythmogenic disorder in the structurally normal heart presenting with QT prolongation that is often associated with peculiar ST-T-wave morphology, syncope, and sudden death (Fig. 16.14). The LQTS can be inherited or acquired and is of particular interest and concern at present. Patients with LQTS are predisposed to the ventricular tachyarrhythmia, torsades de pointes (TdP) which causes syncope and sudden death. Inherited LQTS is the prototype of the "primary cardiac arrhythmias" or "cardiac ion channelopathies". Drug-

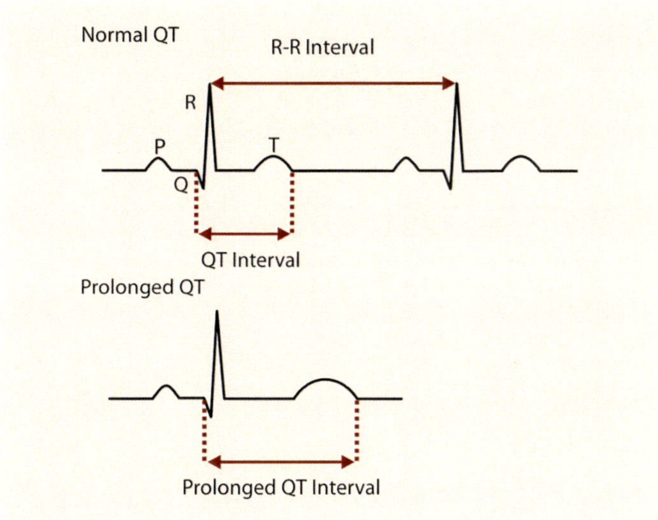

Fig. 16.14: Normal versus long QT interval. The QT interval is the time between the start of the QRS complex and the end of the T wave in the ECG.

induced LQTS is the most common cause of acquired LQTS, and is a pressing public health issue.

Long QT syndrome is caused by mutations of genes which encode for cardiac ion channels. The genes have been numbered in the order of discovery as LQT1, LQT2, etc. Five genes (LQT1, 2, 3, 5, and 6) with over 200 mutations have thus far been discovered.[29] Approximately 60% of LQTS patients have the LQT1 form. Exercise and emotion are the triggers for over 90% of cardiac events. The common triggers are running, swimming, startle, anger and fright.[30] The prevalence of inherited LQTS is estimated at about 1:7,000 persons. The Romano-Ward variant accounts for over 90% of cases. Jervell and Lange-Nielsen syndrome is rare, well less than 1% of currently diagnosed cases. LQTS affects all races and ethnic groups, but it is unknown whether the prevalence is the same in all groups.[31,32]

Different Varieties of Inherited Long QT Syndrome

Romano-Ward Syndrome

With autosomal dominant transmission, males and females are equally affected. Each child of an affected parent has a 50% chance of receiving the abnormal allele. It is the most common form of inherited LQTS.

Jervell and Lange-Nielsen Syndrome

The inheritance of the full Jervell and Lange-Nielsen syndrome (LQTS plus deafness) is recessive and males and females are equally affected.[32] This usually occurs in consanguineous (blood relative) marriage. Each child of this marriage has a 25% chance of inheriting the abnormal allele from each parent, thus being homozygous or compound heterozygous for LQT1 type mutations. These children have Jervell and Lange-Nielsen syndrome, with more severe LQTS than Romano-Ward patients, and profound congenital deafness.[32]

Andersen-Tawil Syndrome

Andersen-Tawil syndrome manifests with QT prolongation associated with facial dysmorphisms and hypokalemic periodic paralysis. It is a rare genetic disorder, and is inherited in an autosomal dominant pattern.[33]

Timothy Syndrome

Timothy syndrome, which shows marked QT prolongation, syndactyly, paroxysmal hypoglycemia, atrioventricular block, congenital heart defects, developmental disorders/ autism spectrum disorders, reduced immune response, and life-threatening arrhythmias.[34]

Acquired Long QT Syndrome

Acquired LQTS is much more frequent than the inherited form. The most common cause is medication induced. Since then, many medications, and also illicit drugs, have been demonstrated to have this adverse property. A number of medications have been withdrawn from the market, most notably perhaps terfenadine in 2000 and cisapride in 2001, amongst a lot of publicity and concern by physicians and medical organizations, the pharmaceutical industry, the Food and Drug Administration (FDA), and the legal profession. Currently, more than 50 commonly prescribed medications cause QT prolongation and/or have been associated with TdP or sudden death. The risk of acquired LQTS from these medications varies widely, ranging from well less than 1% of patients to whom the medication is given, to over 10%.[32] The mechanism of drug-induced QTc prolongation is believed to be usually due to blockade of cardiac potassium channels. A long QT interval is most frequently seen with class I and class III AADs. Other classes of drugs those cause QTc prolongation include antihistamines (terfenadine, astemizole), antidepressants (amitriptyline, imipramine), antibiotics (azithromycin, clarithromycin, erythromycin), antifungal drugs (fluconazole, ketoconazole), and antipsychotics (risperidone, fluphenazine, haloperidol). The prolongation of the QTc interval by these drugs is usually seen within several days of starting them. The class Ia AADs (quinidine, procainamide) and class III drugs (sotalol, amiodarone) prolong the repolarization phase of the cardiac action potential.[35] A sudden rise in intracranial pressure (e.g. due to subarachnoid hemorrhage) may produce characteristic T-wave changes (cerebral T waves): widespread, deep T-wave inversions with a prolonged QTc (Fig. 16.15). Acute myocardial ischemia has been shown to modify the duration of the QT interval, and prolong the duration of the maximum electrocardiographic QT interval (Fig. 16.16).

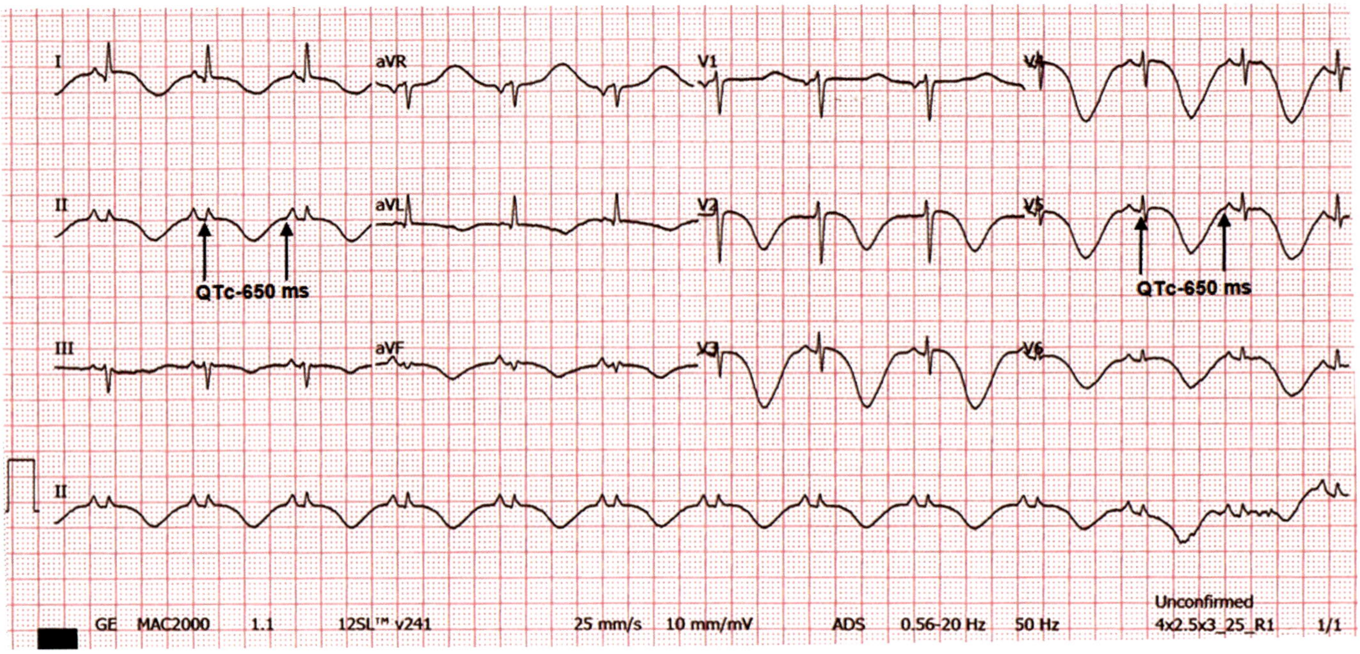

Fig. 16.15: ECG displaying long QT interval (650 ms) in a patient with raised intracranial pressure.

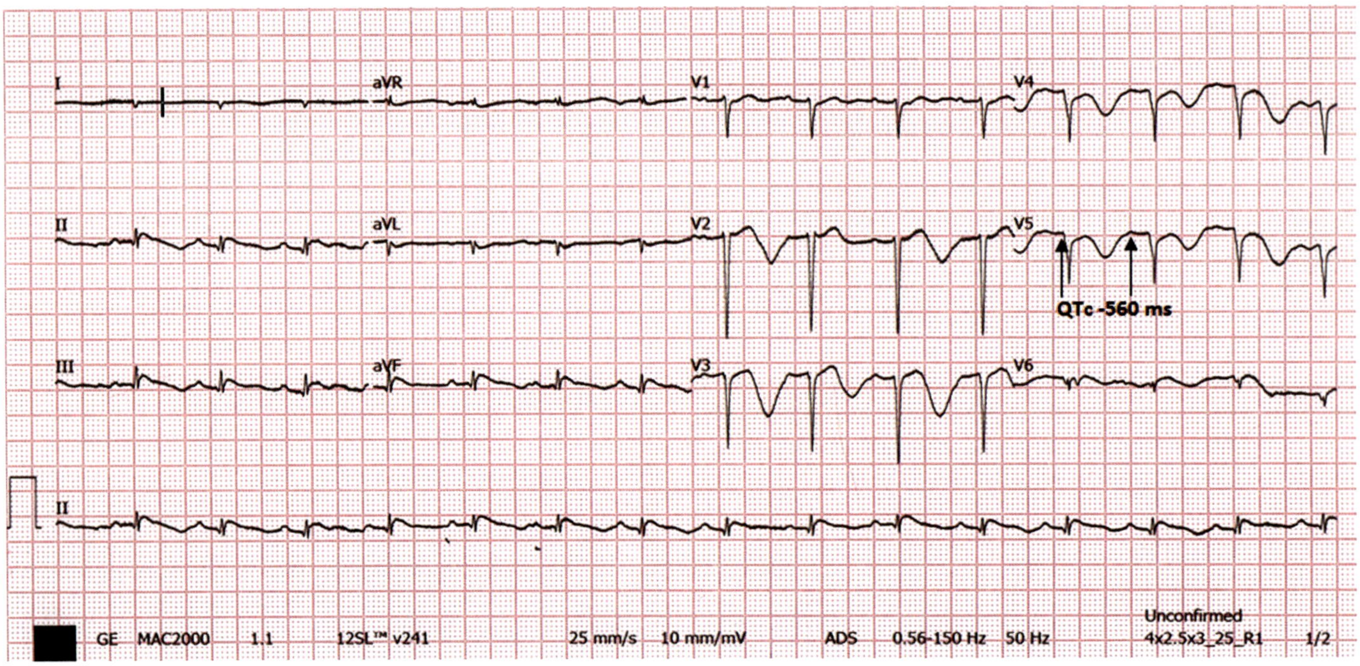

Fig. 16.16: ECG displaying prolonged QT interval (560 ms) in a patient with recent anterior myocardial infarction.

QT and QTc Interval

The QT interval is the time between the start of the QRS complex and the end of the T wave in the ECG. It represents the duration between the onset of depolarization and the completion of repolarization of the myocardium. There is commonly a variation in the QT interval measured in the various leads of the ECG. When multiple leads are used, the longest QT interval is considered to be the true QT interval. The QT interval is dependent on heart rate, age, and gender. A diurnal variation of the QT interval associated with the variations in sympathetic tone has also been described. The observed QT (QTo) interval can be corrected (QTc) for heart rate by using the Bazett's formula where RR is the interval in seconds between two successive R waves on the ECG.[36]

The standard clinical correction is to use Bazett's formula, named after physiologist Bazett, calculating the heart rate-corrected QT interval.

Bazett's formula is:[36]

$QT_C = QT/\sqrt{RR}$

Where QTc is the QT interval corrected for heart rate, and RR is the interval from the onset of one QRS complex to the onset of the next QRS complex, measured in seconds. A QTc interval of 440 ms is accepted as the upper limit of normal for men and 460 ms as the upper limit of normal for women. In children up to the age of 15, the upper limit of normal is 440 ms.[34-37]

The diagnosis of LQTS is based primarily on QT prolongation on the ECG. Current data suggests a confidant diagnosis of LQTS can be made with a QTc of greater than 470 ms in males and greater than 480 ms in females in the absence of drugs, cardiac disease, or other diseases/factors which could independently lengthen the QT interval. Conversely, LQTS is very unlikely with a QTc less than or equal to 400 ms. QTcs between 441 ms and 470 ms in male and between 461 ms and 480 ms in female are indeterminant and these patients require further investigation.[32]

T-Wave Morphology in Long QT Syndrome

Different T-wave patterns characteristics for each genotype have been proposed. These T patterns can be helpful for predicting the correct genotype in families, and can be of assistance in the diagnosis of LQTS in cases of borderline QT duration. Ten typical ST-T-wave patterns were identified: four in LQT1, four in LQT2, and two in LQT3. In patients with LQT1 patterns, the T wave generally appears broad-based, peaked, and asymmetrical but may be "bifid T" or normal appearing T waves. Obvious bifid T waves, subtle bifid T waves and low-amplitude and widely split bifid T waves have been noted in LQT2 patients. LQT3 patterns are associated with late-onset, peaked, and/or biphasic T waves or asymmetrical peaked T wave.[38]

How to Measure QT Interval on Electrocardiogram

The QT interval is most commonly measured in lead II for evaluation of serial ECGs, with leads I and V5 being comparable alternatives to lead II (Fig. 16.14). Leads III, aVL and V1 are generally avoided for measurement of QT interval. The accurate measurement of the QT interval is subjective because the end of the T wave is not always clearly defined and usually merges gradually with the baseline.[39,40] QT interval in an ECG complex can be measured manually by different methods:[41,42]

1. Threshold method
2. Tangent method
3. Superimposed median beat method.

In the threshold method, the end of the T wave is determined by the point at which the component of the T wave merges with the isoelectric baseline. In the tangent method, the end of the T wave is determined by the intersection of a tangent line extrapolated from the T wave at the point of maximum downslope to the isoelectric baseline. In the superimposed median beat method, a median ECG complex is constructed for each of the 12 leads. The 12 median beats are superimposed on each other and the QT interval is measured either from the earliest onset of the Q wave to the latest offset of the T wave or from the point of maximum convergence for the Q wave onset to the T-wave offset.

Schwartz criteria for the diagnosis of LQTS have been shown in Box 16.2.[37]

Arrhythmias in Long QT Syndrome

The long QT interval is responsible for the development of fatal ventricular arrhythmia, torsades de pointes (TdP) which is regarded as harbinger of death (Figs. 16.17A and B). Originally described by Dessertenne the term "torsades de pointes", or twisting of the points, was used to describe cycles of VT with alternating electric polarity and amplitude, such that the peaks of the QRS complexes appeared to be twisting around the isoelectric line of the recording.[43-45] It is almost universally accepted that QT prolongation is a prerequisite for the diagnosis of TdP. In the absence of QT prolongation, the term "polymorphic ventricular tachycardia" should be used instead. By definition, TdP is paroxysmal and nonsustained, but it may progress to VF and sudden death. Exercise and emotion are the triggers for over 90% of cardiac events.[32]

Drugs Associated with QTc Prolongation (Table 16.2)[35]

Once diagnosis is established, beta-blocker therapy is recommended. LQT1 patients respond very well to beta-

Box 16.2: Schwartz criteria for the diagnosis of long QT syndrome.[37]

The Schwartz criteria are diagnostic criteria for long QT syndrome (LQTS) and are distinct from the criteria used to risk-stratify patients with known LQTS. *Patients with 4 or more points have a high probability of having LQTS, those with 2 or 3 points have an intermediate probability, and those with 1 or no point have a low probability of having LQTS*

ECG findings:

Corrected QT interval (calculated by Bazett's formula, where QTc = QT/√RR):
- – ≥480 ms = 3 points
- – 460–479 ms = 2 points
- – 450–459 (in males) = 1 point.
- Torsades de pointes = 2 points
- Visible T-wave alternans = 1 point
- Notched T wave in at least 3 leads = 1 point
- Low heart rate for age (children) = 0.5 point

Clinical history:
- Syncope (cannot receive points for both syncope and torsades de pointes)
  - – With stress = 2 points
  - – Without stress = 1 point.
- Congenital deafness = 0.5 point

Family history (the same family member cannot be counted for LQTS and sudden death):
- Family members with definite LQTS = 1 point
- Unexplained sudden cardiac death under age 30 years among immediate family members = 0.5 point

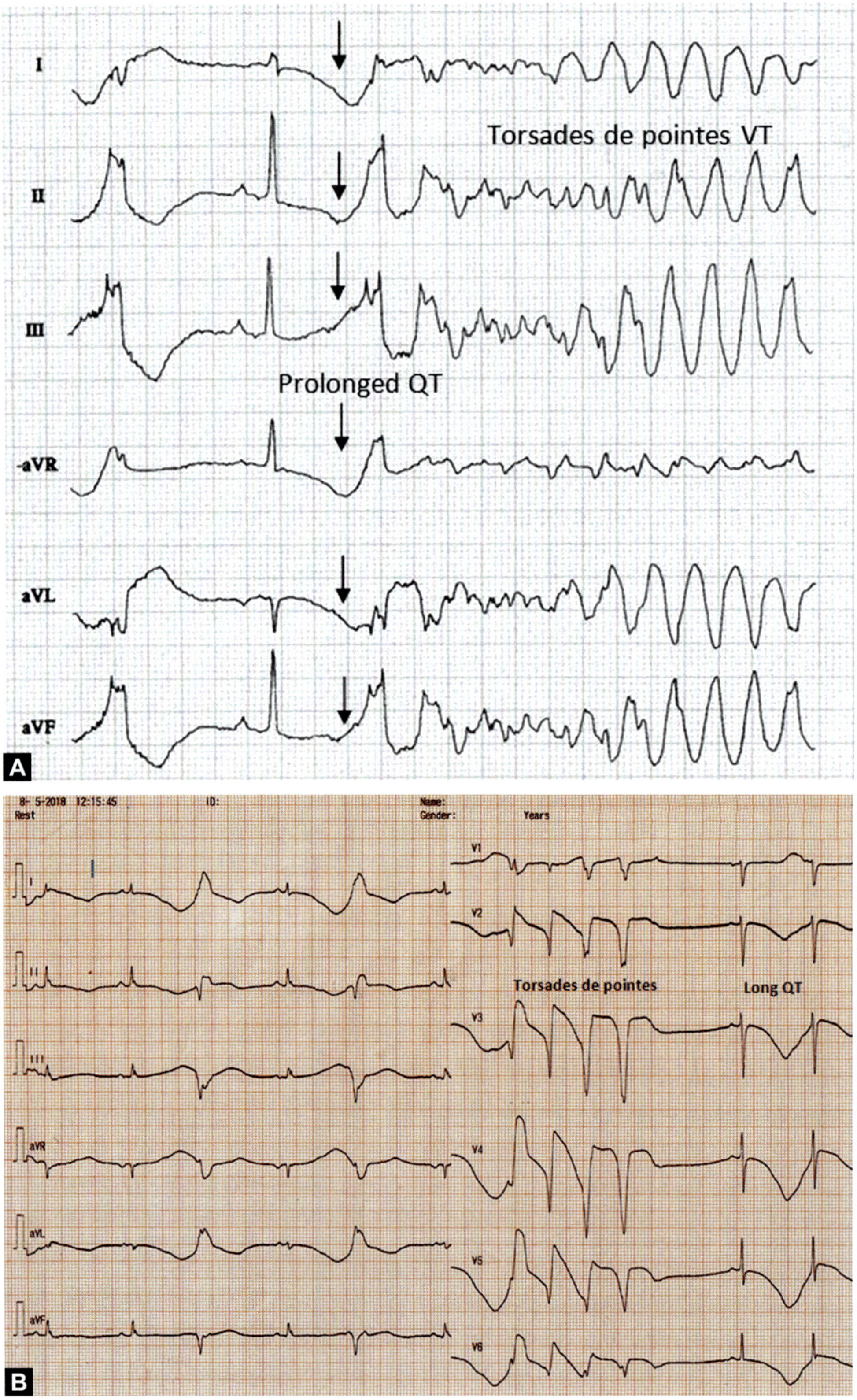

Figs. 16.17A and B: (A) ECG tracing is suggestive of torsades de pointes VT in the presence of marked QT prolongation. Note prolonged QT preceding torsades de pointes VT (arrows); (B) This 12 lead ECG shows torsades de pointes (TdP) VT in a patient with drug induced prolonged QT.

Table 16.2: Drugs associated with QTc prolongation.

Antibiotics		Terfenadine
Azithromycin	*Antiarrhythmics*	Astemizole
Clarithromycin	Disopyramide	
Erythromycin	Procainamide	*Others*
Roxithromycin	Quinidine	Probucol
Metronidazole	Amiodarone	Cisapride
(with alcohol)	Sotalol	
Moxifloxacin	*Antidepressants*	
	Amitriptyline	
Antifungals	Clomipramine	
Fluconazole	Imipramine	
(in cirrhosis)	Dothiepin	
Ketoconazole	Doxepin	
Antiviral	*Antipsychotics*	
Nelfinavir	Risperidone	
	Fluphenazine	
	Haloperidol	
	Clozapine	
Antimalarials	Thioridazine	
Chloroquine	Ziprasidone	
Mefloquine	Pimozide	
Anesthetic	Droperidol	
Halothane	*Antihistamines*	

blockers; interestingly, lack of compliance is the most important cause of events occurring during antiadrenergic treatment in LQT1.[46,47] Compared with LQT1 patients, LQT2 and LQT3 patients have a higher recurrence rate of arrhythmic events while on therapy.[46]

Beta-blockers should be given to patients who have significant QTc interval prolongation. Beta-blockers are effective in preventing cardiac events in approximately 70% of patients, whereas cardiac events continue to occur despite beta-blocker therapy in the remaining 30%. An ICD should be used in survivors of cardiac arrest and is recommended for patients with syncope while receiving beta-blockers. Additionally, left cardiac sympathetic denervation may be an option to reduce the number of recurrences in highly symptomatic patients.[48-54] The use of an ICD may be considered as primary therapy if the patient has a strong family history of SCD.[52,53]

SHORT QT SYNDROME

Short QT syndrome (SQTS) is best defined as a congenital, inherited, primary electric disorder of the heart characterized by abnormally short QT intervals on the surface ECG (<350 ms) and an increased proclivity to develop atrial and/or ventricular tachyarrhythmias. By definition, secondary causes of short QT interval such as hyperkalemia, acidosis, hypercalcemia, hyperthermia, effect of drugs like digitalis, effect of acetylcholine or catecholamine, and abbreviation of QT interval related to activation of ATP-sensitive potassium channel (K_{ATP}) current must be ruled out before considering the diagnosis of SQTS.[55]

In fact, SQTS is a clinically malignant entity characterized by a short QT interval, with tall, symmetric and peaked T waves (Fig. 16.18) leading to atrial fibrillation (AF), ventricular arrhythmias, and SCD.[55,56] It may cause SCD in neonates, because clinical manifestations may appear early in life. Most patients have a family history of SCD with an autosomal dominant pattern of transmission and a high penetrance.[57] Patients with SQTS may develop "idiopathic ventricular fibrillation (IVF)" and SCD.[58]

The presence of high-amplitude, peaked T waves, which are frequently observed on ECG in SQTS subjects, are also included in the diagnostic scorecard of SQTS.[58-60] A high prevalence of early repolarization abnormality in ECG has been observed in SQTS patients.[58]

The QT response to exercise is also considered for use in the diagnostic criteria. The normal physiologic response of the QT interval to an increasing heart rate is to shorten and can be evaluated using the QT/heart rate (QT/HR) ratio during accelerating heart rate.[61] Conventional doctrine states that the QT interval is related to heart rate in an inverse exponential relationship, so that with increasing heart rate the QT interval shortens. The presence of a markedly blunted slope of the QT/HR relationship during exercise has been observed in patients with SQTS.[62,63] This finding suggests a lesser degree of QT shortening response with exercise and accelerating heart rate, possibly reflecting a lack of repolarization reserve due to already enhanced repolarizing currents in the setting of SQTS.[58]

Approximately 62% of the patients are symptomatic and the remaining 38% patients are asymptomatic and are diagnosed on the basis of strong family history. Cardiac arrest is the most frequently (34%) reported symptom, and in 28% of patients it is the first clinical presentation. The available data suggest that patients are at risk of fatal/nonfatal ventricular arrhythmias throughout lifetime. Palpitations are the second most frequently reported symptom (31%), followed by syncope (24%). AF is the first presenting symptom in 17% of patients. Many patients are diagnosed to have SQTS during evaluation of frequent ventricular extrasystoles.[64]

An ICD is recommended as first-line treatment for secondary prevention of SCD and may be useful for primary prevention as well. There is a paucity of information concerning the long-term effectiveness of pharmacological therapy; hence, it might best be reserved as an adjunct to ICD treatment. Quinidine has thus far proved to be the most effective pharmacotherapeutic agent.[64]

CATECHOLAMINERGIC POLYMORPHIC VENTRICULAR TACHYCARDIA

Catecholaminergic polymorphic ventricular tachycardia (CPVT) is a familial arrhythmogenic disorder characterized by the presence of SCD, sometimes associated with bidirectional polymorphic VT. Patients show a normal resting ECG although adrenergic stimulation (vigorous exercise, fear) may induce syncope and/or SCD in a structurally normal heart.[65,66] The mean age of onset of

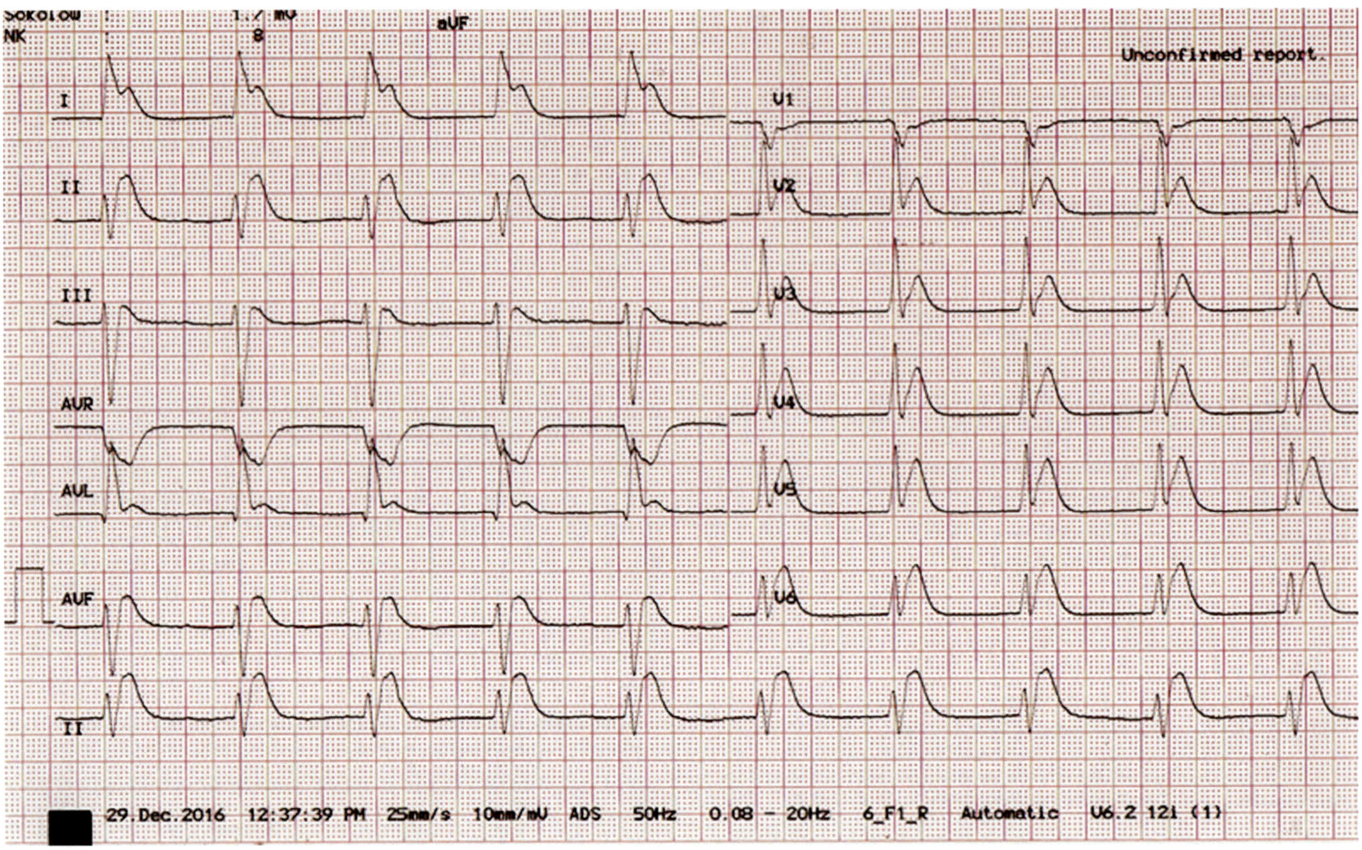

Fig. 16.18: ECG of short QT syndrome (QT interval around 290 ms). Also note symmetric and peaked T waves in chest leads. Symmetric and peaked T waves are frequently observed on ECG in short QT syndrome. Note in this ECG, ST segments appear very short and in many complexes T waves originate directly from the S waves.

symptoms (usually a syncopal episode) of CPVT is between age 7 years and 12 years; onset as late as the fourth decade of life has been reported. If untreated, CPVT is highly lethal, as approximately 30% of affected individuals experience at least one cardiac arrest and up to 80% one or more syncopal spells. Sudden death may be the first manifestation of the disease.

Two genetic forms have been identified, one autosomal dominant form and another a recessive form responsible for CPVT. Both genes are therefore implicated in the mediation of excitation-contraction coupling. In general, mutations lead to increased intracellular Ca^{2+}, leading to late depolarizations which predispose to arrhythmias.[67-69] This condition is due to mutations in genes encoding a voltage-gated calcium channel or proteins related to this channel.

Electrocardiographic Diagnosis of CPVT[70-76]

- The resting ECG of individuals with CPVT is usually normal, although some authors have reported a lower-than-normal resting heart rate and others have observed a high incidence of prominent U waves. Overall these features are inconstant and not sufficiently specific to allow diagnosis. Therefore, in many instances, the origin of the syncope may be erroneously attributed to a neurologic disorder. The exercise stress test is the single most important diagnostic test.
- ECG during exercise stress test allows ventricular arrhythmias to be reproducibly elicited in the majority of affected individuals (Figs. 16.19 and 16.20).
- With increase in workload, the complexity of arrhythmias progressively increases from isolated premature beats to bigeminy and runs of nonsustained VT. If the affected individual continues exercising, the duration of the runs of VT progressively increases and VT may become sustained. Polymorphic VT is common in this condition.
- An alternating 180° QRS axis on a beat-to-beat basis, so-called bidirectional VT, is often the distinguishing presentation of CPVT-related arrhythmias.
- Some individuals with CPVT may also present with irregular polymorphic VT without a "stable" QRS vector alternans.
- Exercise-induced supraventricular arrhythmias (supraventricular tachycardia and AF) are also common.
- Ventricular fibrillation may occur in the setting of acute stress.

Beta-blockers are the first therapeutic choice of proven efficacy for about 60% of individuals with CPVT. Treatment with beta-blockers is currently recommended in all clinically diagnosed patients. The dose of beta-blockers should be titrated up to an effective level. The addition of flecainide seems to be a promising approach in patients where arrhythmias are not completely suppressed by beta-blockers. An ICD or left cervical sympathetic denervation

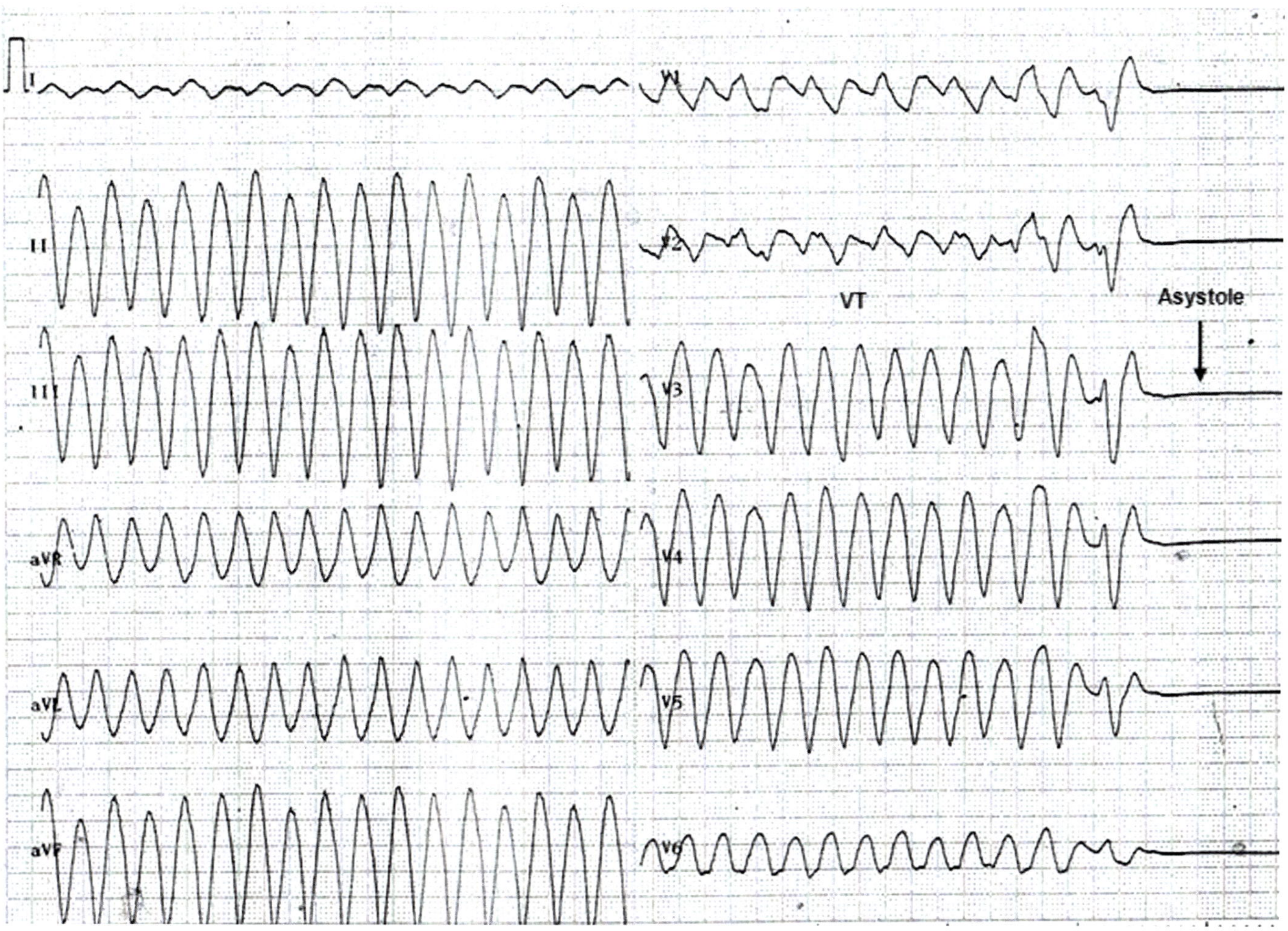

Fig. 16.19: Catecholaminergic polymorphic ventricular tachycardia during exercise with asystole (arrow).

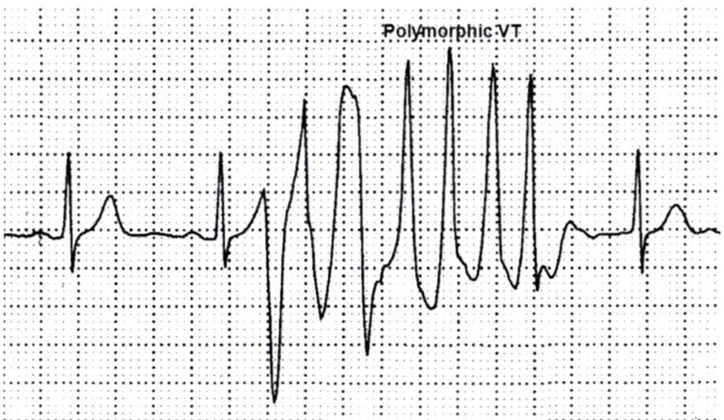

Fig. 16.20: ECG showing self-terminating polymorphic VT in catecholaminergic polymorphic ventricular tachycardia.

might be considered under special circumstances. Genetic counseling is recommended and all first-degree relatives should be properly evaluated.[77-80]

SUMMARY

Our heart beats regularly as the result of an elegant interplay of ions at the cellular level. Ion channels for Na^+, K^+, and Ca^{2+} in the myocardial cellular membrane are responsible for allowing this interplay across the membrane. When genetic abnormalities cause these channels to be dysfunctional, the resulting cardiac channelopathies can predispose to life-threatening arrhythmias. Cardiac channelopathies include BrS, LQTS, SQTS, and CPVT.

Brugada Syndrome

Brugada syndrome (BrS) is characterized by ST-segment elevation in right precordial leads (V1-V3) that is unrelated to ischemia, electrolyte disturbances, or obvious structural heart disease. The BrS is a familial disease that displays an autosomal dominant mode of transmission, with incomplete penetrance. BrS is more common in the regions of Southeast Asia.

Electrocardiographic features of typical BrS include:

- ST-segment elevation with "coved" morphology in the right precordial leads
- Complete or incomplete right bundle branch block pattern ECG.

Three patterns of ECG have been recognized:

Type 1: Coved ST-segment elevation ≥2 mm in right precordial leads V1-V3 (>1 lead) followed by a negative T wave is the only ECG abnormality that is potentially diagnostic. This has been referred to as *Brugada sign*. The other two types of Brugada ECGs are nondiagnostic but possibly warrant further investigation.

Type 2: Brugada pattern, is characterized by a "saddleback" ST-segment elevation, that is, greater than or equal to 1 mm in the right precordial leads V1-V2 or V3.

Type 3: This pattern reveals right precordial ST-segment elevation of less than 1 mm of saddleback type, coved type, or both.

Electrocardiographic diagnosis of BrS has been shown in Box 16.3.

This ECG pattern may be intermittent and may be unmasked by pharmacological challenge with sodium channel blockers such as procainamide, flecainide or ajmaline. The onset of ventricular arrhythmias causes the occurrence of syncope and may lead to sudden death, usually at rest.

Electrocardiographic Criteria: Brugada Pattern versus Right Bundle Branch Block

Complete RBBB and type 1 BrS are characterized by the presence of positive terminal deflections of the QRS and negative T waves in leads V1-V2. However, unlike in BrS, ST-segment in RBBB is not elevated and is accompanied by an S wave in leads I, V5, and V6, with a wider QRS (≥120 ms). By contrast, in BrS, there is no wide and slurred S wave in left precordial leads.

But the distinction between type 2 and type 3 BrP and incomplete RBBB are problematic. But in BrP the r' wave is broad, rounded and generally of low voltage, with a slow descent. In contrast, that of incomplete RBBB is pointed. The QRS duration in leads V1-V2 is the same as in lead V6 in incomplete RBBB, as occurs in athletes who may also present with this pattern, whereas in type 2 BrP usually is longer in leads V1-V2 although often is difficult to determine. For further confirmation, AAD challenge is helpful. Sodium channel blockers can be used effectively to unmask BrS.

Box 16.3: ECG diagnosis of Brugada syndrome.

Three repolarization abnormalities are associated with Brugada pattern, when found in more than one right precordial leads (V1-V3):

1. *Type 1*: It is characterized by a prominent coved ST-segment elevation displaying J-point amplitude or ST-segment elevation greater than or equal to 2 mm, followed by a negative T wave
2. *Type 2*: Greater than or equal to 1 mm ST-segment elevation and a saddleback appearance, followed by a positive or biphasic T wave
3. *Type 3*: It has either a saddleback or coved appearance, but with an ST-segment elevation less than 1 mm

Note: It should be stressed that type 1 is the only ECG diagnostic pattern of BrS while types 2 and 3 should only be considered suggestive of the disease

Arrhythmias in Brugada Syndrome

- Ventricular fibrillation
- Polymorphic ventricular tachycardia
- Atrial fibrillation.
- Other supraventricular tachyarrhythmias
- Monomorphic VT (very rare).

The ECG may show a marked variation over time, ranging from the typical pattern to a completely normal ECG and back again. In subjects with a nondiagnostic ECG, a pharmacological test with sodium channel blockers may disclose the typical BrP. In order to establish the diagnosis, several conditions those can mimic BrP must be excluded. These include RBBB, early repolarization, acute myocardial ischemia, pericarditis, hypercalcemia, hyperkalemia, hypothermia and primary right ventricular diseases, particularly arrhythmogenic right ventricular cardiomyopathy/dysplasia (ARVC/D). Some drugs (e.g. some AADs, psychotropic agents or antihistamines), fever, and enhanced vagal tone, as it occurs after a full meal, may render BrP more evident on the ECG.

No pharmacologic therapy has been proven to reduce the occurrence of ventricular arrhythmias or sudden death. At present, implantation of an automatic ICD is the only treatment proven effective in treating VT and VF and preventing sudden death in patients with BrS.

Conditions other than BrS those can lead to ST-segment elevation in the right precordial leads have been shown in Box 16.4.

Key points of Brugada syndrome have been shown in Box 16.5.

Long QT Syndrome

Patients with LQTS are predisposed to the ventricular tachyarrhythmia, torsades de pointes (TdP) which causes

Box 16.4: ST elevation in leads V1-V3 other than Brugada syndrome.

Conditions other than Brugada syndrome those can lead to ST-segment elevation in the right precordial leads:[18]

- Left ventricular hypertrophy
- Acute myocardial ischemia or infarction
- Acute myocarditis
- Left bundle branch block
- Right ventricular ischemia or infarction
- Dissecting aortic aneurysm
- Acute pulmonary thromboemboli
- Antidepressant overdose
- Duchenne muscular dystrophy
- Friedreich's ataxia
- Thiamine deficiency
- Hypercalcemia
- Hyperkalemia
- Mediastinal tumor compressing right ventricular outflow tract (RVOT)
- Arrhythmogenic right ventricular cardiomyopathy / dysplasia
- Long QT syndrome
- Early repolarization syndrome
- Normal variants

Box 16.5: Brugada syndrome—key points.

- Brugada syndrome (BrS) is an ECG abnormality with a high incidence of sudden death in patients with structurally normal hearts
- First described in 1992 by Brugada brothers (Josep Brugada, Pedro Brugada, and Ramon Brugada)
- The syndrome has been linked to mutations in the cardiac sodium channel genes
- Diagnosis depends on a characteristic ECG finding and clinical criteria. ECG looks like RBBB pattern with coved- or saddle-shaped ST-elevation limited to right precordial leads V1-V3
- *Type 1*: Coved ST-segment elevation greater than or equal to 2 mm in leads V1-V3 (>1 lead) followed by a negative T wave, is the only ECG abnormality that is potentially diagnostic of BrS
- This ECG abnormality must be associated with one of the following clinical criteria to confirm the diagnosis:
  - Documented ventricular fibrillation (VF) or polymorphic ventricular tachycardia (PVT)
  - Family history of sudden cardiac death at young age, less than 45 years
  - Coved-type ST-elevation in ECGs in family members
  - History of syncope
  - Inducible VT
  - Nocturnal agonal respiration.
- *Type 2* and *type 3* ECG criteria are nondiagnostic but possibly warrant further investigation and these ECGs are termed as Brugada pattern (BrP). Type 2 has greater than or equal to 1 mm of saddleback-shaped ST elevation. Brugada type 3 can be the morphology of either type 1 or type 2, but with less than 1 mm of ST-segment elevation
- The typical ST-segment elevation in the right precordial leads that characterize BrS electrocardiographically can be transitory, vary over time, or be modified by various factors such as vagal tone, body temperature, and medications
- The type 1 (coved) ECG pattern is diagnostic for BrS; types 2 and 3 require antiarrhythmic drug challenge to confirm its presence
- Only definitive treatment of BrS is implantation of ICD

syncope and sudden death. The QT interval is the time between the initiation of the QRS complex and the termination of the T wave in the ECG. Prolongation of the QTc interval is either acquired or due to a congenital long QTc syndrome. Drugs are by far the most common cause for an acquired long QTc interval. Women are more susceptible than men to drug-induced QTc prolongation. Renal failure, cardiac failure, and hepatic failure are also risk factors. Many distinct forms of congenital LQTS have been described. Most cases fall into the first three subgroups: (1) LQT1, (2) LQT2, and (3) LQT3. LQT1 is the most common genetic subtype.

QTc criteria of Long QT Syndrome (Table 16.3)

The LQTS may be either genetic or acquired. The Romano-Ward variant accounts for over 90% of cases of genetic

Table 16.3: QTc criteria of long QT syndrome.

QTc (ms)	*Male*	*Female*
Normal	<440	<460
Borderline	441–470	461–480
Prolonged	>470	>480

Box 16.6: Causes of long QTc interval.[35]

Congenital
- Romano-Ward syndrome
- Jervell and Lange-Nielsen syndrome
- Andersen-Tawil syndrome
- Timothy syndrome

Acquired
- Drug induced
- Cardiac pathology (heart failure, ischemia, myocarditis)
- Electrolyte abnormality (hypokalemia, hypomagnesemia)
- Cerebrovascular disease (subarachnoid hemorrhage, ischemic stroke)
- Severe bradycardia (especially complete heart block)
- Hyperthyroidism/hypothyroidism

LQTS. Acquired LQTS usually results from drug therapy, hypokalemia, or hypomagnesemia. Hypokalemia, hypomagnesemia, and bradycardia can increase the risk of drug-induced LQTS.

The class Ia AADs (quinidine, procainamide), class III drugs (sotalol, amiodarone), antihistamines (terfenadine, astemizole), antidepressants (amitriptyline, imipramine), antibiotics (azithromycin, clarithromycin, erythromycin), antifungal drugs (fluconazole, ketoconazole) and antipsychotics (risperidone, fluphenazine, haloperidol) may precipitate fatal arrhythmias by prolonging QT interval.

The QT interval should be measured in lead II, because the influence of a possible U-wave is smallest in this lead. If lead II cannot be used for measurements, then leads LI or V5 can be used alternatively.

The causes of long QTc interval have been shown in Box 16.6.

Patients with LQTS are predisposed to develop TdP which may cause sudden death. TdP is a specific form of polymorphic VT in patients with a long QT interval. It is characterized by rapid, irregular QRS complexes, which appear to be twisting around the ECG baseline. The phrase "torsades de pointes" is French and literally means "twisting of the points", referring to the characteristic appearance of the ECG during the rhythm abnormality. TdP usually occurs in the setting of a prolonged QT interval on the ECG. This arrhythmia may cease spontaneously or degenerate into VF. It causes significant hemodynamic compromise and often death.

Beta-blockers are effective in preventing cardiac events in approximately 70% of patients. The ICD has been shown to be highly effective in preventing SCD in high-risk patients.

Short QT Syndrome

Short QT syndrome is an inheritable primary electric disease of the heart characterized by abnormally short

QT intervals on the ECG (QT interval <350 ms) and an increased propensity to develop atrial and ventricular tachyarrhythmias. It is a relatively recent addition to the list of inherited channelopathies responsible for SCD in individuals with structurally normal hearts.

Electrocardiogram in SQTS is characterized by:

- Abnormally short QT intervals, commonly ranging between 220 ms and 350 ms
- Another common finding on ECG of SQTS patient is tall, peaked, symmetrical, or asymmetrical T waves in the precordial leads
- In most cases, the ST-segment is short or even absent and the T wave originates from the S wave.

Patterns of arrhythmia includes:

- Cardiac arrest
- Nonsustained polymorphic VT
- Ventricular fibrillation
- Atrial fibrillation.

Short QT syndrome patients are at a high risk of SCD because of malignant ventricular arrhythmia. ICD implantation is strongly recommended for secondary prevention of SCD.

Catecholaminergic Polymorphic Ventricular Tachycardia

Catecholaminergic polymorphic ventricular tachycardia is characterized by episodic syncope occurring during exercise or acute emotion in individuals without structural cardiac abnormalities. Arrhythmias may be well tolerated, with only mild symptoms such as dizziness or lipothymia. The underlying cause of these episodes is the onset of fast VT (bidirectional or polymorphic). Spontaneous recovery occurs when these arrhythmias self-terminate. In other instances, VT may degenerate into VF and cause sudden death.

Electrocardiographic Diagnosis of CPVT

- The resting ECG is usually normal.
- The most important diagnostic test is the exercise stress test, which can reproducibly evoke the typical VT during acute adrenergic activation (e.g. exercise, acute emotion).
- Polymorphic ventricular tachycardia and the bidirectional VT are common arrhythmias complicating CPVT.
- Ventricular tachycardia may progress to VF and sudden death.

The use of beta-blockers is the mainstay of CPVT therapy. An ICD may be necessary for those with recurrent cardiac arrest while on beta-blocker therapy or for those unable to take beta-blockers.

REFERENCES

1. Campuzano O, Beltran-Alvarez P, Iglesias A, et al. Genetics and cardiac channelopathies. Genet Med. 2010;12:260-7.
2. Roden DM, Lazzara R, Rosen M, et al. Multiple mechanisms in the long-QT syndrome. Current knowledge, gaps, and future directions. The SADS Foundation Task Force on LQTS. Circulation. 1996;94:1996-2012.
3. Brugada R, Hong K, Dumaine R, et al. Sudden death associated with short-QT syndrome linked to mutations in HERG. Circulation. 2004;109:30-5.
4. Hong K, Brugada J, Oliva A, et al. Value of electrocardiographic parameters and ajmaline test in the diagnosis of Brugada syndrome caused by SCN5A mutations. Circulation. 2004;110:3023-7.
5. Coronel R, Casini S, Koopmann TT, et al. Right ventricular fibrosis and conduction delay in a patient with clinical signs of Brugada syndrome: a combined electrophysiological, genetic, histopathologic, and computational study. Circulation. 2005;112:2769-77.
6. Frustaci A, Priori SG, Pieroni M, et al. Cardiac histological substrate in patients with clinical phenotype of Brugada syndrome. Circulation. 2005;112:3680-7.
7. Frustaci A, Russo MA, Chimenti C. Structural myocardial abnormalities in asymptomatic family members with Brugada syndrome and SCN5A gene mutation. Eur Heart J. 2009;30:1763.
8. Ohkubo K, Watanabe I, Okumura Y, et al. A new criteria differentiating type 2 and 3 Brugada patterns from ordinary incomplete right bundle branch block. Int Heart J. 2011;52(3):159-63.
9. Hoogendijk MG, Opthof T, Postema PG, et al. The Brugada ECG pattern: a marker of channelopathy, structural heart disease or neither? Towards a unifying mechanism of the Brugada syndrome. Circ Arrhythm Electrophysiol. 2010;3:283-90.
10. Mizusawa Y, Wilde AA. Brugada syndrome. Circ Arrhythm Electrophysiol. 2012;3:606-16.
11. Antzelevitch C, Brugada P, Brugada J, et al. Brugada syndrome: 1992–2002: a historical perspective. J Am Coll Cardiol. 2003;41:1665-71.
12. Antzelevitch C, Brugada P, Borggrefe M, et al. Brugada syndrome: report of the second consensus conference. Circulation. 2005;111:659-70.
13. Satish OS, Yeh KH, Wen MS. Brugada syndrome—an update. Chang Gung Med J. 2005;28(2):69-76.
14. Vatta M, Dumaine R, Varghese G, et al. Genetic and biophysical basis of sudden unexplained nocturnal death syndrome (SUNDS), a disease allelic to Brugada syndrome. Hum Mol Genet. 2002;11:337-45.
15. Chen Q, Kirsch GE, Zhang D, et al. Genetic basis and molecular mechanism for idiopathic ventricular fibrillation. Nature. 1998;392:293-6.
16. de Luna AB, García-Niebla J, Baranchuk A. New electrocardiographic features in Brugada syndrome. Curr Cardiol Rev. 2014;10(3):175-80.
17. Oreto G, Corrado D, Delise P, et al. The Brugada syndrome. Doubts of the cardiologist regarding an electrocardiogram presenting QRS V1-V2 complexes with positive terminal wave and ST segment elevation. Consensus Conference promoted by the Italian Cardiology Society. G Ital Cardiol. 2010;11(11 Suppl 2):3S-22S.
18. Wilde AA, Antzelevitch C, Borggrefe M, et al. Proposed diagnostic criteria for the Brugada syndrome. Consensus report. Circulation. 2002;106:2514-9.

19. Priori SG, Napolitano C, Gasparini M, et al. Clinical and genetic heterogeneity of right bundle branch block and ST-segment elevation syndrome: a prospective evaluation of 52 families. Circulation. 2000;102:2509-15.
20. Chevallier S, Forclaz A, Tenkorang J, et al. New electrocardiographic criteria for discriminating between Brugada types 2 and 3 patterns and incomplete right bundle branch block. J Am Coll Cardiol. 2011;58(22):2290-8.
21. Brugada R, Brugada J, Antzelevitch C, et al. Sodium channel blockers identify risk for sudden death in patients with ST-segment elevation and right bundle branch block but structurally normal hearts. Circulation. 2000;101:510-5.
22. Shimizu W, Matsuo K, Takagi M, et al. Body surface distribution and response to drugs of ST segment elevation in Brugada syndrome: clinical implications of eighty-seven-lead body surface potential mapping and its application to twelve-lead electrocardiograms. J Cardiovasc Electrophysiol. 2000;11:396-404.
23. Eckardt L, Kirchhof P, Loh P, et al. Brugada syndrome and supraventricular tachyarrhythmias: a novel association? J Cardiovasc Electrophysiol. 2001;12:680-5.
24. Shimada M, Miyazaki T, Miyoshi S, et al. Sustained monomorphic ventricular tachycardia in a patient with Brugada syndrome. Jpn Circ J. 1996;60:364-70.
25. Boersma LV, Jaarsma W, Jessurun ER, et al. Brugada syndrome: a case report of monomorphic ventricular tachycardia. Pacing Clin Electrophysiol. 2001;24:112-5.
26. Viskin S, Rosso R. Risk of sudden death in asymptomatic Brugada syndrome. J Am Coll Cardiol. 2010;56(19):1585-8.
27. Matsuo K, Kurita T, Inagaki M, et al. The circadian pattern of the development of ventricular fibrillation in patients with Brugada syndrome. Eur Heart J. 1999;20:465-70.
28. Ruan Y, Liu N, Priori SG. Sodium channel mutations and arrhythmias. Nat Rev Cardiol. 2009;6:337-48.
29. Splawski I, Shen J, Timothy KW, et al. Spectrum of mutations in long-QT syndrome genes KVLQT1, HERG, SCN5A, KCNE1, and KCNE2. Circulation. 2000;102:1178-85.
30. Schwartz PJ, Priori SG, Spazzolini C, et al. Genotype-phenotype correlation in the long QT syndrome. Gene-specific triggers for life-threatening arrhythmias. Circulation. 2001;103:89-95.
31. Crotti L, Celano G, Dagradi F, et al. Congenital long QT syndrome. Orphanet J Rare Dis. 2008;3:18.
32. Vincent GM. The long QT syndrome. Indian Pacing Electrophysiol J. 2002;2(4):127-42.
33. Tristani-Firouzi M, Jensen JL, Donaldson MR, et al. Functional and clinical characterization of KCNJ2 mutations associated with LQT7 (Andersen syndrome). J Clin Invest. 2002;110(3):381-8.
34. Marks M, Trippel D, Keating M. Long QT syndrome associated with syndactyly identified in females. Am J Cardiol. 1995;76(10):744-5.
35. Jayasinghe R. Drugs and the QTc interval. Aust Prescr. 2002;25:63-5.
36. Bazett HC. An analysis of the time-relations of electrocardiograms. Heart. 1920;(7):353-70.
37. Schwartz PJ, Moss AJ, Vincent GM, et al. Diagnostic criteria for the long QT syndrome. An update. Circulation. 1993;88:782-4.
38. Zhang L, Timothy KW, Vincent GM, et al. Spectrum of ST-T-wave patterns and repolarization parameters in congenital long-QT syndrome: ECG findings identify genotypes. Circulation. 2000;102:2849-55.
39. Panicker GK, Salvi V, Karnad DR, et al. Drug-induced QT prolongation when QT interval is measured in each of the 12 ECG leads in men and women in a thorough QT study. J Electrocardiol. 2014;47(2):155-7.
40. Panicker GK, Karnad DR, Joshi R, et al. Z-score for bench-marking reader competence in a central ECG laboratory. Ann Noninvasive Electrocardiol. 2009;14(1):19-25.
41. Panicker GK, Karnad DR, Natekar M, et al. Intra- and inter-reader variability in QT interval measurement by tangent and threshold methods in a central electrocardiogram laboratory. J Electrocardiol. 2009;42(4):348-52.
42. Salvi V, Karnad DR, Panicker GK, et al. Comparison of 5 methods of QT interval measurements on electrocardiograms from a thorough QT/QTc study: effect on assay sensitivity and categorical outliers. J Electrocardiol. 2011;44(2): 96-104.
43. Dessertenne F. Ventricular tachycardia with two variable opposing foci. Arch Mal Coeur Vaiss. 1966;59:263-72.
44. Passman R, Kadish A. Polymorphic ventricular tachycardia, long QT syndrome and torsades de pointes. Med Clin North Am. 2003;85(2):321-41.
45. Napolitano C, Bloise R, Monteforte N, et al. Long QT, Brugada, short QT, catecholaminergic polymorphic ventricular tachycardia, and idiopathic ventricular fibrillation. Circulation. 2012;125:2027-34.
46. Priori SG, Napolitano C, Schwartz PJ, et al. Association of long QT syndrome loci and cardiac events among patients treated with beta-blockers. JAMA. 2004;292:1341-4.
47. Vincent GM, Schwartz PJ, Denjoy I, et al. High efficacy of beta-blockers in long-QT syndrome type 1: contribution of noncompliance and QT-prolonging drugs to the occurrence of beta-blocker treatment "failures". Circulation. 2009;119:215-21.
48. Zipes DP, Camm AJ, Borggrefe M, et al. ACC/AHA/ESC 2006 Guidelines for management of patients with ventricular arrhythmias and the prevention of sudden cardiac death: a report of the American College of Cardiology/American Heart Association Task Force and the European Society of Cardiology Committee for Practice Guidelines (writing committee to develop Guidelines for management of patients with ventricular arrhythmias and the prevention of sudden cardiac death): developed in collaboration with the European Heart Rhythm Association and the Heart Rhythm Society. Circulation. 2006;114(10): e385-484.
49. Roden DM. Long QT Syndrome. N Engl J Med. 2008;358(2):169-76.
50. Goldenberg I, Thottathil P, Lopes CM, et al. Trigger-specific ion-channel mechanisms, risk factors, and response to therapy in type 1 long QT syndrome. Heart Rhythm. 2012;9(1):49-56.
51. Zareba W, Moss AJ, Daubert JP, et al. Implantable cardioverter-defibrillator in high-risk long QT syndrome patients. J Cardiovasc Electrophysiol. 2003;14(4):337-41.
52. Goldenberg I, Moss AJ, Peterson DR, et al. Risk factors for aborted cardiac arrest and sudden cardiac death in children with the congenital long-QT syndrome. Circulation. 2008;117(17):2184-91.
53. Goldenberg I, Moss AJ. Long QT syndrome. J Am Coll Cardiol. 2008;51(24):2291-300.

54. Schwartz PJ, Priori SG, Cerrone M, et al. Left cardiac sympathetic denervation in the management of high-risk patients affected by the long-QT syndrome. Circulation. 2004;109:1826-33.
55. Gussak I, Brugada P, Brugada J, et al. Idiopathic short QT interval: a new clinical syndrome?. Cardiology. 2000;94:99-102.
56. Gaita F, Giustetto C, Bianchi F, et al. Short QT syndrome: pharmacological treatment. J Am Coll Cardiol. 2004;43:1494-9.
57. Bellocq C, van Ginneken AC, Bezzina CR, et al. Mutation in the KCNQ1 gene leading to the short QT-interval syndrome. Circulation. 2004;109:2394-7.
58. Gollob MH, Redpath CJ, Roberts JD. The short QT syndrome: proposed diagnostic criteria. J Am Coll Cardiol. 2011;57(7):802-12.
59. Anttonen O, Junttila J, Giustetto C, et al. T-wave morphology in short QT syndrome. Ann Noninvasive Electrocardiol. 2009;14:262-7.
60. Anttonen O, Junttila J, Maury P. Differences in twelve-lead electrocardiogram between symptomatic and asymptomatic subjects with short QT interval. Heart Rhythm. 2009;6:267-71.
61. Magnano AR, Holleran S, Ramakrishnan R, et al. Autonomic nervous system influences on QT interval in normal subjects. J Am Coll Cardiol. 2002;39:1820-6.
62. Redpath CJ, Green MS, Birnie DH, et al. Rapid genetic testing facilitating the diagnosis of short QT syndrome. Can J Cardiol. 2009;25:e133-5.
63. Wolpert C, Schimpf R, Giustetto C. Further insights into the effect of quinidine in short QT syndrome caused by a mutation in HERG. J Cardiovasc Electrophysiol. 2005;16:54-8.
64. Patel C, Yan GX, Antzelevitch C. Short QT syndrome: from bench to bedside. Circ Arrhythm Electrophysiol. 2010;3:401-8.
65. Wehrens XH, Lehnart SE, Huang F, et al. FKBP12.6 deficiency and defective calcium release channel (ryanodine receptor) function linked to exercise-induced sudden cardiac death. Cell. 2003;113:829-40.
66. Coumel P. Catecholaminergic polymorphic ventricular tachyarrhythmias in children. Card Electrophysiol Rev. 2002;6:93-5.
67. Medeiros-Domingo A, Bhuiyan ZA, Tester DJ, et al. The RYR2-encoded ryanodine receptor/calcium release channel in patients diagnosed previously with either catecholaminergic polymorphic ventricular tachycardia or genotype negative, exercise-induced long QT syndrome: a comprehensive open reading frame mutational analysis. J Am Coll Cardiol. 2009;54:2065-74.
68. Laitinen PJ, Brown KM, Piippo K, et al. Mutations of the cardiac ryanodine receptor (RyR2) gene in familial polymorphic ventricular tachycardia. Circulation 2001;103:485-490.
69. Priori SG, Napolitano C, Tiso N, et al. Mutations in the cardiac ryanodine receptor gene (hRyR2) underlie catecholaminergic polymorphic ventricular tachycardia. Circulation. 2001;103:196-200.
70. Postma AV, Denjoy I, Kamblock J, et al. Catecholaminergic polymorphic ventricular tachycardia: RYR2 mutations, bradycardia, and follow-up of the patients. J Med Genet. 2005;42:863-70.
71. Aizawa Y, Komura S, Okada S, et al. Distinct U wave changes in patients with catecholaminergic polymorphic ventricular tachycardia (CPVT). Int Heart J. 2006;47:381-9.
72. Priori SG, Wilde AA, Horie M, et al. HRS/EHRA/APHRS expert consensus statement on the diagnosis and management of patients with inherited primary arrhythmia syndromes: document endorsed by HRS, EHRA, and APHRS in May 2013 and by ACCF, AHA, PACES, and AEPC in June 2013. Heart Rhythm. 2013a;10:1932-63.
73. Priori SG, Wilde AA, Horie M, et al. Executive summary: HRS/EHRA/APHRS expert consensus statement on the diagnosis and management of patients with inherited primary arrhythmia syndromes. Europace. 2013b;15:1389-406.
74. Priori SG, Napolitano C, Grillo M. Concealed arrhythmogenic syndromes: the hidden substrate of idiopathic ventricular fibrillation? Cardiovasc Res. 2001a;50:218-23.
75. Priori SG, Napolitano C, Memmi M, et al. Clinical and molecular characterization of patients with catecholaminergic polymorphic ventricular tachycardia. Circulation. 2002;106:69-74.
76. Watanabe H, Knollmann BC. Mechanism underlying catecholaminergic polymorphic ventricular tachycardia and approaches to therapy. J Electrocardiol. 2011;44(6):650-5.
77. Pflaumer A, Davis AM. Guidelines for the diagnosis and management of catecholaminergic polymorphic ventricular tachycardia. Heart Lung Circ. 2012;21(2):96-100.
78. van der Werf C, Kannankeril PJ, Sacher F, et al. Flecainide therapy reduces exercise-induced ventricular arrhythmias in patients with catecholaminergic polymorphic ventricular tachycardia. J Am Coll Cardiol. 2011;57:2244-54.
79. Liu N, Denegri M, Ruan Y, et al. Short communication: flecainide exerts an antiarrhythmic effect in a mouse model of catecholaminergic polymorphic ventricular tachycardia by increasing the threshold for triggered activity. Circ Res. 2011;109:291-5.
80. Postma AV, Denjoy I, Kamblock J, et al. Catecholaminergic polymorphic ventricular tachycardia: RYR2 mutations, bradycardia, and follow-up of the patients. J Med Genet. 2005;42:863-70.

Chapter 17

Preexcitation Syndromes

INTRODUCTION

Preexcitation syndromes are conditions where the ventricles of the heart become depolarized too early, which leads to their partial premature contraction. Normally, the atria and the ventricles are electrically isolated, and electrical contact between them exists only at the *atrioventricular node* (AV node). In all preexcitation syndromes, at least one more conductive pathway is present. Physiologically, the normal electrical depolarization wave is delayed at the AV node to allow the atria to contract before the ventricles. However, there is no such delay in the abnormal pathway, so the electrical stimulus passes to the ventricle by this tract faster than via normal AV/bundle of His system, so the ventricles are depolarized (excited) before (preexcitation) normal conduction system (Fig. 17.1).

Historically, the possibility of the existence of AV accessory pathways (APs) was first raised by Stanley Kent in 1913.[1] In 1930, Wolff, Parkinson, and White reported on 11 young patients with paroxysms of tachycardia or atrial fibrillation (AF) that had a functional bundle branch block and an abnormally short PR interval on electrocardiograms (ECGs) recorded during sinus rhythm.[2] In 1933, Holzmann and Scherf reported that the mechanism in Wolff-Parkinson-White (WPW) syndrome consisted of an acceleration of passage of the impulse from the atria to the ventricles and not a block, as had been proposed by Wolff, Parkinson, and White.[3] In 1944, Ohnell introduced the term "preexcitation" to the medical literature, and along with Wood et al., confirmed the presence of APs by histologic studies.[4,5]

Anatomically, the atria and ventricles are in apposition, separated by an invagination known as the AV groove. APs that cross the groove and electrically link the atria and ventricles, can produce paroxysmal tachycardias. Although the most common site of insertion is between the lateral aspect of the left atrium and left ventricular myocardium, pathways can cross the AV groove anywhere in its course (except the region between the aortic and mitral valves) to connect the left or right atrium to its respective ventricle. APs are mostly located in the left free wall, posteroseptal space, right free wall, and in the anteroseptal space (Fig. 17.2 and Box 17.1). Each location produces a distinct ECG pattern.

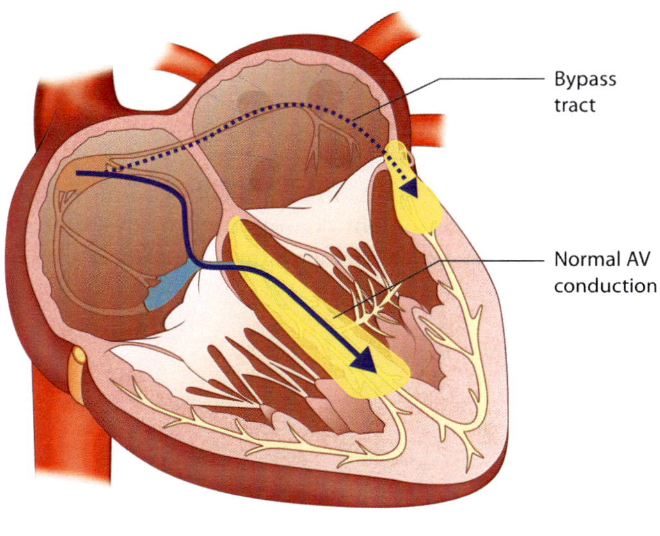

Fig. 17.1: Diagram showing conduction through normal and accessory pathway (bypass tract).

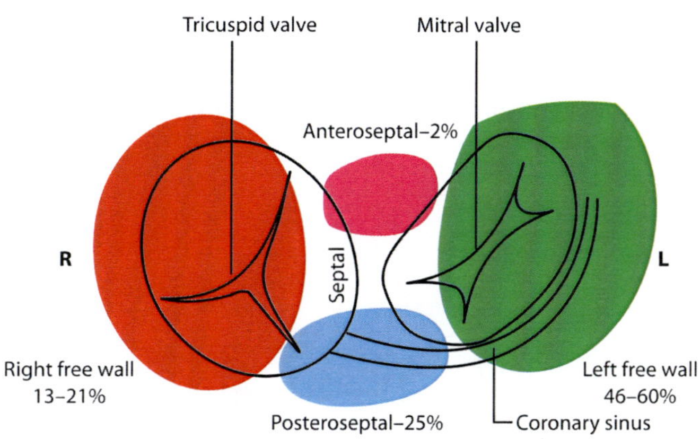

Fig. 17.2: Diagram showing locations of the accessory pathways at the level of atrioventrcicular (AV) valve plane of the heart.

Box 17.1: Location of the accessory pathways.

- *Left free wall:* 46–60%
- *Posteroseptal:* 25%
- *Right free wall:* 13–21%
- *Anteroseptal:* 2%
- *Multiple pathways:* 10%.

TYPES OF PREEXCITATION SYNDROMES (FIGS. 17.3A to D)[6]

- Wolff-Parkinson-White syndrome
- Lown-Ganong-Levine (LGL) syndrome
- Mahaim-type preexcitation.

Wolff–Parkinson–White Syndrome

In the normal heart electrical impulses generated from the sinoatrial (SA) node in the right atrium pass to the AV node. Physiological slowing occurs at this point before conduction to the His-Purkinje system and the ventricular muscle. The PR interval represents the time taken for the atria to depolarize and the wave of depolarization to travel down the AV node and through the His-Purkinje system. In preexcitation syndromes the accessory pathway permits the impulse to bypass the AV node (thus avoiding the associated delay) and permitting early depolarization of the ventricular myocardium. This is reflected on the ECG as a shortened PR interval. Nonspecialized ventricular myocardium conducts at a slower rate. Its direct depolarization in preexcitation syndrome generates an initial slurring or "delta wave" at the start of the QRS complex. Simultaneous activation of the ventricles occur as normal through the AV node and His-Purkinje system and hence the remainder of the QRS complex appears relatively normal. The mechanism of ventricular depolarization in sinus rhythm in patients with WPW syndrome is a combination of preexcitation and normal conduction giving rise to a short PR interval and a delta wave (Fig. 17.4) followed by a relatively broad QRS complex.[7]

The AP is congenital in origin and results from a failure of complete separation of the atria and ventricles. It consists of a thin filamentous structure (bundle of Kent) situated anywhere along the AV groove and the left lateral pathway is the most common (Box 17.2).[7] In around 10% of cases multiple pathways exist.[8]

Delta waves detectable on an ECG have been reported to be present in 0.15–0.25% of the general population.[9] The prevalence of WPW syndrome in the population is about 0.1–0.4% with an associated risk of sudden death of around 0.5–4% (average 1%). A higher prevalence of 0.55% has been reported in first-degree relatives of patients with APs. WPW syndrome is more commonly diagnosed in men than in women, although this sex difference is not observed in children. Among those with the WPW syndrome, 3.4% has first-degree relatives with preexcitation.[8] The familial form is usually inherited as a Mendelian autosomal dominant trait.[10-14]

Most patients with the WPW syndrome have otherwise normal hearts, but some have concomitant congenital heart disease (CHD). The association of ventricular preexcitation (WPW syndrome) with CHD is well known.[15-18] The incidence of associated congenital abnormalities ranges from 7% to 20%.[15-19] Ventricular preexcitation is most often associated with Ebstein anomaly (25%) of cases.[19-23] But WPW syndrome has also been described in patients with hypertrophic cardiomyopathy (HCM), dextro-transposition of the great arteries (d-TGA), levo-transposition of the great arteries (l-TGA), pulmonary atresia/intact ventricular septum, patent ductus arteriosus (PDA), parachute mitral valve, tetralogy of Fallot (TOF), total anomalous pulmonary venous connection (TAPVC), and ventricular septal defect (VSD).[18-20,23]

Electrocardiogram Criteria

The classic ECG findings that are associated with WPW syndrome include: (1) Presence of a short PR interval less than 120 ms (<0.12 seconds), (2) A wide QRS complex longer than 120 ms (>0.12 seconds) with a slurred onset of the QRS waveform producing a delta wave in the early part of QRS, and (3) Secondary ST-T wave changes (Fig. 17.5).

Whether preexcitation is full or not, it cannot be determined from the body surface ECG, but the following criteria are suggestive of full preexcitation:[24]

- PR interval (assuming no intra-atrial or interatrial conduction block) less than 120 ms during sinus rhythm in adults and less than 90 ms in children.
- Slurring of initial portion of the QRS complex (delta wave), which either interrupts the P wave or arises immediately after its termination (Fig. 17.6).

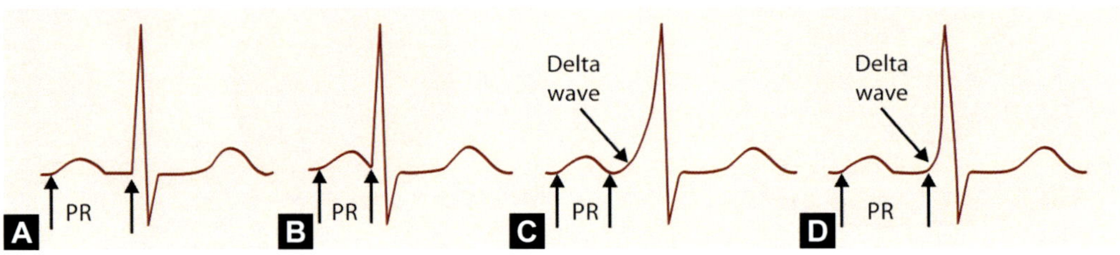

Figs. 17.3A to D: Diagrams showing electrocardiogram (ECG) features of different preexcitation syndromes compared to normal ECG. (A) Normal ECG with normal PR interval, normal QRS configuration, and no delta wave; (B) ECG of Lown–Ganong–Levine (LGL) syndrome: 1. Short PR interval, 2. No delta wave, 3. Normal QRS morphology; (C) ECG of Wolff–Parkinson–White (WPW) syndrome: 1. Short PR interval, 2. Presence of delta wave, 3. Broad QRS complex; and (D) ECG of Mahaim preexcitation: 1. Normal PR interval, 2. Presence of delta wave, 3. Broad QRS complex.

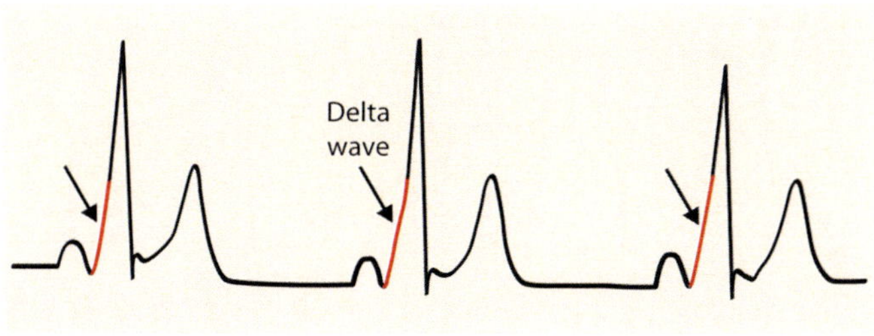

Fig. 17.4: Diagram showing delta waves (*arrows*). The slurred upstroke at the beginning of the QRS complex is called delta wave.

Box 17.2: Types of accessory pathways.

- *Bundle of Kent:* The classic accessory pathway is the AV bypass tract or bundle of Kent in WPW syndrome that directly connects atrial and ventricular myocardium, bypassing the AV node/His-Purkinje system.
- *James fibers:* Connect atrium to distal or compact AV node or atria to bundle of His. (Lown–Ganong–Levine syndrome).
- *Mahaim fibers:* Connect the atrium (atriofascicular pathways), AV node (nodoventricular pathways) or His bundle (fasciculoventricular pathways) to distal Purkinje fibers or ventricular myocardium (Mahaim fiber preexcitation).

(AV: atrioventricular; WPW: Wolff–Parkinson–White)

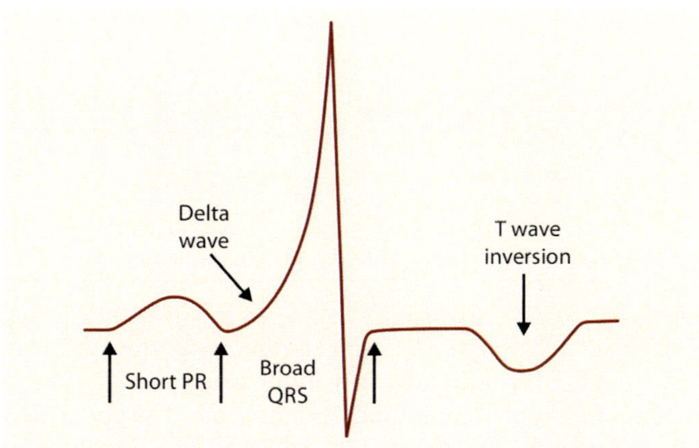

Fig. 17.5: Diagram showing four typical ECG features of WPW syndrome: 1. Short PR interval, 2. A wide QRS complex, 3. Delta wave, and 4. Secondary T wave inversion. Secondary ST depression is also frequently seen in WPW syndrome. (ECG: electrocardiogram; WPW: Wolff–Parkinson–White)

- QRS duration greater than 120 ms (0.12 seconds) in adults and greater than 90 ms in children.
- Secondary ST and T wave changes.

The classic ECG criteria for WPW syndrome include shortened PR interval, delta wave, and increased QRS duration owing to simultaneous fusion of activation of the ventricles via normal AV nodal conduction and via the accessory pathway (Fig. 17.7). The degree of preexcitation is dependent on the conduction time in the atria, over the AV node, the His-Purkinje system, and over the AP. It also varies depending on the location of the AP and left-sided

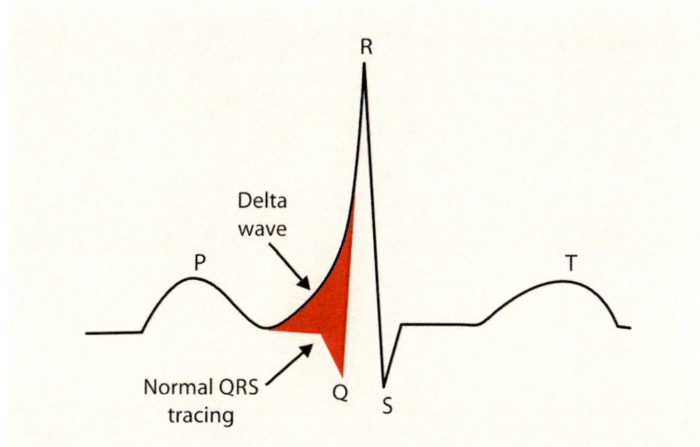

Fig. 17.6: Normal and WPW syndrome ECGs are superimposed on each other. *Note:* Delta wave (slurring at the beginning of the QRS complex) of WPW syndrome and smooth upstroke of initial part of QRS complex (*red*) of normal ECG tracing without any delta wave. In this tracing delta wave starts just at the point of termination of the P wave. (ECGs: electrocardiograms; WPW: Wolff–Parkinson–White)

pathways are more easy to be missed.[25] These factors may result in a spectrum of findings including no apparent preexcitation. In addition, some alternative diagnoses such as HCM and previous Q-wave myocardial infarction, may cause the ECG changes mimicking preexcitation.[26,27] Because of an increased risk of sudden cardiac death in patients with ventricular preexcitation, it is important to recognize it on a surface ECG.[28] Equally, excluding ventricular preexcitation avoids unnecessary invasive procedures and X-ray exposure. A septal Q wave in lead V6 was claimed to exclude ventricular preexcitation.[29] However, apart from the classic triad no other ECG criteria have been described to diagnose preexcitation. But recently in absence of classical triad a new algorithm to diagnose preexcitation has been suggested. A logistic regression analysis showed the combination of the following criteria to be powerful in the confirmation of the diagnosis in patients with suspected preexcitation: (1) Presence of both PR interval less than or equal to 120 ms and PR dispersion more than or equal to 20 ms, (2) Absence of initial positive deflection (septal R wave) in lead aVR, and (3) Horizontal QRS transition in lead V1 or before. PR dispersion is defined as a difference between maximum and minimum PR intervals on a single 12-lead ECG.[30]

Wolff-Parkinson-White syndrome is classified into two types according to the ECG findings:

1. *Type A:* The delta wave and QRS complex are predominantly upright in the precordial leads, producing a dominant R wave in lead V1 (Figs. 17.8A and B).
2. *Type B:* The delta wave and QRS complex are predominantly negative in leads V1 and V2 and positive in the other precordial leads (Figs. 17.9A and B).

The delta wave expressed as a vector may be directed ahead or back. If the wave is directed ahead, there is a tall R wave at V1, initially thought may be due to insertion of the bypass in the left ventricle. This is called type A. If the delta vector is directed back, a QRS complex is predominantly

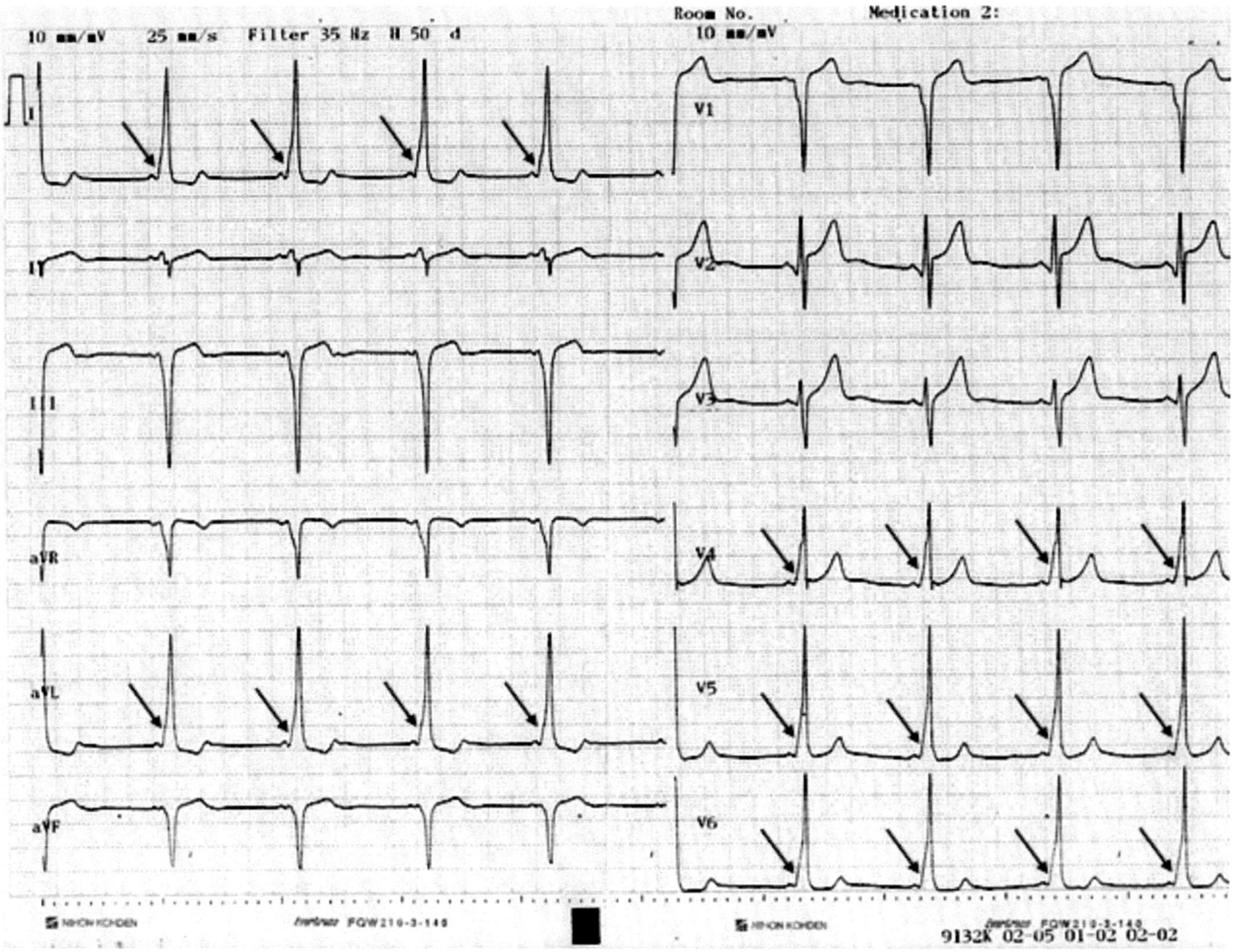

Fig. 17.7: Typical ECG of WPW syndrome, PR 80 ms (0.08 seconds), QRS duration 140 ms (0.14 seconds), and presence of delta wave. Delta waves are present in all the leads but more prominent in L1, aVL, and V4–V6 (*arrows*). (ECG: electrocardiogram; WPW: Wolff–Parkinson–White)

negative at V1 and is classified as type B, initially thought to indicate a right ventricular bypass.

More recently, it has been shown that bypass tracts are widely distributed and transmit impulses at any point around the AV ring or in the septum. The latter may result in delta waves directed ahead or back. The location of bypass cannot be accomplished accurately by the usual surface ECG but requires intracardiac and epicardial mapping. The type A may be confused with true posterior infarction or right ventricular hypertrophy and the type B with anteroseptal infarction. Careful measurement of the P-R interval and close inspection of the QRS morphology will avoid this confusion.

In preexcitation syndromes, APs may be of two types:

1. Manifest APs
2. Concealed APs.

Manifest accessory pathways: Those APs capable of anterograde conduction are called "manifest", demonstrating preexcitation on a standard ECG. Manifest APs usually conduct in both anterograde and retrograde directions.[31]

Concealed accessory pathways: Defined as pathways those are capable of conduction only in the retrograde direction at rates similar or greater than the sinus rate. The concealed APs are noted in between 15% and 42% of patients with AP.[32] Approximately one-third of atrioventricular reentrant tachycardias (AVRTs) are due to concealed APs. The clinical presentation of patients who have a concealed AP is similar to the classic presentation of WPW syndrome with the exception that rapid preexcited responses are not observed during AF. Concealed pathways are more frequently localized to the left free wall (64%), and less frequently in septal (31%) and right free wall locations.[31,32]

Arrhythmias in Wolff–Parkinson–White Syndrome

Among patients with WPW syndrome, AVRT is the most common arrhythmia, accounting for 95% of reentrant tachycardias. AF is a potentially life-threatening arrhythmia in patients with WPW syndrome as it can degenerate to ventricular fibrillation (VF).[33]

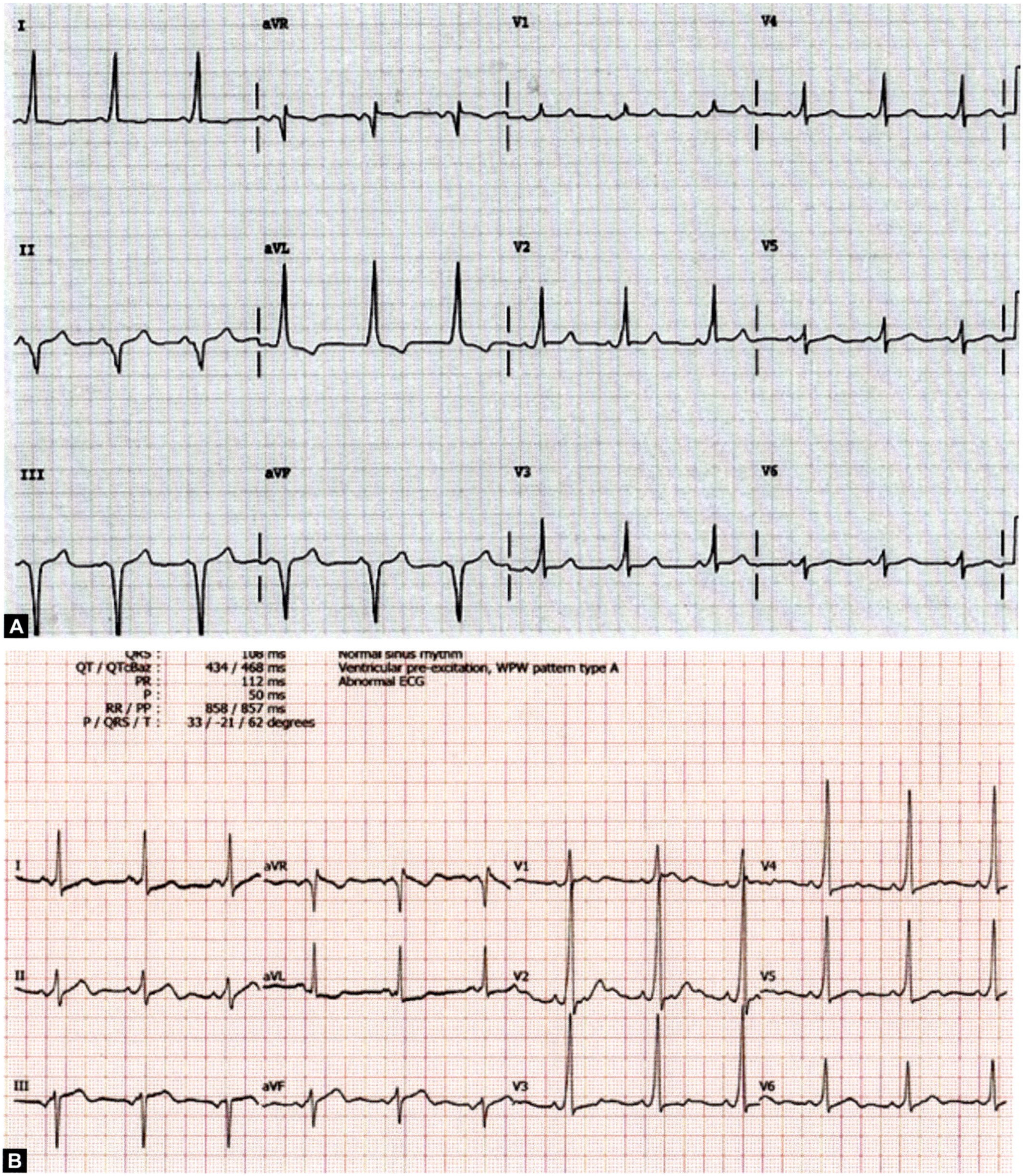

Figs. 17.8A and B: (A) Type A WPW syndrome with tall R waves in leads V1 and V2. This ECG may be confused with true posterior infarction as it shows tall R waves in V1 and V2 with upright T waves. But presence of delta waves confirm the diagnosis of type A WPW syndrome (This pattern of ECG may indicate a possible left-sided accessory pathway); and (B) ECG illustrates the features of type A WPW syndrome with tall R waves in leads V1 and V2 with presence of delta waves in all the limb and precordial leads. (ECG: electrocardiogram; WPW: Wolff–Parkinson–White)

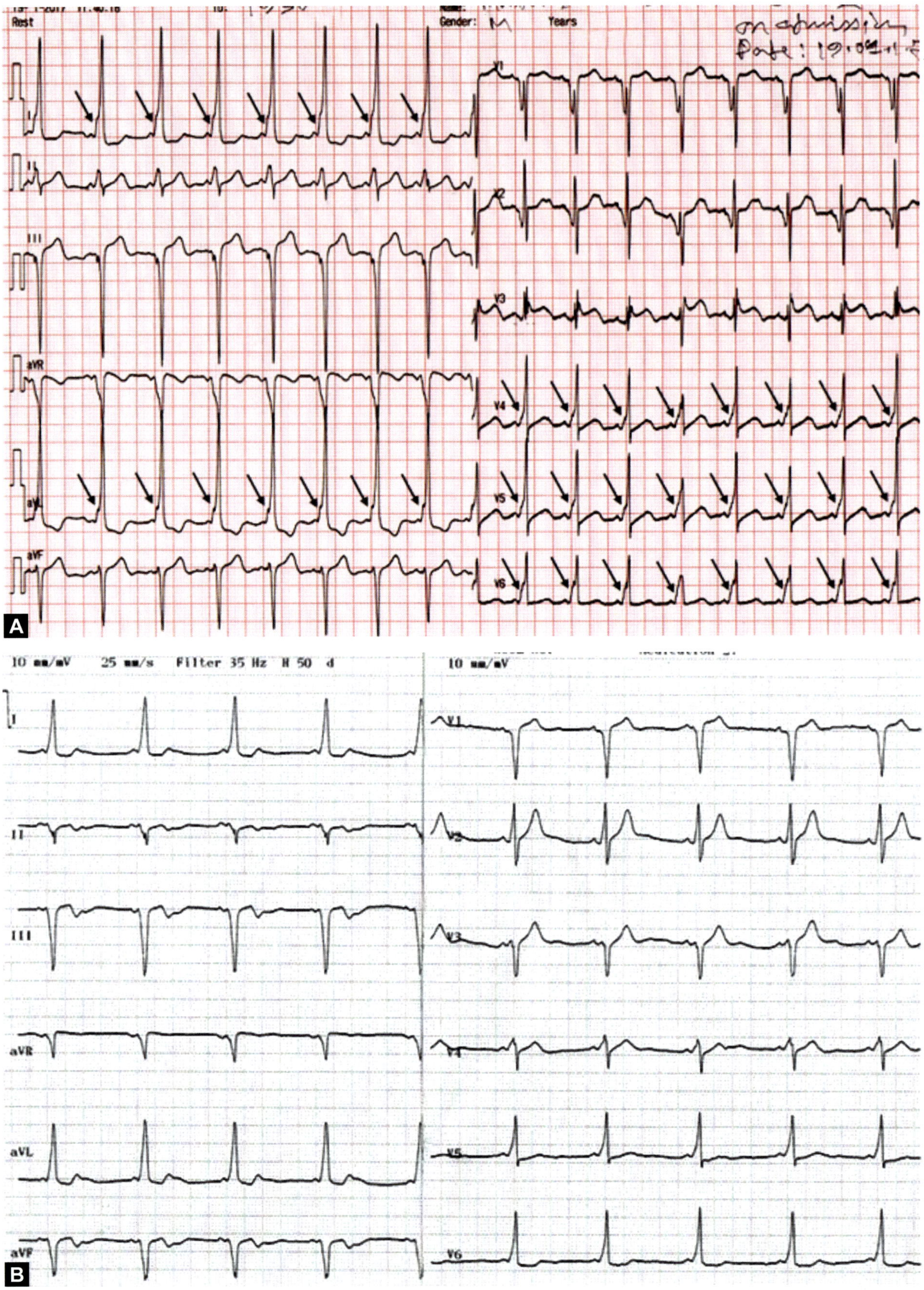

Figs. 17.9A and B: (A) ECG illustrates the typical features of type B WPW syndrome with dominant S wave in V1 and prominent delta waves in most of the limb and precordial leads, most prominent in LI, aVL, and V4–V6 (*arrows*). Also note short PR interval (PR interval 80 ms) with broad QRS complex (QRS duration 140 ms); and (B) ECG is suggestive of type B WPW syndrome with dominant S wave in V1 and prominent delta waves in multiple leads (indicates a possible right-sided accessory pathway). (ECG: electrocardiogram; WPW: Wolff–Parkinson–White)

The most frequently encountered tachycardia in WPW syndrome is an AVRT. The arrhythmia uses the AV node and AP to form a reentry circuit triggered by an appropriately timed ectopic. This reentry circuit may be classified as either orthodromic or antidromic depending on whether the ventricles are activated via the normal conduction system or the AP (Fig. 17.10). Orthodromic AVRTs account for most tachycardias in WPW syndrome (90%). Conduction occurs down the AV node and retrogradely up the AP producing a narrow complex tachycardia. The QRS morphology is normal (that is, with no delta wave) during the arrhythmia because ventricular activation has occurred through the normal pathway. The rate is usually between 140 beats per minute and 280 beats per minute. P waves may be buried in QRS complex or may appear after QRS complex as a retrograde wave. So P waves may or may not be visible on surface ECG (Figs. 17.11 and 12). Retrograde P waves immediately preceding the T waves or inverted P waves may be visible deforming the ST segment indicating that atrial depolarization occurs later than ventricular depolarization.[7] In a patient with a narrow complex tachycardia, the presence of such late P waves are frequently the only ECG evidence that the patient has an AP rather than a much more common atrioventricular nodal reentrant tachycardia (AVNRT). Classically on surface ECG of narrow complex tachycardia, visibility of P waves favor AVRT and is suggestive of the presence of an AP with anterograde conduction via the AV node and retrograde conduction via AP (Figs. 17.13 and 14A and B), though this pattern may occur in the common form of AVNRT.

Antidromic tachycardias occur when the AP conducts anterogradely and the impulse returns to the atria via the AV node. The resulting QRS is broadened reflecting the abnormal ventricular activation. These broad complex tachycardias (Fig. 17.15) can be difficult to distinguish from a ventricular tachycardia (VT) and are less common, occurring in around 10% of patients with WPW syndrome.[7]

In most parts of the world, AVRT, due to WPW syndrome or a concealed AP, is the second most common cause of supraventricular tachycardia (SVT) (after AVNRT), and accounts for up to one-third of all SVT.[34] Though SVT is the most common tachyarrhythmia observed in patients with symptomatic WPW syndrome, but AF is also observed in about 20–30% of this group of patients. Life-threatening malignant ventricular arrhythmias (VT/VF) and sudden cardiac deaths have also been documented in this group of patients.[35-37]

Diagnosis of Coronary Artery Disease in Presence of Wolff–Parkinson–White Syndrome

Diagnosis of coronary artery disease may be difficult in the presence of WPW syndrome. It is known that WPW syndrome may either simulate acute myocardial infarction (AMI) or mask the electrocardiographic abnormalities of AMI.[38] The negative delta waves in the inferior leads, may be morphologically identical to Q-wave infarction and are present in 16% of patients with WPW syndrome (Figs. 17.16A and B).[39] Confusing the negative delta waves of WPW syndrome with a myocardial infarction is a common error. It is not possible to reliably differentiate negative delta waves from myocardial infarction based solely on ECG. If there is doubt whether the inferior Q waves represent infarction or negative delta waves, an echocardiogram may be needed to study inferior wall motion. The sensitivity of an echocardiogram is sufficient to rule out old inferior myocardial infarction if no wall motion abnormalities are seen.[38,40] WPW syndrome may also mask the ECG abnormalities of AMI. It is difficult to recognize AMI in patients with WPW syndrome because preexcitation masks the Q waves of transmural infarction.[41] So WPW syndrome may produce pseudoinfarction pattern due to negatively deflected delta waves in the inferior/anterior leads (pseudo Q waves), or as a prominent R wave in V1–3 mimicking posterior infarction.

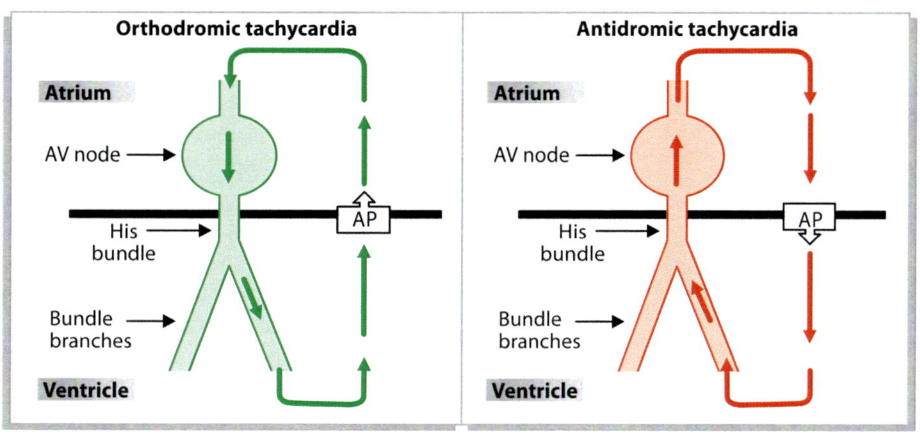

Fig. 17.10: Diagram showing basic mechanism of atrioventricular reentrant tachycardia (AVRT). AVRT may be orthodromic or antidromic. An accessory pathway (AP) can conduct impulses either anterograde, towards the ventricle, retrograde, away from the ventricle, or in both directions. In orthodromic AVRT antegrade conduction occurs via the AV node with retrograde conduction occurring via the AP (*left-sided panel*) and produces narrow complex tachycardia. In antidromic AVRT anterograde conduction occurs via the AP with retrograde conduction via the AV node (*right-sided panel*) and results in wide QRS tachycardia due to abnormal ventricular depolarization via AP.

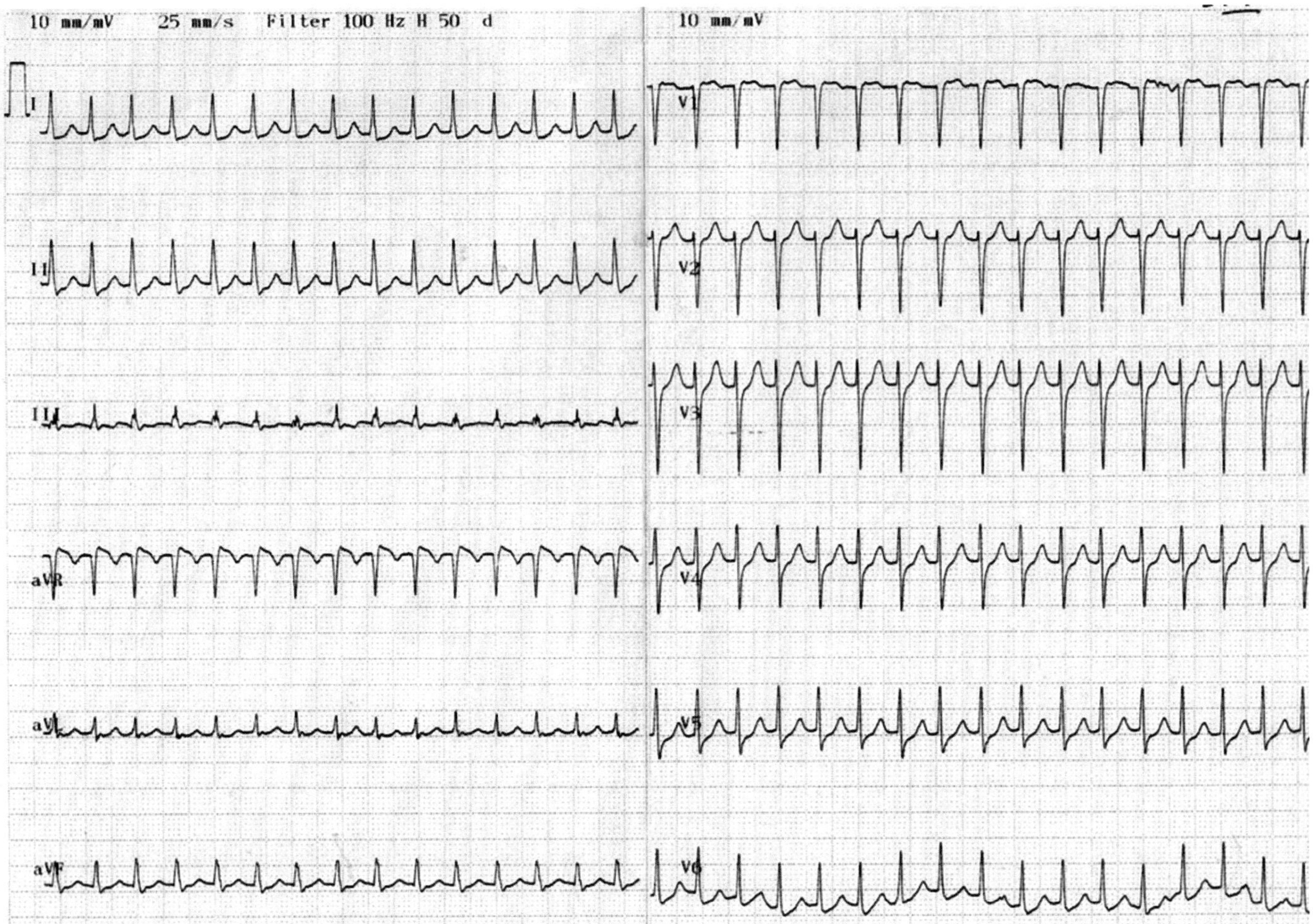

Fig. 17.11: Electrocardiogram (ECG) is suggestive of atrioventricular reentrant tachycardia (AVRT) with regular, narrow complex tachycardia at 192 bpm with no discernible P waves. The QRS complexes are narrow because impulses are being transmitted in an orthodromic direction, antegrade conduction via the AV node with retrograde conduction occurring via the accessory pathway. This rhythm is indistinguishable from atrioventricular nodal reentrant tachycardia (AVNRT).

Localization of the Accessory Pathway

The main electrocardiographic features of preexcitation are a short PR interval less than 120 ms (<0.12 seconds), a prolonged QRS complex more than 120 ms (>0.12 seconds), and a slurred, slow rising onset of the QRS complex that is known as the delta wave.

Localization of the AP is generally of value only when considering catheter ablation. The pathway localization or the degree of preexcitation otherwise does not predict the clinical course. Various algorithms have been used for predicting AP location using different ECG criteria.[33,42] An algorithm developed by Arruda et al. utilizing the surface ECG has an overall sensitivity of 90% and specificity of 99%.[43] AP can be localized using following steps:[33,43]

- *Step 1:* If the delta wave in lead 1 is negative or isoelectric or the R wave is greater in amplitude than the S wave in V1 a left free-wall AP is present. If these criteria are fulfilled then lead aVF is examined. If the delta wave in lead aVF is positive, a left lateral, anterolateral AP is identified. If the delta wave in lead aVF is isoelectric or negative then the AP is located at the left posterior or posterolateral region.
- *Step 2:* Lead II is examined. A negative delta wave in lead II identifies the subepicardial posteroseptal AP. If the delta wave in lead II is isoelectric or positive, proceed to step 3.
- *Step 3:* Lead V1 is examined. A negative or isoelectric delta wave in lead V1 identifies a septal AP. If these criteria are fulfilled, lead aVF is examined. If the delta wave is negative, an AP is identified, which is located at the posteroseptal tricuspid annulus. If the delta wave is isoelectric in lead aVF, the AP may be located to either the posteroseptal tricuspid annulus or the posteroseptal mitral annulus. A positive delta wave in aVF identifies a pathway located within the anteroseptal/right anterior paraseptal or midseptal tricuspid annulus regions. If the delta wave in V1 is positive after having excluded patients with a left free-wall AP in step 1, a right free-wall accessory AV pathway is identified. Proceed to step 4.

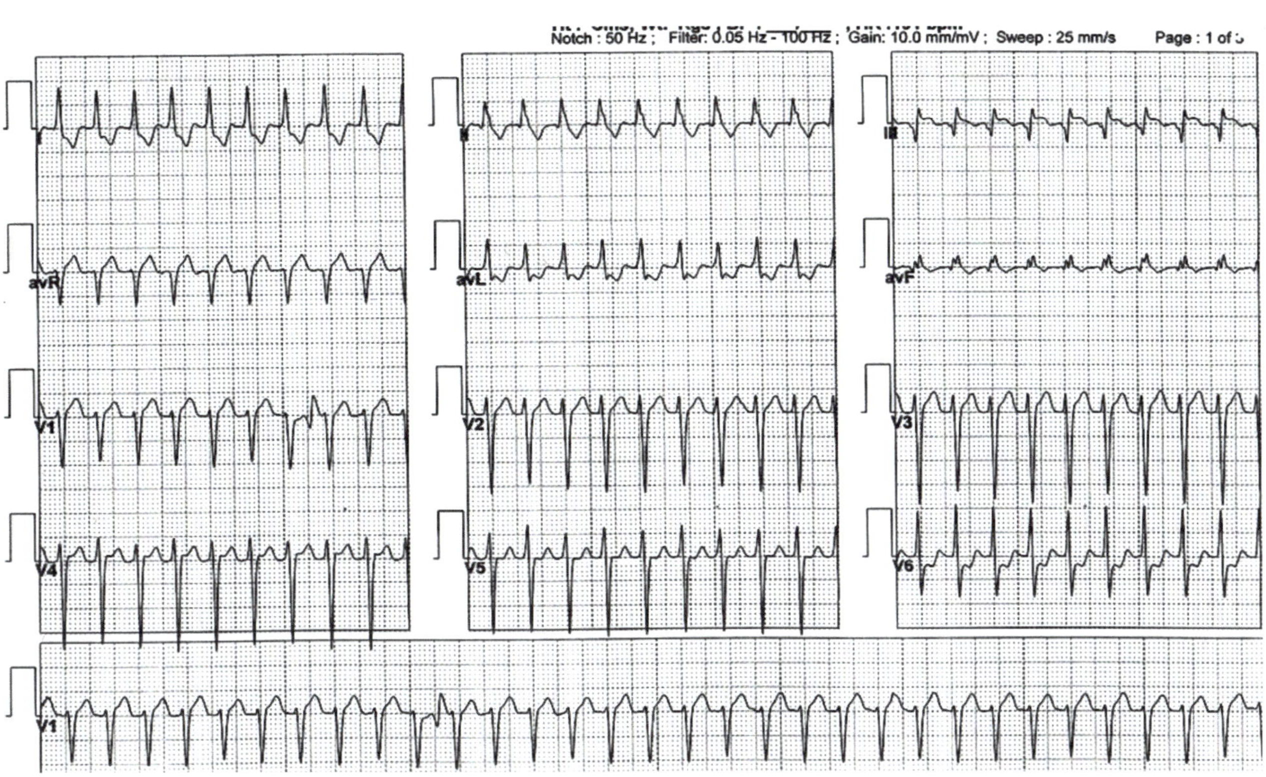

Fig. 17.12: ECG is suggestive of atrioventricular reentrant tachycardia (AVRT) with regular, narrow complex tachycardia at 190 bpm with no discernible P waves. The QRS complexes are narrow because impulses are being transmitted in an orthodromic direction (atrium > ventricle) via the AV node. *Note:* Significant ST segment depression (rate-related change) in multiple leads; this is common in SVT and does not necessarily indicate myocardial ischemia. (ECG: electrocardiogram; SVT: supraventricular tachycardia)

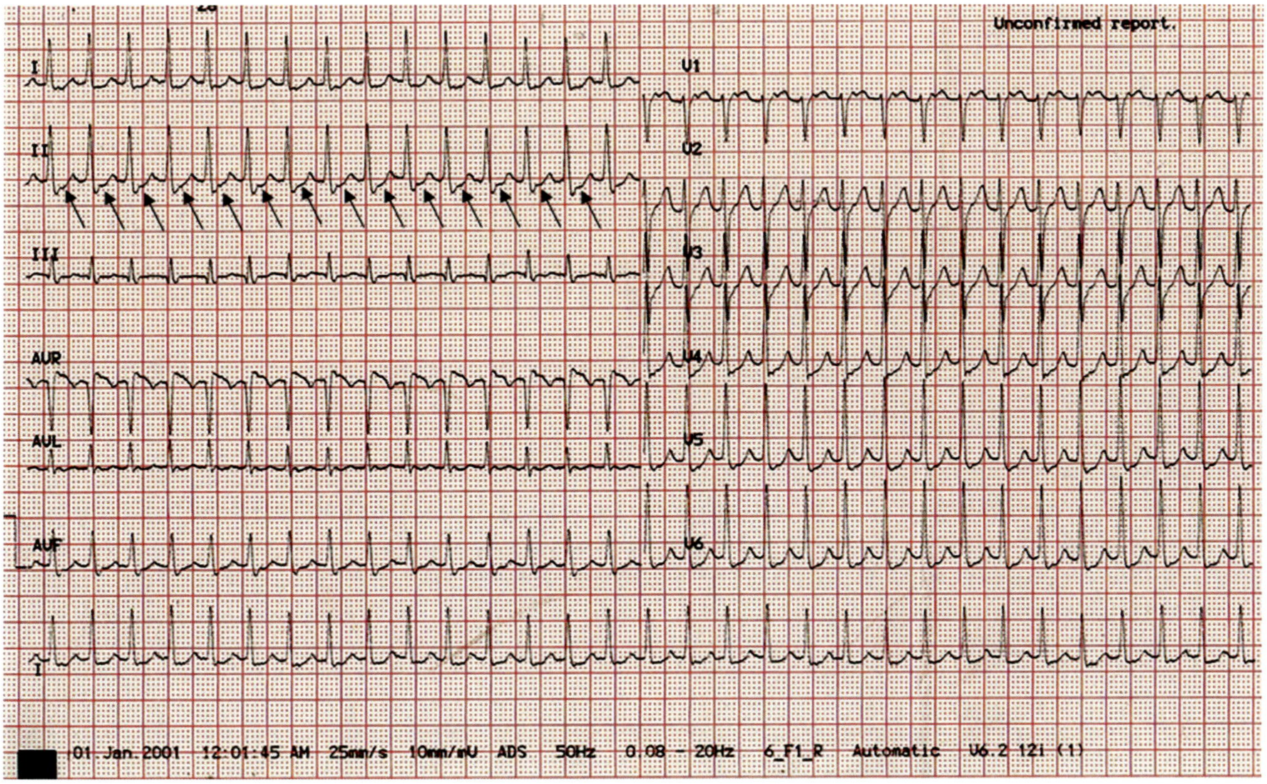

Fig. 17.13: Electrocardiogram (ECG) is suggestive of atrioventricular reentrant tachycardia (AVRT) with regular, narrow complex tachycardia at 186 bpm with discernible retrograde P waves in multiple leads, most prominent in LII (*arrows*). Classically on surface ECG of narrow complex tachycardia, visibility of P waves favor AVRT and is suggestive of the presence of an accessory pathway (AP) with antegrade conduction via the AV node and retrograde conduction via AP.

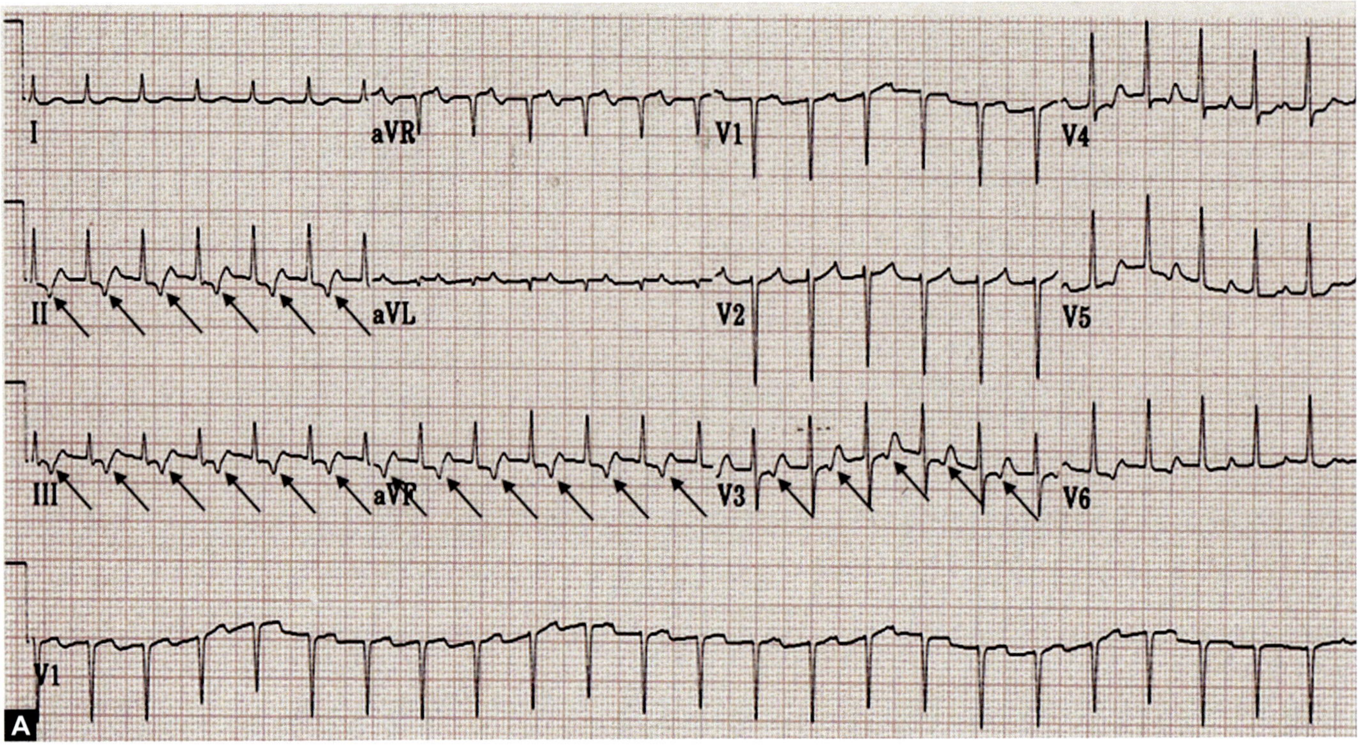

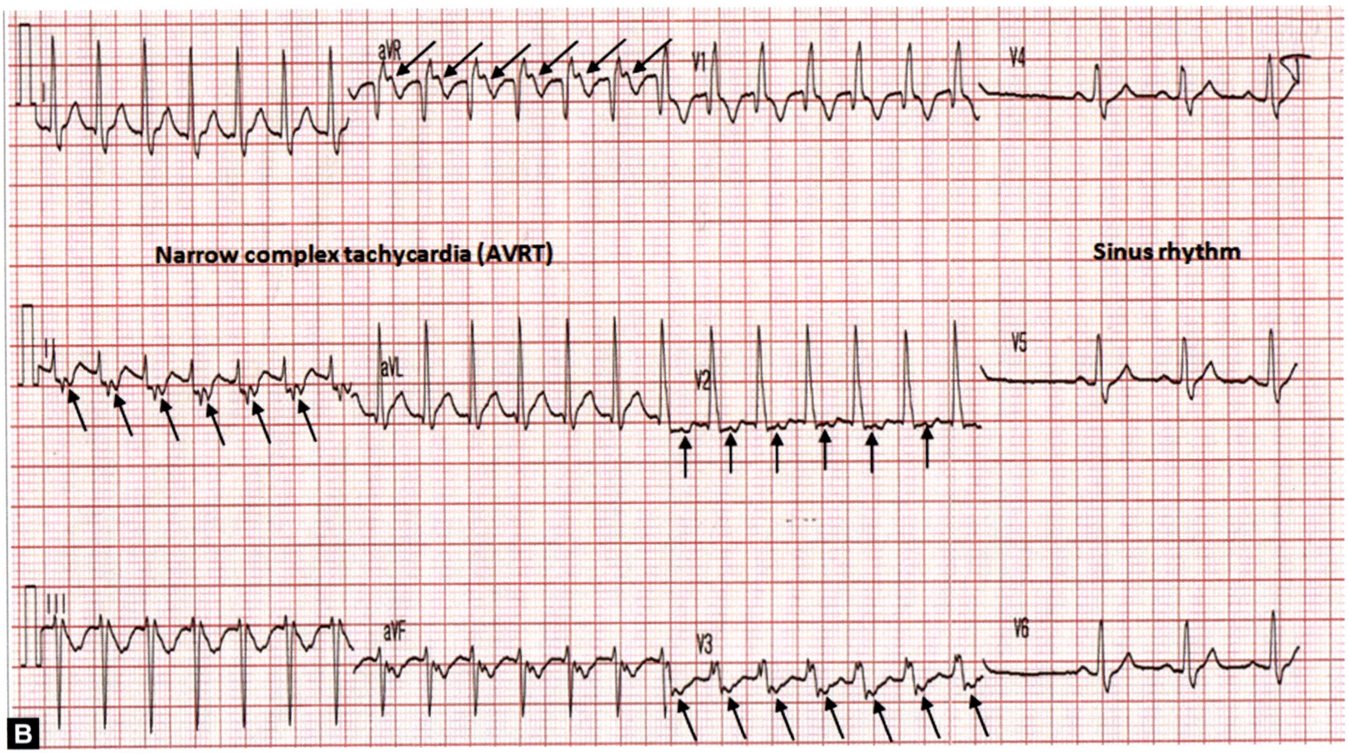

Figs. 17.14A and B: (A) ECG illustrates narrow complex regular tachycardia [atrioventricular reentrant tachycardia (AVRT)], at a rate 150 bpm and shows distortion of the ST segments by the P waves immediately preceding the T waves and the retrograde P waves are best seen in LII, LIII, aVF, and lead V3 (*arrows*). The pattern seen in this ECG is most suggestive of the presence of an accessory pathway (AP) with antegrade conduction via the AV node and retrograde conduction via the AP. Visibility of the retrograde P waves favor the diagnosis of AVRT, though this pattern may occur in the common form of AVNRT; and (B) ECG illustrates spontaneous conversion of AVRT into sinus rhythm during taking 12-lead ECG in emergency department. LI, LII, LIII, aVR, aVL, aVF, and V1–V3 shows regular, narrow complex tachycardia at 156 bpm with discernible retrograde P waves in multiple leads, most prominent in LII, aVR, V2, and V3 (*arrows*). *Note:* AVRT converts to sinus rhythm during ECG taking in leads V4–V6. All QRS complexes in leads V4–V6 are preceded by a P wave of normal morphology with heart rate 96 bpm. (AVNRT: atrioventricular nodal reentrant tachycardia; ECG: electrocardiogram)

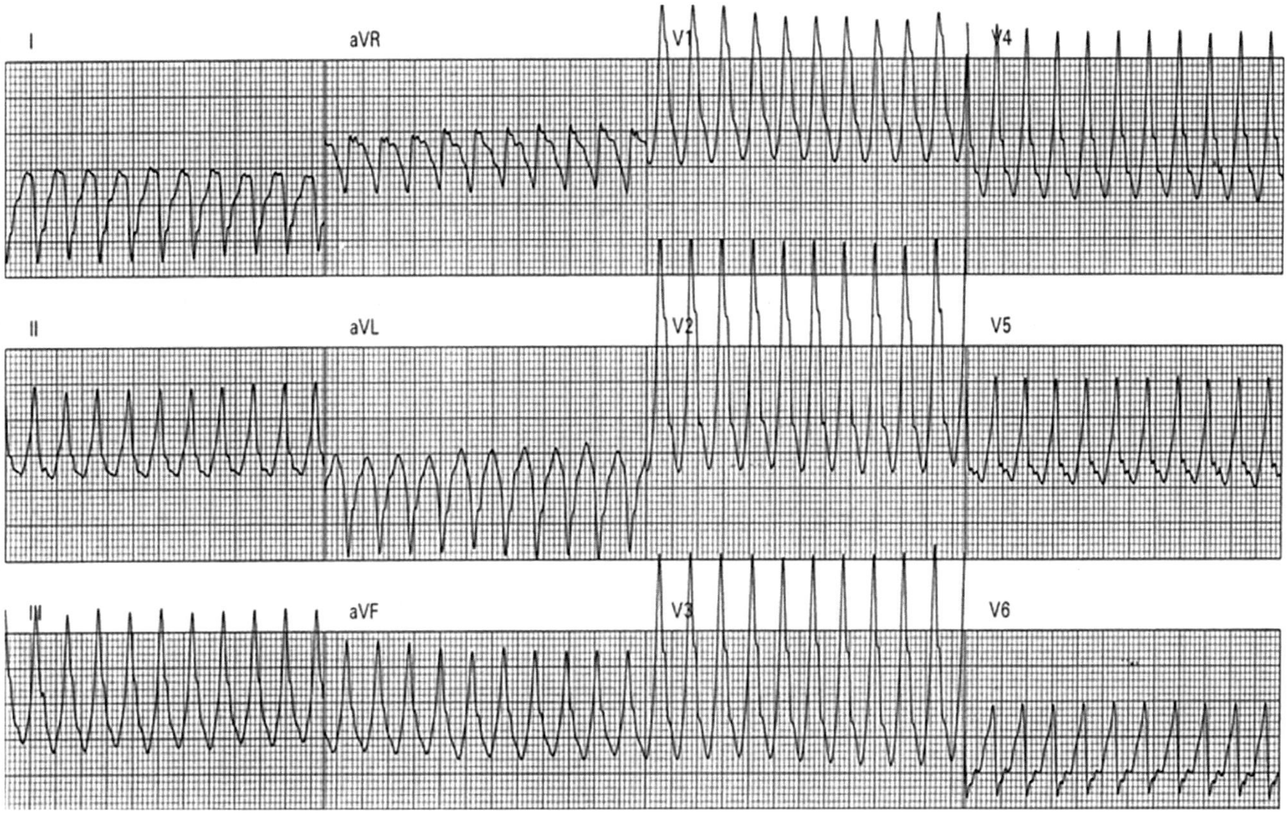

Fig. 17.15: This ECG illustrates an example of antidromic atrioventricular reentrant tachycardia (AVRT) in a patient with known WPW syndrome. This tracing shows a wide complex tachycardia at a rate 216 bpm with right bundle branch block morphology in lead V1 with a rightward QRS frontal axis. The main differential diagnosis of this type of wide complex tachycardia is ventricular tachycardia (VT). However absence of left axis deviation and absence of AV dissociation in this particular tracing do not support the diagnosis of VT. (ECG: electrocardiogram; WPW: Wolff–Parkinson–White)

- *Step 4:* In patients with a right free-wall APs, examine aVF. A positive delta wave in aVF identifies a right anterior/anterolateral AP. If the delta wave in aVF is isoelectric or negative, examine lead II. A positive delta wave in lead II identifies a right lateral AP, and an isoelectric delta wave in lead II identifies a right posterior/posterolateral pathway.

The predictive accuracy of all these algorithms are significantly reduced in the presence of multiple pathways. Coexistent anomalies such as AMI or left ventricular hypertrophy (LVH) may alter the QRS morphology.

Atrial Fibrillation in Wolff–Parkinson–White Syndrome

Atrial fibrillation is not very uncommon in patients with WPW syndrome.[36] The presence of multiple APs is often associated with an increased incidence of AF in patients with WPW syndrome. The characteristic features include an irregular ventricular response due to AF, an unusually rapid response due to conduction over an AP, and predominantly wide and variable QRS morphology because of variable rate-related degrees of preexcitation and varying degrees of fusion of conduction over the normal and APs (Fig. 17.17). QRS complexes of normal duration and morphology often occur in this rhythm when conduction fails in the AP and pure AV node conduction occurs. Even in hemodynamically stable patients, AF with WPW syndrome should be recognized and treated urgently because of its tendency to degenerate to VF.[36]

Preexcitation alternans: In preexcitation alternans, a QRS complex manifesting a delta wave alternates with a normal QRS complex (Fig. 17.18A). This is also a marker for an AP with a relatively long antegrade refractory period.

Intermittent preexcitation: True intermittent preexcitation is characterized by abrupt loss of the delta wave, normalization of the QRS duration, and an increase in the PR interval during a continuous ECG recording in the absence of any significant change in heart rate (Fig. 17.18B). This finding is generally a reliable sign that the AV bypass tract has a relatively long antegrade refractory period and is not capable of frequent impulse conduction.

Concertina effect: Another situation in which the AP is likely to have a relatively long refractory period is the "concertina" form of preexcitation. In this phenomenon, PR intervals and QRS complex durations show a cyclic pattern, e.g. preexcitation becomes progressively more prominent over a number of QRS complex cycles followed by a gradual diminution in the degree of preexcitation over several QRS cycles despite a fairly constant heart rate.

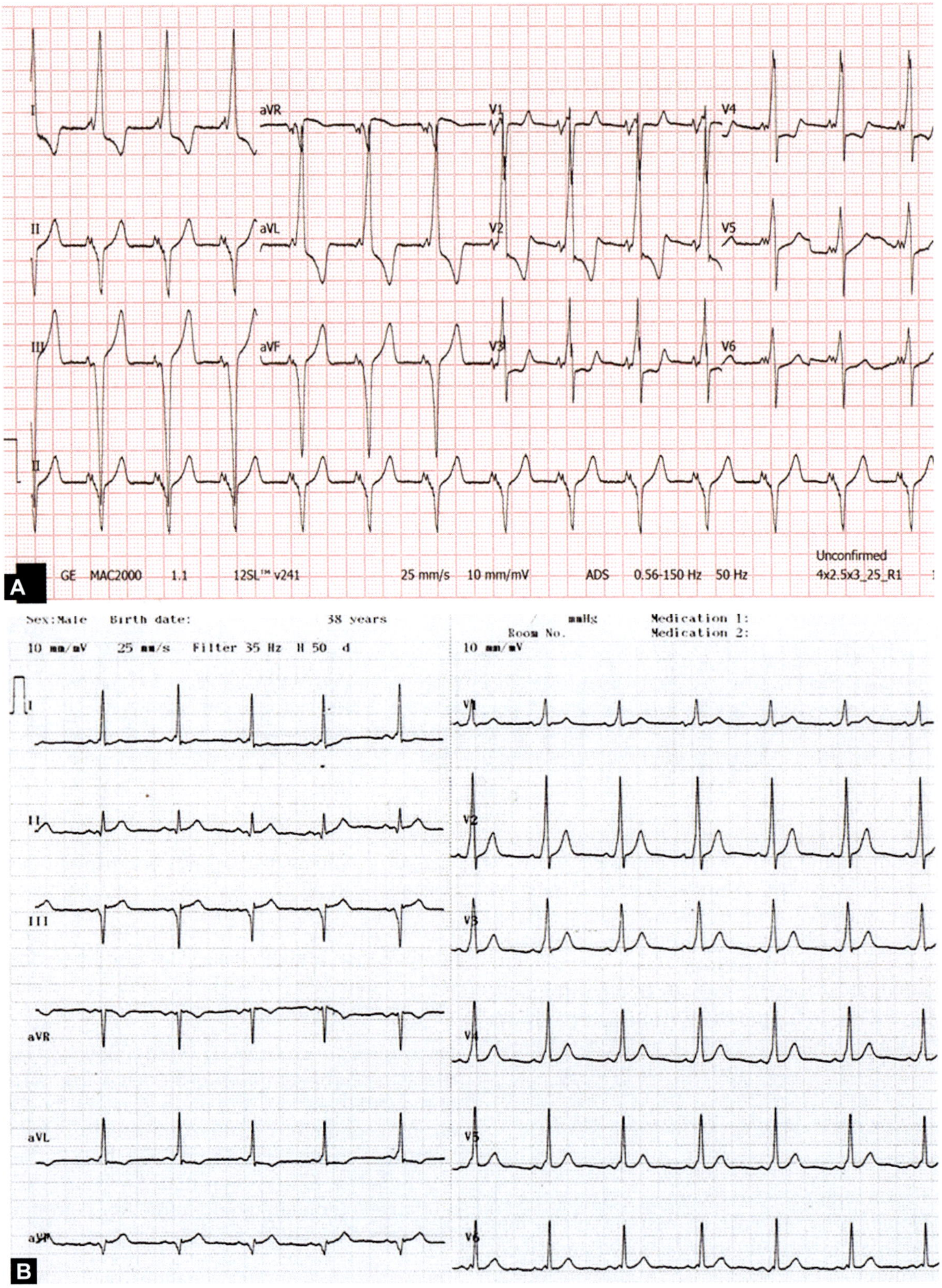

Figs. 17.16A and B: (A) This ECG illustrates an example of pseudoinfarction pattern in the ECG of WPW syndrome (type B). Presence of deep Q waves in LII, LIII, and aVF mimics old inferior myocardial infarction. But short PR interval (80 ms), presence of delta waves, and broad QRS complexes confirm the diagnosis of WPW syndrome. WPW syndrome may produce pseudoinfarction pattern due to negatively deflected delta waves in the inferior/anterior leads and these Q waves are called pseudo Q waves; and (B) ECG illustrates pseudoinfarction pattern in a patient with WPW syndrome (type A), mimicking old inferior myocardial infarction (Q in LII, LIII, and aVF). *Note:* Tall R waves in leads V1–V2 with upright T waves (mimicking posterior infarction). Pseudoinfarction pattern is due to negatively deflected delta waves in the inferior leads (pseudo Q waves). (ECG: electrocardiogram; WPW: Wolff–Parkinson–White)

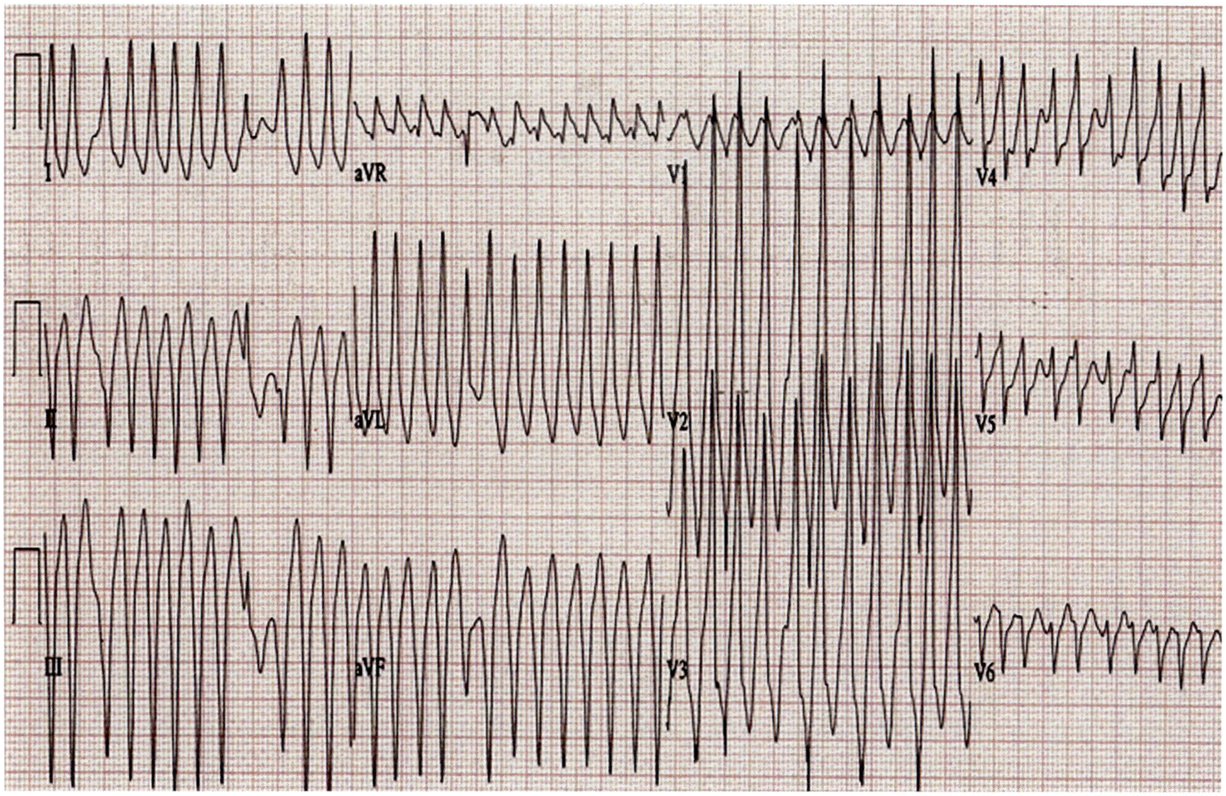

Fig. 17.17: This ECG tracing illustrates atrial fibrillation (AF) in the presence of WPW syndrome. ECG features include an irregular rapid ventricular response due to AF, an unusually rapid heart rate due to conduction over an accessory pathway, and predominantly wide and variable QRS morphology because of variable rate-related degrees of preexcitation and varying degrees of fusion of conduction over the normal and accessory pathway. (ECG: electrocardiogram; WPW: Wolff–Parkinson–White)

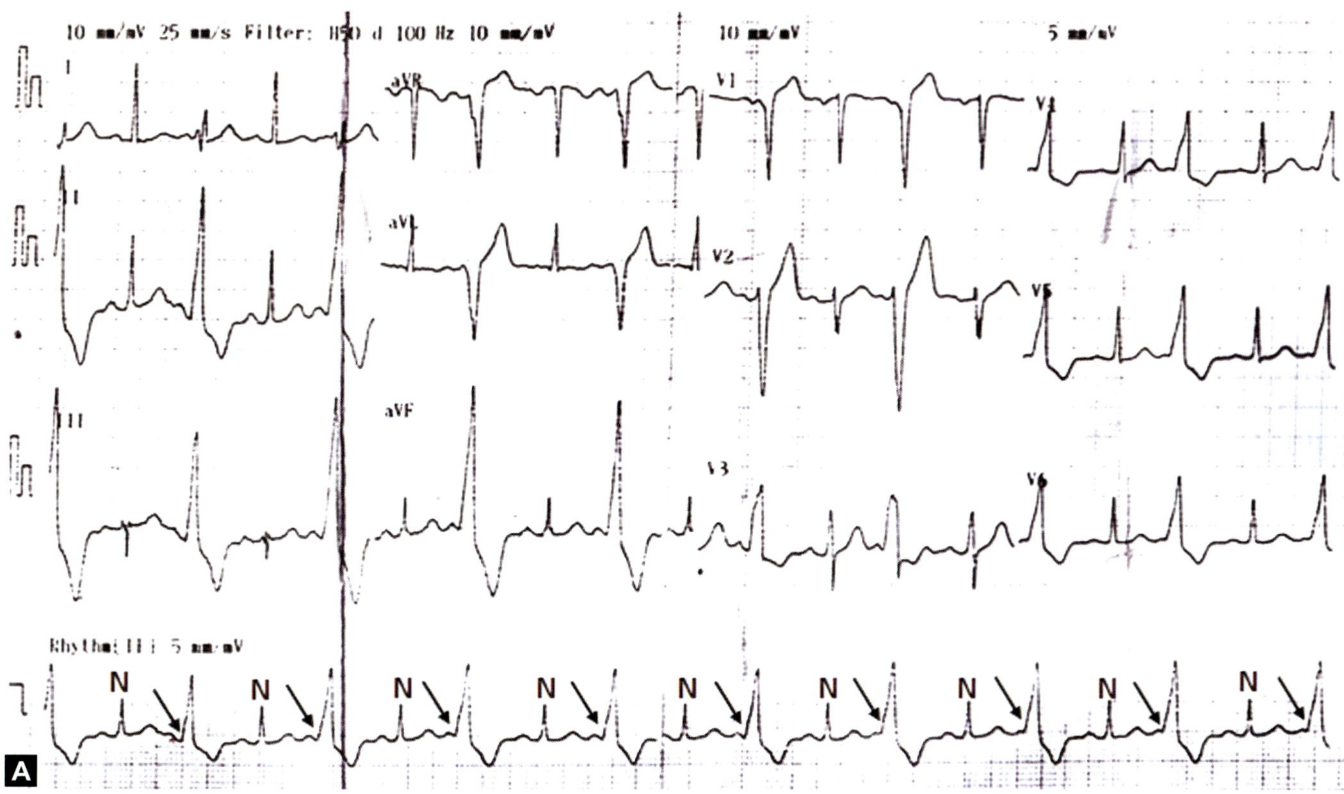

Fig. 17.18A: This electrocardiogram (ECG) illustrates an example of preexcitation alternans. *Note:* A QRS complex manifesting a delta wave (*arrows*) alternates with a normal QRS complex (*N*) without any delta wave with normal QRS configuration (*Courtesy:* Dr Mokaddas Hossain Sadi, Labaid Cardiac Hospital).

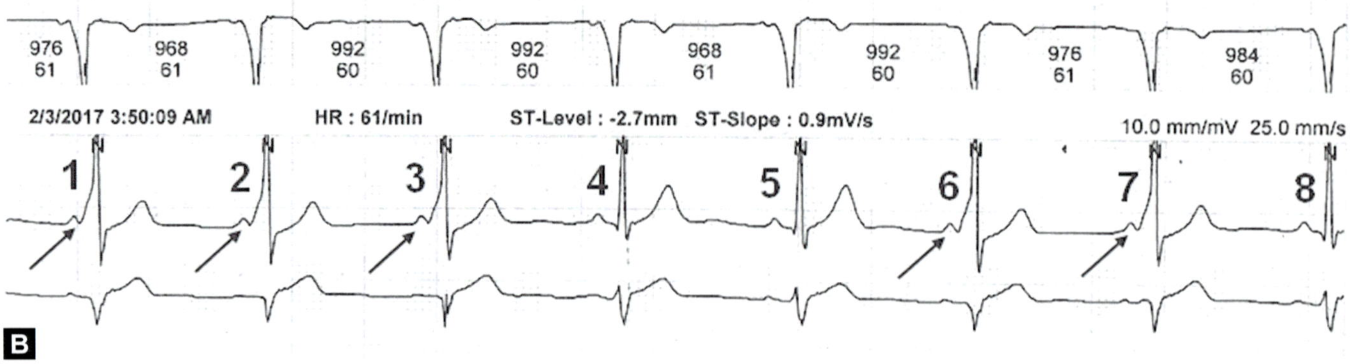

Fig. 17.18B: This ECG strip illustrates an example of intermittent preexcitation. *Note:* 1st, 2nd, 3rd, 6th, and 7th complexes show features of preexcitation (*arrows*) with short PR interval, delta wave, and broad QRS complexes but 4th, 5th, and 8th complexes show normal conduction without any preexcitation with normal PR interval, normal QRS duration, and without any delta wave.

Sudden Death in Wolff–Parkinson–White Syndrome

Several clinical observational studies of patients with ventricular preexcitation have been conducted with long follow-up periods. The main conclusions are: (a) The prevalence of ventricular preexcitation in the general population ranges between 0.1% and 0.4%; (b) Between 10% and 50% of patients are asymptomatic at the beginning of the follow-up period; (c) During long follow-up periods of between 5 years and 15 years, a minority of patients (up to one-third if they are aged less than 40 years at the beginning of the study) will experience supraventricular tachyarrhythmias, typically SVT, although a few will experience AF; (d) Sudden death is a very rare event; and (e) When sudden death occurs it is characteristically preceded by symptomatic tachyarrhythmias, such that it is virtually nonexistent in previously asymptomatic subjects as the first manifestation of the disease.[6,33,44-51] WPW syndrome accounted for approximately 1% of deaths in a long-term registry of sudden death in athletes.[52,53]

Lown–Ganong–Levine Syndrome

The LGL syndrome is a clinical syndrome consisting of paroxysms of tachycardia and ECG findings of a short PR interval and normal QRS duration (Figs. 17.19 and 20). LGL syndrome is usually categorized in a class of preexcitation syndromes that includes the WPW syndrome, LGL syndrome, and Mahaim-type preexcitation.[54] Less is known regarding the structural anomalies underlying LGL syndrome. Theories proposed to explain LGL have centered around the possible existence of intranodal or paranodal fibers that bypass all or part of the AV node. In 1938, Clerc, Levy, and Critesco first described the occurrence of frequent paroxysms of tachycardia in patients with a short PR interval and normal QRS duration.[55] This syndrome was again described in 1952 by Lown, Ganong, and Levine, whose names form the eponym now used to describe it.[56] James described fibers that originate in the low atrium and terminate low in the AV node.[57]

Historically, some authors have referred to patients with a short PR interval and normal QRS duration as having LGL syndrome. However, this practice has been largely abandoned as more evidence has accumulated demonstrating that such patients without a history of tachycardia likely fall into a class of normal variants. Patients with an isolated finding of short PR interval may be characterized as having enhanced atrioventricular nodal conduction (EAVNC).[58]

Criteria for LGL syndrome include a PR interval less than or equal to 120 ms (0.12 seconds), normal QRS complex duration of less than 120 ms (0.12 seconds) without any delta wave, and occurrence of a clinical tachycardia.

Mahaim-type Preexcitation

In 1937, during pathologic examination of the heart, Mahaim and Benatt identified islands of conducting tissue extending from the His bundle tissue into the ventricular myocardium. These fibers were termed Mahaim or fasciculoventricular fibers.[59] This description was subsequently expanded to include connections between the AV node and the ventricular myocardium (nodoventricular fibers). These findings have been confirmed by other investigators, but true continuity of these pathways is less common than was initially suspected.[60,61]

Patients with Mahaim fibers form a distinct subgroup of the preexcitation syndromes (less than 3% of all preexcitation syndromes).[62] Originally, Mahaim fibers have been classified into two main groups: (1) Nodoventricular and (2) Fasciculoventricular fibers. The preexcited tachycardia (antidromic reentrant tachycardia) is distinctive with a left bundle branch block (LBBB) pattern.[62] Paroxysmal tachycardia with widened QRS complexes have been documented with Mahaim fibers preexcitation.[63] The majority of these patients do not have episodes of narrow QRS complex, due to the absence of retrograde conduction of the AP. Mahaim preexcitation gives rise to LBBB pattern tachycardia.[61]

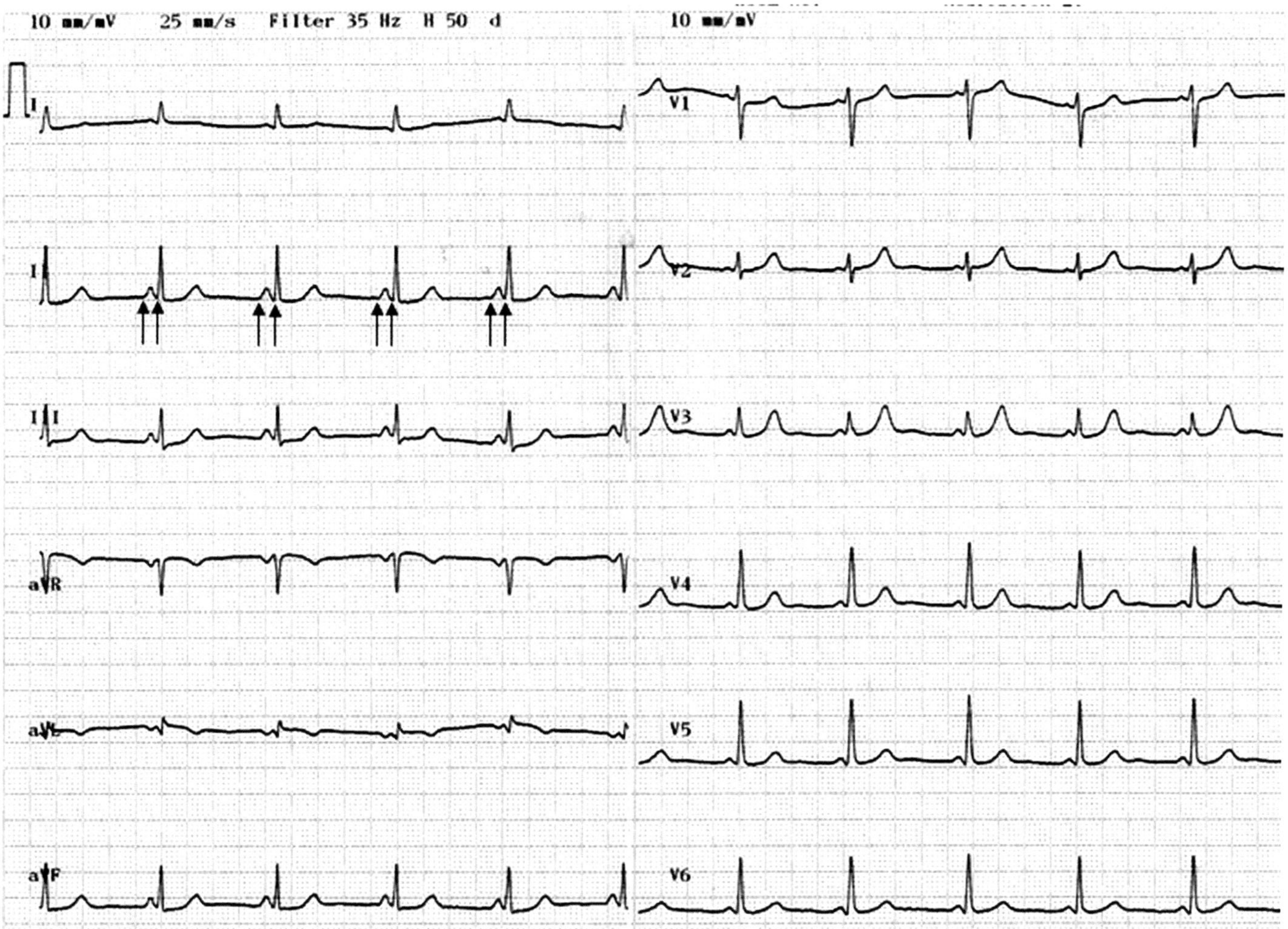

Fig. 17.19: ECG of LGL syndrome with short PR interval, 80 ms (0.08 seconds) (*arrows*), without any delta wave. QRS morphology is normal. (ECG: electrocardiogram; LGL: Lown–Ganong–Levine)

If Mahaim fibers are present, the ECG findings are a normal or long PR interval and an abnormally wide QRS complex with a delta wave (Figs. 17.21A and B). Preexcitation may not be apparent during sinus rhythm but can be demonstrated with premature right atrial stimulation, so presence of delta wave may be intermittent.

During sinus rhythm overt pre-excitation may be absent. Only subtle ECG abnormalities, such as an rS pattern in lead III, absence of septal Q waves in leads I and V6, and terminal QRS slurring or notching, suggest the presence of Mahaim conduction. However, patients with short, rapidly conducting fibres may have typical pre-excitation.[64]

Characteristics of Mahaim Tachycardia

- Right-sided APs connecting either AV node to ventricles, fascicles to ventricles, or atria to fascicles.
- Decremental conduction—usually antegrade only.
- Delta wave may be permanent or intermittent on surface ECG.
- Can support an antidromic reciprocating tachycardia using Mahaim fibers as the antegrade limb and AV node as the retrograde limb, resulting in a wide QRS tachycardia of LBBB morphology.

SUMMARY

Preexcitation syndromes are defined as a congenital condition involving abnormal conductive tissue between the atria and the ventricles that provides a pathway for a reentrant tachycardia circuit. The prevalence of ventricular preexcitation in the general population ranges between 0.1 and 0.4%.

Wolff–Parkinson–White syndrome is the most common of the ventricular preexcitation syndromes. Others include LGL syndrome and Mahaim-type preexcitation. They are important because of the association with paroxysmal tachycardias that can result in serious cardiovascular complications and sudden death. In ECG terms they are important to recognize, because of the risk of misdiagnosis. Investigations into WPW syndrome have revealed that an AP for conduction, called a bundle of Kent, from the atria to the ventricles underlies the preexcitation observed in patients with WPW syndrome.

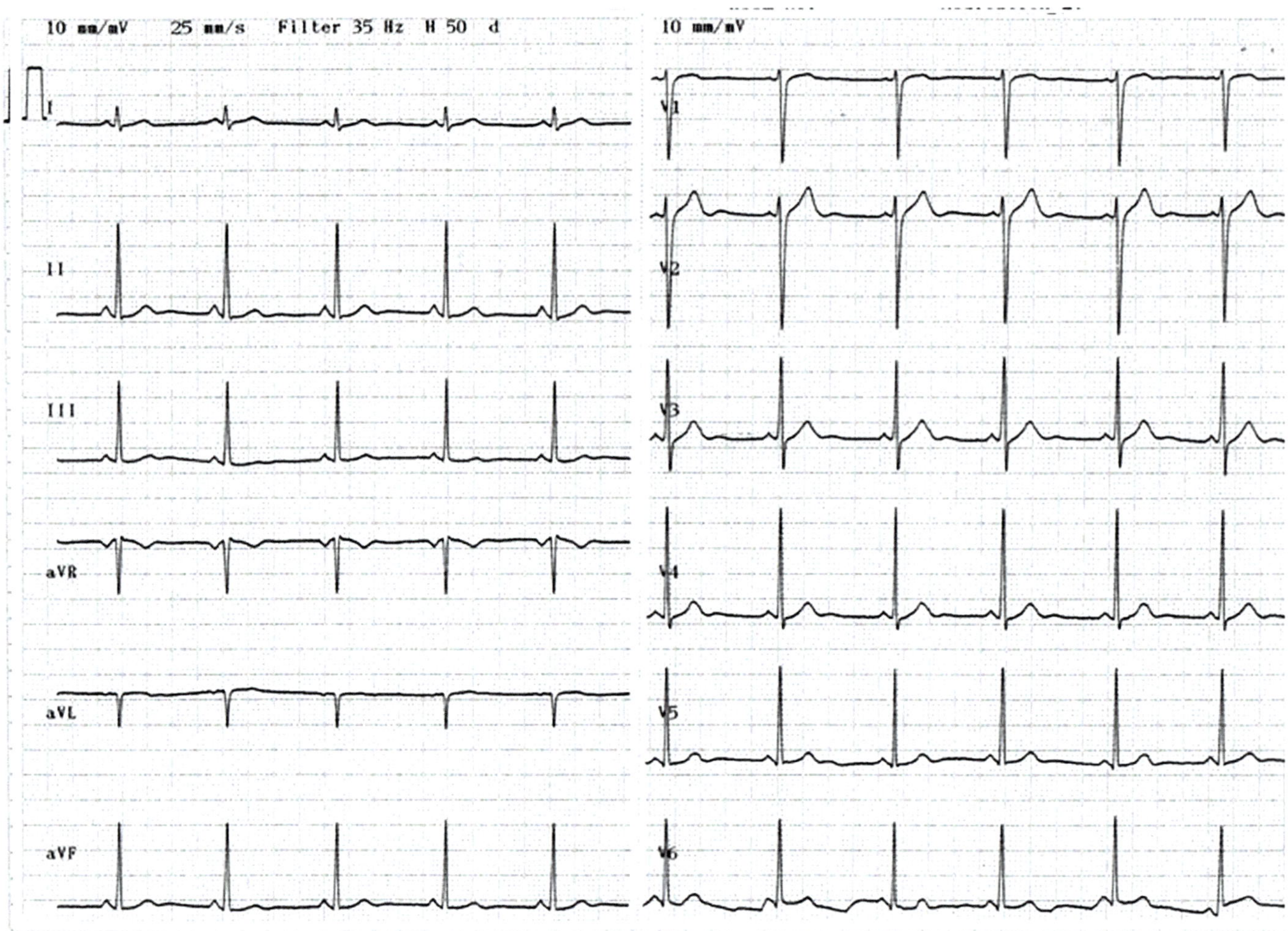

Fig. 17.20: This ECG illustrates a typical LGL syndrome with short PR interval, normal QRS complex morphology, and no delta wave. (ECG: electrocardiogram; LGL: Lown–Ganong–Levine)

Most of the subjects with preexcitation syndromes do not have any structural heart disease but 7–20% of patients with this condition are associated with CHD. Ventricular preexcitation is most often associated with Ebstein anomaly, HCM, d-TGA, l-TGA, pulmonary atresia/intact ventricular septum, PDA, parachute mitral valve, TOF, TAPVC, and VSD.

Diagnostic Criteria of Different Patterns of Preexcitation Syndromes

The diagnostic ECG criteria of different patterns of preexcitation syndromes are illustrated in Table 17.1.

Although the ECG morphology varies widely, the classic ECG features of WPW syndrome are as follows:

- A shortened PR interval, less than 120 ms (<0.12 seconds).
- A slurring and slow rise of the initial upstroke of the QRS complex (delta wave).
- A widened QRS complex, total duration more than 120 ms (>0.12 seconds).
- ST segment-T wave changes, generally directed opposite the major delta wave and QRS complex.

Accessory pathways those are capable of only retrograde conduction are referred to as "concealed", whereas those capable of antegrade conduction are "manifest", demonstrating preexcitation on a standard ECG. Manifest APs usually conduct in both antegrade and retrograde directions. It is important to note that if the AP only conducts retrogradely (ventriculoatrial) the resting ECG will be normal in sinus rhythm with no evidence of preexcitation. This is known as a concealed pathway.

Supraventricular tachycardia is the most common type of arrhythmia documented in WPW syndrome. It can be orthodromic or antidromic. Orthodromic tachycardia has a narrow QRS complex and is the most common variety accounting for 90%. The remaining 10% is antidromic and has a wide QRS. In orthodromic tachycardia the impulse travels down the normal AV pathway into the ventricle and back into the atrium through the AP. Vice versa occurs in antidromic tachycardia. Antidromic tachycardia is often mistaken for VT due to the wide QRS. It may be noted that preexcitation (delta wave) does not manifest during orthodromic tachycardia. Hence a diagnosis of WPW syndrome usually cannot be made during the tachycardia. An ECG taken after termination of the tachycardia will

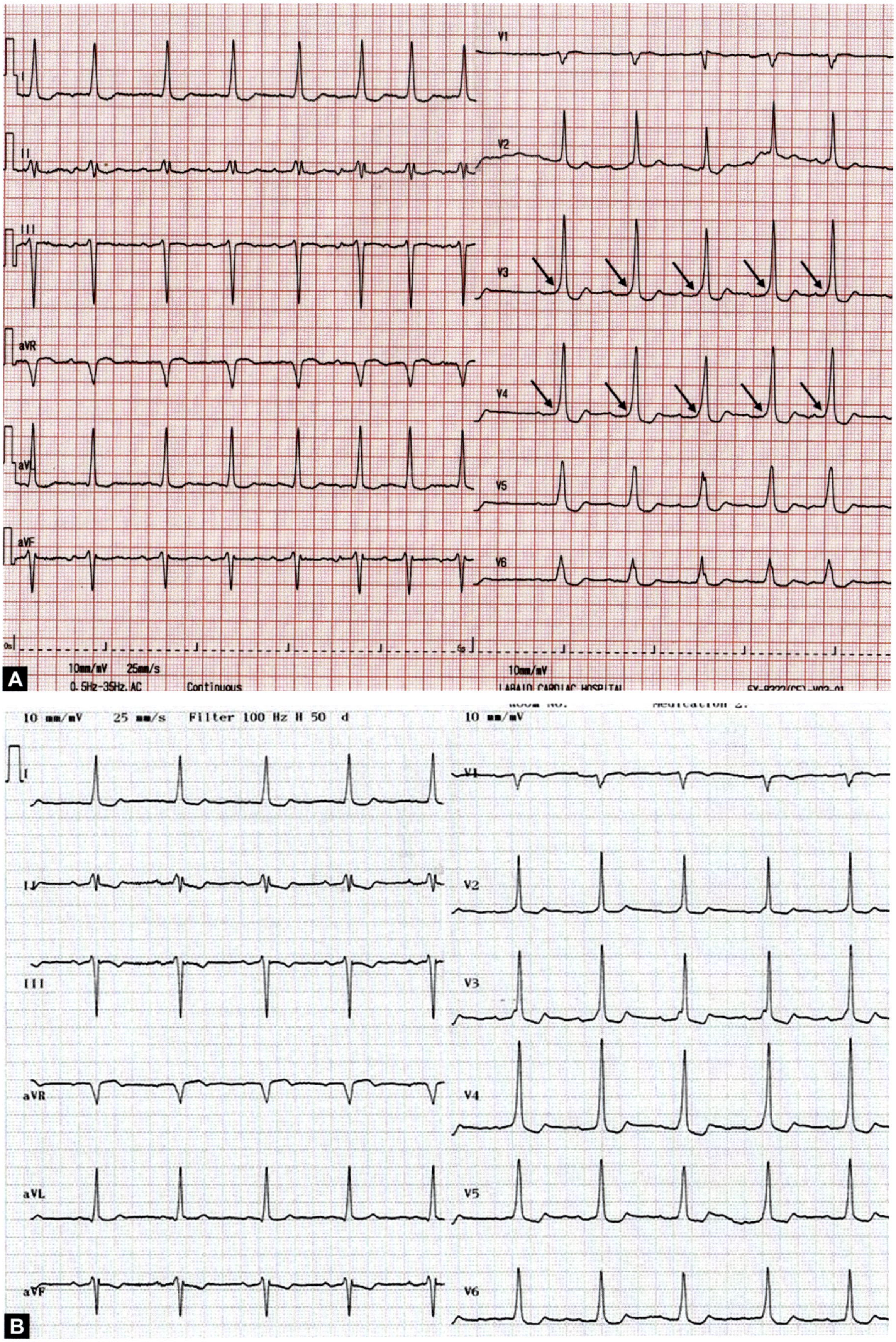

Figs. 17.21A and B: (A) This electrocardiogram (ECG) illustrates Mahaim preexcitation pattern with prolonged PR interval (PR 240 ms) with delta waves (*arrows*) and broad QRS complex (QRS duration 135 ms); and (B) This ECG illustrates possible Mahaim preexcitation with normal PR interval 180 ms (0.18 seconds) with delta waves and mildly broad QRS complex.

Table 17.1: Diagnostic criteria of different patterns of preexcitation syndromes.

Type	*Accessory pathway*	*PR interval*	*QRS duration*	*Delta wave*
Wolff–Parkinson–White syndrome	Bundle of Kent (atria to ventricles)	Short	Long	Yes
Lown–Ganong–Levine syndrome	James bundle [atria to low atrioventricular (AV) node or bundle of His]	Short	Normal	No
Mahaim-type preexcitation	Mahaim fibers (atriofascicular, nodoventricular, and fasciculoventricular pathways)	Normal or prolonged	Long	Yes

show the delta wave so that it is mandatory to take an ECG after termination of SVT. AF is the next common type of arrhythmia documented.

Wolff–Parkinson–White syndrome may be described as type A or B.

- Type A has a positive delta wave in precordial leads, producing a dominant R wave in lead V1 (R/S > 1 in V1).
- Type B has a negative delta wave in leads V1 and V2 and QRS complexes are predominantly negative in leads V1 and V2.

The type A may be confused with true posterior infarction or right ventricular hypertrophy and the type B with anteroseptal infarction. Type A pattern was initially thought to indicate a left ventricular bypass tract and type B, right ventricular bypass. But more recently, it has been shown that bypass tracts are widely distributed and transmit impulses at any point around the AV ring or in the septum and the location of bypass cannot be accomplished accurately by merely documenting type A or type B pattern.

Arrhythmias in Patients with Wolff–Parkinson–White Syndrome

- Supraventricular tachycardia—most common
- Atrial fibrillation
- Malignant ventricular arrhythmias (VT/VF)—rare.

Orthodromic Supraventricular Tachycardia

- Regular and narrow complex rhythm. Most common tachyarrhythmia documented in WPW syndrome.
- Conduction down the normal AV nodal pathway and back up to atrium through an AP.

Antidromic Supraventricular Tachycardia

- Regular and wide complex rhythm.
- Conduction down the AP and back up to atrium through the AV node.

Electrocardiogram Difference between Atrioventricular Reentrant Tachycardia (AVRT) and Atrioventricular Nodal Reentrant Tachycardia (AVNRT)

A visible P wave is usually uncommon in AVNRT. Classically on surface ECG of narrow complex tachycardia, visibility of P waves favor AVRT and is suggestive of the presence of an AP with antegrade conduction via the AV node and retrograde conduction via AP. Retrograde P waves immediately preceding the T waves or inverted P waves may be visible deforming the ST segment in AVRT. In a patient with a narrow complex tachycardia the presence of such late P waves is frequently the only ECG evidence that the patient has AVRT rather than AVNRT.

Pseudoinfarction Pattern of Electrocardiogram in Presence of Wolff–Parkinson–White Syndrome

In presence of WPW syndrome ECG diagnosis of coronary artery disease may be difficult. This is because WPW syndrome may mask the underlying electrocardiographic abnormalities or may simulate other cardiac disorders.

Wolff–Parkinson–White syndrome may produce pseudoinfarction pattern due to negatively deflected delta waves in the inferior/anterior leads (pseudo Q waves), or as a prominent R wave in V1–3 mimicking posterior infarction. Bedside echocardiogram may confirm the diagnosis if the ECG interpretation proves misleading in this situation.

The incidence of sudden cardiac death in patients with the WPW syndrome is very rare. It is unusual for cardiac arrest to be the first symptomatic manifestation of WPW syndrome.

Lown–Ganong–Levine Syndrome

The LGL syndrome is characterized by the presence of:

- Short PR interval
- Normal QRS complex on the ECG
- No delta wave.

This finding may represent a perinodal AP or enhanced AV nodal conduction. The incidence of paroxysmal SVT is significantly higher in these patients when compared to a control group with a normal PR interval.

Mahaim-type Preexcitation

Right-sided APs connecting either AV node to ventricles, fascicles to ventricles, or atria to fascicles.

Electrocardiogram features include:

- Normal or prolonged PR interval.
- Delta wave is usually present but delta wave may be intermittent.

- Broad QRS complex. May result in variation in QRS morphology.
- Reentry tachycardia typically of wide complex and has LBBB morphology.

REFERENCES

1. Kent AF. The structure of cardiac tissues at the auricular ventricular junction: proceedings of the Physiological Society. J Physiol (Lond). 1913;47:17-9.
2. Wolff L, Parkinson J, White PD. Bundle-branch block with short P-R interval in healthy young people prone to paroxysmal tachycardia. Am Heart J. 1930;5(6):685-704.
3. Holzman M, Scherf D. Uber Elektrokardiogramme met verkurzter vorhof-kammer distanz und positiven P zachen. Ztschr Klin Med. 1932;121:404-23.
4. Öhnell RF. Pre-excitation, cardiac abnormality, patho-physiological, patho-anatomical and clinical studies of excitatory spread phenomenon bearing upon the problem of the WPW (Wolff, Parkinson, and White) electrocardiogram and paroxysmal tachycardia. Acta Med Scand. 1944;152:1-167.
5. Wood FC, Wolferth CC, Geckeler GD. Histologic demonstration of accessory muscular connections between auricle and ventricle in a case of short P-R interval and prolonged QRS complex. Am Heart J. 1943;25(4):454-62.
6. Almendral J, Castellanos E, Ortiz. M. Paroxysmal supraventricular tachycardias and preexcitation syndromes. Rev Esp Cardiol. 2012;65(5):456-69.
7. Keating L, Morris FP, Brady WJ. Electrocardiographic features of Wolff-Parkinson-White syndrome. Emerg Med J. 2003;20(5):491-3.
8. Colovita PG, Packer DL, Pressley JC, et al. Frequency, diagnosis and clinical characteristics of patients with multiple accessory atrioventricular pathways. Am J Cardiol. 1987;59:601-6.
9. Blomström-Lundqvist C, Scheinman MM, Aliot EM, et al. ACC/AHA/ESC guidelines for the management of patients with supraventricular arrhythmias—executive summary. Eur Heart J. 2003;24:1857-97.
10. Deal BJ, Keane JF, Gillette PC, et al. Wolff-Parkinson-White syndrome and supraventricular tachycardia during infancy: management and follow-up. J Am Coll Cardiol. 1985;5(1):130-5.
11. Massumi RA. Familial Wolff-Parkinson-White syndrome with cardiomyopathy. Am J Med. 1967;43(6):951-5.
12. Vidaillet HJ, Pressley JC, Henke E, et al. Familial occurrence of accessory atrioventricular pathways (preexcitation syndrome). N Engl J Med. 1987;317(2):65-9.
13. MacRae CA, Ghaisas N, Kass S, et al. Familial hypertrophic cardiomyopathy with Wolff-Parkinson-White syndrome maps to a locus on chromosome 7q3. J Clin Invest. 1995;96(3):1216-20.
14. Gollob MH, Green MS, Tang AS, et al. Identification of a gene responsible for familial Wolff-Parkinson-White syndrome. N Engl J Med. 2001;344(24):1823-31.
15. Al-Khatib SM, Pritchett EL. Clinical features of Wolff-Parkinson-White syndrome. Am Heart J. 1999;138(3 Pt 1):403-13.
16. Gaita F, Giustetto C, Riccardi R, et al. Wolff-Parkinson-White syndrome. Identification and management. Drugs. 1992;43(2):185-200.
17. Hummel JD, Kalbfleisch SJ, Dillon JM. Pocket Guide for Cardiac Electrophysiology, 1st edition. Philadelphia: Saunders; 1999.
18. Ehtisham J, Watkins H. Is Wolff-Parkinson-White syndrome a genetic disease? J Cardiovasc Electrophysiol. 2005;16(11):1258-62.
19. Katritsis DG, Camm AJ. Atrioventricular nodal reentrant tachycardia. Circulation. 2010;122(8):831-40.
20. Van Hare GF, Lesh MD, Stanger P. Radiofrequency catheter ablation of supraventricular arrhythmias in patients with congenital heart disease: results and technical considerations. J Am Coll Cardiol. 1993;22(3):883-90.
21. Pressley JC, Wharton JM, Tang AS, et al. Effect of Ebstein's anomaly on short- and long-term outcome of surgically treated patients with Wolff-Parkinson-White syndrome. Circulation. 1992;86(4):1147-55.
22. Delhaas T, Sarvaas GJ, Rijlaarsdam ME, et al. A multicenter, long-term study on arrhythmias in children with Ebstein anomaly. Pediatr Cardiol. 2010;31(2):229-33.
23. Levine JC, Walsh EP, Saul JP. Radiofrequency ablation of accessory pathways associated with congenital heart disease including heterotaxy syndrome. Am J Cardiol. 1993;72(9):689-93.
24. Surawicz B, Childers R, Deal BJ, et al. AHA/ACCF/HRS recommendations for the standardization and interpretation of the electrocardiogram: part III: intraventricular conduction disturbances: a scientific statement from the American Heart Association Electrocardiography and Arrhythmias Committee, Council on Clinical Cardiology; the American College of Cardiology Foundation; and the Heart Rhythm Society: endorsed by the International Society for Computerized Electrocardiology. Circulation. 2009;119(10):e235-40.
25. Robinson K, Rowland E, Krikler DM. Latent pre-excitation: exposure of anterograde accessory pathway conduction during atrial fibrillation. Br Heart J. 1988;59(1):53-5.
26. Perosio AM, Suarez LD, Bunster AM, et al. Pre-excitation syndrome and hypertrophic cardiomyopathy. J Electrocardiol. 1983;16(1):29-40.
27. Goldberger AL. Pseudo-infarct patterns in the Wolff-Parkinson-White syndrome: importance of Q wave-T wave vector discordance. J Electrocardiol. 1980;13(2):115-8.
28. Klein GJ, Bashore TM, Sellers TD, et al. Ventricular fibrillation in the Wolff-Parkinson-White syndrome. N Engl J Med. 1979;301:1080-5.
29. Bogun F, Kalusche D, Li YG, et al. Septal Q waves in surface electrographic lead V6 exclude minimal ventricular preexcitation. Am J Cardiol. 1999;84(1):101-4.
30. Eisenberger M, Davidson NC, Todd DM, et al. A new approach to confirming or excluding ventricular pre-excitation on a 12-lead ECG. Europace. 2010;12(1):119-23.
31. Kulig J, Koplan BA. Wolff-Parkinson-White syndrome and accessory pathways. Circulation. 2010;122:e480-3.
32. Kuck KH, Friday KJ, Kunze KP, et al. Sites of conduction block in accessory atrioventricular pathways. Basis for concealed accessory pathways. Circulation. 1990;82(2):407-17.
33. Sethi KK, Dhall A, Chadha DS, et al. WPW and preexcitation syndromes. J Assoc Physicians India. 2007;55 Suppl:10-5.
34. Katritsis DG. Wolff–Parkinson–White syndrome and antidromic atrioventricular reentrant tachycardia. Europace. 2013;15(6):779-80.

35. Erdem A, Madak N, Yilmaz A, et al. Development of malignant ventricular arrhythmias in a young male with WPW pattern. Indian Pacing Electrophysiol J. 2010;10(4): 195-200.
36. Rahman MM, Khan MM, Kamal N, et al. Clinical and demographic characteristics of WPW syndrome attending arrhythmia clinic of NICVD. Bangladesh Med J. 2012;41(2): 50-3.
37. Pappone C, Vicedomini G, Manguso F, et al. Risk of malignant arrhythmias in initially symptomatic patients with Wolff-Parkinson-White syndrome: results of a prospective long-term electrophysiological follow-up study. Circulation. 2012;125(5):661-8.
38. Butcovan D. Myocardial infarction in an individual with Wolff-Parkinson-White syndrome. Rom J Leg Med. 2013;21:1-4.
39. Lustik SJ, Wojtczak J, Chhibber AK. Wolff-Parkinson-White syndrome simulating inferior myocardial infarction in a cocaine abuser for urgent dilation and evacuation of the uterus. Anesth Analg. 1999;89(3):609-12.
40. Yusuf A. Wolff-Parkinson-White syndrome mimicking ischemia of inferolateral wall. In: Weyman AE (Ed). Principles and Practice of Echocardiography, 2nd edition. Philadelphia: Lippincott Williams & Wilkins; 1993. pp. 656-86.
41. Mark DG, Brady WJ, Pines JM. Preexcitation syndromes: diagnostic consideration in the ED. Am J Emerg Med. 2009;27(7):878-88.
42. Taguchi N, Yoshida N, Inden Y, et al. A simple algorithm for localizing accessory pathways in patients with Wolff-Parkinson-White syndrome using only the R/S ratio. J Arrhythmia. 2014;30(6):439-43.
43. Arruda MS, McClelland JH, Wang X, et al. Development and validation of an ECG algorithm for identifying accessory pathway ablation site in Wolff-Parkinson-White syndrome. J Cardiovasc Electrophysiol. 1998;9(1):2-12.
44. Berkman NL, Lamb LE. The Wolff-Parkinson-White electrocardiogram. A follow-up study of five to twenty-eight years. N Engl J Med. 1968;278(9):492-4.
45. Soria R, Guize L, Chretien JM, et al. The natural history of 270 cases of Wolff-Parkinson-White syndrome in a survey of the general population. Arch Mal Coeur Vaiss. 1989;82(3):331-6.
46. Munger TM, Packer DL, Hammill SC, et al. A population study of the natural history of Wolff-Parkinson-White syndrome in Olmsted County, Minnesota, 1953-1989. Circulation. 1993;87(3):866-73.
47. Goudevenos JA, Katsouras CS, Graekas G, et al. Ventricular pre-excitation in the general population: a study on the mode of presentation and clinical course. Heart. 2000;83(1):29-34.
48. Fitzsimmons PJ, McWhirter PD, Peterson DW, et al. The natural history of Wolff-Parkinson-White syndrome in 228 military aviators: a long-term follow-up of 22 years. Am Heart J. 2001;142(3):530-6.
49. Todd DM, Klein GJ, Krahn AD, et al. Asymptomatic Wolff-Parkinson-White syndrome: is it time to revisit guidelines? J Am Coll Cardiol. 2003;41(2):245-8.
50. Santinelli V, Radinovic A, Manguso F, et al. Asymptomatic ventricular preexcitation: a long-term prospective follow-up study of 293 adult patients. Circ Arrhythm Electrophysiol. 2009;2(2):102-7.
51. Santinelli V, Radinovic A, Manguso F, et al. The natural history of asymptomatic ventricular pre-excitation a long-term prospective follow-up study of 184 asymptomatic children. J Am Coll Cardiol. 2009;53(3):275-80.
52. Maron BJ, Doerer JJ, Haas TS, et al. Sudden deaths in young competitive athletes: analysis of 1866 deaths in the United States, 1980-2006. Circulation. 2009;119(8):1085-92.
53. Pediatric and Congenital Electrophysiology Society (PACES), Heart Rhythm Society (HRS), American College of Cardiology Foundation (ACCF), et al. PACES/HRS expert consensus statement on the management of the asymptomatic young patient with a Wolff-Parkinson-White (WPW, ventricular preexcitation) electrocardiographic pattern: developed in partnership between the Pediatric and Congenital Electrophysiology Society (PACES) and the Heart Rhythm Society (HRS). Endorsed by the governing bodies of PACES, HRS, the American College of Cardiology Foundation (ACCF), the American Heart Association (AHA), the American Academy of Pediatrics (AAP), and the Canadian Heart Rhythm Society (CHRS). Heart Rhythm. 2012;9(6):1006-24.
54. Derejko P, Szumowski LJ, Sanders P, et al. Atrial fibrillation in patients with Wolff-Parkinson-White syndrome: role of pulmonary veins. J Cardiovasc Electrophysiol. 2012;23(3):280-6.
55. Clerc A, Levy R, Critesco C. A propos du raccourcissement permanent de l'espace P-R de l'electrocardiogramme sans deformation du complex ventriculaire. Arch Mal Coeur. 1938;31:569.
56. Lown B, Ganong WF, Levine SA. The syndrome of short P-R interval, normal QRS complex and paroxysmal rapid heart action. Circulation. 1952;5(5):693-706.
57. James TN. Morphology of the human atrioventricular node, with remarks pertinent to its electrophysiology. Am Heart J. 1961;62:756-71.
58. Jackman WM, Prystowsky EN, Naccarelli GV, et al. Reevaluation of enhanced atrioventricular nodal conduction: evidence to suggest a continuum of normal atrioventricular nodal physiology. Circulation. 1983;67(2):441-8.
59. Mahaim I, Benatt A. Nouvelles recherches sur les connexions supérieures de la branche gauche du faisceau de His-Tawara avec la cloison interventriculaire. Cardiologia. 1937;1:61-73.
60. Anderson RH, Becker AE, Brechenmacher C, et al. Ventricular preexcitation. A proposed nomenclature for its substrates. Eur J Cardiol. 1975;3(1):27-36.
61. Lev M, Lerner R. The theory of Kent; a histologic study of the normal atrioventricular communications of the human heart. Circulation. 1955;12(2):176-84.
62. Aliot E, de Chillou C, Revault d'Allones G, et al. Mahaim tachycardias. Eur Heart J. 1998;19 Suppl E:E25-31, E52-3.
63. Komatsu C, Ito K, Ishinaga T, et al. AV nodal reentrant tachycardia with Mahaim fiber conduction. Jpn Heart J. 1989;30(6):817-25.
64. Katritsis DG, Wellens HJ, Josephson ME. Mahaim Accessory Pathways.Arrhythm Electrophysiol Rev. 2017; 6(1):29-32.

Chapter

18

Electrocardiographic Diagnosis of Cardiomyopathies

INTRODUCTION

In 1980, the World Health Organization (WHO) defined cardiomyopathies as "heart muscle diseases of unknown cause" to distinguish cardiomyopathy from cardiac dysfunction due to known cardiovascular entities such as hypertension, ischemic heart disease, or valvular disease. In strict sense, cardiomyopathies are primary heart muscle diseases of unknown causes and current major society definitions of cardiomyopathy exclude heart diseases secondary to known cardiovascular disorders. But in clinical practice, however, the term "cardiomyopathy" has also been applied to diseases of known cardiovascular cause, e.g. "ischemic cardiomyopathy" and "hypertensive cardiomyopathy".[1,2] As a result, the 1995 WHO/International Society and Federation of Cardiology (ISFC) task force on the definition and classification of the cardiomyopathies expanded the classification to include all diseases affecting heart muscle and to take into consideration etiology as well as the dominant pathophysiology.[1-4] In this 1995 classification, the cardiomyopathies were defined as "diseases of the myocardium associated with cardiac dysfunction".

Cardiomyopathies are classified into the following types:[5]

1. Hypertrophic cardiomyopathy (HCM)
2. Dilated cardiomyopathy (DCM)
3. Restrictive cardiomyopathy (RCM)
4. Arrhythmogenic right ventricular cardiomyopathy/dysplasia (ARVC/D).
5. Unclassified, e.g. left ventricular noncompaction (LVNC), Takotsubo cardiomyopathy.

HYPERTROPHIC CARDIOMYOPATHY

Hypertrophic cardiomyopathy is a genetic disorder of cardiac muscle with a prevalence of 1 in 500 of the general population. In most adults, HCM is inherited as an autosomal dominant trait caused by mutations in genes encoding cardiac sarcomere proteins. The disease is clinically defined by left ventricular hypertrophy (LVH) unexplained by abnormal loading conditions, and is often associated with left ventricular outflow tract (LVOT) obstruction caused by the systolic anterior movement of the mitral valve. Histologically, HCM is characterized by cardiomyocyte hypertrophy and disarray, myocardial fibrosis, and small vessel disease.[6-8] HCM is associated with sudden cardiac death (SCD). The mortality rate is approximately 1%.[9] HCM is the most common cause of SCD in young people.[10] In 75–95% of HCM patients, electrocardiogram (ECG) shows changes in the form of LVH.[9,10] The clinical diagnosis of HCM is conventionally made with cardiac imaging, most commonly with echocardiography (Figs. 18.1 and 18.2). There are three patterns of HCM and include (1) asymmetrical septal hypertrophy (ASH)—70%, (2) concentric hypertrophy—20%, and (3) apical cardiomyopathy—10%. When HCM is associated with LVOT obstruction then it is called hypertrophic obstructive cardiomyopathy (HOCM). Around 75% of HCM is not associated with LVOT obstruction.

Over 90% of patients with HCM will have an abnormal ECG.[11,12] ECG abnormalities include voltage criteria of LVH associated with ST- and T-wave changes, T-wave inversions (TWIs), ST-segment depression, pathological Q waves, conduction delay, left-axis deviation (LAD), and left atrial enlargement (LAE) (Figs. 18.3A to C). There is an association between HCM and Wolff-Parkinson-White (WPW) syndrome. ECG features of WPW syndrome are seen in up to 5–10% of patients with HCM (Fig. 18.4).[13]

ST-segment elevation has also been documented in ECG of patients with HCM but it is rare.[14-17]

1. *Voltage criteria for LVH*: Voltage criteria for LVH are commonly identified in individuals with HCM (Figs. 18.3A to C and 18.4). However, the presence of isolated increased QRS voltage in the absence of other ECG abnormalities is uncommon and present in less than 2% of individuals with the HCM. The isolated presence of high QRS voltages fulfilling voltage criterion for LVH is regarded as a normal finding in athletes related to physiological increases in cardiac chamber size and/or wall thickness and does not in itself require

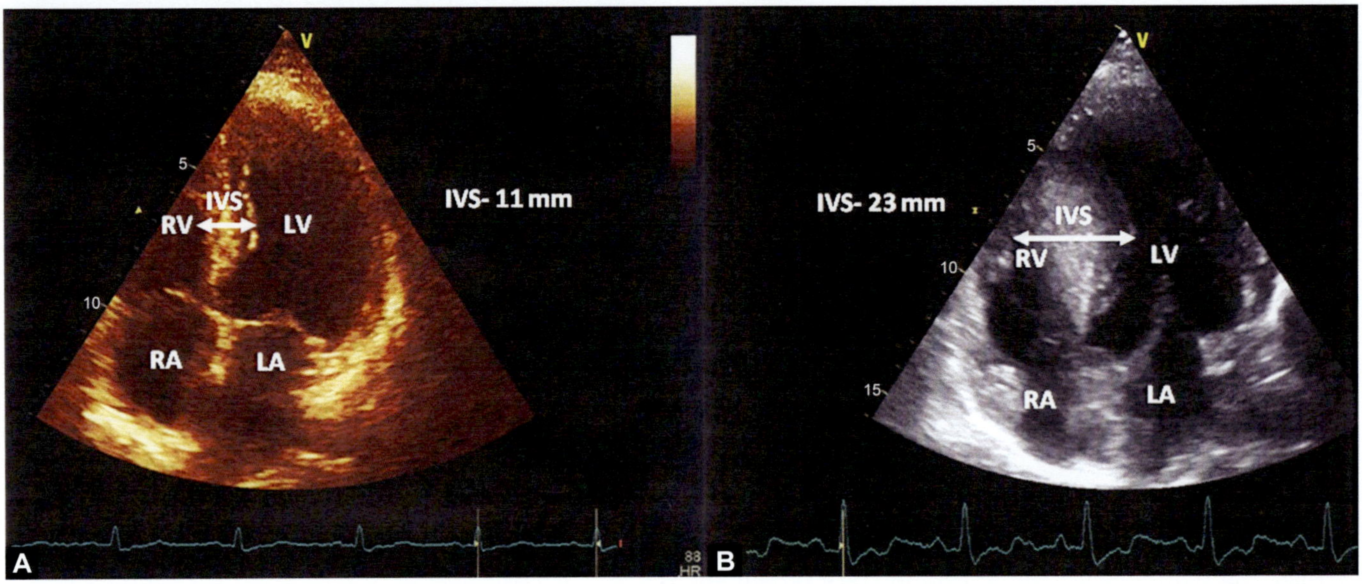

Figs. 18.1A and B: Two-dimensional echocardiography (apical 4-chamber view) showing interventricular septum (IVS) thickness (arrows) in (A) normal and (B) hypertrophic cardiomyopathy. (*Source:* Courtesy of Dr AHM Abul Monsur)

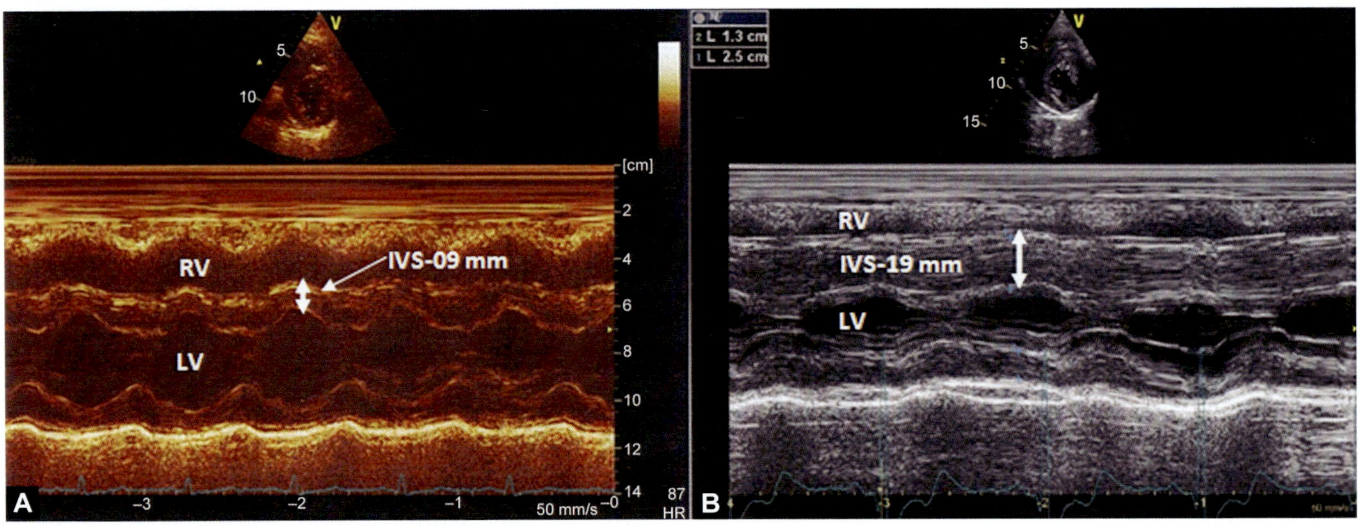

Figs. 18.2A and B: M-mode echocardiography showing interventricular septum (IVS) thickness (arrows) in (A) normal and (B) hypertrophic cardiomyopathy. (*Source:* Courtesy of Dr AHM Abul Monsur)

additional evaluation.[18-20] But voltage criteria of LVH associated with coexisting ECG abnormalities such as TWI, ST-segment depression, pathological Q waves, intraventricular conduction delay (IVCD), LAD or LAE suggest the diagnosis of HCM.[21-26]

2. *ST-segment depression*: ST-segment depression is a common abnormality in HCM (Figs. 18.3A to C and 18.4), but extremely rare in otherwise healthy athletes, making it a concerning indicator of disease if identified on an athlete's ECG. ST-segment depression is reported in 46–50% of patients with HCM, but in less than 1% of apparently healthy athletes or adolescents undergoing ECG screening. Any degree of ST depression beyond 0.5 mm in two or more leads is significant and requires further investigation for HCM.[13]
3. *T-wave inversion (TWI):* T-wave inversion in the lateral or inferolateral leads is seen commonly in HCM and this ECG abnormality has been documented in up to 62% patients with this condition (Figs. 18.3A to C and 18.4).[25] TWI occurs more commonly in the lateral leads (77%) and less frequently in the inferior leads (2%).[22,23] Abnormal TWI is defined as greater than 1 mm in depth in two or more leads V2-V6, II and aVF, or I and aVL (excludes leads III, aVR and V1). Deep TWI in the mid-precordial to lateral precordial leads (V4-V6) should raise the possibility of apical HCM.
4. *Pathological Q waves*: Pathological Q waves mimicking old myocardial infarction may be present in the ECG of HCM. In HCM, abnormal Q waves are often seen, especially in the left precordial leads and lead I. These

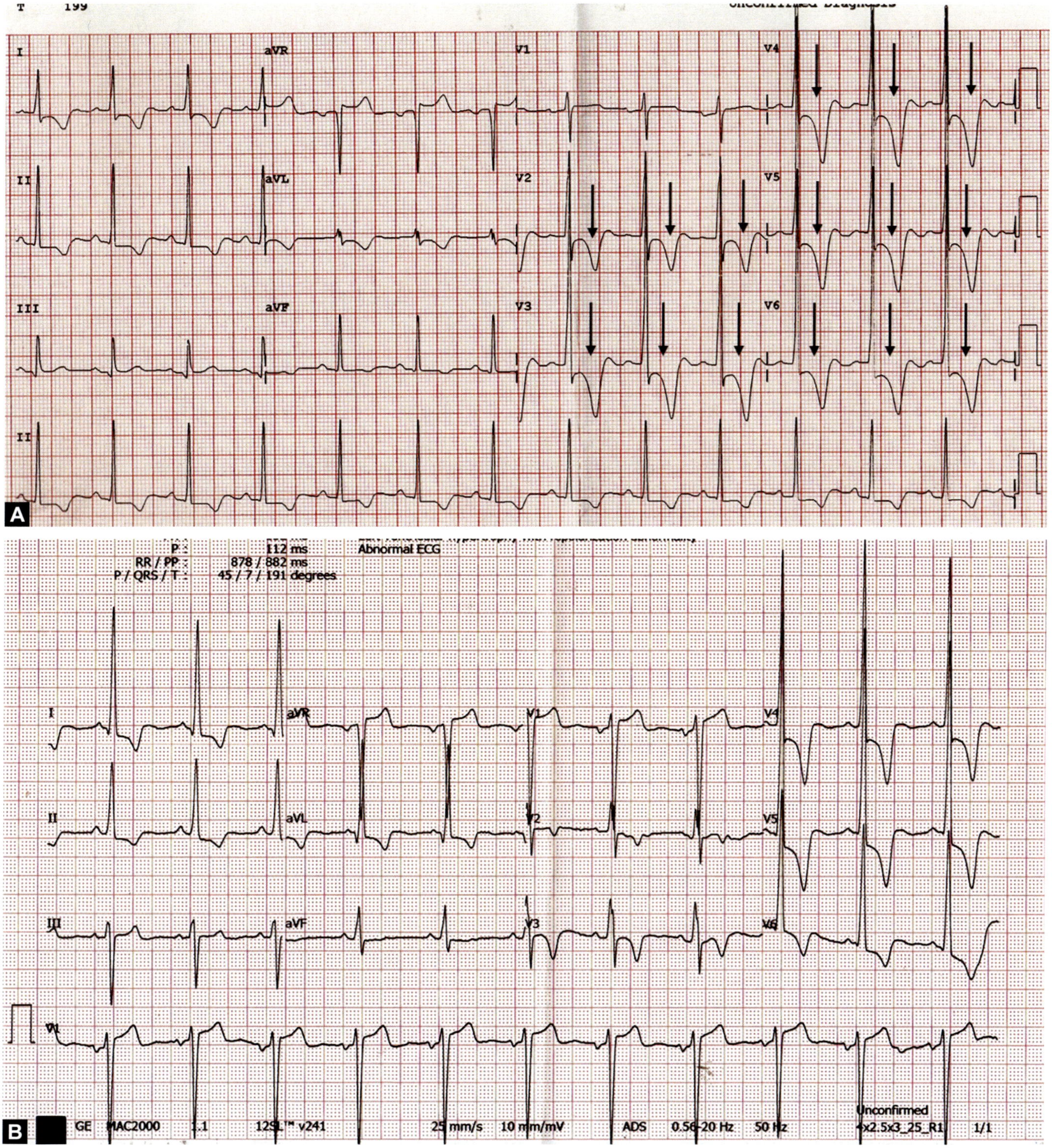

Figs. 18.3A and B: (A) This ECG illustrates the typical features of hypertrophic cardiomyopathy (HCM) with voltage criteria of LVH, marked ST-segment depression with deep asymmetrical T-wave inversions (arrows); (B) This ECG illustrates the typical features of hypertrophic cardiomyopathy (HCM) with LVH systolic overload pattern with deep asymmetrical T-wave inversions in leads V4 and V5. Also note ECG sign of LA enlargement in lead V1.

Q waves have been attributed to ventricular septal hypertrophy and produces pseudoinfarction pattern. In patients with HCM, pathological Q waves are reported in 32–42% of patients.[21,27] In one series of asymptomatic patients with HCM, 42% demonstrated pathological Q waves.[25] The consensus of this group is to define Q waves for HCM as greater than 3 mm in depth or greater than 40 ms in duration in at least two leads (excluding leads III and aVR) (Figs. 18.5A to D). This detects HCM with a sensitivity of 35% and a specificity of 95% in patients

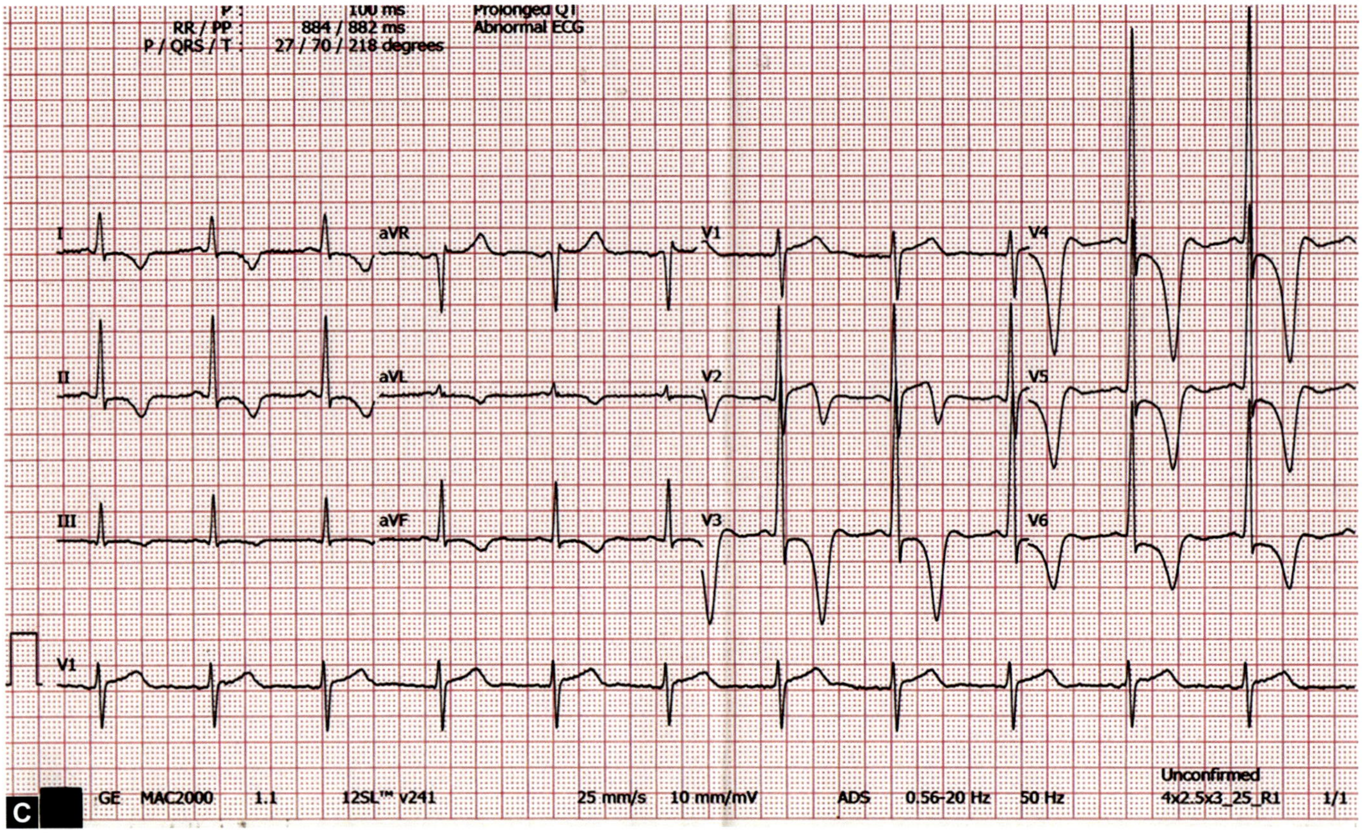

Fig. 18.3C: This ECG shows the typical features of hypertrophic cardiomyopathy (HCM). Note the LVH systolic overload pattern with marked ST-segment depression with deep asymmetrical T-wave inversions more prominent in lateral chest leads V3-V6

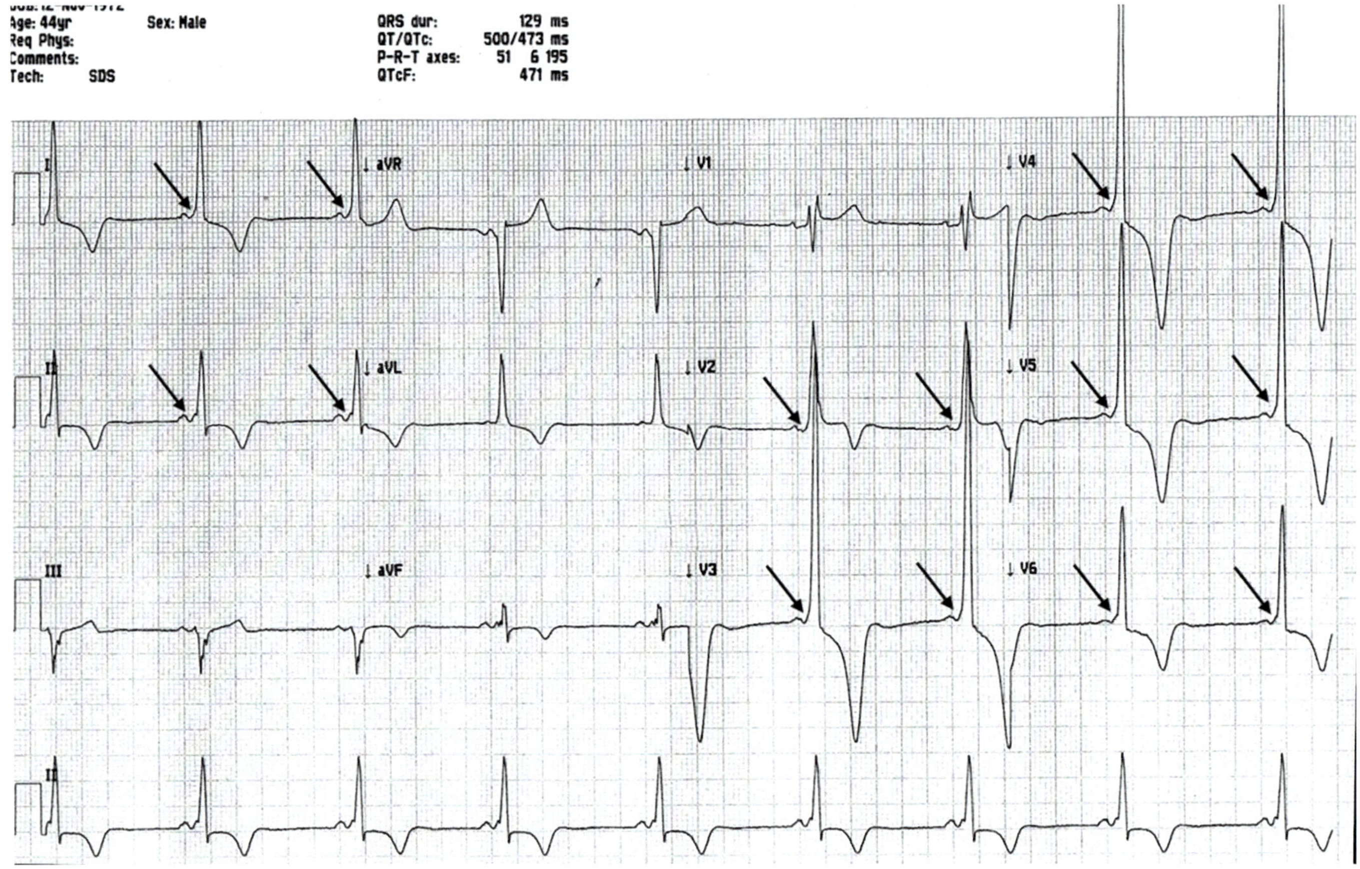

Fig.18.4: ECG is consistent with the features of HCM with Wolff-Parkinson-White (WPW) syndrome. Note short PR interval with presence of delta waves (arrows) in multiple leads with wide QRS complex (QRS duration = 128 ms). (*Source:* Courtesy of Dr Ziaul Kabir, Labaid Cardiac Hospital)

with preclinical HCM based on molecular genetic diagnosis.[26]

5. *Intraventricular conduction delay (IVCD):* The significance of a nonspecific IVCD with normal QRS morphology is uncertain but, marked nonspecific IVCD greater than 120 ms is considered abnormal and should prompt further evaluation to exclude HCM (Fig. 18.6).[13] Left bundle branch block (LBBB) is an abnormal finding detected in 2% of patients with HCM.[21,24,28] Right bundle branch block (RBBB) is found more commonly in HCM than in athletes (Fig. 18.7).[13]
6. *Left-axis deviation (LAD):* Left-axis deviation, defined as –30 to –90°, is present in almost 12% of HCM patients (Fig. 18.8) but less than 1% of normal athletes without any pathological heart disease. LAD can be a secondary marker for pathological LVH and if present warrants additional evaluation.[22,24,28]
7. *Left atrial enlargement (LAE):* ECG findings suggestive of LAE have been defined in different ways. Overall, LAE on ECG is present in approximately 10–21% of HCM patients (Fig. 18.9) but has been reported in up to 44% of black patients with HCM. LAE is defined as a prolonged P wave duration of greater than 120 ms in leads I or II with negative portion of the P wave greater than or equal to 1 mm in depth and greater than or equal to 40 ms in duration in lead V1. LAE on ECG is an uncommon finding in athletes and should prompt additional investigation.[13,21,22]
8. *ST-segment elevation*: Most patients with HCM have ST-segment depression and TWI on resting ECGs probably due to marked LVH but ST-segment elevation mimicking acute myocardial infarction (AMI) is a very unusual findings in patients with HCM. However, ST-segment elevation in patients with HCM has been reported in literature (Figs. 18.10 and 18.11).[14-17] But ST elevation in HCM is always static and is not associated with ECG evidence of reciprocal ST depression.[14] ST elevation in the setting of AMI usually shows dynamic changes. But if confusion still arises the possibilty of AMI can be excluded by bedside echocardiography and serial enzyme study.

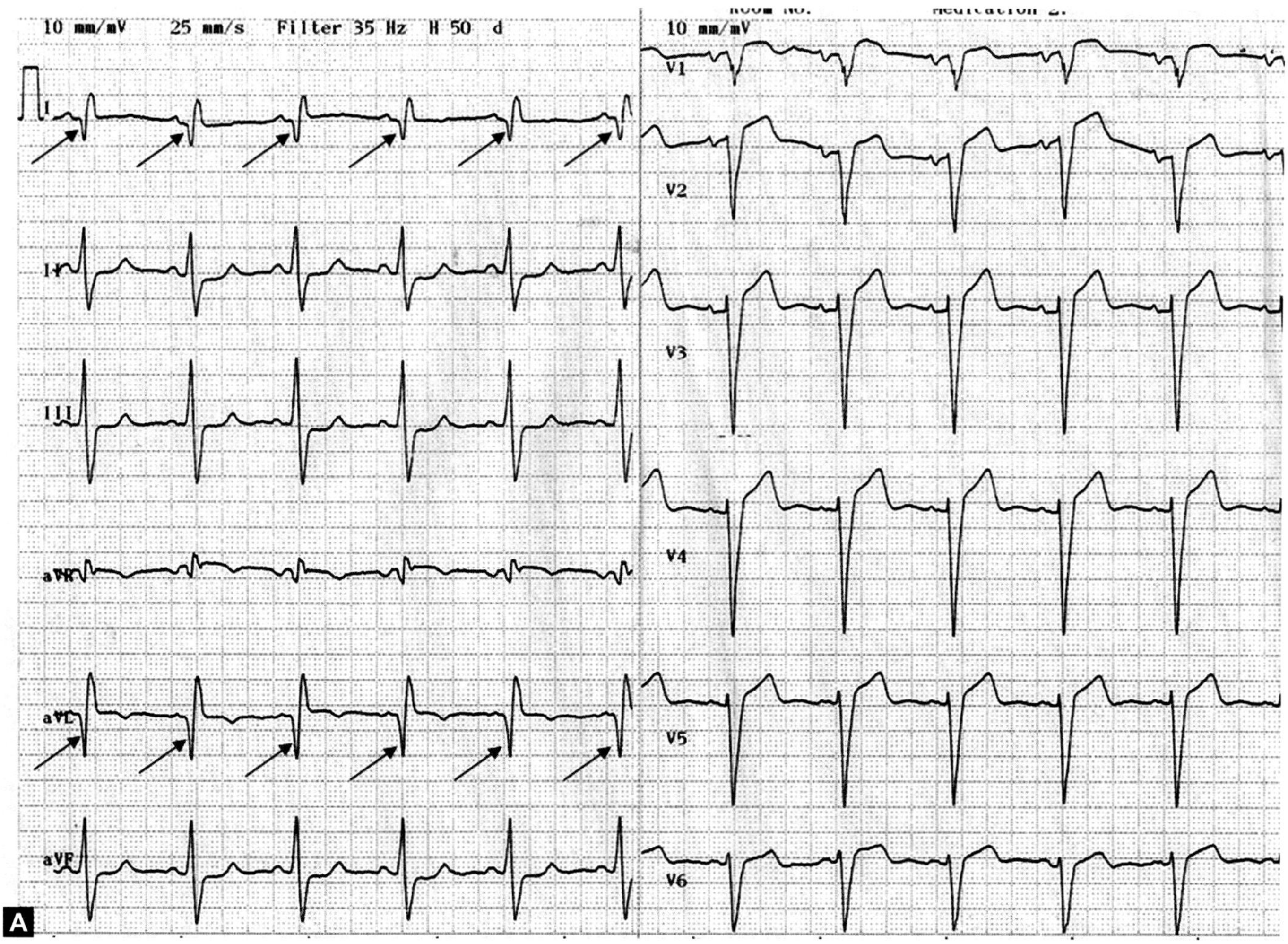

Fig. 18.5A: ECG of HCM with LBBB pattern, showing pathological Q waves in LI and aVL (arrows). Also note ECG sign of LA enlargement in lead V1;

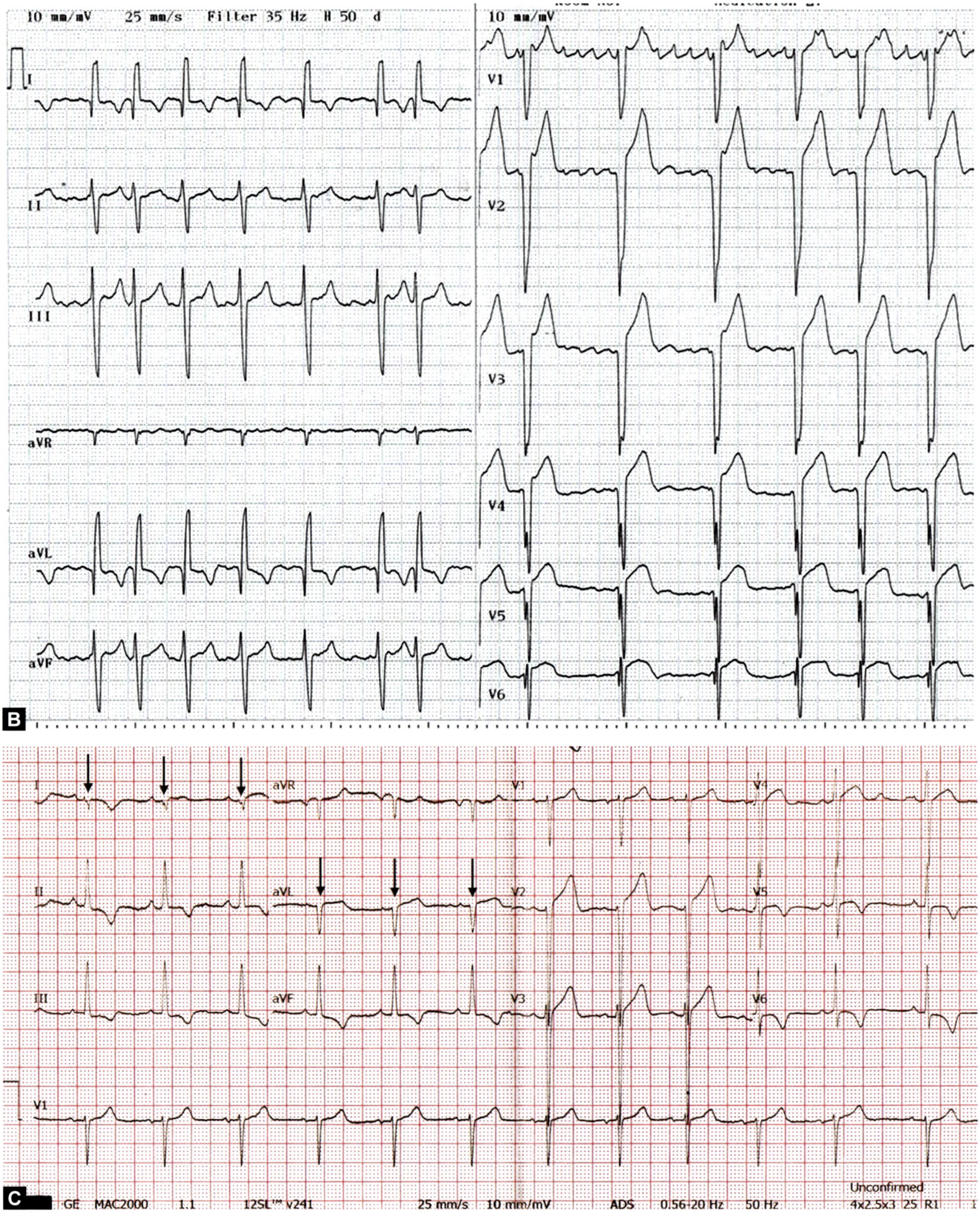

Figs. 18.5B and C: (B) ECG showing pathological Q waves in LI, aVL, and V2-V6 mimicking anterior myocardial infarction in a patient with hypertrophic obstructive cardiomyopathy (pseudoinfarction pattern). Also note some ST-segment elevations in anterior leads with AF; (C) ECG of a 24-year-old young man with HCM. Note pathological Q waves in LI and aVL, mimicking old high lateral myocardial infarction (arrows); Also note T wave inversions in leads LII, LIII, aVF, V5 and V6.

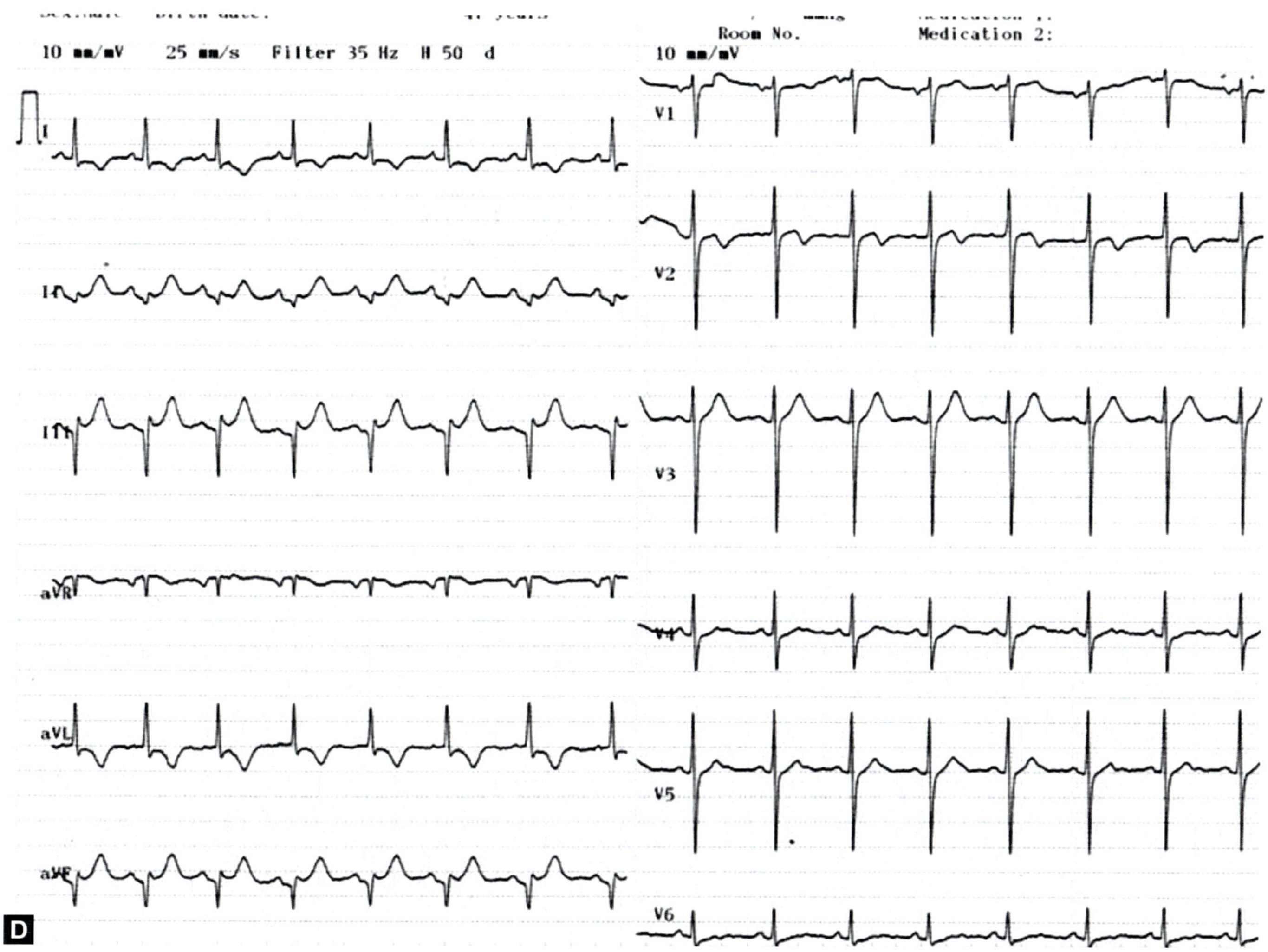

Fig. 18.5D: ECG showing pathological Q waves in LII, LIII and aVF with some ST segment elevation in the same leads mimicking recent inferior myocardial infarction in a patient with hypertrophic cardiomyopathy (pseudo-infarction pattern). These ECG abnormalities remained static over several years and coronary angiogram was normal. Also note T wave inversions in LI and aVL with deep S waves in leads V4 and V5.

Basic Criteria for ECG Diagnosis of Hypertrophic Cardiomyopathy

Left ventricular hypertrophy voltage criteria with ST-segment depression with TWI in chest leads give clues to the diagnosis of HCM. In the absence of hypertension and aortic stenosis, the ECG features of HCM (particularly ASH) as proposed by Anis Waiz and Baren Chakraborty (Anis-Baren triad), may suggest the diagnosis of HCM.[29-37] They proposed the following three ECG criteria suggestive of HCM (Figs. 18.12 and 18.13):

1. ECG criteria suggestive of LVH systolic overload pattern
2. T-wave inversion in LII
3. Upright T in aVR and LIII.

In the normal ECG, the T wave is always upright in leads I, II, V3-V6, and always inverted in lead aVR. The other leads are variable depending on the direction of the QRS and the age of the patient. TWI in LII is an uncommon ECG finding in normal population but TWI in lead III is considered as a normal variant. But the reverse is true in HCM. In HCM, T wave is usually inverted in LII but upright in LIII and aVR (Figs. 18.14 and 18.15). Sometimes instead of inversion, T wave may be biphasic in LIII. This pattern of T-wave polarity (inverted T in LII and upright T in LIII and aVR) as described by Anis-Baren may also be seen in many cases of apical cardiomyopathy with or without ECG evidence of LVH.[29-31,36,37]

Apical Cardiomyopathy

The most commonly observed pattern of HCM is called ASH and this pattern produces asymmetrical thickening of the anterior interventricular septum (IVS). ASH is classically associated with systolic anterior motion (SAM) of the mitral valve and dynamic LVOT obstruction. However, in the majority of cases (75%), HCM is not associated with LVOT obstruction. Less common patterns of HCM include concentric hypertrophy and apical hypertrophic cardiomyopathy (AHCM).[38-43]

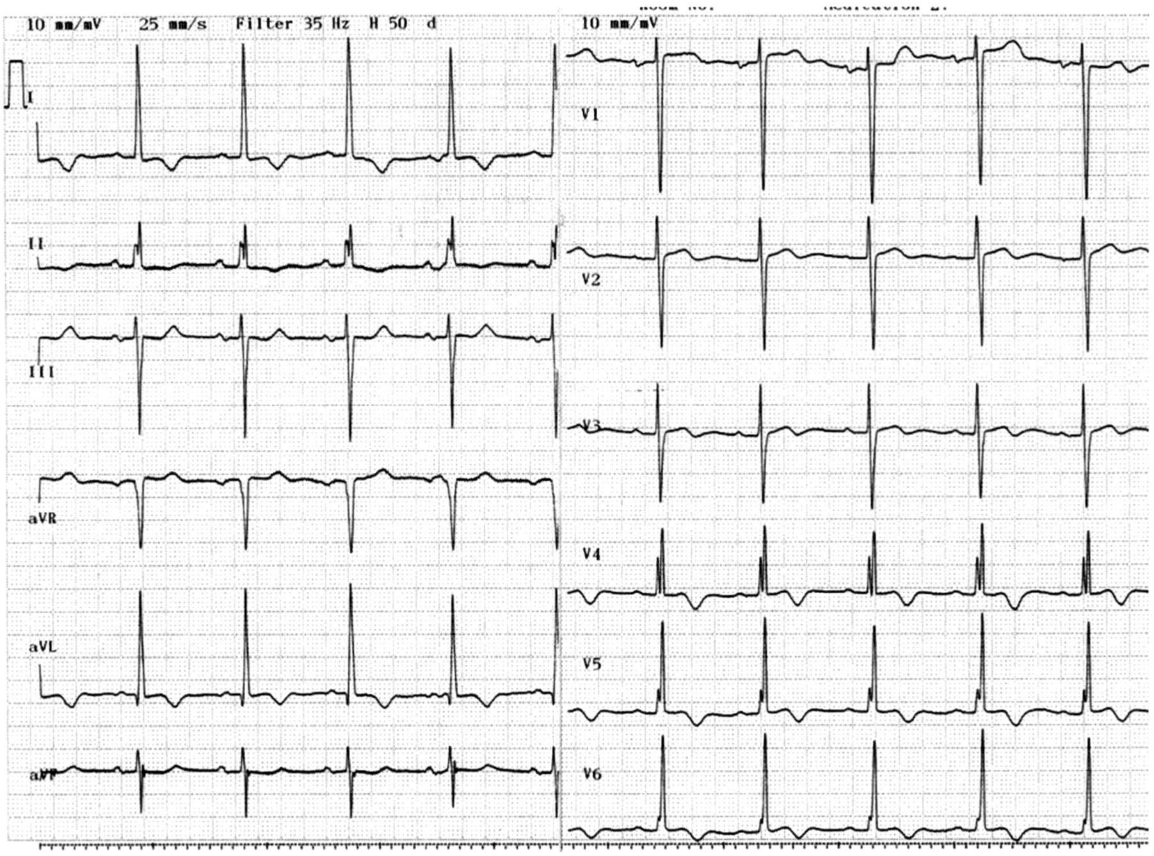

Fig. 18.6: ECG of HCM, showing features of intraventricular conduction delay, slurred QRS complexes in LII, V4-V6 (QRS duration 120 ms). Note voltage criteria of LVH with ST- and T-wave changes.

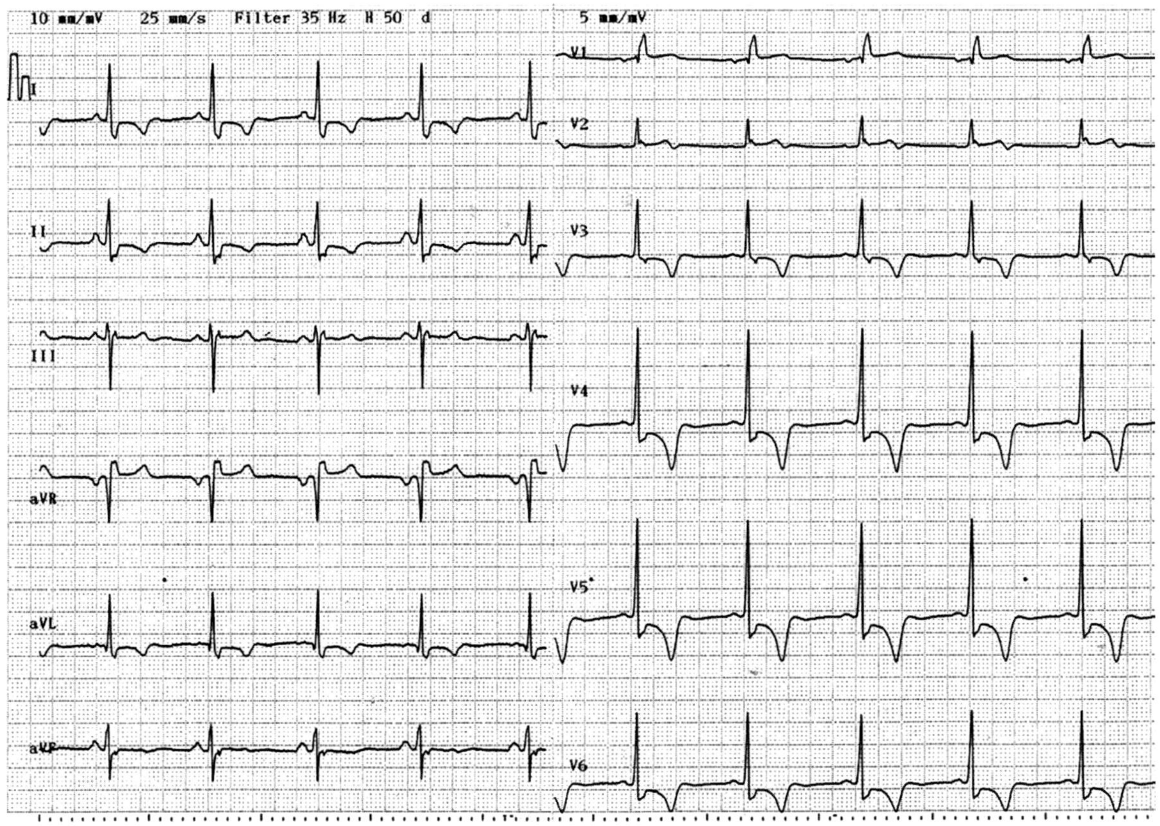

Fig. 18.7: ECG of HCM with right bundle branch block pattern (rSR pattern in V1 with slurred S waves in lateral leads). Note asymmetrical T-wave inversions with ST depression in leads V4-V6.

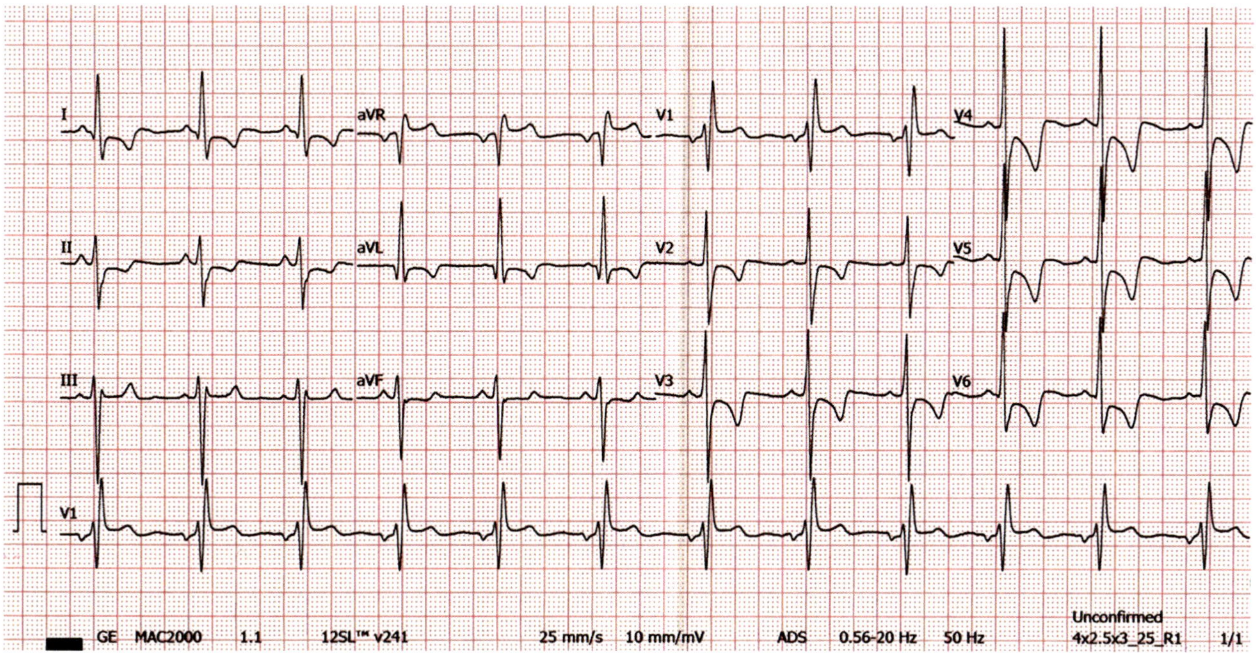

Fig. 18.8: ECG illustrates presence of left-axis deviation in the electrocardiogram of HCM. Note the asymmetrical T inversion in leads V4-V6 with marked ST-segment depression. Also note the presence of RBBB.

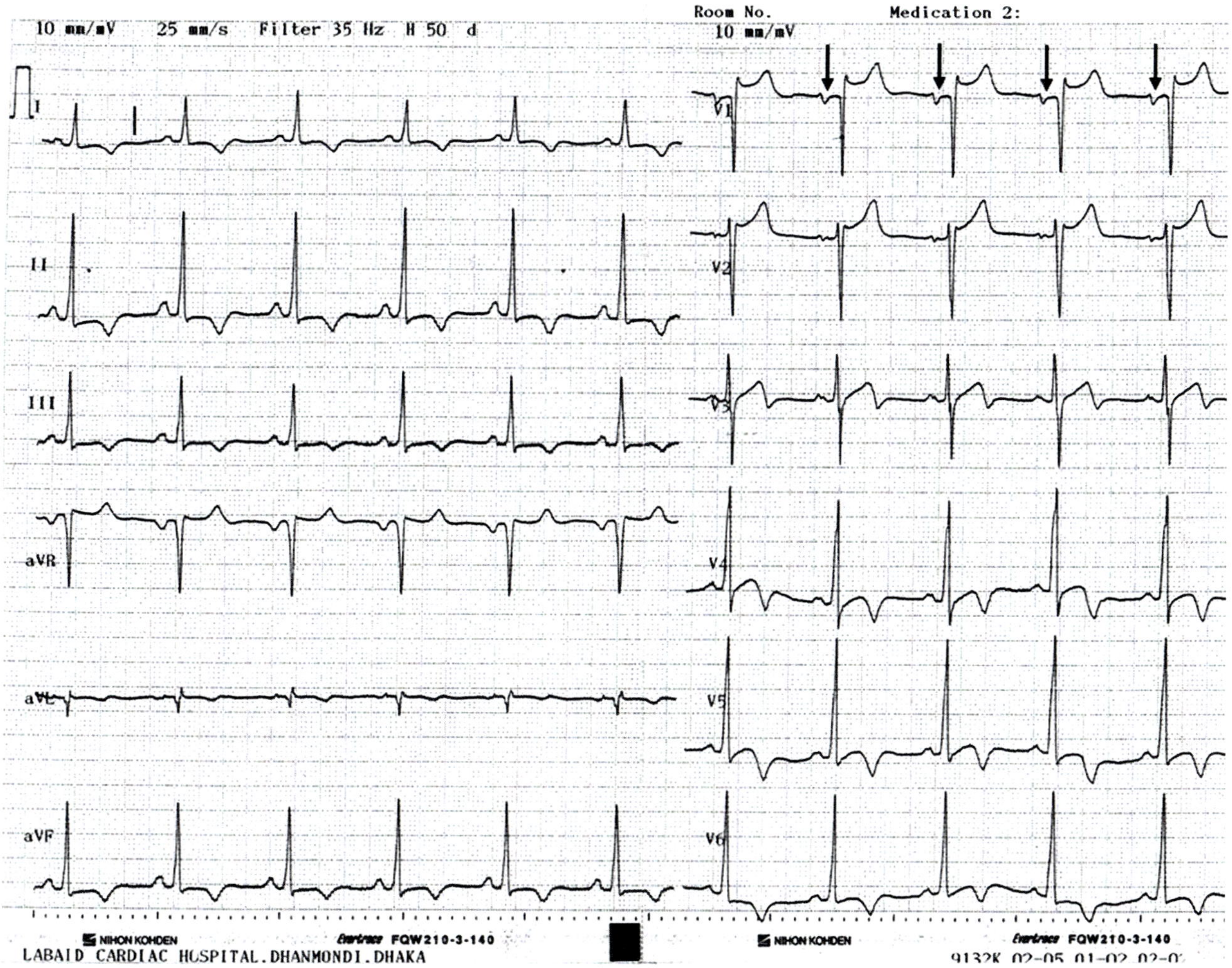

Fig. 18.9: ECG of HCM showing features of left atrial enlargement. Note biphasic P wave with terminal negative portion greater than 1 mm deep in lead V1 (arrows). Also note bifid P wave in leads LII, and V2-V5.

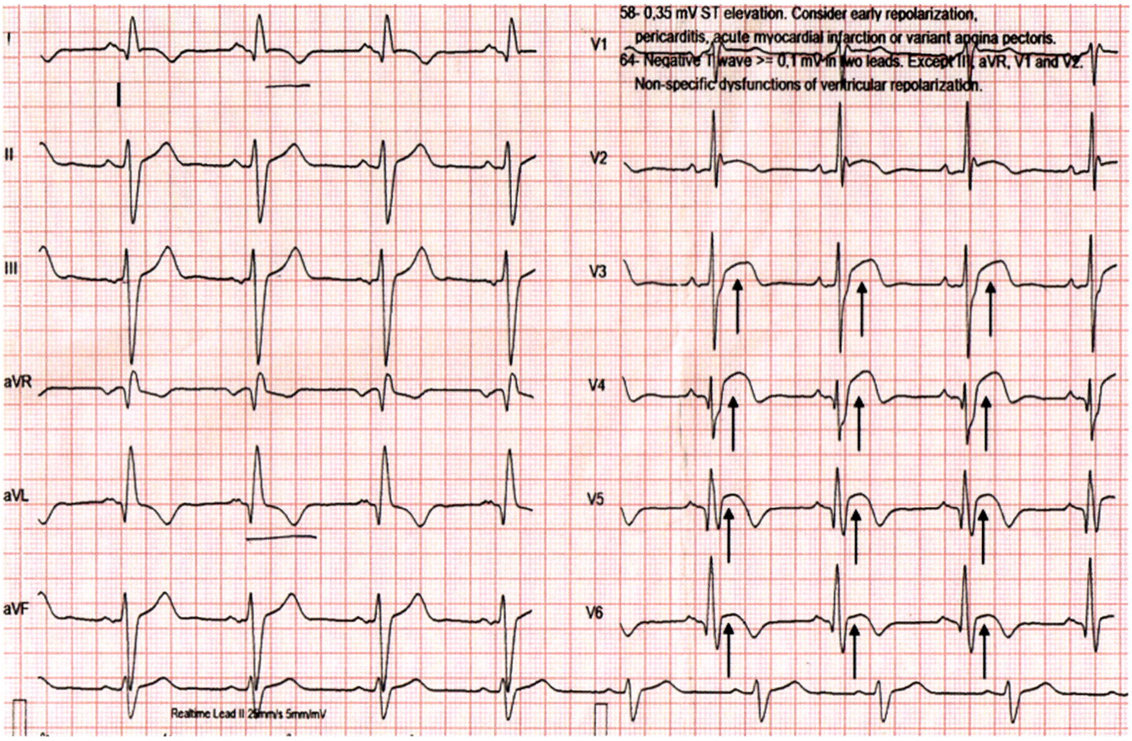

Fig. 18.10: ECG of HCM showing coved ST elevation mimicking acute anterior ST-segment elevation myocardial infarction (STEMI) in leads V3-V6 (arrows). Note there is no reciprocal ST-segment depression in inferior leads (LII, LIII, and aVF) suggesting acute anterior STEMI. Also note RBBB with left-axis deviation with Q waves in LI, aVL, and V4-V6. ST elevation in acute MI is dynamic but in HCM is static without any reciprocal ST-segment depression.

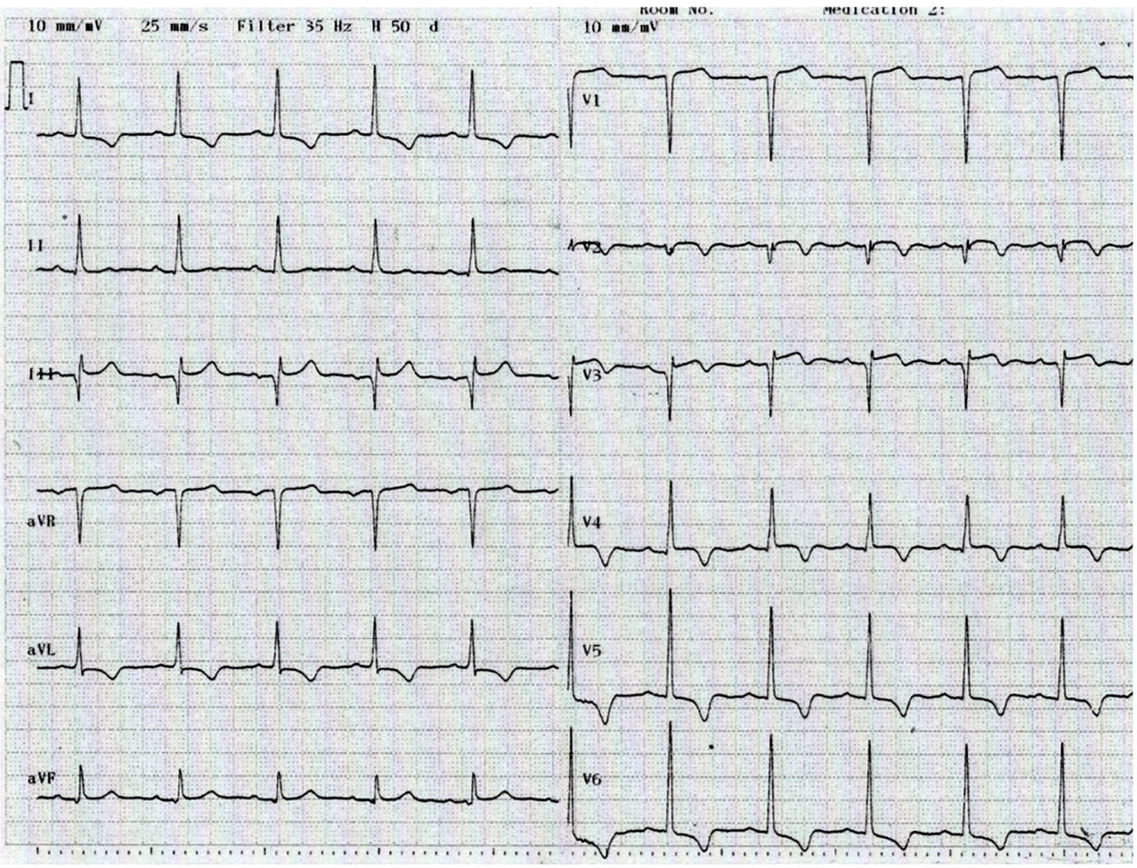

Fig. 18.11: ECG of HCM showing ST segment elevation in leads V1-V3 and LIII along with biphasic T and pathological Q waves. Also note voltage criteria of LVH with asymmetrical T wave inversions in L1, aVL and V4-V6.

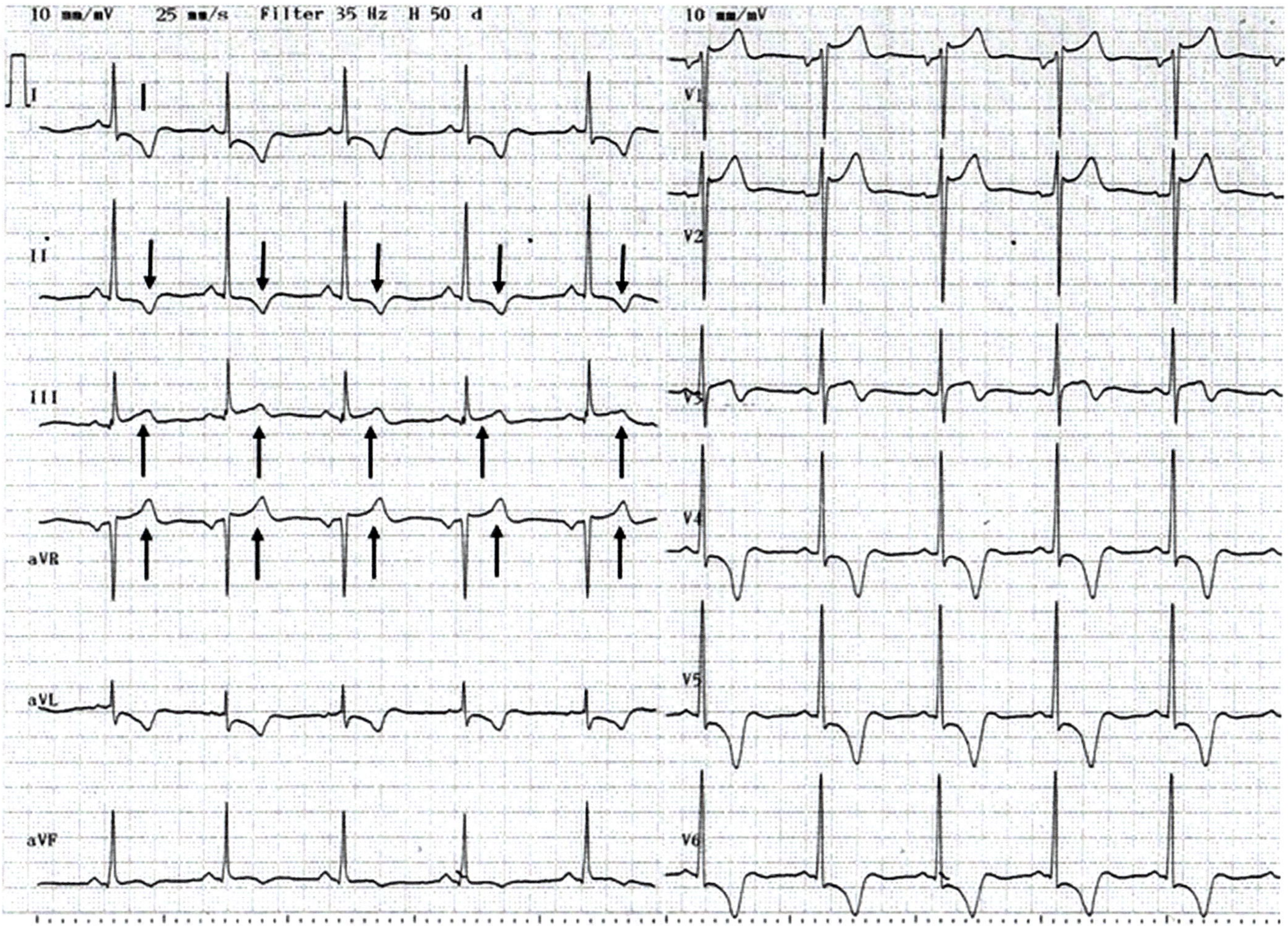

Fig. 18.12: This ECG illustrates all the features of Anis-Baren triad for the ECG diagnosis of hypertrophic cardiomyopathy (HCM). ECG shows (1) LVH systolic overload pattern with voltage criteria of LVH with marked ST-segment depression with T-wave inversion in leads LI, aVL, and V4-V6; (2) T-wave inversion in LII (arrows); and (3) upright T in aVR and LIII (arrows). Note also the sign of left atrial enlargement in V1.

AHCM is a rare form of HCM which usually involves the apex of the left ventricle and rarely involves the right ventricular (RV) apex or both. Historically, this condition was thought to be confined to the Japanese population but it is also found in other populations. Of all the HCM patients in Japan, the prevalence of AHCM was 15–25%, whereas in the United States of America the prevalence was only 3%.[44-46]

The most frequent ECG findings are deeply inverted T waves in the precordial leads which are found in 93% of patients (Figs. 18.16 and 18.17), followed by LVH in 65% of patients (Fig. 18.18). Negative T waves with a depth greater than 10 mm are found in 47% of patients with AHCM (Figs. 18.19A and B).[45,46] Patients with this condition may remain asymptomatic, with the condition detected by chance as a result of an abnormal ECG. In general, the condition carries a benign prognosis, although complications including ventricular fibrillation (VF), atrial fibrillation (AF) (Figs. 18.20A and B), apical myocardial infarction, and apical aneurysm can occur in rare instances.[47-49]

Sudden Cardiac Death in Hypertrophic Cardiomyopathy

Sudden cardiac death, heart failure, and thromboembolism are the main causes of death in patients with HCM. The annual SCD rate is less than 1%, but within the general population with HCM there are subgroups with much higher incidence. SCD in HCM is mediated primarily by VF.[6] Numerous cardiac arrhythmias have been reported in association with SCD in HCM, including asystole, atrioventricular (AV) block, pulseless electrical activity, and supraventricular arrhythmias. Data from chance electrocardiographic recordings and stored intracardiac electrograms suggest that SCD in HCM is most commonly caused by VF. Most of the presently reported data suggest that implantable cardioverter-defibrillators (ICDs) can prevent SCD and there is a clinical need to identify accurately individual patients at high risk.[6,50]

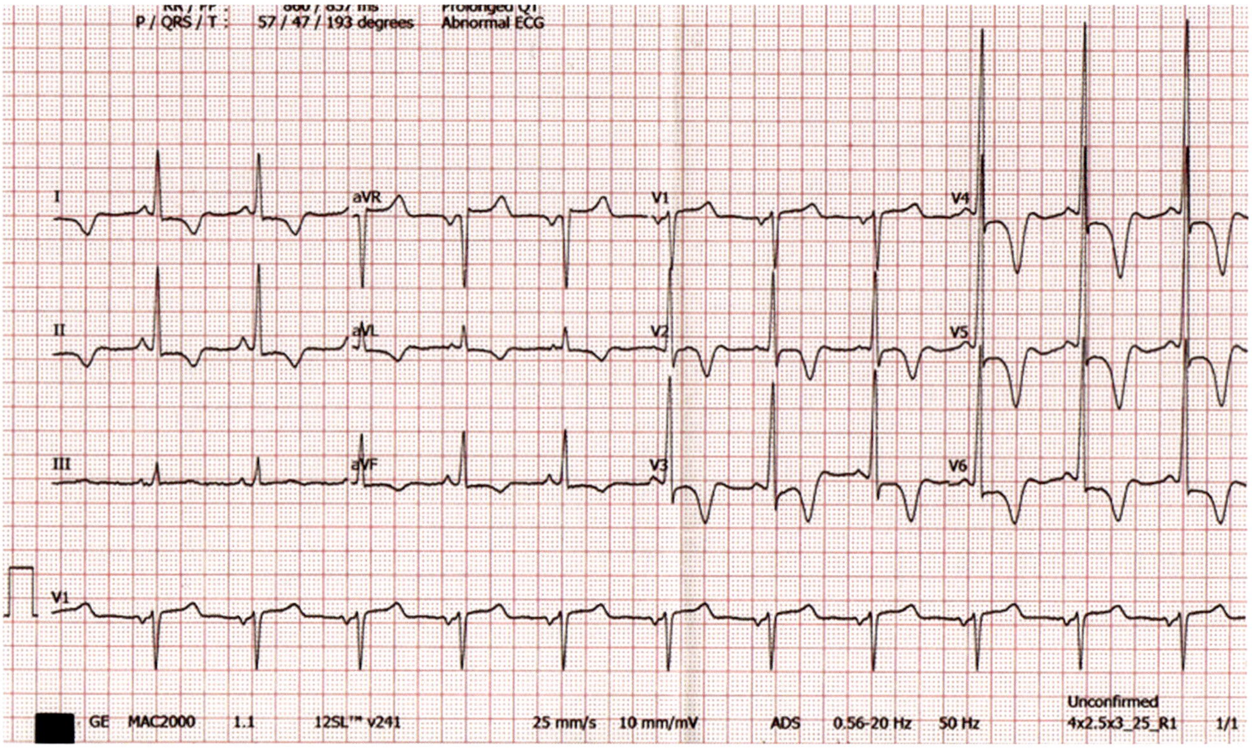

Fig. 18.13: This ECG shows typical features of HCM with presence of Anis-Baren triad: (1) LVH systolic overload pattern; (2) T-wave inversion in LII; and (3) upright T in aVR and LIII. For the ECG diagnosis of HCM by using Anis-Baren triad possibility of aortic stenosis and hypertension should be excluded.

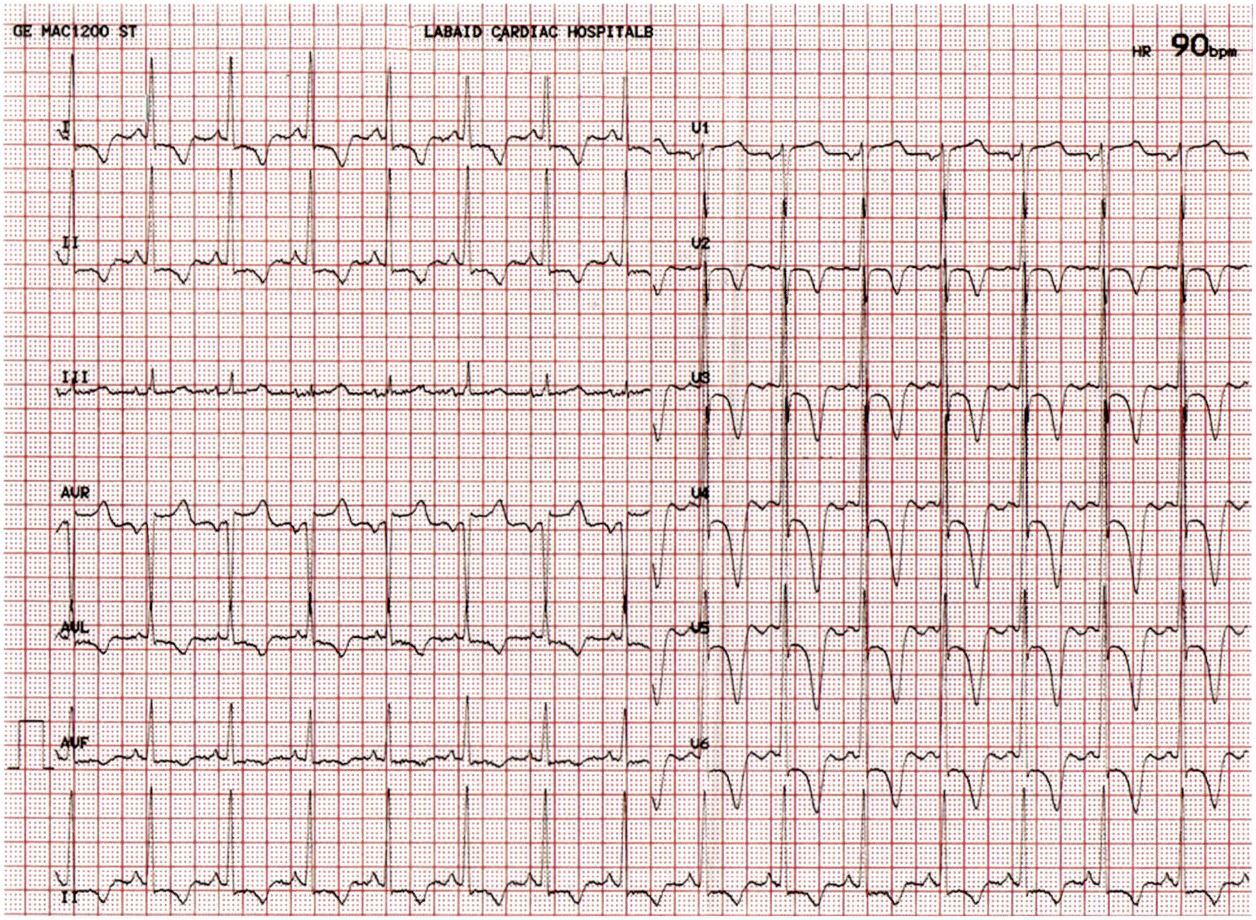

Fig. 18.14: ECG of HCM showing Anis-Baren triad: (1) LVH systolic overload pattern; (2) T-wave inversion in LII; and (3) upright T in aVR and LIII.

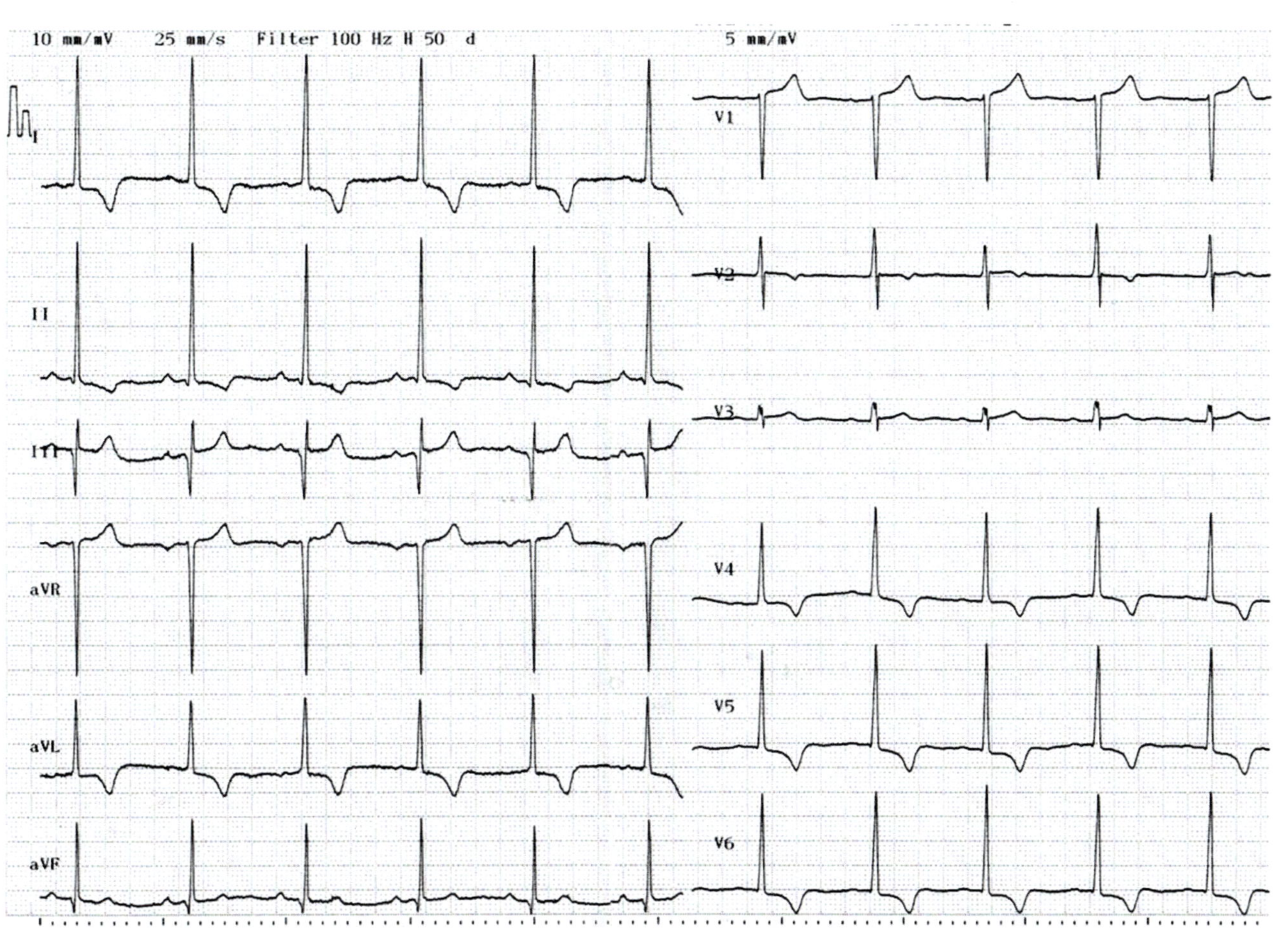

Fig. 18.15: ECG of hypertrophic cardiomyopathy (HCM) illustrating Anis-Baren triad [(1) LVH systolic overload pattern; (2) T-wave inversion in LII; and (3) upright T in aVR and LIII] for the electrocardiographic diagnosis of HCM. Note also the presence of isolated pathological Q wave in LIII.

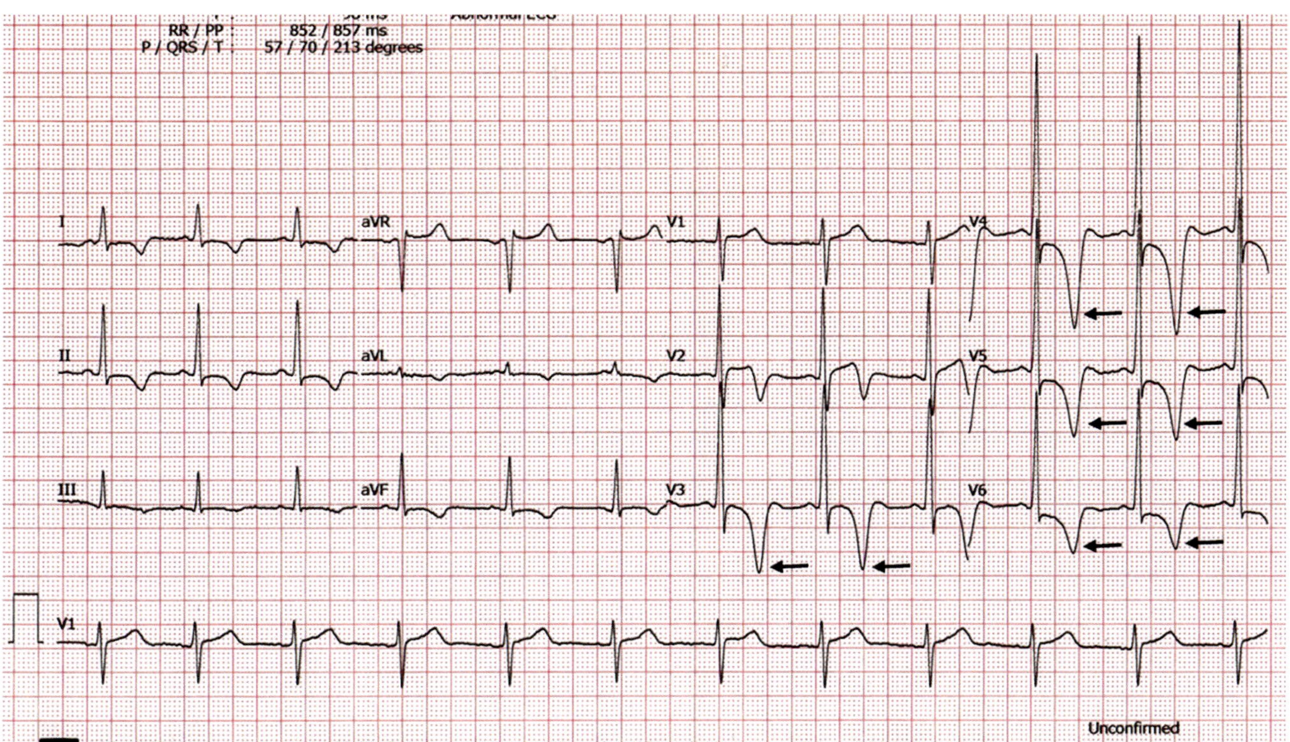

Fig. 18.16: This ECG illustrates the features of apical cardiomyopathy with deep asymmetrical T-wave inversions in leads V3-V6 (arrows) with marked ST-segment depression.

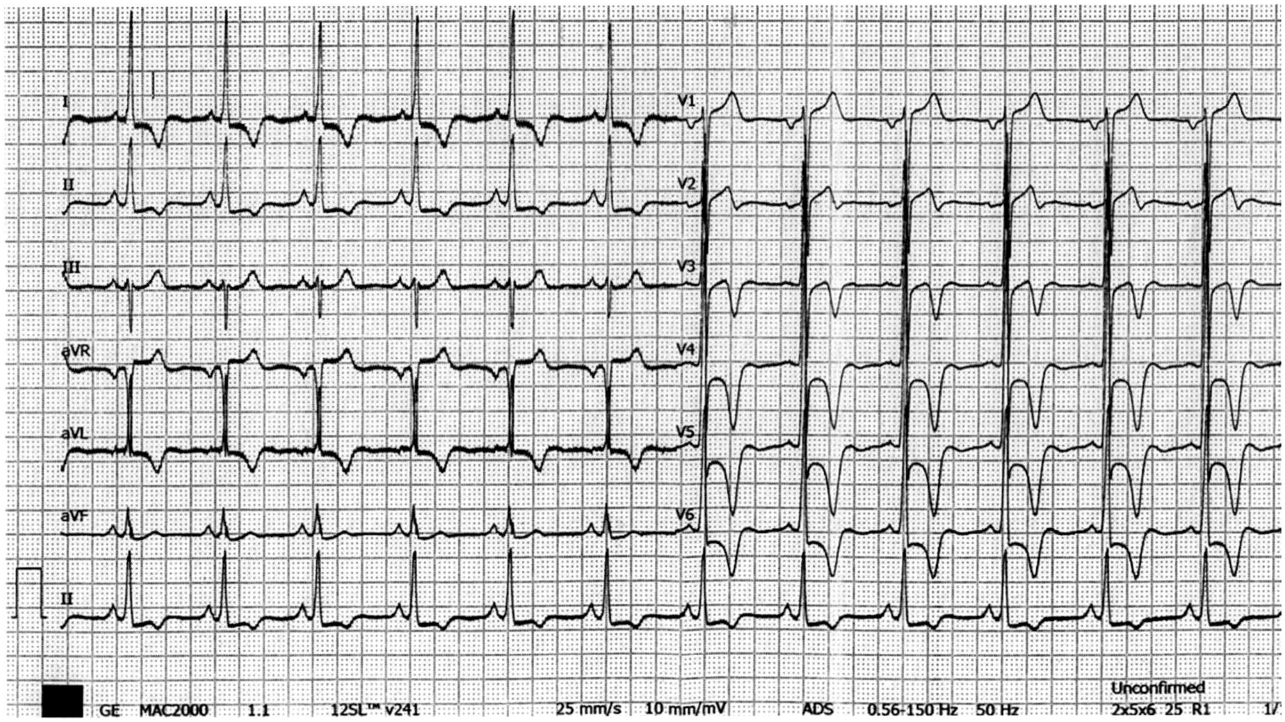

Fig. 18.17: This ECG illustrates the features of apical cardiomyopathy with deep asymmetrical T-wave inversions in leads V4-V6 with marked ST-segment depression.

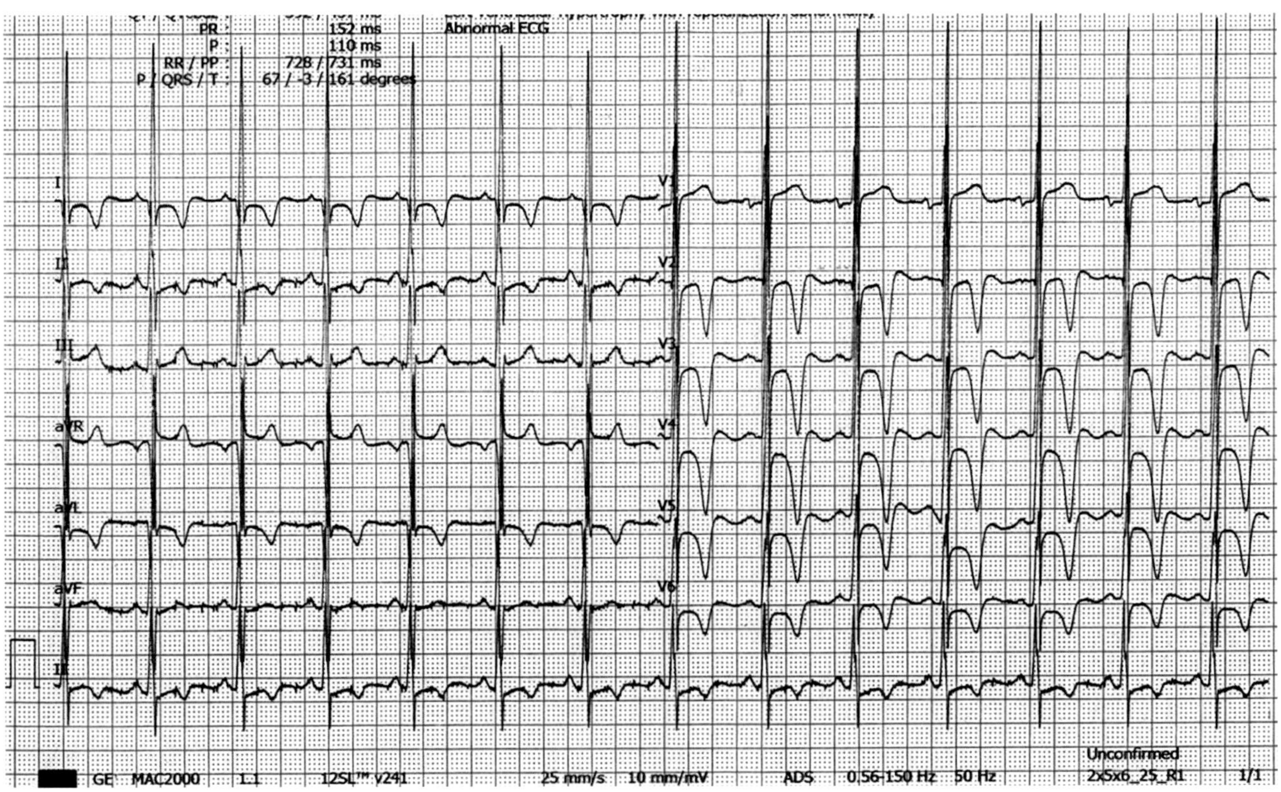

Fig. 18.18: This ECG illustrates the features of apical cardiomyopathy with ECG criteria of LVH. Note deep asymmetrical T-wave inversions in leads V2-V6 with marked ST-segment depression.

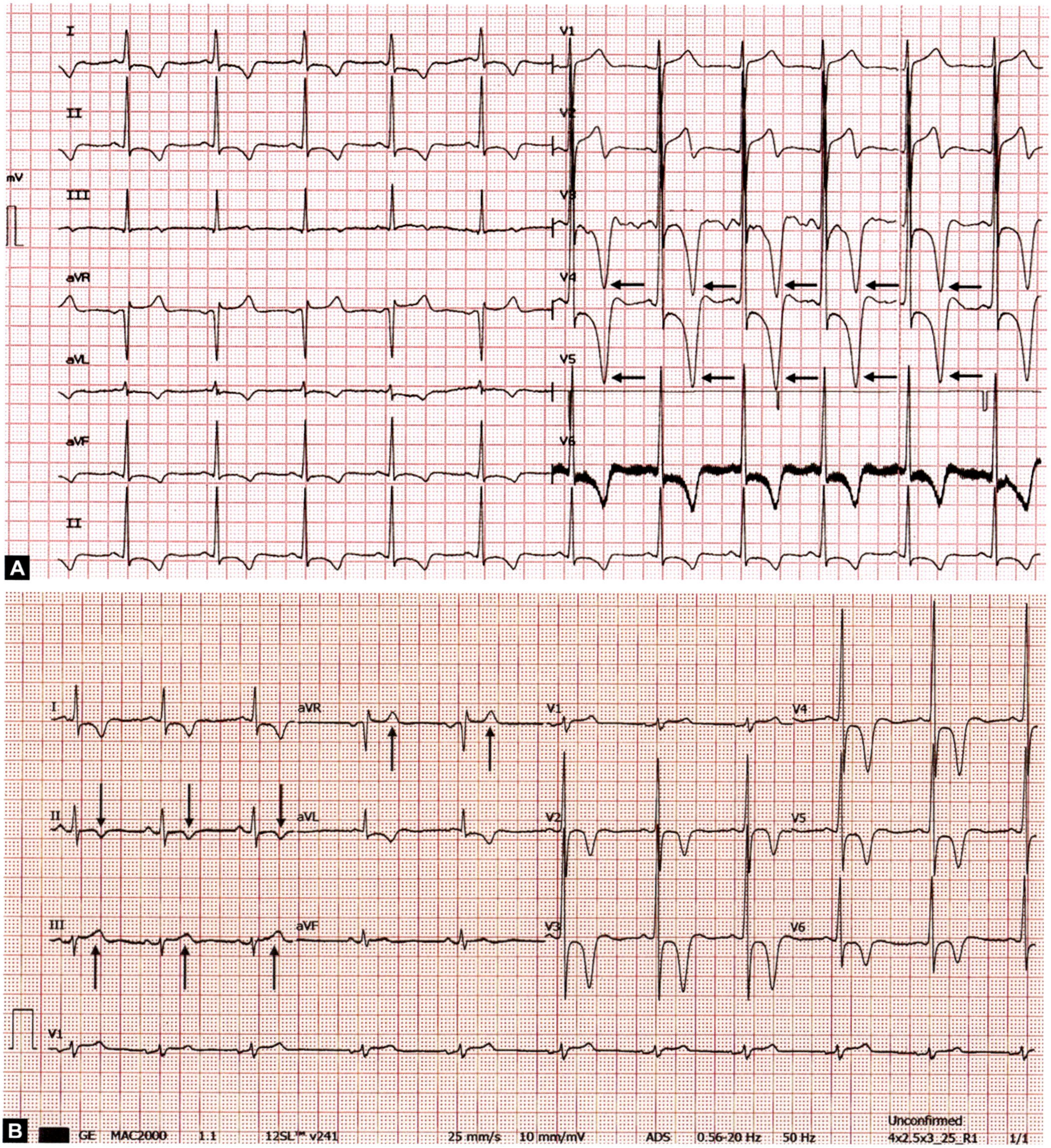

Figs. 18.19A and B: (A) ECG showing deep negative T waves with a depth greater than 10 mm in leads V3 and V4 (arrows), typical of apical cardiomyopathy. Note also the voltage criteria of LVH; (B) ECG showing deep negative T waves with a depth greater than 10 mm in leads V3 and V4, typical of apical cardiomyopathy without any voltage criteria of LVH. Note also the presence of T-wave inversion in LII and upright T wave in LIII and aVR (arrows), as a part of Anis-Baren triad for the ECG diagnosis of HCM (asymmetrical septal hypertrophy). This pattern of T-wave polarity (inverted T in LII and upright T in LIII and aVR) may also be seen in the ECGs of apical cardiomyopathy.

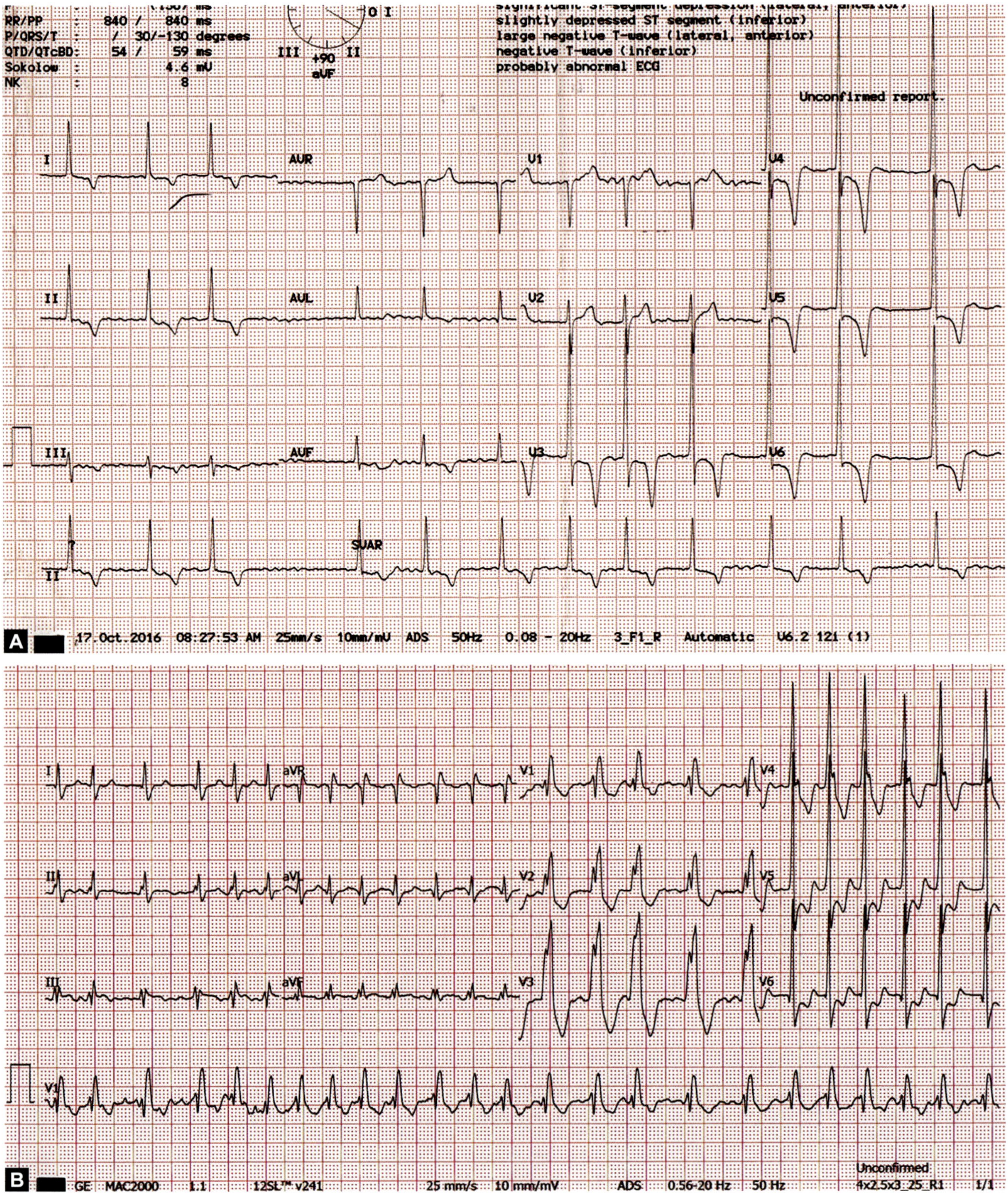

Figs. 18.20A and B: (A) ECG is suggestive of atrial fibrillation in a patient with apical cardiomyopathy; (B) Fast AF (heart rate 142 bpm) in a patient with apical HCM with right bundle branch block (RBBB). Note high QRS voltage in the lateral chest leads with marked ST depression with T-wave changes.

DILATED CARDIOMYOPATHY

Dilated cardiomyopathy (DCM) is a myocardial disease characterized by ventricular dilatation and global myocardial dysfunction (left vetricular ejection fraction <40%). Patients usually present with symptoms of biventricular failure, e.g. fatigue, dyspnea, orthopnea, ankle edema.

Dilated cardiomyopathy can be divided into two subgroups: (1) ischemic and (2) nonischemic.

1. *Ischemic*: Ischemic DCM commonly occurs following massive anterior myocardial infarction due to extensive myocardial necrosis and loss of contractility.
2. *Nonischemic*: Nonischemic DCM is mostly idiopathic but up to 25% are familial. A small proportion of cases may occur due to: viral myocarditis (coxsackie B/adenovirus), alcoholism, drug induced (e.g. doxorubicin and daunorubicin), autoimmune disease. Pregnancy-associated DCM is termed as peripartum cardiomyopathy. Development of heart failure during last trimester of pregnancy or first 6 months postpartum is called peripartum cardiomyopathy.

Overall, approximately 90% of individuals with DCM have abnormal ECG findings.[51-54] The ECG may show sinus tachycardia and nonspecific ST-segment depression with low voltage or inverted T waves (Fig. 18.21). Sometimes pathologic Q waves are present in the precordial leads, simulating previous myocardial infarction. LBBB and AF are common. Patients with prior myocardial infarction may manifest pathological Q waves (Fig. 18.22).[53-55]

In 1982, Goldberger described a novel ECG triad that was highly specific for patients with DCM and congestive heart failure (attributable to various etiologic factors), with a sensitivity of 70%, a specificity of 99%, and a positive predictive value of 91%. For unknown reasons, ventricular dilatation causes the QRS vector to shift towards the transverse plane and away from the frontal plane, resulting in differential effects on QRS voltages in the chest and the limb leads.[56,57]

Goldberger's triad (Fig. 18.23) which consists of:

- High precordial QRS voltages (LVH), defined as (SV1 or SV2) + (RV5 or RV6) greater than or equal to 3.5 mV (35 mm)

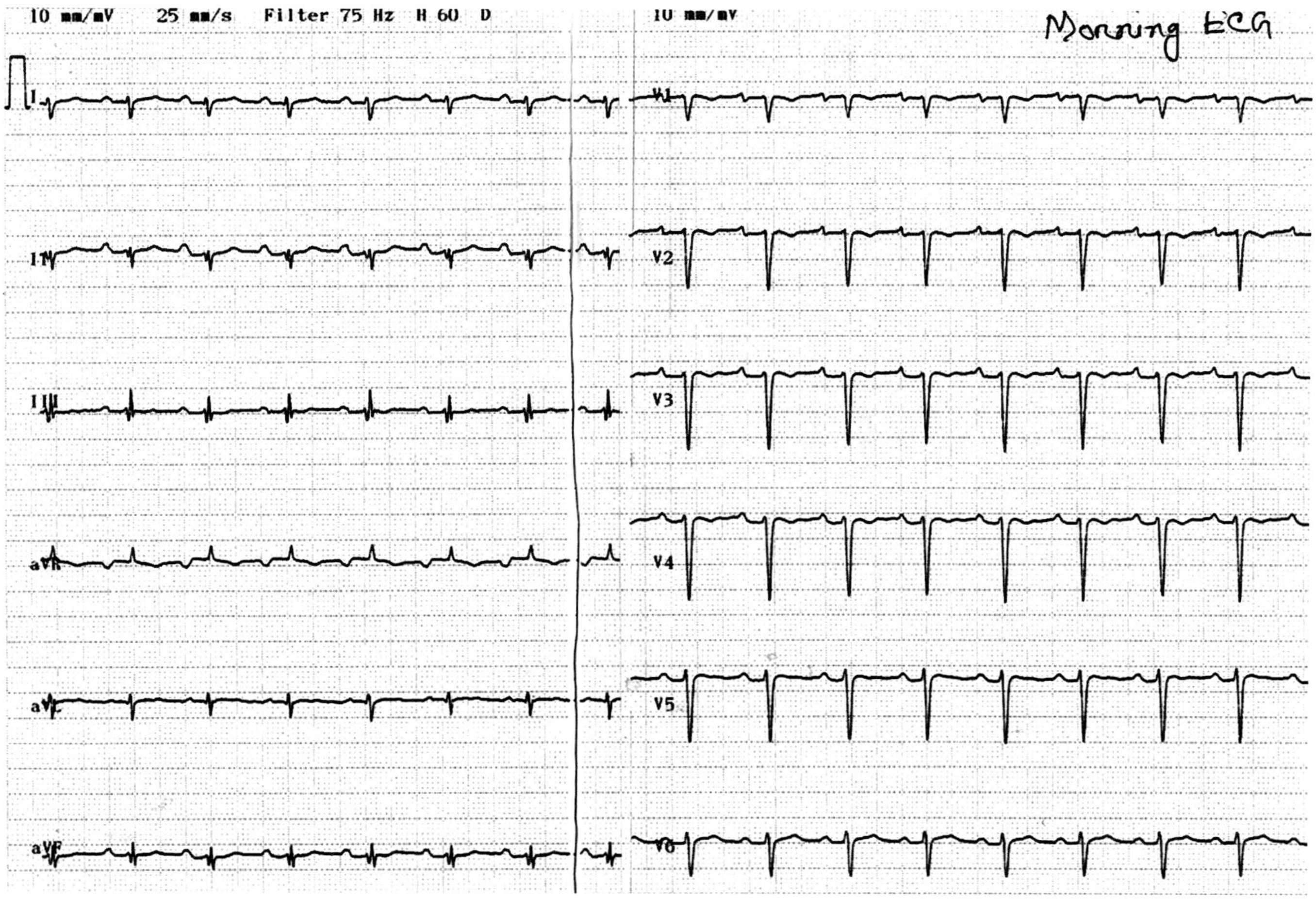

Fig. 18.21: This ECG illustrates the electrocardiographic features of dilated cardiomyopathy (DCM). Note low voltage (QRS voltage <5 mm) in the first six leads with poor R-wave progression from V1-V6 with nonspecific ST- and T-wave changes.

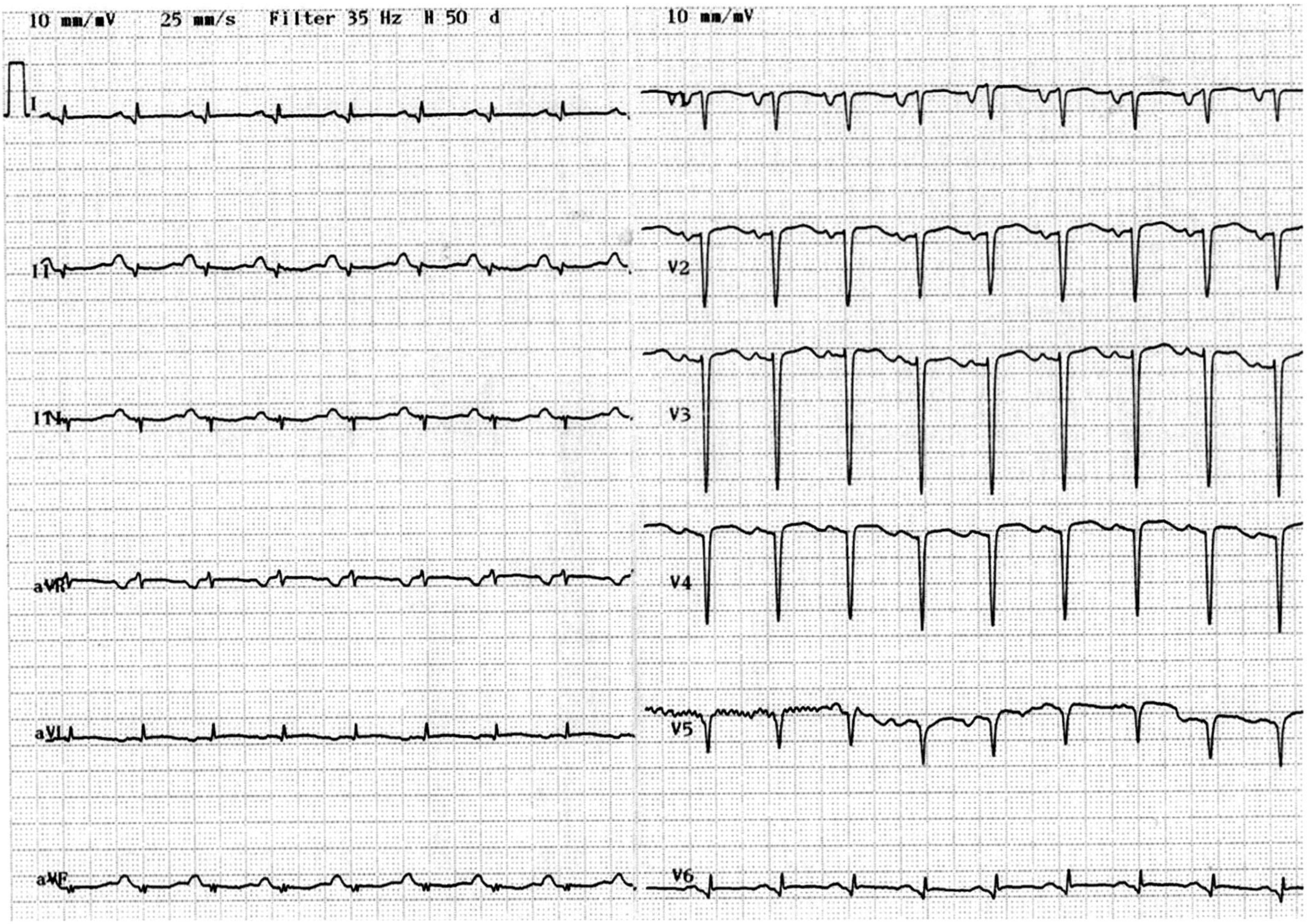

Fig. 18.22: This ECG illustrates the electrocardiographic features of ischemic dilated cardiomyopathy (IDCM). Note low voltage in the first six leads with sinus tachycardia (heart rate 110 bpm) with Q waves in LI and V4-V6. Also note poor R-wave progression V1 to V3 along with ECG sign of left atrial enlargement in V1. Presence of pathological Q waves in multiple leads indicate prior myocardial infarction.

- Relatively low limb lead QRS voltages, defined as total QRS amplitude (i.e. R + S) less than or equal to 0.8 mV (8 mm) in each of the limb leads
- Poor R-wave progression in the precordial leads V1 to V3 ± V4.

Goldberger's triad is a specific ECG sign for DCM, it is not reflective of the severity of left ventricular dysfunction.[58]

The ECG abnormalities of ischemic DCM usually include:

- Presence of pathological Q waves suggesting old myocardial infarction (Figs. 18.24 and 18.25)
- Diffuse ST-segment depression and TWI
- Bundle branch block pattern or IVCD
- Voltage criteria of LVH.

The ECG abnormalities those are frequently seen in patients with nonischemic DCM (Fig. 18.26) are:

- Left ventricular hypertrophy pattern: even if the wall thickness is not increased, the LVH pattern may be seen due to increased left ventricular mass of the dilated heart
- LBBB (more frequent), IVCD, RBBB (less frequent)
- Left atrial abnormality, biatrial abnormality: due to increased ventricular end-diastolic pressure and the resultant atrial dilatation
- Abnormal Q waves (pseudoinfarction pattern): due to myocardial fibrosis
- Poor R-wave progression in chest leads particularly in leads V1-V4
- Nonspecific ST-segment depression with widespread T inversion
- Sinus tachycardia: due to increased sympathetic activity in heart failure
- Supraventricular arrhythmias (AF, etc.)
- Ventricular arrhythmias [isolated premature ventricular contraction (PVC), couplets, bigeminy, trigeminy, etc.]
- First-degree AV block.

Among individuals with nonischemic cardiomyopathy, the most common abnormalities seen include; voltage criteria for LVH (33–40%), widespread TWI (25–45%), LAE (15–33%), LAD (15–25%), pathological Q waves (10–25%), LBBB (9–25%), PVCs (5–10%), and RBBB (4%).[59] But unfortunately these findings are nonspecific for DCM.

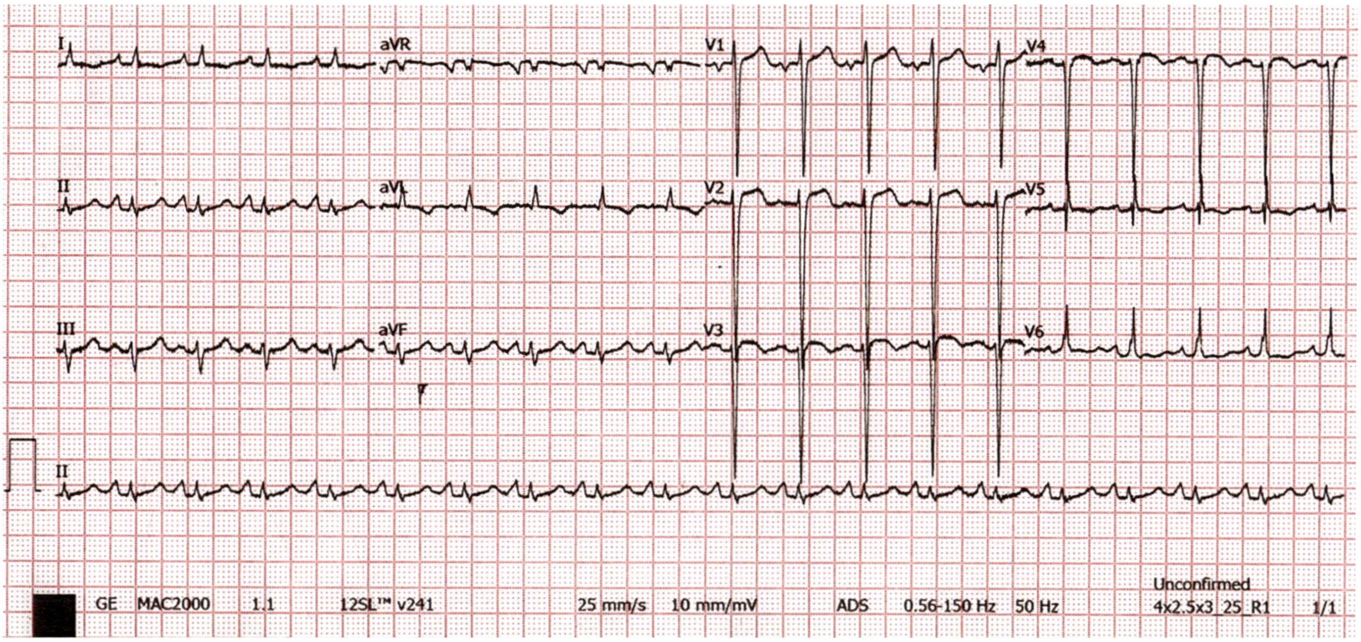

Fig. 18.23: This ECG illustrates all the features of Goldberger's triad for the diagnosis of dilated cardiomyopathy: (1) LVH in the anterior precordial leads (SV1 + RV6 = 35 mm and S in V2 = 32 mm); (2) Low voltage ECG in limb leads (R + S) less than 8 mm; and (3) Poor R-wave progression in leads V1-V4.

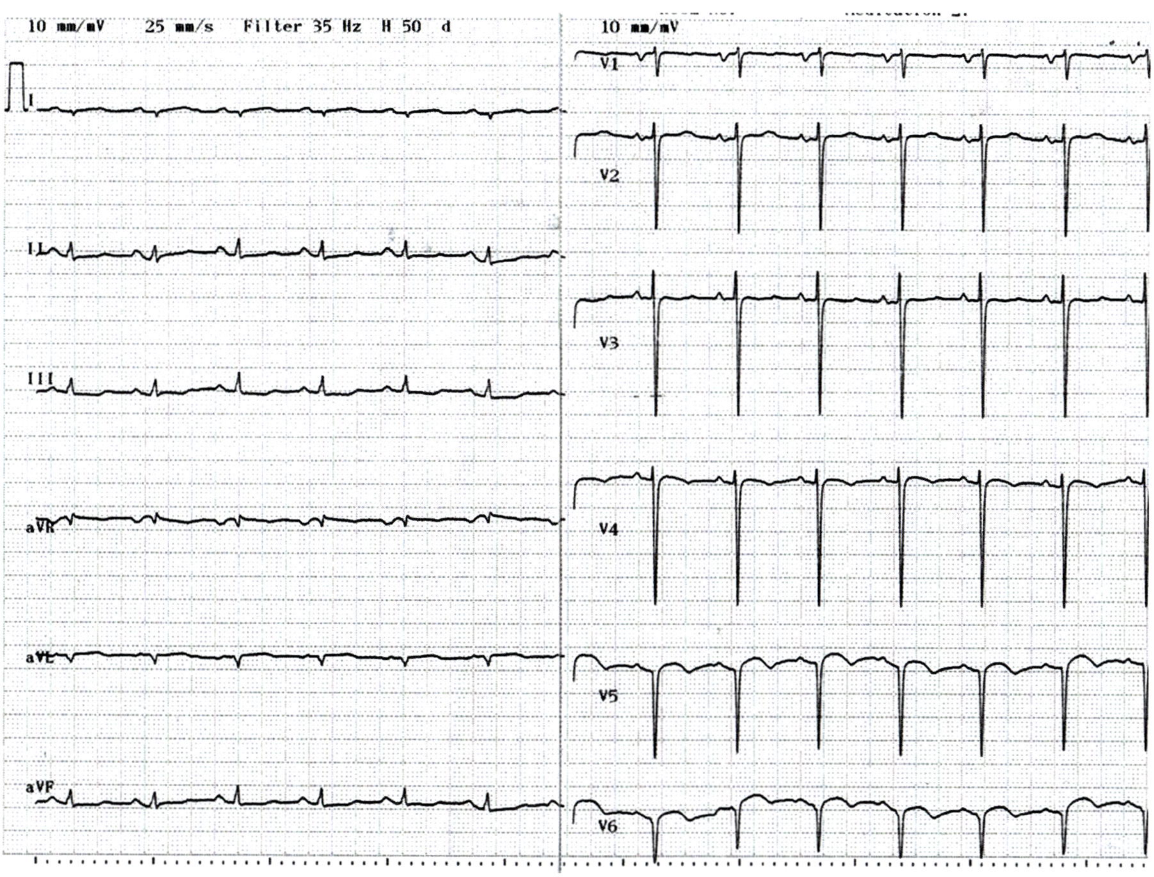

Fig. 18.24: This ECG illustrates the electrocardiographic features of ischemic dilated cardiomyopathy (IDCM). Note pathological Q waves in LI, aVL, V5-V6 along with low voltage in the first six leads. Also note poor R-wave progression V1 to V4 along with ECG sign of left atrial enlargement in V1. Presence of pathological Q waves suggesting old anterior myocardial infarction.

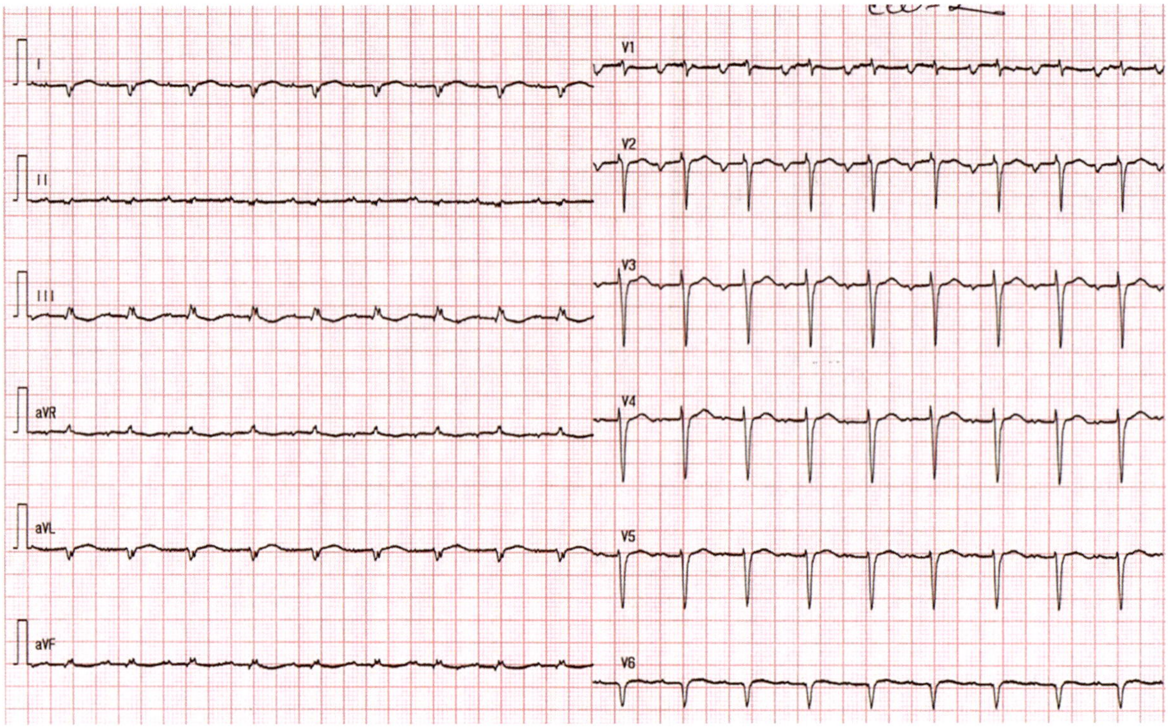

Fig. 18.25: This ECG illustrates the typical ECG features of ischemic dilated cardiomyopathy (IDCM). Note pathological Q waves in LI, aVL, and V6 along with low voltage in the first six leads. Also note poor R-wave progression V1 to V5 along with ECG sign of left atrial enlargement in V1 with sinus tachycardia (heart rate 106 bpm). Presence of pathological Q waves indicate prior myocardial infarction.

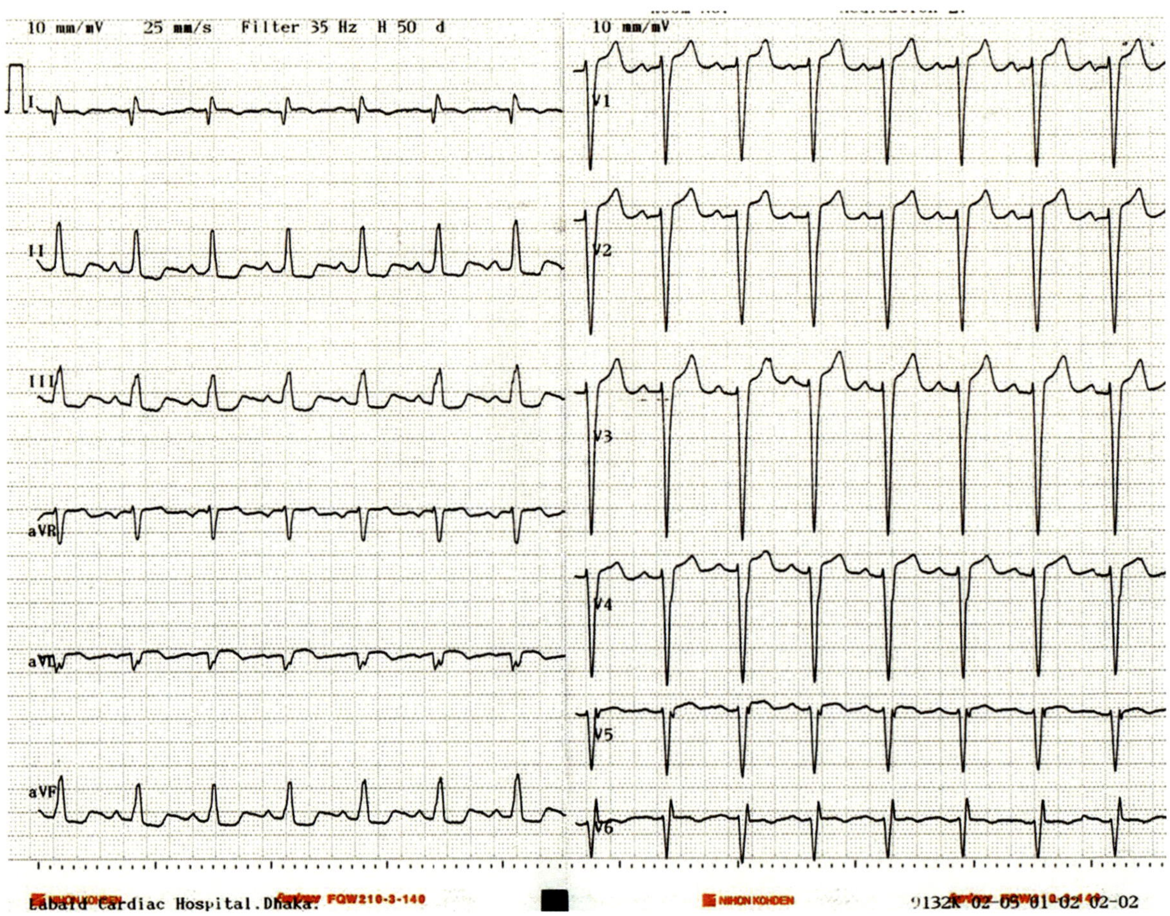

Fig. 18.26: This ECG illustrates the typical ECG features of nonischemic dilated cardiomyopathy (DCM) with LBBB pattern with poor R-wave progression V1-V6 with abnormal Q waves (pseudoinfarction pattern) in LI and aVL with nonspecific ST-segment depression and T-wave changes. Abnormal Q waves (pseudoinfarction pattern) in the ECG of DCM are due to myocardial fibrosis.

RESTRICTIVE CARDIOMYOPATHY

Restrictive cardiomyopathy (RCM) is a primary abnormality of diastolic function caused by derangement in the dynamics of ventricular filling, resulting in an increase in ventricular end-diastolic pressures and dilated atria. Systolic function is preserved in most cases, depending on the underlying cause.[59,60]

Restrictive cardiomyopathy commonly results from myocardial or endomyocardial diseases of diverse causes which "stiffen" the heart by infiltration or fibrosis. RCM may be classified as primary or secondary. The primary RCMs include endomyocardial fibrosis, Loeffler endocarditis, and idiopathic cardiomyopathy. The secondary forms of RCM are more common and include specific heart muscle diseases in which the heart is affected as part of a multisystem disorder. These can be subclassified as noninfiltrative (e.g. carcinoid heart disease), infiltrative (e.g. amyloidosis, sarcoidosis, or postirradiation therapy), or as storage disorders (hemochromatosis, glycogen storage disease, Fabry disease).[61]

The 12-lead ECG at the time of the initial diagnosis was reviewed in one series of 94 patients and demonstrated AF in 70 patients (74%), sinus rhythm in 20 (21%), and paced rhythm in 4. Of those in sinus rhythm, 4 patients had a history of paroxysmal AF. Eighteen patients (19%) had an IVCD. Nonspecific ST-T wave abnormalities were noted in 75 patients (79.8%), premature ventricular beats in 13 (13.8%), and premature atrial beats in 5 (5.3%). Two patients (2.1%) had a normal ECG.[59,60]

Diffuse myocardial infiltration leads to low voltage QRS complexes (the amplitudes of all the QRS complexes in the limb leads are <5 mm; or the amplitudes of all the QRS complexes in the precordial leads are <10 mm). AF usually occurs due to atrial enlargement (Fig. 18.27) but ventricular arrhythmias are also common. Infiltration of the cardiac conducting system (e.g. due to septal granuloma formation in sarcoidosis) may lead to conduction disturbance—e.g. bundle branch blocks and AV block and healing granulomas, e.g. sarcoidosis may produce "pseudoinfarction" Q waves.[59-61] In echocardiogram the atriums appear dilated and the ECG may exhibits large P waves indicating biatrial enlargement (Figs. 18.28 and 18.29) accompanied by various ST-segment and T-wave abnormalities.[62,63]

ARRHYTHMOGENIC RIGHT VENTRICULAR CARDIOMYOPATHY/DYSPLASIA

Unlike HCM, DCM, and RCM, ARVC/D is defined histologically by the presence of progressive replacement of RV myocardium with adipose and fibrous tissue often confined to a "triangle of dysplasia" comprising the RV inflow, outflow, and apex.[5] ARVC/D is defined by the presence of RV dysfunction (global or regional), with or without left ventricular disease, in the presence of histological evidence for the disease. Although uncommon (estimated prevalence 1:5,000), ARVC/D is a frequent cause of sudden death in young people in some areas of Europe.[5,64]

Ninety percent of individuals with ARVC/D have some ECG abnormality and the *epsilon wave* is the typical ECG finding (Figs. 18.30 and 18.31). The most common ECG abnormality seen in ARVC/D is TWI in leads V1 to V3 (Fig. 18.32). However, this is a nonspecific finding, and may be considered a normal variant in RBBB, women, and children under 12 years old. RBBB itself is seen frequently in individuals with ARVC/D. This may be due to delayed activation of the right ventricle, rather than any intrinsic abnormality in the right bundle branch. The *epsilon wave* is found in about 50% of those with ARVC/D. This is described as a terminal notch in the QRS complex. It is due to slowed intraventricular conduction. Ventricular ectopy seen on a

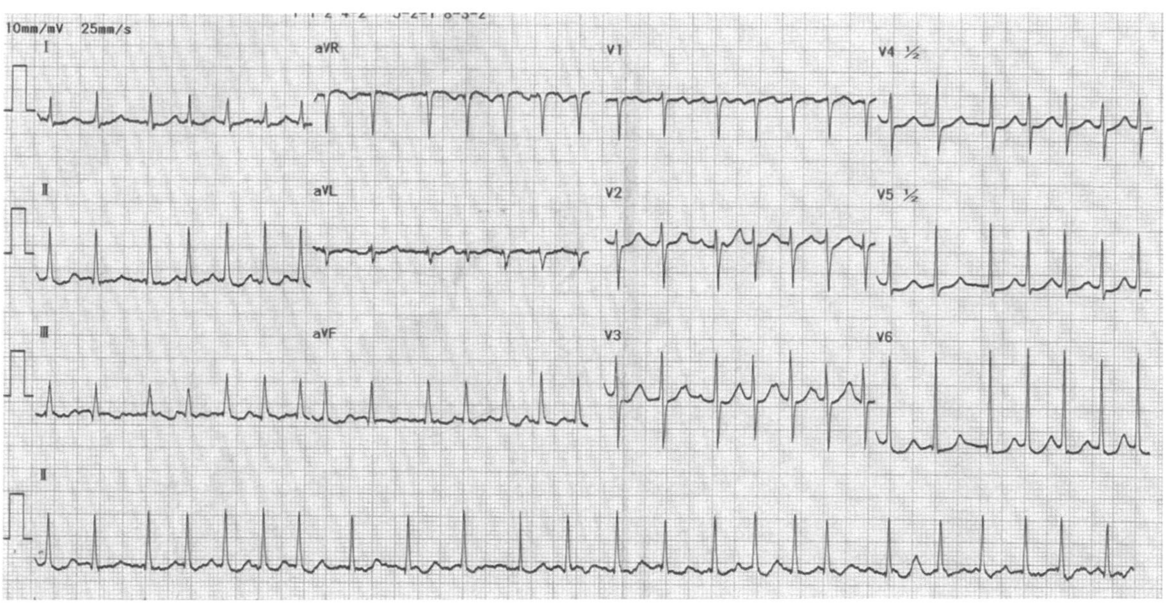

Fig. 18.27: ECG showing fast AF (heart rate 143 bpm) in a patient with restrictive cardiomyopathy. AF is a frequently seen arrhythmia in patients with restrictive cardiomyopathy.

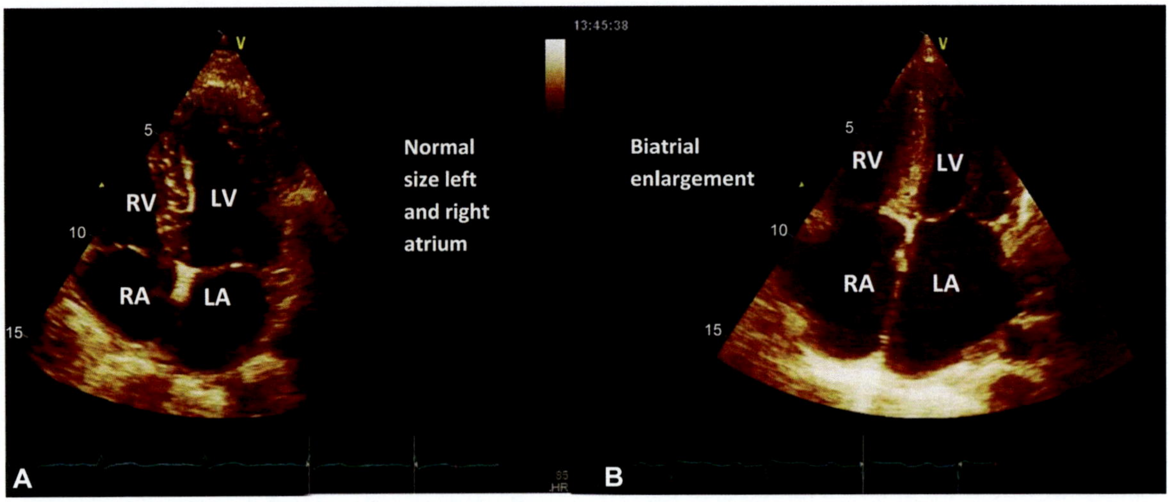

Figs. 18.28A and B: Two-dimensional (2D) echocardiogram, apical 4-chamber view showing (A) normal left and right atrium and (B) biatrial enlargement in a patient with restrictive cardiomyopathy. (LA: left atrium; RA: right atrium; LV: left ventricle; RV: right ventricle). (*Source:* Courtesy of Dr Azizur Rahman)

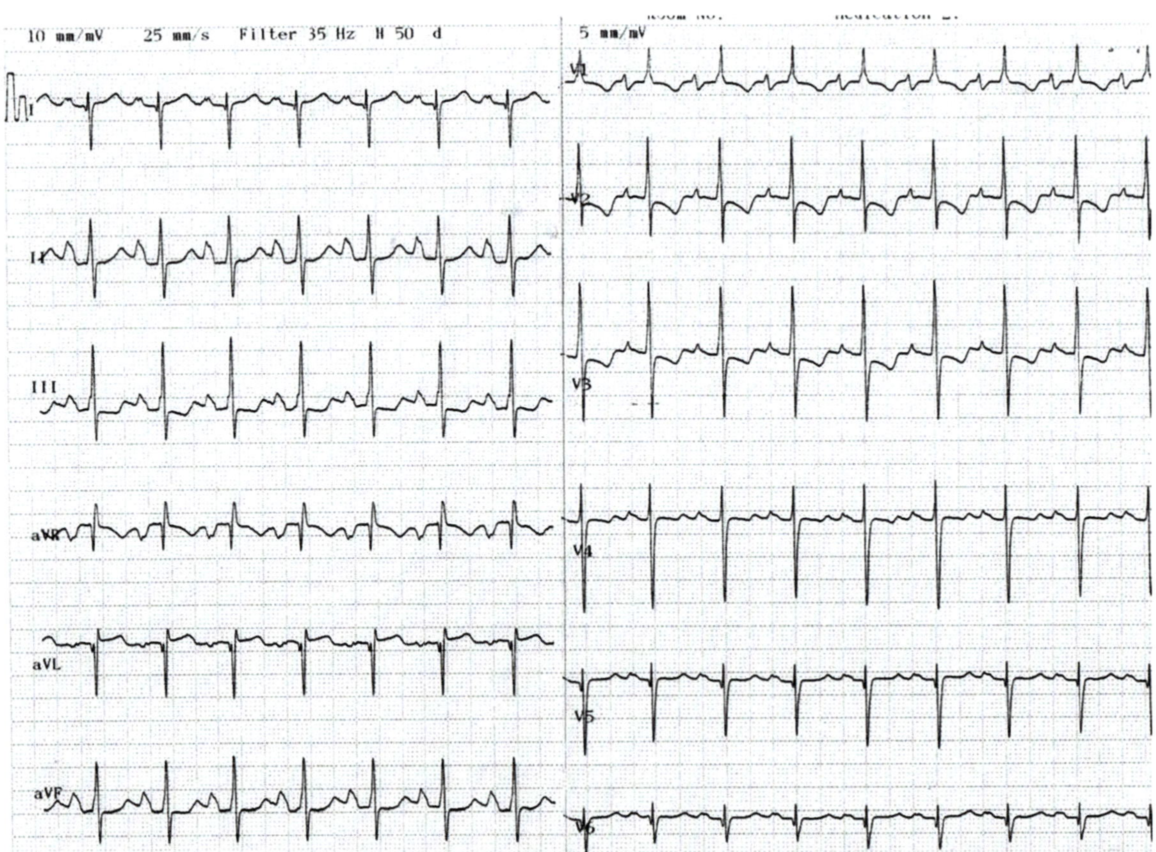

Fig. 18.29: ECG illustrates biatrial enlargement in restrictive cardiomyopathy. This ECG shows biphasic P waves in V1 with a tall positive deflection (1.5 mm in height), suggestive of right atrial enlargement and a negative deflection that is both deep (>1 mm) and wide (>40 ms), suggestive of left atrial enlargement. Also note ECG evidence of P pulmonale in LII (amplitude of P wave >2.5 mm) and bifid P waves in LI, V4-V6 suggestive of P mitrale. ECG also shows partial right bundle branch block with diffuse ST depression and T-wave changes with right axis deviation.

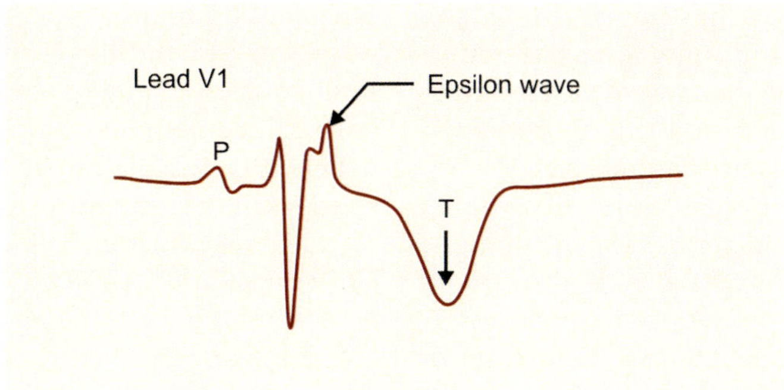

Fig. 18.30: ECG in lead V1 showing *Epsilon wave*. Note the epsilon wave as a small positive deflection (blip) between end of QRS complex to onset of the T wave (arrow).

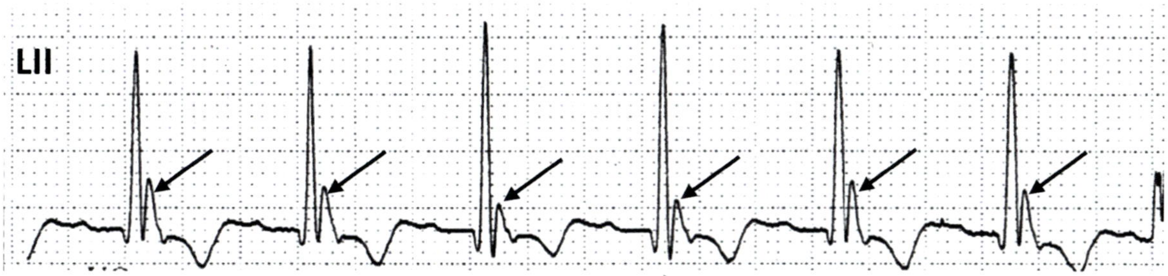

Fig. 18.31: ECG displaying *Epsilon waves* (arrows) with T-wave inversions.

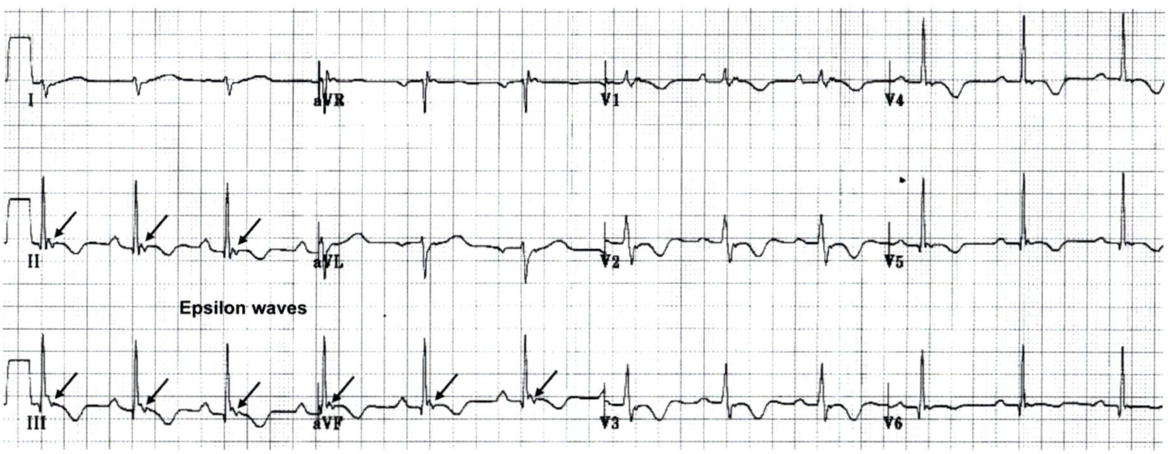

Fig. 18.32: ECG displaying the classical electrocardiographic features of arrhythmogenic right ventricular cardiomyopathy/dysplasia (ARVC/D). Note the presence of *Epsilon wave* in multiple leads (arrows) more marked in inferior leads and T-wave inversion in leads V1-V3. This particular ECG also shows T-wave inversion in multiple limb and precordial leads with partial RBBB pattern.

surface ECG in the setting of ARVC/D is typically of LBBB morphology, with a QRS axis of –90° to +110°. The origin of the ectopic beats is usually from one of the three regions of fatty degeneration: (1) the RV outflow tract, (2) the RV inflow tract, and (3) the RV apex. The specific ECG abnormalities reflect the pathophysiology of the disease including TWI due to scarring of the free wall of the RV, localized right precordial QRS prolongation, prolonged S-wave duration due to slow depolarization of the terminal part of the QRS because the RV is the last part of the heart to undergo depolarization, and epsilon waves due to slow conduction in the RV.[65-67] In ARVC/D patients with complete RBBB, possibly the most sensitive and specific parameter is an r'/s ratio less than 1 in V1.[68]

LEFT VENTRICULAR NONCOMPACTION

Left ventricular noncompaction is reported to be the most common cause of unclassified cardiomyopathies.[69] LVNC is frequently familial, with at least 25% of asymptomatic relatives having a range of echocardiographic abnormalities. LVNC is characterized by prominent left ventricular trabeculae and deep intertrabecular recesses. The myocardial wall is often thickened with a thin, compacted epicardial layer and a thickened endocardial layer.[5,70]

A high prevalence of ECG abnormalities has been noted in this condition. In a published series, 75% of patients of LVNC had ECG abnormalities. The most prominent features are biventricular hypertrophy, extreme QRS voltage, isolated or diffuse TWI.[71] But there are no ECG features or patterns specific for this disease. Sometimes ECGs of LVNC are associated with WPW syndrome, premature atrial and ventricular contractions.[71]

TAKOTSUBO CARDIOMYOPATHY

Takotsubo cardiomyopathy, also called "apical ballooning syndrome (ABS)", "broken heart syndrome", and "stress-induced cardiomyopathy", is an increasingly reported syndrome generally characterized by transient systolic dysfunction of the apical and/or mid segments of the left ventricle that mimics myocardial infarction, but in the absence of obstructive coronary artery disease.[72-77] Takotsubo cardiomyopathy was first described in Japan,[72,74] and was subsequently reported in non-Asian populations, including the United States and Europe.[76,78,79] More than 90% of reported cases are in women ages 58–75.

Takotsubo cardiomyopathy is a unique cardiomyopathy characterized by chest pain, ECG, and regional wall motion abnormalities closely mimicking AMI, in the absence of significant coronary artery disease. Classic ECG changes of Takotsubo cardiomyopathy include ST elevation or TWI.[80] Currently, the criteria proposed by the Mayo Clinic group are widely used for the diagnosis of Takotsubo cardiomyopathy. About a third of patients with Takotsubo cardiomyopathy have ST-segment elevation (Fig. 18.33) and another third have TWIs. ECG is normal or shows minor nonspecific changes in the remaining third.[73,81,82]

Electrocardiographic findings in patients with Takotsubo cardiomyopathy vary at presentation. ST-segment elevation is present in approximately one-third of patients, with the anterior leads most commonly involved.[83] However, deep TWI and nonspecific ST-T wave changes may also be seen on the ECG at presentation. Common changes observed with serial ECGs include prolongation of the QT interval and deep, symmetric TWI that may take several weeks or months to resolve.[83] Despite the long QT interval, torsades de pointes rarely is reported.[84,85]

Differentiation between Acute Anterior Myocardial Infarction and Takotsubo Cardiomyopathy

Because clinical features of Takotsubo cardiomyopathy mimics those of acute anterior myocardial infarction, the differential diagnosis is important in selecting the appropriate treatment strategy, especially in the acute phase.[86,87]

The absence of abnormal Q waves, absence of reciprocal changes, ST-segment depression in lead aVR, and absence of ST-segment elevation in lead V1 can identify Takotsubo cardiomyopathy (Fig. 18.34) with sensitivities of 42%, 94%, 97%, and 94%, specificities of 74%, 49%, 75%, and

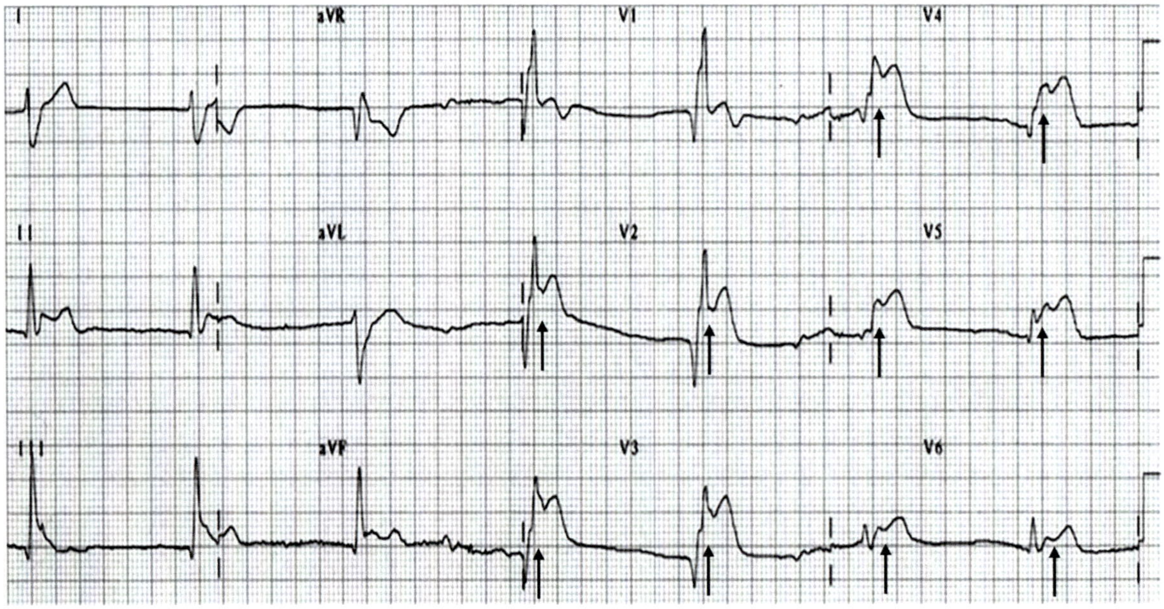

Fig. 18.33: ECG illustrates classical features of Takotsubo cardiomyopathy with ST-segment elevation in chest leads V2-V6 mimicking acute anterior ST-segment elevation myocardial infarction (STEMI). Absence of reciprocal ST depression in inferior leads and ST segment depression in lead aVR suggest the diagnosis of Takotsubo cardiomyopathy rather than anterior STEMI. Note there is no reciprocal ST depression in LII, LIII and aVF, rather ST-segment appears elevated in these inferior leads.

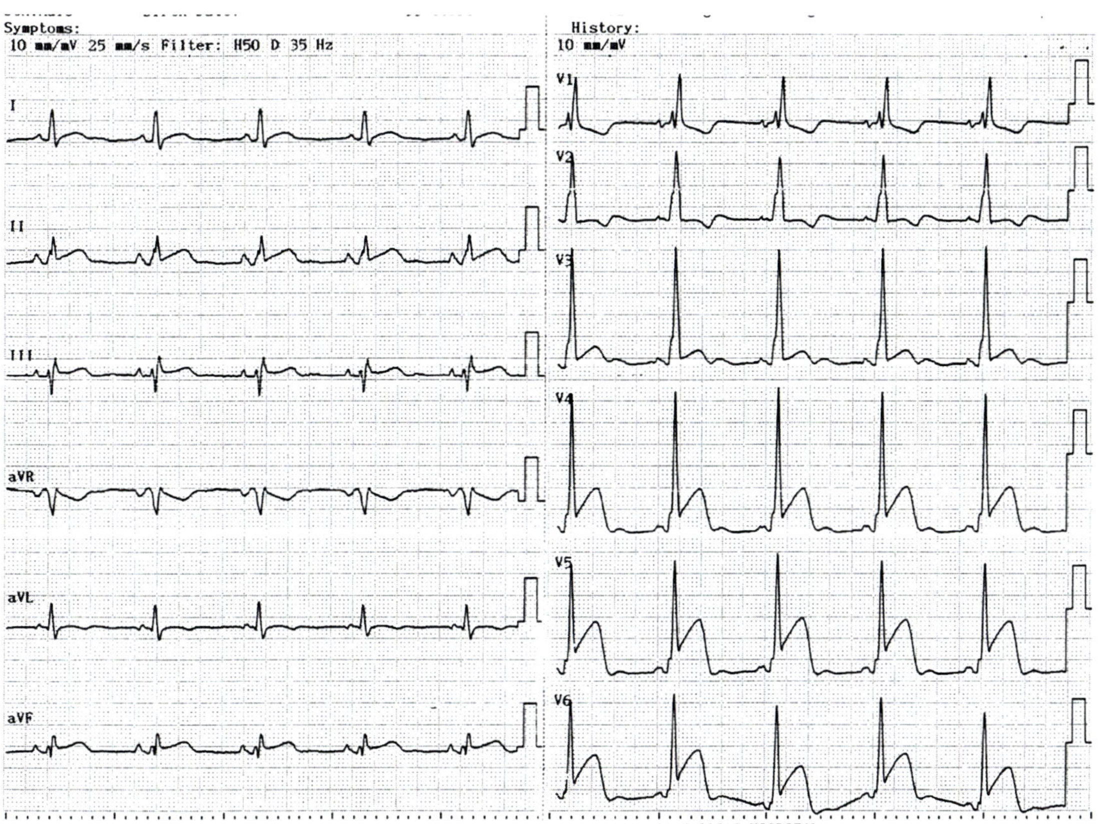

Fig. 18.34: ECG of a 60-year-old lady displaying typical features of Takotsubo cardiomyopathy. Note ST-segment elevation in leads V4-V6 mimicking acute anterior ST-segment elevation myocardial infarction (STEMI) without any reciprocal ST depression in inferior leads. Absence of reciprocal changes, ST-segment depression in lead aVR and absence of ST-segment elevation in lead V1 are suggestive of Takotsubo cardiomyopathy rather than acute anterior STEMI.

71%, and predictive accuracies of 71%, 53%, 77%, and 73%, respectively.[88] The combination of the presence of ST-segment depression in lead aVR and the absence of ST-segment elevation in lead V1 can identify Takotsubo cardiomyopathy with 91% sensitivity, 96% specificity, and 95% predictive accuracy, which is superior to any other electrocardiographic findings.[88] Compared with anterior AMI, Takotsubo cardiomyopathy is associated with less ST-segment elevation and more frequent absence of abnormal Q waves, suggesting less myocardial damage. Nevertheless, in Takotsubo cardiomyopathy, ST-segment elevation was more extensive, involving not only the anterior region.[74,82,88]

SUMMARY

Cardiomyopathy is a progressive disease of the myocardium. In cardiomyopathy, the heart muscle becomes thick, enlarged, or rigid. In rare cases, the muscle tissue in the heart is replaced with scar tissue.

Cardiomyopathies are classified into five different types: (1) HCM, (2) DCM, (3) RCM, (4) ARVC/D, and (5) unclassified, e.g. LVNC, Takotsubo cardiomyopathy.

Hypertrophic Cardiomyopathy

Hypertrophic cardiomyopathy is a genetic disorder of cardiac muscle with a prevalence of 1 in 500 of the general population. In most adults, HCM is inherited as an autosomal dominant trait. HCM is one of the most common inherited cardiac disorders and is the number one cause of SCD in young athletes. Annual mortality is around 1%. HCM may be associated with WPW syndrome and features of both the conditions may be reflected on the ECG.

Patterns of HCM have been shown in Box 18.1.

Electrocardiograms of HCM usually reveal LVH voltage criteria with nonspecific ST-segment and T-wave abnormalities along with deep, narrow (dagger-like) Q waves in the lateral (V5-V6, I, aVL) and inferior (II, III, aVF) leads. These may mimic prior myocardial infarction. Lateral Q waves are more common than inferior Q waves in HCM.

Box 18.1: Patterns of hypertrophic cardiomyopathy.

- Asymmetrical septal hypertrophy (ASH)—70%
- Concentric hypertrophy—20%
- Apical cardiomyopathy—10%

Electrocardiograms of HCM usually show the following abnormalities:

- Voltage criteria of LVH
- ST-segment depression
- T-wave inversion
- Pathological Q waves
- Intraventricular conduction delay
- Left-axis deviation
- Left atrial enlargement
- ST-segment elevation (rarely).

In absence of hypertension and aortic stenosis, HCM, particularly ASH, can be diagnosed easily by using Anis-Baren ECG triad which includes ECG evidence of LVH systolic overload pattern along with TWI in LII with upright T in aVR and LIII (Box 18.2).

Apical hypertrophic cardiomyopathy is an atypical phenotype of nonobstructive HCM with an indistinguishable histology. In Japan, this apical variant constitutes approximately 15–25% of patients with HCM, although it is uncommon in other parts of the world, accounting for only 3% of patients with HCM.

Electrocardiographic features of apical hypertrophic cardiomyopathy include:

- The presence of giant (over 10 mm) inverted T waves in anterolateral leads particularly in leads V4 and V5 of the resting ECG
- Voltage criteria of LVH, the electrocardiographic sum RV5 + SV1 greater than 35 mm.

Though Anis-Baren ECG triad is more specific for electrocardiographic diagnosis of ASH variety of HCM but inverted T in LII and upright T in LIII, and aVR may also be seen in many cases of apical cardiomyopathy with or without ECG evidence of LVH.

Dilated Cardiomyopathy

Dilated cardiomyopathy is a disease of the heart muscle with impaired systolic function (impaired contractility) which involves one or both ventricles.

There are no ECG features unique to DCM, although the ECG is usually abnormal. The most common ECG abnormalities are those associated with atrial and ventricular hypertrophy—typically, left-sided changes are seen but there may be signs of biatrial or biventricular hypertrophy. The following ECG features may suggest the diagnosis of DCM:

Box 18.2: Anis-Baren triad for the diagnosis of hypertrophic cardiomyopathy (HCM).

In the absence of hypertension and aortic stenosis, the following three ECG features are suggestive of HCM:

1. Left ventricular hypertrophy (LVH) systolic overload pattern
2. T-wave inversion in LII
3. Upright T in aVR and LIII

- Sinus tachycardia with diffuse ST-T wave changes
- Left ventricular hypertrophy or biventricular enlargement
- Poor R-wave progression with QS complexes in V1-V4 (pseudoinfarction pattern)
- Left bundle branch block or IVCD. But RBBB can also occur
- Left-axis deviation
- Left atrial enlargement or biatrial enlargement
- Arrhythmias like AF or frequent ventricular ectopics and ventricular bigeminy may be seen.

Dilated cardiomyopathy is of two types:

1. *Ischemic*: Following massive anterior myocardial infarction or due to diffuse coronary artery disease.
2. *Nonischemic*: Nonischemic DCM is mostly idiopathic but up to 25% are familial. It may be due to viral myocarditis, alcoholism, drug-induced or due to autoimmune diseases. Pregnancy-associated DCM is termed as peripartum cardiomyopathy.

Goldberger ECG triad of DCM includes:

- LVH in the anterior precordial leads (SV1 or SV2) + (RV5 or RV6) greater than or equal to 3.5 mV (35 mm)
- Low limb lead voltage (i.e. R + S) less than or equal to 0.8 mV (8 mm)
- Poor precordial R-wave progression in leads V1 to V4.

Restrictive Cardiomyopathy

Restrictive cardiomyopathy is the least common form of cardiomyopathy. It may be primary or secondary. As a secondary phenomenon, it may occur in the advanced stages of myocardial infiltrative diseases—e.g. due to hemochromatosis, amyloidosis or sarcoidosis.

The ECG criteria of restrictive cardiomyopathy include:

- Nonspecific ST-segment/T-wave changes
- Low voltage QRS complexes
- Atrial and ventricular dysrhythmias. AF is a common ECG finding
- ECG evidence of biatrial enlargement
- Atrioventricular block (even third-degree AV block may occur in sarcoidosis)
- Pathological Q waves
- Bundle branch block pattern.

Arrhythmogenic Right Ventricular Cardiomyopathy/Dysplasia

The ECG provides important information to aid in the diagnosis of ARVC/D. The ECG changes may be explained by the pathophysiology of the disease. The proximity of the right ventricle to the anterior chest leads V1 to V3, explains why the characteristic ECG abnormalities are most prominent in those leads. The extent of ECG abnormalities correlates with the degree of structural change in the right ventricle.

The important ECG features of ARVC/D include:

- T-wave inversion in leads V1 to V3
- The *epsilon wave* is found in about 50% cases
- A prolonged S-wave upstroke in V1 through V3 is a frequent ECG finding in ARVC/D
- RBBB is seen frequently in individuals with ARVC/D
- Localized right precordial QRS prolongation
- Ventricular ectopy with typical LBBB morphology.

Takotsubo Cardiomyopathy

Takotsubo cardiomyopathy is a novel cardiomyopathy that has been recently recognized as an important consideration in the differential diagnosis of acute coronary syndrome particularly anterior ST-elevation myocardial infarction (STEMI). The presenting features of Takotsubo cardiomyopathy are similar to those of myocardial ischemia but without epicardial coronary occlusion. A preceding emotional or physical stressor is common. Although the acute presentation can include life-threatening symptoms and hemodynamic compromise, the long-term prognosis is more benign than that of traditional acute coronary syndrome.

In acute setting, it is very difficult to differentiate Takotsubo cardiomyopathy from STEMI. So acute extensive STEMI-in-evolution is often the initial diagnosis. Takotsubo cardiomyopathy is also known as "transient ventricular ballooning syndrome", "stress-induced cardiomyopathy", "ampulla cardiomyopathy", and "broken heart syndrome".

The ECG features of Takotsubo cardiomyopathy include:

- ST-segment elevation mimicking acute anterior myocardial infarction is present in approximately one-third of patients
- Deep TWI and nonspecific ST-T wave changes may also be seen in another one-third of patients
- ECG is normal or shows minor nonspecific changes in the remaining one-third of patients.

In the acute phase, ECG of Takotsubo cardiomyopathy may be confused with acute anterior myocardial infarction and these two conditions may be differentiated with reasonable certainty from the ECGs. The differentiating points are:

- Reciprocal ST depression is an important ECG finding in the setting of evolving acute ST elevation anterior myocardial infarction, which is absent in the ECG of Takotsubo cardiomyopathy.
- Absence of abnormal Q waves goes in favor of the diagnosis of Takotsubo cardiomyopathy.
- Compared with anterior STEMI, Takotsubo cardiomyopathy is associated with less ST-segment elevation and more frequent absence of abnormal Q waves.
- In Takotsubo cardiomyopathy, ST-segment elevation is more extensive, involving not only the anterior region.
- In ECG, the presence of ST-segment depression in lead aVR and the absence of ST-segment elevation in lead V1 are suggestive of Takotsubo cardiomyopathy.

REFERENCES

1. Abelmann WH. Classification and natural history of primary myocardial disease. Prog Cardiovasc Dis. 1984;27:73-94.
2. Report of the WHO/ISFC task force on the definition and classification of cardiomyopathies. Br Heart J. 1980;44:672-3.
3. Richardson P, McKenna W, Bristow M, et al. Report of the 1995 World Health Organization/International Society and Federation of Cardiology task force on the definition and classification of cardiomyopathies. Circulation. 1996;93:841-2.
4. Maron BJ, Towbin JA, Thiene G, et al. Contemporary definitions and classification of the cardiomyopathies: an American Heart Association Scientific Statement from the Council on Clinical Cardiology, Heart Failure and Transplantation Committee; Quality of Care and Outcomes Research and Functional Genomics and Translational Biology Interdisciplinary Working Groups; and Council on Epidemiology and Prevention. Circulation. 2006;113:1807-16.
5. Elliott P, Andersson B, Arbustini E, et al. Classification of the cardiomyopathies: a position statement from the European Society Of Cardiology Working Group on myocardial and pericardial diseases. Eur Heart J. 2008;29:270-6.
6. O'Mahony C, Elliott PM. Prevention of sudden cardiac death in hypertrophic cardiomyopathy. Heart. 2014;100:254-60.
7. Maron BJ, Contemporary insights and strategies for risk stratification and prevention of sudden death in hypertrophic cardiomyopathy. Circulation. 2010;121:445-56.
8. Gersh BJ, Maron BJ, Bonow RO, et al. 2011 ACCF/AHA guideline for the diagnosis and treatment of hypertrophic cardiomyopathy: a report of the American College of Cardiology Foundation/American Heart Association Task Force on practice guidelines. Developed in collaboration with the American Association for Thoracic Surgery, American Society of Echocardiography, American Society of Nuclear Cardiology, Heart Failure Society of America, Heart Rhythm Society, Society for Cardiovascular Angiography and Interventions, and Society of Thoracic Surgeons, J Am Coll Cardiol. 2011;58:e212-60.
9. Maron BJ, Maron MS, Wigle ED, et al. The 50-year history, controversy, and clinical implications of left ventricular outflow tract obstruction in hypertrophic cardiomyopathy from idiopathic hypertrophic subaortic stenosis to hypertrophic cardiomyopathy. J Am Coll Cardiol. 2009;54:191-200.
10. Maron BJ, Maron MS, Danielson GK, et al. American College of Cardiology/European Society of Cardiology clinical expert consensus document on hypertrophic cardiomyopathy: a report of the American College of Cardiology Foundation Task Force on Clinical Expert Consensus Documents and the European Society of Cardiology Committee for Practice Guidelines, J Am Coll Cardiol. 2003;42:1687-713.
11. Ryan MP, Cleland JG, French JA, et al. The standard electrocardiogram as a screening test for hypertrophic cardiomyopathy. Am J Cardiol. 1995;76:689-94.
12. Rowin EJ, Maron BJ, Appelbaum E, et al. Significance of false negative electrocardiograms in preparticipation screening of athletes for hypertrophic cardiomyopathy. Am J Cardiol. 2012;110:1027-32.
13. Drezner JA, Ashley E, Baggish AL, et al. Abnormal electrocardiographic findings in athletes: recognising changes

suggestive of cardiomyopathy. Br J Sports Med. 2013;47: 137-52.
14. Chakraborty B, Khair A, Zaman F, et al. Hypertrophic cardiomyopathy (HCM) with marked ST segment elevation mimicking acute anterior myocardial infarction: a case report. Bangladesh J Cardiol. 2014;1:682-4.
15. Olearczyk B, Gollol-Raju N, Menzies DJ. Apical hypertrophic cardiomyopathy mimicking acute coronary syndrome: a case report and review of the literature. Angiology. 2008;59(5):629-31.
16. Luzza F, Carerj S, Oreto G. Hypertrophic cardiomyopathy with persistent ST segment elevation simulating acute myocardial infarction. Heart. 2004;90(4):380.
17. Daralammouri Y, El Garhy M, Same K, et al. Hypertrophic cardiomyopathy mimicking acute anterior myocardial infarction associated with sudden cardiac death. Case Rep Med. 2012;2012:236154.
18. Corrado D, Pelliccia A, Heidbuchel H, et al. Recommendations for interpretation of 12-lead electrocardiogram in the athlete. Eur Heart J. 2010;31:243-59.
19. Uberoi A, Stein R, Perez MV, et al. Interpretation of the electrocardiogram of young athletes. Circulation. 2011;124:746-57.
20. Williams ES, Owens DS, Drezner JA, et al. Electrocardiogram interpretation in the athlete. Herzschrittmacherther Elektrophysiol. 2012;23:65-71.
21. Lakdawala NK, Thune JJ, Maron BJ, et al. Electrocardiographic features of sarcomere mutation carriers with and without clinically overt hypertrophic cardiomyopathy. Am J Cardiol. 2011;108:1606-13.
22. Papadakis M, Carre F, Kervio G, et al. The prevalence, distribution, and clinical outcomes of electrocardiographic repolarization patterns in male athletes of African/Afro-Caribbean origin. Eur Heart J. 2011;32:2304-13.
23. Papadakis M, Basavarajaiah S, Rawlins J, et al. Prevalence and significance of T-wave inversions in predominantly Caucasian adolescent athletes. Eur Heart J. 2009;30:1728-35.
24. Le VV, Wheeler MT, Mandic S, et al. Addition of the electrocardiogram to the preparticipation examination of college athletes. Clin J Sport Med. 2010;20:98-105.
25. Groeneweg JA, van der Heijden JF, Dooijes D et al. Arrhythmogenic cardiomyopathy: diagnosis, genetic background, and risk management. Neth Heart J. 2014;22:316-25.
26. Konno T, Shimizu M, Ino H, et al. Diagnostic value of abnormal Q waves for identification of preclinical carriers of hypertrophic cardiomyopathy based on a molecular genetic diagnosis. Eur Heart J. 2004;25:246-51.
27. Steinvil A, Chundadze T, Zeltser D. Mandatory electrocardiographic screening of athletes to reduce their risk for sudden death proven fact or wishful thinking? J Am Coll Cardiol. 2011;57:1291-6.
28. Marek J, Bufalino V, Davis J, et al. Feasibility and findings of large-scale electrocardiographic screening in young adults: data from 32,561 subjects. Heart Rhythm. 2011;8:1555-9.
29. Waiz A, Chakraborty B. Diagnostic value of ECG as screening test for hypertrophic cardiomyopathy. Bangladesh Armed Forces Med J. 1990;14(1):31-40.
30. Waiz A, Chakraborty B. ECG diagnosis and treatment outcome of 96 patients with hypertrophic cardiomyopathy. Abstract book, VI World Congress of Cardiac Rehabilitation, Buenos Aires, Argentina; 1996. page 94.
31. Waiz A, Chakraborty B. An analysis of 48 cases of hypertrophic cardiomyopathy. Abstract book, German-Bangladesh Joint Conference on Cardiology, 1990, page 7.
32. Chakraborty B, Perveen S, Ali ML. Determinants of left atrial size in apical cardiomyopathy. J Bangladesh Assoc Physicians. 2004;12:213-7.
33. Waiz A, Chakraborty B. Natural history of hypertrophic cardiomyopathy—our experience. Abstract book, Annual Scientific Meetings of Association of Physicians of Bangladesh, March 2000, page 27.
34. Chakraborty B, Perveen S, Ali ML, et al. Left atrial size in hypertrophic cardiomyopathy—the impact of mitral regurgitation and left ventricular outflow tract gradient. Chest Heart J. 2003;27(1):27-30.
35. Chakraborty B, Perveen S, Ali ML, et al. Impact of left ventricular outflow tract obstruction on the clinical outcome of patients with hypertrophic cardiomyopathy. Indian Heart J. 2003;55(5):554-5.
36. Chakraborty B, Waiz A. Verapamil versus propranolol in hypertrophic cardiomyopathy—our experience. J Bangladesh Assoc Physicians. 1997;2:143-6.
37. Chakraborty B, Waiz A. Hypertrophic cardiomyopathy: an analysis. J Univ Sci Tech. Bangladesh. 1996;1:70-80.
38. Sakamoto T. Apical hypertrophic cardiomyopathy (apical hypertrophy): an overview. J Cardiol. 2001;37(Suppl 1):161-78.
39. Ates M, Kwong RY, Lipton MJ, et al. Apical hypertrophic cardiomyopathy: diagnosed by cardiac magnetic resonance imaging. Tex Heart Inst J. 2006;33(3):408-9.
40. McLeod CJ, Ackerman MJ, Nishimura RA, et al. Outcome of patients with hypertrophic cardiomyopathy and a normal electrocardiogram. J Am Coll Cardiol. 2009;54(3):229-33.
41. Hansen MW, Merchant N. MRI of hypertrophic cardiomyopathy: part I, MRI appearances. Am J Roentgenol. 2007;189(6):1335-43.
42. Kelly BS, Mattu A, Brady WJ. Hypertrophic cardiomyopathy: electrocardiographic manifestations and other important considerations for the emergency physician. Am J Emerg Med. 2007;25(1):72-9.
43. Maron BJ. Hypertrophic cardiomyopathy. Lancet. 1997;350(9071):127-33.
44. Kitaoka H, Doi Y, Casey SA, et al. Comparison of prevalence of apical hypertrophic cardiomyopathy in Japan and the United States. Am J Cardiol. 2003;92:1183-6.
45. Eriksson MJ, Sonnenberg B, Woo A, et al. Long-term outcome in patients with apical hypertrophic cardiomyopathy. J Am Coll Cardiol. 2002;39:638-45.
46. Yusuf SW, Bathina JD, Banchs J, et al. Apical hypertrophic cardiomyopathy. World J Cardiol. 2011;3(7):256-9.
47. Sakamoto T, Tei C, Murayama M, et al. Giant T wave inversion as a manifestation of asymmetrical apical hypertrophy (AAH) of the left ventricle. Echocardiographic and ultrasono-cardiotomographic study. Jpn Heart J. 1976;17(5):611-29.
48. Moon JC, Fisher NG, McKenna WJ, et al. Detection of apical hypertrophic cardiomyopathy by cardiovascular magnetic resonance in patients with non-diagnostic echocardiography. Heart. 2004;90(6):645-9.

49. Zachariah S, Davis GK. A patient with recurrent syncope. Postgrad Med J. 2004;80(940):117, 120-1.
50. O'Mahony C, Elliott P, McKenna W. Sudden cardiac death in hypertrophic cardiomyopathy. Circ Arrhythm Electrophysiol. 2013;6:443-51.
51. Wang TJ, Evans JC, Benjamin EJ, et al. Natural history of asymptomatic left ventricular systolic dysfunction in the community. Circulation. 2003;108:977-82.
52. Baig MK, Goldman JH, Caforio AL, et al. Familial dilated cardiomyopathy: cardiac abnormalities are common in asymptomatic relatives and may represent early disease. J Am Coll Cardiol. 1998;31:195-201.
53. Grunig E, Tasman JA, Kucherer H, et al. Frequency and phenotypes of familial dilated cardiomyopathy. J Am Coll Cardiol. 1998;31:186-94.
54. Mahon NG, Murphy RT, MacRae CA, et al. Echocardiographic evaluation in asymptomatic relatives of patients with dilated cardiomyopathy reveals preclinical disease. Ann Intern Med. 2005;143:108-15.
55. Jefferies JL, Towbin JA. Dilated cardiomyopathy. Lancet. 2010;375:752-62.
56. Goldberger AL. A specific ECG triad associated with congestive heart failure. Pacing Clin Electrophysiol. 1982;5:593-9.
57. Goldberger AL, Dresselhaus T, Bhargava V. Dilated cardiomyopathy: utility of the transverse: frontal plane QRS voltage ratio. J Electrocardiol. 1985;18:35-40.
58. Tan RS, Lau KW, Ding ZP, et al. Goldberger's triad in dilated cardiomyopathy—can it predict the severity of left ventricular dysfunction? Ann Acad Med Singapore. 1998;27:786-8.
59. Surwicz B, Knilan T. Chou's Electrocardiography in Clinical Practice. Philadelphia: WB Saunders Company; 2001. pp. 256-8.
60. Ammash NM, Seward JB, Bailey KR, et al. Clinical profile and outcome of idiopathic restrictive cardiomyopathy. Circulation. 2000;101:2490-6.
61. Dec GW, Fuster V. Idiopathic dilated cardiomyopathy. N Engl J Med. 1994;331(23):1564-75.
62. Mogensen J, Arbustini E. Restrictive cardiomyopathy. Curr Opin Cardiol. 2009;24:214-20.
63. Edhouse J, Thakur RK, Khalil JM. ABC of clinical electrocardiography. Conditions affecting the left side of the heart. BMJ. 2002;324(7348):1264-7.
64. McKenna WJ, Thiene G, Nava A, et al. Diagnosis of arrhythmogenic right ventricular dysplasia/cardiomyopathy. Task Force of the Working Group Myocardial and Pericardial Disease of the European Society of Cardiology and of the Scientific Council on Cardiomyopathies of the International Society and Federation of Cardiology. Br Heart J. 1994;71:215-8.
65. Marcus FI, Zareba W. The electrocardiogram in right ventricular cardiomyopathy/dysplasia. How can the electrocardiogram assist in understanding the pathologic and functional changes of the heart in this disease? J Electrocardiol. 2009;42(2):136.e1-5.
66. Peters S, Trümmel M, Koehler B, et al. The value of different electrocardiographic depolarization criteria in the diagnosis of arrhythmogenic right ventricular dysplasia/cardiomyopathy. J Electrocardiol. 2007;40(1):34-7.
67. Nasir K, Bomma C, Tandri H, et al. Electrocardiographic features of arrhythmogenic right ventricular dysplasia/cardiomyopathy according to disease severity: a need to broaden diagnostic criteria. Circulation. 2004;110(12):1527-34.
68. Jain R, Dalal D, Daly A, et al. Electrocardiographic features of arrhythmogenic right ventricular dysplasia. Circulation. 2009;120(6):477-87.
69. Nugent AW, Daubeney PE, Chondros P, et al. National Australian Childhood Cardiomyopathy Study. Clinical features and outcomes of childhood hypertrophic cardiomyopathy: results from a national population-based study. Circulation. 2005;112:1332-8.
70. Jenni R, Oechslin EN, van der Loo B. Isolated ventricular non-compaction of the myocardium in adults. Heart. 2007;93:11-5.
71. Pignatelli RH, McMahon CJ, Dreyer WJ, et al. Clinical characterization of left ventricular noncompaction in children. Circulation. 2003;108:2672-8.
72. Dote K, Sato H, Tateishi H, et al. Myocardial stunning due to simultaneous multivessel coronary spasms: a review of 5 cases. J Cardiol. 1991;21(2):203-14.
73. Bybee KA, Kara T, Prasad A, et al. Systematic review: transient left ventricular apical ballooning: a syndrome that mimics ST-segment elevation myocardial infarction. Ann Intern Med. 2004;141(11):858-65.
74. Tsuchihashi K, Ueshima K, Uchida T, et al. Transient left ventricular apical ballooning without coronary artery stenosis: a novel heart syndrome mimicking acute myocardial infarction. Angina Pectoris-Myocardial Infarction Investigations in Japan. J Am Coll Cardiol. 2001;38(1):11-8.
75. Abe Y, Kondo M, Matsuoka R, et al. Assessment of clinical features in transient left ventricular apical ballooning. J Am Coll Cardiol. 2003;41(5):737-42.
76. Sharkey SW, Lesser JR, Zenovich AG, et al. Acute and reversible cardiomyopathy provoked by stress in women from the United States. Circulation. 2005;111(4):472-9.
77. Bybee KA, Prasad A. Stress-related cardiomyopathy syndromes. Circulation. 2008;118(4):397-409.
78. Desmet WJ, Adriaenssens BF, Dens JA. Apical ballooning of the left ventricle: first series in white patients. Heart. 2003;89(9):1027-31.
79. Kurowski V, Kaiser A, von Hof K, et al. Apical and midventricular transient left ventricular dysfunction syndrome (Takotsubo cardiomyopathy): frequency, mechanisms, and prognosis. Chest. 2007;132(3):809-16.
80. Chauhan K, Sontineni SP, Alla VM, et al. Electrocardiographic abnormalities of takotsubo cardiomyopathy in a patient with paced ventricular rhythm. Cardiol Res Pract. 2010.
81. Dib C, Asirvatham S, Elesber A, et al. Clinical correlates and prognostic significance of electrocardiographic abnormalities in apical ballooning syndrome (Takotsubo/stress-induced cardiomyopathy). Am Heart J. 2009;157(5):933-8.
82. Ogura R, Hiasa Y, Takahashi T, et al. Specific findings of the standard 12-lead ECG in patients with 'Takotsubo' cardiomyopathy: comparison with the findings of acute anterior myocardial infarction. Circ J. 2003;67:687-90.
83. Hurst RT, Prasad A, Askew JW, et al. Takotsubo cardiomyopathy: a unique cardiomyopathy with variable ventricular morphology. J Am Coll Cardiol Img. 2010;3(6):641-9.

84. Elkhateeb OE, Beydoun HK. Recurrent long QT syndrome and syncope in transient apical ballooning syndrome (takotsubo cardiomyopathy). Can J Cardiol. 2008;24:917-9.
85. Dib C, Prasad A, Friedman PA. Malignant arrhythmia in apical ballooning syndrome: risk factors and outcomes. Indian Pacing Electrophysiol J. 2008;8:182-92.
86. Prasad A, Lerman A, Rihal CS. Apical ballooning syndrome (Tako-Tsubo or stress cardiomyopathy): a mimic of acute myocardial infarction. Am Heart J. 2008;155(3):408-17.
87. Antonopoulos A, Kyriacou C. Apical ballooning syndrome or Takotsubo cardiomyopathy: a new challenge in acute cardiac care. Cardiol J. 2008;15(6):572-7.
88. Kosuge M, Ebina T, Hibi K, et al. Simple and accurate electrocardiographic criteria to differentiate takotsubo cardiomyopathy from anterior acute myocardial infarction. J Am Coll Cardiol. 2010;55(22):2514-6.

Chapter

19

Electrocardiogram Diagnosis of Pericarditis and Other Cardiac Inflammatory Conditions

INTRODUCTION

The heart is made up of three basic layers: (1) Outer layer (pericardium), (2) Middle layer (myocardium), and (3) An inner layer (endocardium). Inflammation of the heart may affect only one layer, or may extend from one layer to the next. When inflammation only affects pericardium it is called pericarditis, if myocardium is only affected the condition is called myocarditis, and when inflammation affects endocardium only, the condition is termed as endocarditis. If all the layers are simultaneously involved the condition is called pancarditis.

PERICARDITIS

Pericarditis accounts for 5% of emergency department visits for chest pain in the absence of myocardial infarction.[1] Infectious pericarditis constitutes two-thirds of cases and remaining one-third of cases are due to noninfectious causes. Viral pericarditis are mostly due to echovirus and coxsackievirus but influenza, Epstein–Barr virus (EBV), hepatitis B virus (HBV), hepatitis C virus (HCV), human immunodeficiency virus (HIV), cytomegalovirus (CMV), adenovirus, varicella, rubella, mumps, parvovirus B19, and human herpes virus 6 may also cause acute pericarditis. Tuberculosis is the most common cause of bacterial pericarditis (4–5%). Pneumococcus, meningococcus, gonococcus, haemophilus, and staphylococci rarely may cause pericarditis. Fungus and parasitic infection rarely give rise to pericarditis. Autoimmune pericarditis (<10%), e.g. systemic lupus erythematosus, Sjögren syndrome, rheumatoid arthritis, systemic sclerosis, systemic vasculitides, and neoplastic pericarditis (5–7%) are the common causes of noninfectious pericarditis. Metabolic conditions like uremia, myxedema, trauma, postmyocardial infarction syndrome (Dressler's syndrome), and postpericardiotomy inflammation may also cause pericarditis.[2-6] Dressler's syndrome is also known as postmyocardial infarction syndrome and the term is also sometimes used to refer to postpericardiotomy pericarditis.

The diagnosis of acute pericarditis is based on the presence of typical symptoms of chest pain, pericardial rub, and characteristic electrocardiographic changes. Acute pericarditis classically presents with progressive, frequently severe, chest pain that is sharp and pleuritic. The pain is generally worse when lying supine, is relieved by sitting, and might radiate to the neck, arms, or left shoulder, making differentiation from myocardial ischemia difficult. A pericardial friction rub is pathognomonic for pericarditis, but is frequently not present. Best heard in end expiration when the patient is leaning forward.[6-12]

Electrocardiogram (ECG) is perhaps the most useful diagnostic test for acute pericarditis and classically shows widespread saddle-shaped or upward concave ST-segment elevation that reflects subepicardial inflammation.[6,8,13-15] PTa segment depression or PR-segment depression can accompany or precede ST changes (The PTa segment is the part between the P wave and the Q or R wave. The PTa segment is also called PR or PQ or PTp segment) (Fig. 19.1). Electrocardiographic abnormalities in acute pericarditis may evolve through several phases.[6] Unlike pericarditis, the ST-segment changes in acute myocardial infarction are characteristically regional. There is no Q-wave formation or

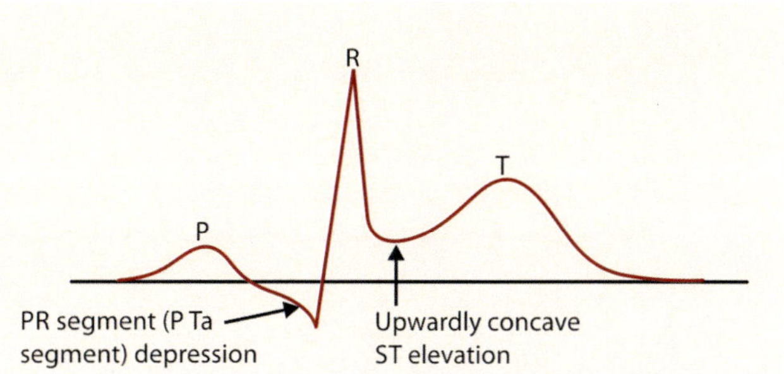

Fig. 19.1: Diagram shows classical electrocardiogram (ECG) changes in acute pericarditis. Upwardly concave ST-segment elevation and PR-segment (PTa segment) depressions are the typical ECG signs of acute pericarditis (*arrows*).

loss of R wave in acute pericarditis. The electrocardiographic changes of pericarditis can be differentiated from the early repolarization pattern, which rarely shows widespread PR-segment depression with PR elevation in aVR.[6,10,16,17]

Electrocardiogram of acute pericarditis classically shows sinus tachycardia with widespread saddle-shaped (upward concave) ST-segment elevation in the precordial and limb leads (Figs. 19.2 and 19.3). In pericarditis the degree of ST elevation is typically modest usually in the range of 0.5–1 mm (2.5 mm at most). PTa-segment depression or PR-segment depression (Fig. 19.4) (with PR-segment elevation in lead aVR) can accompany or precede the ST changes and is known as the "discordant ST-PR segment sign". These changes are seen in 60% of patients.[8] A distinctive feature of acute pericarditis is the ratio of ST elevation to T-wave amplitude in leads I, V4, V5, and V6. If the ratio exceeds 0.25, acute pericarditis is present. The end of the PR segment is used as the baseline for the ST-segment onset and T-wave maximal amplitude.[8] Reciprocal ST depression and PR elevation in lead aVR (± V1) is common in acute pericarditis (Fig. 19.5).

The ECG changes of acute pericarditis develop in stages, making them easy to differentiate from early repolarization and, more significantly, from myocardial infarction. Four stages are apparent (Fig. 19.6). These findings occur in progressive stages, all of which are seen in about 50% of cases of pericarditis.[9-13]

1. *Stage I (acute phase):* Diffuse upwardly concave ST-segment elevation in most of the leads, PR depression in most leads (may be subtle), and sometimes notching at the end of the QRS complex (during the first 2 weeks).
2. *Stage II:* ST-segment elevation and PR depression have resolved. T waves may be normal or flattened (1–3 weeks).
3. *Stage III:* T waves are inverted and the ECG is otherwise normal (3 to several weeks).
4. *Stage IV:* The T waves return to the upright position thus the ECG is back to normal (several weeks onwards).

In the acute phase of pericarditis (stage I) *Spodick's sign* is found in around 80% of cases. Spodick's sign signifies to a downsloping TP segment in patients with acute pericarditis (Figs. 19.7. and 19.8).[10,13,16] This sign is often best visualized in lead II and lateral precordial leads. In addition, Spodick's sign may also serve as an important distinguishing electrocardiographic tool between the acute pericarditis and acute coronary syndrome. PR-segment depression when used alone can sometimes be a masquerader, as it can be seen in both acute pericarditis and in some cases acute

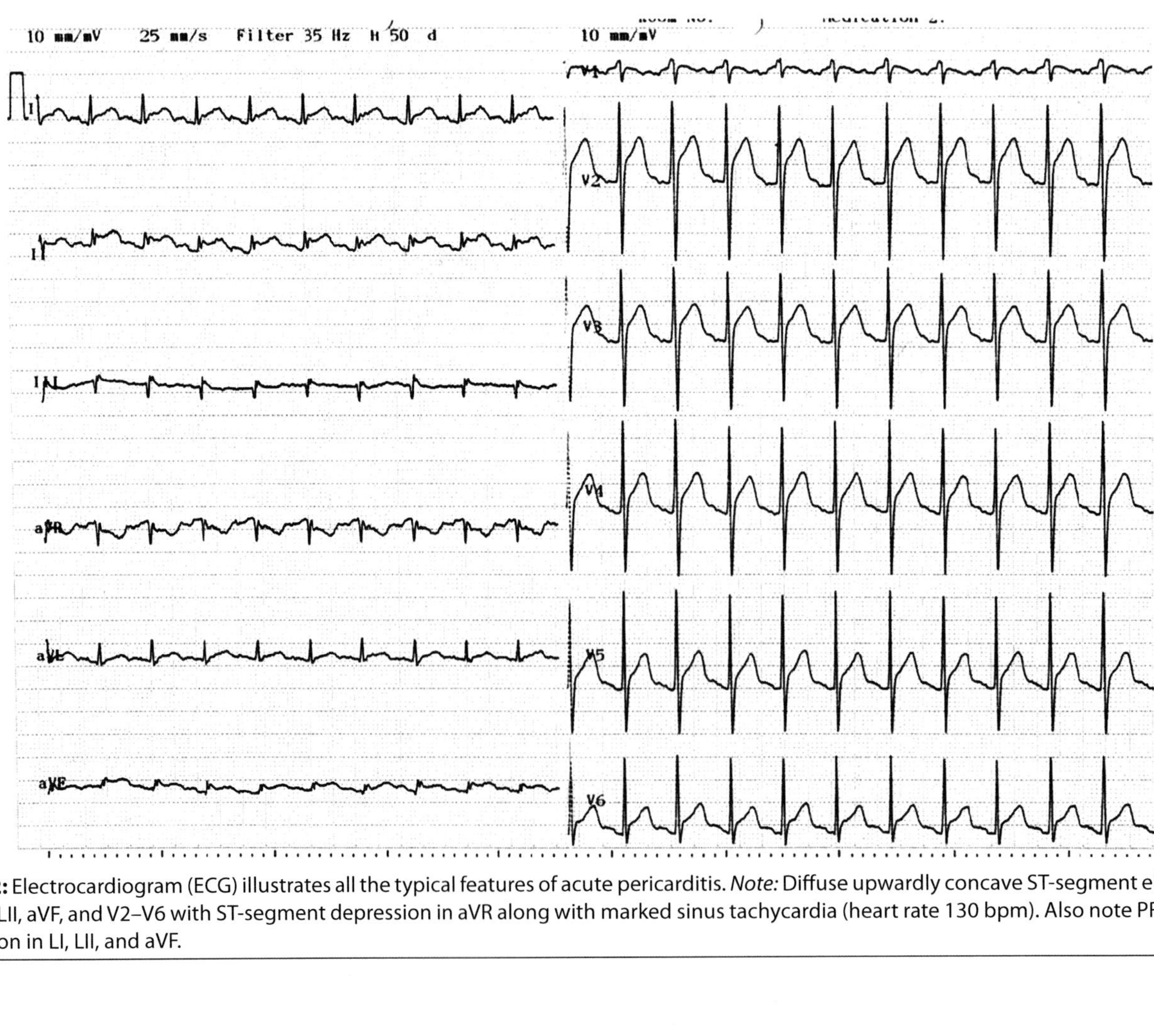

Fig. 19.2: Electrocardiogram (ECG) illustrates all the typical features of acute pericarditis. *Note:* Diffuse upwardly concave ST-segment elevation in leads LI, LII, aVF, and V2–V6 with ST-segment depression in aVR along with marked sinus tachycardia (heart rate 130 bpm). Also note PR-segment depression in LI, LII, and aVF.

coronary syndrome. However, simultaneous presence of PR-segment depression and Spodick's sign may confirm the diagnosis of acute pericarditis.[10,13,16]

The ECG changes of pericarditis vary widely from one patient to another, depending on the extent and severity of pericardial inflammation and the timing of the patient's presentation. Changes vary in duration. In some cases, ST elevation returns to baseline within a few days without T-wave inversions; in other cases, T-wave inversions can persist for weeks to months. Sometimes the abnormalities resolve by the time symptoms develop.[8]

PTa-segment (PR segment) depression in pericarditis is thought to be due to atrial wall injury. Later in the course of pericarditis the T waves can become inverted. This needs to be differentiated from early repolarization, a normal variant where the PR segment is not depressed. ECG changes of acute pericarditis mimic acute ST-elevation myocardial infarction (STEMI) and the ECG should be reviewed carefully to avoid misdiagnosis and wrong treatment. In STEMI, the ST-segment elevation is localized to the distribution of the affected coronary artery.[18] Acute pericarditis, early repolarization pattern (ERP), and acute STEMI, all three conditions give rise to ST-segment elevations but can be differentiated from each other from the varying patterns of ST-segment elevations and other specific ECG criteria (Fig. 19.9).

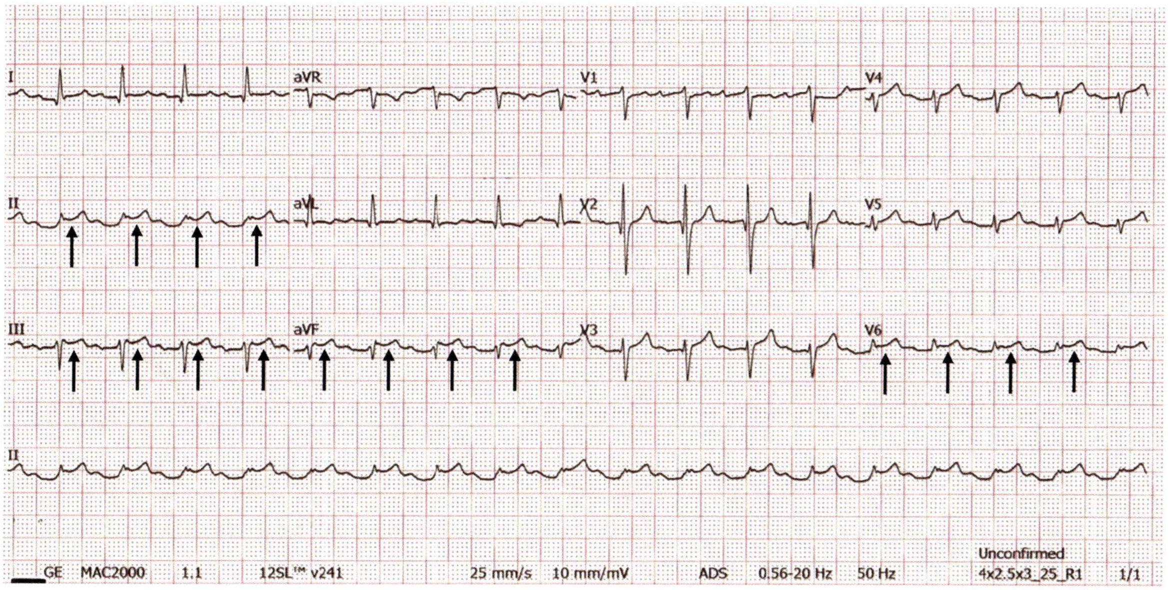

Fig. 19.3: Electrocardiogram (ECG) illustrates classical upwardly concave ST-segment elevation in leads LII, LIII, aVF, and V6 (*arrows*) with sinus tachycardia (heart rate 110 bpm). Also note marked PR-segment depression in LII.

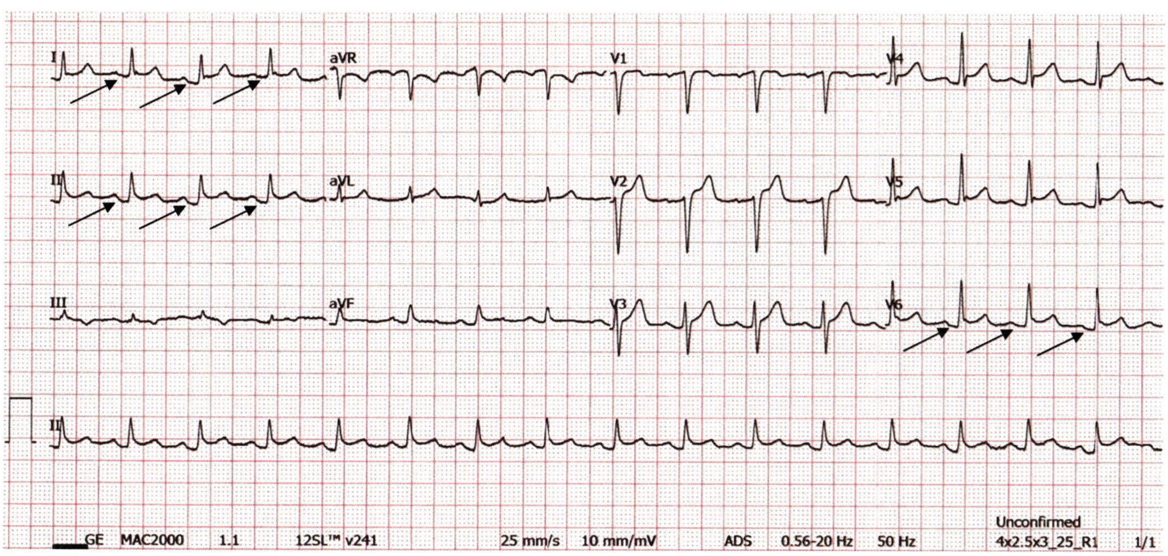

Fig. 19.4: This electrocardiogram (ECG) shows PR-segment depression in LI, LII, and V6 (arrows) along with diffuse ST-segment elevation with upward concavity in both limb and chest leads.

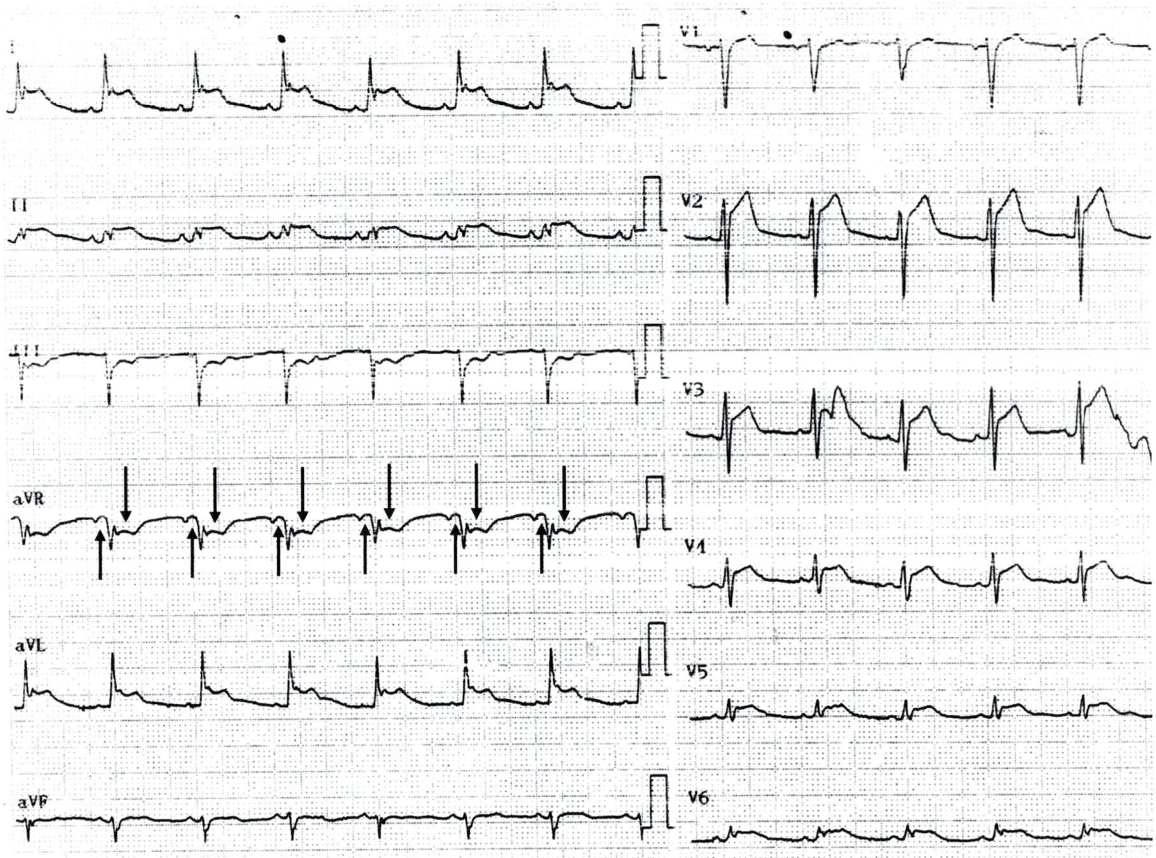

Fig. 19.5: This electrocardiogram (ECG) shows marked ST-segment depression and PR-segment elevation in lead aVR (*arrows*), typical of acute pericarditis with diffuse upwardly concave ST-segment elevation in both limb and precordial leads.

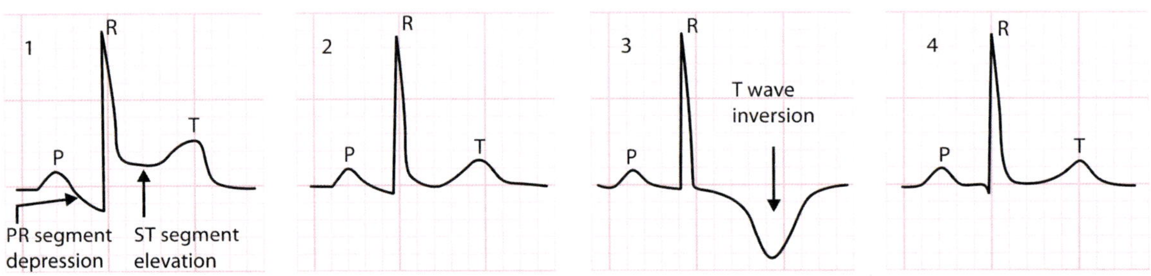

Fig. 19.6: This diagram illustrates the four phases of electrocardiogram (ECG) changes in acute pericarditis. Panel 1 shows ECG features of stage I pericarditis with upwardly concave ST-segment elevation and PR depression (*arrows*). Panel 2 shows almost normalization of ST-segment elevation and PR-segment depression as it occurs in stage II. Panel 3 shows features of stage III pericarditis with appearance of T-wave inversion. Panel 4 is suggestive of stage IV pericarditis where the T waves return to the upright position thus the ECG is back to normal. Practically, stage I is the only diagnostic phase because stage II and stage IV looks normal and stage III mimics ischemia.

Differentiation of Acute Pericarditis from Acute ST-elevation Myocardial Infarction

Electrocardiogram changes in acute pericarditis differ from those in STEMI in many ways. ST-segment elevation with upward convexity suggests STEMI but ST-segment elevation with upward concavity is suggestive of acute pericarditis. ST-segment elevation in pericarditis rarely exceeds 2.5 mm (usually 0.5–1.0 mm), in contrast to acute myocardial infarction, in which ST elevation is more marked and has to be more than 2 mm and in two anatomically contiguous leads.[19] Amplitude of ST elevation in STEMI usually more than 2.0 mm but can reach upto 8–10 mm. In pericarditis, the ECG changes occur more slowly and in stages, reflecting the evolving inflammation of different areas of the pericardium. The ST segment is elevated diffusely in the precordial and limb leads in pericarditis, indicating involvement of

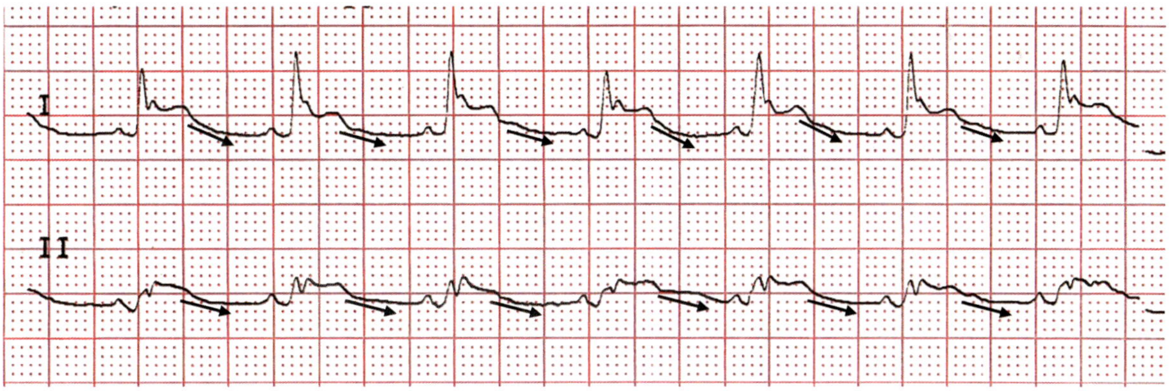

Fig. 19.7: Electrocardiogram (ECG) showing Spodick's sign in LI and LII in the acute phase of pericarditis (stage I). Spodick's sign signifies to a downsloping TP segment (*arrows*) in patients with acute pericarditis.

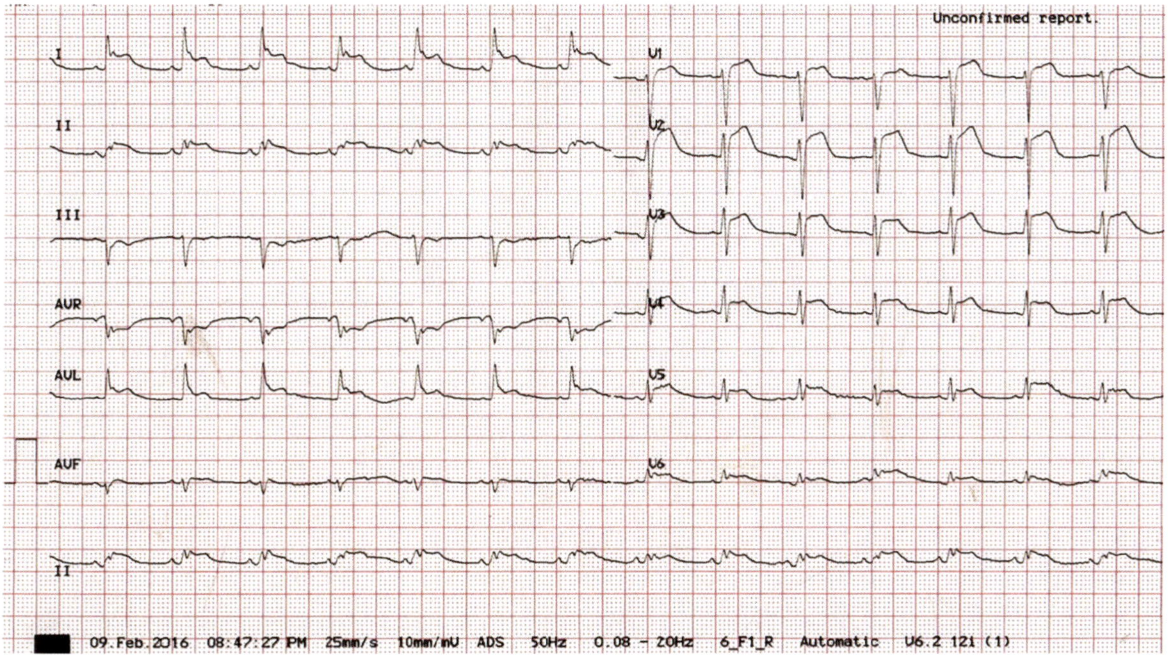

Fig. 19.8: This electrocardiogram (ECG) illustrates classical Spodick's sign (downsloping TP segment) in LI, LII, aVL, and V2–V6 with diffuse upwardly concave ST-segment elevation in both limb and precordial leads. Also note ST-segment depression in aVR. *Courtesy:* Dr M Jalaluddin, Labaid Cardiac Hospital

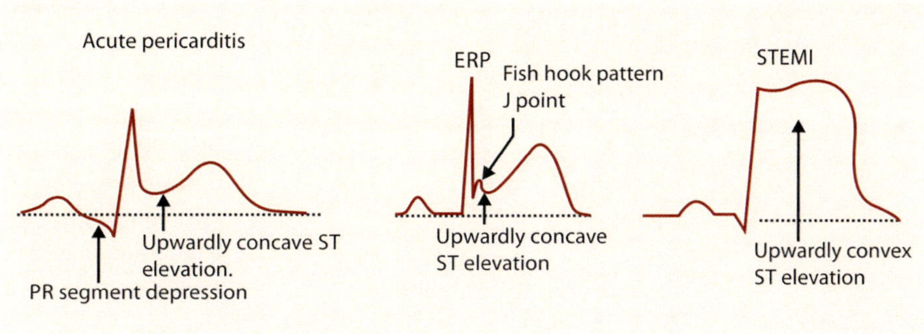

Fig. 19.9: Diagrams showing basic electrocardiogram (ECG) features of acute pericarditis with PR-segment depression with upwardly concave ST-segment elevation, early repolarization pattern (ERP) with upwardly concave ST-segment elevation along with fish hook pattern J point, and acute ST-elevation myocardial infarction (STEMI) with marked upwardly convex ST-segment elevation.

more than one coronary vascular territory, differentiating it from characteristic regional changes in myocardial infarction.[19,20] Reciprocal ST depressions are absent in acute pericarditis, although they are frequently found with acute myocardial infarction. Pathologic Q waves or high-grade heart block reflects acute myocardial infarction, not seen in ECGs of acute pericarditis. PR-segment depression is a common ECG finding in acute pericarditis which is unusual in acute myocardial infarction.[8] Loss of R-wave progression may occur with acute myocardial infarction, but this feature is not present with acute pericarditis.[21]

Acute STEMI usually presents with upwardly convex ST-segment elevations and acute pericarditis with upwardly concave ST elevations. But acute STEMI may produce ST elevation with either upwardly convex, obliquely straight, or upwardly concave morphology (Figs. 19.10A to C). So, if STEMI presents with upwardly concave ST elevation then it may be confused with the diagnosis of acute pericarditis. If ECG features are equivocal then bedside echocardiogram can establish the correct diagnosis.

Electrocardiographic Differences between Acute ST-elevation Myocardial Infarction and Acute Pericarditis

The electrocardiographic differences between acute ST-elevation myocardial infarction and acute pericarditis are described in Table 19.1.

Differentiation of Acute Pericarditis from Early Repolarization Pattern

Early repolarization pattern (ERP) also known as benign early repolarization (BER) is a common ECG variant, characterized by J-point elevation manifested either as terminal QRS slurring (the transition from the QRS segment to the ST segment) or notching (a positive deflection inscribed on terminal QRS complex) associated with concave upward ST-segment elevation and prominent T waves in at least two contiguous leads (Fig. 19.11).[21-23] Early repolarization is sometimes seen in healthy young people, especially in black men.

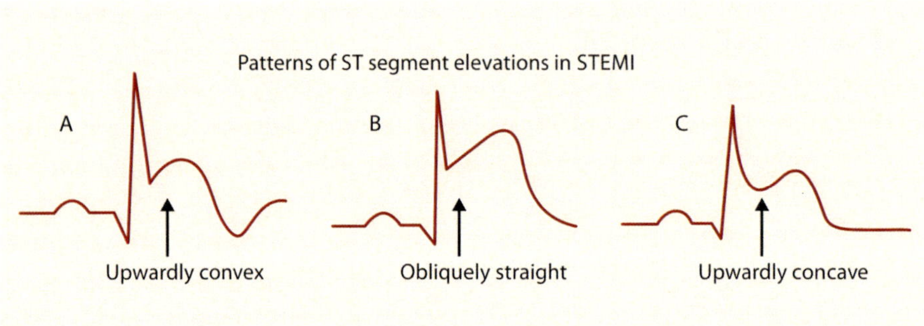

Figs. 19.10A to C: Diagram showing different patterns of ST-segment elevations in acute ST-elevation myocardial infarction (STEMI). (A) Upwardly convex; (B) Obliquely straight; and (C) Upwardly concave morphology.

Table 19.1: Electrocardiographic differences between acute ST-elevation myocardial infarction and acute pericarditis.

ECG features	*Acute pericarditis*	*STEMI*
Patterns of ST-segment elevation	Upwardly concave	Usually upwardly convex
Location of ST-segment elevations	Diffuse, involves both limb and precordial leads	Area of the involved arterial territory
PR-segment depression	Commonly seen and is regarded as the typical ECG finding	Usually not seen
Reciprocal ST-segment depression	Not seen	Commonly seen
Q waves	Not seen	Usually present
Loss of R-wave voltage	Not seen	Loss of R-wave voltage is a common phenomenon in STEMI
T-wave inversion	Appears after ST normalization	Appears concomitantly with ST changes
Spodick's sign (downsloping TP segment)	Spodick's sign is found in around 80% of cases	Not seen
Amplitude of ST elevation	Typically modest, usually in the range of 0.5–1 mm (2.5 mm at most)	Marked, ST elevation, usually > 2.0 mm but can reach up to 8–10 mm

(ECG: electrocardiogram; STEMI: ST-elevation myocardial infarction)

Early repolarization is characterized by elevation of the J point (i.e. the junction between the end of the QRS complex and the beginning of the ST segment). Elevation of the J point causes elevation of the ST segment in the mid to lateral precordial leads (V3–V6) with a tall peak upright T wave.[24-26] Notched J-point elevation in V4 with a "fish hook" morphology is a characteristic sign of ERP (Fig. 19.12). Acute pericarditis tends to cause ST-segment elevation in both the limb and precordial leads, whereas ST elevation in early repolarization mainly involves the mid and lateral precordial leads. The PR-segment depression is more prominent in acute pericarditis which is not seen in ERP. Acute pericarditis develops in stages, where ECG changes are dynamic which makes it easy to differentiate from ERP where ECG changes are almost static.

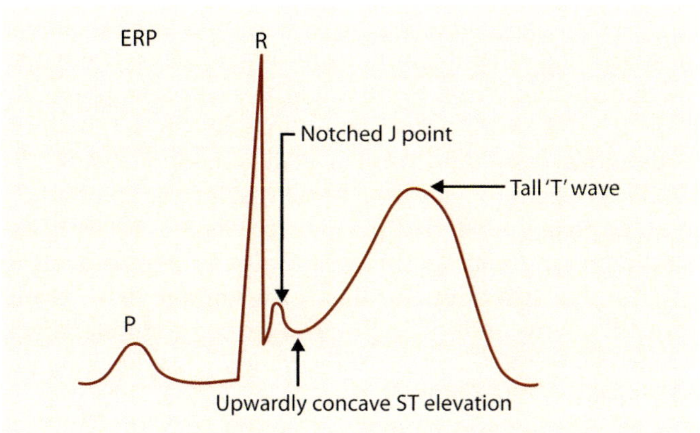

Fig. 19.11: Diagram showing typical electrocardiogram (ECG) features of early repolarization pattern (ERP) with notched J-point elevation, tall and peak T wave with upwardly concave ST-segment elevation (*arrows*).

It may be difficult to differentiate acute pericarditis from ERP as both the conditions are associated with upwardly concave ST elevation. However, three things may help to distinguish pericarditis from ERP:[8,21,23]

1. The ratio of the ST-segment elevation and T-wave amplitude can differentiate pericarditis from ERP. ST elevation is less than 25% of the T-wave amplitude in ERP but it is more than 25% in acute pericarditis. In other words, the T wave in ERP is usually more than four times the amplitude of the ST elevation.
2. In ERP, ST elevations are mostly confined to the precordial leads but ST elevations in acute pericarditis are usually diffuse.
3. Early repolarization pattern, unlike acute pericarditis usually is a benign ECG finding that should not be associated with any symptoms.

ST segment/T-wave ratio (Fig. 19.13)

One useful way to distinguish between acute pericarditis and ERP is to look at the ST segment/T-wave ratio:

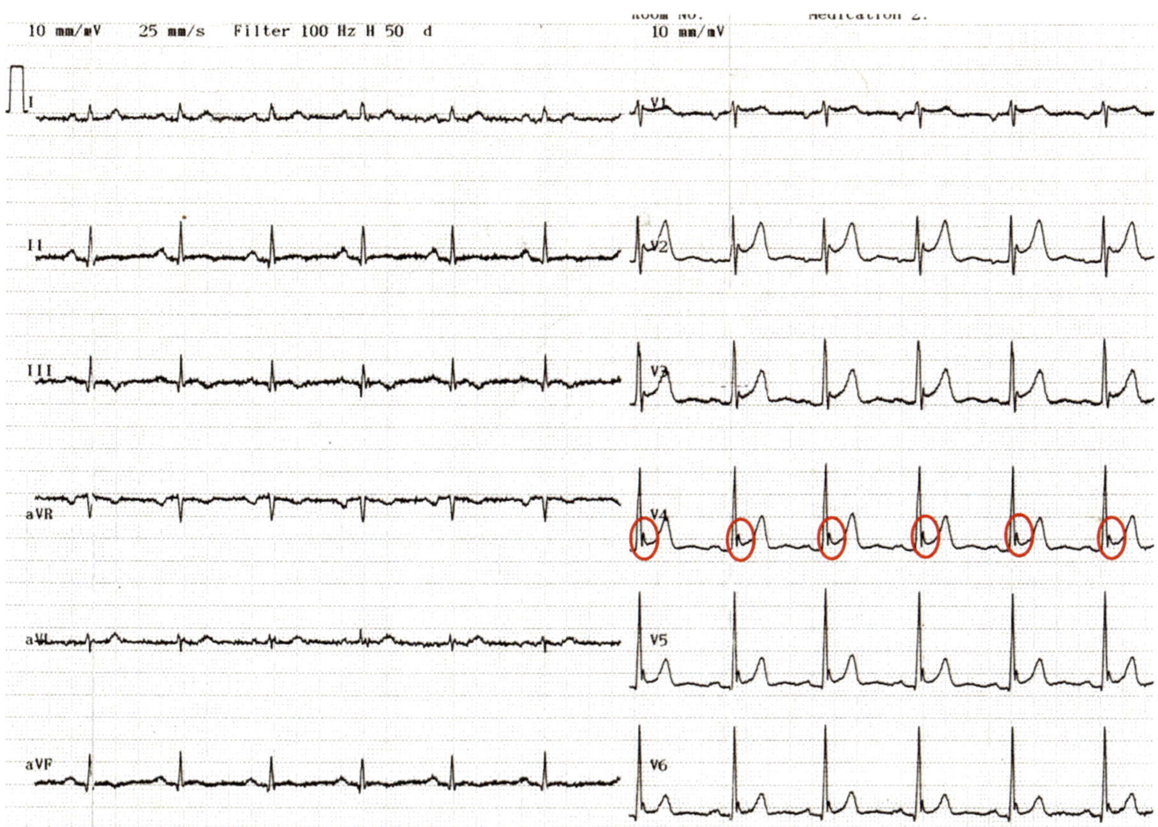

Fig. 19.12: This electrocardiogram (ECG) illustrates the typical features of early repolarization pattern (ERP) with notched J point with upwardly concave ST-segment elevations in leads V2–V6. *Note:* Notched J-point elevations with a "fish hook" morphology in leads V3–V6, most prominent in V4, a characteristic sign of ERP (*red circles*).

- The vertical height of the ST-segment elevation (from the end of the PR segment to the J point) is measured and compared to the amplitude of the T wave in V6.
- A ratio of more than 0.25 suggests acute pericarditis.
- A ratio of less than 0.25 suggests ERP.

Electrocardiographic Differences between Acute Pericarditis and Early Repolarization Pattern

The electrocardiographic differences between acute pericarditis and early repolarization pattern are illustrated in Table 19.2.

Electrocardiogram Changes in Pericardial Effusion

A pericardial effusion occurs when a significant amount of fluid fills the pericardial space. Normal individuals have a small amount of pericardial fluid (15–50 mL) which helps to promote cardiac chamber interaction by allowing the heart to move freely without restriction. Pericardial effusion can be caused by multiple disease states and include any process that results in pericarditis or myocarditis. Both viral infection (e.g. coxsackievirus) and bacterial infection (e.g. tuberculosis) may be the cause of pericardial effusion. Inflammatory disorders such as systemic lupus erythematosus, rheumatoid arthritis, postmyocardial infarction pericarditis (Dressler's syndrome), malignancy, congestive heart failure, myxedema, and nephrotic syndrome are also associated with pericardial effusion.

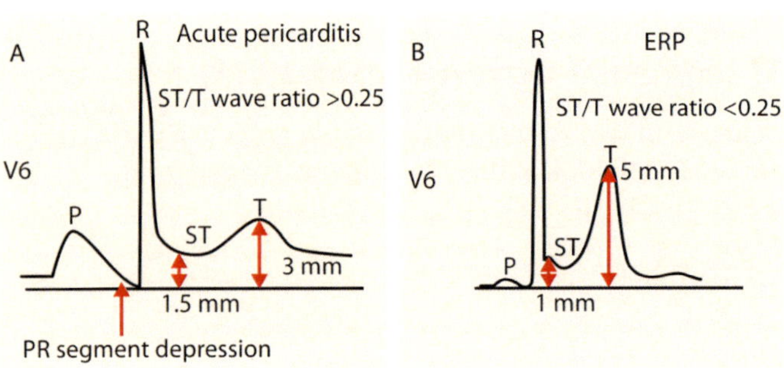

Fig. 19.13: Diagram showing ST/T-wave ratio in the electrocardiogram (ECG) of acute pericarditis and early repolarization pattern (ERP) in lead V6. In *panel A*, ST segment height 1.5 mm and T wave height 3.0 mm and ST/T-wave ratio = 0.5 which is more than 0.25 and consistent with the diagnosis of acute pericarditis. In *panel B*, ST segment height 1.0 mm and T wave height 5.0 mm and ST/T-wave ratio = 0.2 which is less than 0.25 and consistent with the diagnosis of ERP *(The vertical height of the ST-segment elevation is usually measured at the level of the end of the PR segment to the J point and compared to the amplitude of the T wave in V6).*

Low voltage is an electrocardiographic manifestation of pericardial effusion, but this finding is neither sensitive nor specific. Low voltage on the ECG is defined as a peak-to-peak QRS amplitude of less than 5 mm in all the limb leads and/or less than 10 mm in all the precordial leads (Fig. 19.14). ST-segment elevation and PR-segment depression, in an appropriate distribution, are reasonably accurate for diagnosing pericarditis, but their value for detecting effusion has not been studied. Low voltage ECG, along with PR-segment depression and ST-segment elevation are suggestive but are not confirmatory in establishing the diagnosis of pericardial effusion, because low voltage ECG may be seen in many clinical conditions (Box 19.1). In one series of pericardial effusion low voltage was detected in 26% patients, PR-segment depression in 26%, and ST-segment elevation in 7% patients.[27]

Box 19.1: Important causes of low voltage ECG.

- Hypothyroidism
- Obesity
- Emphysema
- Pericardial effusion
- Pneumothorax or pneumopericardium
- Old large anterior MI
- Dilated cardiomyopathy (DCM)
- Infiltrative/restrictive diseases such as amyloidosis or hemochromatosis.

(ECG: electrocardiogram; MI: myocardial infarction)

Table 19.2: Electrocardiographic differences between acute pericarditis and early repolarization pattern.

Electrocardiogram (ECG) features	*Acute pericarditis*	*Early repolarization pattern (ERP)*
Location of ST-segment elevations	Diffuse, involves both limb and precordial leads	Mostly limited to precordial leads
PR-segment depression	Present	Absent
Evolution of ST segment and T waves	ST segment and T wave changes are dynamic	Static and nonprogressive
T-wave morphology	Normal amplitude	Prominent and sometimes appear tall and peak
J-point elevation with "fish hook" appearance in lead V4	Absent	Usually present
ST segment/T-wave ratio	>0.25	<0.25

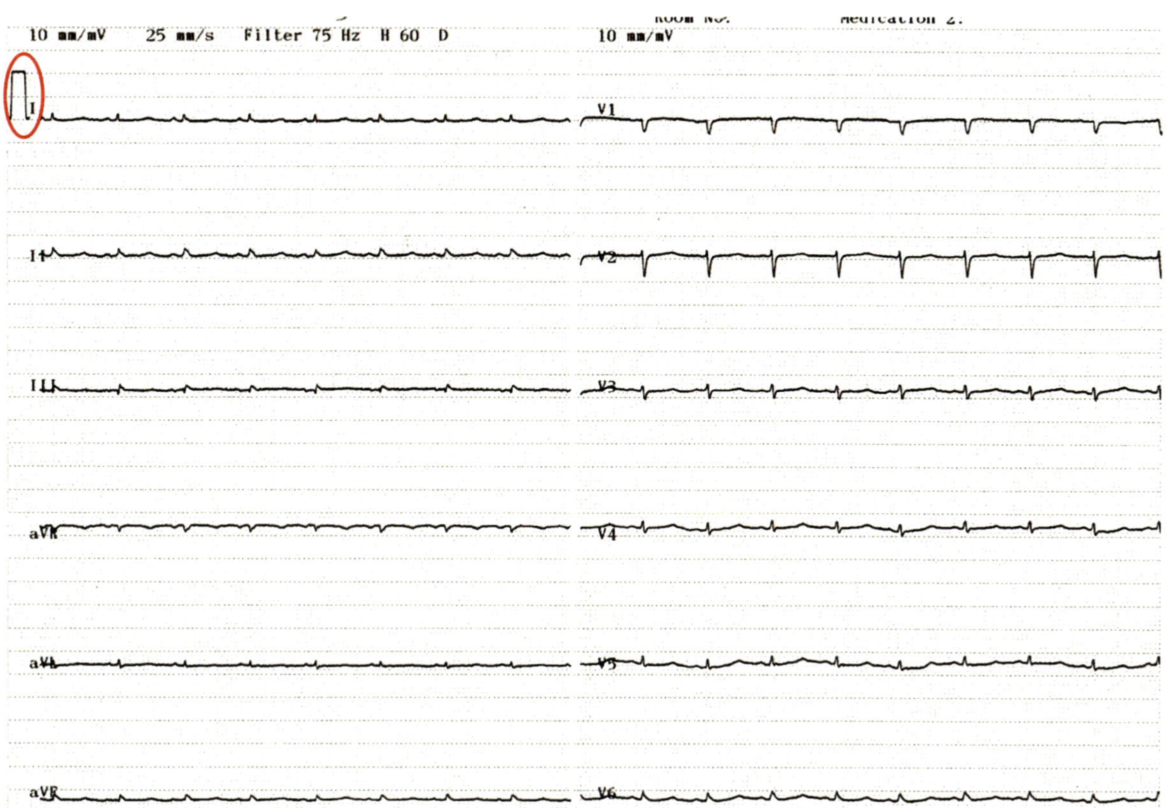

Fig. 19.14: This electrocardiogram (ECG) illustrates low voltage ECG with sinus tachycardia (heart rate 106 bpm). *Note:* Peak-to-peak QRS amplitude of less than 5 mm in the limb leads and less than 10 mm in the precordial leads. *Before diagnosing low voltage ECG, the clinician must judge, whether the standardization of voltage on the ECG paper is proper or not (red circle). If standardization is not proper then ECG interpretation will be wrong. Standard calibration of ECG machine is 10 mm (10 small boxes = two large squares) equals 1 mV.*

The ECG of pericardial effusion may show:

- Sinus tachycardia
- Low-voltage QRS complexes (low voltage ECG)
- Alternation of the QRS complexes, usually in a 2:1 ratio. Electrical alternans can also be seen in myocardial ischemia, acute pulmonary embolism, and tachyarrhythmias
- PR-segment depression (this can also be observed in an atrial infarction).

In pericardial effusion the ECG usually shows sinus tachycardia and low voltage (Fig. 19.15).[28-30] Pericardial effusion and cardiac tamponade have long been associated with low voltage of the 12-lead ECG, and the diagnostic accuracy, sensitivity, and specificity of this ECG finding have previously been reported. Different mechanisms have been proposed to explain low QRS voltage associated with pericardial effusion and cardiac tamponade. Mechanisms proposed to explain low QRS voltage associated with pericardial effusion include internal short-circuiting of the electrical currents by accumulated fluids within the pericardial sac, greater distance of the heart from body surface electrodes, reduced cardiac size caused by effusion, and change in the generation and propagation of electrical current in the myocardium.[8,30] Electrical alternans, defined as the alteration of the QRS complex amplitude or axis between beats, is specific but not very sensitive for cardiac tamponade. Electrical alternans reflects the swinging motion of the heart in pericardial fluid.[31] PR-segment depression is a relatively common ECG sign associated with pericardial effusion, and it is an ECG indicator of inflammatory pericardial involvement.[1]

Cardiac Tamponade

In case of tamponade, fluid collects in the pericardium. Because the pericardium is stiff, the heart is compressed, resulting in filling difficulties. This is a potentially life-threatening situation and should be treated with pericardiocentesis, drainage of the fluid. Tamponade can be the result of pericarditis or myocarditis. Sinus tachycardia and electrical alternans are specific but not sensitive signs of pericardial tamponade. Electrical alternans is characterized by beat-to-beat alterations in amplitude and the axis of QRS complexes in the limb and precordial leads as a result of the mechanical swinging of the heart in a large pericardial effusion. There is evidence to suggest that low QRS voltage is more the result of the tamponade than the effusion (Figs. 19.16A and B).[8,32]

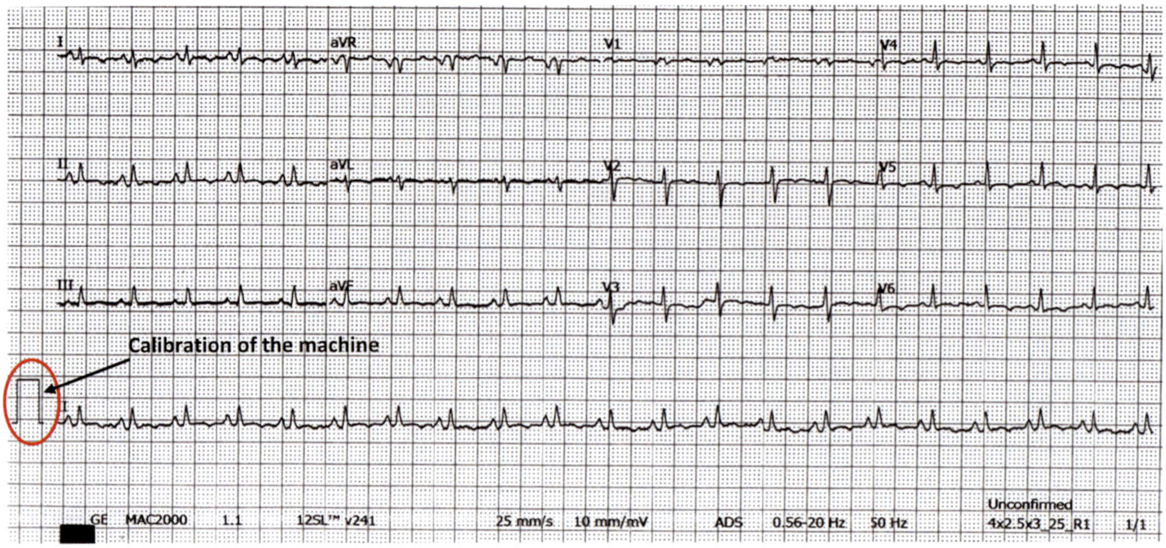

Fig. 19.15: Electrocardiogram (ECG) of pericardial effusion showing features of low voltage ECG with sinus tachycardia (heart rate 125 bpm). *Note:* Peak-to-peak QRS amplitude of less than 5 mm in the limb leads and less than 10 mm in the precordial leads, suggestive of low voltage ECG. *Note also* optimal calibration of the ECG machine (red circle). *Standard calibration of ECG machine is 10 mm (10 small boxes = two large squares) equals 1 mV. Before starting ECG interpretation the clinician must judge, whether the standardization of voltage and timing intervals on the ECG paper are proper or not. If standardization is not proper then ECG interpretation will be wrong.*

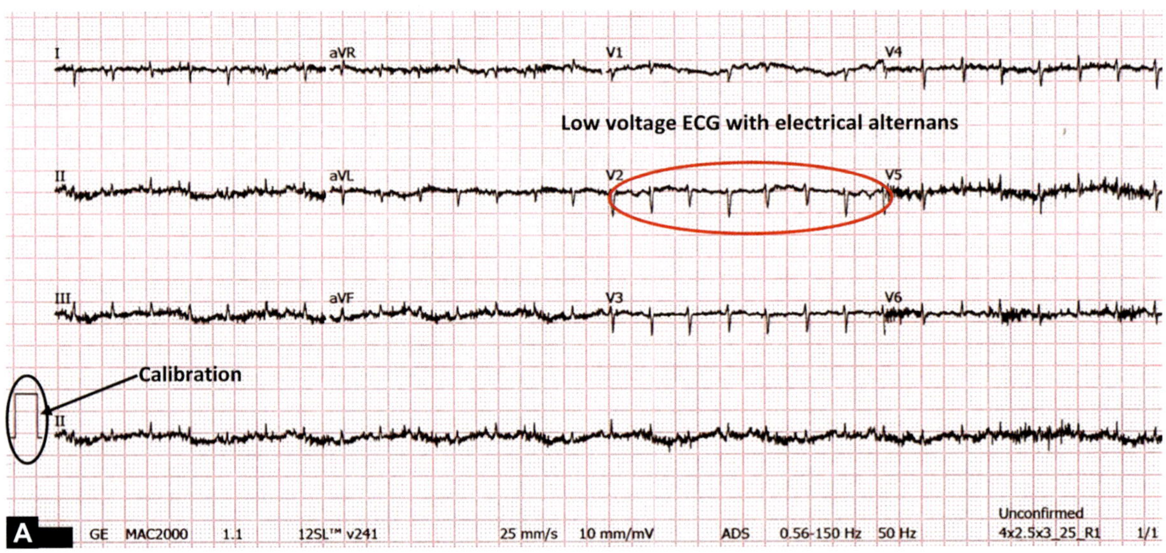

Fig. 19.16A: Electrocardiogram (ECG) illustrates the features of cardiac tamponade (before aspiration of pericardial fluid) with low voltage ECG with marked sinus tachycardia (heart rate 172 bpm) with some features of electrical alternans best seen in lead V2 (red circle). Also note some motion artifacts obscuring some ECG waveforms due to tremor and shivering as the patient was restless during taking the ECG.

Courtesy: Dr Elias Ali, Labaid Cardiac Hospital

ELECTROCARDIOGRAPHIC DIAGNOSIS OF MYOCARDITIS

Myocarditis is clinically and pathologically defined as "inflammation of the myocardium". Clinical presentations of the disease range from nonspecific systemic symptoms (fever, myalgias, palpitations, or exertional dyspnea) to fulminant hemodynamic collapse and sudden death. Prospective postmortem data have implicated myocarditis in sudden cardiac death of young adults at rates of 8.6–12% and it has been identified as a cause of dilated cardiomyopathy in 9% of cases in a large prospective series.[33,34] A broad array of etiologies have been implicated as causes of myocarditis but viral myocarditis remains the prototype for the study of the disease and its evolution. Enteroviruses, specifically coxsackie group B serotypes, have traditionally been perceived as the predominant viral cause.[35] HCV, HIV, adenovirus, rubella virus, and CMV may also cause myocarditis. Bacteria like brucella, corynebacterium diphtheriae, and gonococcus may cause

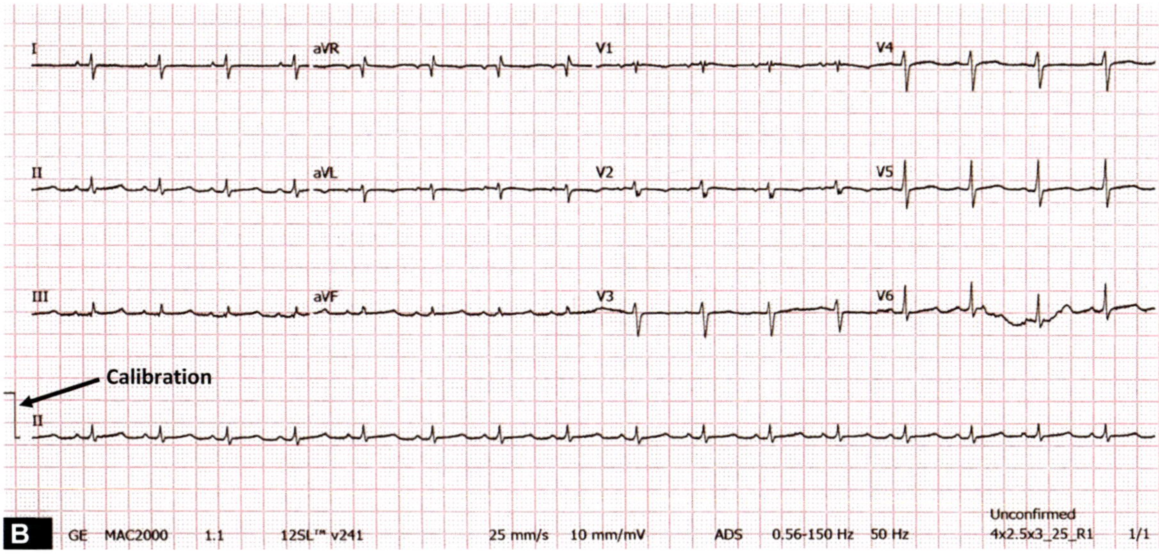

Fig. 19.16B: ECG of the same patient with cardiac tamponade (Fig. 19.16A) (*taken immediately after aspiration of pericardial fluid*). ECG after aspiration still shows the features of low voltage but heart rate came down from 172 bpm to 100 bpm and ECG evidence of electrical alternans has disappeared.

Courtesy: Dr Elias Ali, Labaid Cardiac Hospital

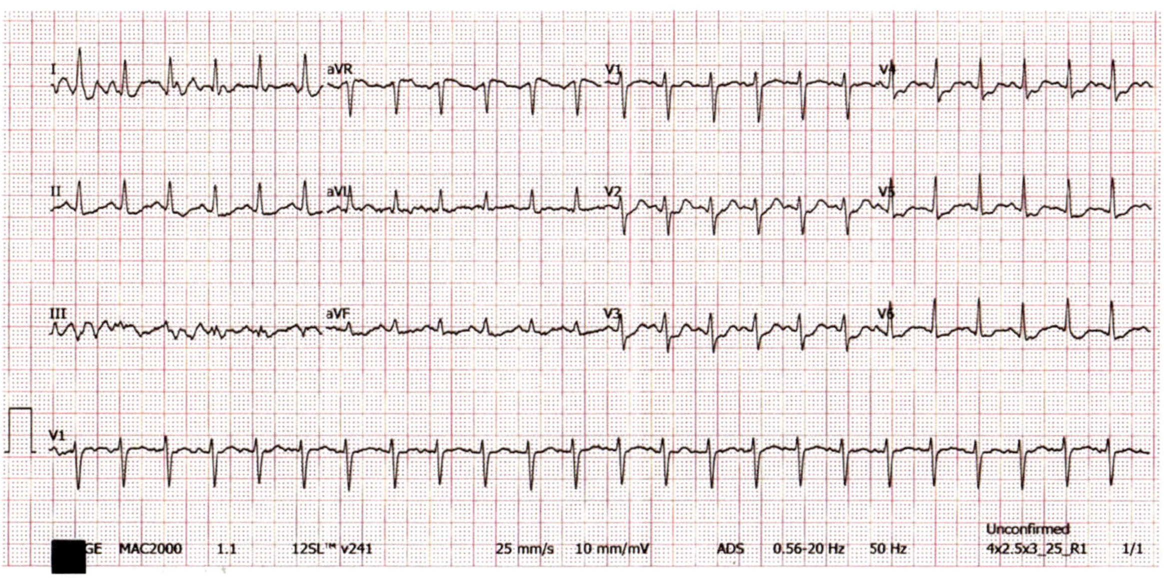

Fig. 19.17: Electrocardiogram (ECG) of myocarditis showing marked sinus tachycardia (heart rate 150 bpm) with diffuse nonspecific ST segment and T-wave changes.

myocarditis. Autoimmune diseases those are associated with active myocarditis include rheumatoid diseases such as systemic lupus erythematosus, mixed connective tissue disease and systemic sclerosis, celiac disease, and Whipple's disease.[36] Numerous medications have been implicated in hypersensitivity myocarditis including antidepressants (tricyclics), antibiotics (penicillins, cephalosporins, sulfonamides), and antipsychotics (clozapine).[36]

Electrocardiogram is widely used as a screening tool despite low sensitivity.[37] The ECG findings in patients with myocarditis vary from sinus tachycardia with nonspecific T-wave and ST-segment changes (Fig. 19.17) to ST-segment elevation mimicking an acute myocardial infarction.[38,39] Also, atrial or ventricular conduction delays (Fig. 19.18) as well as supraventricular and ventricular arrhythmias can occur in patients with inflammatory heart disease. The presence of Q waves or a new left bundle branch block are associated with higher rates of cardiac death or heart transplantation.[40] The prognostic role of ECG parameters was investigated in patients with suspected myocarditis. A QTc prolongation more than 440 ms, an abnormal QRS axis, and ventricular ectopic beats were associated with poor clinical outcome. A prolonged QRS duration of more than or equal to 120 ms was found to be an independent predictor for cardiac death. Hence, the ECG represents an easily available tool for risk stratification in patients with suspected myocarditis.[41,42]

Myocarditis masquerading as an acute coronary syndrome has also been well described.[43-46] When inflammation involves the adjacent pericardium, ECG features of pericarditis can also been seen and then the condition is termed as myopericarditis. Diseases like diphtheria, typhoid, HIV infection, dengue fever, Lyme disease, and tetanus can produce various forms of cardiac inflammatory conditions varying from endocarditis, myocarditis to pancarditis (Box 19.2).[47-51]

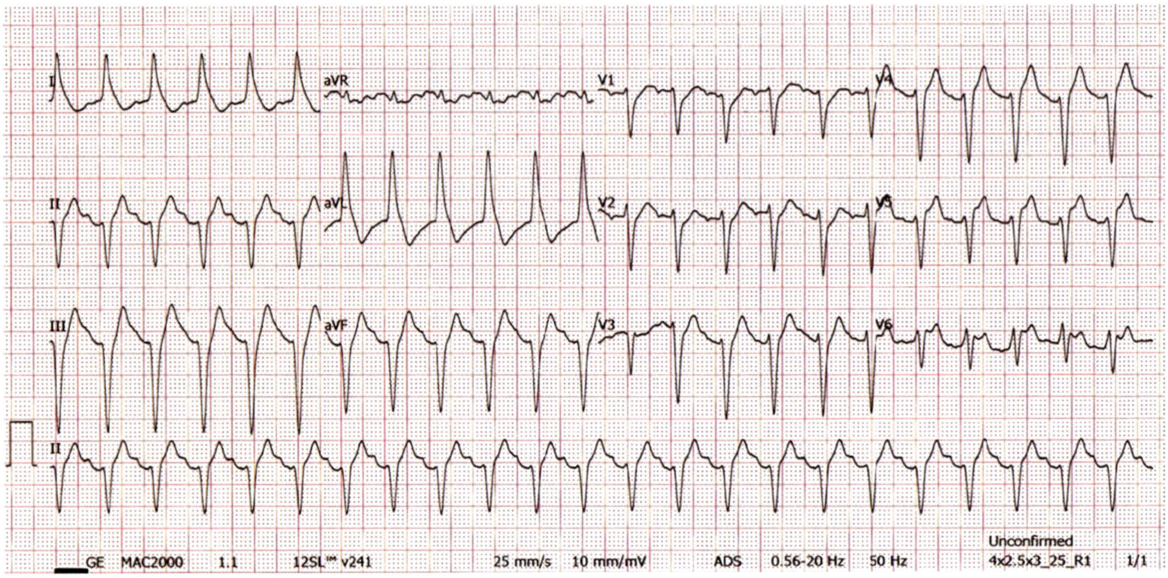

Fig. 19.18: Electrocardiogram (ECG) of myocarditis showing sinus tachycardia (heart rate 140 bpm) with intraventricular conduction delay mimicking ventricular tachycardia (VT). *Note:* All the QRS complexes are preceded by a P wave, suggesting sinus tachycardia.

Box 19.2: ECG changes in different infectious diseases.[48-51]

- *Diphtheria:* Inappropriate sinus tachycardia, ST-segment depression in precordial leads, PR interval prolongation, T-wave changes, intraventricular conduction defects, and AV conduction blocks.
- *Typhoid:* First-degree AV block, QT prolongation, ST-segment depression, and T-wave inversion are not uncommon. If typhoid myocarditis develops then the most common ECG abnormalities along with sinus tachycardia are QTc prolongation (29%) followed by ST-T changes (20%), bundle branch block (7%), and arrhythmia (2%). All the ECG changes are transient except bundle branch block which persist for long time. Relative bradycardia has been described as a characteristic feature of typhoid fever in the 1st week of disease *(When body temperature rises by 1°C, the heart rate increases on the average by 8 beats per minute. In a febrile patient if the pulse rate does not increase according to this rule and appears relatively slower, this is called relative bradycardia or Faget sign or pulse-temperature dissociation).*
- *Tetanus:* Sinus tachycardia, prolonged QT interval, nonspecific ST-T abnormalities, and P-wave changes are common. Other less common abnormalities include short PR interval, supraventricular tachycardia, intraventricular conduction delay, inappropriate sinus bradycardia, first-degree AV block, abnormal axis deviation, right ventricular hypertrophy, and sinoatrial Wenckebach phenomenon.
- *Rubella:* Nonspecific ST-segment and T-wave changes.
- *HIV infection:* Approximately 51% of the patients with HIV infection show some ECG abnormalities either minor or major changes. ECG of 8% of patients show major ECG abnormalities, and 49% develop minor abnormalities. Major ventricular conduction defects, QT prolongation, major Q/QS abnormalities, and major isolated ST/T abnormalities are the most common major abnormalities. Minor isolated ST/T abnormalities, sinus tachycardia, high R waves, and incomplete bundle branch block are the most common minor ECG abnormalities.
- *Pertussis:* Sinus node and AV nodal blocks.
- *Dengue fever:* Electrocardiographic abnormalities as a result of dengue infection are common and have been reported to be in the range of 34–75%. These are predominantly sinus bradycardia and conduction defects, all of which are transient. Abnormal ECG findings like sinus tachycardia, supraventricular tachycardia, left bundle branch block, ST depression, and poor progression of R wave are also noted. Rarely atrial fibrillation (AF) is seen.
- *Lyme disease:* PR interval prolongation.
- *Chagas disease:* Right bundle branch block, left anterior hemiblock, and varying degrees AV blocks.
- *Leptospirosis:* First-degree heart block, ECG evidences of pericarditis.

(AV: atrioventricular; ECG: electrocardiogram; HIV: human immunodeficiency virus)

ELECTROCARDIOGRAPHIC DIAGNOSIS OF ENDOCARDITIS

Electrocardiogram should be recorded at the very beginning of infectious endocarditis. It provides information on the origin and complications of possible organic disease. Moreover regular follow-up of ECG tracings can reveal changes signalizing spread of the infection beyond the endocardium.

Sinus tachycardia is the most common finding, seen in approximately 53% of patients. Other observed findings are low QRS voltage (44%), varying degrees of heart blocks (9%), ST elevation, atrial fibrillation, ventricular tachycardia, and supraventricular tachycardia (Fig. 19.19).[47-50] Conduction abnormalities can also suggest that the disease is extending into the perivalvular region. Thus the conduction system may be affected, may give rise to bundle branch block, atrioventricular (AV) blocks, first degree to third degree. Extrasystoles are common. Typical ECG changes of acute myocardial infarction may develop after embolization of the vegetation into the coronary artery. Last but not least, the pericardium may be involved after spreading of the infection into the pericardial cavity and may display diffuse ST segment elevations on the ECG tracing.

ELECTROCARDIOGRAM CHANGES IN RHEUMATIC CARDITIS

Sinus tachycardia is usual in rheumatic fever (Fig. 19.20), although some children develop bradycardia. ECG may show a prolonged PR interval. ST elevation suggests pericarditis.[52-54] First-degree AV block (prolonged PR interval) is a common finding associated with rheumatic fever (Fig. 19.21). Clarke and Keith documented prolonged PR intervals in 84% of 508 children with rheumatic fever, and arrhythmias were identified in one-eighth of the cases with abnormal ECG findings; among these cases, three children had complete heart block, and one required artificial pacing for Stokes-Adams attacks.[55] Advanced AV block is rare during the course of rheumatic carditis but second-degree and complete AV block have been documented in rheumatic fever.[52,56-58] Ventricular arrhythmias are uncommon in acute rheumatic carditis. But rheumatic carditis may cause prolonged QT interval, and torsades de pointes.[59] When advanced heart block occurs with rheumatic fever, it appears to be a transient event, resolving over a period of days with anti-inflammatory treatment.

SUMMARY

The pericardium is a thin layer that covers the heart and separates it from other structures in the mediastinum. Pericardial syndromes include acute, recurrent, constrictive, and effusive-constrictive pericarditis, as well as pericardial effusion with or without tamponade. Causes include viral (echovirus, coxsackievirus, HIV, etc.) or bacterial (tuberculous, staphylococcal, pneumococcal, meningococcal infection), postmyocardial infarction syndrome (Dressler's syndrome), postpericardiotomy pericarditis, primary and metastatic tumors, trauma, uremia, radiation, and autoimmune diseases, but pericardial syndromes can also be idiopathic. Acute pericarditis is the most common pericardial syndrome and occurs in all age groups. Pericarditis classically presents with positional chest pain, a pericardial friction rub, sinus tachycardia, diffuse ST-segment elevation with concavity upwards, and PR-segment depression.

Acute pericarditis develops in stages, which makes it easy to differentiate from early repolarization and, more significantly, myocardial infarction.

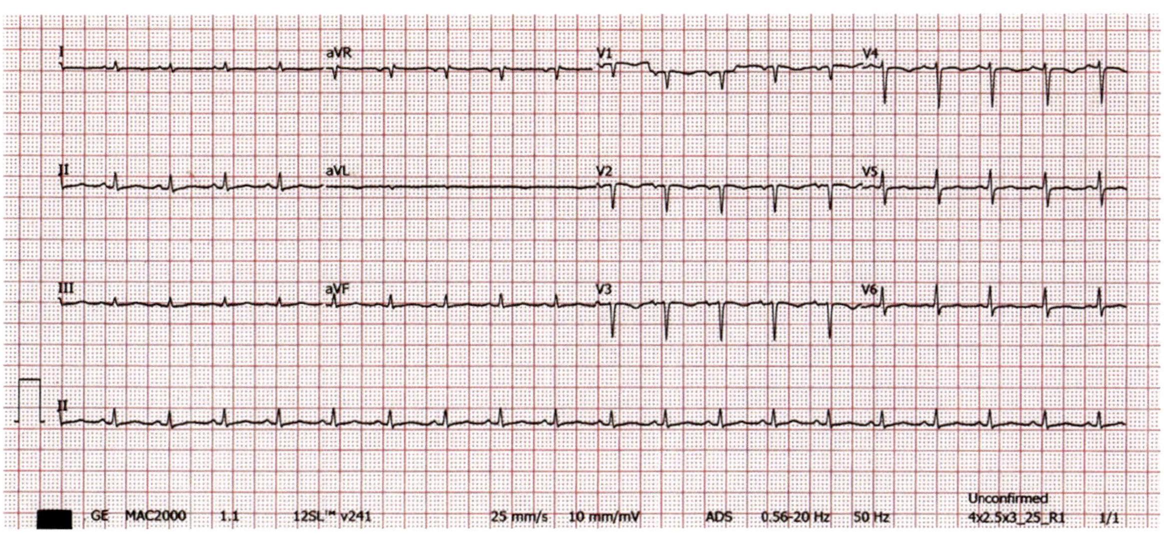

Fig. 19.19: This electrocardiogram (ECG) illustrates the ECG features of endocarditis with low voltage (peak-to-peak QRS amplitude of less than 5 mm in the limb leads and less than 10 mm in the precordial leads) and sinus tachycardia (heart rate 118 bpm).

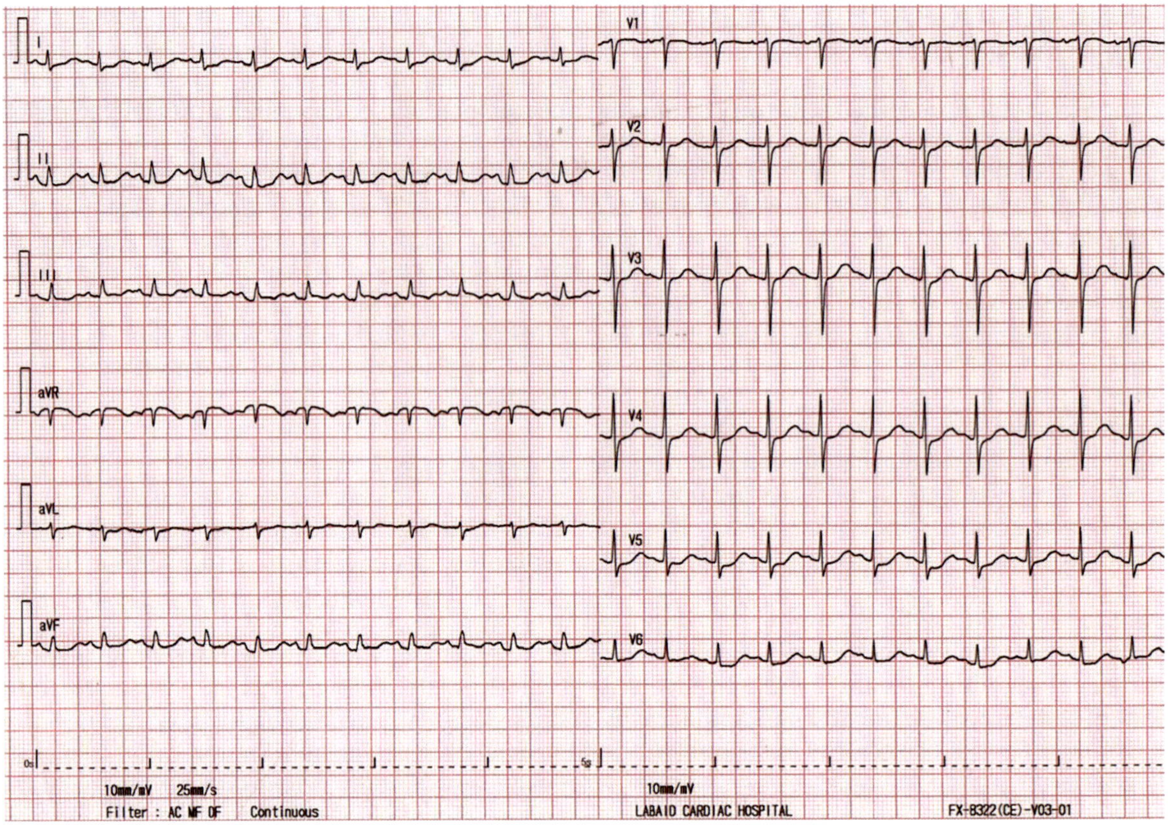

Fig. 19.20: Electrocardiogram (ECG) shows marked sinus tachycardia (heart rate 146 bpm) in a patient of rheumatic carditis.

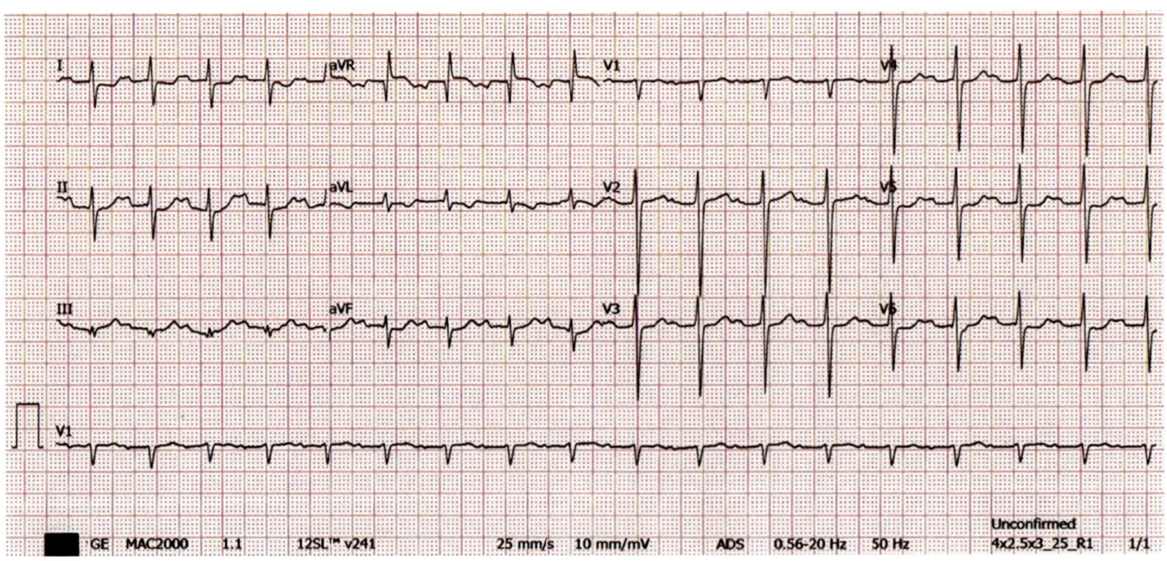

Fig. 19.21: Electrocardiogram (ECG) shows first-degree heart block (PR interval 220 ms) with sinus tachycardia (heart rate 106 bpm) suggestive of rheumatic carditis. *Note:* T wave and P waves are fused together giving a biphasic appearance.

Courtesy: Dr Samiron Kumar Saha, Labaid Specialized Hospital

Electrocardiogram Criteria of Acute Pericarditis

- *Stage I:* ST elevation with concavity upwards in both limb and precodial leads. PR-segment depression (also called PTa depression) (depression between the end of the P wave and the beginning of the QRS complex) is the typical ECG sign of acute pericarditis.
- *Stage II:* Pseudonormalization (transition), the ST and PR segments normalize.
- *Stage III:* Widespread T-wave inversion.
- *Stage IV:* Normalization of the T waves.

- In stage I Spodick's sign is found in around 80% of cases. Spodick's sign signifies to a downsloping TP segment in patients with acute pericarditis.

The duration for evolution of ST segment and T wave changes through each of the four ECG stages is highly variable ranging from hours to weeks. Practically, stage I is the only diagnostic phase because stage II looks normal and stage III mimics myocardial ischemia.

The ECG changes of pericarditis must be distinguished from those of acute myocardial infarction and ERP. ST-segment elevation with upward convexity suggests acute STEMI but ST-segment elevation with upward concavity is suggestive of acute pericarditis.

In pericarditis ST segment is elevated diffusely in the precordial and limb leads, differentiating it from characteristic regional changes in STEMI. Reciprocal ST depression and Q waves are absent in ECGs of acute pericarditis. Both acute pericarditis and early repolarization pattern give rise to ST-segment elevation with upward concavity, so differentiating these two conditions sometimes may be difficult. Acute pericarditis tends to cause ST-segment elevation in both the limb and precordial leads, whereas ST elevation in early repolarization mainly involves the precordial leads. ST-segment elevation in early repolarization pattern is associated with tall and peak T waves, which is not seen in case of acute pericarditis. PTa (PR segment) depression is common in acute pericarditis but it is uncommon in early repolarization abnormality.

Acute pericarditis develops in stages, where ECG changes are dynamic which makes it easy to differentiate from early repolarization pattern where ECG changes are almost static.

Comparison of Electrocardiogram Features of Acute Pericarditis, ST-elevation Myocardial Infarction and Early Repolarization Pattern

The comparison of electrocardiogram features of acute pericarditis, ST-elevation myocardial infarction and early repolarization pattern are given in Table 19.3.

Table 19.3: Comparison of electrocardiogram features of acute pericarditis, ST-elevation myocardial infarction and early repolarization pattern.

Electrocardiogram (ECG) findings	*Acute pericarditis*	*Acute ST-elevation myocardial infarction (STEMI)*	*Early repolarization pattern (ERP)*
Pattern of ST-segment elevation	Upwardly concave	Upwardly convex	Upwardly concave
Reciprocal ST-segment depression	Absent	Present	Absent
PR-segment depression	Present	Absent	Absent
Presence of pathological Q waves	Absent	May be present	Absent
Location of ST-segment elevations	Diffuse, both limb and precordial leads	Area of culprit arterial territory	Mostly in precordial leads
Loss of R-wave voltage	Absent	Present	Absent
ST/T ratio in lead V6	>0.25	Not applicable	<0.25

Pericardial Effusion and Tamponade

Sinus tachycardia with low voltage ECG is commonly seen in ECG of pericardial effusion. Low voltage ECG is defined as a peak-to-peak QRS amplitude of less than 5 mm in the limb leads and/or less than 10 mm in the precordial leads. Electrical alternans defined as the alteration of the QRS complex amplitude or axis between beats, is specific but not very sensitive for cardiac tamponade.

Myocarditis

Myocarditis is defined as inflammation of the heart muscle (myocardium).

Viral (e.g. coxsackievirus, HIV), bacterial (e.g. corynebacterium diphtheriae, brucella, gonococcus) and various protozoal, parasitic, and fungal infection may cause myocarditis. Fever, palpitation, chest pain, and congestive heart failure are the usual presenting features.

The most common abnormality seen in myocarditis is sinus tachycardia with nonspecific ST segment and T-wave changes. The ECG may show ventricular arrhythmias or varying degrees of heart blocks, or it may mimic the findings in acute myocardial infarction or pericarditis.

Electrocardiographic features of myocarditis are mostly nonspecific but ECG usually displays the following findings:

- Sinus tachycardia.
- Diffuse T-wave inversion.
- Ventricular and supraventricular arrhythmias.
- Atrioventricular conduction defects.
- QRS/QT prolongation.
- ST-segment elevation mimicking an acute myocardial infarction.
- New left bundle branch block.

ECG diagnosis of various cardiac inflammatory conditions are given in Box 19.3.

Endocarditis

Sinus tachycardia is the most common ECG finding in patients with endocarditis. Other findings include low QRS

Box 19.3: ECG diagnosis of various cardiac inflammatory conditions.

Acute pericarditis:
- Sinus tachycardia
- Widespread upwardly concave ST-segment elevation
- PR-segment depression (I, II, III, aVF, and V4–6)
- Reciprocal ST depression and PR elevation in aVR and V1.

Pericardial effusion:
- Low voltage ECG
- Sinus tachycardia.

Cardiac tamponade:
- Low voltage ECG
- Sinus tachycardia
- Electrical alternans.

Myocarditis:
- Sinus tachycardia with nonspecific ST segment and T-wave changes (most common abnormality)
- QRS/QT prolongation
- AV conduction defects
- Diffuse T-wave inversion
- Ventricular arrhythmias.

Endocarditis:
- Sinus tachycardia
- Low QRS voltage
- Varying degrees of heart blocks.

Rheumatic fever:
- Sinus tachycardia
- First-degree heart block.

(AV: atrioventricular; ECG: electrocardiogram)

voltage, varying degrees of heart blocks, both ventricular and supraventricular arrhythmias.

Rheumatic Carditis

Sinus tachycardia and first-degree AV block (prolonged PR interval) are common ECG findings in rheumatic fever. High-grade AV block (second-degree heart block or complete heart block) and ventricular arrhythmias are very rare.

REFERENCES

1. Khandaker MH, Espinosa RE, Nishimura RA, et al. Pericardial disease: diagnosis and management. Mayo Clin Proc. 2010;85(6):572-93.
2. Imazio M, Spodick DH, Brucato A, et al. Controversial issues in the management of pericardial diseases. Circulation. 2010;121(7):916-28.
3. Zayas R, Anguita M, Torres F, et al. Incidence of specific etiology and role of methods for specific etiologic diagnosis of primary acute pericarditis. Am J Cardiol. 1995;75(5):378-82.
4. Maisch B, Seferović PM, Ristić AD, et al. Guidelines on the diagnosis and management of pericardial diseases executive summary; the Task Force on the diagnosis and management of pericardial diseases of the European society of cardiology. Eur Heart J. 2004;25(7):587-610.
5. Lilly LS. Treatment of acute and recurrent idiopathic pericarditis. Circulation. 2013;127(16):1723-6.
6. Troughton RW, Asher CR, Klein AL. Pericarditis. Lancet. 2004;363(9410):717-27.
7. Oakley CM. Myocarditis, pericarditis and other pericardial diseases. Heart. 2000;84(4):449-54.
8. Alraies MC, Klein AL. Should we still use electrocardiography to diagnose pericardial disease? Cleveland Clin J Med. 2013;80(2):97-100.
9. Imazio M, Trinchero R. Triage and management of acute pericarditis. Int J Cardiol. 2007;118(3):286-94.
10. Spodick DH. Acute pericarditis: current concepts and practice. JAMA. 2003;289(9):1150-3.
11. Shabetai R. Acute pericarditis. Cardiol Clin. 1990;8(4):639-44.
12. Baljepally R, Spodick DH. PR-segment deviation as the initial electrocardiographic response in acute pericarditis. Am J Cardiol. 1998;81(12):1505-6.
13. Spodick DH. Diagnostic electrocardiographic sequences in acute pericarditis. Significance of PR segment and PR vector changes. Circulation. 1973;48(3):575-80.
14. Ginzton LE, Laks MM. The differential diagnosis of acute pericarditis from the normal variant: new electrocardiographic criteria. Circulation. 1982;65(5):1004-9.
15. Brady WJ, Perron A, Ullman E. Errors in emergency physician interpretation of ST-segment elevation in emergency department chest pain patients. Acad Emerg Med. 2000;7(11):1256-60.
16. Spodick DH. Differential characteristics of the electrocardiogram in early repolarization and acute pericarditis. N Engl J Med. 1976;295(10):523-6.
17. Bonnefoy E, Godon P, Kirkorian G, et al. Serum cardiac troponin I and ST-segment elevation in patients with acute pericarditis. Eur Heart J. 2000;21(10):832-6.
18. Rathore S, Dodds PA. Diagnosing chest pain: characteristic ECG changes in acute pericarditis. Heart. 2007;93(9):1063.
19. Wang K, Asinger RW, Marriott HJ. ST-segment elevation in conditions other than acute myocardial infarction. N Engl J Med. 2003;349(22):2128-35.
20. Chaubey VK, Chhabra L. Spodick's sign: a helpful electrocardiographic clue to the diagnosis of acute pericarditis. Perm J. 2014;18(1):e122.
21. Mehta M, Jain AC, Mehta A. Early repolarization. Clin Cardiol. 1999;22(2):59-65.
22. Klatsky AL, Oehm R, Cooper RA, et al. The early repolarization normal variant electrocardiogram: correlates and consequences. Am J Med. 2003;115(3):171-7.
23. Derval N, Shah A, Pierre JP. Definition of early repolarization. Circulation. 2011;124:2185-6.
24. Kambara H, Phillips J. Long-term evaluation of early repolarization syndrome (normal variant RS-T segment elevation). Am J Cardiol. 1976;38(2):157-6.
25. Perez MV, Friday K, Froelicher V. Semantic confusion: the case of early repolarization and the J point. Am J Med. 2012;125(9):843-4.
26. Patton KK, Ellinor PT, Ezekowitz M, et al. Electrocardiographic Early Repolarization: A Scientific Statement From the American Heart Association. Circulation. 2016;133(15):1520-9.

27. Kudo Y, Yamasaki F, Doi T, et al. Clinical significance of low voltage in asymptomatic patients with pericardial effusion free of heart disease. Chest. 2003;124(6):2064-7.
28. Setty NS, Sadananda KS, Nanjappa MC, et al. Massive pericardial effusion and cardiac tamponade due to cholesterol pericarditis in a case of subclinical hypothyroidism: a rare event. J Am Coll Cardiol. 2014;63(14):1451.
29. Lee J, Rinehart S. Pericardial effusion with tamponade: physiology secondary to high grade B-cell lymphoma. J Am Coll Cardiol. 2014;63(12):A630.
30. Bruch C, Schmermund A, Dagres N, et al. Changes in QRS voltage in cardiac tamponade and pericardial effusion: reversibility after pericardiocentesis and after anti-inflammatory drug treatment. J Am Coll Cardiol. 2001;38(1):219-26.
31. Spodick DH. Acute cardiac tamponade. N Engl J Med. 2003;349(7):684-90.
32. Eisenberg MJ, de Romeral LM, Heidenreich PA, et al. The diagnosis of pericardial effusion and cardiac tamponade by 12-lead ECG. A technology assessment. Chest. 1996;110(2):318-24.
33. Doolan A, Langlois N, Semsarian C. Causes of sudden cardiac death in young Australians. Med J Aust. 2004;180(3):110-2.
34. Felker GM, Hu W, Hare JM, et al. The spectrum of dilated cardiomyopathy. The Johns Hopkins experience with 1,278 patients. Medicine (Baltimore). 1999;78(4):270-83.
35. Baboonian C, Treasure T. Meta-analysis of the association of enteroviruses with human heart disease. Heart. 1997;78(6):539-43.
36. Magnani JW, Dec GW. Myocarditis: current trends in diagnosis and treatment. Circulation. 2006;113(6): 876-90.
37. Morgera T, Di Lenarda A, Dreas L. Electrocardiography of myocarditis revisited: clinical and prognostic significance of electrocardiographic changes. Am Heart J. 1992;124(2): 455-67.
38. Pauschinger M, Noutsias M, Lassner D, et al. Inflammation, ECG changes and pericardial effusion: whom to biopsy in suspected myocarditis? Clin Res Cardiol. 2006;95(11): 569-83.
39. Cooper LT. Myocarditis. N Engl J Med. 2009;360(15): 1526-38.
40. Nakashima H, Katayama T, Ishizaki M, et al. Q wave and non-Q wave myocarditis with special reference to clinical significance. Jpn Heart J. 1998;39(6):763-74.
41. Ukena C, Mahfoud F, Kindermann I, et al. Prognostic electrocardiographic parameters in patients with suspected myocarditis. Eur J Heart Fail. 2011;13(4):398-405.
42. Kindermann I, Barth C, Mahfoud F, et al. Update on myocarditis. J Am Coll Cardiol. 2012;59(9):779-92.
43. Dec GW, Waldman H, Southern J, et al. Viral myocarditis mimicking acute myocardial infarction. J Am Coll Cardiol. 1992;20(1):85-9.
44. Angelini A, Calzolari V, Calabrese F, et al. Myocarditis mimicking acute myocardial infarction: role of endomyocardial biopsy in the differential diagnosis. Heart. 2000;84(3):245-50.
45. Sarda L, Colin P, Boccara F, et al. Myocarditis in patients with clinical presentation of myocardial infarction and normal coronary angiograms. J Am Coll Cardiol. 2001;37(3):786-92.
46. Feldman AM, McNamara D. Myocarditis. N Engl J Med. 2000;343(19):1388-98.
47. Meine TJ, Nettles RE, Anderson DJ, et al. Cardiac conduction abnormalities in endocarditis defined by the Duke criteria. Am Heart J. 2001;142(2):280-5.
48. Mahmod M, Darul ND, Mokhtar I, et al. Atrial fibrillation as a complication of dengue hemorrhagic fever: non-self-limiting manifestation. Int J Infect Dis. 2009;13(5):e316-8.
49. Mitra RC, Gupta RD, Sack RB. Electrocardiographic changes in tetanus: a serial study. J Indian Med Assoc. 1991;89(6):164-7.
50. Nalmas S, Nagarakanti R, Slim J, et al. Electrocardiographic Changes in Infectious Diseases. Wayne: Turner White Communications Inc.; 2007. pp. 15-27.
51. Soliman EZ, Prineas RJ, Roediger MP, et al. Prevalence and Prognostic Significance of ECG Abnormalities in HIV-infected Patients: Results from the Strategies for Management of Antiretroviral Therapy (SMART) Study. J Electrocardiol. 2011;44(6):779-85.
52. Yoo GH. Complete Atrioventricular Block in an Adolescent With Rheumatic Fever. Korean Circ J. 2009;39(3):121-3.
53. Jeong EY, Jun BJ, Kim NS, et al. A study of clinical manifestations of acute rheumatic fever. J Korean Pediatr Cardiol Soc. 2007;11:116-23.
54. Kumar RK, Tandon R. Rheumatic fever & rheumatic heart disease: the last 50 years. Indian J Med Res. 2013;137(4): 643-58.
55. Clarke M, Keith JD. Atrioventricular conduction in acute rheumatic fever. Br Heart J. 1972;34(5):472-9.
56. Zalzstein E, Maor R, Zucker N, et al. Advanced atrioventricular conduction block in acute rheumatic fever. Cardiol Young. 2003;13(6):506-8.
57. Uemura A, Morimoto S, Hiramitsu S, et al. Endomyocardial biopsy findings in 50 patients with idiopathic atrioventricular block: presence of myocarditis. Jpn Heart J. 2001;42(6):691-700.
58. Malik JA, Hassan C, Khan GQ. Transient complete heart block complicating acute rheumatic fever. Indian Heart J. 2002;54(1):91-2.
59. Liberman L, Hordof AJ, Alfayyadh M, et al. Torsade de pointes in a child with acute rheumatic fever. J Pediatr. 2001;138(2):280-2.

Chapter 20

Electrocardiographic Manifestations of Electrolyte Abnormalities

INTRODUCTION

As cardiac myocyte depolarization and repolarization depend on intra and extracellular shifts in ion gradients, abnormal serum electrolyte levels can have profound effects on cardiac conduction and electrocardiogram (ECG). Changes in extracellular potassium, calcium, and magnesium levels can change myocyte membrane potential gradients and alter the cardiac action potential. These changes can result in incidental findings on the 12-lead ECG or precipitate potentially life-threatening dysrhythmias.

Electrolyte abnormalities may generate or facilitate clinical arrhythmias, even in the setting of normal cardiac tissue. Furthermore, electrolyte aberrations are more likely to interact with abnormal myocardial tissue to generate their own cadre of cardiac arrhythmias. Electrolyte disorders exert their actions by modulating the conduction of ions across specific cardiac membrane channels; and this in turn can result in antiarrhythmic or proarrhythmic sequelae.[1]

HYPERKALEMIA

Hyperkalemia is defined as serum potassium concentration greater than 5.5 mmol/L (Normal potassium level is 3.5–5.5 mmol/L). The prevalence of hyperkalemia in the general population is unknown, but it is thought to occur in 1–10% of patients admitted to hospital.[2] Hyperkalemia can induce deadly cardiac arrhythmias. Electrocardiographic manifestations of hyperkalemia vary from the classic sine-wave rhythm, which occurs in severe hyperkalemia, to nonspecific repolarization abnormalities seen with mild elevations of serum potassium.[1] Renal insufficiency, medications those interfere with urinary excretion, e.g. angiotensin converting enzyme (ACE) inhibitors and angiotensin receptor blockers (ARBs), potassium-sparing diuretics (e.g. amiloride and spironolactone), nonsteroidal anti-inflammatory drugs (NSAIDs), such as ibuprofen, naproxen, or celecoxib, Addison's disease, aldosterone deficiency, etc. may produce the state of hyperkalemia.[1-4]

As the myocardium is highly sensitive to any changes in potassium ion concentration, the imbalance of the potassium concentration gradient in hyperkalemia can cause a progression of ECG changes, such as increased T-wave amplitude (peaked T waves), prolongation of the PR interval and QRS duration, loss of P waves, atrioventricular (AV) conduction delay, culminating in the merging of the QRS complex with the T-wave producing a sine-wave pattern, and asystole (Figs. 20.1A to D).[3,4] Clinically, patients can present with palpitations, syncope, and sudden cardiac death.

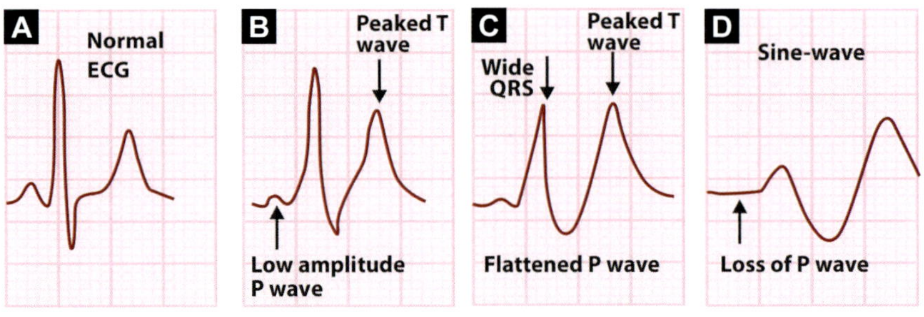

Figs. 20.1A to D: Schematic representation of the electrocardiograms (ECGs) at various phases of hyperkalemia. (A) Normal ECG; (B) ECG of mild hyperkalemia showing tall peak T-wave with low amplitude P-wave; (C) ECG changes in moderate hyperkalemia showing more peaked T-wave with wide QRS complex with flattened P-wave; (D) ECG features of severe hyperkalemia illustrating *sine wave* (QRS complex and T-wave fused together) along with disappearance of P-wave.

Different Stages of Hyperkalemia[5-9] (Table 20.1)

1. Mild levels of hyperkalemia (5.5–6.0 mmol/L) are associated with acceleration of terminal repolarization, resulting in T-wave changes. The most common changes seen in the T waves are "tenting" or "peaking", they are considered to be the earliest abnormalities seen in the ECG (Fig. 20.2).
2. Moderate hyperkalemia (6.1–7.0 mmol/L) causes depression of conduction between adjacent cardiac myocytes; this results in prolongation of the PR and QRS intervals as potassium levels rise (Fig. 20.3). Amplitude of the P waves gradually decreases and P waves eventually disappear (Fig. 20.4). P-wave amplitude disappears early because of the sensitivity of atrial myocytes to hyperkalemia.
3. Severe hyperkalemia (>7.0 mmol/L) causes suppression of sinoatrial and atrioventricular conduction, resulting in the appearance of escape beats and escape rhythms (Fig. 20.5). The QRS complex will continue to widen and may blend with the T-wave, creating a *sine-wave appearance* to the ECG (Figs. 20.6 and 20.7A and B). If the potassium level is allowed to rise without treatment, sinus arrest will occur. Serum potassium level of greater than 9.0 mmol/L causes cardiac arrest due to ventricular fibrillation (VF), pulseless electrical activity (PEA) rhythm, and asystole.

These classic ECG changes, which have been well described in the literature, are not always present.[10,11] The relation between ECG changes and serum potassium will vary between people. It is therefore important to realize that the ECG is not always a reliable test for mild to moderate hyperkalemia. Even in severe hyperkalemia, only minimal changes may be seen on the ECG.[10,11]

Table 20.1: Electrocardiogram (ECG) features during different phases of hyperkalemia.

Degree of hyperkalemia	*Serum potassium level in mmol/L*	*ECG features*
Mild	5.5–6.0	1. Tall, peak, and tented T waves 2. Flattening of P waves.
Moderate	6.1–7.0	1. Low amplitude P-wave and P waves eventually disappear. 2. Prolonged PR interval 3. Widening of QRS complex. 4. ST-segment elevation.
Severe	>7.0	1. Bizarre widening of QRS complex. 2. Bradycardia or nodal rhythm 3. Sine wave 4. Ventricular fibrillation 5. Asystole.

In general, hyperkalemia produces a gradual depression of the excitability, conduction velocity of the specialized pacemaker cells, and conducting tissues throughout the heart. High serum potassium levels are thought to impair the conduction in the Purkinje fibers and ventricles more than in the AV node, although complete atrioventricular block can occur. In addition to the classic ECG manifestations there have been other ECG changes resulting from hyperkalemia reported in the literature. These include complete heart block, trifascicular block, and QRS axis shift.[12,13] Second-degree heart block and complete heart

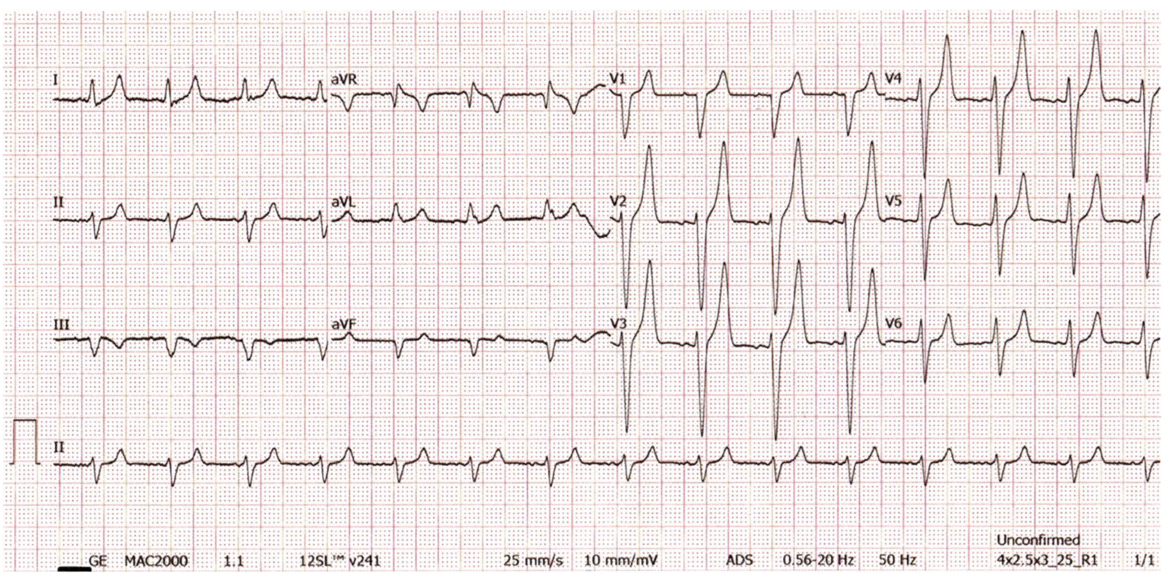

Fig. 20.2: Electrocardiogram illustrating the features of mild hyperkalemia. Note tall and peak T waves (>10 mm in height) in leads V2–V5 with low amplitude P waves in both limb and chest leads.

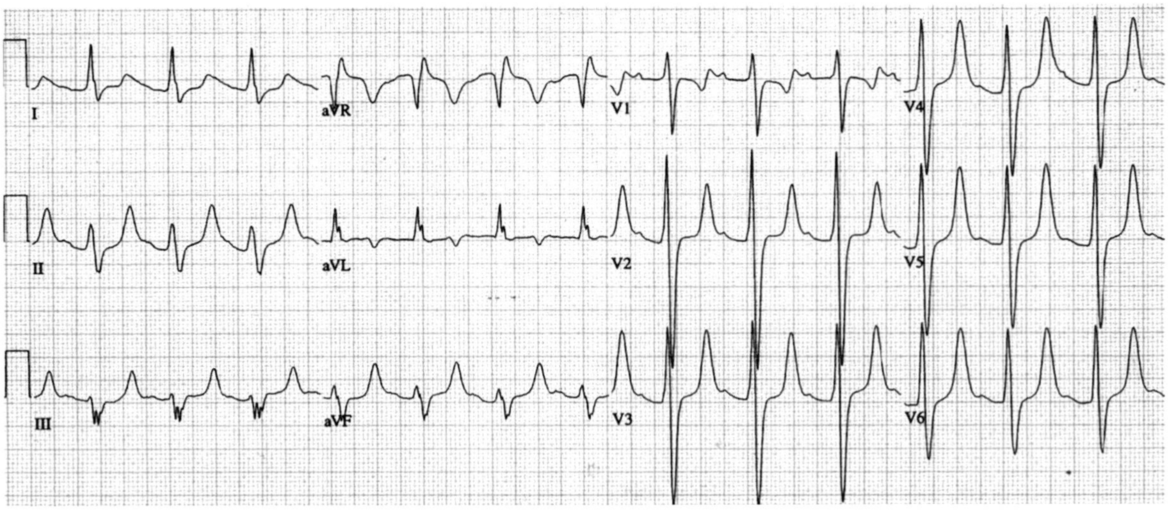

Fig. 20.3: Electrocardiogram illustrating the features of moderate degree hyperkalemia. Note tall and peak T waves (>10 mm in height) in leads V2–V6 with prolonged PR interval (PR is 240 ms) with broad QRS complex (QRS duration is 160 ms).

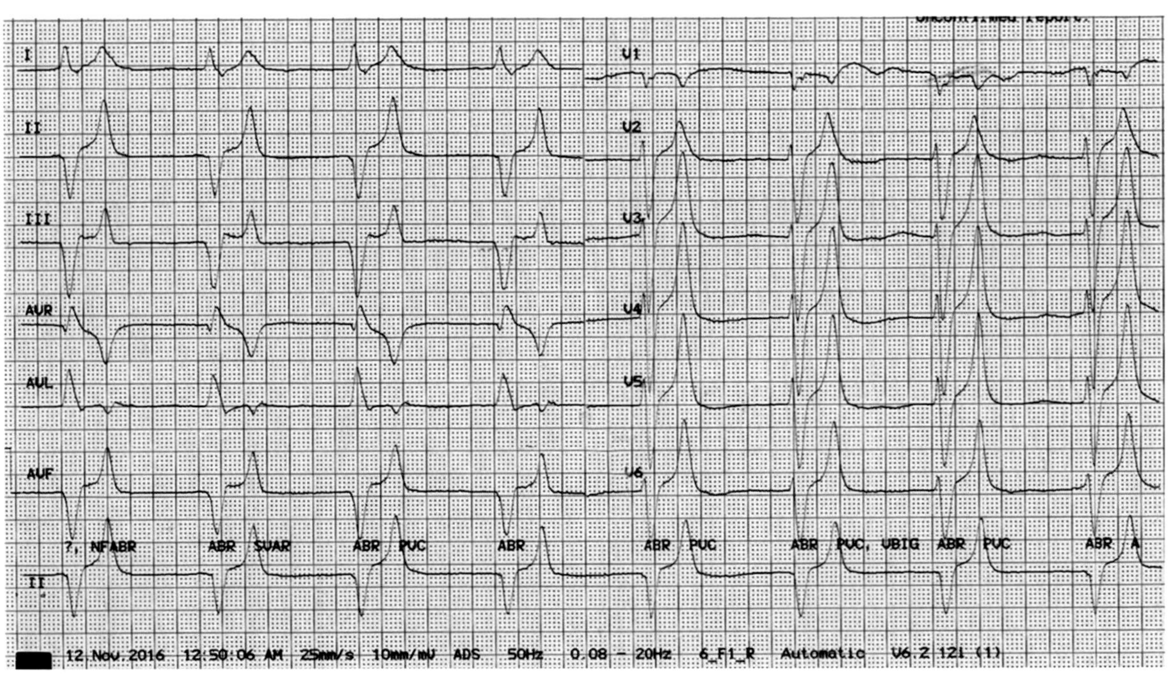

Fig. 20.4: Electrocardiogram illustrating the features of moderate degree hyperkalemia. Note tall and peak T waves (>10 mm in height) in almost all the leads along with loss of P waves with broad QRS complex (QRS duration is 160 ms). Also note marked bradycardia. (*Courtesy:* Dr AK Miah, Labaid Cardiac Hospital).

block have been documented in severe hyperkalemia and may require temporary pacing during the course of treatment.[14-18] Hyperkalemia may also produce ECG changes that mimic acute myocardial infarction. This is of particular importance to the emergency physician as it may result in the administration of inappropriate treatment such as thrombolysis/coronary angiogram with a view to primary percutaneous coronary intervention. The changes mimicking infarction or ischemia will resolve with the treatment of hyperkalemia.[19]

There is no clear correlation between levels of potassium and the likelihood of an arrhythmia; however, arrhythmia is more likely if the increase in potassium is rapid.

HYPOKALEMIA

Hypokalemia is defined as a potassium level less than 3.5 mmol/L. Mild hypokalemia is a serum level of 3.0–3.5 mmol/L, moderate hypokalemia is a serum level of 2.5–2.9 mmol/L, and severe hypokalemia is defined as a level less than 2.5 mmol/L. Gastrointestinal tract losses, e.g. diarrhea, vomiting, laxative abuse, and renal losses; salt-losing nephropathy, renal tubular acidosis, diuretic drugs, e.g. thiazides, loop diuretics, and osmotic diuretics are the common causes of hypokalemia.

The electrocardiographic manifestation of hypokalemia is due to its effects on repolarization and those emanating

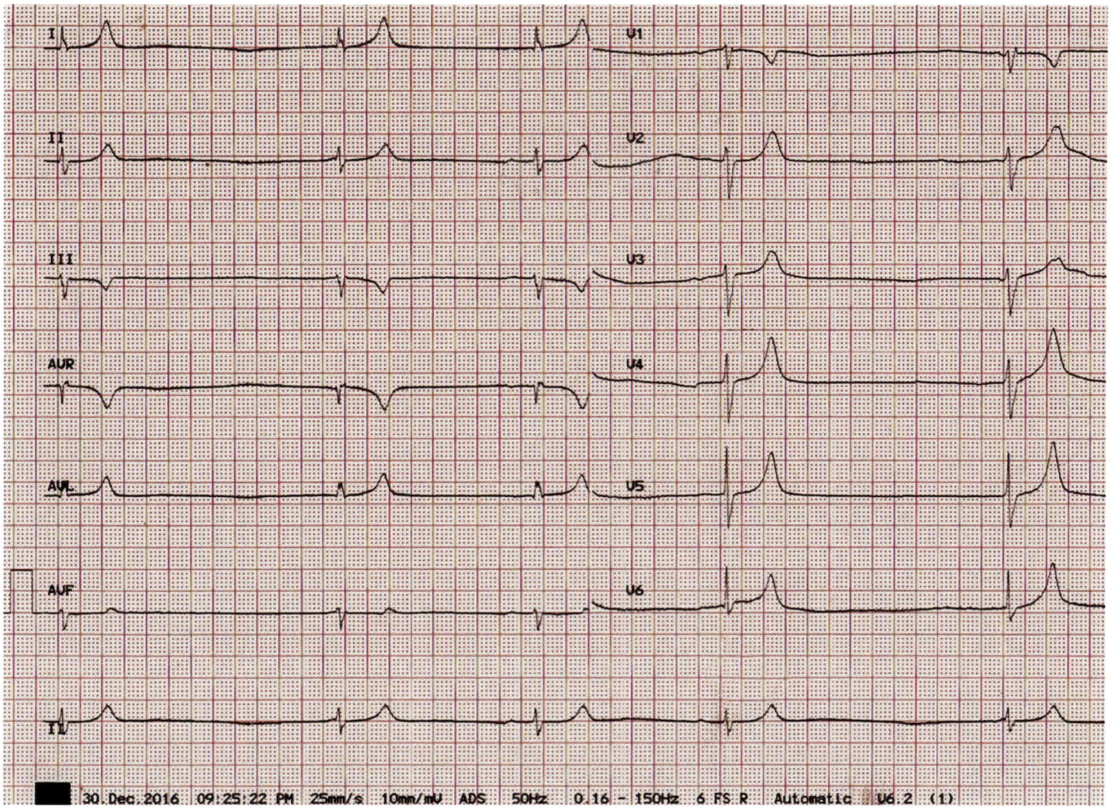

Fig. 20.5: This ECG illustrates marked junctional bradycardia (heart rate is 28 bpm) as an electrocardiographic manifestation of severe hyperkalemia. At the time of taking this ECG, potassium level was 8.1 mmol/L. (*Courtesy:* Dr Nur Mohammad, Labaid Cardiac Hospital).

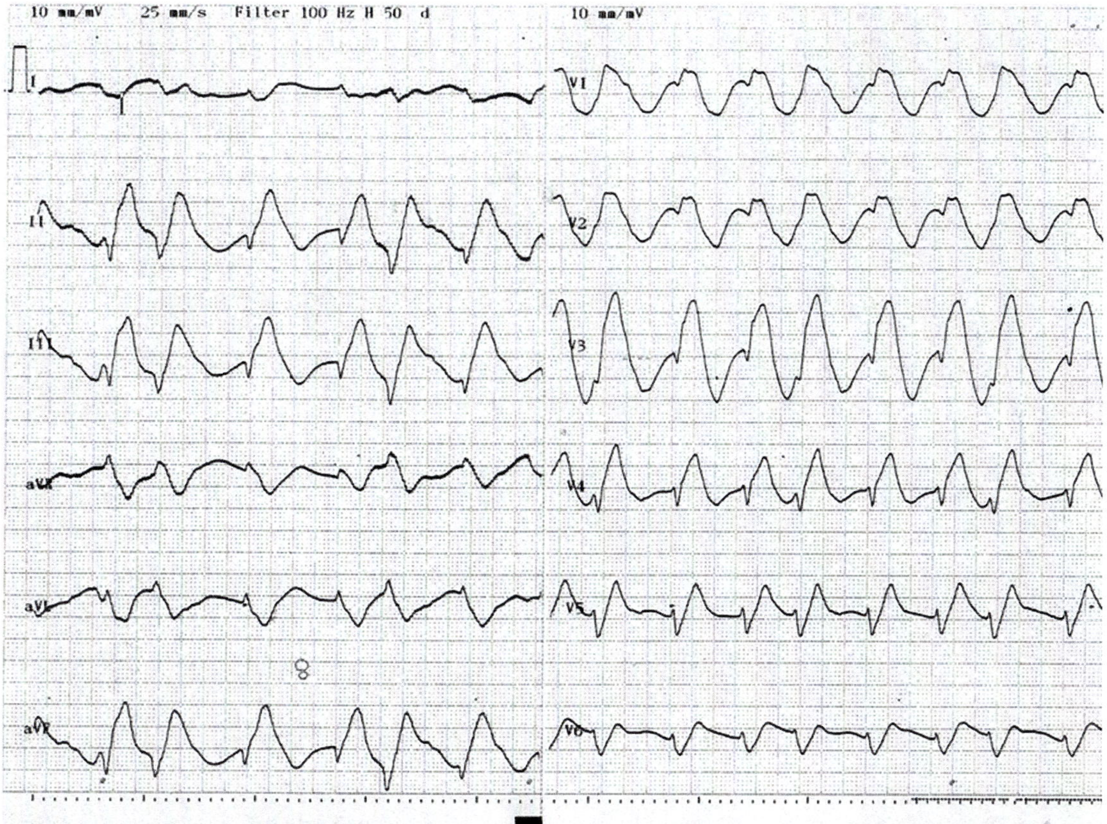

Fig. 20.6: This ECG shows a bizarre rhythm with a widened QRS complex in a *sine-wave* configuration, and there are no discernible P waves. The T waves have been fused with the widened QRS complexes to form the sine-wave pattern, raising suspicion of severe hyperkalemia. The patient's serum potassium level was 8.7 mmol/L at the time of taking this ECG. (*Courtesy:* Dr Habibur Rahman, Labaid Cardiac Hospital).

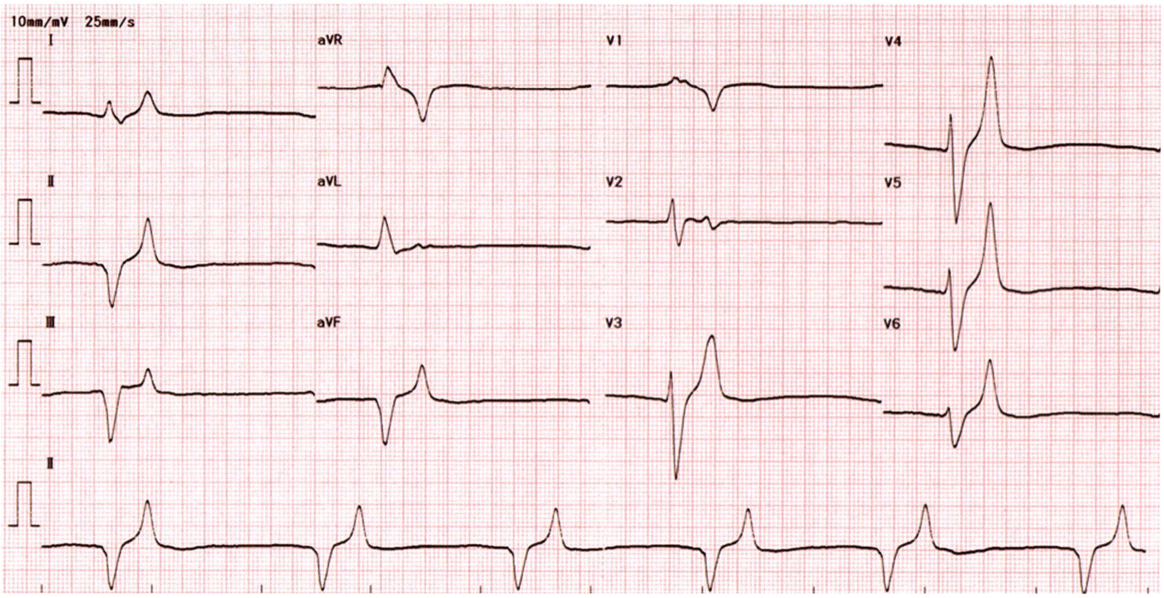

Fig. 20.7A: This ECG shows huge peaked T waves in precordial leads with almost sine-wave appearance with marked bradycardia. This patient had severe hyperkalemia (K^+- 9.0 mmol/L) secondary to chronic renal failure. (*Courtesy:* Dr Rafiqul Alam, Bangabandhu Sheikh Mujib Medical University, Dhaka).

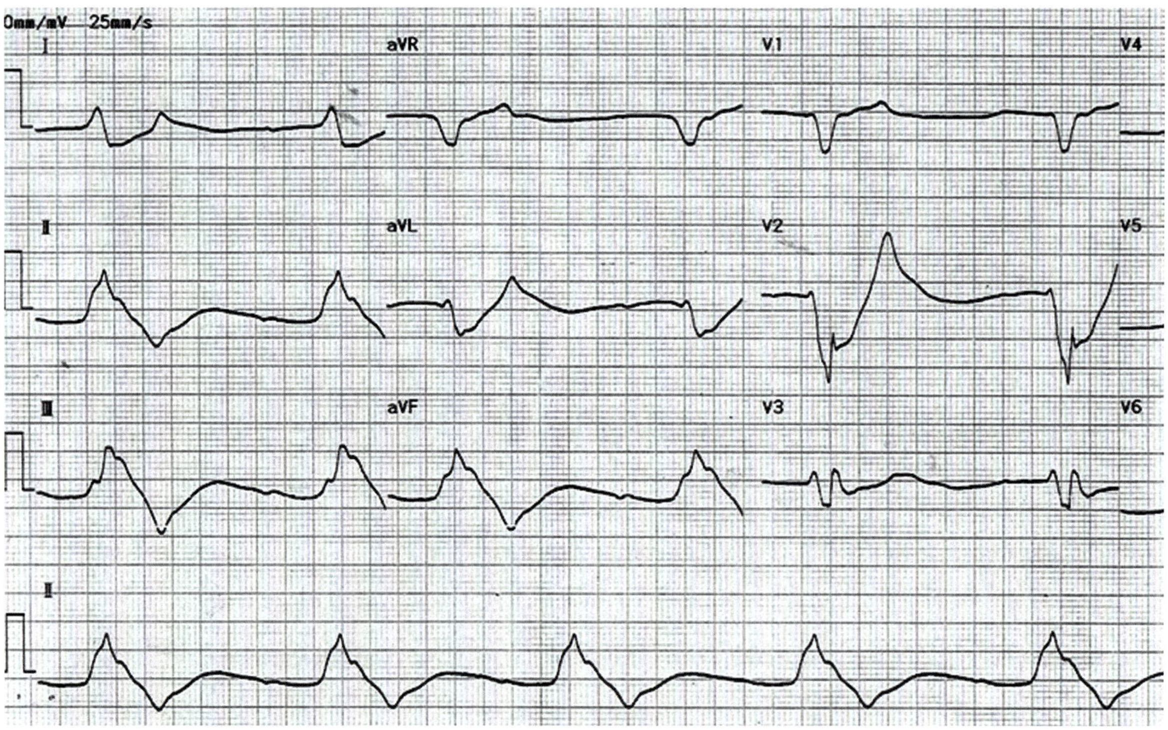

Fig. 20.7B: This ECG shows a bizarre wide complex rhythm with severe bradycardia in a *sine-wave* configuration. Note there is no discernible P wave. The QRS complexes and T waves have been fused together to form the sine-waves. This patient, a known case of chronic kidney disease was brought to the emergency department in collapsed state and her BP was nonrecordable during initial assessment. Temporary pacemaker was inserted immediately after admission and her first potassium level was 8.8 mmol/L. Her ECG reverted back to normal sinus rhythm within 12 hours of initiation of treatment of hyperkalemia. (*Courtesy:* Dr Atiquzzaman Sohel, Labaid Cardiac Hospital).

from its effects on conduction (Table 20.2). Hypokalemia causes decrease in conduction velocity, shortening of the effective refractory period, prolongation of the relative refractory period, and increased automaticity. Hypokalemia enhances the propensity for VF in the normal, as well as the ischemic heart.[1]

The earliest ECG change associated with hypokalemia is a decrease in the T-wave amplitude and prominent U wave. The U-wave is described as a positive deflection after the T-wave, often best seen in the mid-precordial leads (e.g. V2 and V3). The U-wave amplitude is usually less than one-third of T-wave amplitude in same lead and maximum

Table 20.2: Electrocardiogram features during different phases of hypokalemia.

Degree of hypokalemia	*Serum potassium level in mmol/L*	*ECG changes*
Mild	3.0–3.5	1. Decrease in the T-wave amplitude. 2. U-wave becomes prominent.
Moderate	2.5–2.9	1. U-wave exceeds the T-wave amplitude. 2. ST-segment depression and T-wave inversions appear. 3. PR interval can be prolonged. 4. An increase in the amplitude of the P-wave may be noted.
Severe	<2.5	1. T and U-wave fusion with giant U-wave formation (pseudo-prolonged QT interval) with an absent T-wave. 2. Atrial fibrillation (AF), frequent ventricular or supraventricular ectopics 3. Ventricular tachycardia/fibrillation and rarely atrioventricular block.

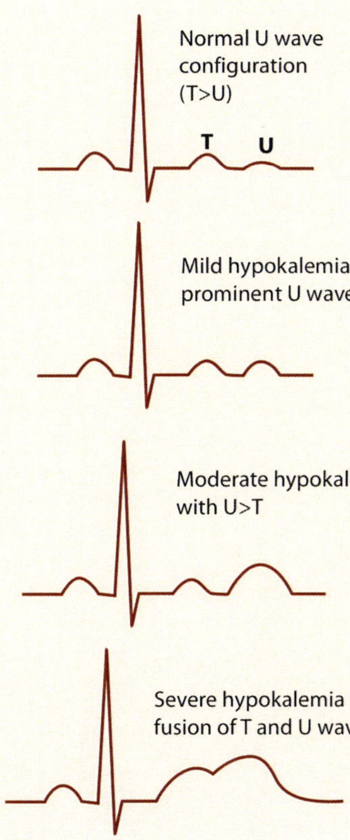

Fig. 20.8: Schematic representation of the U-wave configuration in different phases of hypokalemia, compared to normal U-wave. In normal ECG, T-wave amplitude is always more than the amplitude of the U-wave in the same lead but as the hypokalemia worsens U waves get bigger than the amplitude of the T waves and ultimately in severe hypokalemia T and U waves blend together with pseudo prolongation of QT interval.

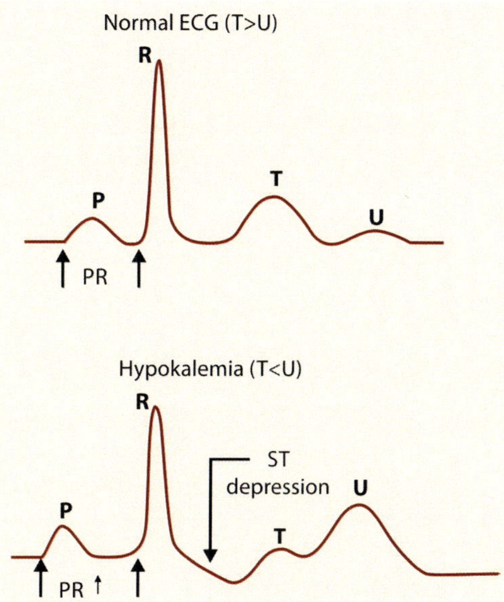

Fig. 20.9: Schematic representation of normal and ECG features of hypokalemia. Note disproportionally large U-wave in the ECG of hypokalemia. Also note ST-segment depression, an increase in the amplitude of the P-wave and mild prolongation of PR interval in the ECG of hypokalemia.

normal amplitude of the U-wave is 1–2 mm. Configuration of U-wave changes according to severity of hypokalemia (Fig. 20.8). Disproportionally large U waves are abnormal and it is an important ECG evidence of hypokalemia (Fig. 20.9). As potassium levels decline, ST-segment depression, biphasic T waves or T-wave inversions are seen, while the PR interval can be prolonged along with an increase in the amplitude of the P-wave (Figs. 20.10A to D).[20-23] Normal U-wave amplitude is always less than the amplitude of the preceding T-wave, so normally T is greater than U (Fig. 20.11). Mild degree of hypokalemia is reflected by prominent U waves along with the decrease in the amplitude of T waves (Fig. 20.12). When the U-wave exceeds the T-wave amplitude, the serum potassium level is less than 3.0 mmol/L.[23] Moderate degree of hypokalemia is reflected by biphasic or flattening or inversion of T waves, ST-segment depression, prominent U waves, and sometimes prolongation of the PR interval (Fig. 20.13).

Abnormally prominent U waves are characteristically seen in severe hypokalemia. In severe hypokalemia, T-and U-waves fusion with giant U waves masking the smaller preceding T waves become apparent on the ECG (Figs. 20.14A and B).[22-24] A pseudo-prolonged QT interval may be seen, which is actually the QU interval with an absent T-wave. Severe hypokalemia can also cause a variety of arrhythmias, including frequent supraventricular and ventricular ectopics, atrial fibrillation (AF), atrial flutter, atrial tachycardia, ventricular tachycardia/fibrillation, and rarely atrioventricular block.[22,23]

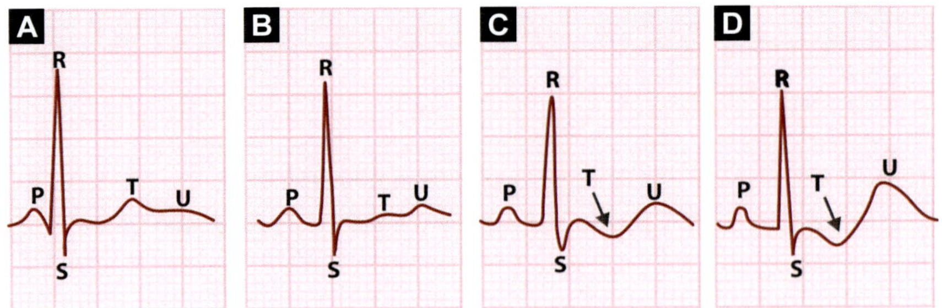

Figs. 20.10A to D: Schematic representation of the ECGs at various phases of hypokalemia. (A) Normal ECG; (B) ECG of mild hypokalemia showing prominent U-wave with decrease in the T-wave amplitude suggestive of mild hypokalemia; (C) ECG changes in moderate hypokalemia showing ST-segment depression with biphasic T-wave with high amplitude U-wave; (D) ECG features of severe hypokalemia illustrating giant U-wave almost merging with preceding T-wave with pseudoprolongation of QT interval. Also note ST segment depression with an increase in the amplitude of P-wave with prolonged PR interval.

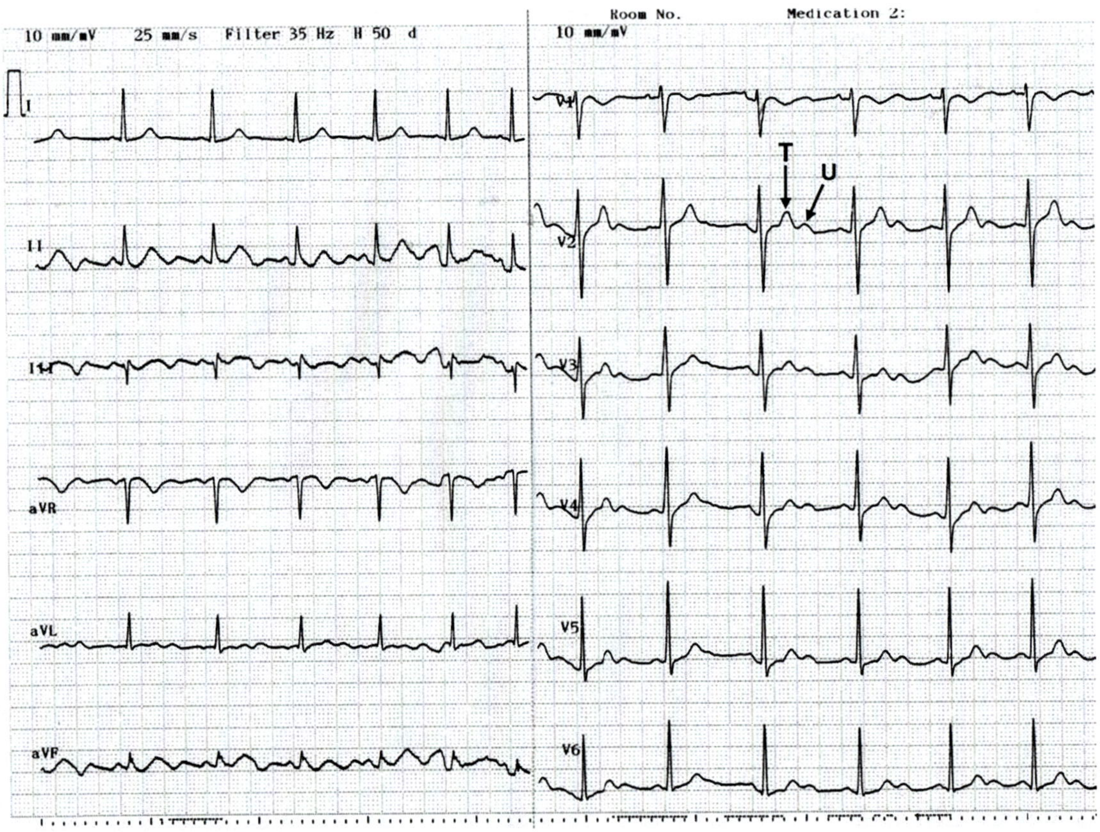

Fig. 20.11: Electrocardiogram showing normal U waves configuration. Normal U-wave amplitude is always less than the amplitude of the preceding T-wave, so normally T is greater than U (*arrows*).

HYPERCALCEMIA

Hypercalcemia, means high calcium (Ca^{2+}) level in the blood serum. The normal range is 2.1–2.6 mmol/L (8.8–10.7 mg/dL) with levels greater than 2.6 mmol/L defined as hypercalcemia. Primary hyperparathyroidism and malignancy account for about 90% of cases of hypercalcemia.

The effect of calcium on the surface ECG can be explained by its effect on the action potential within the myocyte. The role of calcium is most prominent in phase 2 of the action potential and corresponds to the ST segment on the surface ECG. As the action potential shortens, the ST-segment shortens and vice versa. When hypercalcemia is present, the duration of phase 2 is lessened and therefore the ST segment is shortened resulting in the characteristic short QT interval of hypercalcemia. In some cases, there is apparently no ST segment and the T-wave comes immediately off of the S-wave.

Hypercalcemia can result in an increase in heart rate and a positive inotropic effect (increase in contractility). But hypercalcemia does not typically cause bradycardia. But sometimes hypercalcemia may give rise to severe bradyarrhythmia leading to asystole. Hypercalcemia seems to decrease atrial activity and increase ventricular activity, as evidenced by the appearance of bradycardia, sinus arrest, and ectopic ventricular beats.

The main ECG abnormality seen with hypercalcemia is shortening of the QT interval (Fig. 20.15). In severe

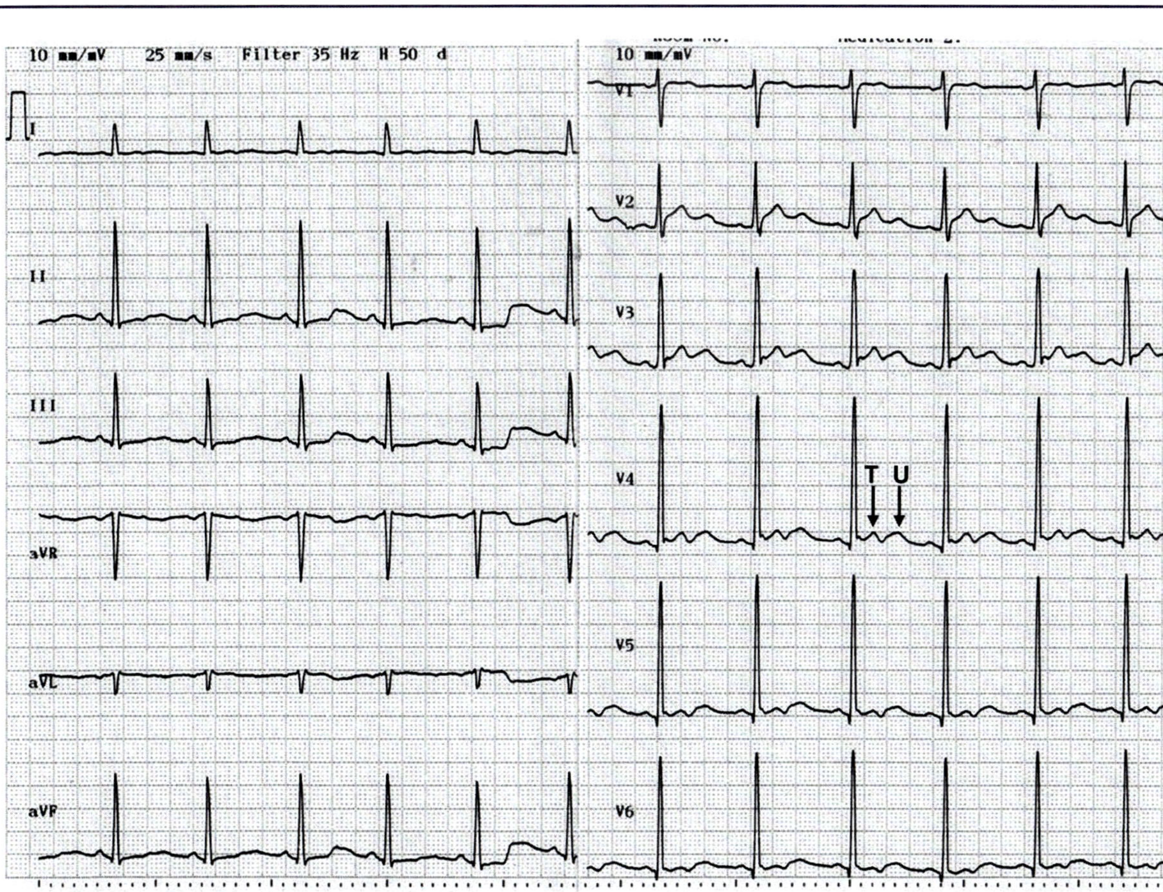

Fig. 20.12: Electrocardiogram is suggestive of mild degree of hypokalemia with very prominent U waves. Note U-wave amplitudes are almost equal to the amplitudes of the T waves and in some precordial leads amplitude of U waves exceed the amplitudes of the preceding T waves (*arrows*).

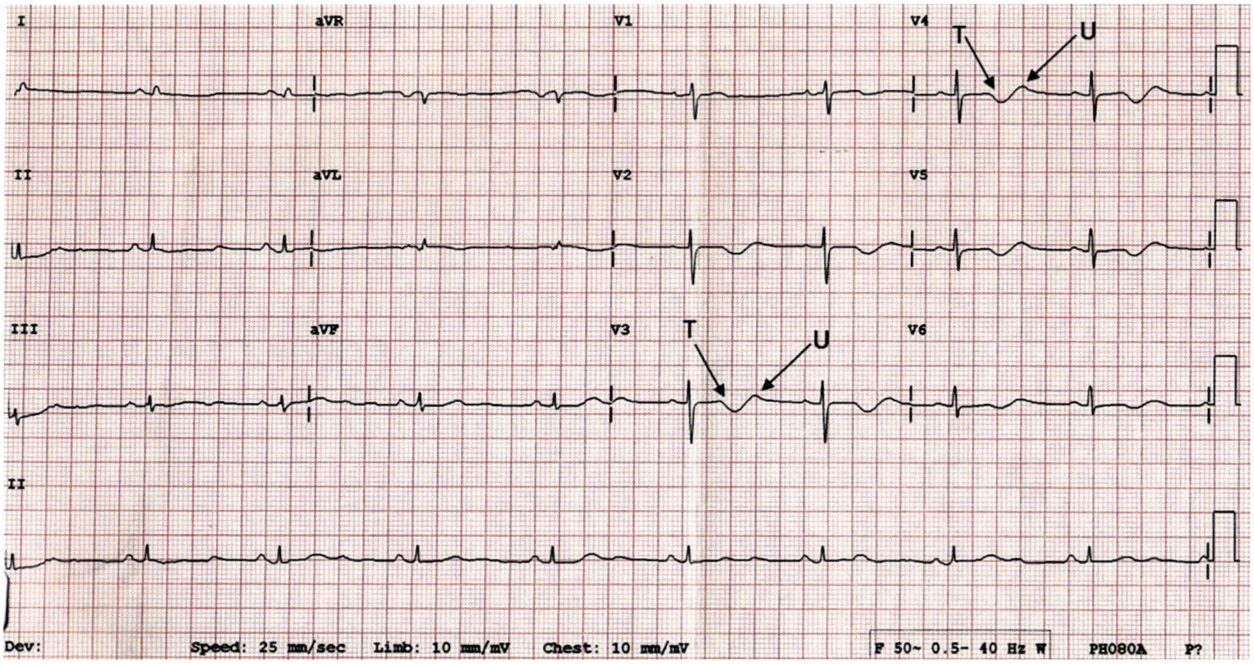

Fig. 20.13: Electrocardiogram illustrates the features of moderate hypokalemia. Note biphasic T waves merging with the following U waves producing pseudo-prolongation of QT interval (QTc is 523 ms) in precordial leads (*arrows*). Also note amplitude of the U waves exceed the amplitude of preceding T waves in almost all the precordial leads. (*Courtesy*: Dr Atikuzzaman Sohel, Labaid Cardiac Hospital).

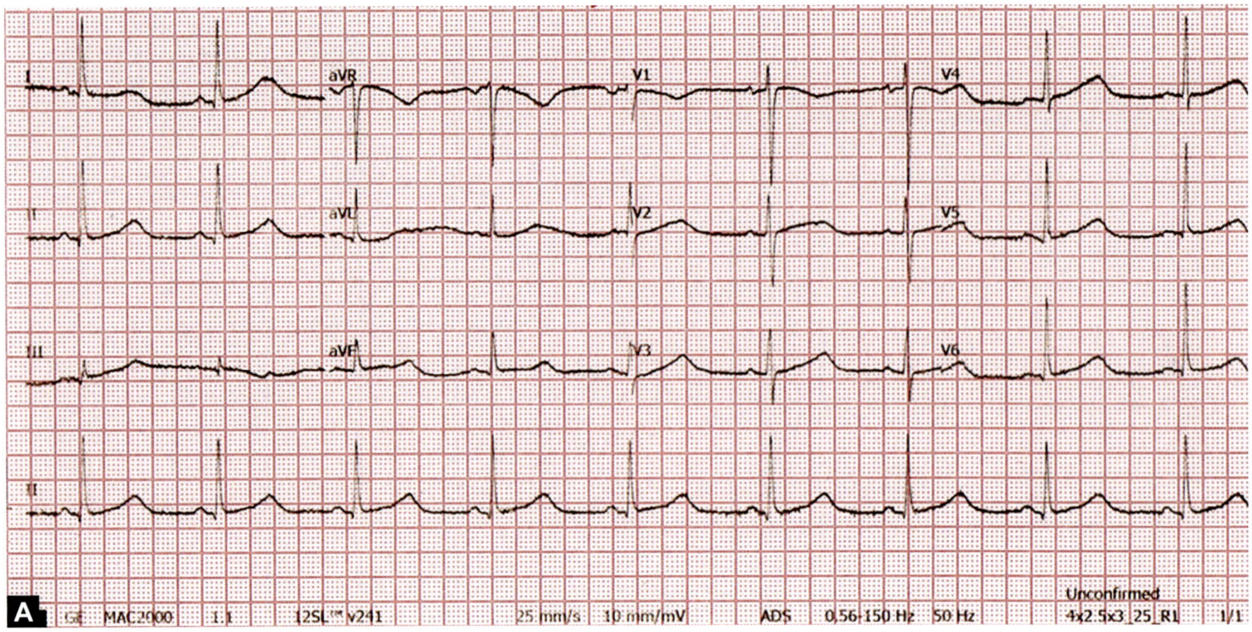

Fig. 20.14A: Electrocardiogram shows features of severe hypokalemia. Note fusion of T and U waves with giant U waves formation along with pseudo-prolonged QT interval (QTc is 576 ms). In severe hypokalemia (serum potassium level < 2.5 mmol/L), T and U waves fusion, with giant U waves masking the smaller preceding T waves become apparent on the ECG.

(*Courtesy: Dr Habibur Rahman , Labaid Cardiac Hospital*).

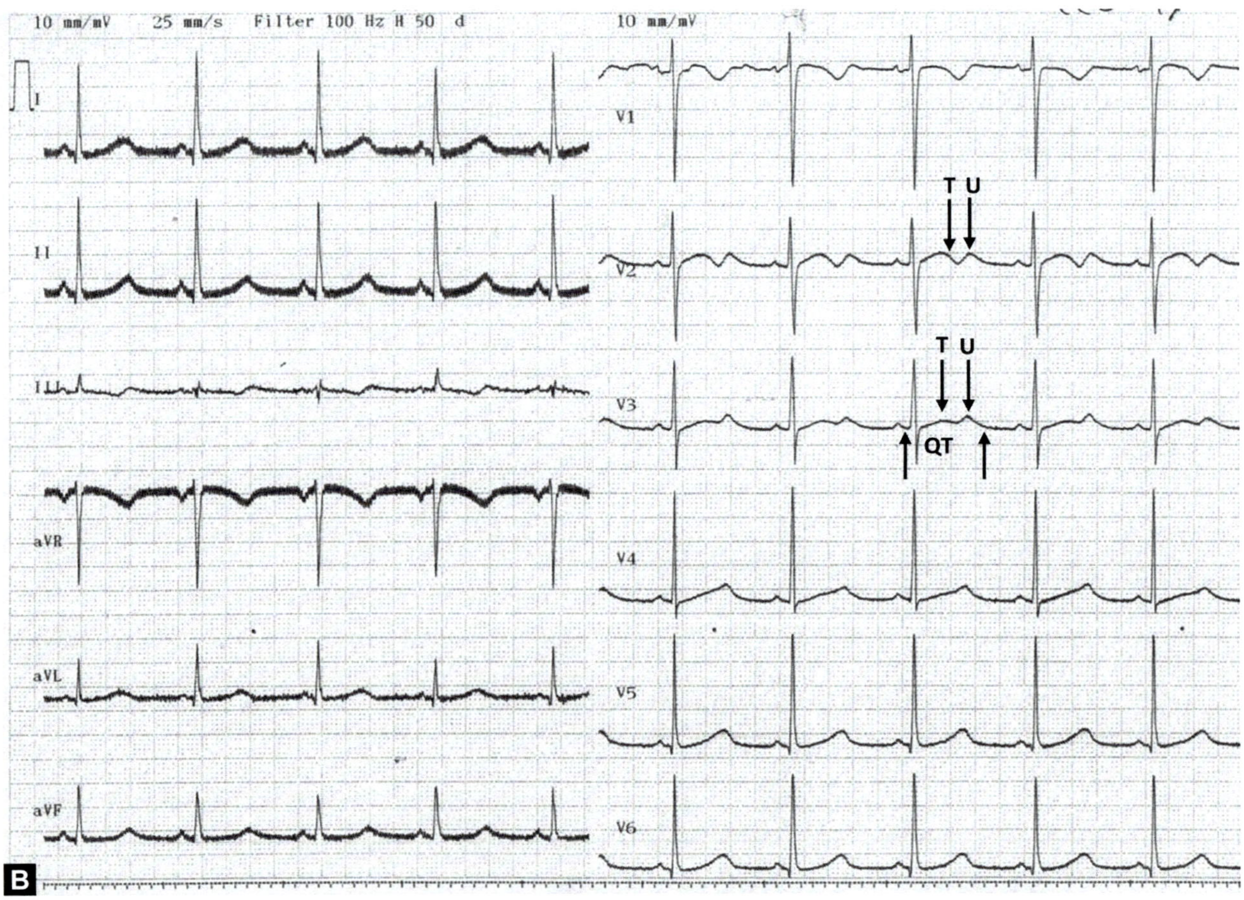

Fig. 20.14B: ECG shows features of severe hypokalemia. Note biphasic T with prominent U waves (*arrows*) in precordial leads. Also note fusion of T and U waves with single U-wave formation along with pseudo-prolongation of QT interval (QTc is 590 ms) in leads V4–V6. Serum potassium level of the patient during the time of taking this ECG was 1.9 mmol/L. (*Courtesy: Dr AK Miah, Labaid Cardiac Hospital*).

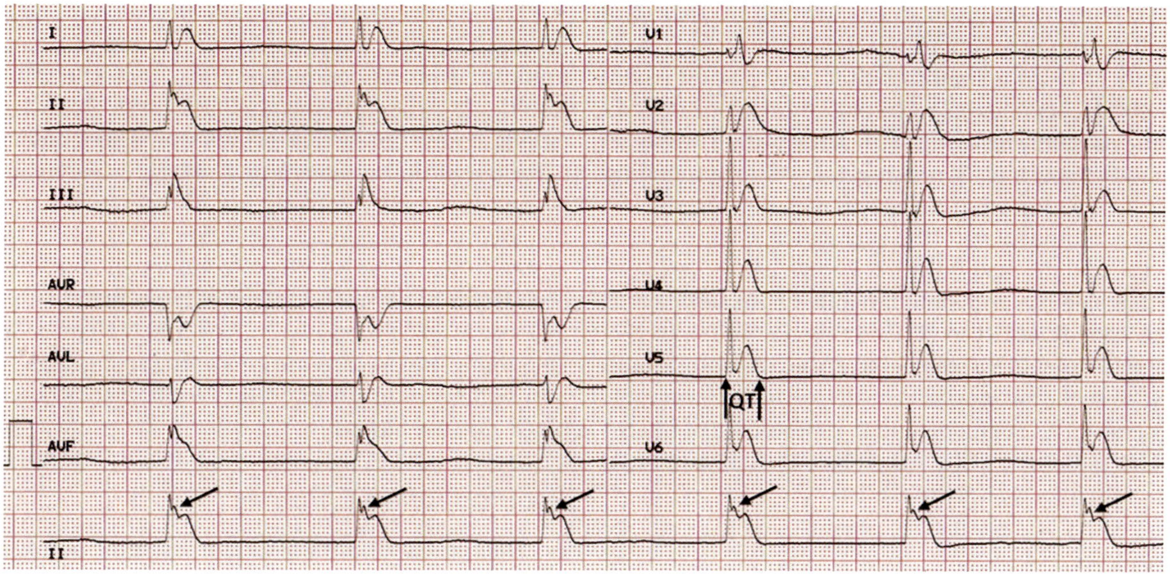

Fig. 20.15: Electrocardiogram illustrates the features of severe hypercalcemia in a patient with malignancy with diffuse bony metastasis. Note short QT interval (280 ms) with apparently no ST segment and the T-wave comes immediately off of the QRS complex. Also note possible *Osborn waves* in LII (*arrows*). Osborn waves are positive deflections occurring at the junction between the QRS complex and the ST segment. This ECG also shows marked bradycardia but hypercalcemia does not typically cause bradycardia. However, sometimes hypercalcemia may give rise to severe bradyarrhythmia leading to asystole. At the time of taking this ECG, serum calcium level of the patient was 6.0 mmol/L and the patient developed cardiac arrest within few minutes after taking this ECG. (*Courtesy:* Dr Shiblee Sadik Pathan, Labaid Cardiac Hospital).

hypercalcemia, Osborn waves may be seen. The Osborn wave is a positive deflection at the J-point [negative in augmented vector right (aVR) and V1]. It is usually most prominent in the precordial leads. Ventricular irritability, VF, and cardiac arrest have been reported with extreme hypercalcemia. Significant hypercalcemia can cause ECG changes mimicking an acute myocardial infarction.[25-29]

HYPOCALCEMIA

Common causes of hypocalcemia include hypoparathyroidism, vitamin D deficiency, and chronic kidney disease (CKD). Symptoms of hypocalcemia include neuromuscular irritability (including tetany and bronchospasm), electrocardiographic changes, and seizures.

The ECG hallmark of hypocalcemia remains the prolongation of the QTc interval because of lengthening of the ST segment, which is directly proportional to the degree of hypocalcemia. The exact opposite holds true for hypercalcemia.[30] Intermittent QT prolongation on the ECG has been documented. The implications of intermittent QTc prolongation predisposes to life-threatening cardiac electrical instability. This type of electrical instability puts the patient at high-risk of torsades de pointes and VF.[30-34]

HYPERMAGNESEMIA

Hypermagnesemia (normal serum magnesium = 0.8 – 1.0 mmol/L) is a serum magnesium (Mg) concentration greater than 1.05 mmol/L. The major cause is renal failure. Symptoms include hypotension, respiratory depression, and cardiac arrest. At serum Mg concentrations of 2.5–5.0 mmol/L, the ECG shows prolongation of the PR interval, prolonged QTc, widening of the QRS complex, and increased T-wave amplitude. In severe hypermagnesemia, a patient may develop complete AV block and asystole.

HYPOMAGNESEMIA

Hypomagnesemia means serum Mg level is less than 0.8 mmol/L. Hypomagnesemia usually results from decreased absorption or increased loss of magnesium from either the kidneys or intestines (diarrhea). Hypomagnesemia is far more common than hypermagnesemia. Magnesium depletion in general is associated with changes in the ECG. Widening of the QRS complex and peaking of T waves have been described with modest magnesium loss, whereas more severe magnesium depletion can lead to prolongation of the PR and QT intervals, progressive widening of the QRS complex, and diminution of the T-wave.[35-37] Hypomagnesemia is a well-known cause for an acquired prolonged QTc interval.[38] Atrial and ventricular ectopy, atrial tachyarrhythmias, and torsades de pointes are seen in the context of hypomagnesemia.

Electrocardiogram Features of Multiple Electrolyte Imbalances

The surface ECG has been used as a useful method for detection of metabolic disturbances for a long time. However, it may be difficult to distinguish the exact disturbance when more than one metabolic abnormality exists in a patient simultaneously. Although, "classic" ECG characterizations of common electrolyte disturbances are well-described, multiple concurrent electrolyte disturbances may lead to ECG abnormalities that may not be easily detectable.[39,40] Hyperkalemia, with concurrent hypocalcemia and hypomagnesemia results in (1) peaking of the T-wave, (2) a prominent U-wave, and (3) prolongation of the descending limb of the T-wave such that it overlaps with the next P-wave and the unusual appearance of this segment between the peak of the T-wave and the next P-wave is known as the "tee-pee" sign.[39] Hypercalcemia and simultaneous hypokalemia and hypomagnesemia give rise to: (1) Flattening of the T-wave, (2) a prominent U-wave, (3) prolongation of the descending limb of the T-wave such that it overlaps with the next U-wave, (4) virtual absence of ST segment, and (5) shortening of the QT interval. This pattern of ECG change has been documented in patients with hyperparathyroid crisis.[40]

SUMMARY

Hyperkalemia

Hyperkalemia is defined as a potassium level greater than 5.5 mmol/L (Normal potassium level is 3.5–5.5 mmol/L). Progressively worsening hyperkalemia leads to suppression of impulse generation by the SA node and reduced conduction by the AV node and His-Purkinje system, resulting in bradycardia, conduction blocks, "Sine-Wave" appearance, and ultimately cardiac arrest. Acute kidney injury (AKI), CKD, medicines those interfere with the renin-angiotensin axis—e.g. ACE inhibitors, ARBs, NSAIDs, medicines those interfere with potassium excretion—e.g. amiloride, spironolactone are the common causes of hyperkalemia.

Classic teaching of the chronological ECG changes of hyperkalemia include:

- Tall and peaked T waves
- Prolongation of PR interval
- Widening QRS Complex
- Loss of P-wave
- "Sine Wave"
- Asystole.

Electrocardiogram changes according to serum potassium level:

- *Serum K 5.5–6.0 mmol/L*: Tall and peaked T waves; flattening of P waves.
- *Serum K 6.1–7.0 mmol/L*: Loss of P-wave, prolonged PR interval, prolonged QRS complex, and ST-segment elevation.
- *Serum K is greater than 7.0 mmol/L*: Progressive widening of QRS complex, ectopic beats and escape rhythms, sine wave, VF, and asystole.

Hypokalemia

Hypokalemia is defined as a potassium level less than 3.5 mmol/L. Hypokalemia is the most common electrolyte abnormality encountered in clinical practice. Diarrhea, vomiting, and diuretic use are the common causes of hypokalemia.

The electrocardiographic manifestations of hypokalemia is due to its effects on repolarization and those emanating from its effects on conduction (Box 20.1). The ECG changes resulting from its effects on repolarization include—decreased amplitude and broadening of the T waves; prominent U waves; ST-segment depression; and T- and U-wave fusion, which is seen in severe hypokalemia. *When the U-wave exceeds the T-wave in amplitude, the serum potassium is less than 3 mmol/L.* ECG changes due to conduction abnormalities are seen in more advanced stages of hypokalemia and include increase in QRS duration without a concomitant change in the QRS configuration; increase in P-wave amplitude and duration; and slight prolongation of the PR interval, atrioventricular block, and cardiac arrest.

Repolarization Changes

- Decreased amplitude and broadening of the T waves
- Prominent U waves
- ST-segment depression
- T- and U-waves fusion (in severe hypokalemia).

Conduction Abnormalities

- Increase in QRS duration
- Slight prolongation of the PR interval.
- Atrioventricular block
- Cardiac arrest.

Hypercalcemia

Electrocardiogram manifestations of hypercalcemia include:

- Short QT interval
- Bizarre-looking QRS complexes
- Osborn waves may be seen (Osborn waves are positive deflections occurring at the junction between the QRS complex and the ST segment).

Box 20.1: Electrocardiogram features of hypokalemia.

ECG changes in hypokalemia:

- Decrease in T-wave amplitude. T-wave flattening and inversion.
- Increased amplitude and width of the P-wave
- Prolongation of the PR interval
- ST-segment depression
- Prominent U waves (best seen in the precordial leads). Amplitude of U-wave exceeds the amplitude of preceding T-wave.
- Fusion of T and U waves with apparent prolongation of QT interval (pseudo-prolonged QT).

Arrhythmias in hypokalemia:

With worsening hypokalemia patient may develop:

- Atrial fibrillation (AF)
- Frequent ventricular or supraventricular ectopics
- Life-threatening ventricular arrhythmias, e.g. ventricular tachycardia (VT), torsades de pointes and even ventricular fibrillation (VF).

Severe hypercalcemia may cause significant ST elevation mimicking an acute myocardial infarction.

Hypocalcemia

- QTc prolongation primarily by prolonging the ST segment.
- Torsades de pointes may occur.
- Rarely AF.

Hypermagnesemia

- Prolonged PR interval
- Widened QRS complex
- Complete AV block and asystole.

Hypomagnesemia

- Prolonged QTc
- Atrial tachyarrhythmias
- Torsades de pointes is also seen.

REFERENCES

1. El-Sherif N, Turitto G. Electrolyte disorders and arrhythmogenesis. Cardiol J. 2011;8(3):233-45.
2. Nyirenda MJ, Tang JI, Padfield PL, et al. Hyperkalaemia. BMJ. 2009;339:b4114.
3. Spodick D. Effects of severe hyperkalemia. Am Heart Hosp J. 2008;6(1):68.
4. Mushiyakh Y, Dangaria H, Qavi S, et al. Treatment and pathogenesis of acute hyperkalemia. J Community Hosp Intern Med Perspect. 2011;1(4):7372.
5. Webster A, Brady W, Morris F. Recognising signs of danger: ECG changes resulting from an abnormal serum potassium concentration. Emerg Med J. 2002;19(1):74-7.
6. Przybojewski JZ, Knott-Craig CJ. Hyperkalaemic complete heart block. A report of 2 unique cases and a review of the literature. S Afr Med J. 1983;63(11):413-20.
7. Pick A. Arrhythmias and potassium in man. Am Heart J. 1966;72(3):295-306.
8. Yu AS. Atypical electrocardiographic changes in severe hyperkalemia. Am J Cardiol. 1996;77(10):906-8.
9. Levis JT. ECG Diagnosis: Hyperkalemia. Perm J. 2013;17(1):69.
10. Wrenn KD, Slovis CM, Slovis BS. The ability of physicians to predict hyperkalemia from the ECG. Ann Emerg Med. 1991;20(11):1229-32.
11. Martinez-Vea A, Bardaji A, Garcia C. Severe hyperkalemia with minimal electrocardiographic manifestations: a report of seven cases. J Electrocardiol. 1999;32(1):45-9.
12. Lichstein E, Gupta PK, Grunwald AA. Hyperkalemic fascicular block. Chest. 1976;70(2):290-1.
13. Ewy GA, Karliner J, Bedynek JL Jr. Electrocardiographic QRS axis shift as a manifestation of hyperkalemia. JAMA. 1971;215(3):429-32.
14. Kim NH, Oh SK, Jeong JW. Hyperkalaemia induced complete atrioventricular block with a narrow QRS complex. Heart. 2005;91(1):e5.
15. Parham W, Mehdirad A, Biermann KM, et al. Hyperkalemia revisited. Tex Heart Inst J. 2006;33(1):40-7
16. Sohoni A, Perez B, Singh A. Wenckebach block due to hyperkalemia: a case report. Emerg Med Int. 2010;2010.
17. Ohmae M, Rabkin SW. Hyperkalemia-induced bundle branch block and complete heart block. Clin Cardiol. 1981;4(1):43-6.
18. Chakraborty B, Rahman M, Ahmed QS, et al. Life threatening hyperkalemia requiring prolonged temporary pacing support: our experience. Orion Med J. 2006;25:411-4.
19. Chawla KK, Cruz J, Kramer NE, et al. Electrocardiographic changes simulating acute myocardial infarction caused by hyperkalemia: report of a patient with normal coronary arteriograms. Am Heart J. 1978;95:637-40.
20. Surawicz B, Braun HA, Crum WB, et al. Quantitative analysis of the electrocardiographic pattern of hypopotassemia. Circulation. 1957;16(5):750-63.
21. Surawicz B. Relationship between electrocardiogram and electrolytes. Am Heart J. 1967;73(6):814-34.
22. Levis JT. ECG diagnosis: hypokalemia. Perm J. 2012;16(2):57.
23. Diercks DB, Shumaik GM, Harrigan RA, et al. Electrocardiographic manifestations: electrolyte abnormalities. J Emerg Med. 2004;27(2):153-60.
24. Gennari FJ. Disorders of potassium homeostasis. Hypokalemia and hyperkalemia. Crit Care Clin. 2002;18(2);273-88.
25. Wesson L, Suresh V, Parry R. Severe hypercalcaemia mimicking acute myocardial infarction. Clin Med. 2009;9(2):186-7.
26. Donovan J, Jackson M. Hypercalcaemia mimicking STEMI on electrocardiography. Case Rep Med. 2010;2010:3.
27. Sado DM, Greaves K. Severe hypercalcaemia mimicking acute myocardial infarction. Clin Med. 2009;9(5):503.
28. Falk RH. Severe hypercalcaemia mimicking acute myocardial infarction. Clinical Med. 2009;9(5):503-4.
29. Nishi SPE, Barbagelata NA, Atar S, et al. Hypercalcemia-induced ST-segment elevation mimicking acute myocardial infarction. J Electrocardiol. 2006;39(3):298-300.
30. RuDusky BM. ECG abnormalities associated with hypocalcemia. Chest. 2001;119(2):668-9.
31. Nijjer S, Ghosh AK, Dubrey SW. Hypocalcaemia, long QT interval and atrial arrhythmias. BMJ Case Rep. 2010;2010.
32. Eryol NK, Colak R, Ozdogru I, et al. Effects of calcium treatment on QT interval and QT dispersion in hypocalcemia. Am J Cardiol. 2003;91(6):750-2.
33. Bradley TJ, Metzger DL, Sanatani S. Long on QT and low on calcium. Cardiol Young. 2004;14(6):667-70.
34. Mangat JS, Till J, Bridges N. Hypocalcaemia mimicking long QT syndrome: a case report. Eur J Pediatr. 2008;167(2):233-5.
35. van den Bergh WM, Algra A, van der Sprenkel JW, et al. Hypomagnesemia after aneurysmal subarachnoid hemorrhage. Neurosurgery. 2003;52(2):276-82.
36. Dyckner T. Serum magnesium in acute myocardial infarction. Relation to arrhythmias. Acta Med Scand. 1980;207(1-2):59-66.
37. van den Bergh WM, Algra A, Gabriel JE, et al. Electrocardiographic abnormalities and serum magnesium in patients With subarachnoid hemorrhage. Stroke. 2004;35:644-8.
38. Haverkamp W, Breithardt G, Camm AJ, et al. The potential for QT prolongation and proarrhythmia by non-antiarrhythmic drugs: clinical and regulatory implications. Report on a policy conference of the European Society of Cardiology. Eur Heart J. 2000;21(15): 1216-31.
39. Johri AM, Baranchuk A, Simpson CS, et al. ECG manifestations of multiple electrolyte imbalance: peaked T wave to P wave ("tee-pee sign"). Ann Noninvasive Electrocardiol. 2009;14(2):211-4.
40. Hajsadeghi S, Chitsazan M, Miresmail SJ. A rare electrocardiographic manifestation of a rare form of multiple electrolyte disturbances: hyperparathyroid crisis. Acta Med Iran. 2011;49(12):824-7.

Chapter 21

Electrocardiograms in Specific Clinical Conditions

CHRONIC OBSTRUCTIVE PULMONARY DISEASE

Electrocardiograms (ECGs) are routinely obtained on patients presenting with signs and symptoms suggestive of chronic obstructive pulmonary disease (COPD) and are recommended by consensus guidelines. As with chest X-ray, this is largely to identify comorbid or confounding illness that may be the underlying cause of the patient's decompensation, especially acute coronary syndromes.

ECG abnormalities associated with COPD include signs of right atrial enlargement (P pulmonale, a "P"-wave with height > 2.5 mm in leads II, III, and aVF) and right ventricular hypertrophy (RVH; right axis deviation, prominent R in V1 and V2, right precordial ST depression and T-wave inversion, and rS pattern in V5–V6) (Fig. 21.1). The lung hyperinflation associated with COPD can cause rightward rotation of the heart (associated with poor R-wave progression) as well as low voltages.[1-3]

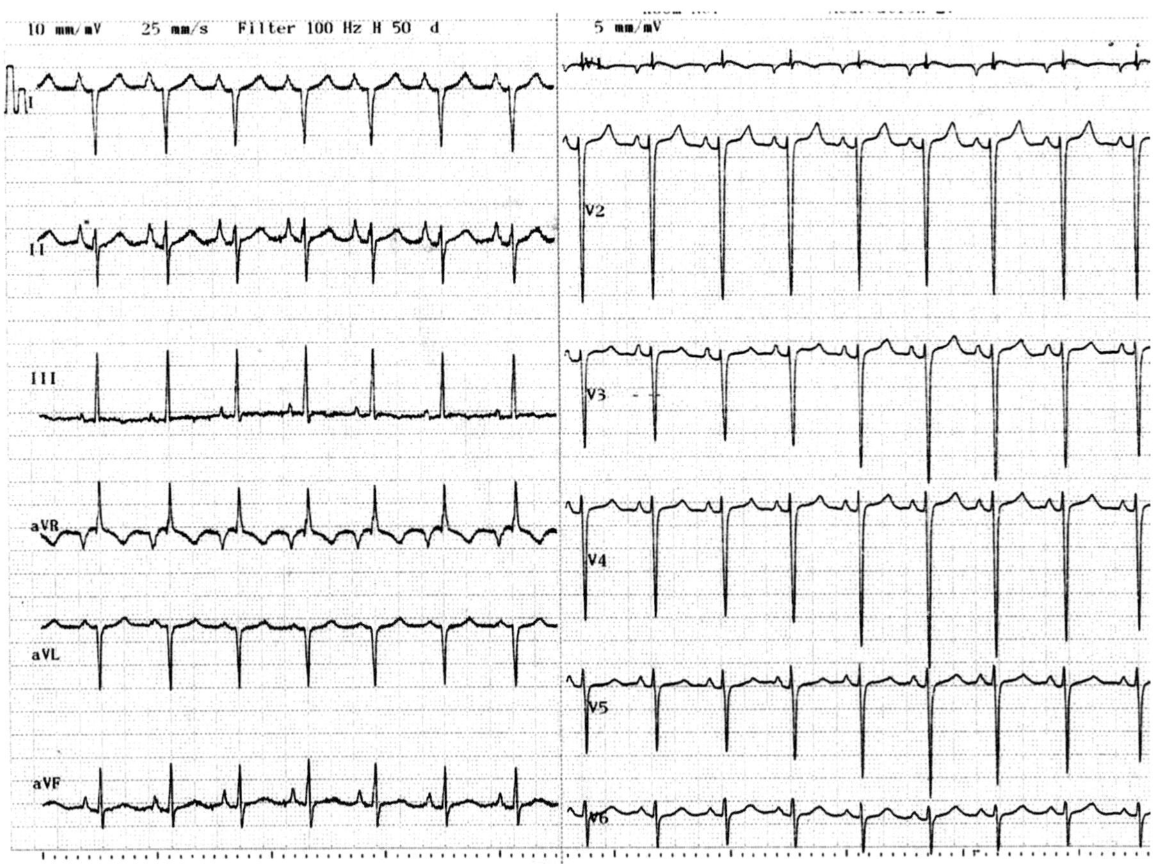

Fig. 21.1: Electrocardiogram illustrates the typical features of COPD showing electrocardiographic evidence of right atrial enlargement (P pulmonale, a "P"-wave with height greater than 2.5 mm) in lead II and aVF, prominent R in V1 with right axis deviation. Also note poor progression of R-wave from V2–V6 with rS pattern in V5–V6 characteristic of ECG of COPD.

Chronic obstructive pulmonary disease is a progressive disease characterized by airflow limitation/obstruction, i.e. either not reversible at all or only partially reversible. Chronic bronchitis and emphysema are grouped together as COPD as these conditions cannot be separated easily. In COPD, hyperinflation of the lungs lead to depression of the diaphragm, and this is associated with clockwise rotation of the heart along its longitudinal axis. This clockwise rotation means that the transitional zone (defined as the progression of rS to qR in the chest leads) shifts toward the left with persistence of an rS pattern as far as V5 or even V6 (Fig. 21.2). This may give rise to a "pseudoinfarct" pattern, with deep S waves in the right precordial leads simulating the appearance of the QS waves and poor R-wave progression seen in anterior myocardial infarction (MI). The amplitude of the QRS complexes may be small in patients with COPD as the hyperinflated lungs are poor electrical conductors.

The typical ECG changes in COPD are (Figs. 21.3A and B)—(1) Prominent P waves in leads II, III, and aVF; (2) rightward shift of the QRS axis in the frontal plane; (3) poor progression of the R-wave in the precordial leads; (4) low voltage of the QRS complexes especially in the left precordial leads (V4–V6), and (5) the "lead I sign" (Schamroth's sign) consists of isoelectric or flat P-wave in lead I combined with a very small QRS complex of less than 1.5 mm total deflection and a T-wave of less than 0.5 mm in lead I.[4-7]

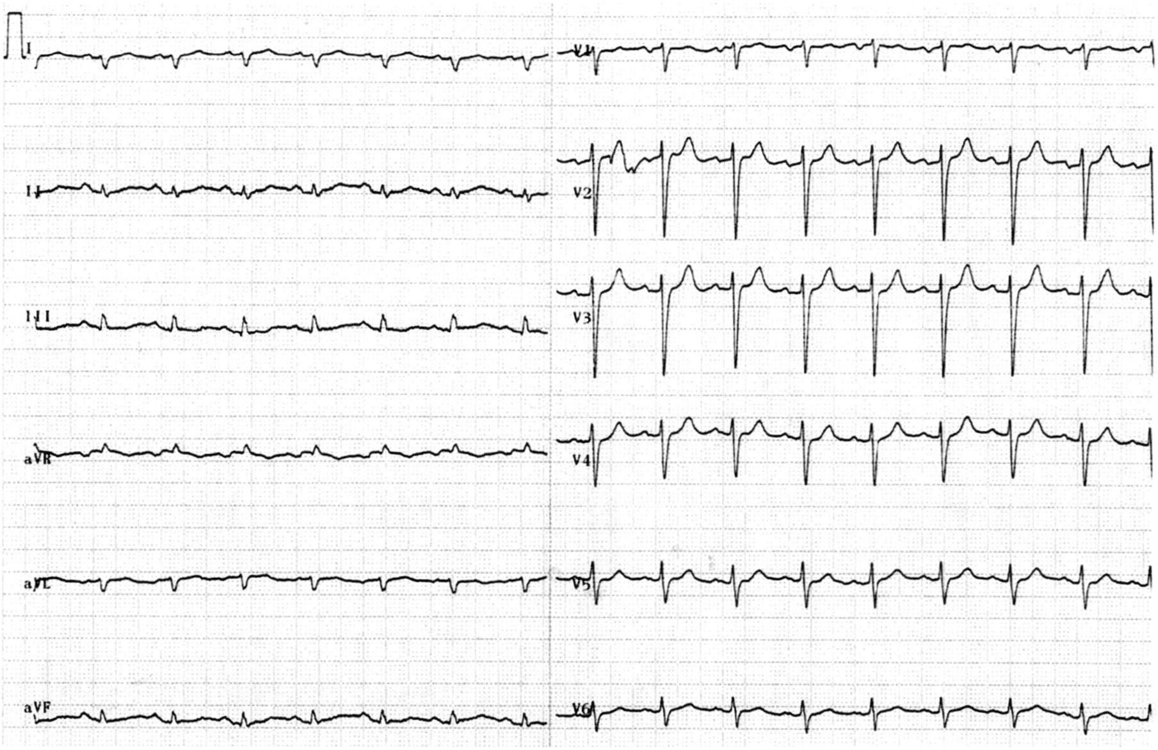

Fig. 21.2: Electrocardiogram illustrates the features of COPD with clockwise rotation (transitional zone shifted towards the left with persistence of an rS pattern as far as V6) with low voltage ECG (amplitude of all the QRS complexes in all the limb leads are less than 5 mm). (*Courtesy*: Dr. Md.Ali Hossain, National Institute of Diseases of the Chest & Hospital, NIDCH)

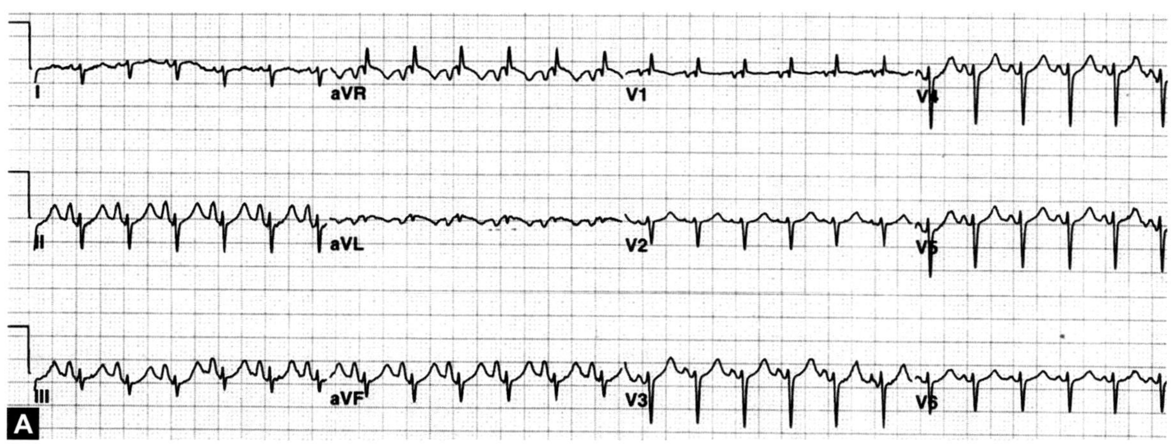

Fig. 21.3A: Electrocardiogram illustrates the features of COPD with prominent P waves in leads II, III, and aVF with poor progression of the R-wave in the precordial leads V2–V6 with partial RBBB pattern. (RBBB: right bundle branch block)

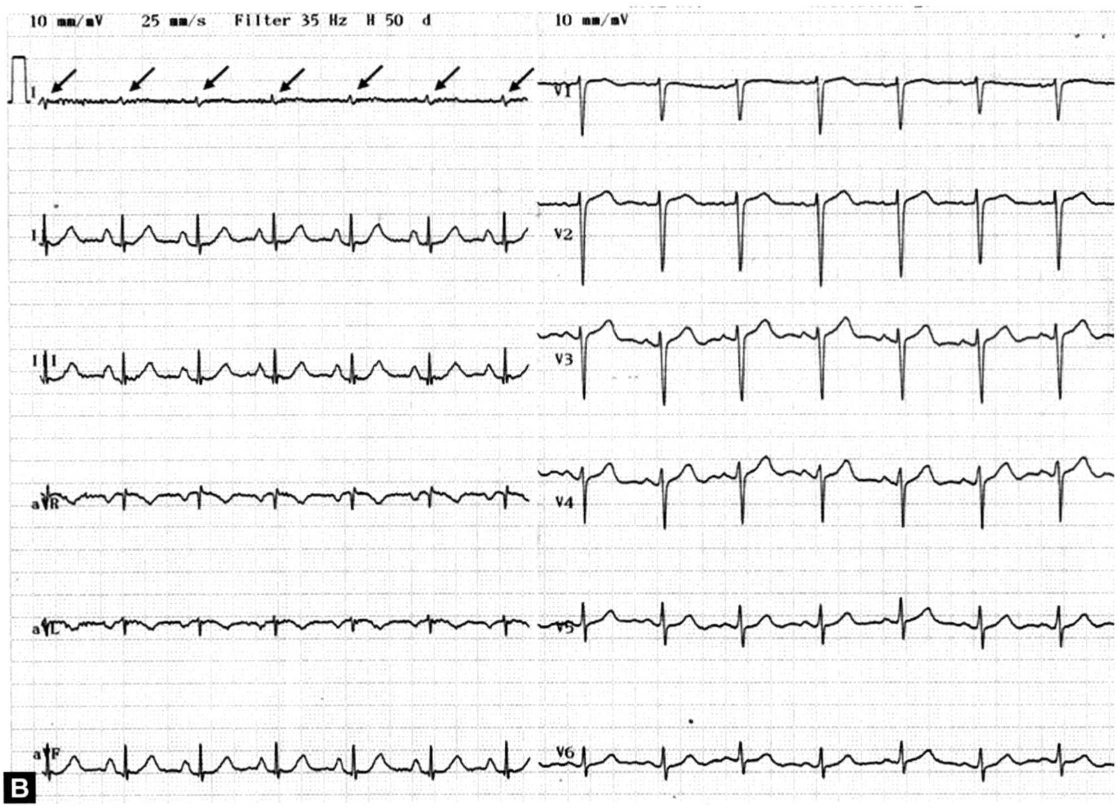

Fig. 21.3B: This ECG illustrates the typical Lead I sign (*Schamroth's Sign*) of COPD with all three main complexes the P, QRS, and T-waves with tiny amplitude in lead I (*arrows*). Schamroth's Sign includes three features: 1. Flat or Isoelectric P wave in lead I; 2.Very small QRS complex of less than 1.5 mm total deflection and 3.T wave of less than 0.5 mm in lead I. Also note peaked P waves in the LII,LIII & aVF > 2.5 mm (P pulmonale) with a rightward P-wave axis (inverted in aVL) and clockwise rotation of the heart with a delayed R/S transition point (transitional lead = V5). (*Courtesy:* Dr Md. Sayedul Islam, National Institute of Diseases of the Chest & Hospital, NIDCH).

About three quarters of patients with COPD have electrocardiographic abnormalities. P pulmonale is often but not invariably present and may occur with or without clinical evidence of cor pulmonale.[3] Various ECG changes in COPD and their possible mechanism have been well-described. Low voltage ECG (low voltage on the ECG is defined as the amplitudes of all the QRS complexes in the limb leads are <5 mm and/or <10 mm in the precordial leads) is due to insulating effect of hyperinflated lungs and lowered position of the heart (tubular) with respect to electrodes. Right axis deviation of QRS with clockwise rotation is due to rotation of the heart on horizontal and frontal plane. Right atrial enlargement (P pulmonale) and RVH (tall R in leads V1 and V2 with R:S > 1) is secondary to development of pulmonary hypertension (PHT) and subsequent development of cor pulmonale. ECG of COPD usually displays poor progression of R-wave in chest leads from V1 to V6 (Fig. 21.2). This occurs due to clockwise rotation of heart shifting the transition zone leftward resulting in poor voltage in precordial leads.[4]

Cardiac arrhythmias may occur in patients with COPD, particularly in association with an acute respiratory tract infection, respiratory failure, or pulmonary embolism (PE). Arrhythmias are sometimes the result of the underlying disease process but may also occur as side effects of the drugs used to treat the disease. The arrhythmias are mostly supraventricular in origin and include atrial extrasystoles, atrial fibrillation (AF) or atrial flutter, and multifocal atrial tachycardia (MAT). Ventricular extrasystoles and ventricular tachycardia may also occur.

PULMONARY EMBOLISM

Acute pulmonary embolism (PE) is the most serious clinical presentation of venous thromboembolism (VTE). PE is, in most cases, the consequence of deep vein thrombosis (DVT). Major trauma, surgery, lower limb fractures and joint replacements, and spinal cord injury, are strong provoking factors for VTE.[8-10] Malignancy is a well-recognized predisposing factor for VTE leading to PE. The risk of VTE varies with different types of cancer; hematological malignancies, lung cancer, gastrointestinal cancer, pancreatic cancer, and brain cancer carry the highest risk.[11-14] In fertile women, oral contraception is the most frequent predisposing factor for VTE.[15,16]

Pulmonary embolism remains an important clinical problem with a high mortality rate. The most common symptoms at the time of diagnosis are dyspnea (82%) and chest pain (49%).[17]

The ECG is abnormal in over 70% of patients with PE.[18] The greatest utility of the ECG in a patient with suspected PE is ruling out other life-threatening diagnoses (e.g. acute MI). ECG findings in PE may include sinus tachycardia, dominant R-wave in lead V1, right bundle branch block (RBBB), right axis deviation (deep S-wave in lead I), Q-wave

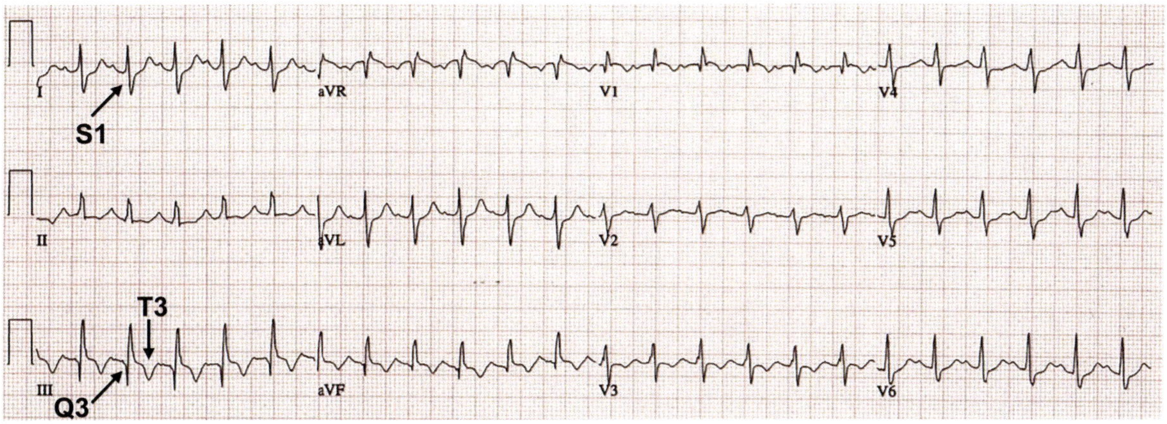

Fig. 21.4: Electrocardiogram illustrates the typical features of pulmonary embolism with "S1Q3T3" sign with prominent S-wave in lead I, Q-wave and inverted T-wave in lead III (*arrows*). Also note marked sinus tachycardia with partial RBBB.

and inverted T-wave in lead III (when combined with a deep S-wave in lead I, this gives the S1Q3T3 pattern suggestive of right ventricular strain), T-wave inversion in leads V1–V4, P pulmonale, supraventricular arrhythmias, and clockwise rotation (persistent S-wave in lead V6). The 12-lead ECG provides important prognostic information in patients with PE. The presence of premature ventricular extrasystoles, AF, and low voltage QRS complexes are associated with increased 30-day mortality.[19]

Common Electrocardiographic Features of Pulmonary Embolism

The electrocardiographic features of acute PE depend on the size of the embolus and its hemodynamic effects and on the underlying cardiopulmonary reserve of the patient. The timing and frequency of the ECG recording is also important as changes may be transient. Patients who present with a small pulmonary embolus are likely to have a normal ECG or a trace showing only sinus tachycardia. If the embolus is large and associated with pulmonary artery obstruction, acute right ventricular dilatation may occur. This may produce an S-wave in lead I and a Q-wave in lead III. T-wave inversion in lead III may also be present, producing the well-known S1Q3T3 pattern (Fig. 21.4). However, classical ECG changes are usually found in more severe cases of PE.[20]

Sinus Tachycardia

For PE, the ECG has been described to be neither sensitive nor specific, with the most commonly seen ECG abnormality in patients with PE is sinus tachycardia (Fig. 21.4). In milder cases of PE, the only anomaly may be sinus tachycardia, present in 40% of patients.[8,21]

S1, Q3, T3 Pattern

Though the most common ECG finding in the setting of a PE is sinus tachycardia, however, the "S1Q3T3" pattern of acute cor pulmonale is classic. This is termed as the *McGinn-White sign*. "S1Q3T3" pattern was first described by McGinn and White in 1935.[22] The "S1Q3T3" sign (prominent S-wave in lead I, Q-wave and inverted T-wave in lead III) is a sign of acute cor pulmonale (acute pressure and volume overload of the right ventricle because of PHT) and reflects right ventricular strain.[23,24] But unfortunately this classic ECG finding is present in only 15–25% of patients with confirmed diagnosis of PE (Figs. 21.5A and B).[25] Any cause of acute cor pulmonale can result in the S1Q3T3 findings on ECG, including PE, acute bronchospasm, pneumothorax, and other acute lung disorders.[23] S1Q3T3 pattern disappears after successful treatment.

New Right Bundle Branch Block

Electrocardiogram findings noted during the acute phase of a PE include new RBBB (complete or incomplete), rightward shift of the QRS axis, ST-segment elevation in V1 and aVR, generalized low amplitude QRS complexes.[21] Right ventricular dilatation may lead to right sided conduction delays, which manifest as incomplete or complete RBBB. There may be some rightward shift of the frontal plane QRS axis.

Acute Right Heart Strain

When the ECG shows features of RVH accompanied by ST-segment depression and T-wave inversion, a ventricular "strain" pattern is said to exist. Ventricular strain is seen mainly in leads V1 and V2. The mechanism is unclear. A strain pattern is sometimes seen in acute massive PE but is also seen in patients with RVH in the absence of any detectable stress on the ventricle. Both pneumothorax and massive pleural effusion with acute right ventricular dilatation may also produce a strain pattern.[3] "S1Q3T3" pattern is also suggestive of acute right ventricular strain. Right ventricular strain pattern on ECG is associated with adverse short-term outcome.[26]

Anterior T-wave Inversion

Anterior T-wave inversion (T-wave inversions in leads V1–V4) has been observed in patients with PE (Fig. 21.5B).

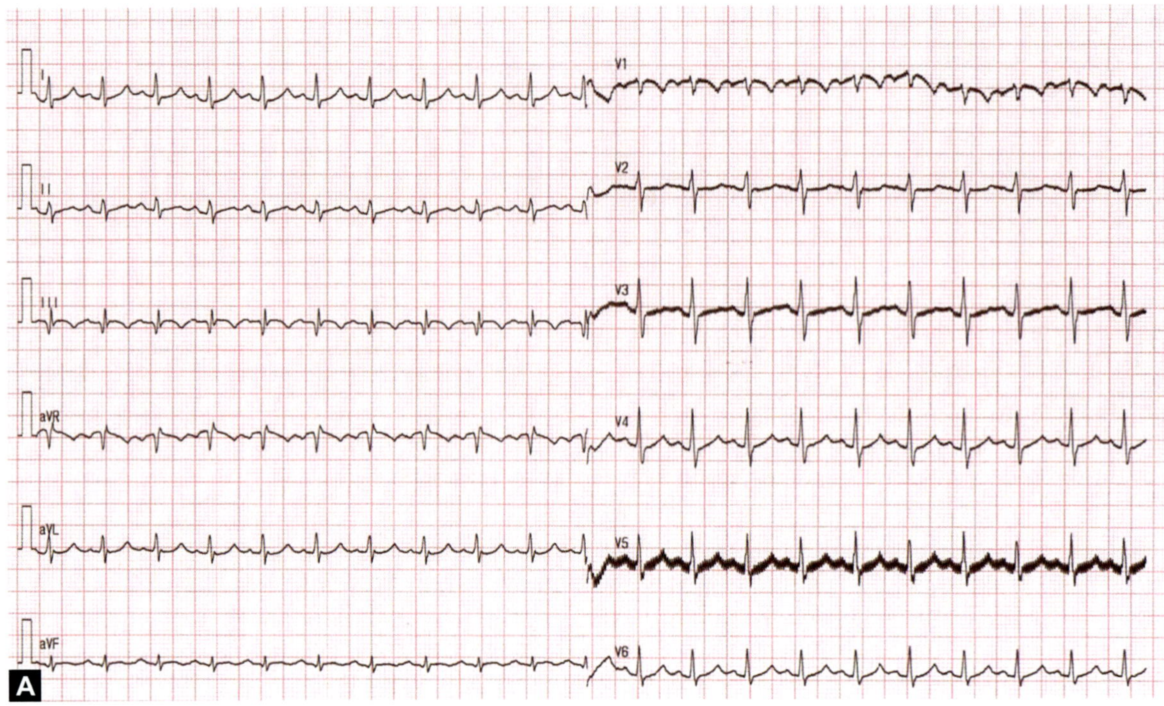

Fig. 21.5A: Electrocardiogram illustrates the features of pulmonary embolism with sinus tachycardia (heart rate is 130 bpm) with "S1Q3T3" sign with S-wave in lead I, Q-wave and inverted T-wave in lead III (ECG taken on the day of admission). (*Courtesy*: Dr APM Sohrabuzzaman, Labaid Cardiac Hospital)

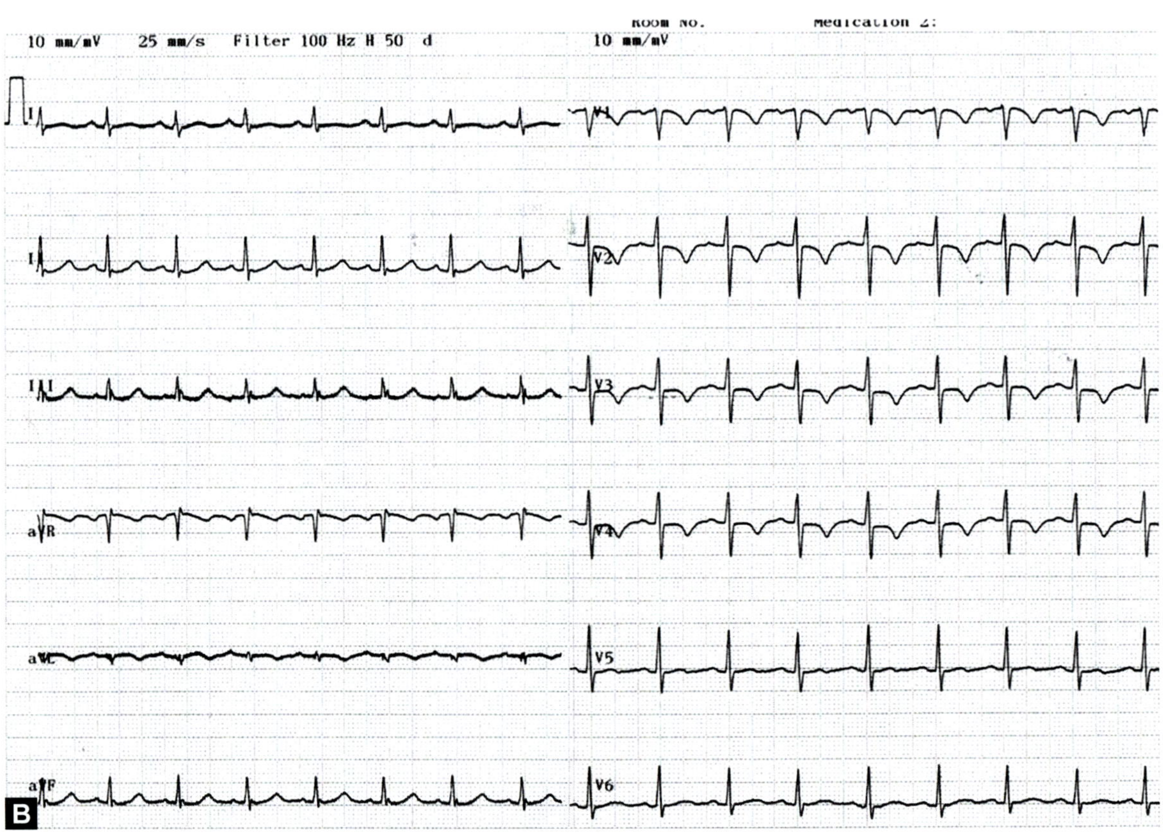

Fig. 21.5B: Electrocardiogram of the same patient (Fig. 21.5A) taken on the 3rd day of admission after treatment with thrombolysis. This ECG shows disappearance of "S1Q3T3" sign and new appearance of anterior T-wave inversions with sinus tachycardia (heart rate is 106 bpm). Anterior T-wave inversions (T-wave inversions in leads V1–V4) have been observed in patients with PE. (*Courtesy*: Dr APM Sohrabuzzaman, Labaid Cardiac Hospital)

Ferrari et al. observed that anterior T-wave inversion was present in 85% of cases of massive PE and 19% of cases of nonmassive PE, and that its reversibility before the 60th day pointed to a good outcome.[22,27]

P pulmonale

Right atrial dilatation in PE may lead to prominent P waves in the inferior leads. One study documented that ECG finding of sinus tachycardia and P pulmonale as determined by amplitude of P waves greater than or equal to 0.25 mV (2.5 mm) in lead II each had 100% specificity and 100% positive predictive value in assessing the severity of PE but had poor sensitivity and negative predictive value.[27,28] The gradual reduction in P-wave amplitude may reflect a reduction in right atrial strain after treatment.

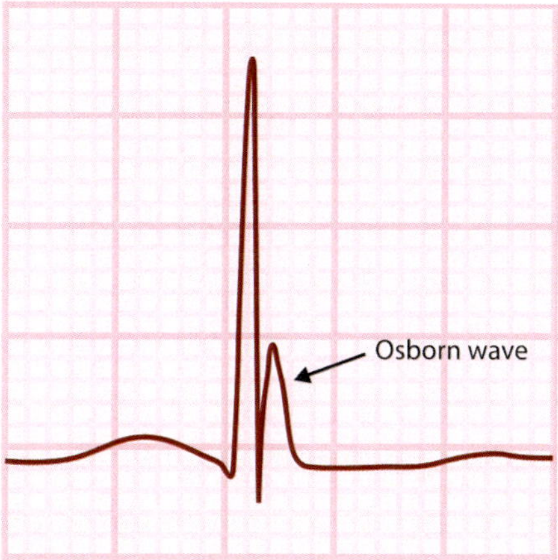

Fig. 21.6: Schematic representation of Osborn wave (*arrow*). Osborn waves are positive deflections occurring at the junction between the QRS complex and the ST segment.

Arrhythmias

Atrial arrhythmias including atrial flutter and AF are common in PE. Premature ventricular extrasystoles are also seen. The 12-lead ECG provides important prognostic information in patients with PE. The presence of premature ventricular extrasystoles, AF, and low voltage QRS complexes are associated with increased 30-day mortality.[19]

The clinical presentation of PE is believed to be dependent on the clot size and lung function, with a variable ranging from an asymptomatic patient to cardiogenic shock and cardiopulmonary arrest. Signs of right ventricular strain and hemodynamic instability in the setting of a PE are described as indications for emergency thrombolysis and or embolectomy.[29]

HYPOTHERMIA

Hypothermia, defined as core body temperature less than 35°C (<95°F), is associated with ECG changes of diagnostic and prognostic importance. Hypothermia affects virtually all organ systems. Perhaps the most significant effects are seen in the cardiovascular system and the central nervous system (CNS). Hypothermia results in decreased depolarization of cardiac pacemaker cells, causing bradycardia. Since this bradycardia is not vagally mediated, it can be refractory to standard therapies such as atropine. Mean arterial pressure and cardiac output decrease, and an ECG may show characteristic J or Osborn waves (Fig. 21.6).[30,31]

In the initial stages of hypothermia, a sinus tachycardia develops as part of the general stress reaction. Hypothermia also has an influence on the conduction of the heart. As the temperature drops below 32.2°C (90°F), a sinus bradycardia supervenes, associated with progressive prolongation of the PR interval, prolongation of QRS complex, prolonged QT interval, and shivering artifacts (Fig. 21.7). Slow junctional rhythms and varying degrees of AV block (first to third) have also been documented. With temperature approaching 30°C (86°F), atrial ectopic activity is often noted and can progress to AF. At this level of hypothermia, ECG also shows *Osborn waves* that consist of an extra deflection at the end of the QRS complex.[30-33]

Osborn waves are positive deflections occurring at the junction between the QRS complex and the ST segment (Fig. 21.8). These waves were definitively described in 1953 by Dr John J Osborn and were named in his honor. The prominent J deflection attributed to hypothermia was first reported in 1938 by Tomaszewski. Over time, the wave has increasingly been referred to as an Osborn wave, in most part due to Osborn's 1953 article on experimental hypothermia.[32-34] John Osborn described the J-wave as an "injury current" resulting in ventricular fibrillation (VF) during experimental hypothermia. More recent findings suggest that hypothermia increases the epicardial potassium current relative to the current in the endocardium during ventricular repolarization. This transmural voltage gradient is reflected on the surface ECG as a prominent J, or Osborn wave. The differential diagnosis of prominent Osborn waves include early repolarization, hypercalcemia, and the Brugada syndrome.[32,33]

J waves or Osborn waves appear secondary to an exaggerated outward potassium current leading to repolarization abnormality. These waves are detectable in 80% of the patients when core body temperature is lower than 30°C (86°F).[34-39] Osborn waves, also known as J waves, camel-hump waves, and hypothermic waves, are best seen in the inferior and lateral precordial leads. They become more prominent as the body temperature drops, and they regress gradually with rewarming. With temperature less than 30°C (<86°F), a progressive widening of the QRS complex increases the risk of VF. Fatal VF or asystole can occur when core body temperature is below 28°C (<82.4°F).[35-40]

THYROTOXICOSIS

The cardiovascular system is very sensitive to increased levels of circulating thyroid hormones. Increase in cardiac output and heart rate are early features in thyrotoxicosis. The most common ECG changes seen in thyrotoxicosis are sinus

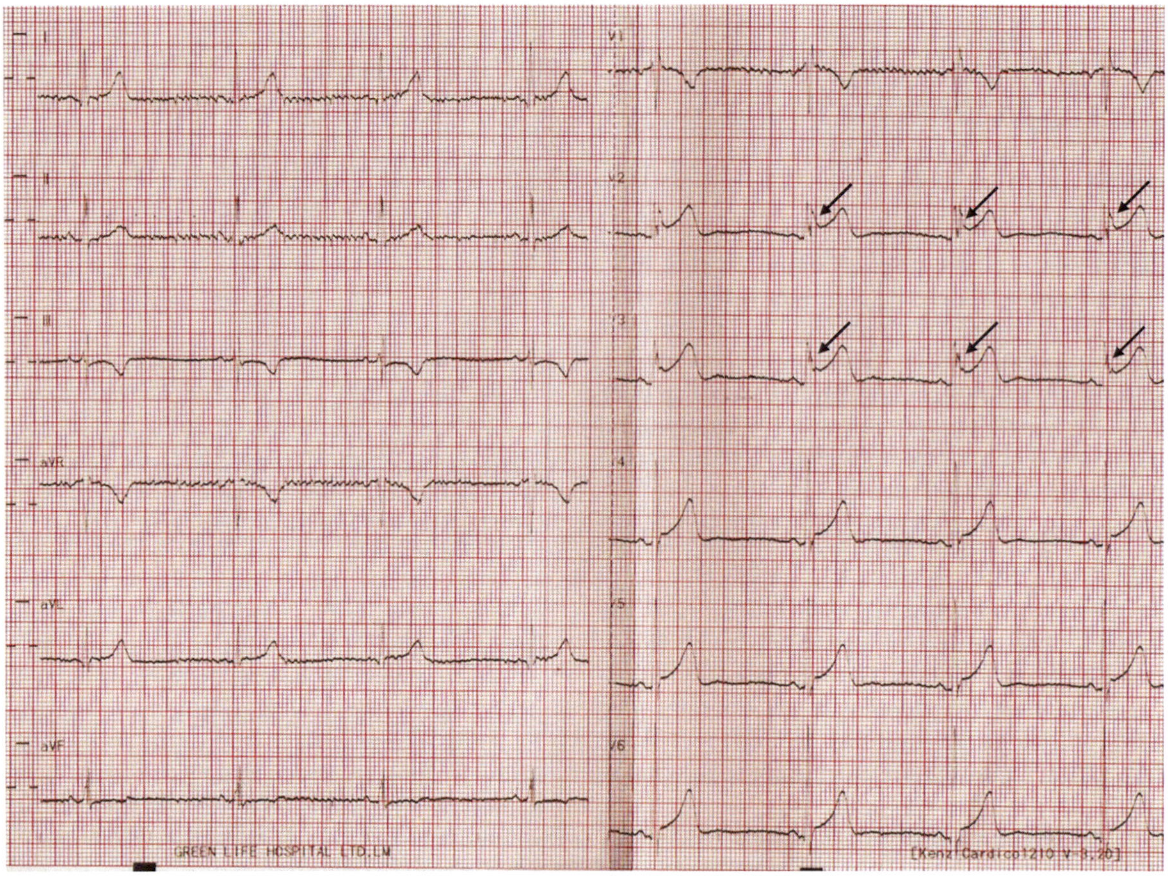

Fig. 21.7: Electrocardiogram illustrates the features of hypothermia showing marked sinus bradycardia (heart rate is 46 bpm) with Osborn waves (*arrows*). Also note shivering artifacts due to low body temperature.

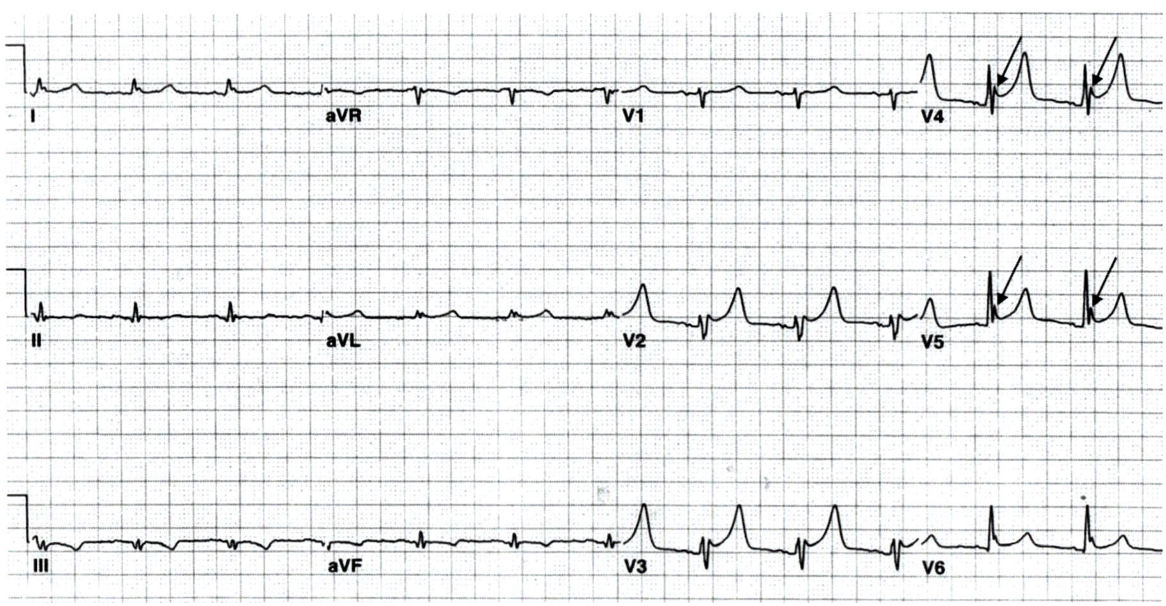

Fig. 21.8: Electrocardiogram showing Osborn waves (an extra deflection at the end of the QRS complex) in a patient with hypothermia.

tachycardia (Fig. 21.9), an increased electrical amplitude of all deflections, and AF. The other common ECG changes are—higher voltage of P and T waves, elevated amplitude of QRS complex, prolonged P-Q, and shortened Q-T intervals. In 20% of cases atrial fibrillation is evidenced.[41]

About 50% of thyrotoxic patients have a resting pulse rate above 100 beats/min. Atrial tachyarrhythmias are common as the atrias are very sensitive to the effects of thyroid hormones. Patients with thyrotoxicosis may develop paroxysmal supraventricular tachycardia with rates exceeding 200 beats/min (Fig. 21.10). Increased voltage is a common ECG finding but nonspecific ST and T-wave changes on ECG are also seen.

Atrial fibrillation is the most common sustained arrhythmia in thyrotoxicosis (Fig. 21.11) but MAT and atrial flutter with 2:1 conduction, and even 1:1 conduction, may also be seen. Ventricular arrhythmias may be seen, though much less frequently than atrial arrhythmias. Thyrotoxic patients have two or three times the normal number of premature ventricular contractions.[41,42]

HYPOTHYROIDISM

Hypothyroidism causes slowing of the metabolic rate and affects almost all bodily functions, including heart rate and contractility. It causes slowing of electrical conduction throughout the heart. It has various cardiovascular manifestations including impaired diastolic function, reduced contractility and infrequently pericardial effusion, and heart failure. ECG changes in hypothyroidism are bradycardia, low voltage ECG, RBBB, flat or inverted T-wave, QRS prolongation, QT prolongation and infrequently ventricular arrhythmia, torsades de pointes (Fig. 21.12).[43,44] Low voltage ECG (low voltage on the ECG is defined as a QRS amplitude of <5 mm in all the limb leads and/or <10 mm in the precordial leads) is possibly due to myxedematous deposits of gelatinous connective tissue within the myocardium and decreased activity of the sympathetic nervous system (Fig. 21.13).

Patients with severe hypothyroidism and those with preexisting heart disease may also develop increasing degrees of heart block or bundle-branch block (especially RBBB). Conduction abnormalities due to hypothyroidism resolve with thyroid hormone therapy. Depolarization, like all phases of the action potential, is slowed in hypothyroidism, and it results in a prolonged QT interval. Torsades de pointes ventricular tachycardia has been reported in hypothyroid patients and is related to prolongation of the QT interval.[45] Severe hypothyroidism patients may present with presyncope/syncope as prolongation of the QT interval may lead to polymorphic ventricular tachycardia (torsades de pointes).[43,44] Uncommonly, patients may develop large pericardial effusion, which give rise to electrical alternans (beat-to-beat variation in QRS voltages). Myxedema coma

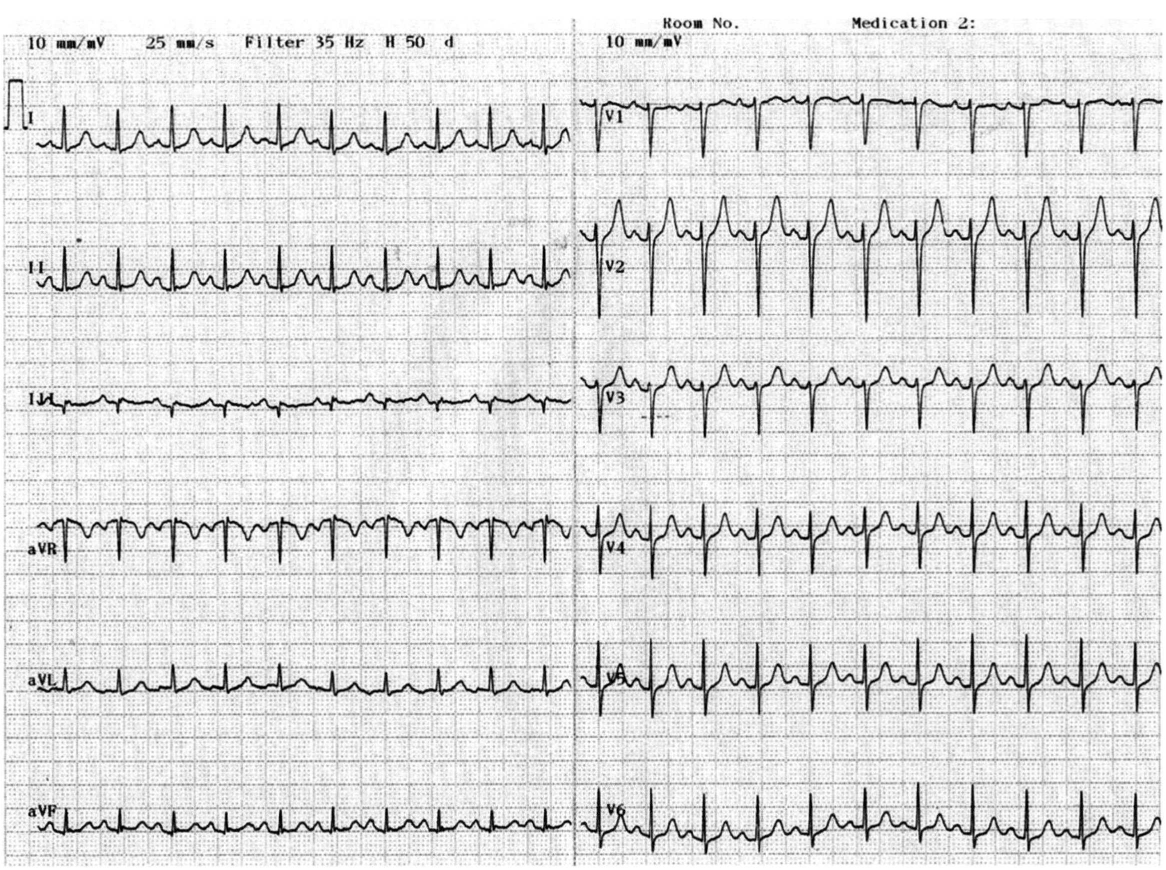

Fig. 21.9: Electrocardiogram showing marked sinus tachycardia (heart rate is 132 bpm) due to thyrotoxicosis.

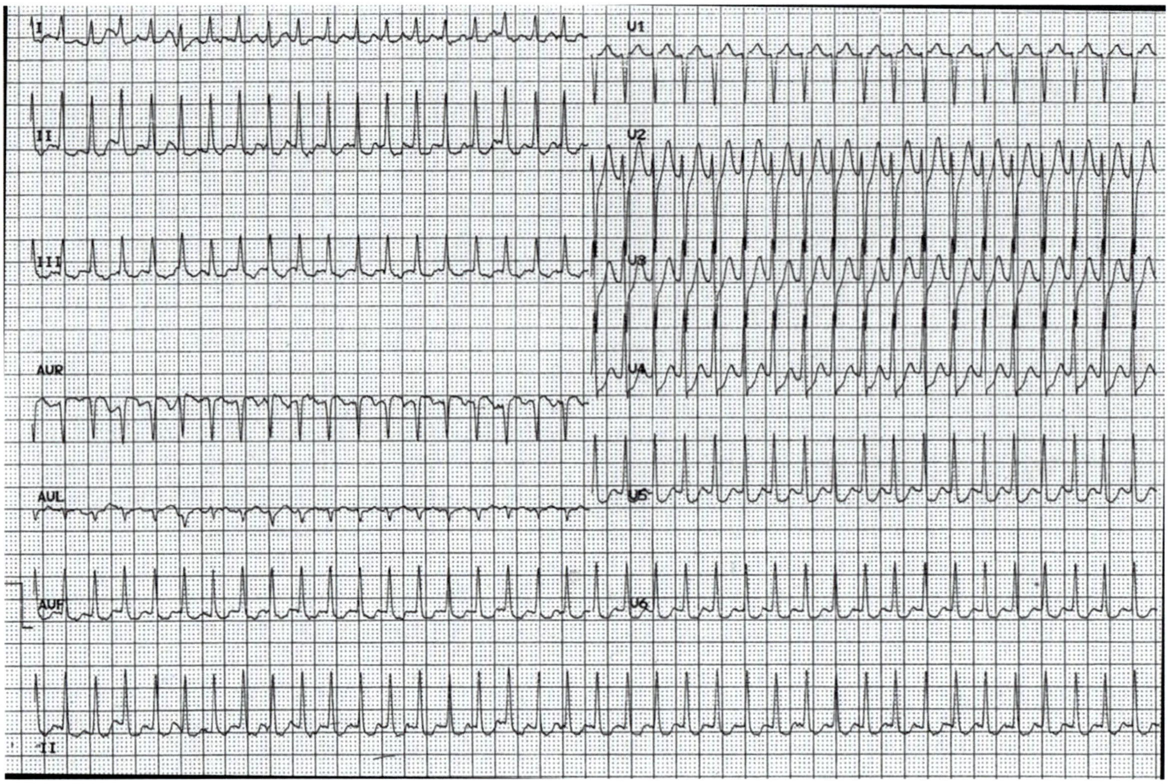

Fig. 21.10: Electrocardiogram of supraventricular tachycardia (rate is 226 bpm) in a patient with thyrotoxicosis.

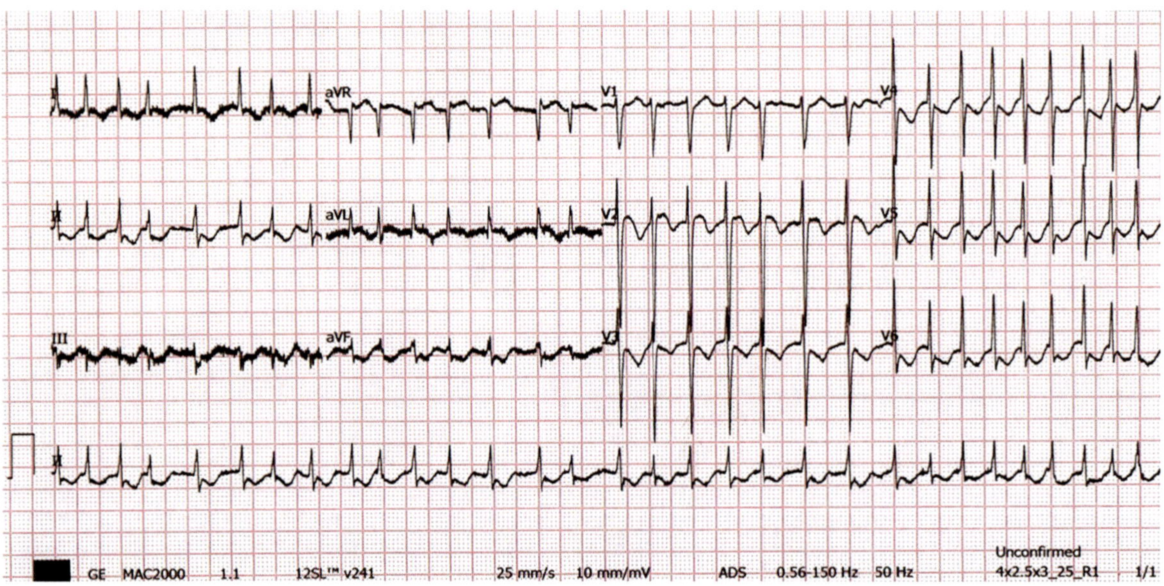

Fig. 21.11: Electrocardiogram is suggestive of fast atrial fibrillation (rate 185 bpm) in a patient with thyrotoxicosis.

should always be suspected in patients with altered mental states who have bradycardia and low voltage ECG.[45]

ELECTROCARDIOGRAM FEATURES OF INCREASED INTRACRANIAL PRESSURE

Various electrocardiographic changes are found in patients with increased intracranial pressure (ICP). The most common findings are sinus bradycardia, QT prolongation, ST-segment changes, and T- or U-wave abnormalities. The presence of J-wave is reported rarely.[46]

The association of electrocardiographic abnormalities with intracranial damage has been known for decades. Burch et al. were the first to describe its association with acute cerebrovascular accidents (CVAs).[47] These electrocardiographic changes can occur in patients with a

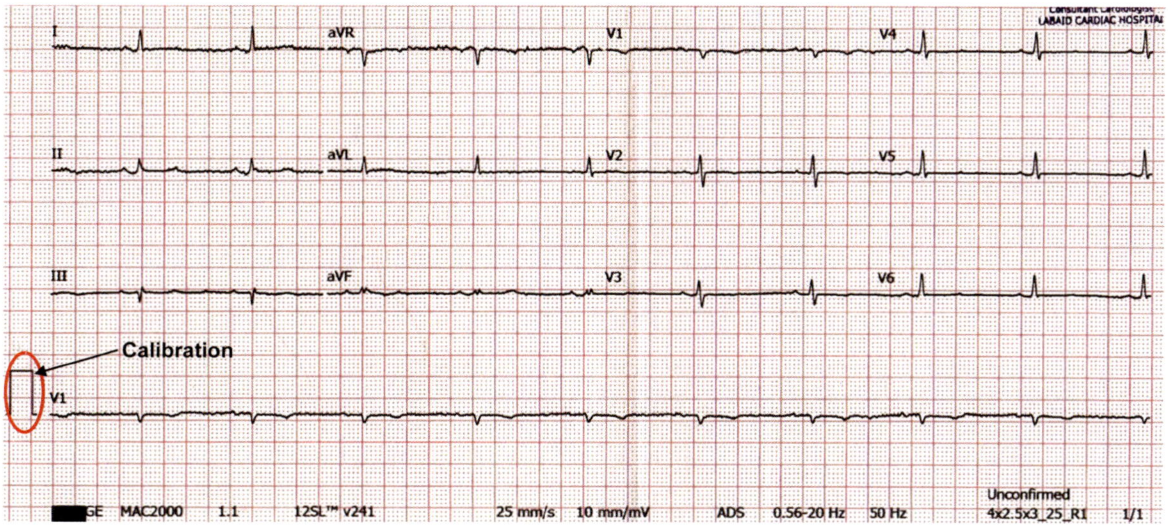

Fig. 21.12: This electrocardiogram illustrates the features of hypothyroidism showing low voltage with sinus bradycardia (heart rate is 58 bpm). Note peak-to-peak QRS amplitude of less than 5 mm in the limb leads and less than 10 mm in the precordial leads, suggestive of low voltage ECG. Note also the optimal calibration of the ECG machine (red circle). *Standard calibration of ECG machine is 10 mm (10 small boxes = 2 large squares) equals 1 mV. Before starting ECG interpretation the clinician must judge, whether the standardization of voltage and timing intervals on the ECG paper are proper or not. If standardization is not proper then ECG interpretation will be wrong.* (*Courtesy:* Dr. Khwaja Nazim Uddin, BIRDEM General Hospital)

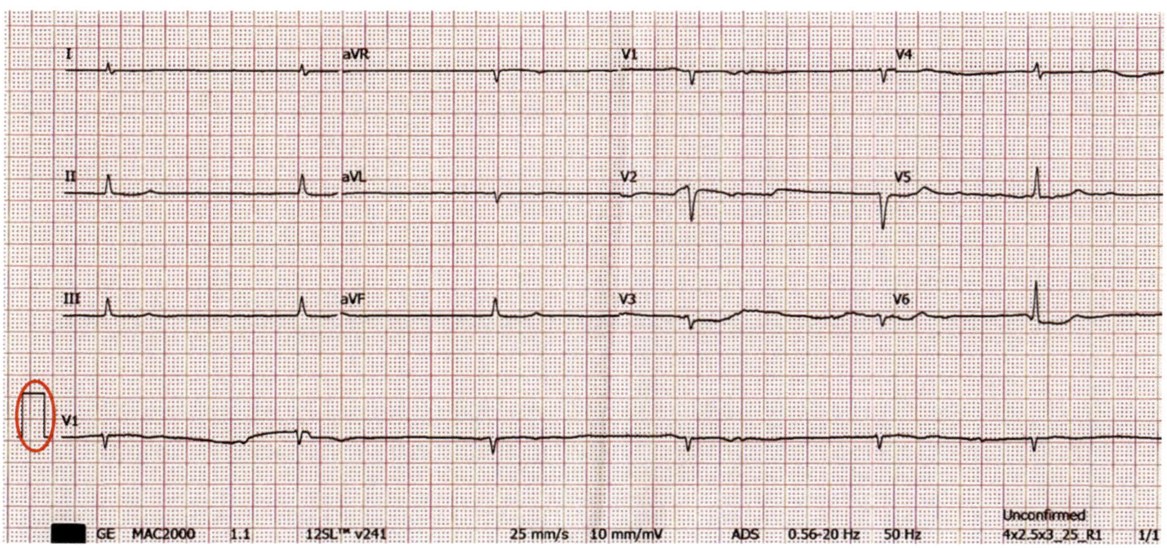

Fig. 21.13: This electrocardiogram illustrates the features of hypothyroidism showing low voltage with severe bradycardia (heart rate is 36 bpm). Note also the optimal calibration of the ECG machine (red circle).

previously normal ECG and they can occur at any age, even adolescence.[40,48] Electrocardiographic anomalies can also be found in 42% of patients with tumors of the brainstem and 56% with intracerebral tumors.[49]

Other than sinus bradycardia, disorders of the CNS usually cause abnormalities in ventricular repolarization. The most common findings are—elevated or depressed ST-segment, deeply inverted T waves, prolonged QT interval, and presence of U waves (Fig. 21.14). These alterations can be transient or may remain for several weeks.[48] Sinus bradycardia due to Cushing reflex, is a physiological nervous system response to increased ICP that results in Cushing's triad of increased blood pressure, irregular breathing, and sinus bradycardia.

The pathophysiology of ECG changes in presence of raised ICP is still unclear. Several different mechanisms have been proposed, including elevated ICP, vagal tonicity, and excessive stimulation of the sympathetic nervous system with catecholamine production. The predominating theory involves the neurohormonal system. Damage to the CNS can result in increased catecholamine levels and sympathetic outflow, which would not only cause electrical problems, but also could lead to physical myocardial damage. Catecholamines probably have a direct toxic effect

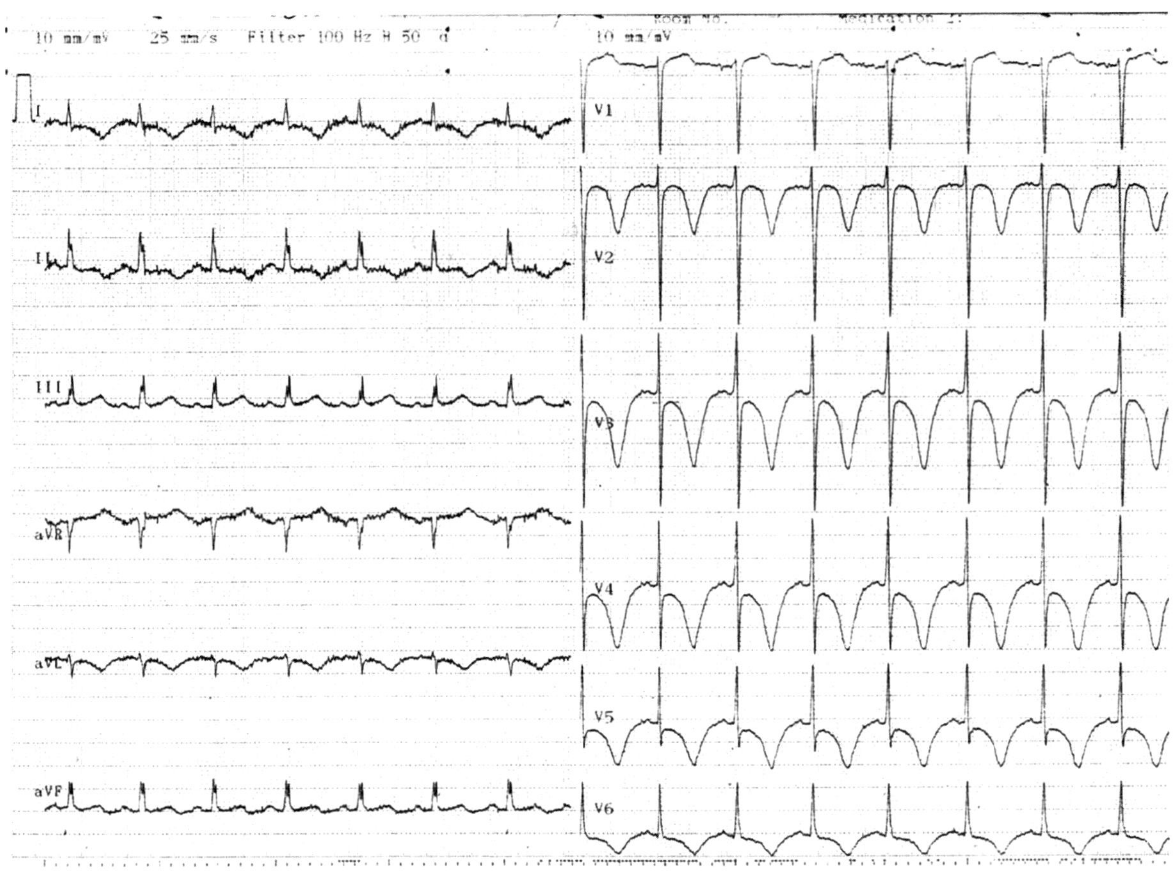

Fig. 21.14: This electrocardiogram illustrates the features of raised intracranial pressure with giant T-wave inversions in precordial leads with prolonged QT interval (QTc is 530 ms) along with ST-segment depressions.

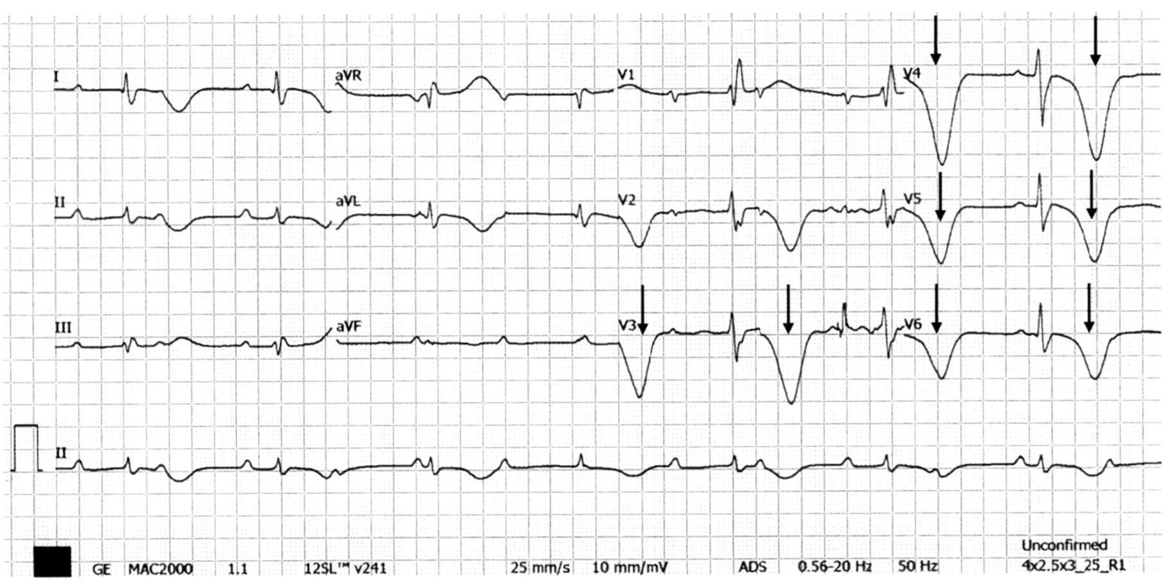

Fig. 21.15: Electrocardiogram of a patient with complete heart block with subarachnoid hemorrhage (SAH). Note giant T-wave inversions and the T wave inversions are diffuse with a widely splayed appearance with a prolonged QT interval (*arrows*), typical of SAH. (*Courtesy*: Dr Abduz Zaher, Labaid Cardiac Hospital)

on myocardial cells or mediate a vasoconstrictive effect on the coronaries.[50-52]

Giant T-wave inversions are also seen in CVAs especially in subarachnoid hemorrhage (SAH). T waves are diffuse with a widely splayed appearance with a prolonged QT interval (Figs. 21.15 and 16). The proposed pathogenesis is cardiomyocytolysis from excessive sympathetic stimulation. Presence of giant T waves should generally prompt investigations for apical variant of hypertrophic cardiomyopathy, raised ICP, severe myocardial ischemia and post-tachycardia syndrome.[53] T-wave inversions produced by MI are classically narrow and symmetric

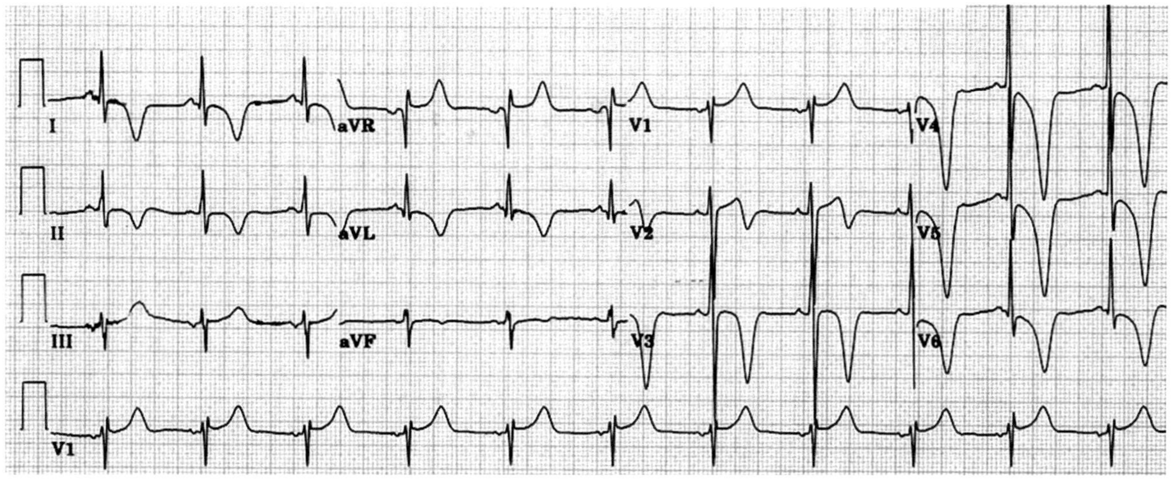

Fig. 21.16: Electrocardiogram of a patient with SAH. Note giant T-wave inversions and ST-segment depressions in both limb and precordial leads.

but deep, symmetric T-wave inversions in all vascular distributions, consistent with neurogenic T waves.[54,55]

Raised ICP may display ST-segment elevation mimicking acute ST-segment elevation MI (STEMI). Without significant coronary artery stenosis, ischemic electrocardiographic changes including ST-segment elevation may develop after CNS injuries, such as subarachnoid, intracranial, or subdural hemorrhage. Misdiagnosing these patients as STEMI may result in catastrophic outcomes.[56-58]

Electrocardiogram changes in SAH usually show widespread giant T-wave inversions along with QT prolongation and bradycardia (due to Cushing reflex). Sometimes, ECG of SAH may reflect changes suggestive of coronary artery disease including ST-segment elevation. ST elevations seem to resolve while "T"-wave inversions appear to persist—even for months/years. Hypothalamic stimulation as well as autonomic dysregulations has been implicated as causative for the ECG changes in SAH without corroborative conclusive evidence.[59]

PARKINSON'S DISEASE

Electrocardiogram from a patient with Parkinson's disease usually shows a regular rhythm with regular high frequency activity which could readily be mistaken for atrial activity. Patient's P waves are usually remain obscured by the artifacts. These regular and high frequency artifacts are characteristic of Parkinson's disease ECG (Figs. 21.17 and 18). Similar patterns of electrical artifacts can also be seen in patients with other causes of muscle tremor, shivering, seizure activity, or hiccough.

Other common causes of motion artifacts in ECG include fever (due to rigors), hypothermia (due to shivering), cardiopulmonary resuscitation (CPR) (due to chest compressions), noncompliant patient (due to restlessness), talkative patient (due to movement), etc. Motion artifacts due to tremor or shivering can obscure the waveforms of the ECG or simulate pathology, making ECG interpretation difficult.

ELECTROCARDIOGRAM CHANGES IN NEUROMUSCULAR DISORDERS

Electrocardiogram changes are seen in most of the cases of muscular dystrophies. The most frequent abnormalities are T-wave changes, tall R waves in right precordial leads and deep Q waves in inferior and lateral leads. These changes, probably due to myocardial fibrosis of the posterolateral wall of the left ventricle, resemble pseudoinfarction pattern of HCM or old MI.[60-62] *Duchenne muscular dystrophy* is an X-linked, recessive form of muscular dystrophy. Cardiac involvement is present in about 90% of the patients and 20% of patients die from cardiac complications. Cardiac involvement is due to progressive replacement of cardiomyocytes and Purkinje system by connective tissue or fat.[62] ECG abnormalities include sinus tachycardia, tall R waves in leads V1, V2 (R/S ratio >1), abnormal Q waves in lateral leads. Prolonged QT interval, short PR interval, RVH, atrial premature beats, supraventricular arrhythmias, ventricular premature beats, and conduction abnormalities are also reported. Sinus tachycardia is the most frequent cardiac abnormality.[63-66] Tachycardia may be attributed to cardiac autonomic nervous system function impairment.[67] Arrhythmias are attributed to progressive fibrosis of the cardiac conduction system and impairment in the cardiac autonomic nervous system function.[63] Atrophy and scarring of the posterobasal region and the adjacent lateral wall of the left ventricle are reported and may explain the ECG pattern with abnormal Q waves.[63-65]

FRIEDREICH'S ATAXIA: CEREBELLAR ATAXIA

Friedreich's ataxia is an autosomal recessive inherited disease that causes progressive degeneration of nerve tissue in the spinal cord, in particular sensory neurons (through connections with the cerebellum) essential for directing muscle movement of the arms and legs. This condition may

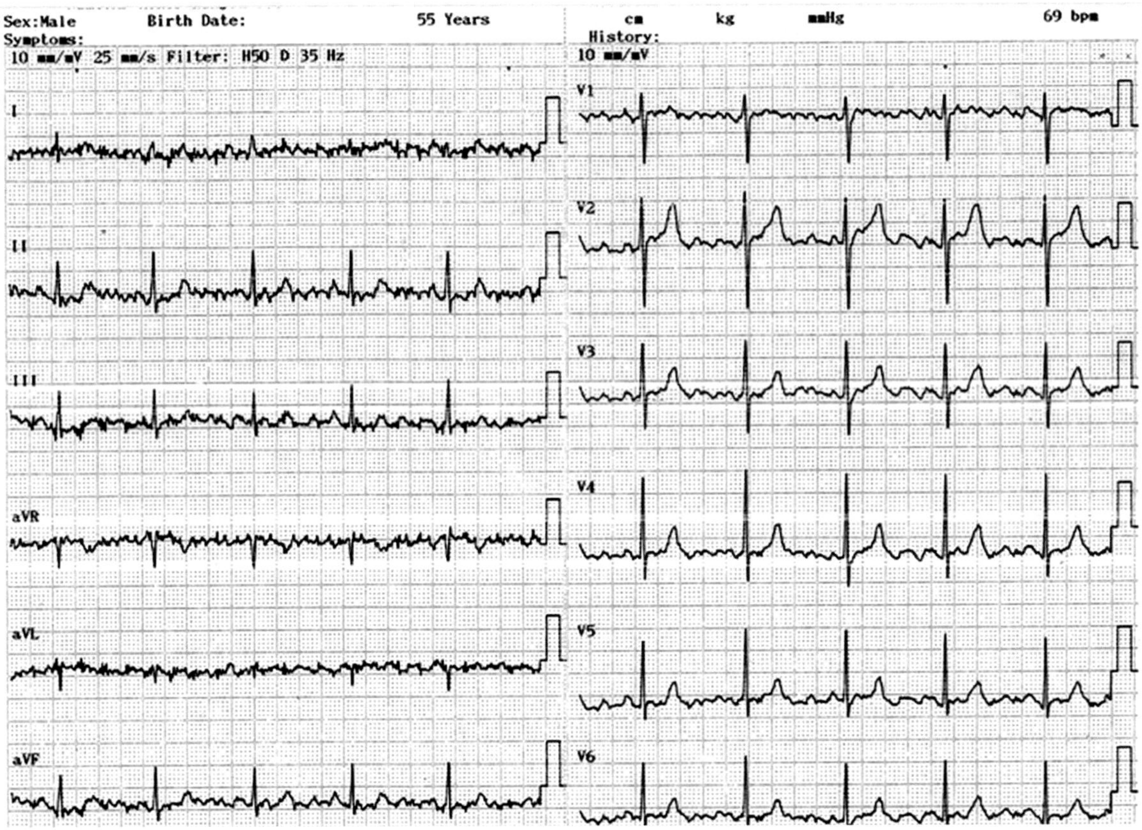

Fig. 21.17: Electrocardiogram from a patient with Parkinson's disease showing motion artifacts along the baseline almost obscuring the P waves. These motion artifacts could readily be mistaken for atrial activity. (*Courtesy*: Dr Ashraf Ali, Labaid Specialized Hospital)

be associated with hypertrophic cardiomyopathy, muscular subaortic stenosis and dilated cardiomyopathy.[68-71]

Between 30% and 90% of individuals with Friedreich ataxia have ECG abnormalities that include nonspecific ST-T wave abnormalities, ventricular hypertrophy, or right axis deviation. Other abnormalities include a short PR interval in up to 24% of patients and interatrial block in up to 48% of patients.[72-80] One study examined, 114 patients with Friedreich ataxia, with 75.4% having an abnormal ECG tracing. Eighty percent of patients with an abnormal ECG had nonspecific T-wave changes. Other commonly reported abnormalities included right axis deviation, right ventricular hypertrophy and left ventricular hypertrophy.[75] In another study, electrocardiographic and vectorcardiographic abnormalities occurred in 69 patients (92%) of the 75 patients. ECGs revealed ST-T wave abnormalities in 79%, right axis deviation in 40%, short PR interval in 24%, abnormal R-wave in lead V1 in 20%, abnormal inferolateral Q waves in 14%, and left ventricular hypertrophy (voltage and repolarization criteria) in 16%.[79] Hypertrophic cardiomyopathy and left ventricular hypertrophy develop in about 75% of patients and conduction disturbances in 10%.[79] There can be abnormal Q waves in the inferior and lateral leads, simulating old inferior and lateral wall MI. Myocardial fibrosis is often responsible for the pseudoinfarction pattern in patients with Friedreich's ataxia.[81]

ELECTROCARDIOGRAM AFTER HEART TRANSPLANTATION

There are two types of heart transplantation: (1) Orthotopic heart transplantation and (2) heterotopic transplantation. In orthotopic heart transplantation, the patient's own heart is mostly removed (the cardiectomy for the recipient) and replaced with the donor heart or less commonly, the recipient's diseased heart is left in place to support the donor heart (heterotopic transplantation).

Electrocardiogram of a patient with orthotopic heart transplantation may show a second set of "P" waves which are dissociated from the underlying QRS complexes. This is a common ECG finding following heart transplantation which represents atrial activity from the recipient atrial remnant (Fig. 21.19). Recipient atrial activity is present in 40% of patients in the first 2 weeks after transplantation, but decreases to 16% at 1 year and 3% at 5 years. Nonspecific repolarization abnormalities are commonly seen, but are not prognostically important. New onset of incomplete or complete RBBB may be seen in transplant patients (16–69%) but are not indicative of adverse outcome.[82-84]

In heterotopic heart transplantation, the recipient's native heart is left in place and the allograft is implanted in the right chest. The post transplantation ECG shows two QRS complexes with different axis.[85]

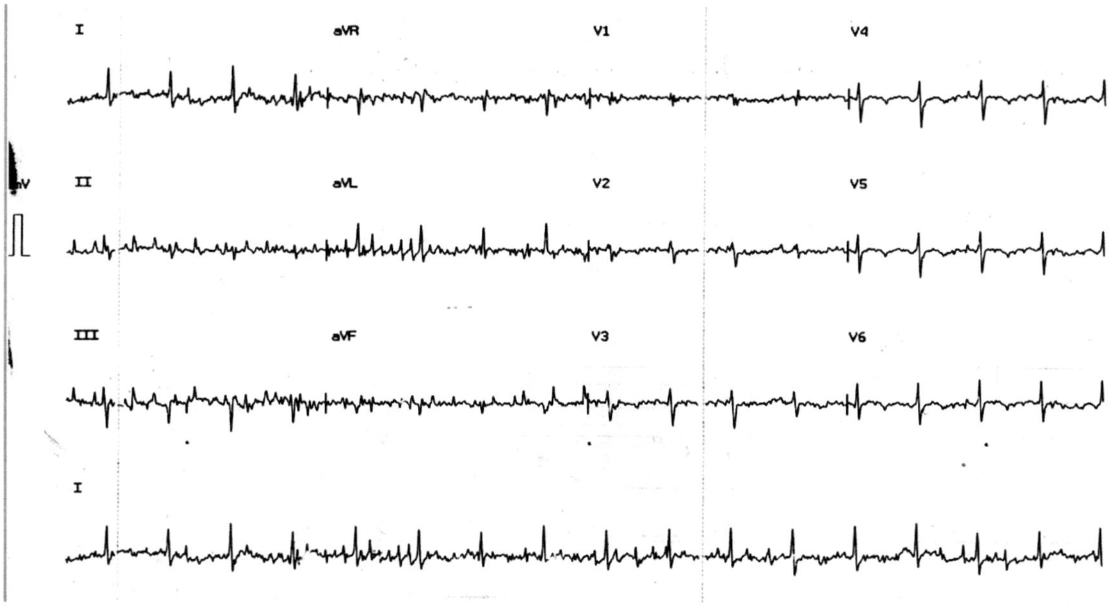

Fig. 21.18: Electrocardiogram of a patient with Parkinson's disease displaying regular rhythm high frequency motion artifacts. These motion artifacts look like atrial activity. Note the patient's P waves are obscured by the artifacts.

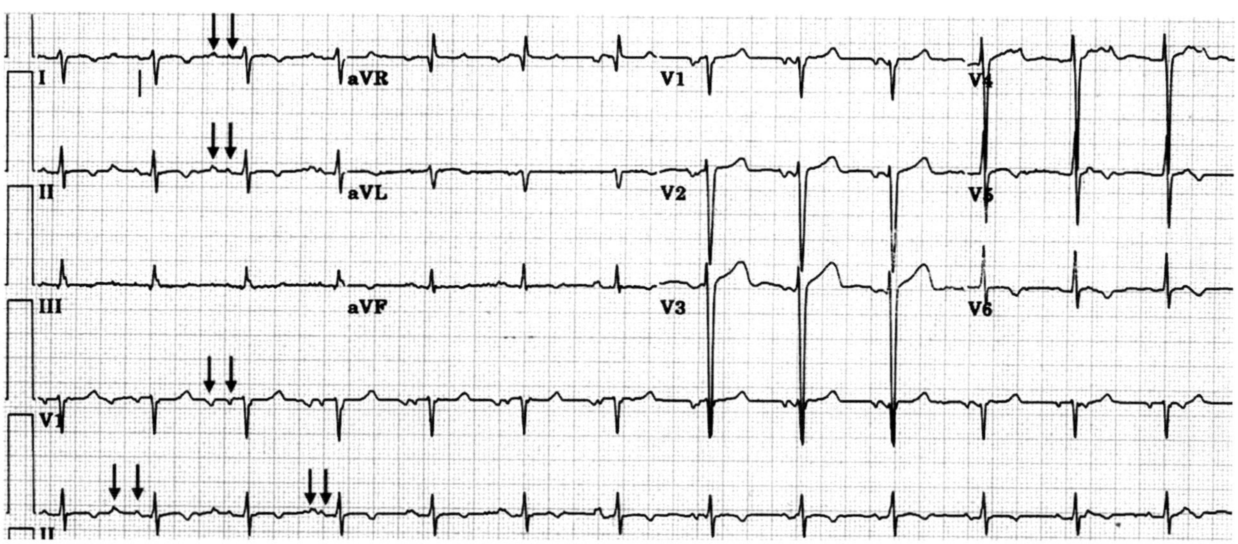

Fig. 21.19: This electrocardiogram illustrates the features of orthotopic heart transplantation with two sets of P waves (*arrows*). The second set of "P" waves are dissociated from the QRS complexes. This is a common ECG finding following heart transplantation and these second set of P waves represent atrial activity from the recipient atrial remnant.

ELECTROCARDIOGRAM FEATURES OF PRIMARY PULMONARY HYPERTENSION (PPH)

Pulmonary hypertension (PHT) may be primary or secondary. Primary PHT is a relatively rare idiopathic condition. PHT is present when mean pulmonary artery pressure exceeds 25 mm Hg at rest or 30 mm Hg with exercise. Secondary PHT is more common and is usually due to cardiac or respiratory causes. Important causes of secondary PHT include—COPD, interstitial lung disease (ILD), obstructive sleep apnea syndrome (OSAS), valvular heart disease, e.g. mitral stenosis, mitral regurgitation, multiple valvular heart disease, systemic disorders, e.g. sarcoidosis, vasculitis, connective tissue diseases, e.g. scleroderma, HIV infection, and chronic thromboembolic PHT, etc. ECG features of primary and secondary PHT are almost identical.

Electrocardiographic features are often abnormal in primary PHT and include (Figs. 21.20 and 21.21):

- Right atrial enlargement
- Right axis deviation
- Right ventricular hypertrophy
- Characteristic ST depression in right precordial leads
- T-wave inversions in the anterior leads
- Sometimes, an incomplete RBBB may be seen.

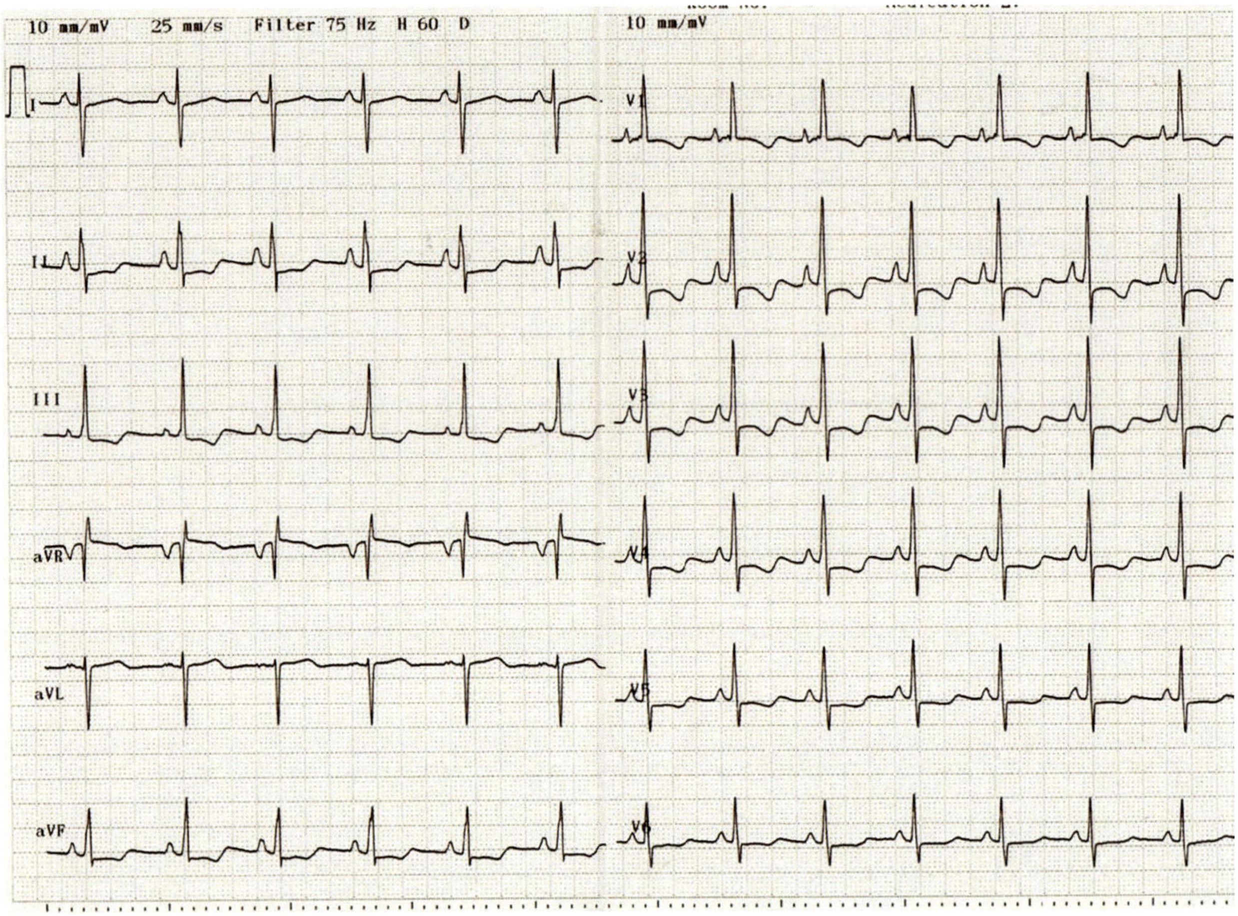

Fig. 21.20: Electrocardiogram illustrates the features of primary pulmonary hypertension (PPH). Note tall R in V1 with ST-segment depression and biphasic T waves in precordial leads (V1–V5) and inferior leads with electrocardiographic evidence of P pulmonale (tall and peak P waves greater than 2.5 mm in LII). Also note right axis deviation. (*Courtesy*: Dr Md Elias Ali, Labaid Cardiac Hospital)

Many clinical conditions may produce electrocardiographic manifestations of RVH, including mitral stenosis, atrial septal defects, COPD, endocardial cushion defect, pulmonary valve stenosis, etc. but extremely tall monophasic R-wave in lead V1 is characteristic of PPH (Fig. 21.22).

SUMMARY

Chronic Obstructive Pulmonary Disease

Electrocardiogram changes occur in COPD due to the presence of hyperexpanded emphysematous lungs within the chest and the long-term effects of hypoxic pulmonary vasoconstriction upon the right side of the heart, causing PHT and subsequent right atrial enlargement and RVH. Low voltage ECG (low voltage on the ECG is defined as QRS amplitude of less than 5 mm in all the limb leads and/or less than 10 mm in the precordial leads) is due to hyperinflated lungs and P pulmonale and RVH are due to PHT.

Chronic obstructive pulmonary disease can induce typical ECG features and they include:

- P pulmonale
- Low voltage ECG
- Clockwise rotation of the heart with a delayed R/S transition point
- Poor R-wave progression V1–V6
- Right axis deviation
- Right ventricular hypertrophy/RBBB.
- S1-S2-S3 pattern.
- Lead I sign (Schamroth's Sign):
  - Flat or Isoelectric P wave in lead I
  - Very small QRS complex of less than 1.5 mm total deflection
  - T wave of less than 0.5 mm in lead I.

In COPD, the ECG evidence of right atrial enlargement (P pulmonale) and RVH indicate presence of cor pulmonale.

Supraventricular arrhythmias: Atrial premature complexes (APCs), atrial flutter, AF, paroxysmal atrial tachycardia, and MAT are commonly seen during acute exacerbation of COPD.

Pulmonary Embolism

Pulmonary embolism is, in most cases, the consequence of DVT. Major trauma, surgery, lower limb fractures and joint replacements, spinal cord injury, malignancies and oral

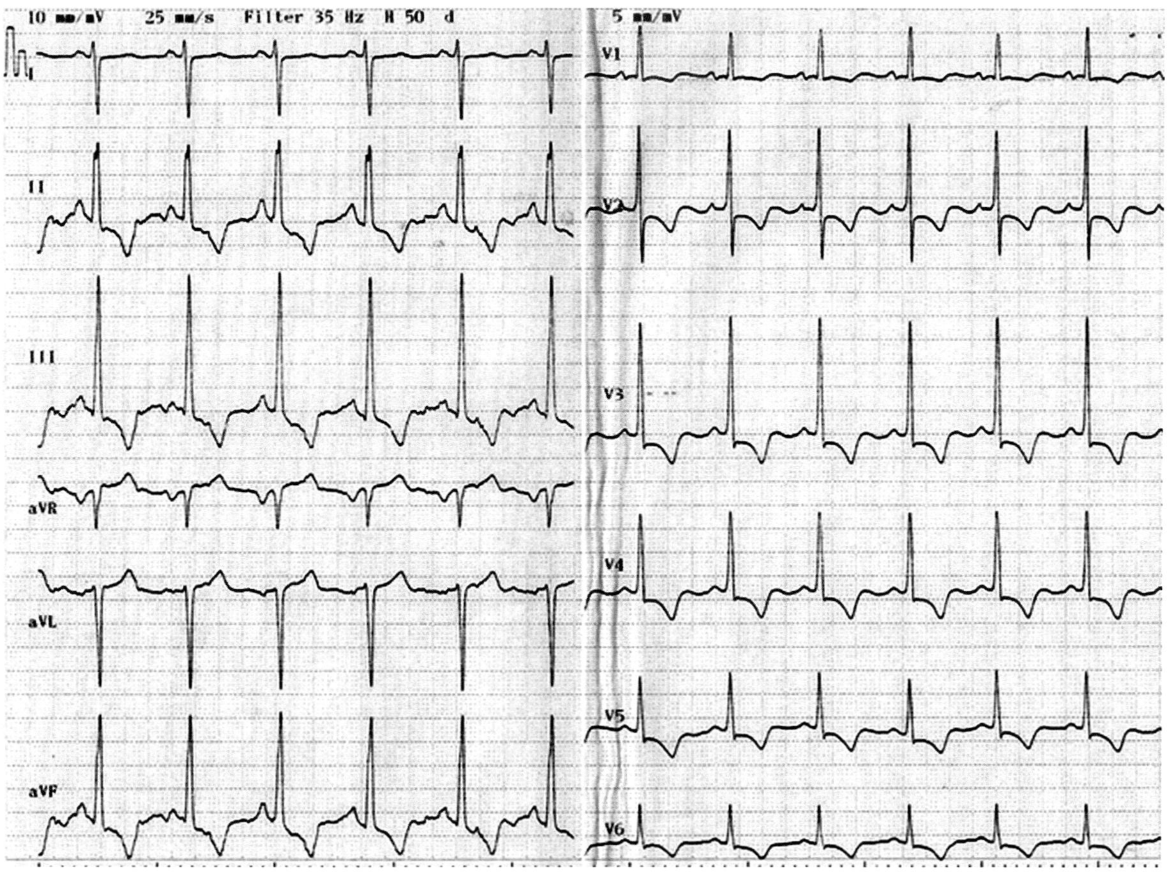

Fig. 21.21: Electrocardiogram illustrates the features of PPH. Note tall R in V1 with ST depression and T-wave inversions in precordial leads (V1–V6) and inferior leads with electrocardiographic evidence of P pulmonale (tall and peak P waves greater than 2.5 mm in LII, LIII, and aVF). Also note right axis deviation.

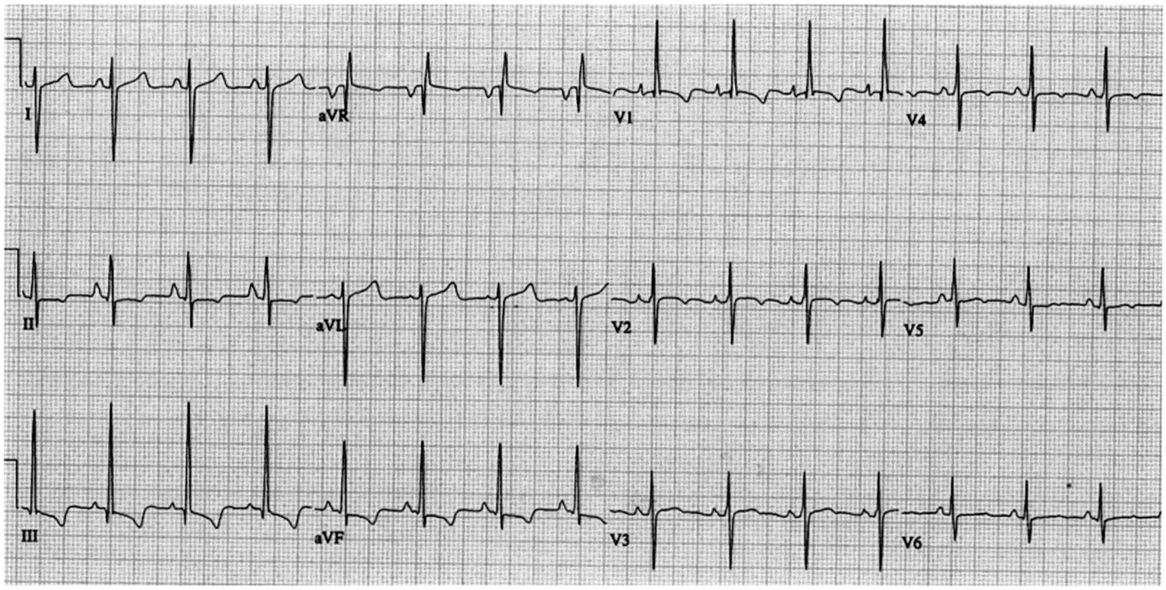

Fig. 21.22: Electrocardiogram illustrates the features of PPH. Note extremely tall monophasic R-wave in lead V1, which is characteristic of PPH. Also note other ECG features of RVH (deep terminal S waves in lateral precordial leads, right axis deviation, and evidence of right atrial enlargement).

contraceptive pills are well-recognized predisposing factor for DVT leading to PE. The ECG is a poor diagnostic test for PE.

Electrocardiogram features of pulmonary embolism include:

- Sinus tachycardia
- New onset of right bundle branch block (incomplete or complete)
- S1Q3T3 pattern
- T-wave inversion in the right precordial leads
- P pulmonale
- Right axis deviation
- Atrial flutter or fibrillation.

The most common ECG abnormality in PE is sinus tachycardia which is present in at least 40% of cases. S1Q3T3 pattern is a classic ECG sign of PE but this pattern is present in only 15–25% of patients with confirmed diagnosis of PE.

Hypothermia

Hypothermia, defined as core body temperature less than 35°C (<95°F). Hypothermia may show ECG features of sinus bradycardia, slow junctional rhythms, varying degrees of AV block (first to third), shivering artifact, prolonged PR, QRS, and QT intervals, Osborn waves (J waves), AF, ventricular ectopics and if the condition remains unabated leads to cardiac arrest due to VT, VF, or asystole (Box 21.1).

Electrocardiogram features change according to the severity of hypothermia:

Below 32.2°C (<90°F)

- Sinus bradycardia
- Progressive prolongation of the PR interval
- Prolongation of QRS complex
- Prolonged QT interval.

Below 30.0°C (<86°F)

- Osborn waves
- Atrial fibrillation.

Below 28°C (<82.4°F)

- Ventricular fibrillation
- Asystole.

Osborn waves (J waves) are positive deflections at junction between the QRS complex and ST segment (Box 21.2). This wave is a repolarization abnormality caused by exaggerated outward K^+ current, usually observed in patients with hypothermia but may be seen in early repolarization, hypercalcemia, and the Brugada syndrome. These waves are detectable in 80% of the patients when core body temperature is lower than 30.0°C (86°F).

Box 21.1: Basic electrocardiogram changes during hypothermia.

- Sinus bradycardia
- Classic Osborn waves
- Prolonged PR, QRS, and QT intervals
- Varying degrees of AV block
- Shivering artifacts
- VF or asystole.

Box 21.2: Osborn wave.

The Osborn wave (J-wave) is a positive deflection at the J-point, most prominent in the precordial leads (negative in aVR and V1). It is characteristically seen in hypothermia when core body temperature is lower than 30.0°C (86°F).

Causes of Osborn wave on ECG:

- Hypothermia
- Hypercalcemia
- Early repolarization pattern (ERP)
- Brugada syndrome
- Severe head injury
- Subarachnoid hemorrhage
- Normal variant.

Thyrotoxicosis

The cardiovascular system is very sensitive to increased levels of circulating thyroid hormones. Increase in cardiac output and heart rate are early features in thyrotoxicosis. The most common ECG changes seen in thyrotoxicosis are:

- Sinus tachycardia
- Increased electrical amplitude of all waves
- Atrial fibrillation (20%)
- Paroxysmal supraventricular tachycardia
- Nonspecific ST and T-wave changes
- Ventricular extrasystole.

Hypothyroidism

Patients with overt hypothyroidism show several ECG changes including sinus bradycardia, low amplitude QRS complexes, QT interval prolongation, and alterations in T-wave morphology. Atrioventricular and intraventricular conduction disturbances are also commonly seen. Ventricular tachyarrhythmias, e.g. polymorphic ventricular tachycardia (torsades de pointes) associated with prolonged QT interval have been documented.

Electrocardiographic Features of Hypothyroidism

Hypothyroidism (myxedema) classically causes a triad of ECG findings as follows:

- Sinus bradycardia
- Low QRS voltage
- Widespread T-wave inversions (usually without ST deviation).

Common findings

- Sinus bradycardia
- Low voltage ECG
- Flat or inverted T waves
- Prolonged QT interval.

Less common

- Bundle branch block
- First degree heart block
- Intraventricular conduction defects
- Ventricular extrasystoles
- Rarely polymorphic ventricular tachycardia (torsades de pointes).

Electrocardiogram Features of Increased Intracranial Pressure (ICP)

Electrocardiogram changes due to increased ICP are most commonly seen with massive intracranial hemorrhage:

- Subarachnoid hemorrhage
- Intraparenchymal hemorrhage (hemorrhagic stroke).

Raised ICP is associated with certain characteristic ECG changes.

Common ECG findings

- Sinus bradycardia
- Widespread giant T-wave inversions (cerebral T waves).
- QT prolongation.

Possible ECG findings

- ST-segment elevation/depression which may mimic myocardial ischemia or acute STEMI or pericarditis.
- Prominent U-wave.
- Junctional rhythms, premature ventricular contractions, and AF.

The ST-segment and T-wave abnormalities are caused by an abrupt elevation of serum catecholamine levels. An excess of catecholamines can damage myocytes directly and can also lead to generalized spasm of the coronary arteries.

T-wave inversions produced by MI are classically narrow and symmetric but deep and symmetric T-wave inversion often with broadening are usually seen in raised intracranial pressure. The T waves of myocardial ischemia are typically not very broad but severe CNS disorders produce excessive broadening of T waves.

Central nervous system injuries such as subarachnoid, intracranial or subdural hemorrhage and head injury may display ST-segment elevation mimicking acute STEMI. Misdiagnosing these patients as STEMI may result in catastrophic outcomes.

Box 21.3: Common causes of motion artifacts in electrocardiogram.

- Fever (due to rigors)
- Parkinsonism (due to resting tremor)
- Hypothermia (due to shivering)
- Cardiopulmonary resuscitation (due to chest compressions)
- Noncompliant patient (due to restlessness)
- Talkative patient (due to movement).

Parkinson's Disease

Regular and high frequency motion artifacts are characteristic of Parkinson's disease ECG (Box 21.3). Patient's P waves are usually remain obscured by the artifacts.

Electrocardiogram Changes in Neuromuscular Disorders

Duchenne muscular dystrophy is an X-linked, recessive form of muscular dystrophy. Cardiac involvement is present in about 90% of the patients. Sinus tachycardia is the most frequent cardiac abnormality. Tachycardia may be attributed to cardiac autonomic nervous system function impairment.

Electrocardiogram changes in Duchenne's muscular dystrophy

- Tall R waves in the right-sided chest leads (V1 and V2)
- Short PR interval
- Pathological Q waves in the lateral chest leads (V5 and V6) and limb leads.

Friedreich's ataxia is an autosomal recessive disease with spinocerebellar disorder and cardinal features include progressive limb and gait ataxia, dysarthria, and loss of joint position. This condition is frequently associated with hypertrophic cardiomyopathy.

Between 30% and 90% of individuals with Friedreich's ataxia have ECG abnormalities that include:

- Nonspecific ST–T wave abnormalities
- Ventricular hypertrophy
- Right axis deviation
- Tall R-wave in V1
- Pathological Q-wave mimicking old myocardial infarction.

Electrocardiogram after Heart Transplantation

Electrocardiogram of a patient with orthotopic heart transplantation may show a second set of "P" waves which are dissociated from the underlying QRS complexes. These second set of "P" waves represent electrical activity from the recipient atrial remnant. ECG of heterotopic heart transplantation patients display two QRS complexes with different axis.

Electrocardiogram Features of Primary Pulmonary Hypertension (PPH)

Pulmonary hypertension may be primary or secondary. PHT is present when mean pulmonary artery pressure exceeds 25 mm Hg at rest or 30 mm Hg with exercise. Primary PHT is a relatively rare idiopathic condition. PHT is mostly secondary and due to COPD, valvular heart disease, connective tissue disorders, etc. ECG features of primary PHT include—right atrial enlargement, right axis deviation, RVH, ST depression in right precordial leads, and T-wave inversions in the anterior leads. Very tall monophasic R-wave in lead V1 is characteristic of PPH.

REFERENCES

1. Rabe K, Hurd S, Anzueto A, et al. Global strategy for the diagnosis, management, and prevention of chronic obstructive pulmonary disease: GOLD executive summary. Am J Respir Crit Care Med. 2007;176(6):532-55.
2. Celli B, MacNee W. Standards for the diagnosis and treatment of patients with COPD: a summary of the ATS/ERS position paper. Eur Respir J. 2004;23(6):932-46.
3. Harrigan R, Jones K. ABC of clinical electrocardiography. Conditions affecting the right side of the heart. BMJ. 2002;324(7347):1201-4.
4. Banker H, Verma A. Electrocardiographic changes in COPD. NHL J Med Sci. 2013;2(2):55-8.
5. Yip JW, Chia BL, Tan WC. The ECG "lead I sign" in cardiac disease--an indicator of coexisting obstructive pulmonary disease. Singapore Med J. 1999;40(4):281-3.
6. Agrawal RI, Kumar D, Gurpreet, et al. Diagnostic values of electrocardiogram in chronic obstructive pulmonary disease (COPD). Lung India. 2008;25(2):78-81.
7. Incalzi RA, Fuso L, Rosa MD, et al. Electrocardiographic signs of chronic cor pulmonale. A negative prognostic finding in chronic obstructive pulmonary disease. Circulation. 1999;99(12):1600-5.
8. Konstantinides SV, Torbicki A, Agnelli G, et al. 2014 ESC guidelines on the diagnosis and management of acute pulmonary embolism. The Task Force for the Diagnosis and Management of Acute Pulmonary Embolism of the European Society of Cardiology (ESC). Eur Heart J. 2014;35(43):3033-69.
9. Anderson FA Jr., Spencer FA. Risk factors for venous thromboembolism. Circulation. 2003;107(23 Suppl 1):I9-I16.
10. Rogers MA, Levine DA, Blumberg N, et al. Triggers of hospitalization for venous thromboembolism. Circulation. 2012;125(17):2092-9.
11. Ku GH, White RH, Chew HK, et al. Venous thromboembolism in patients with acute leukemia: incidence, risk factors, and effect on survival. Blood. 2009;113(17):3911-7.
12. Chew HK, Wun T, Harvey D, et al. Incidence of venous thromboembolism and its effect on survival among patients with common cancers. Arch Intern Med. 2006;166(4):458-64.
13. Blom JW, Doggen CJ, Osanto S, et al. Malignancies, prothrombotic mutations, and the risk of venous thrombosis. JAMA. 2005;293(6):715-22.
14. Timp JF, Braekkan SK, Versteeg HH, et al. Epidemiology of cancer-associated venous thrombosis. Blood. 2013;122(10):1712-23.
15. Blanco-Molina A, Rota LL, Di Micco P, et al. Venous thromboembolism during pregnancy, postpartum or during contraceptive use. Thromb Haemost. 2010;103(2):306-11.
16. Blanco-Molina A, Trujillo-Santos J, Tirado R, et al. Venous thromboembolism in women using hormonal contraceptives. Findings from the RIETE Registry. Thromb Haemost. 2009;101(3):478-82.
17. Goldhaber SZ, Visani L, De Rosa M. Acute pulmonary embolism: clinical outcomes in the international cooperative pulmonary embolism registry (ICOPER). Lancet. 1999;353(9162):1386-9.
18. Stein PD, Terrin ML, Hales CA, et al. Clinical, laboratory, roentgenographic, and electrocardiographic findings in patients with acute pulmonary embolism and no pre-existing cardiac or pulmonary disease. Chest. 1991;100:598-603.
19. Sallach JA, Sallach SM, Thomas JD, et al. Prognostic value of electrocardiographic abnormalities in patients with acute pulmonary embolism. Chest. 2003;124(4):S239.
20. Geibel A, Zehender M, Kasper W, et al. Prognostic value of the ECG on admission in patients with acute major pulmonary embolism. Eur Respir J. 2005;25(5):843-8.
21. Rodger MA, Makropoulos D, Turek M, et al. Diagnostic value of the electrocardiogram in suspected pulmonary embolism. Am J Cardiol. 2000;86(7):807-9.
22. McGinn S, White PD. Acute cor pulmonale resulting from pulmonary embolism: its clinical recognition. JAMA. 1935;104(17):1473-80.
23. Levis JT. ECG diagnosis: pulmonary embolism. Perm J. 2011;15(4):75.
24. Chan TC, Vilke GM, Pollack M, et al. Electrocardiographic manifestations: pulmonary embolism. J Emerg Med. 2001;21(3):263-70.
25. Ullman E, Brady WJ, Perron AD, et al. Electrocardiographic manifestations of pulmonary embolism. Am J Emerg Med. 2001;19(6):514-9.
26. Vanni S, Polidori G, Vergara R, et al. Prognostic value of ECG among patients with acute pulmonary embolism and normal blood pressure. Am J Med. 2009;122(3):257-64.
27. Ferrari E, Imbert A, Chevalier T, et al. The ECG in pulmonary embolism: predictive value of negative T waves in precordial leads: 80 case reports. Chest. 1997;111(3):537-43.
28. Cheng ASH, Money-Kyrle A. Instructive ECG series in massive bilateral pulmonary embolism. Heart. 2005;91(7):860-2.
29. Baez A, Goyal D. Acute cor pulmonale from massive bilateral pulmonary emboli. Int J Emerg Med. 2005;3(1):1-3.
30. Alhaddad IA, Khalil M, Brown EJ Jr., Osborn waves of hypothermia. Circulation. 2000;101(25):e233-e244.
31. Saadlla H. Electrocardiographic changes in extreme hypothermia. N Engl J Med. 2004;351:e4.
32. Maruyama M, Kobayashi Y, Kodani E, et al. Osborn waves: history and significance. Indian Pacing Electrophysiol J. 2004;4(1): 33-9.
33. Osborn JJ. Experimental hypothermia: respiratory and blood pH changes in relation to cardiac function. Am J Physiol. 1953;175(3):389-98.

34. Aydin M, Gursurer M, Bayraktaroglu T, et al. Prominent J wave (Osborn wave) with coincidental hypothermia in a 64-year-old woman. Tex Heart Inst J. 2005;32(1):105.
35. Mareedu RK, Grandhe NP, Quinn DL. Classic EKG changes of hypothermia. Clin Med Res. 2008;6(3-4):107-8.
36. Alsafwah S. Electrocardiographic changes in hypothermia. Heart Lung. 2001;30:161-3.
37. Olgers TJ, Ubels FL. The ECG in hypothermia: Osborn waves. Neth J Med. 2006;64(9):350, 353.
38. Nolan J, Soar J. Images in resuscitation: the ECG in hypothermia. Resuscitation. 2005;64(2):133-4.
39. Graham CA, McNaughton GW, Wyatt JP. The electrocardiogram in hypothermia. Wilderness Environ Med. 2001;12(4):232-5.
40. Van Mieghem C, Sabbe M, Knockaert D. The clinical value of the ECG in noncardiac conditions. Chest. 2004;125(4): 1561-76.
41. Malenkovic V, Paunovic I, Milosevic M, et al. Cardiovascular manifestations of hyperthyroidism. Clinical significance and preoperative preparation. Srp Arh Celok Lek. 2000;128(11-12): 379-83.
42. Osman F, Franklyn JA, Holder RL, et al. Cardiovascular Manifestations of Hyperthyroidism Before and After Antithyroid Therapy; A Matched Case-Control Study. J Am Coll Cardiol. 2007;49(1):71-81.
43. Shojaie M, Eshraghian A. Primary hypothyroidism presenting with Torsades de pointes type tachycardia: a case report. Cases J. 2008;1:298.
44. Schenck JB, Rizvi AA, Lin T. Severe primary hypothyroidism manifesting with torsades de pointes. Am J Med Sci. 2006;331(3):154-6.
45. Slovis C, Jenkins R. ABC of clinical electrocardiography: Conditions not primarily affecting the heart. BMJ. 2002;324(7349):1320-3.
46. Milewska A, Guzik P, Rudzka M, et al. J-wave formation in patients with acute intracranial hypertension. J Electrocardiol. 2009;42(5):420-3.
47. Burch GE, Meyers R, Abildskov JA. A new electrocardiographic pattern observed in cerebrovascular accidents. Circulation. 1954;9(5):719-23.
48. Koepp M, Kern A, Schmidt D. Electrocardiographic changes in patients with brain tumors. Arch Neurol. 1995;52(2):152-5.
49. Rodehill A, Olsonn Gl, Sundquist K, et al. ECG abnormalities in patients with subarachnoid haemorrhage and intracranial tumours. J Neurol Neurosurg Psychiatry. 1987;50(10): 1375-81.
50. Goldstein LB, El Husseini N. Neurología y cardiología: puntos de contacto. Rev Esp Cardiol. 2011; 64(4):319-27.
51. Lopez-Lluva MT, Arizon-Munoz JM, Gonzalez-Ruiz de la Herran F, et al. Electrocardiographic changes underlying central nervous system damage. Rev Esp Cardiol. 2012;65(10):958-60.
52. Abdulhadi M, Alfitori G, Mennim P. A non-cardiac cause of an abnormal ECG. Acute Med. 2009;8(2):70-2.
53. Pillarisetti J, Gupta K. Giant Inverted T waves in the emergency department: case report and review of differential diagnoses. J Electrocardiol. 2010;43(1):40-2.
54. Catanzaro JN, Meraj PM, Zheng S, et al. Electrocardiographic T-wave changes underlying acute cardiac and cerebral events. Am J Emerg Med. 2008;26(6):716-20.
55. Lindberg DM, Jauch EC. Neurogenic T Waves Preceding Acute Ischemic Stroke. Circulation. 2006;114(9):e369-e370.
56. Hahn TH, Doo YC, Seo YM, et al. A case of ST-segment elevation in a patient with subarachnoid hemorrhage. Korean Circ J. 1995;25(1):106-9.
57. Cropp GJ, Manning GW. Electrocardiographic changes simulating myocardial ischemia and infarction associated with spontaneous intracranial hemorrhage. Circulation. 1960;22:25-38.
58. Heo WJ, Kang JH, Jo SW. Subarachnoid hemorrhage misdiagnosed as an acute ST elevation myocardial infarction. Korean Circ J. 2012;42(3):216-9.
59. Chatterjee S. ECG changes in subarachnoid haemorrhage: a synopsis. Neth Heart J. 2011;19(1):31-4.
60. Slucka C. The electrocardiogram in Duchenne progressive muscular dystrophy. Circulation. 1968;38(5):933-40.
61. Khan MA, Almashham Y, Almoukirish A, et al. Electrocardiographic changes in cases of Duchenne muscular dystrophy. J Saudi Heart Assoc. 2013;25(2):154-5.
62. Finsterer J, Stollberger C. The heart in human dystrophinopathies. Cardiology. 2003;99(1):1-19.
63. Fayssoil A. Electrocardiogram's particularities in Duchenne muscular dystrophy. J Clinic Experiment Cardiol. 2011;2:115.
64. Thrush PT, Allen HD, Viollet L, et al. Re-examination of the electrocardiogram in boys with Duchenne muscular dystrophy and correlation with its dilated cardiomyopathy. Am J Cardiol. 2009;103(2):262-5.
65. Thrush PT, Edward N, Flanigan KM, et al. Precordial R wave height does not correlate with echocardiographic findings in boys with Duchenne muscular dystrophy. Congenit Heart Dis. 2013;8(6):561-7.
66. Takami Y, Takeshima Y, Awano H, et al. High incidence of electrocardiogram abnormalities in young patients with Duchenne muscular dystrophy. Pediatr Neurol. 2008;39(6):399-403.
67. Lanza GA, Dello Russo A, Giglio V, et al. Impairment of cardiac autonomic function in patients with Duchenne muscular dystrophy: relationship to myocardial and respiratory function. Am Heart J. 2001;141(5): 808-12.
68. Weidemann F, Scholz F, Florescu C, et al. Heart involvement in Friedreich's ataxia. Herz. 2015;40(Suppl 1):85-90.
69. Weidemann F, Stork S, Liu D, et al. Cardiomyopathy of Friedreich ataxia. J Neurochem. 2013;126 (Suppl 1):88-93.
70. Bourke T, Keane D. Friedreich's Ataxia: a review from a cardiology perspective. Ir J Med Sci. 2011;180(4):799-805.
71. Steinsapir K, Lewis W. Dilated cardiomyopathy associated with Friedreich's ataxia. Arch Pathol Lab Med. 1985;109(5):454-6.
72. Schadt KA, Friedman LS, Lin KY. Cross-sectional analysis of electrocardiograms in a large heterogeneous cohort of Friedreich ataxia subjects. J Child Neurol. 2012;27(9): 1187-92.
73. Albano LM, Nishioka SA, Moyses RL, et al. Friedreich's ataxia. Cardiac evaluation of 25 patients with clinical diagnosis and literature review. Arq Bras Cardiol. 2002;78(5):448-51.
74. Payne RM. The heart in Friedreich's Ataxia: Basic Findings and Clinical Implications. Prog Pediatr Cardiol. 2011; 31(2): 103–109.
75. Harding AE, Hewer RL. The heart disease of Friedreich's ataxia: a clinical and electrocardiographic study of 115 patients, with an analysis of serial electrocardiographic changes in 30 cases. Q J Med. 1983;52(208):489-502.
76. Giunta A, Maione S, Biagini R, et al. Noninvasive assessment of systolic and diastolic function in 50 patients with Friedreich's ataxia. Cardiology. 1988;75(5):321-7.

77. Panas M, Gialafos E, Spengos K, et al. Prevalence of interatrial block in patients with Friedreich's ataxia. Int J Cardiol. 2010;145(2):386-7.
78. Lagedrost SH, Sutton MSJ, Cohen MS, et al. Idebenone in Friedreich ataxia cardiomyopathy—results from a 6-month phase III study (IONIA). Am Heart J. 2011;161(3):639-45.
79. Child JS, Perloff JK, Bach PM, et al. Cardiac involvement in Friedreich's ataxia: A clinical study of 75 patients. J Am Coll Cardiol. 1986;7(6):1370-78.
80. Schulz JB, Boesch S, Burk K, et al. Diagnosis and treatment of Friedreich ataxia: a European perspective. Nat Rev Neurol. 2009;5(4):222-34.
81. Cheng TO. Pseudoinfarctions. Circulation. 2001;103(12):e69.
82. Butman SM, Phibbs B, Wild J. One heart, two bodies: insight from the transplanted heart and its new electrocardiogram. Am J Cardiol. 1990;66(5):632-5.
83. Gao SZ, Hunt SA, Wiederhold V, et al. Characteristics of serial electrocardiograms in heart transplant recipients. Am Heart J. 1991;122(3 Pt 1):771-4.
84. Glshayan D, Seydoux C, Berguer DG, et al. Incidence and prognostic value of electrocardiographic abnormalities after heart transplantation. Clin Cardiol. 1998;21(9):680-4.
85. Ghany RA, de Marchena E. Two Hearts. N Engl J Med. 2007;356:e6.

Chapter 22

Effects of Various Drugs on the Electrocardiogram

INTRODUCTION

The use of various medications is associated with characteristic changes on electrocardiogram (ECG). These changes may occur with either therapeutic or toxic blood levels. Probably the most classic of these medications is digoxin, the use of which is known to cause different ECG changes with different blood levels. β-Blockers (BBs), antiarrhythmic medications, calcium-channel blockers, several antibiotics, and tricyclic antidepressants (TCAs) may have profound effects on the surface electrocardiogram.

DIGITALIS

Digitalis (Digoxin) is widely used for patients with heart failure and atrial fibrillation (AF). Digoxin is usually indicated in patients with heart failure with impaired left ventricular (LV) systolic function. Digoxin is also indicated in patients with AF, with or without heart failure and a rapid ventricular response. Therapeutic doses of digoxin have a predominantly parasympathomimetic action on atrial myocardium, slowing conduction, and prolonging atrioventricular (AV) node refractory period. There are practically no electrophysiological effects on the Purkinje system. Although digoxin intoxication may produce lethal arrhythmias, therapeutic doses do not appear to increase arrhythmias in the absence of ischemia.[1,2]

A distinction should be made between a digoxin effect (sagging of the ST segments), digoxin excess (second degree AV block), and digoxin intoxication (ventricular arrhythmias). The usual therapeutic range for digoxin is 0.5–2 ng/mL. Its half-life: 36 hours and toxic level: more than 2 ng/mL. Serum levels of digitalis (digoxin) usually do not correlate with toxicity or with therapeutic effect. The patient may be toxic at low levels but response may be subtherapeutic even at high levels. So history and ECG findings are very important to make the proper diagnosis of digitalis toxicity.[2,3]

Digoxin Effect[4-6]

There are six findings on ECG those are consistent with the presence of digoxin (e.g., digoxin effect), yet do not correlate with digoxin toxicity.

1. The earliest finding is that of T-wave changes of virtually any form, from flattening to inversion (that can simulate acute ischemia or pericarditis).
2. The second finding is QT-interval shortening from a decrease in ventricular repolarization time.
3. The third finding is the classic "sagging" or "scooped" appearance of the ST segment with concomitant ST-segment depression (Figs. 22.1 and 22.2). This finding is more pronounced in leads with tall R waves, such as the lateral leads. ST-segment changes are also seen as a downward sloping ST-segment depression, which is often associated with T-wave flattening. This classic digoxin effect is called the "reverse tick sign" (Figs. 22.3 to 22.5A and B) phenomenon (resembles the tick made by a left-handed person).

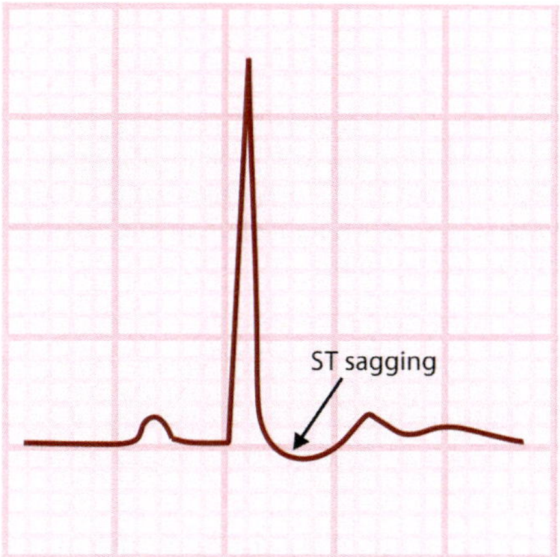

Fig. 22.1: Schematic representation of ST-segment sagging. This type of downsloping ST depression with a characteristic "sagging" appearance is a sign of digoxin effect.

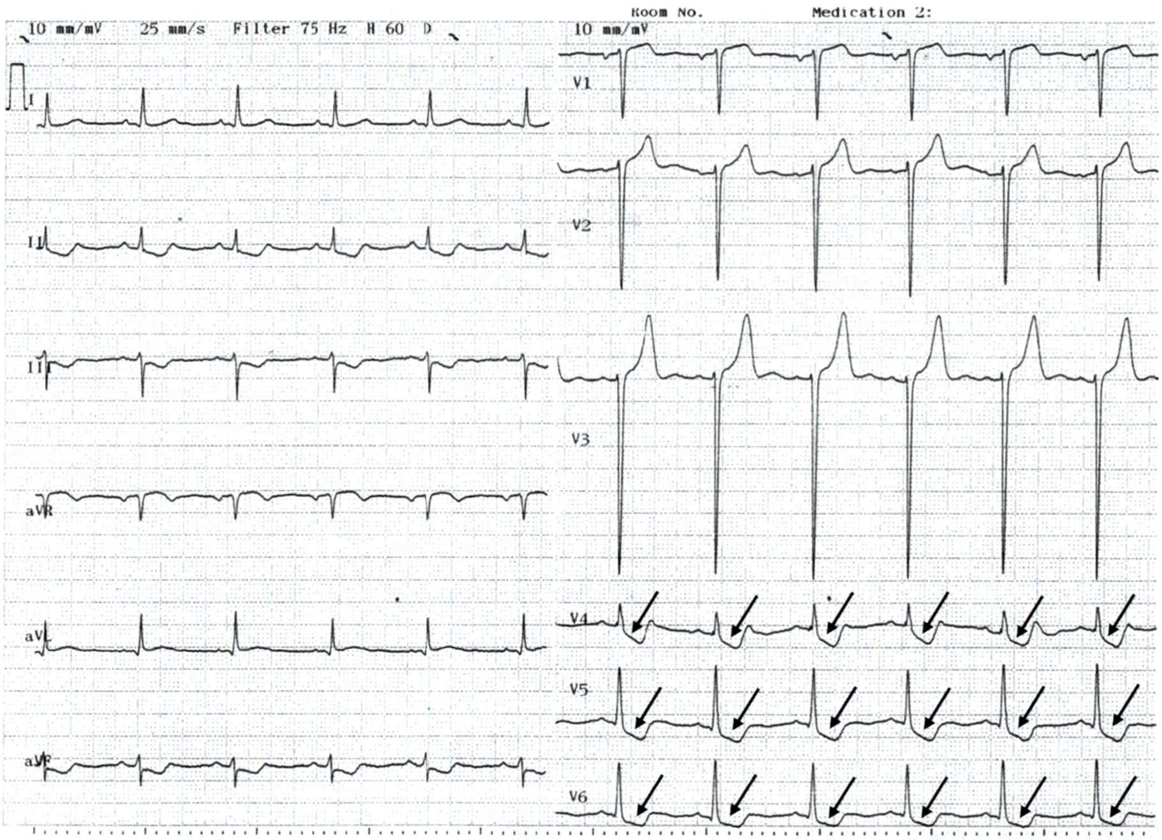

Fig. 22.2: Electrocardiogram (ECG) illustrates the features of ST-segment "sagging" as a sign of digoxin effect. Note "scooped" appearance of the ST segment with concomitant ST-segment depression in leads V4–V6 (arrows) on the ECG of a patient of dilated cardiomyopathy who was on digoxin. ST sagging is a sign of digoxin effect not toxicity.

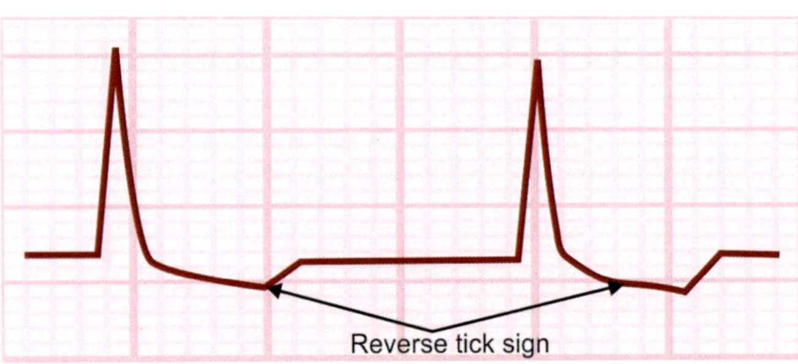

Fig. 22.3: Schematic representation of "reverse tick sign". ST segment changes are seen as a downward sloping ST-segment depression, which is often associated with T-wave flattening. This classic digoxin effect is called the "reverse tick sign" phenomenon (resembles the tick made by a left-handed person).

4. Digitalis can result in PR-interval prolongation as a result of slowing conduction through the AV node (Fig. 22.6).
5. Electrocardiogram may display an increase in the U-wave amplitude.
6. Sinus bradycardia (Fig. 22.6).

In patients with ventricular hypertrophy or bundle-branch block, the above repolarization abnormalities may be masked. However, a definite sagging of the ST segment with an upward concavity is still highly suggestive of digitalis effect even in this setting (Fig. 22.7). Additionally, in left bundle branch block or LV hypertrophy where the QT interval is prolonged, a shortened or normal interval suggests digitalis effect.[4]

The presence of digoxin effect on the ECG is not a marker of digoxin toxicity. It merely indicates that the patient is taking digoxin.

ECG Manifestations of Digitalis Toxicity

Digitalis can produce virtually any type of cardiac arrhythmia, although rapid atrial fibrillation/flutter and bundle-branch block are rare.

Increased Automaticity

As a result of increased automaticity, ectopy is a common manifestation of digitalis toxicity. Premature ventricular complexes (PVCs), both unifocal and multifocal, are often the earliest dysrhythmia associated with digitalis intoxication, and account for half of the arrhythmias associated with digoxin (Fig. 22.8).[4]

Conduction Block

Depressed conduction is a predominant feature of digoxin toxicity. Conduction block in this setting can be of any

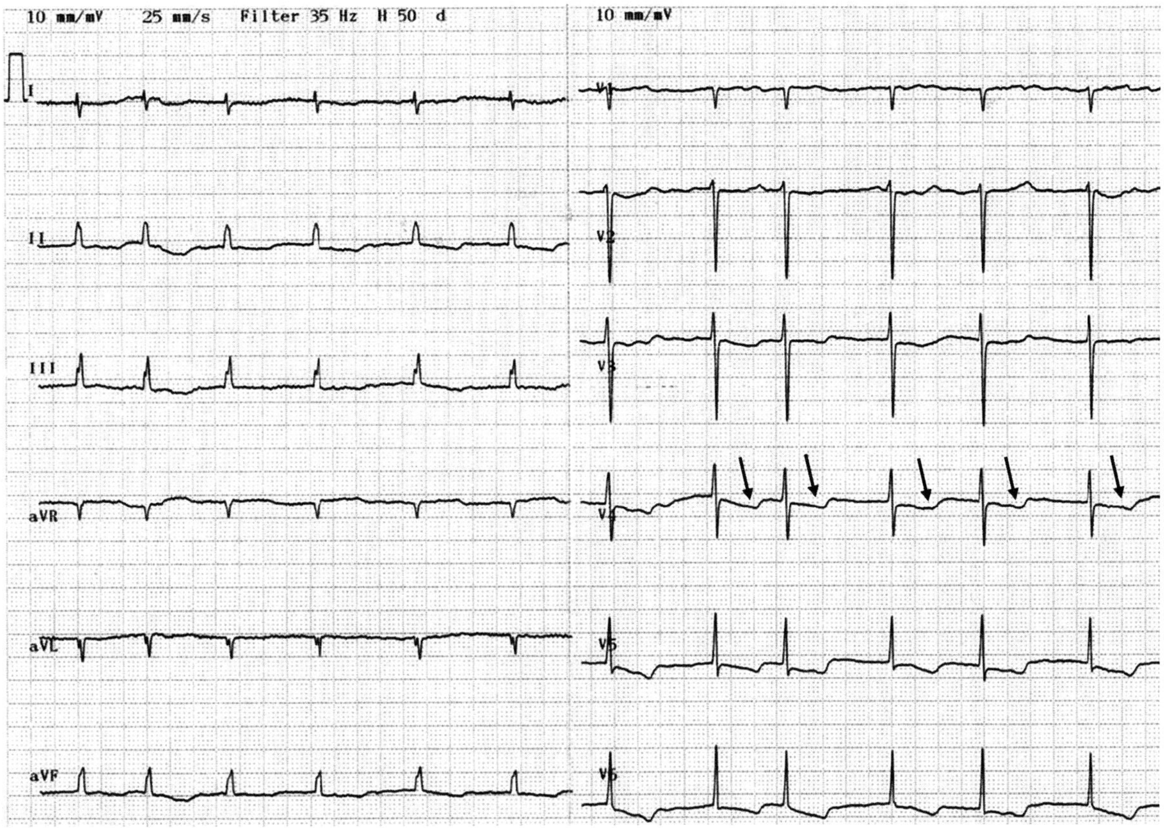

Fig. 22.4: Electrocardiogram displaying "reverse tick sign" (arrows) with atrial fibrillation. Patient was on digoxin for heart failure. Reverse tick sign is a sign of digitalis effect not toxicity.

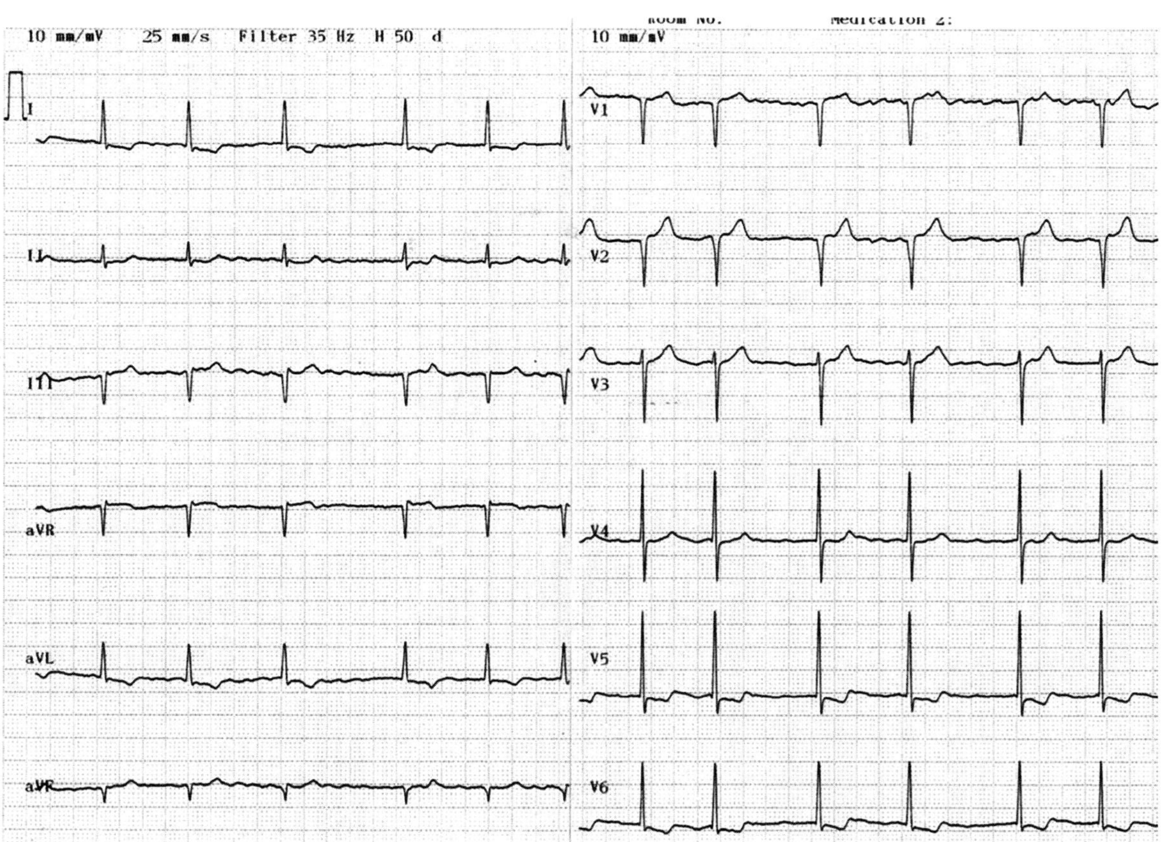

Fig. 22.5A: Electrocardiogram displaying "reverse tick sign," most prominent in leads L1, aVL, and V5–V6 in a patient with atrial fibrillation who was on digoxin.

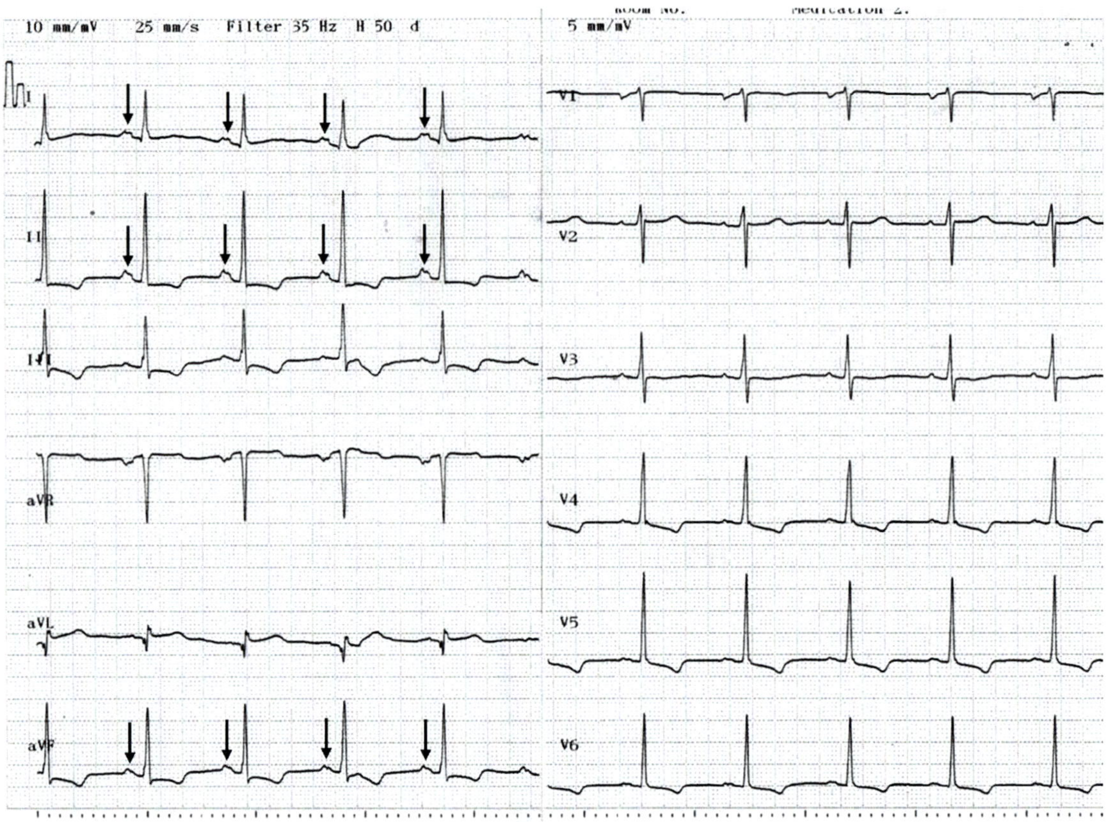

Fig. 22.5B: ECG displaying "reverse tick sign" on the ECG of a patient with mitral stenosis who was on digoxin. Note prominent reverse tick sign in LII, LIII, aVF, and V4–V6. Also note ECG evidence of P mitrale [broad and bifid P waves in LI, LII, and aVF (arrows) along with biphasic P-wave with terminal negative portion > 1 mm deep in lead V1)]

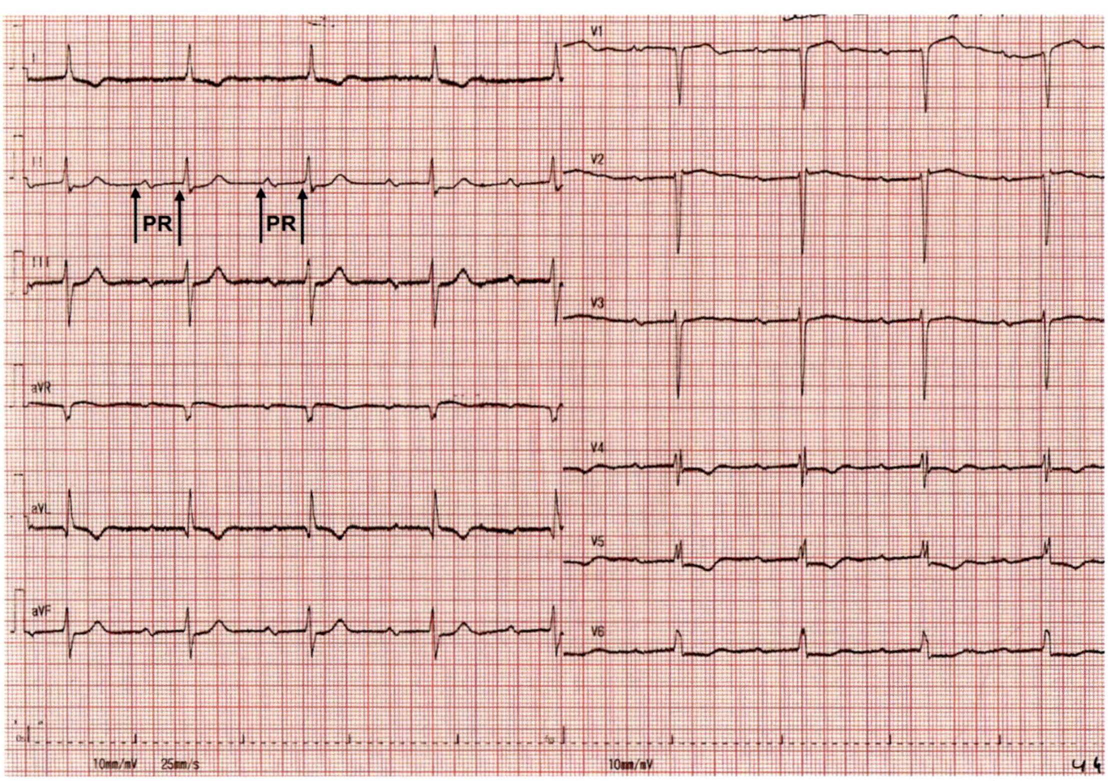

Fig. 22.6: Electrocardiogram is consistent with marked sinus bradycardia (heart rate is 44 bpm) with first-degree heart block (PR interval is 360 ms). Sinus bradycardia with PR-interval prolongation are signs of digitalis effect not toxicity.

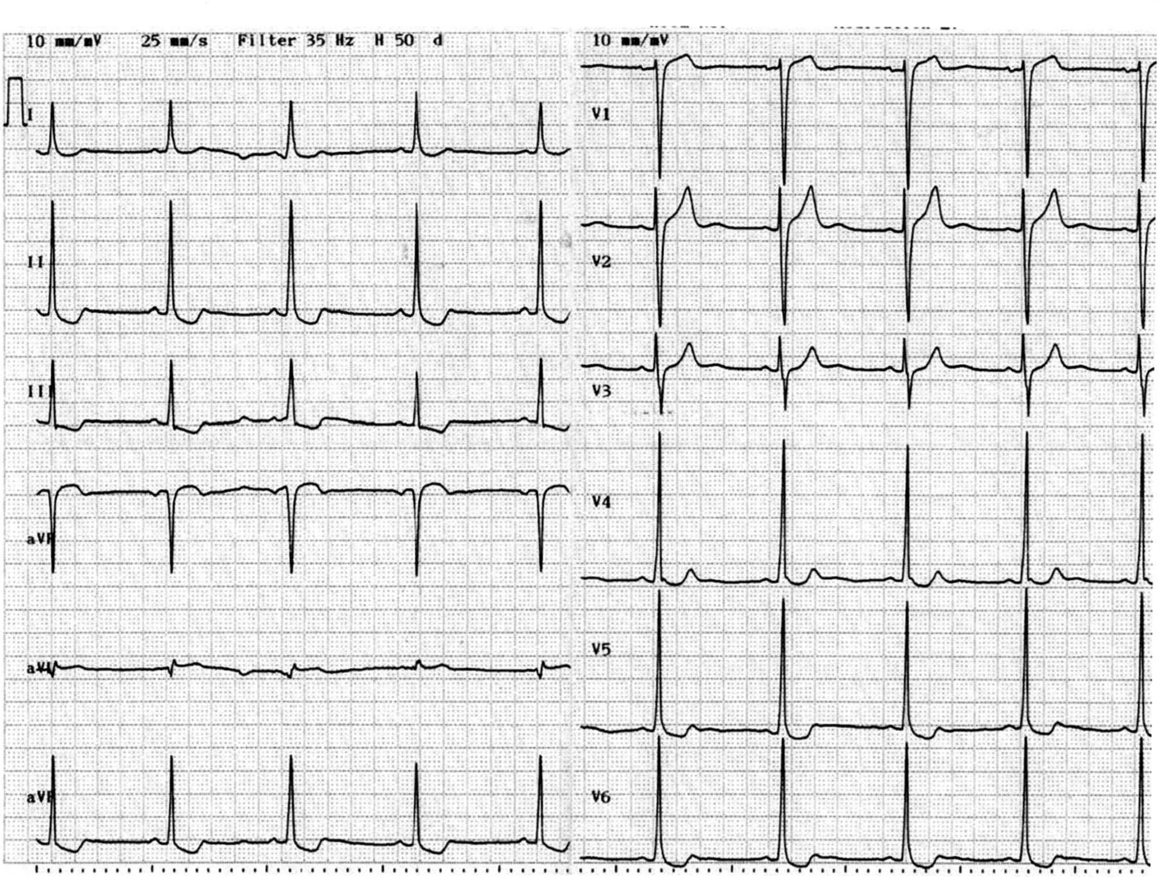

Fig. 22.7: Electrocardiogram illustrates the features of ST-segment "sagging" in presence of left ventricular hypertrophy (LVH) voltage criteria. Note "scooped" appearance of the ST segment with concomitant ST-segment depression in leads LII, LIII, aVF, and V4–V6 suggestive of digoxin effect.

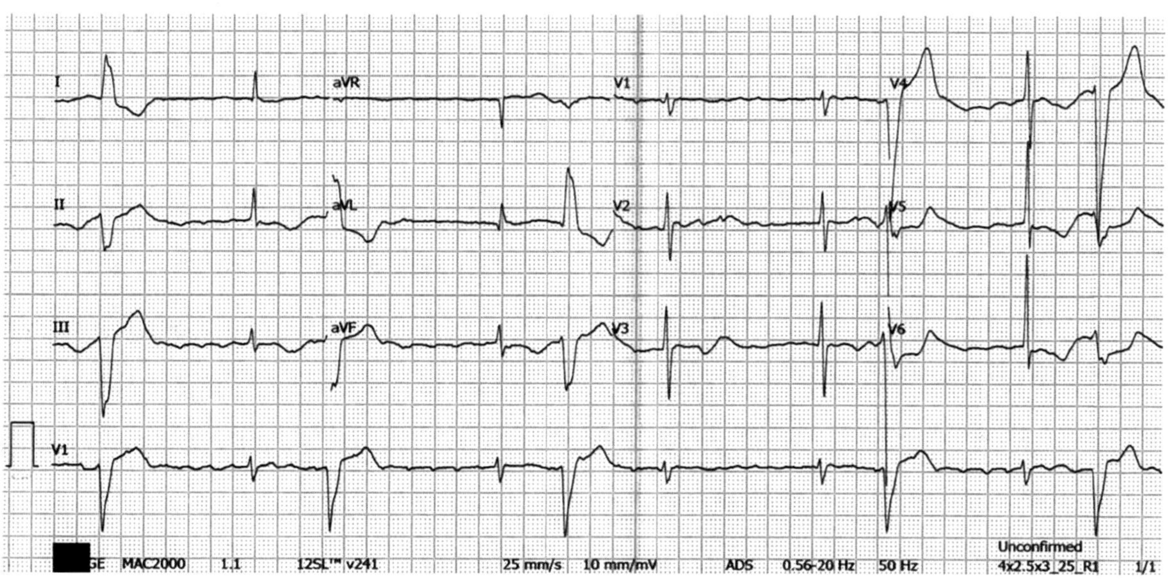

Fig. 22.8: This ECG illustrates the features of digoxin toxicity with marked bradycardia with frequent premature ventricular complexes (PVCs). This patient, a known case of atrial fibrillation with chronic kidney disease was on digoxin 0.125 mg per day. In digoxin toxicity, the finding of frequent PVCs is the most common and the earliest dysrhythmia.

degree from first-degree AV block to complete heart block, though Mobitz type II is considered rare (Fig. 22.9). In addition, sinus bradycardia, from increased vagal tone, and other bradydysrhythmias are very common. Sinoatrial (SA) arrest has been reported, although rarely. Digitalis has little effect on the bundle branches and consequently, bundle-branch block is not believed to be attributable to digoxin.[7]

Along with increased ventricular ectopy and conduction block, the three classically described dysrhythmias that should immediately suggest digitalis intoxication include

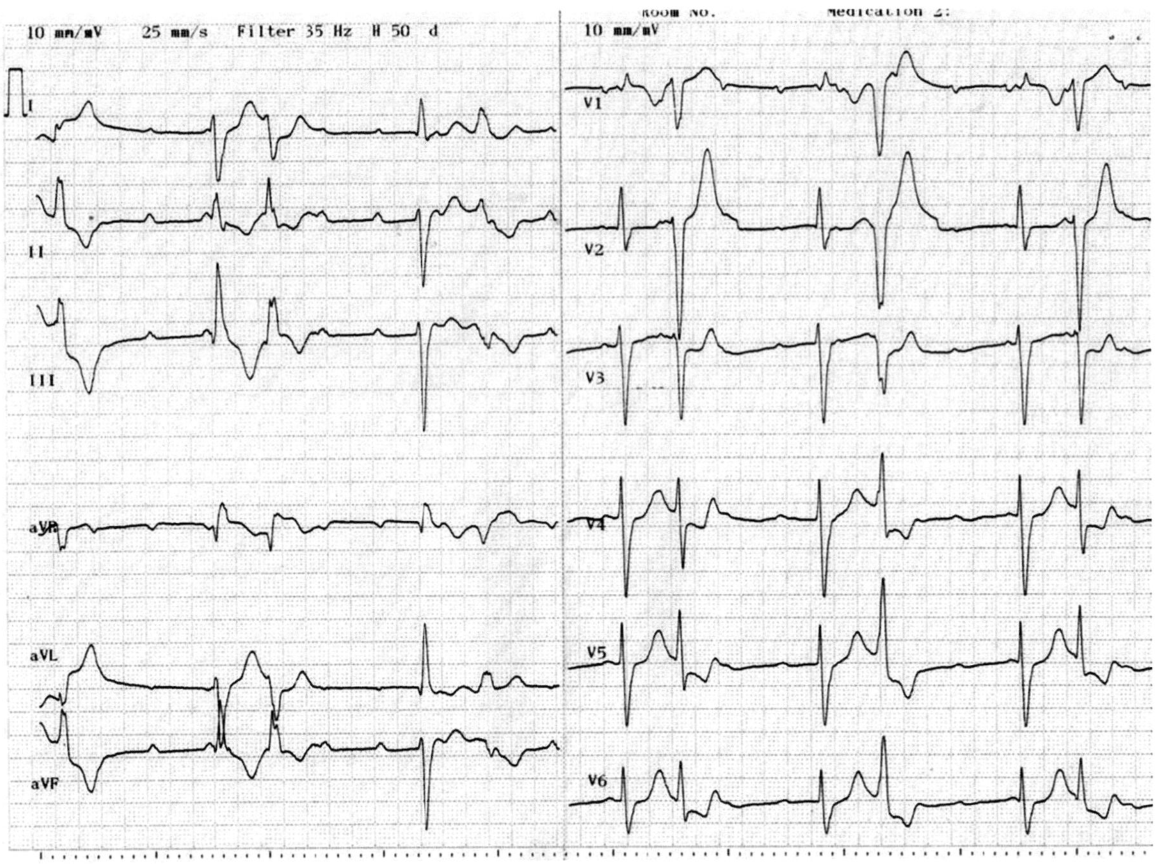

Fig. 22.9: Electrocardiogram demonstrates digoxin induced complete heart block with frequent ventricular escape beats of multifocal origin. Note PP intervals are regular but PR intervals are nor regular. This patient with dilated cardiomyopathy was on digoxin 0.25 mg per day for the treatment of heart failure.

paroxysmal atrial tachycardia (PAT) with block, junctional (AV nodal) tachycardia, and ventricular tachycardia (VT).[8]

In digoxin toxicity, the finding of frequent PVCs is the most common and the earliest dysrhythmia. In addition, depressed conduction is a predominant feature of digoxin toxicity. Other ECG changes that suggest digoxin toxicity include ventricular bigeminal or trigeminal rhythms and bidirectional VT.

TRICYCLIC ANTIDEPRESSANTS

The TCAs, e.g. amitriptyline, imipramine, and nortriptyline are used primarily in the clinical treatment of major depressive disorder. These drugs have profound effects on ECG in high doses. TCAs produce cardiac effects by their sodium-channel blocking properties. Tachycardia, hypotension, and seizures are the common presenting features.

Electrocardiogram findings that can be observed in TCA toxicity include sinus tachycardia, prolongation of the PR interval, QRS prolongation, and long QTc intervals, nonspecific ST-segment, and T-wave changes. Downsloping ST-segment elevation in leads V1–V3 in association with right bundle branch block (Brugada pattern) may also be noted.[9-11] Tall secondary R-wave in aVR (terminal R-wave > 3 mm in aVR), a finding has an 83% sensitivity and 63% specificity for TCA toxicity (Fig. 22.10). The degree of QRS broadening on the ECG is correlated with adverse events—seizures and ventricular arrhythmias, e.g. VT. QRS duration >100 ms is predictive of seizures and arrhythmias.

β-BLOCKERS

Beta-adrenergic antagonists competitively antagonize the effects of catecholamines at the β-adrenergic receptor and blunt the chronotropic and inotropic response to catecholamines.[12] Most beta-blockers (BBs) cause sinus bradycardia and first-degree heart block but ECG changes from BB overdose may include: (1) progressively worsening sinus bradycardia (Fig. 22.11), (2) increased PR intervals, (3) loss of atrial activity, (4) AV junctional rhythm, (5) widening of the QRS complex, (6) AV block, (7) idioventricular rhythm, and (8) rarely asystole.[13]

In acute BB overdose, the most pronounced effects are bradycardia (from decreased SA node function), varying degrees of AV block, and hypotension. Inhibition of the conducting system most commonly causes first-degree AV block, but higher levels of toxicity can promote second- and third-degree AV blocks, junctional rhythms, and intraventricular conduction delays.[12-14]

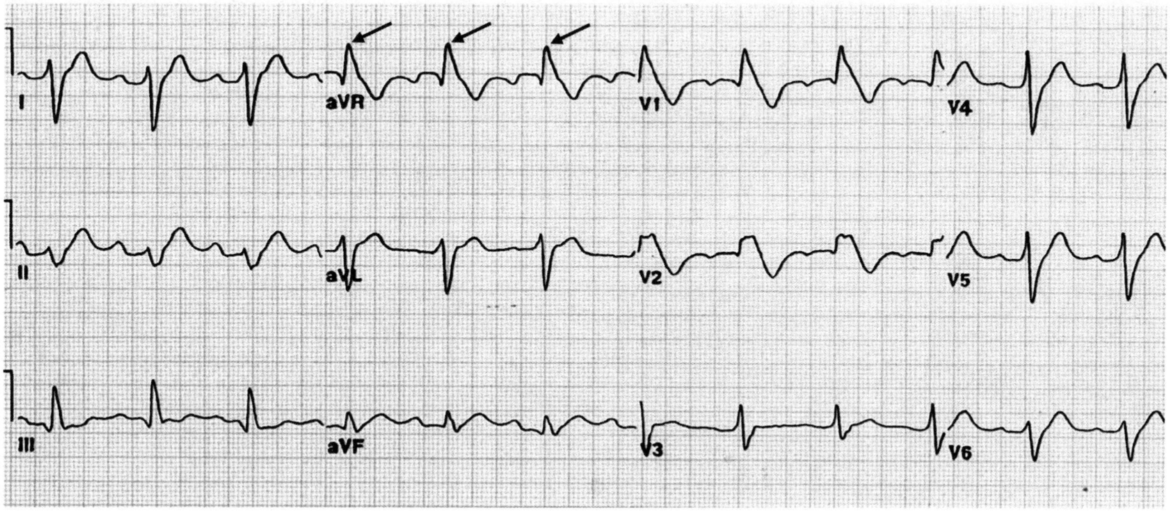

Fig. 22.10: This ECG illustrates the typical electrocardiographic features of tricyclic antidepressant (TCA) drug overdose. ECG shows evidence of first-degree heart block (PR interval is 320 ms), broadening of QRS complexes (QRS duration is 150 ms) with prominent terminal R-wave in aVR (arrows). Sinus tachycardia is not represented on this ECG, which is a common manifestation of TCA overdose. Due to TCA induced QRS prolongation, sinus tachycardia in this setting may be misdiagnosed as ventricular tachycardia. So, clinicians must be cautious during interpreting the ECG of TCA overdose when ECG shows tachycardia with wide QRS complex.

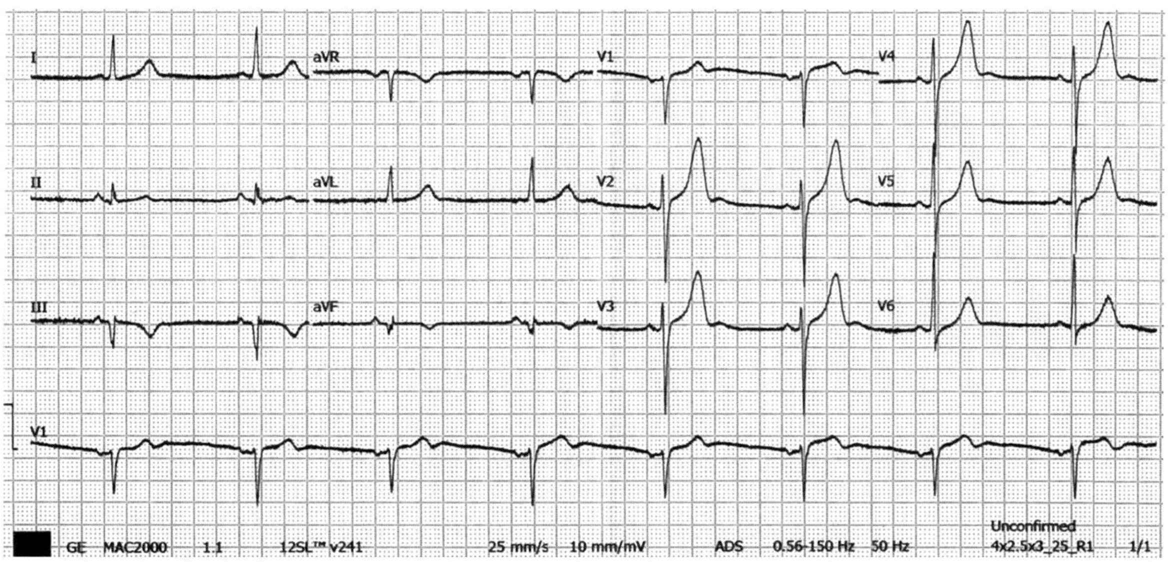

Fig. 22.11: Electrocardiogram is consistent with sinus bradycardia (heart rate is 48 bpm) induced by β-blocker in a patient with previous inferior myocardial infarction. Note pathological Q waves in LII, LIII, and aVF.

Some BB is known to prolong QTc intervals, e.g. sotalol and acebutolol. Sotalol blocks potassium channels, thereby prolong the action potential and the repolarization duration. The prolongation of the QTc interval predisposes the patient to ventricular tachyarrhythmias and torsades de pointes (TdP), which have been described after both sotalol overdose and therapeutic administration.[15-18]

VERAPAMIL

The mechanism of action of this drug is by inhibition of slow calcium channels in the myocardial cell membrane. This causes slowing of the sinus rate, thus bradycardia and AV conduction delay (hence, a prolonged PR interval) (Fig. 22.12). Slow calcium-channel blockers inhibit the slow inward calcium current, which may prolong conduction and refractoriness in the AV node. The increase in PR interval caused by verapamil is minimal, and at doses of less than 480 mg/d, AV block occurs infrequently. When AV block occurs, it is first-degree block in most patients, and it is usually asymptomatic. The electrophysiologic effects of diltiazem are similar to those of verapamil. There is no change in the QRS complex or the corrected QT interval. The effects of verapamil on the SA and AV nodes are additive with β-blocking drugs. The use of these two together can give rise to catastrophic bradycardias.

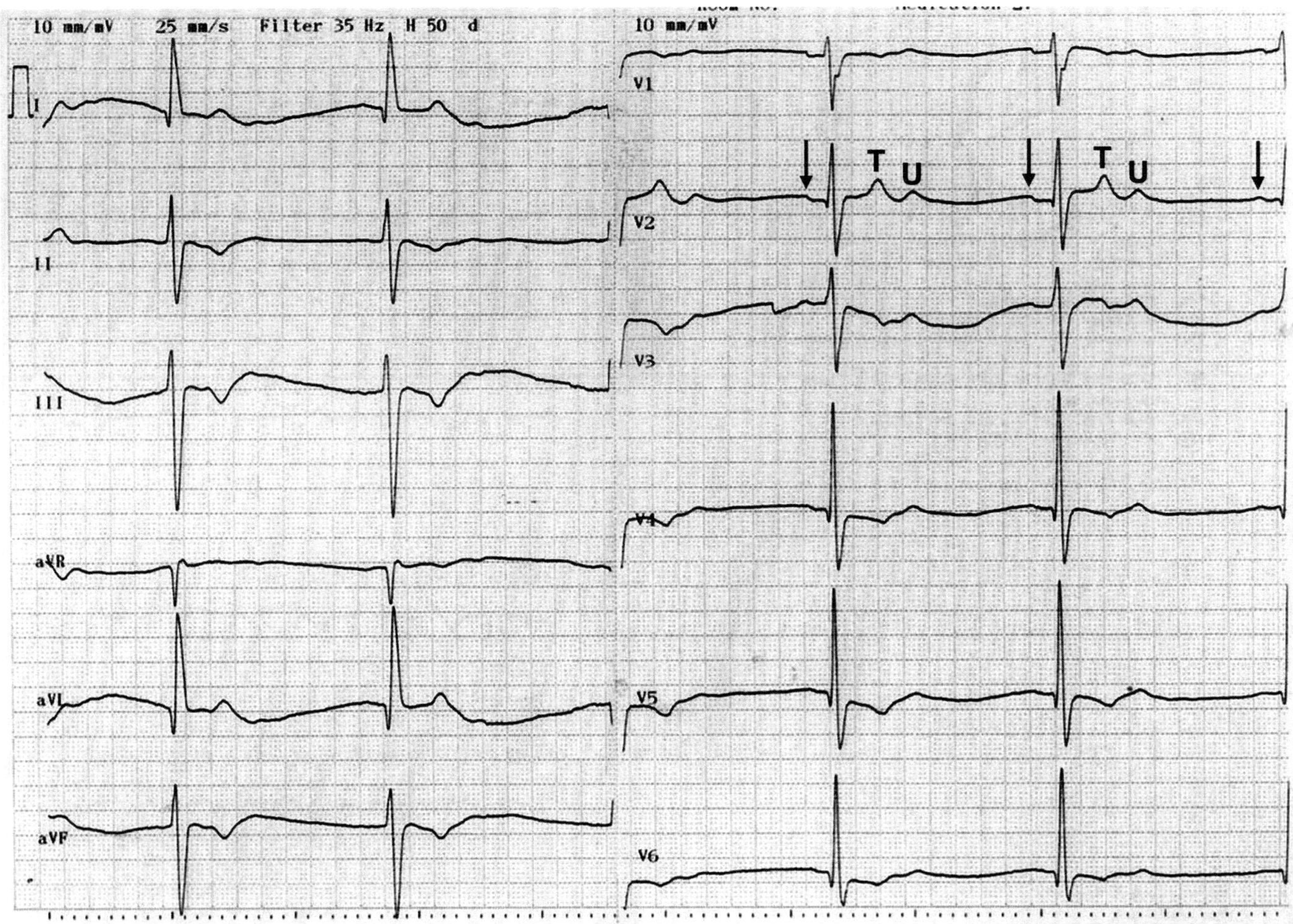

Fig. 22.12: Electrocardiogram shows severe sinus bradycardia (heart rate is 34 bpm) induced by verapamil. Note all the QRS complexes are preceded by a P-wave (arrows), so the rhythm is sinus. Also note prolonged PR interval (PR interval is 240 ms) and prominent U waves in most of the leads.

FLUOROQUINOLONES

Although being very useful agents, fluoroquinolones are associated with a number of adverse events, some with considerable clinical significance. Prolongation of the QT interval, for example, is an adverse effect associated with the use of fluoroquinolones. Fluoroquinolones prolong the QT interval by blocking voltage-gated potassium channels. Moxifloxacin carries the greatest risk of QT prolongation from all available quinolones in clinical practice and it should be used with caution in patients with predisposing factors for TdP. Although gemifloxacin, levofloxacin, and ofloxacin are associated with a lower risk of QT prolongation compared with moxifloxacin, they should also be used with caution in patients at risk for QT prolongation. Ciprofloxacin appears to be associated with the lowest risk for QT prolongation and the lowest TdP rate.[19]

MACROLIDE ANTIBIOTICS

Macrolide antibiotics (erythromycin, clarithromycin, and azithromycin) appear to be associated with the greatest degree of QTc interval prolongation and risk for TdP. A comparative pharmacodynamic study listed the rank order of arrhythmogenic potential to be erythromycin greater than clarithromycin greater than azithromycin.[20]

Macrolides may cause QT prolongation and TdP if used in patients with additional risk factors. Erythromycin has been most frequently implicated, followed by clarithromycin. Azithromycin has less association with QT prolongation. In addition, oral macrolide administration is associated with less risk of QT prolongation because bioavailability is 50%; thus, decreasing the amount of drug exposure.[21]

ANTIARRHYTHMIC DRUGS

Prolongation of the QTc interval has been associated with proarrhythmia, resulting in a potentially fatal form of polymorphic VT (TdP). Class Ia (quinidine, procainamide, and disopyramide), class Ic (flecainide and propafenone), and class III (sotalol, amiodarone, dofetilide, and ibutilide) drugs have been associated with QT prolongation and TdP due to their mechanism of action of delaying repolarization and slowing cardiac conduction.[21-23] Among the antiarrhythmics, amiodarone is known to have a low-risk of TdP because it blocks the potassium channels in concentrations that exceed therapeutic levels and has multiple mechanisms including blockage of calcium channels.[21,23] The risk of TdP was found to be highest within the first few days of initiation of an anti-arrhythmic drug.[24]

SUMMARY

Digitalis (Digoxin) is widely used for patients with heart failure and AF. Electrocardiogram changes typical for digoxin effects:

- Oddly shaped ST-depression with "ST sagging" ("scooped out" appearance of the ST segment).
- Flat, negative or biphasic T-wave
- Short QT interval
- Reverse tick sign
- Prolonged PR interval
- Sinus bradycardia.

Electrocardiogram changes typical for digoxin toxicity:

- Bradyarrhythmias: Atrioventricular block, which includes complete AV block and Wenckebach phenomenon
- Tachyarrhythmias:
  - Junctional tachycardia
  - Atrial tachycardia
  - Ventricular ectopics, bigeminy, monomorphic VT, bidirectional VT, and ventricular fibrillation.

Digoxin effects on the baseline ECG include downward scooping of the ST segment (ST sagging) and inverted T waves. These findings are not indicative of toxicity. New QRS prolongation, varying degrees of AV block, and arrhythmias may signify digoxin toxicity. Comparison with previous ECGs is helpful.

In digoxin toxicity, the finding of frequent premature ventricular complexes (PVCs) is the most common and the earliest dysrhythmia.

Tricyclic Antidepressants

Tricyclic antidepressant produces cardiac effects by their sodium-channel blocking properties. Tachycardia, hypotension, and seizures are the common presenting features. ECG features of TCAs overdose include:

- Sinus tachycardia
- Intraventricular conduction delay(QRS > 100 ms)
- Prolonged QT interval
- Terminal R-wave >3 mm in aVR.

Duration of QRS >100 ms precipitates ventricular arrhythmias.

β-Blockers

Most beta-blockers (BBs) cause sinus bradycardia and first-degree heart block. Though inhibition of the conducting system most commonly causes first-degree AV block, but overdose of BB can promote second- and third-degree AV blocks, junctional rhythms, and intraventricular conduction delays.

A prolonged QT interval has been observed after sotalol use. Sotalol blocks myocardial potassium channels, causing QT prolongation and torsades de pointes (TdP) in overdose.

Verapamil

Verapamil causes slowing of the sinus rate, thus sinus bradycardia and AV conduction defects, hence, a prolonged PR interval. The effects of verapamil on the SA and AV nodes are additive with β-blocking drugs. The use of these two together can give rise to catastrophic bradycardias.

Fluoroquinolones

Fluoroquinolones prolong the QT interval and predispose the patient to polymorphic VT (TdP) and cardiac arrest. Moxifloxacin carries the greatest risk of QT prolongation from all available quinolones and ciprofloxacin appears to be associated with the lowest risk for QT prolongation and the lowest TdP rate.

Macrolide Antibiotics

Macrolide antibiotics (erythromycin, clarithromycin, and azithromycin) appear to be associated with the QTc interval prolongation and risk for TdP. Erythromycin has been most frequently implicated, followed by clarithromycin. Azithromycin has less association with QT prolongation and thus TdP.

Antiarrhythmic Drugs

Antiarrhythmic drugs (e.g. quinidine, sotalol, amiodarone, disopyramide, etc.) have been associated with QT prolongation and TdP due to their mechanism of action of delaying repolarization and slowing cardiac conduction. Among the antiarrhythmics, amiodarone is known to have a low-risk of TdP.

REFERENCES

1. Gheorghiade M, Adams KF, Colucci WS. Digoxin in the management of cardiovascular disorders. Circulation. 2004;109:2959-64.
2. Lown B, Graboys TB, Podrid PJ, et al. Effect of a digitalis drug on ventricular premature beats. N Engl J Med. 1977;296(6):301-6.
3. Ma G, Brady WJ, Pollack M, et al. Electrocardiographic manifestations: Digitalis toxicity. J Emerg Med. 2001;20(2):145-52.
4. Levine HD, Angelakos ET. Late peaking of the T wave as a digitalis effect. Am Heart J. 1964;68(3):320-4.
5. Irons GV, Orgain ES. Digitalis-induced arrhythmias and their management. Prog Cardiovasc Dis. 1996;8:539-69.

6. Kirilmaz B, Saygi S, Gungor H, et al. Digoxin intoxication: An old enemy in modern era. J Geriatr Cardiol. 2012;9(3): 237-42.
7. Fisch C, Knoebel SB. Digitalis cardiotoxicity. J Am Coll Cardiol. 1985;5(5A):91A-8A.
8. Derlet RW, Horowitz BZ. Cardiotoxic drugs. Emerg Med Clin North Am. 1995;13(4):771-91.
9. Thanacoody HK, Thomas SH. Tricyclic antidepressant poisoning: cardiovascular toxicity. Toxicol Rev. 2005;24(3):205-14.
10. Monteban-Kooistra WE, van den Berg MP, Tulleken JE. Brugada electrocardiographic pattern elicited by cyclic antidepressants overdose. Intensive Care Med. 2006;32(2): 281-5.
11. Goldgran-Toledano D, Sideris G, Kevorkian JP. Overdose of cyclic antidepressants and the Brugada syndrome. N Engl J Med. 2002;346(20):1591-2.
12. Wax PM, Erdman AR, Chyka PA, et al. Beta-blocker ingestion: an evidence-based consensus guideline for out-of-hospital management. Clin Toxicol. 2005;43(3):131-46.
13. Love JN, Enlow B, Howell JM, et al. Electrocardiographic changes associated with beta-blocker toxicity. Ann Emerg Med. 2002;40(6):603-10.
14. Anderson AC. Management of beta-adrenergic blocker poisoning. Clin Pediatr Emerg Med. 2008;9(1):4-16.
15. Delk C, Holstege CP, Brady WJ. Electrocardiographic abnormalities associated with poisoning. Am J Emerg Med. 2007;25(6):672-87.
16. Lionte C, Bologa C, Sorodoc L. (2012). Toxic and drug-induced changes of the electrocardiogram. In: Millis R (Ed). Advances in Electrocardiograms-Clinical Applications. Rijeka: InTech; 2012.
17. Yap YG, Camm AJ. Drug induced QT prolongation and torsades de pointes. Heart. 2003;89(11):1363-72.
18. Dapro B. Spectrum of drugs prolonging QT interval and the incidence of torsades de pointes. Eur Heart J. 2001;3(Suppl K):K70-80.
19. Briasoulis A, Agarwal V, Pierce WJ. QT prolongation and torsade de pointes induced by fluoroquinolones: infrequent side effects from commonly used medications. Cardiology. 2011;120(2):103-10.
20. Ohtani H, Taninaka C, Hanada E, et al. Comparative pharmacodynamic analysis of QT interval prolongation induced by the macrolides clarithromycin, roxithromycin, and azithromycin. Chemotherapy. 2000;44:2630-7.
21. Nelson S, Leung J. QTc prolongation in the intensive care unit: a review of offending agents. AACN Adv Crit Care. 2011;22(4):289-95.
22. Heist EK, Ruskin JN. Drug-induced arrhythmia. Circulation. 2010;122(14):1426-35.
23. van Noord C, Eijgelsheim M, Stricker BH. Drug- and non-drug-associated QT interval prolongation. Br J Clin Pharmacol. 2010;70(1):16-23.
24. Al-Khatib SM, LaPointe NM, Kramer JM, et al. What clinicians should know about the QT interval. JAMA.2003;289(16): 2120-7.

Chapter 23

Electrocardiogram Features of Congenital Heart Diseases

INTRODUCTION

Congenital heart diseases are the most common type of birth defects and affect 8 out of every 1,000 newborns. They range from simple defects with no symptoms to complex defects with severe, life-threatening symptoms. Common congenital heart diseases include atrial septal defect (ASD), ventricular septal defect (VSD), tetralogy of Fallot (TOF), Ebstein's anomaly, dextrocardia, patent ductus arteriosus (PDA), coarctation of the aorta, pulmonary valve stenosis (PS), aortic valve stenosis (AS), tricuspid atresia, hypoplastic left heart syndrome, total anomalous pulmonary venous connection, transposition of the great arteries, truncus arteriosus, etc. Electrocardiogram (ECG) may be a valuable aid during the initial steps of diagnosis and evaluation of congenital heart diseases.

ATRIAL SEPTAL DEFECT

Atrial septal defects (ASDs) account for about 10–15% of all congenital cardiac anomalies and are the most common congenital cardiac lesion presenting in adults. There are three major types of ASDs or interatrial communications: ostium secundum, ostium primum, and sinus venosus defects. The ostium secundum is a true defect of the atrial septum and involves the region of the fossa ovalis. The ostium primum defect is within the spectrum of the atrioventricular (AV) septal defects; also known as AV canal defects or endocardial cushion defects, the complete form of which also includes a large ventricular septal defect and a common AV valve. The sinus venosus defect is usually located at the junction of the right atrium and superior vena cava and is almost always associated with partial anomalous pulmonary venous return.[1,2] The ostium secundum type defects account for 70% of ASDs and the remaining ASDs are ostium primum type 20%, sinus venosus type ASDs 10% and unroofed coronary sinus, or coronary sinus septal defects, less than1%.[3-6] ASDs are common and can present at any age. Females constitute 65–75% of patients with secundum ASDs, but the gender distribution is equal for sinus venosus and ostium primum ASDs.[2]

The ECG may be an important clue to diagnosis. Size of ASD determines the shunt flow which in turn results in most of the ECG abnormalities. If the ASD is very small, the ECG may be normal. A common finding in the ECG of ASD patient is the presence of incomplete right bundle branch block (RBBB) (Fig. 23.1). The presence of a right bundle branch block is so characteristic that if it is absent, the diagnosis of ASD should be reconsidered.[7-10] An rSr′ or rsR′ QRS configuration is typically seen on the ECG in right precordial leads (Fig. 23.2). This likely reflects right ventricular overload rather than true conduction delay.

The rhythm may be sinus, atrial fibrillation, or atrial flutter. Inverted P-waves in the inferior leads suggest an absent or deficient sinus node, as may be seen in a sinus venosus defect.[11,12] Right atrial overload is often present. First-degree heart block suggests a primum ASD but may be seen in older patients with a secundum ASD. The QRS axis is typically rightward in secundum ASD, markedly so if pulmonary hypertension is present. The QRS axis is leftward or extremely to the right in ostium primum ASDs. Voltage evidence of right ventricular hypertrophy may be seen in ASD, often in the form of 'incomplete' right bundle-branch block, with the more extreme forms usually found in patients with pulmonary hypertension.[2,8-13]

Patients with a secundum ASD may have peaked P-waves in lead II suggesting right atrial enlargement, but in the majority of patients P-wave amplitude and duration are normal.[14] When the left-to-right shunt is significant, there is almost always right ventricular conduction delay and right ventricular overload with an rSr′ pattern in lead V1 (Fig. 23.3).[15] The QRS axis is typically rightward.[7] PR prolongation is seen in 6–19% of patients and uncommonly progresses toward higher-degree AV block, with complete block rarely reported.[16,17] The prolongation of the PR interval is probably due to the enlargement of the atria that is common in ASDs and the increased distance due to the defect itself (Fig. 23.4). Both of these can cause an increased distance of internodal conduction from the SA node to the AV node.

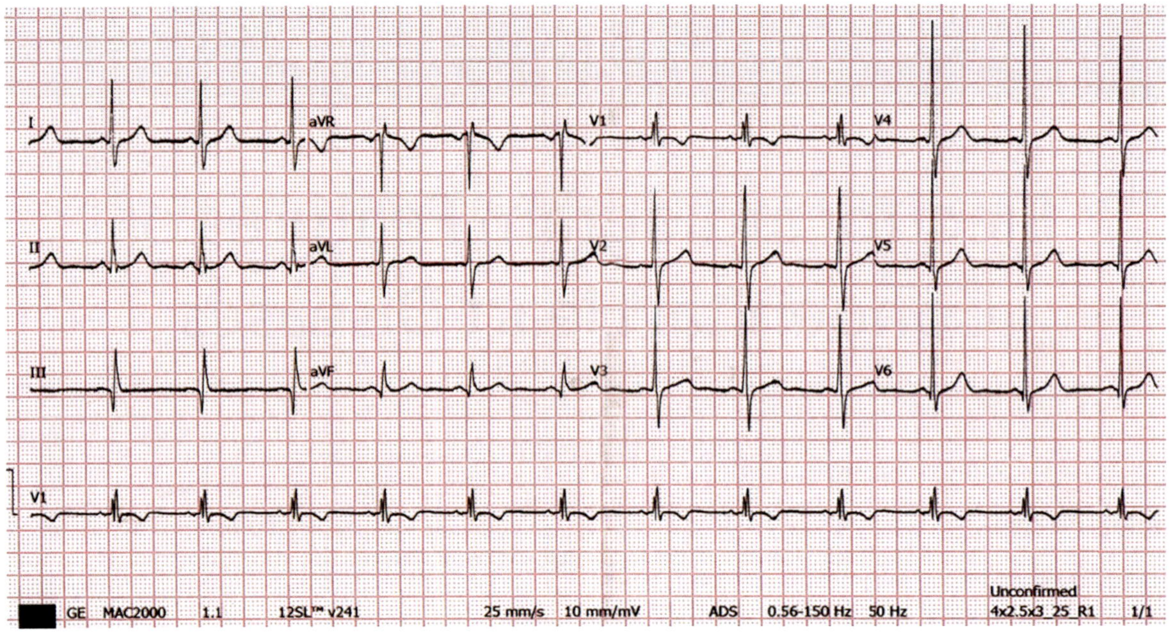

Fig. 23.1: Electrocardiogram (ECG) of a patient with secundum atrial septal defect (ASD) and shows features of incomplete right bundle branch block (RBBB) with rSr' pattern QRS in V1 with QRS duration 96 ms (<120 ms).

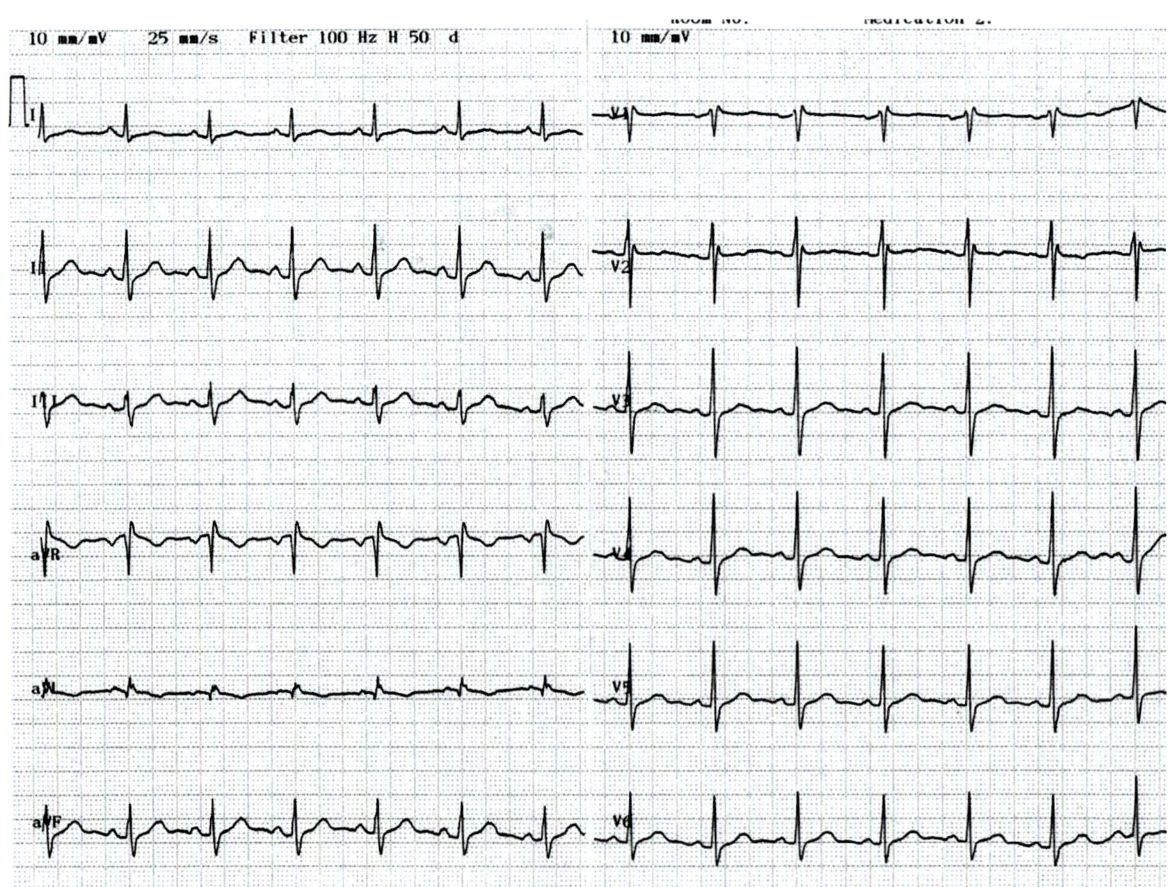

Fig. 23.2: Electrocardiogram of a patient with secundum ASD showing features of incomplete right bundle branch block (RBBB) with rSr' pattern QRS in V1 with QRS duration 90 ms. Also note deep and slurred S waves in leads V5 and V6.

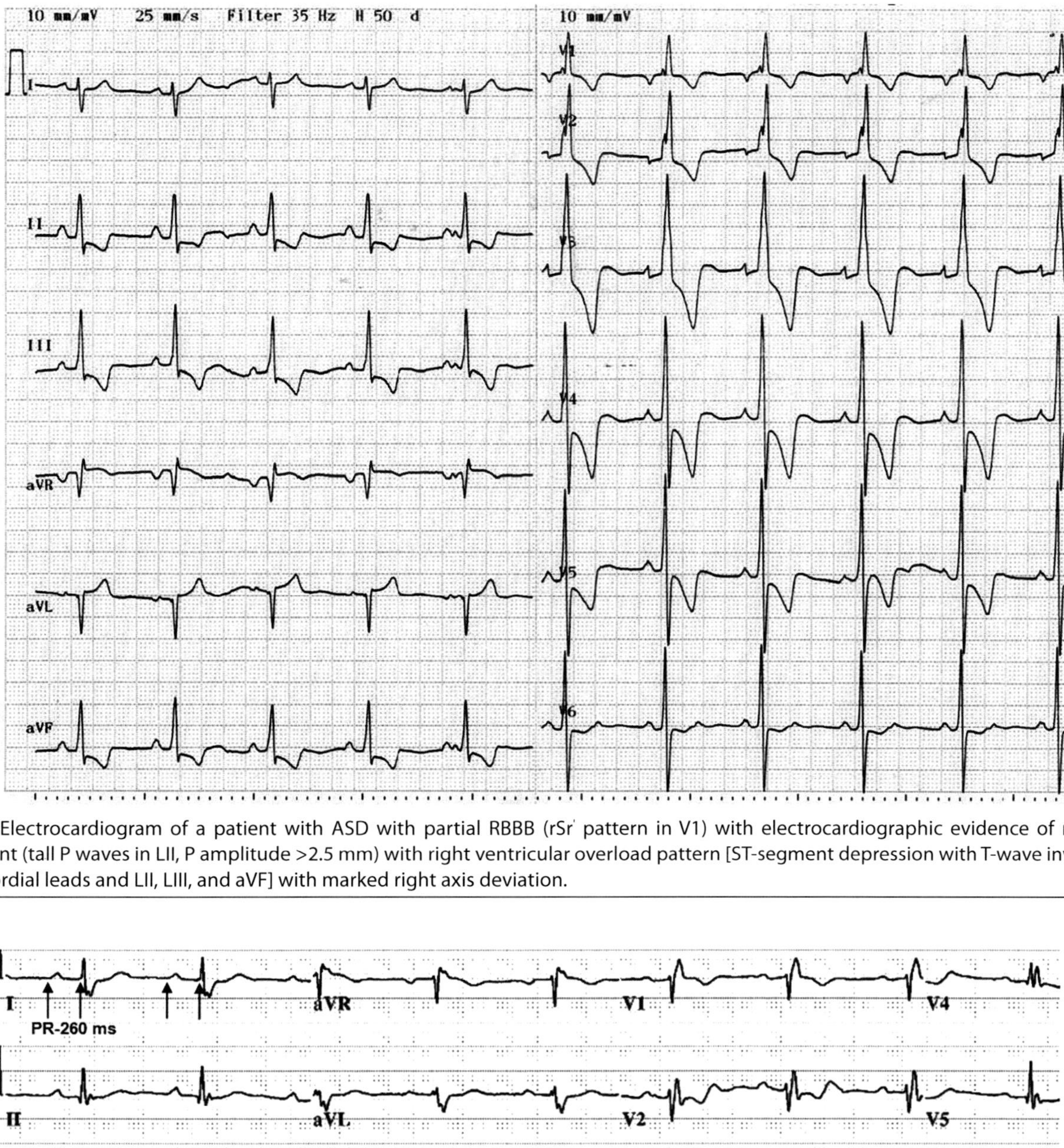

Fig. 23.3: Electrocardiogram of a patient with ASD with partial RBBB (rSr′ pattern in V1) with electrocardiographic evidence of right atrial enlargement (tall P waves in LII, P amplitude >2.5 mm) with right ventricular overload pattern [ST-segment depression with T-wave inversions in right precordial leads and LII, LIII, and aVF] with marked right axis deviation.

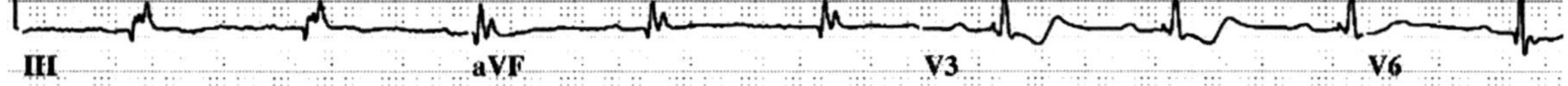

Fig. 23.4: Electrocardiogram of a patient with ASD showing RBBB with first degree AV block (PR interval 260 ms) (arrows). First-degree heart block is probably due to the enlargement of the atria that is common in ASDs and the increased distance due to the defect itself.

Another sign that could be found and which correlates with shunt severity is the 'crochetage sign'.[18,19] In inferior leads, a notch near the apex of the R-wave, coined 'crochetage sign' has been correlated with ASD (Figs. 23.5A and B).[18] In 1,560 adults and adolescents, 73.1% of patients with ASDs displayed this pattern, with a specificity of 92% when present in all inferior limb leads.[19] Its incidence was higher in patients with larger defects and greater left-to-right shunting. Early disappearance was observed in 35.1% of surgically repaired patients, although the right bundle-branch block pattern persisted. In another study, the crochetage sign was observed in at least 1 inferior limb lead in 31.7% of preoperative patients with secundum ASDs. Specificity of the crochetage pattern was 86.1% and >92% when present in at least 1 and in all 3 inferior leads, respectively.[20] On an average this sign involves all 3 inferior leads in 27% of the ASD patients (Figs. 23.6A and B) and involves at least one inferior limb lead in 73% of the patients (Figs. 23.7A and B). Some times Crochetage sign is also noted in the ECGs of ventricular septal defects (VSDs) and pulmonary stenosis (PS).

The ECG can provide clues to differentiate the various types of ASDs (Box 23.1). The distinctive feature of an ostium

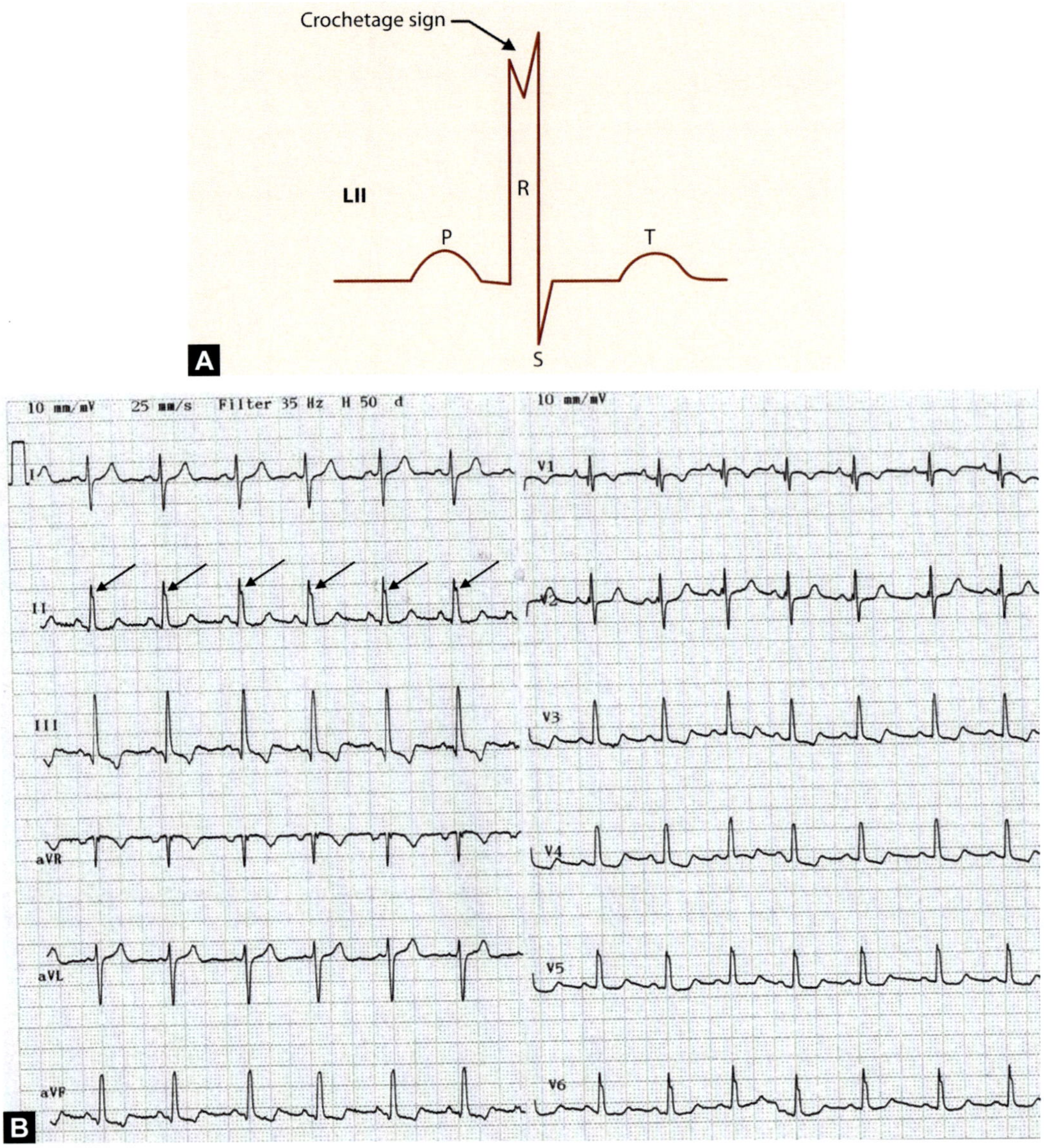

Figs. 23.5A and B: (A) Schematic representation of "Crochetage sign" (arrow). In inferior leads, a notch near the apex of the R-wave, is known as "Crochetage sign" has been correlated with ASD. (B) This ECG illustrates the "Crochetage sign" (notching near the apex of the R wave) in LII (arrows). Also note ECG features of partial RBBB (rSr' pattern in V1, V2, and QRS duration <120 ms) with right axis deviation.

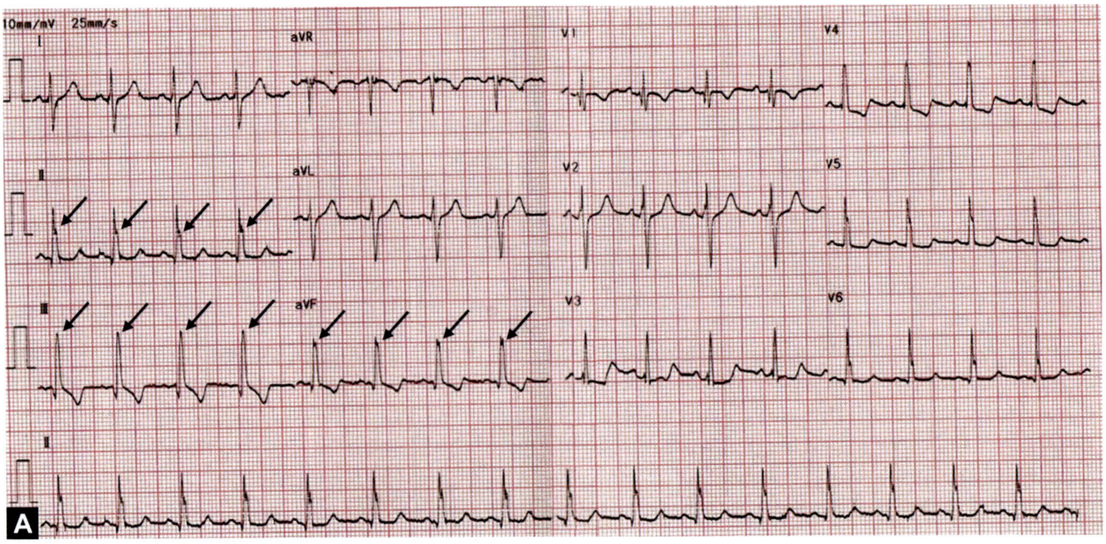

Fig. 23.6A: This ECG illustrates the 'Crochetage sign' at the apex of R waves in all three inferior leads LII, LIII, and aVF (arrows). Also note ECG features of partial RBBB (rSr' pattern in V1 with QRS duration <120 ms) with right axis deviation.

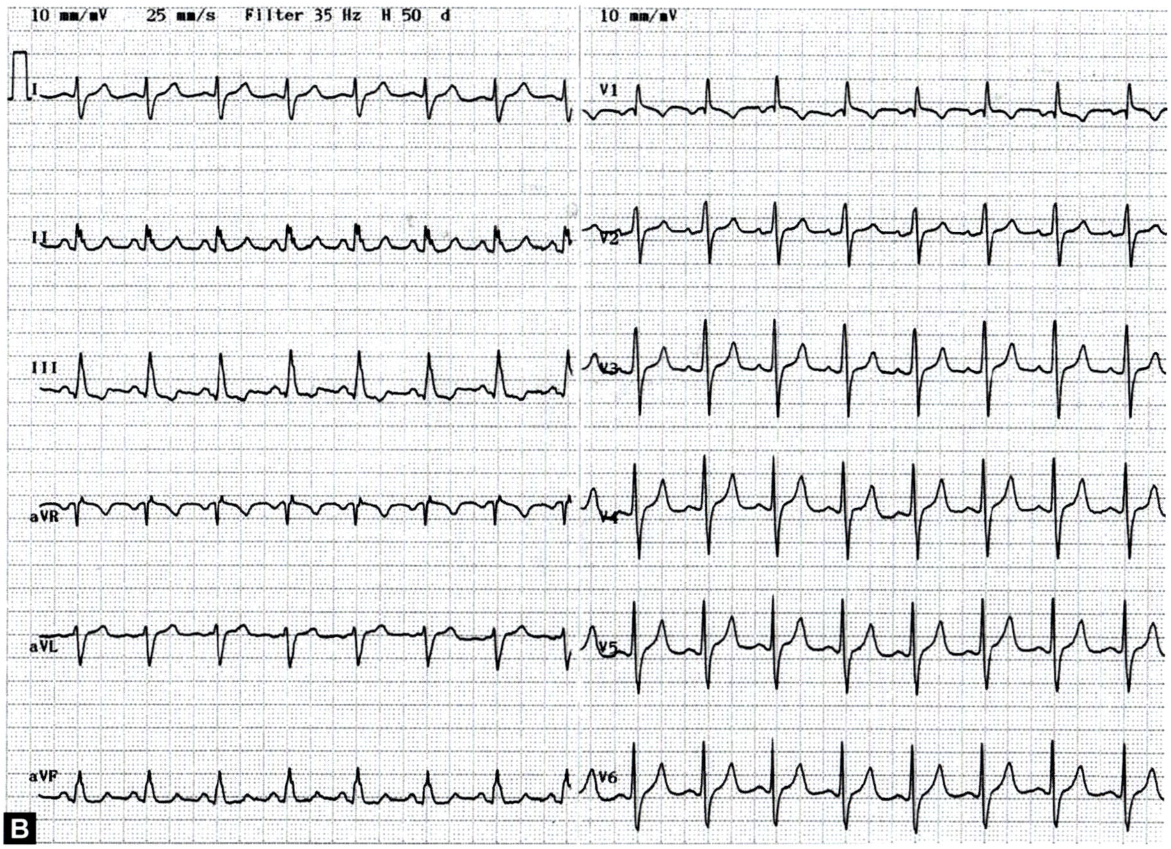

Fig. 23.6B: This ECG illustrates the "Crochetage sign" (notching near the apex of the R wave) in all three inferior leads LII, LIII, and aVF. Also note ECG features of partial RBBB (qR pattern in lead V1 with deep and slurred S waves in V5 and V6) with right axis deviation.

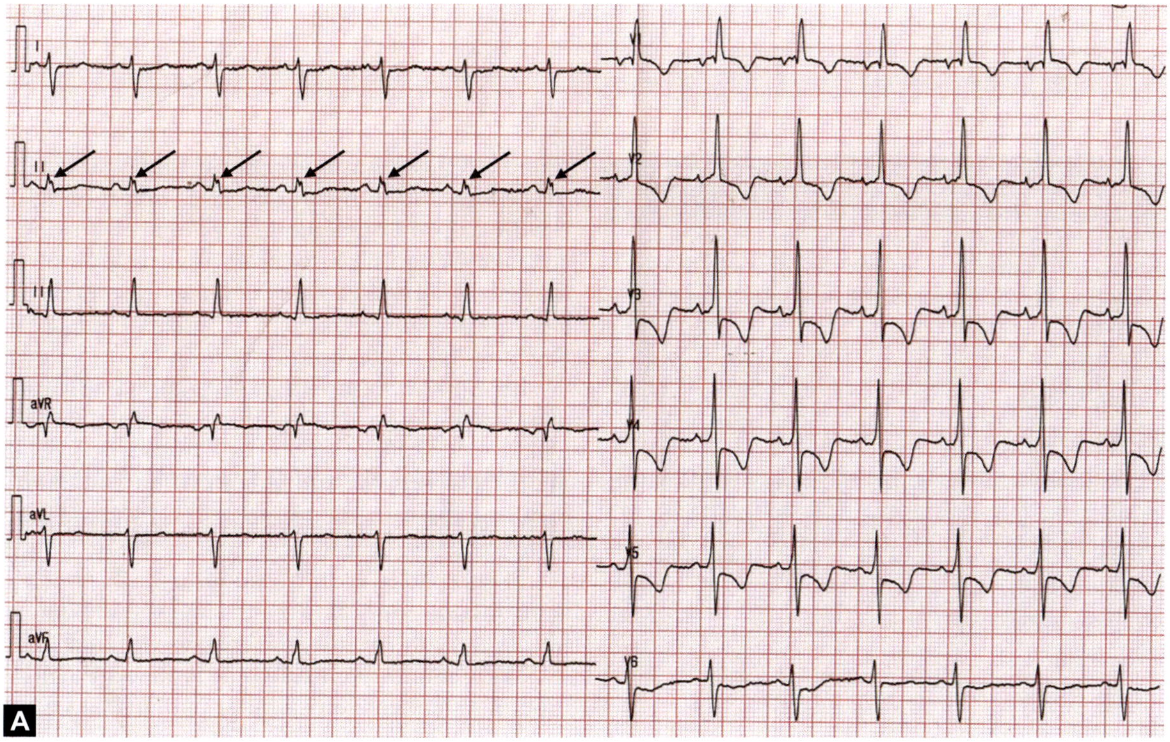

Fig. 23.7A: This ECG illustrates the "Crochetage sign" (notching near the apex of the R-wave) in single inferior lead LII (arrows).Also note ECG features of partial RBBB (qR pattern in lead V1 with deep and slurred S-waves in V5 and V6) with right axis deviation with ST-segment depression with T-wave inversions predominantly in right precordial leads suggestive of severe pulmonary hypertension.

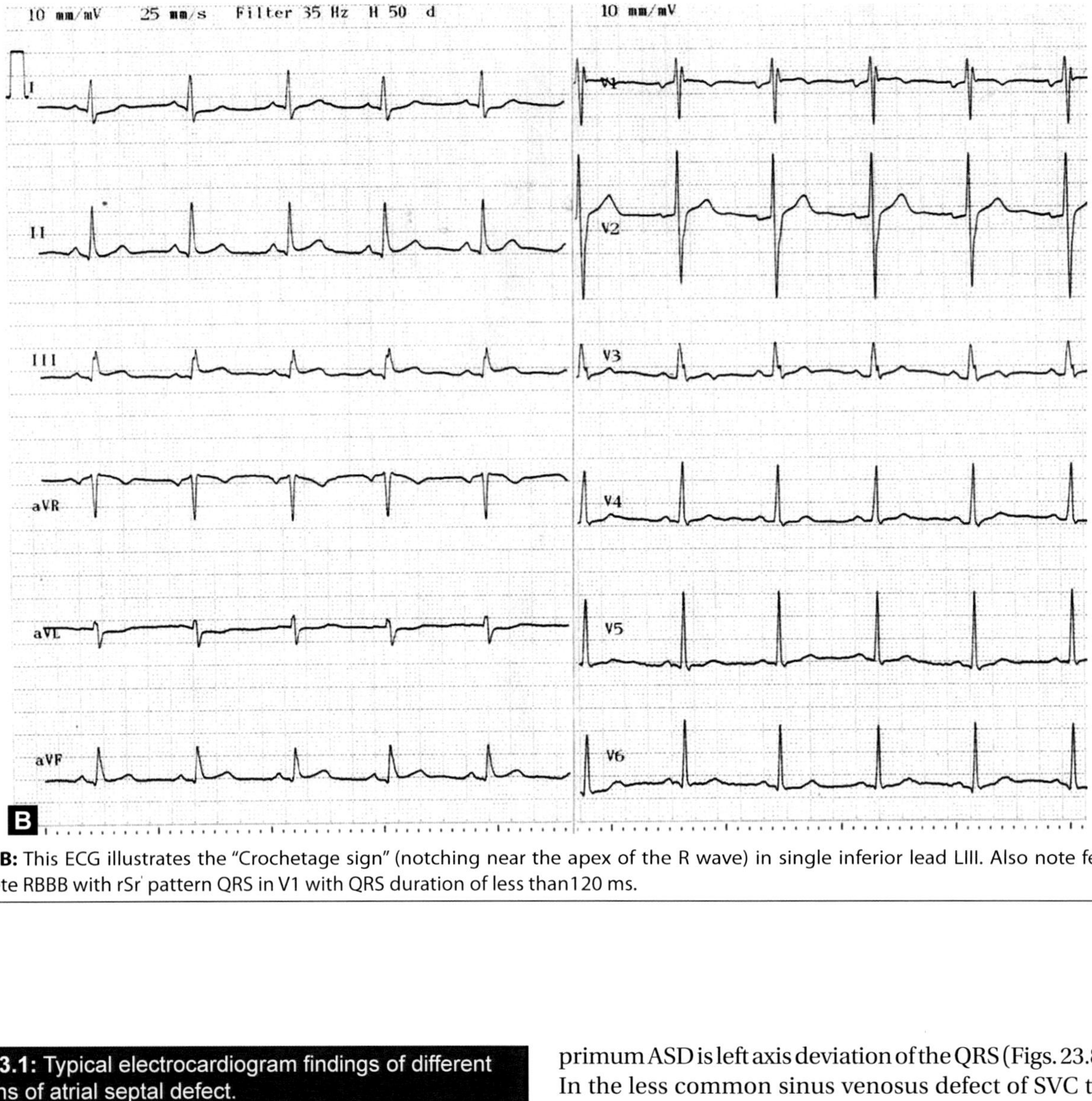

Fig. 23.7B: This ECG illustrates the "Crochetage sign" (notching near the apex of the R wave) in single inferior lead LIII. Also note features of incomplete RBBB with rSr' pattern QRS in V1 with QRS duration of less than120 ms.

Box 23.1: Typical electrocardiogram findings of different patterns of atrial septal defect.

The most frequent ECG abnormality in ASD is incomplete RBBB pattern (rSr' pattern) in lead V1. Complete RBBB is observed less frequently. If the ASD is very small, the ECG may be normal.

Secundum ASD:

1. Incomplete RBBB
2. ±Right axis deviation
3. Crochetage sign

Primum ASD:

1. Incomplete RBBB
2. Left axis deviation
3. ±First-degree AV block

Sinus Venosus ASD:

1. Incomplete RBBB
2. ±Right axis deviation
3. Negative P-waves in inferior leads (II, III, and aVF)

primum ASD is left axis deviation of the QRS (Figs. 23.8A to D). In the less common sinus venosus defect of SVC type, the P-wave axis in frontal plane in patients with sinus rhythm, is either left and superior or normal.[7] Ectopic atrial rhythm may be observed in sinus venosus type defect. Negative P-waves in inferior leads (II, III, and aVF) suggest low atrial rhythm (Figs. 23.9A and B).[14,21,22]

In addition to the PR prolongation, individuals with a primum ASD have a left axis deviation of the QRS complex while those with a secundum ASD have a right axis deviation of the QRS complex. Individuals with a sinus venosus ASD exhibit a left axis deviation of the P-wave (not the QRS complex).[22,23]

In unrepaired ostium secundum ASDs, the ECG rhythm is most commonly sinus, although the incidence of atrial fibrillation and/or flutter increases with age and is found in 20%.[24,25] Surgical closure may reduce atrial arrhythmias, though less effectively in older patients and all persistent arrhythmias may remain as before even after successful transcatheter device closure.[23,26]

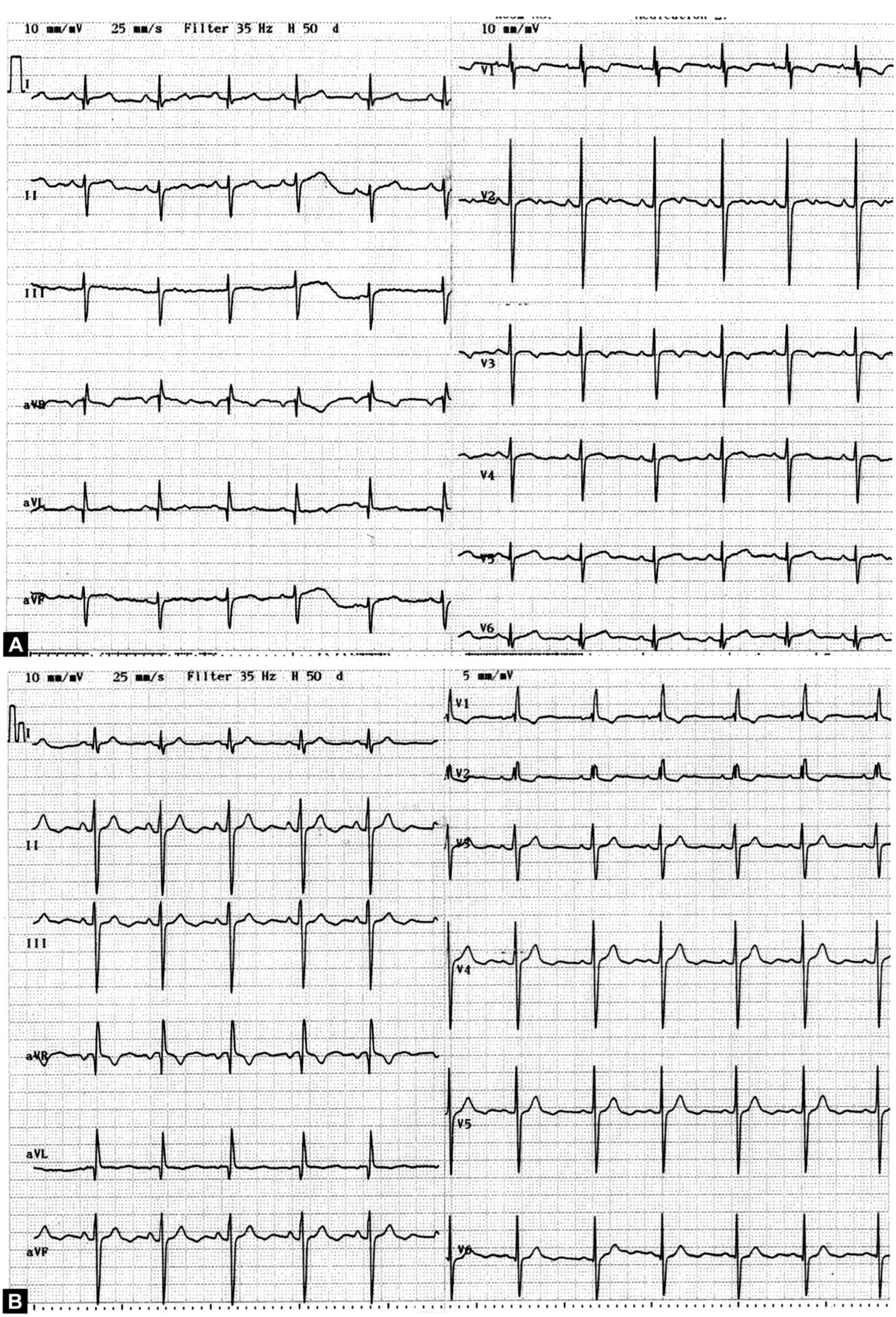

Figs. 23.8A and B: (A) Electrocardiogram of a patient (age-12 years) with primum ASD showing features of incomplete RBBB with rSr' pattern QRS in V1 with QRS duration 90 ms with deep S waves in leads V4–V6 with left axis deviation (tall R in LI and aVL with deep S wave in LII,LIII, and aVF). (B) ECG of a patient (age: 27 years) with primum ASD showing features of incomplete RBBB with rSr' pattern QRS in V1 and V2 with QRS duration 100 ms with deep S-waves in leads V5 and V6 with left axis deviation (tall R in LI and aVL with deep S-wave in LII, LIII, and aVF).

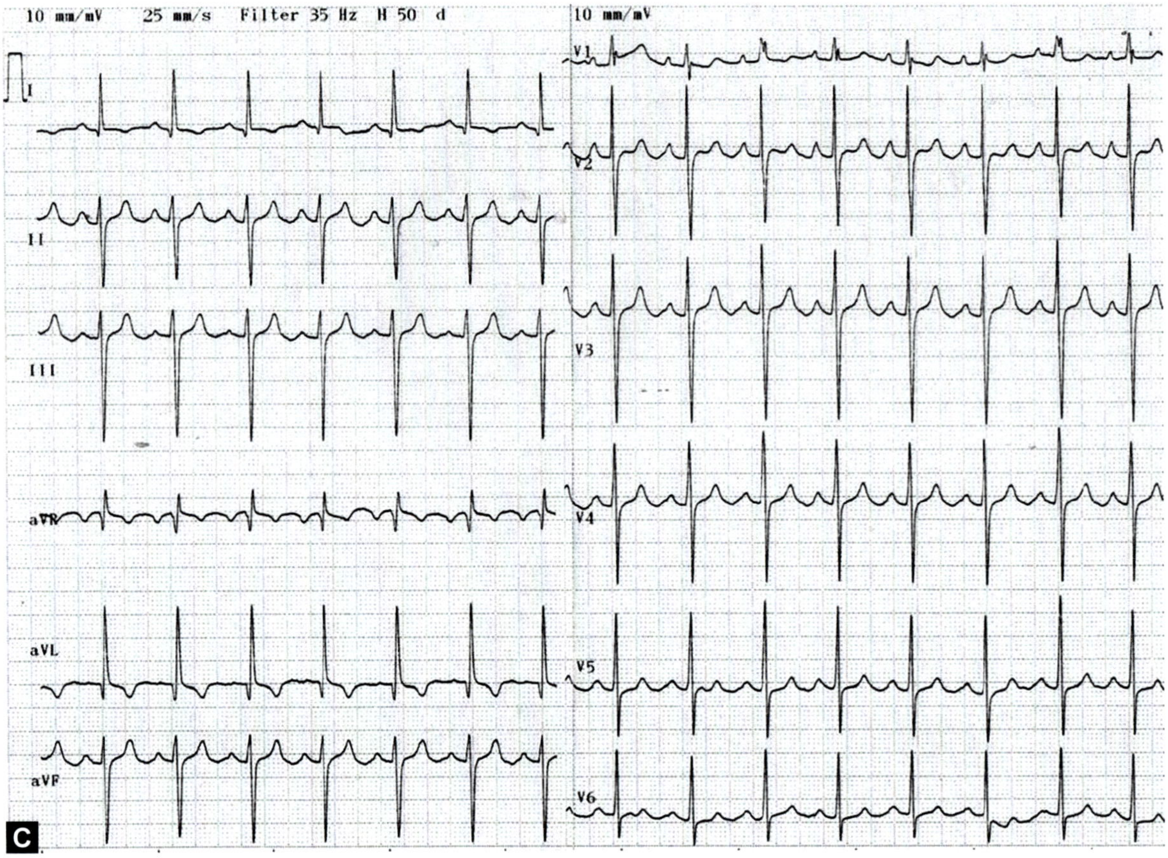

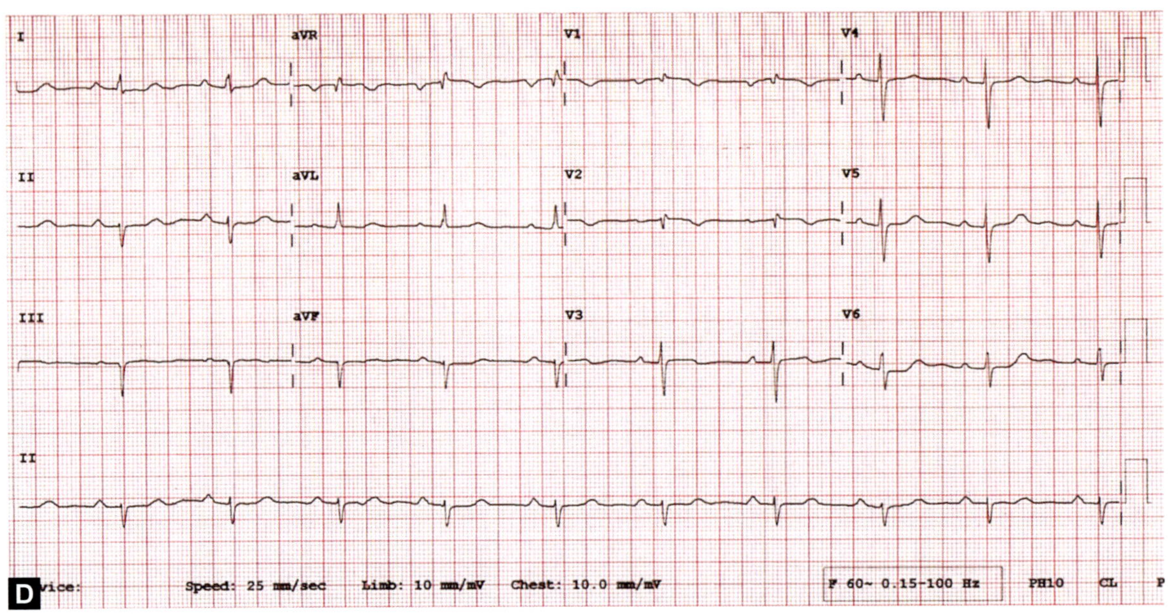

Figs. 23.8C and D: (C) ECG of a female patient (age-28 years) showing all the three typical electrocardiographic features of primum ASD; 1. Incomplete RBBB with rSr′ pattern QRS in V1 with QRS duration 95 ms with deep S waves in leads V5 and V6. 2. Left axis deviation (tall R in LI and aVL with deep S wave in LII,LIII, and aVF). 3. First-degree heart block (PR interval 210 ms). (D) ECG of a patient (age: 19 years) with primum ASD showing features of incomplete RBBB with slurred QRS in V1 and V2 with deep S-waves in leads V5 and V6 with left axis deviation with first-degree heart block (PR interval: 228 ms).

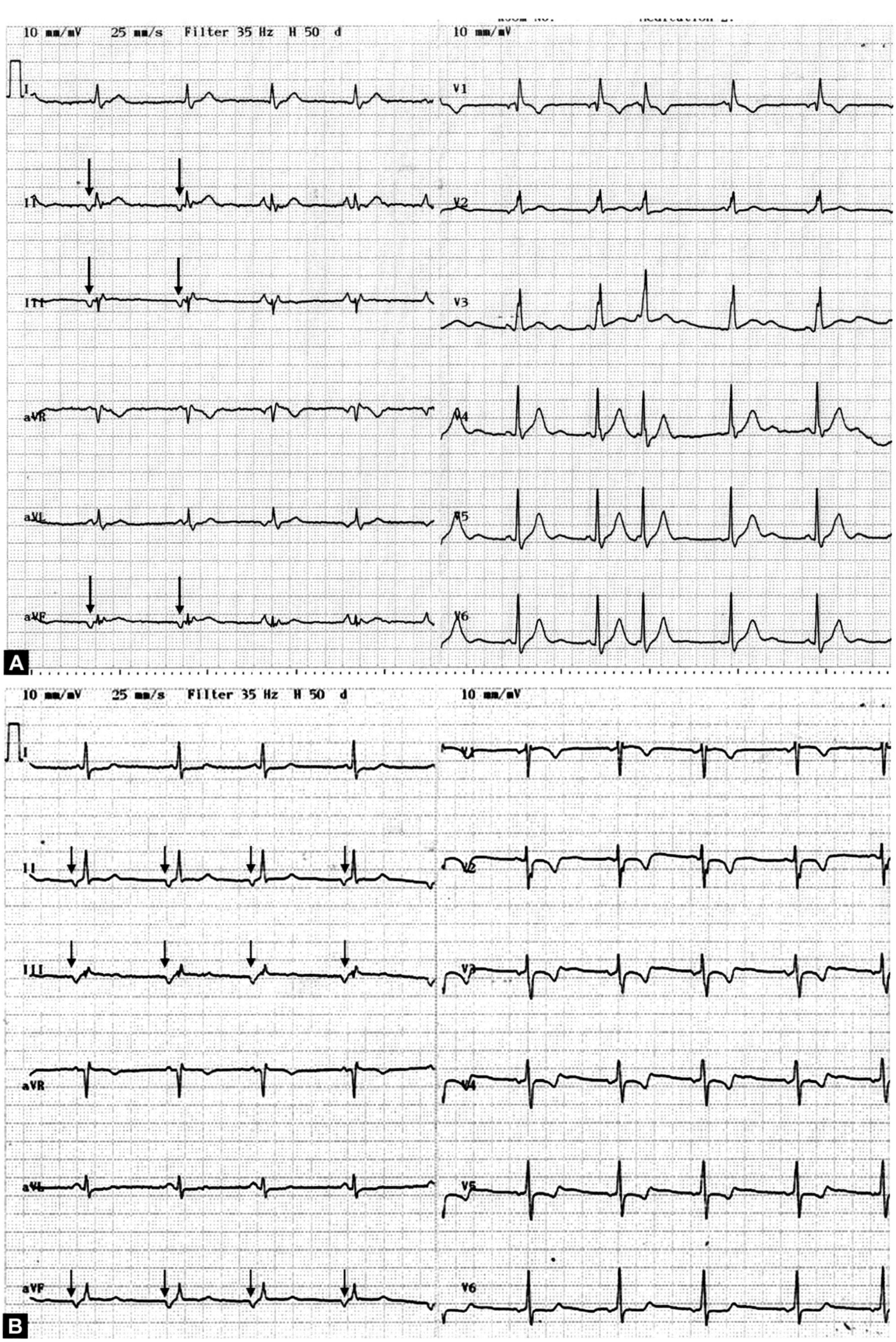

Figs. 23.9A and B: (A) Electrocardiogram of a patient (age: 17 years) with sinus venosus type of ASD showing features of incomplete RBBB with rSr' pattern QRS in V1 with QRS duration 100 ms with slurred S-waves in leads V4–V6 along with frequent low atrial rhythm. Note negative P-waves in inferior leads (II, III, and aVF) (arrows) with frequent low atrial ectopics. Ectopic atrial rhythm is a typical ECG sign of sinus venosus type ASD; (B) ECG of a patient (age: 21 years) with sinus venosus type of ASD showing features of incomplete RBBB with negative P waves in inferior leads (II, III and aVF) (arrows).

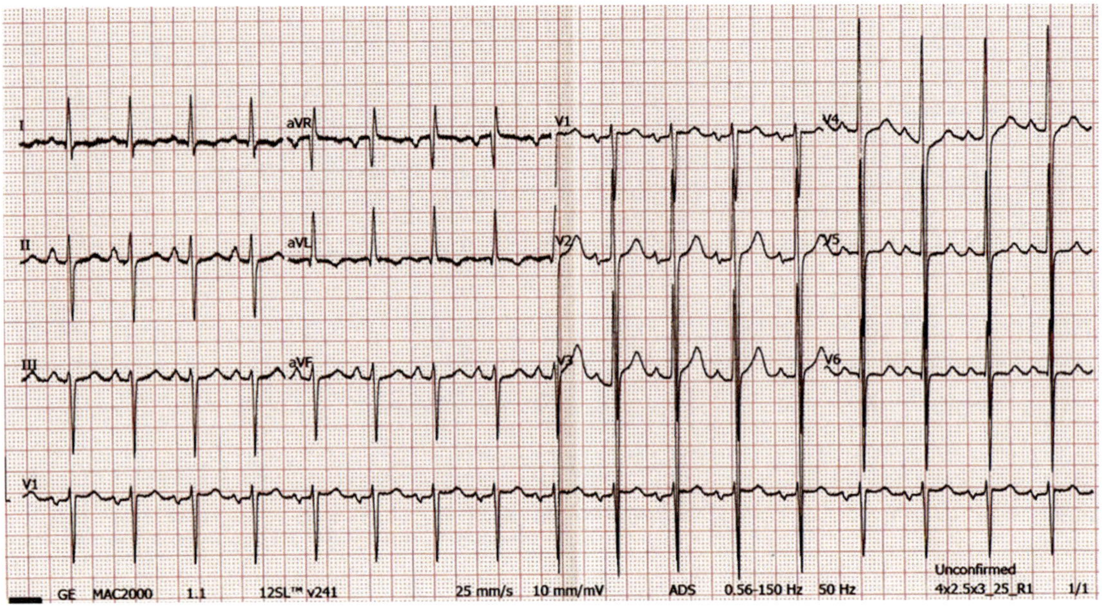

Fig. 23.10: Electrocardiogram showing Katz Wachtel phenomenon pattern in VSD with large diphasic (biphasic) RS complexes in V2–6. This is the classic ECG pattern of biventricular hypertrophy, most commonly seen in children with VSD. Also note the signs of biatrial enlargement.

ECG Findings in Ventricular Septal Defect

In ventricular septal defect (VSD), the ECG mirrors the size of the shunt and the degree of pulmonary hypertension. In patients with small VSD the ECG is generally normal.[27] However, rhythm disturbances such as complete heart block, atrial fibrillation, and flutter have been reported even in small perimembranous VSD's with septal aneurysms. Medium-sized VSDs produce a broad, notched P-wave characteristic of left atrial overload. Signs of LV volume overload—namely, deep Q and tall R-waves with tall T-waves in leads V5 and V6 are sometimes present. Large VSDs are associated with right and sometimes left atrial enlargement, with broad notched P-waves in leads I and II, and negative terminal forces in lead V1 and evidence for biventricular hypertrophy is found in 23–61% of patients.[28,29] The Katz-Wachtel phenomenon may be seen, with large diphasic RS complexes in midprecordial leads.[30] The Katz-Wachtel phenomenon/sign is tall diphasic RS complexes at least 50 mm in height in lead V2, V3, or V4—mid precordial leads. The sign has been described in ventricular septal defect with biventricular hypertrophy in children (Fig. 23.10). It can be seen with isolated ventricular septal defect as well as complex ventricular septal defect.[30] The R-wave amplitude in V1 may meet right ventricular hypertrophy criteria, and deep Q-waves may be present in lateral precordial leads. Right bundle-branch block is found in many patients, independent of whether the VSD was repaired through an atrial or ventricular incision.[28,31] Left-axis deviation is seen in 3–15% of patients. First-degree AV block occurs in about 10% of patients, with a 1–3% incidence of complete heart block on long-term follow-up.[28,32]

In VSD sinus rhythm is the norm but isolated premature ventricular contractions, couplets, and multiform premature ventricular contractions may be noted. Nonsustained or sustained ventricular tachycardia occurs in 5.7% of patients, particularly with higher pulmonary artery pressures.[28,33] Sudden cardiac death is uncommon but has been described in patients with cardiac hypertrophy and progressive fibrosis of the conduction system. After surgical repair, late sudden death occurs in about 4% of patients.[28,32]

ECG abnormalities in adult patients who have been operated for closure of the VSD during their childhood may show right bundle branch block in 50–90% of cases if operated by right ventriculotomy and in 40% patients if operated by right atrial approach. Complete AV block is very rare. Transcatheter VSD closure is an alternative to surgery in selected patients. Complete heart block is a recognized complication of transcatheter device closure.[34]

TETRALOGY OF FALLOT

Tetralogy of Fallot (TOF) is the most common cyanotic heart disease in adults.[35] The original definition consists of four main anatomical features: a large VSD, overriding of aorta, right ventricular outflow tract (RVOT) obstruction, and right ventricular hypertrophy (RVH).

There is also right-sided aortic arch in around 20% of cases and ASD in 8–10%—pentalogy of Fallot. Findings of RVH are the dominant ECG features of TOF and include—(1) Right axis deviation, (2) P pulmonale—peaked P-wave in lead II >2.5 mm, (3) Dominant R-wave in V1 (>7 mm tall; R/S ratio >1), (4) Dominant S-wave in V6 (>7 mm deep; R/S ratio <1), and (5) Right ventricular strain pattern in V1-V3 (Fig. 23.11).[36,37] RVH of TOF is depicted by presence of monophasic R-wave in lead V1, but in lead V2, there is sudden transition to rS pattern (Figs. 23.12A and B). In adult TOF patients, about 0.7% have LVH instead of RVH. Usually

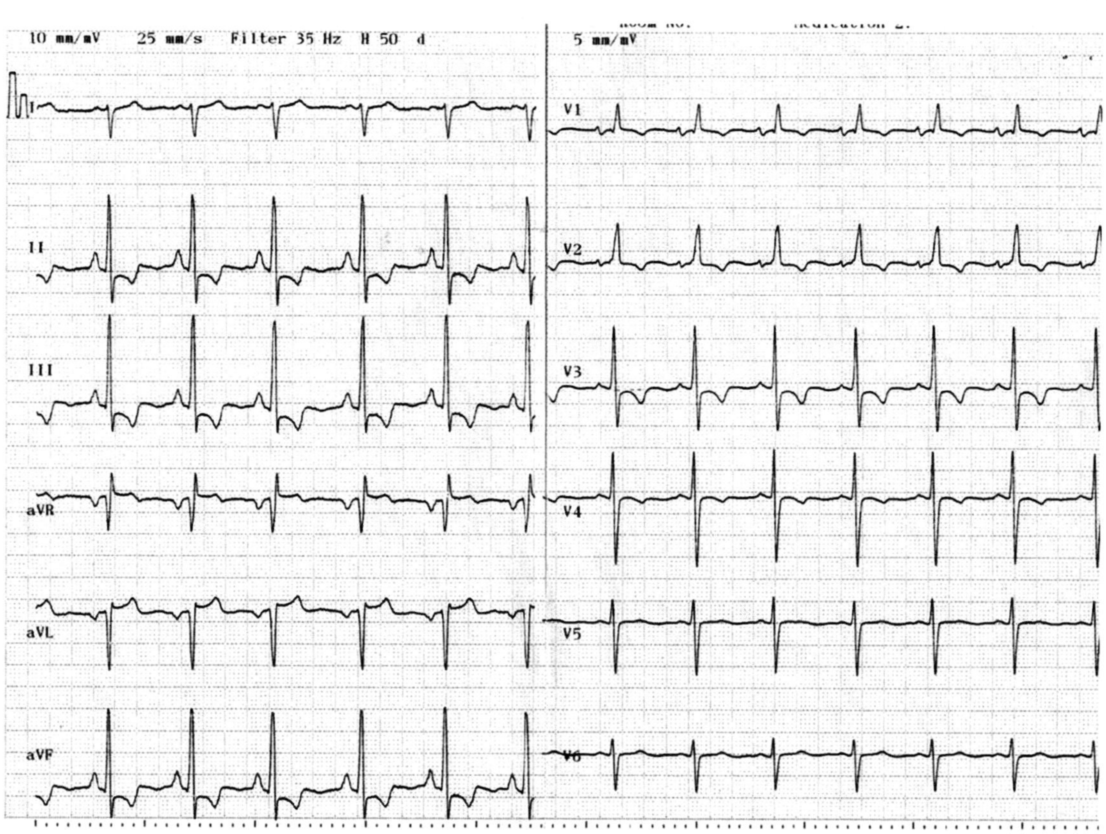

Fig. 23.11: Electrocardiogram showing almost all the typical features of tetralogy of Fallot (TOF) with monophasic R-wave in V1, right axis deviation, P pulmonale (tall and peaked P-wave in lead II >2.5 mm), dominant S-wave in V6 (R/S ratio <1) and right ventricular strain pattern in V1–V3. Note absence of q-waves in lateral leads. Usually in ECG of TOF, q-waves are absent in lateral leads suggesting decreased pulmonary blood flow.
Source: Dr Fahmida Zaman, Labaid Cardiac Hospital.

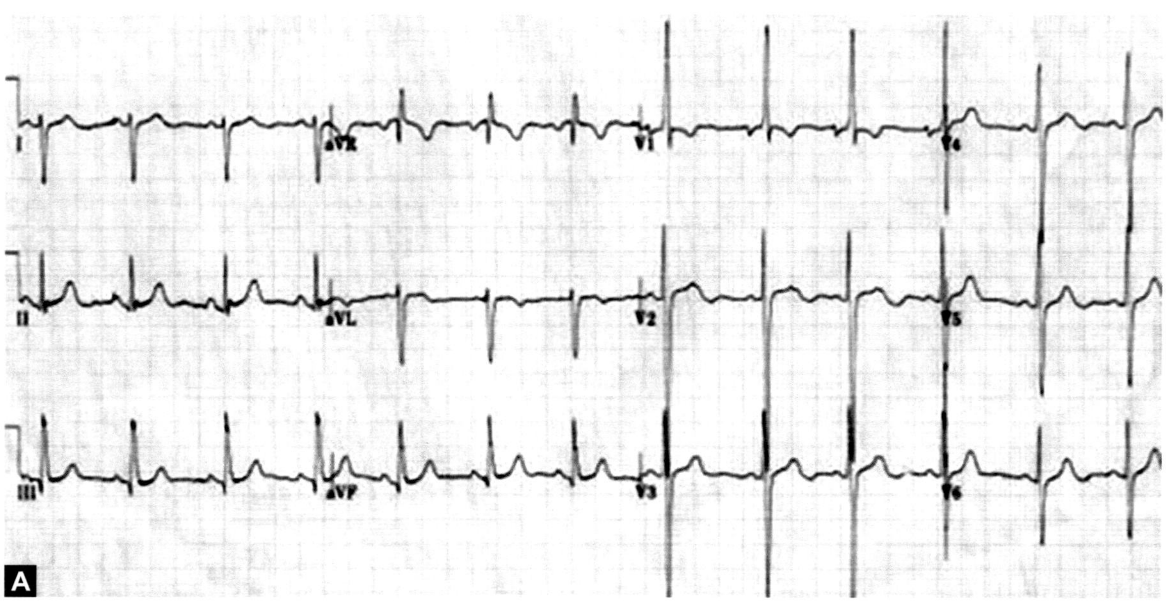

Fig. 23.12A: This ECG illustrates the features of tetralogy of Fallot (TOF) with monophasic R-wave in V1, right axis deviation and dominant S-wave in V6 (R/S ratio <1). Note absence of q-waves in lateral leads.

(*Source:* Dr Mahbubor Rahman, Labaid Cardiac Hospital.)

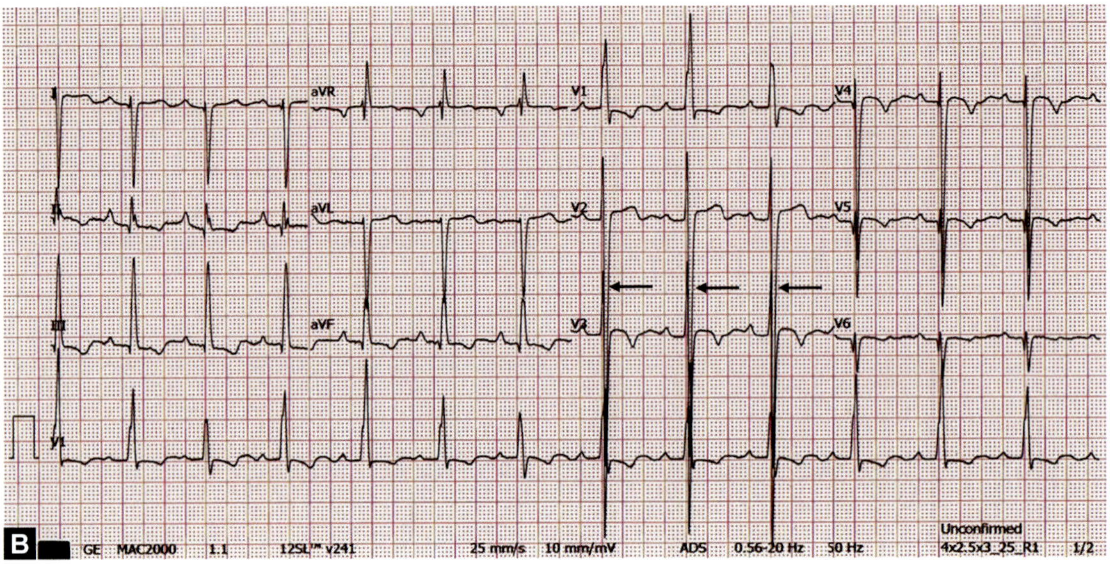

Fig. 23.12B: An ECG illustrating the classic and sudden transition of R-wave in V2 which is typically seen in the tetralogy of Fallot (TOF). RVH of TOF is depicted by presence of monophasic R-wave in lead V1, but in lead V2, there is sudden transition to rS pattern (R<S) (arrows).This sudden transition is typical for TOF ECG. Also note the right axis deviation, P pulmonale (tall and peaked P-wave in lead II >2.5 mm), dominant S wave in V6. Only ECG finding, presence of q-waves in lead V5, V6 are not in agreement with ECG features of TOF. Usually q-waves are absent in lateral leads in the ECG of TOF which suggests decreased pulmonary blood flow. But in presence multiple cardiac pathology q-waves may be seen occasionally in lateral leads but it is uncommon.

(*Source:* Dr Mahbubor Rahman, Labaid Cardiac Hospital.)

q-waves are absent in lateral leads suggesting decreased pulmonary blood flow. Corrective surgery involves atriotomy and/or ventricular incisions and patches, which predisposes patients to the late development of arrhythmias. Intra-atrial reentrant tachycardias may develop after surgery.[38-40] Moreover sudden cardiac death is the most common cause of death late after repair. In a multicenter cohort study, 10% of patients developed atrial flutter, 11.9% of patients experienced sustained ventricular tachycardia (VT), and 8.3% of patients died suddenly.[38]

Ebstein's Anomaly

In Ebstein's anomaly, the tricuspid valve is displaced apically, creating an atrialized portion that is morphologically and electrically right ventricle but functionally right atrium.[41] This anomaly is a rare congenital heart disorder accounting for less than 1% of all cases of congenital heart disease.[42,43]

The ECG is abnormal in most patients with Ebstein's anomaly. It may show tall and broad P-waves as a result of right atrial enlargement, as well as complete or incomplete right bundle-branch block. The R-waves in leads V1 and V2 are small. Bizarre morphologies of the terminal QRS complexes result from infra-Hisian conduction disturbance and abnormal activation of the atrialized right ventricle (Figs. 23.13A and B).[42,44,45] The ECG of Ebstein's patients shows very tall P-waves ≥5 mm (Himalayan P-wave), which is a characteristic finding (Fig. 23.14).

First-degree AV block occurs in 42% of patients because of right atrial enlargement and structural abnormalities of the AV conduction system but complete heart block is rare in Ebstein's anomaly.[42] The downward displacement of the septal leaflet of the tricuspid valve is associated with discontinuity of the central fibrous body and septal AV ring with direct muscular connections, thus creating a potential substrate for accessory AV connections and pre-excitation. Accessory AV or atriofascicular pathways are found in 25% of patients and are frequently right-sided and multiple (Fig. 23.15). From 6–36% of patients with Ebstein's anomaly have ≥1 accessory pathways.[42,46,47] Supraventricular tachyarrhythmias, including AV reciprocating tachycardia, ectopic atrial tachycardia, and atrial fibrillation or flutter, occur in 30–40% of patients, constituting the most common presentation in adolescents and adults.[48] In addition, wide QRS tachycardia over a septal accessory AV pathway, ventricular tachycardia, or flutter, as well as ectopic atrial tachycardia, atrial flutter, and atrial fibrillation, can occur.[42]

Dextrocardia

Dextrocardia situs inversus is a congenital condition characterized by a heart that is horizontally inverse, or mirrored. The anatomic right ventricle is anterior to the left ventricle and the aortic arch curves to the right and posteriorly. The anatomic right lung with its three lobes is on the left side. The gastric fundus gas bubble is on the right and the liver on the left. It is a rare clinical phenomenon with a reported incidence of 1 in 5,000–30,000.[49]

There are several variants of dextrocardia:

1. Dextrocardia and situs inversus (mirror image dextrocardia): in addition to the heart, internal organs of abdomen are also positioned on the opposite side.
2. Dextrocardia and situs solitus: Dextrocardia with situs solitus, is a congenital condition where, the heart is on the right side of the chest, but all of the other internal

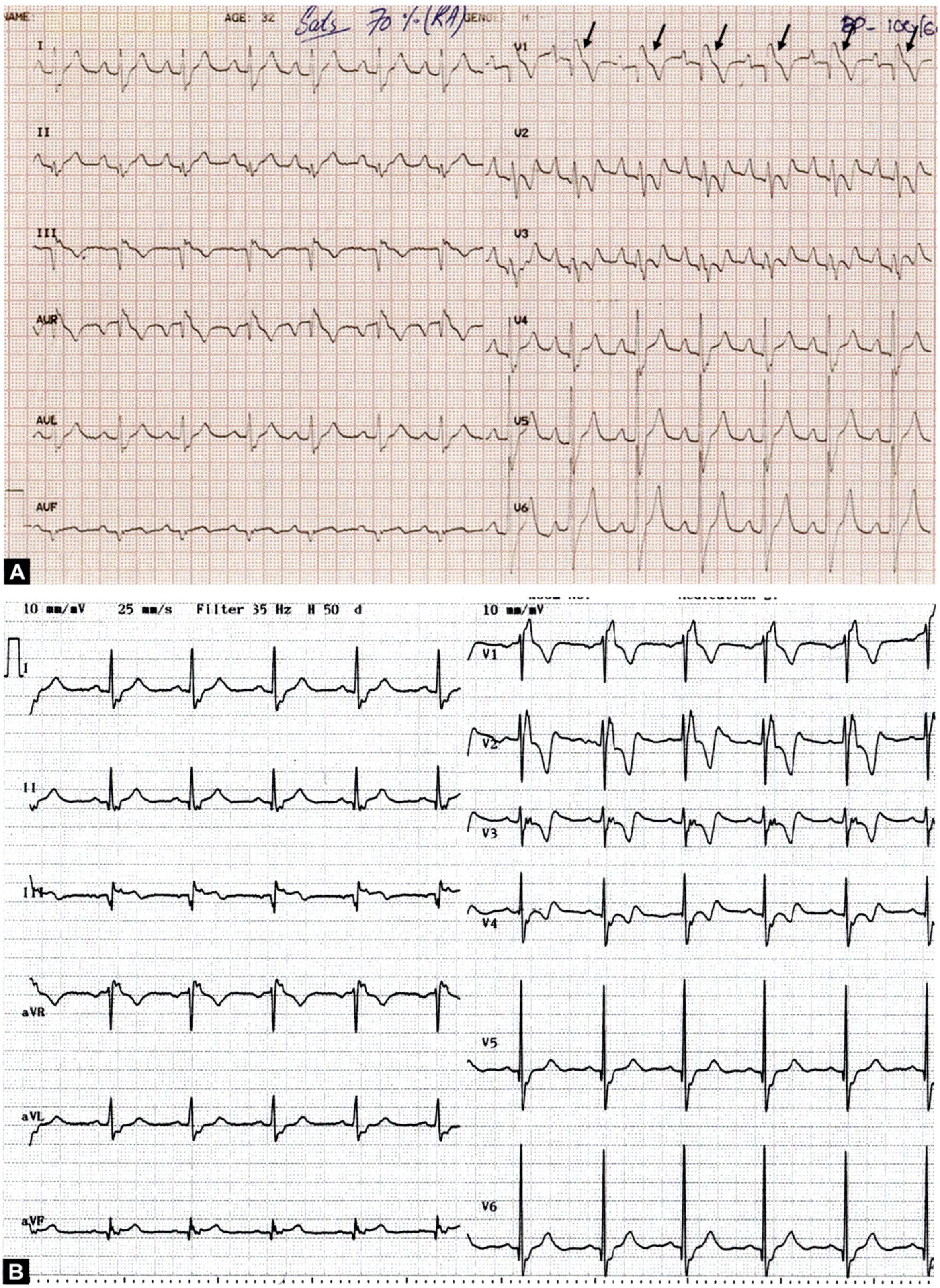

Figs. 23.13A and B: (A) Electrocardiogram of a patient with Ebstein's anomaly (preoperative) showing low-amplitude bizarre pattern atypical RBBB (arrows) with electrocardiographic evidences of right atrial enlargement (RAE). Note P-wave amplitudes greater than 2.5 mm in leads LI, LII, V2–V4, and P-wave height is 5 mm in lead V2. The ECG of Ebstein's anomaly patients may show very tall P waves greater than or equal to 5 mm (Himalayan P-wave), which is a characteristic finding of this congenital defect. Also note first degree heart block (PR interval 220 ms). (B) ECG of the same patient with Ebstein's anomaly as displayed in (A) 4 years after operative treatment. Note bizarre pattern atypical RBBB still persisting but electrocardiographic evidences of right atrial enlargement and first degree heart block disappeared. P waves' height and PR intervals are now normal.

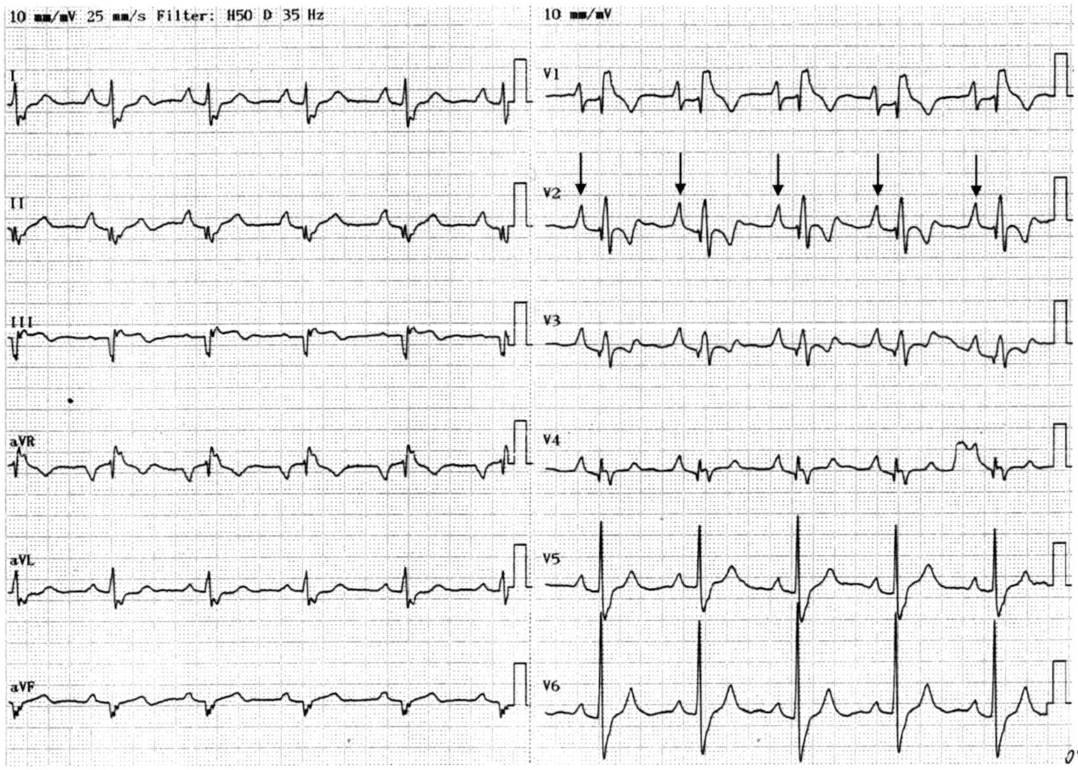

Fig. 23.14: Electrocardiogram illustrates Himalayan P-wave in a patient with Ebstein's anomaly. Note electrocardiographic evidences of right atrial enlargement in leads LII and V1 (the P-wave amplitude in lead II greater than 2.5 mm and the upward deflection of the P-wave in lead V1 greater than 1.5 mm in amplitude). Also note huge P-wave in V2 with height 5 mm (arrows) suggestive of Himalayan P wave. Also note first-degree AV block (PR interval 240 ms). First-degree AV block occurs in 42% of patients with Ebstein's anomaly because of right atrial enlargement and structural abnormalities of the atrioventricular conduction system.

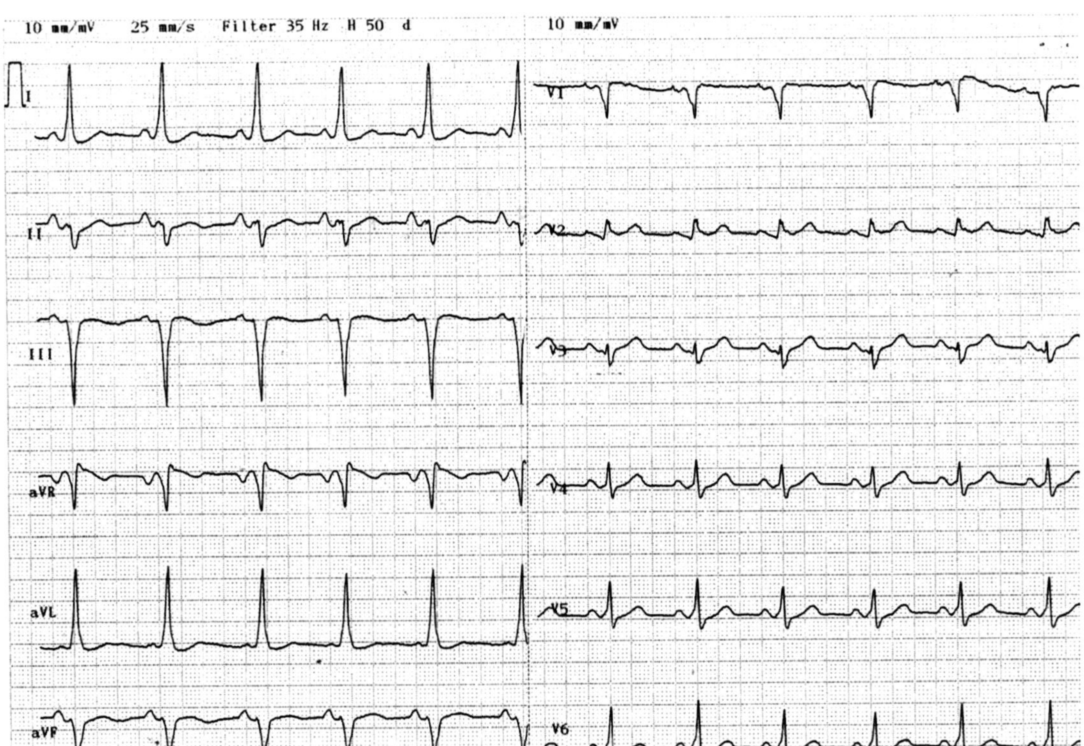

Fig. 23.15: Electrocardiogram showing features of Wolff–Parkinson–White syndrome in a patient with Ebstein's anomaly. Note short PR interval and presence of delta waves in multiple leads (negative in V1) with evidence of right atrial enlargement (P amplitude >2.5 mm in LII) with slurred S-in V5 and V6. Accessory AV or atriofascicular pathways are found in 25% of patients with Ebstein's anomaly which are frequently right-sided and multiple.

organs are in their normal positions. Only heart is on the opposite side; internal organs are not affected.

3. Dextroposition: The anatomically corrected heart is displaced to the right hemithorax. Deformities of chest wall, deformities of diaphragm, postpneumonectomy, hypoplastic right lung, eventration of diaphragm, left hemidiaphragmatic paralysis, pneumomediastinum may give rise to dextroposition. Dextrocardia should be distinguished from dextroposition, in which the heart is located within the right thorax but its apex points to the patient's left.
4. Mesocardia: The heart is placed in the midline of thorax. Apex of the heart is either in the midline or directed towards right.
5. Situs ambiguus (heterotaxy syndrome) is a disturbance in the usual left and right distribution of the thoracic and abdominal organs which does not entirely correspond to the complete or partial mirror image.[50]

Mirror-image dextrocardia is the most common form of cardiac malposition encountered and is almost always associated with situs inversus of the abdominal organs. Twenty-five percent of these patients will have associated sinusitis and bronchiectasis (Kartagener's syndrome). The risk in these patients lies in the atypical presentation of diseases such as angina pectoris, myocardial infarction, acute cholecystitis, acute appendicitis, and diverticulitis where pain is referred to the 'wrong' side. Recognizing the presence of dextrocardia will also help to avoid unnecessary workup for abnormal ECG.[51]

ECG findings of dextrocardia include global negativity in lead I (a negative P-wave, QRS complex and T-wave), positively deflected QRS complex in aVR, reverse R-wave progression in precordial leads, and right axis deviation (Fig. 23.16). To recognize the ECG changes associated with a dextrocardia, it is important to have a clear understanding of the electrical axis. Right axis deviation is normally due to a pathological cause such as left posterior fascicular block. Extreme right axis deviation (ERAD), is normally only seen with ventricular rhythms, such as ventricular tachycardia or paced rhythms. ERAD may be a normal finding with a patient who has dextrocardia.[52]

On a standard ECG with normal heart placement, LI will almost always be positive and lead aVR negative with any supraventricular rhythm. The finding of a positively deflected QRS complex in aVR and a negatively deflected QRS complex in lead I should cause concern. The most common cause for this finding is reversed electrode placement of arm leads (left and right). However, in arm lead reversal, the precordial leads reveal a normal R-wave progression (since the heart is on the left side). In true dextrocardia, since the heart is on the right side of the chest, the left ventricular apex is at the right midclavicular line, the left precordial leads reveal reversed R-wave progression; the R-wave is tallest in V1 and progressively decreases in amplitude in leads V2–V6 (Fig. 23.17).[49,51,53]

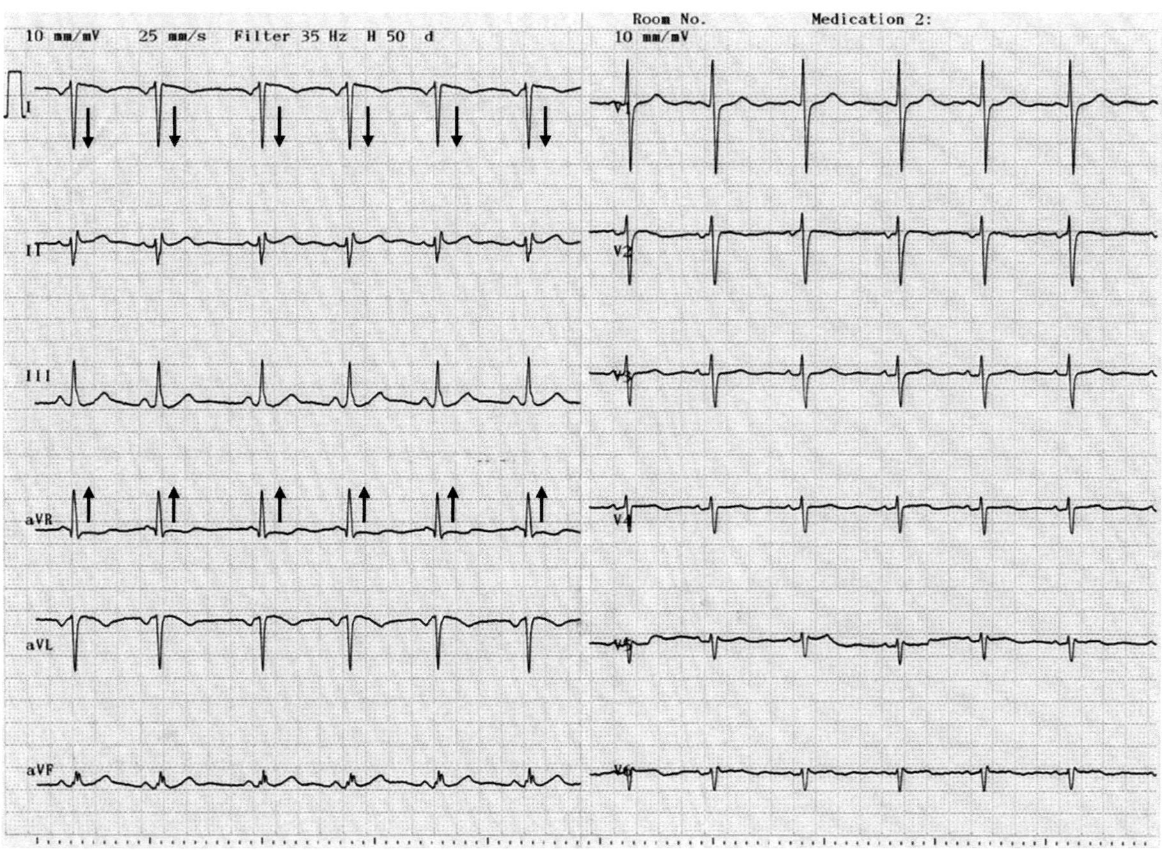

Fig. 23.16: Electrocardiogram illustrates the features of mirror-image dextrocardia and shows inversion of all complexes (global negativity) with inverted P-waves, negative QRS, inverted T-waves in LI and positive QRS complexes (with upright P- and T-waves) in aVR (arrows). Also note absent normal R-wave progression in the chest leads (dominant S-waves throughout) and right-axis deviation.

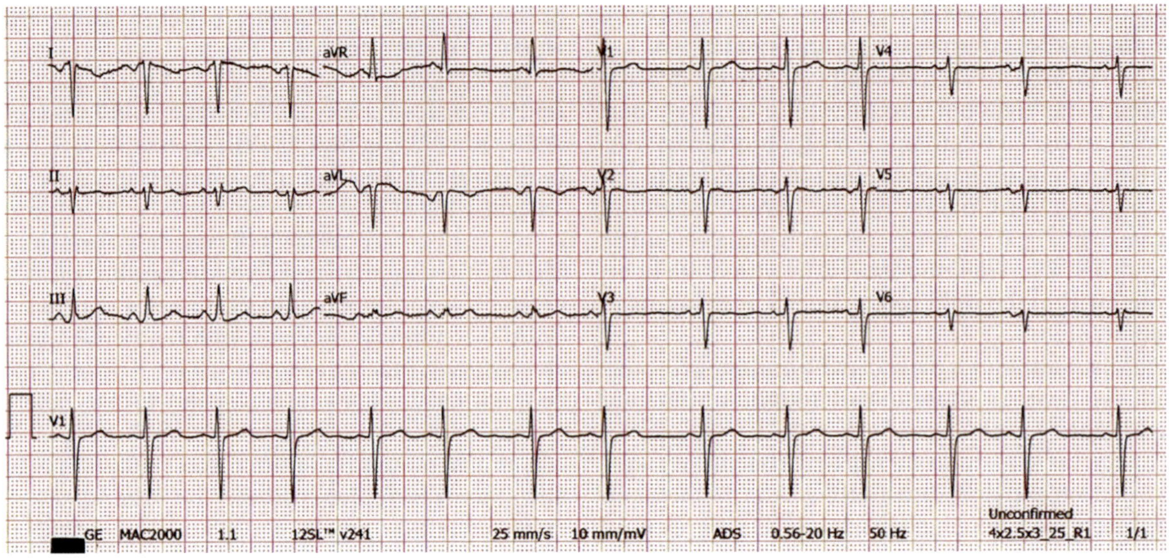

Fig. 23.17: Electrocardiogram shows reversed R-wave progression in precordial leads in true dextrocardia, the R-wave is tallest in V1 and progressively decreases in amplitude in leads V2–V6. Also note ECG findings of mirror image dextrocardia with global negativity in lead I (a negative P-wave, QRS complex, and T-wave), and positively deflected QRS complex in aVR.

Technical Dextrocardia

Technical dextrocardia or arm lead inversion (right arm lead placed on left arm and vice versa) can be recognized by inverted P-waves, negative QRS and T-waves in lead I. The same pattern can be seen in true dextrocardia as well. But in true dextrocardia, the chest electrodes will not show the usual progression of R-waves, instead the QRS amplitude will progressively decrease from V1 to V6 as the heart is on the opposite side. Simple option is to get a repeat ECG for verification, if possible under direct supervision. Arm lead inversion or technical dextrocardia is one of the commonest errors in ECG recording.[53-55]

Accidental lead reversal (technical dextrocardia) specifically reversal of the left and right arm electrodes may produce a similar ECG picture to true dextrocardia in the limb leads but with normal R wave progression (R wave amplitudes progressively increase from V1 to V6) in the precordial leads (Fig 23.18).

Patent Ductus Arteriosus

Most incidentally identified patent ductus arteriosus (PDAs) are small in caliber and associated with a normal ECG, as opposed to moderate or large PDAs that may promote pulmonary hypertension and are accompanied by ECG findings dominated by Eisenmenger's physiology.[28] With a moderately sized PDA, sinus rhythm is usually present, although atrial fibrillation may occur in older individuals.[56] Left atrial enlargement may be present, and PR prolongation is found in 10–20% of patients.[57] The QRS axis is usually normal. Left ventricular volume overload may be characterized by deep S-waves in V1 and tall R-waves in leads V5 and V6, accompanied by nonspecific repolarization changes (Fig. 23.19).[56,57]

Coarctation of Aorta

In aortic coarctation the basic pathology resulting in ECG changes is left ventricular hypertrophy (LVH) due to systemic hypertension. Some patients have accompanying congenital heart diseases, including bicuspid aortic valve or ventricular septal defect (VSD). In aortic coarctation some patients have normal ECG. ECG abnormalities that may be observed in patients with coarctation of the aorta is due to development of LVH manifested by increased QRS voltage, secondary ST segment, or T-wave changes with ECG findings of left atrial enlargement (Fig. 23.20).[58]

Pulmonary Stenosis

Standard criteria for right ventricular hypertrophy (RVH) are applicable to valvular pulmonary stenosis (PS). In general, severity of PS correlates with the R/S ratio in leads V1 and V6 and R-wave amplitude in lead V1.[59] High-amplitude peaked P-waves in lead II are commonly found in severe pulmonary stenosis (Fig. 23.21), but not consistently so. The QRS axis may be normal with mild pulmonary stenosis but is deviated rightward with moderate or severe obstruction. Degree of right-axis deviation is positively correlated with right ventricular pressure.[28]

Eisenmenger Syndrome

Eisenmenger syndrome is a complication of uncorrected large intracardiac left-to-right shunts. Increased pulmonary resistance may develop over time, eventually leading to bidirectional shunting and then to right-to-left shunting. Deoxygenated blood enters the systemic circulation, causing symptoms of hypoxia. Congenital heart anomalies those, if untreated, may result in Eisenmenger syndrome

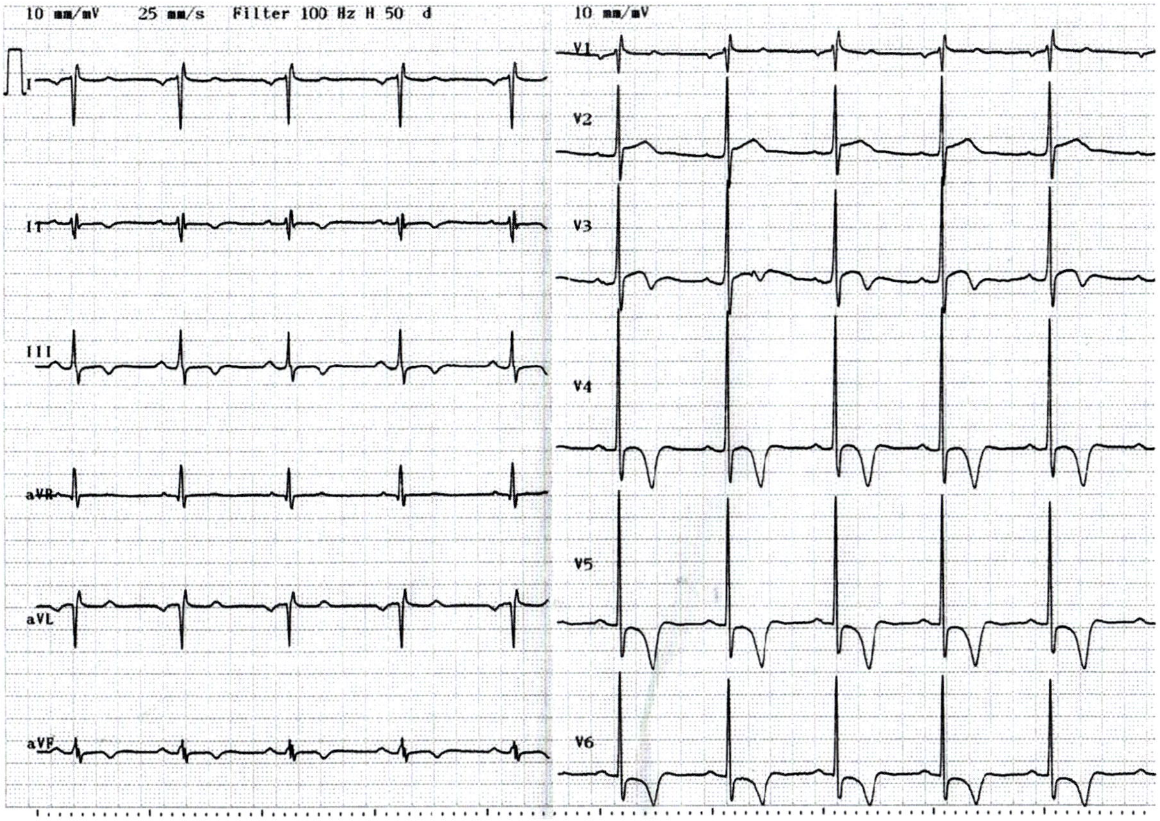

Fig. 23.18: Electrocardiogram illustrates the features of technical dextrocardia and shows inversion of P-waves and negative QRS complexes in LI and positive QRS complexes (with upright P- and T-waves) in aVR suggestive of dextrocardia. But note normal R-wave progression in the precordial leads, an increase in R-wave amplitude from lead V1–V6 (normal R-wave progression). It is possible to distinguish lead reversal (technical dextrocardia) and true (mirror image) dextrocardia by watching the precordial leads. True dextrocardia will not show any R-wave progression in leads V1–V6, whereas lead reversal will. Also note RBBB-type ECG with left ventricular hypertrophy (LVH) systolic overload pattern.

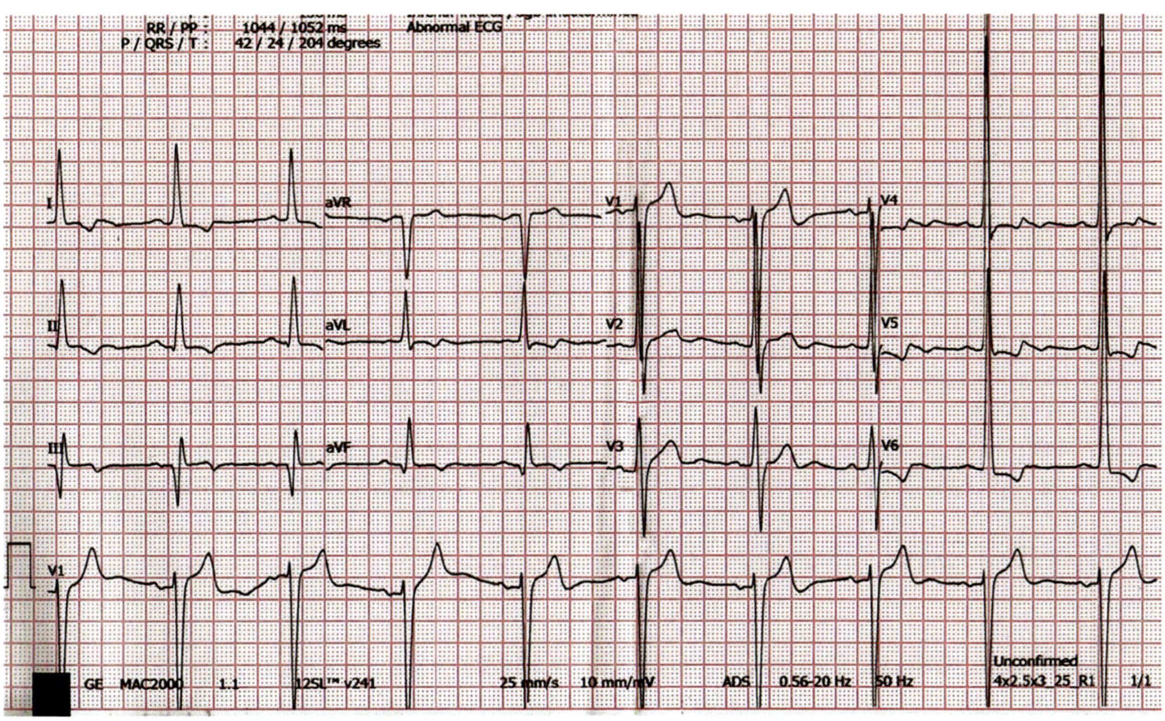

Fig. 23.19: Electrocardiogram illustrates the features of left ventricular volume overload in a patient with PDA characterized by deep S-waves in V1 and very tall R-waves in leads V5 and V6, accompanied by nonspecific repolarization changes. R in V5 (65 mm) + S in V1 (35 mm) = 100 mm.

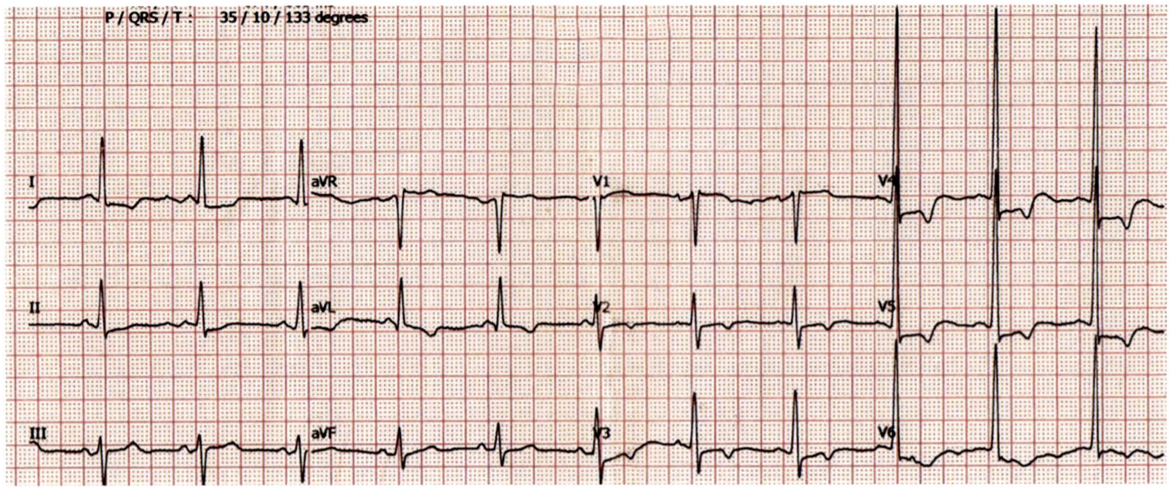

Fig. 23.20: Electrocardiogram shows features of LVH systolic overload pattern in a patient with coarctation of the aorta. Note very high amplitudes of R-waves in leads V4–V6 with secondary ST-segment depressions and T-wave changes in most of the leads.

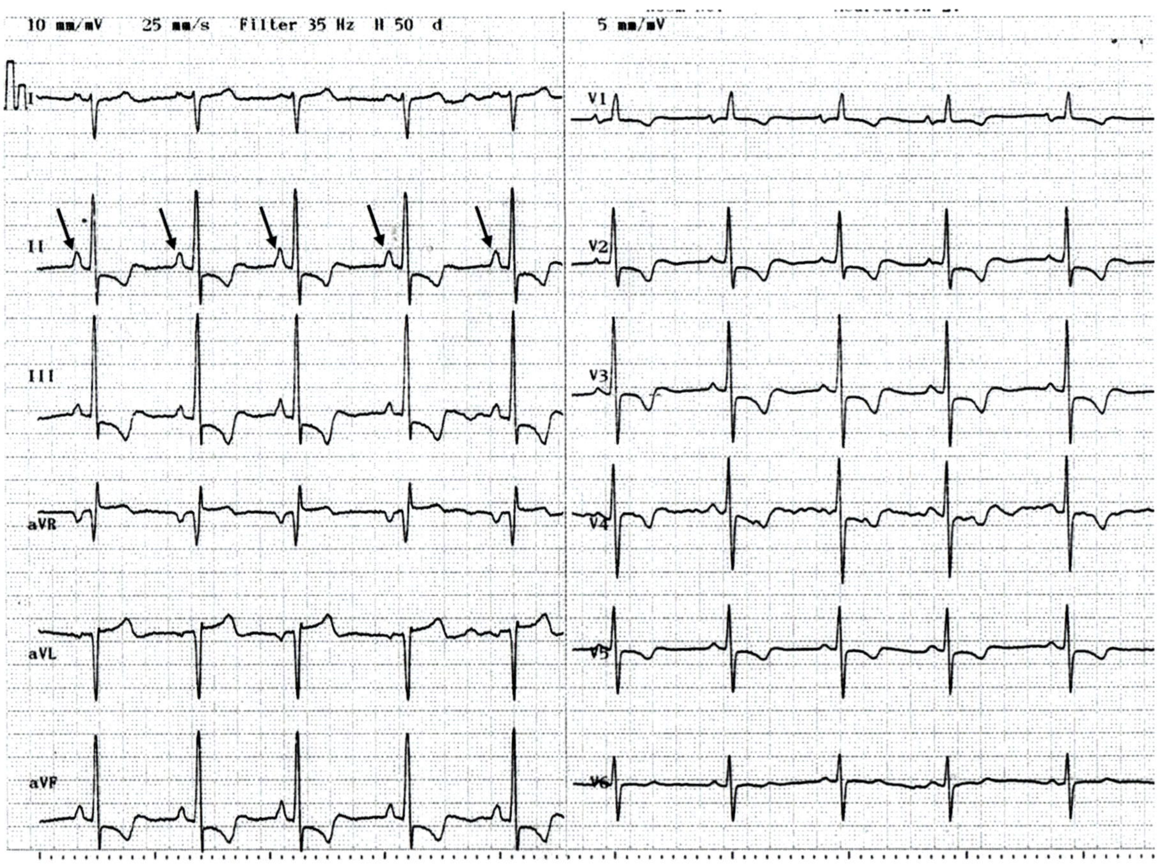

Fig. 23.21: Electrocardiogram features are suggestive of pulmonary stenosis (PS) showing features of right ventricular hypertrophy (RVH) with tall R in V1 with deep S wave in V6 (R/S ratio in V6 is <1) with high-amplitude peaked P-waves in lead II (arrows) and marked right axis deviation which is positively correlated with right ventricular pressure overload.

include ventricular septal defect, AV canal defect, ASD, patent ductus arteriosus, truncus arteriosus, transposition of the great arteries etc.[60,61] ECG is almost always abnormal and shows features suggestive of right ventricular hypertrophy (with tall R-wave in V1, deep S-wave in V6, ST- and T-wave abnormalities, P pulmonale) as well as abnormalities associated with the underlying defect.[60-63] ECG of Eisenmenger syndrome usually shows extreme right axis deviation, biatrial enlargement and right ventricular hypertrophy (RVH) with strain pattern (Fig. 23.22).

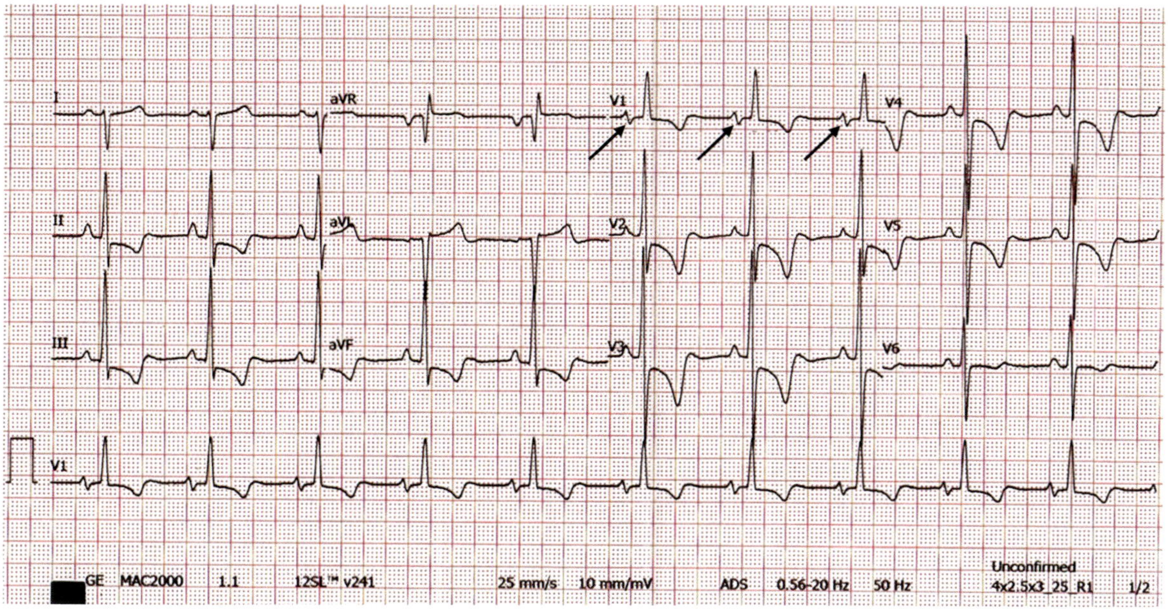

Fig. 23.22: Electrocardiogram shows features of Eisenmenger syndrome with RVH with signs of biatrial enlargement. Note features of RVH strain pattern with tall R-wave in V1 with marked ST-segment depression with T-wave inversions in leads V1–V5 with extreme right axis deviation with signs of biatrial enlargement (tall peak P-waves in inferior leads suggestive of P pulmonale with terminal P negativity in lead V1 with P terminal force duration >40 ms and depth >1 mm, suggestive of left atrial enlargement) (arrows).

Transposition of the Great Arteries

Transposition of the great arteries (TGA) refers to ventriculoarterial discordance. The aorta arises from a morphological right ventricle, and the pulmonary artery arises from a morphological left ventricle. Complete TGA accounts for 5–7% of all congenital cardiac malformations.[64]

The ECG demonstrates right-axis deviation and RV hypertrophy. Bradycardia may represent a slow junctional rhythm or complete heart block. Rhythm abnormalities may be further elucidated by ambulatory rhythm monitoring. Bradycardia and/or syncope may be presenting features related to sinus node dysfunction. After surgery late arrhythmic complications include sinus node dysfunction, atrial tachyarrhythmias, and sudden cardiac death. Sinus node dysfunction and AF are noted in upto 60% and 24% of patients, respectively, at 20 years.[65-69]

Congenitally corrected TGA has been referred to as ventricular inversion, as the ventricles and associated bundle branches are reversed. The sinus node is normally positioned, generating a standard P-wave axis and morphology. However, the ventricular septum is depolarized in the opposite right-to-left direction, contributing to the pathognomonic ECG pattern. Septal Q-waves are absent in left precordial leads and are found over right precordial leads. As the septum is activated in a superior direction, broad Q-waves are seen in leads III and aVF, most pronounced in lead III. Thus, left-axis deviation is the rule. Interestingly, positive T-waves are present over all precordial leads in more than 80%.[28,70] Young adults with isolated congenitally corrected TGA may remain asymptomatic and undetected. The 12-lead ECG can provide the first clue to establish this diagnosis. Given the displaced and fragile AV conduction system, complete AV block is estimated to occur in 2% of patients per year, irrespective of associated anomalies, with a prevalence of 22% on long-term follow-up.[71,72]

Tricuspid Atresia

Tricuspid atresia accounts for 1–3% of congenital heart anomalies. ECG characteristically shows left axis deviation (between 0° and –90°) and left ventricular hypertrophy. Right atrial or combined atrial enlargement is also common. Biatrial hypertrophy with characteristic P 'tricuspidale' is noted in 81% of the electrocardiograms in patients with tricuspid atresia. Sinus rhythm is generally present, with tall P-waves indicative of atrial enlargement. First-degree AV block may be observed. Because of the origin of the left bundle branch from a common bundle, the frontal plane QRS axis may be leftward or superior. An adult pattern of QRS progression over the precordial leads (V1 through V6) is usually present. This pattern of QRS is characterized by absent right ventricular forces and well-developed left ventricular forces consistent with left ventricular hypertrophy. The P-waves are tall (>5 mm) and peaked in lead II. These types of P-waves are called giant P-waves or Himalayan P-waves and are indicative of a dilated right atrium due to a restrictive atrial communication. Presence of Himalayan P-waves have been documented in patients with Tricuspid atresia and Ebstein's anomaly.[73-75]

Mitral Valve Prolapse (MVP)

Mitral valve prolapse (MVP) is a valvular heart disease characterized by the displacement of an abnormally thickened mitral valve leaflet into the left atrium during systole, may be congenital or acquired in origin. The diagnosis of MVP depends upon echocardiography, which uses ultrasound to visualize the mitral valve. The prevalence of MVP is estimated at 2–3% of the population. Echocardiography is the most useful method of diagnosing a prolapsed mitral valve. Thickening of the mitral leaflets >5 mm and leaflet displacement >2 mm indicates classic mitral valve prolapse. The electrocardiogram is often normal in patients with MVP. The most common abnormality is the presence of ST-segment depression or T-wave inversion in the inferior leads (II, III, and aVF).[76] Early repolarization pattern in ECG, presented as a notch in descending arm of QRS and/or ST segment or J-point elevation is more frequent in patients with MVP syndrome.[77] Reverse delta-wave is a possible sign in electrocardiography to diagnose mitral valve prolapse. It is a notch, reverse delta-wave in the descending arm of QRS complex, observed in 79% of patients with MVP, consisting of 58% in inferior leads, and 21% in LI and aVL leads. Reverse delta-wave in ECG may help in the clinical diagnosis of MVP.[78]

SUMMARY

Atrial Septal Defect

Atrial septal defects account for about 10–15% of all congenital cardiac anomalies and are the most common congenital cardiac lesion presenting in adults. Ostium secundum type ASDs account for 70% of all ASDs. The remaining ASDs are ostium primum type (20%), sinus venosus type ASDs 10%, and unroofed coronary sinus, or coronary sinus septal defects (<1%).

Size of ASD determines the shunt flow which in turn results in most of the ECG abnormalities. If the ASD is very small, the ECG may be normal.

Ostium Secundum ASD

1. The most frequent ECG abnormality in ASD is right bundle branch block (RBBB) pattern. RBBB is usually incomplete. However, a complete RBBB pattern is not infrequent with increasing age.
2. Normal axis or right axis deviation due to right ventricular diastolic overload.
3. Crochetage sign: notched R-wave in inferior limb leads. This sign may disappear after closure of the defect (Box 23.2).
4. Right atrial abnormality may or may not be observed (tall and peaked P-waves in lead II suggesting right atrial enlargement may be noted).
5. Prolongation of the PR interval: first degree AV block may be present but less frequent than ostium primum ASD.
6. If the defect is very large then atrial dilatation results in atrial flutter or AF in adults.

Box 23.2: Crochetage sign.

A notch near the apex of the R-wave in inferior leads is known as Crochetage sign. Common in ASD but may be seen in VSD and PS.

Crochetage sign in ASD

1. Involves all three inferior leads in 27% of the ASD patients.
2. Involves at least one inferior limb lead in 73% of the ASD patients.
3. Crochetage pattern is independent of the incomplete right bundle branch block, frequently seen in patients with ASD.
4. Crochetage pattern correlates with shunt severity in patients with ASD.
5. Crochetage sign disappears in approximately 35% of the patients within two weeks after closure of the ASD.

Crochetage sign in VSD

1. Involves all three inferior leads in 2% of the VSD patients.
2. Involves at least one inferior limb lead in 35% of the VSD patients.

Crochetage sign in PS

1. Involves all three inferior leads in 0.7% of the pulmonary stenosis patients.
2. Involves at least one inferior limb lead in 23% of the pulmonary stenosis patients.

Ostium Primum ASD

1. Incomplete or complete RBBB.
2. Left axis deviation.
3. Prolongation of the PR interval (first degree AV block).

Sinus Venosus ASD

1. Incomplete or complete RBBB.
2. Right axis deviation.
3. Ectopic atrial rhythm may be observed. Negative P-waves in inferior leads (II, III, and aVF) suggest low atrial rhythm.

A common finding in the ECG of ASD patient is the presence of incomplete right bundle branch block (RBBB). The presence of a right bundle branch block is so characteristic that if it is absent, the diagnosis of ASD should be reconsidered. The ECG of a patient with ASD should show a right bundle branch block (mostly incomplete) partially due to the right ventricular volume and pressure overload that occurs.

When an ostium primum ASD is present, the ECG reveals left axis deviation. When an ostium secundum ASD is present, the ECG reveals right axis deviation.

The presence of an ectopic atrial pacemaker is suggestive of a sinus venosus ASD. With the development of pulmonary hypertension, right ventricular hypertrophy becomes evident. Atrial arrhythmias such as atrial fibrillation and supraventricular tachycardia may appear in patients in the third or fourth decades of life.

Electrocardiogram Features of Ventricular Septal Defect (VSD)

The ECG is reflective of the size and hemodynamic effect of the VSD.

1. In children with small ventricular communications, the ECG will be normal for age.
2. With increasing defect size and the resulting shunting, there will be left ventricular hypertrophy noted.
3. With unrestrictive large ventricular septal defects which allow the right ventricular pressure to reflect that of the left ventricle, there may also be right ventricular or Bi-ventricular hypertrophy (tall R-waves and deep S-waves in leads V1–V6),on the electrocardiogram.
4. P-wave changes consistent with left atrial enlargement may also become evident.
5. The Katz–Wachtel phenomenon may be seen, with large diphasic RS complexes in midprecordial leads.

ECG in Tetralogy of Fallot

Tetralogy of Fallot is the most common cyanotic congenital heart disease characterized by the presence of four anatomical findings: (1) Ventricular septal defect; (2) Pulmonary stenosis (right ventricular outflow obstruction); (3) Dextroposition of the aorta(overriding aorta); and (4) Right ventricular hypertrophy.

On ECG, patients with TOF will show increased right ventricular forces as evidenced by tall R waves in V1. Additionally right atrial enlargement is manifested by prominent P waves in LII. Right ventricular hypertrophy is demonstrated by a rightward deviated axis.

Classical ECG features of TOF include:

1. Tall monophasic R-wave in lead V1.
2. Tall R-wave in lead V1 with rS in V2 (sudden transition)
3. Right axis deviation
4. Usually no q waves in lateral leads suggesting decreased pulmonary blood flow.

If RV hypertrophy is absent on ECG, the diagnosis of tetralogy of Fallot should be in doubt.

Ebstein's Anomaly

Ebstein's anomaly is a congenital heart defect in which the septal and posterior leaflets of the tricuspid valve are displaced towards the apex of the right ventricle of the heart.

ECG features of Ebstein's anomaly include:

1. Signs of right atrial enlargement or tall and broad "Himalayan" P waves
2. First degree AV block manifesting as a prolonged PR-interval
3. Atypical right bundle branch block (bizarre pattern QRS complex in V1)
4. T wave inversion in V1–V4.
5. About 25% of individuals with Ebstein's anomaly have evidence of Wolff-Parkinson-White syndrome.

Dextrocardia

Dextrocardia is a congenital defect occurs when the heart is positioned in the right side of the chest instead of the left. In patients with this condition, the heart is presented as a mirror image of itself with its apex pointing to the right.

ECG findings of dextrocardia include:

1. Global negativity in lead I (a negative P-wave, QRS complex, and T-wave)
2. Positively deflected QRS complex in aVR
3. Reverse R-wave progression in precordial leads (the R-wave is tallest in V1 and progressively decreases in amplitude in leads V2–V6).
4. Right axis deviation.

Differential diagnosis of true and technical dextrocardia is important. Limb lead reversal or technical dextrocardia usually occurs due to the technical error of reversing the right and left arm electrodes and has become more common as non-experienced personnel replace ECG technicians. When arm leads are reversed the P-waves become negative in lead I and positive in lead aVR. In addition to the P wave, QRS complex and T-wave are also negative in lead I. However, reversal of arm leads does not affect R-wave progression in chest leads and results in an increase in R wave amplitude from lead V1 to V6: normal R-wave progression. Reverse R-wave progression across the precordial leads, with the tallest R-wave in V1 progressively decreasing in amplitude in leads V1–V6, is typical of true (mirror image) dextrocardia. Reverse R-wave progression is never seen in technical dextrocardia.

Patent Ductus Arteriosus

1. Rhythm: normal sinus rhythm, AF may develop with age
2. Prolonged PR interval in 10–20% of patients.
3. LVH: Deep S V1, tall R V5, and V6
4. Left atrial enlargement (LAE)

Coarctation of Aorta

1. LVH, especially by voltage criteria.
2. Atrial enlargement: possible LAE
3. QRS axis: normal or left axis deviation (LAD)
4. QRS configuration: normal

Pulmonary Stenosis

1. RVH; severity correlates with R:S in V1 and V6
2. Right atrial enlargement (RAE).
3. QRS axis: normal if mild; right axis deviation (RAD) with moderate/severe.

Eisenmenger Syndrome

1. RVH manifested by tall R wave in V1, deep S wave in V6
2. ST and T wave abnormalities
3. P pulmonale/ biatrial enlargement.

Complete TGA

1. Sinus bradycardia 60%; junctional rhythm; complete heart block; Intraatrial reentrant tachycardia (IART) 25%.
2. RVH with right axis deviation
3. Right atrial enlargement (RAE)
4. PR interval may be prolonged.

Congenitally Corrected TGA

1. PR interval: first degree AV block >50%; complete AV block 2%/year.
2. Q in Lead III, aVF
3. Absence of septal q waves.

Tricuspid Atresia

1. The P waves are tall (>5 mm) and peaked in lead II. These types of P waves are called giant P waves or Himalayan P waves and are caused by dilated right atrium resulting from pressure overloading.
2. Left axis deviation on electrocardiography and left ventricular hypertrophy.
3. An adult pattern of QRS progression over the precordial leads (V1 through V6) is usually present. This pattern of QRS is characterized by absent right ventricular forces and well-developed left ventricular forces consistent with left ventricular hypertrophy.

Mitral Valve Prolapse (MVP)

1. The most common abnormality is the presence of ST segment depression or T-wave inversion in the inferior leads (II, III and aVF).
2. Early repolarization pattern with J-point elevation is more frequent in patients with MVP syndrome.
3. Reverse delta-wave in descending arm of QRS may be observed in inferior leads, LI and aVL.

REFERENCES

1. Alpendurada F, Wage R, Mohiaddin R. Evaluation of a sinus venosus atrial septal defect by magnetic resonance: a case report. Rev Port Cardiol. 2008;27(10):1317-21.
2. Webb G, Gatzoulis MA. Atrial septal defects in the adult: recent progress and overview. Circulation. 2006;114(15):1645-53.
3. Becker SM, Al Halees Z, Molina C, et al. Consanguinity and congenital heart disease in Saudi Arabia. Am J Med Genet. 2001;99(1):8-13.
4. Samanek M, Voriskova M. Congenital heart disease among 815,569 children born between 1980 and 1990 and their 15-year survival: a prospective Bohemia survival study. Pediatr Cardiol. 1999;20(6):411-7.
5. Botto LD, Correa A, Erickson JD. Racial and temporal variations in the prevalence of heart defects. Pediatrics. 2001;107(3):e32-e34.
6. Borgmann S, Luhmer I, Arslan-Kirchner M, et al. A search for chromosome 22q11.2 deletions in a series of 176 consecutively catheterized patients with congenital heart disease: No evidence for deletions in non-syndromic patients. Eur J Pediatr. 1999;158(12):958-63.
7. Nadrai A. ECG in the diagnostics of atrial septal defect. Acta Paediatr Acad Sci Hung. 1964;65:201-15.
8. Heller J, Hagege AA, Besse B, et al. "Crochetage" (notch) on R wave in inferior limb leads: A new independent electrocardiographic sign of atrial septal defect. J Am Coll Cardiol. 1996;27(4):877-82.
9. Zufelt K, Rosenberg HC, Li MD, et al. The electrocardiogram and the secundum atrial septal defect: A reexamination in the era of echocardiography. Can J Cardiol. 1998;14(2): 227-32.
10. Guray U, Guray Y, Yylmaz MB, et al. Evaluation of P wave duration and P wave dispersion in adult patients with secundum atrial septal defect during normal sinus rhythm. Int J Cardiol. 2003;91(1):75-9.
11. Jost CH, Connolly HM, Danielson GK, et al. Sinus venosus atrial septal defect: long-term postoperative outcome for 115 patients. Circulation. 2005;112(13):1953-8.
12. Davia JE, Cheitlin MD, Bedynek JL. Sinus venosus atrial septal defect: analysis of fifty cases. Am Heart J. 1973;85(2):177-85.
13. Fournier A, Young ML, Garcia OL, et al. Electrophysiologic cardiac function beforeand after surgery in children with atrioventricular canal. Am J Cardiol. 1986;57(13):1137.
14. DiValentino M, Gallino A, Klimusina J, et al. Typical signs of secundum atrial septal defect in a young man. Cardiovas Med. 2011;14(3):98-100.
15. Azhari N, Shihata MS, Al-Fatani A. Spontaneous closure of atrial septal defects within the oval fossa. Cardiol Young. 2004;14(2):148.
16. Anderson PA, Rogers MC, Canent RV Jr, et al. Atrioventricular conduction in secundum atrial septal defects. Circulation. 1973;48:27-31.
17. Emanuel R, O'Brien K, Somerville J, et al. Proceedings: Association of secundum atrial septal defect with abnormalities of atrioventricular conduction or left axis deviation: a new syndrome. Br Heart J. 1976;38(5): 536-41.
18. Rodriguez-Alvarez A, Martinez De Rodriguez G, Goggans AM, et al. The vectorcardiographic equivalent of the "crochetage" of the QRS of the electrocardiogram in atrial septal defect of the ostium secundum type: preliminary report. Am Heart J. 1959;58:388-94.
19. Bhattacharyya PJ. 'Crochetage' sign on ECG in secundum ASD: clinical significance BMJ Case Reports. 2016.
20. Cohen JS, Patton DJ, Giuffre RM. The crochetage pattern in electrocardiograms of pediatric atrial septal defect patients. Can J Cardiol. 2000;16(10):1241-7.
21. Guray U, Guray Y, Mecit B, et al. Maximum p wave duration and p wave dispersion in adult patients with secundum

atrial septal defect: The impact of surgical repair. Ann Noninvasive Electrocardiol. 2004;9(2):136.
22. Davia JE, Cheitlin MD, Bedynek JL. Sinus venosus atrial septal defect: analysis of fifty cases. Am Heart J. 1973;85(2):177-85.
23. Khairy P, Marelli AJ. Clinical use of electrocardiography in adults with congenital heart disease. Circulation. 2007;116(23):2734-46.
24. Gatzoulis MA, Freeman MA, Siu SC, et al. Atrial arrhythmia after surgical closure of atrial septal defects in adults. N Engl J Med. 1999;340(11):839-46.
25. Attie F, Rosas M, Granados N, et al. Surgical treatment for secundum atrial septal defects in patients >40 years old: a randomized clinical trial. J Am Coll Cardiol. 2001;38(7): 2035-42.
26. Silversides CK, Siu SC, McLaughlin PR, et al. Symptomatic atrial arrhythmias and transcatheter closure of atrial septal defects in adult patients. Heart. 2004;90(10):1194-8.
27. Rojas CA, Cruite DM, Chung JH. Traumatic ventricular septal defect: Characterization with electrocardiogram-gated cardiac computed tomography angiography. J Thorac Imaging. 2012;27(6):174-6.
28. Vince DJ, Keith JD. The electrocardiogram in ventricular septal defect. Circulation. 1961;23:225-40.
29. Riggs T, Mehta S, Hirschfeld S, et al. Ventricular septal defect in infancy: A combined vectorgraphic and echocardiographic study. Circulation. 1979; 59(2): 385-94.
30. Katz LN, Wachtel H. The diphasic QRS type of electrocardiogram in congenital heart disease. Am Heart J. 1937;13:22-4.
31. Kidd L, Driscoll DJ, Gersony WM, et al. Second natural history study of congenital heart defects: Results of treatment of patients with ventricular septal defects. Circulation. l993;87(Suppl 1):I38-I59.
32. Moller JH, Patton C, Varco RL, et al. Late results (30 to 35 years) after operative closure of isolated ventricular septal defect from 1954 to 1960. Am J Cardiol. 1991;68:(15)1491-7.
33. Liberman L, Kaufman S, Alfayyadh M, et al. Noninvasive prediction of pulmonary artery pressure in patients with isolated ventricular septal defect. Pediatr Cardiol. 2000;21(3):197-201.
34. Knauth AL, Lock JE, Perry SB, et al. Transcatheter device closure of congenital and postoperative residual ventricular septal defects. Circulation. 2004;110(5):501-7.
35. Brickner ME, Hillis LD, Lange RA. Congenital heart disease in adults: Second of two parts. N Engl J Med. 2000;342(5): 334-42.
36. Monaco M, Williams I. Tetralogy of Fallot: fetal diagnosis to surgical correction. Minerva Pediatr. 2012;64(5): 461-70.
37. Apitz C, Webb GD, Redington AN. Tetralogy of Fallot. Lancet. 2009;374(9699);1462-71.
38. Gatzoulis MA, Balaji S, Webber SA, et al. Risk factors for arrhythmia and sudden cardiac death late after repair of tetralogy of Fallot: S multicentre study. Lancet. 2000;356(9234):975-981.
39. Harrison DA, Siu SC, Hussain F, et al. Sustained atrial arrhythmias in adults late after repair of tetralogy of Fallot. Am J Cardiol. 2001;87(5):584-8.
40. Gillette PC, Garson A. Sudden cardiac death in the pediatric population. Circulation. 1992;85(Suppl): 64-I69.
41. Ho SY, Goltz D, McCarthy K, et al. The atrioventricular junctions in Ebstein malformation. Heart. 2000; 83(4): 444-9.
42. Attenhofer Jost CH, Connolly HM, Dearani JA, et al. Congenital heart disease for the adult cardiologist; Ebstein's anomaly. Circulation. 2007;115(2):277-85.
43. Frescura C, Angelini A, Daliento L, et al. Morphological aspects of Ebstein's anomaly in adults. Thorac Cardiovasc Surg. 2000;48(4):203-8.
44. Giuliani ER, Fuster V, Brandenburg RO, et al. Ebstein's anomaly: the clinical features and natural history of Ebstein's anomaly of the tricuspid valve. Mayo Clin Proc. 1979; 54(3):163-73.
45. Hebe J. Ebstein's anomaly in adults. Arrhythmias: diagnosis and therapeutic approach. Thorac Cardiovasc Surg. 2000;48(4):214-9.
46. Attenhofer Jost CH, Connolly HM, Edwards WD, et al. Ebstein's anomaly—review of a multifaceted congenital cardiac condition. Swiss Med Wkly. 2005;135(19-20):269-81.
47. Edwards WD. Embryology and pathologic features of Ebstein's anomaly. Prog Pediatr Cardiol. 1993;2:5-15.
48. Celemajer D, Bull C, Till J, et al. Ebstein's anomaly: presentation and outcome from fetus to adult. J Am Coll Cardiol. 1994;23(1):170-6.
49. Solzbach U, Beuter M, Hartig B, et al. Isolated dextrocardia with situs solitus (dextroversion). Herz. 2010;35(3):207-10.
50. Martinez-Frias ML. Heterotaxia as an outcome of maternal diabetes: An epidemiological study. Am J Med Genetics. 2001;99(2):142-6.
51. Al-Khadra AS. Mirror-image dextrocardia with situs inversus. Circulation. 1995;91:1602-3.
52. Jones MB, Glancy DL, Jain N. ECG of the month: Right-axis deviation of the QRS complex with precordial R-wave regression. Situs inversus with mirror image dextrocardia, sinus rhythm, and a long P-R interval. J La State Med Soc. 2009;161(3):125-8.
53. Sabah KM, Chowdhury AW, Islam MS, et al. Situs inversus totalis: A rare congenital anomaly and the presence of COPD giving a concept of dextroposition with limb lead reversal in ECG. Bangladesh Heart J. 2016;31(2):100-3.
54. Yin LK, Mohamed AL. Dextrocardia with Situs Inversus. N Engl J Med. 2005;353:933.
55. Amin MG, Chowdhury AW, Ahmed M, et al. Lead-reversal ECG simulating myocardial infarction—a case report and literature review. Bangladesh Heart J. 2016;31(2):104-8.
56. Marquis RM, Miller HC, McCormack RJ, et al. Persistence of ductus arteriosus with left to right shunt in the older patient. Br Heart J. 1982;48(5):469-84.
57. Mirowski M, Arevalo F, Medrano GA, et al. Conduction disturbances in patent ductus arteriosus: a study of 20 cases before and after surgery with determination of the P-R index. Circulation. 1962;25:807-13.
58. Glancy DL, Morrow AG, Simon AL, et al. Juxtaductal aortic coarctation. Analysis of 84 patients studied hemodynamically, angiographically, and morphologically after age 1 year. Am J Cardiol. 1983; 51:537-51.
59. Rasmussen K, Sorland SJ. Prediction of right ventricular systolic pressure in pulmonary stenosis from combined vectorcardiographic data. Am Heart J. 1973;86:318-28.
60. D'Alto M, Mahadevan VS. Pulmonary arterial hypertension associated with congenital heart disease. Eur Respir Rev. 2012;21(126):328-37.

61. Trojnarska O, Plaskota K. Therapeutic methods used in patients with Eisenmenger syndrome. Cardiol J. 2009;16(6):500-6.
62. Beghetti M, Galie N. Eisenmenger syndrome a clinical perspective in a new therapeutic era of pulmonary arterial hypertension. J Am Coll Cardiol. 2009;53(9):733-40.
63. Oya H, Nagaya N, Uematsu M, et al. Poor prognosis and related factors in adults with Eisenmenger syndrome. Am Heart J. 2002;143(4):739-44.
64. Brickner ME, Hillis LD, Lange RA. Congenital heart disease in adults: First of two parts. N Engl J Med. 2000;342(4): 256-63.
65. Gelatt M, Hamilton RM, McCrindle BW, et al. Arrhythmia and mortality after the Mustard procedure: a 30-year single-center experience. J Am Coll Cardiol. 1997;29:(1)194-201.
66. Khairy P, Landzberg MJ, Lambert J, et al. Long-term outcomes after the atrial switch for surgical correction of transposition: a meta-analysis comparing the Mustard and Senning procedures. Cardiol Young. 2004;14:284-92.
67. Puley G, Siu S, Connelly M, et al. Arrhythmia and survival in patients >18 years of age after the Mustard procedure for complete transposition of the great arteries. Am J Cardiol. 1999;83:1080-4.
68. Sarkar D, Bull C, Yates R, et al. Comparison of long-term outcomes of atrial repair of simple transposition with implications for a late arterial switch strategy. Circulation. 1999;(Suppl);100:II176-II181.
69. Kammeraad JA, van Deurzen CH, Sreeram N, et al. Predictors of sudden cardiac death after Mustard or Senning repair for transposition of the great arteries. J Am Coll Cardiol. 2004;44(5):1095-102.
70. Victorica BE, Miller BL, Gessner IH. Electrocardiogram and vectorcardiogram in ventricular inversion (corrected transposition). Am Heart J. 1973;86:733-44.
71. Huhta JC, Maloney JD, Ritter DG, et al. Complete atrioventricular block in patients with atrioventricular discordance. Circulation. 1983;67(6):1374-7.
72. Gillette PC, Busch U, Mullins CE, et al. Electrophysiologic studies in patients with ventricular inversion and "corrected transposition". Circulation. 1979;60(4):939-45.
73. Reddy SC, Zuberbuhler JR. Himalayan P-waves in a patient with tricuspid atresia. Circulation. 2003; 107(3):498.
74. Davutoglu V, Kilinc M, Dinckal MH. Himalayan P waves in a patient with combined tricuspid and pulmonic stenosis. Heart. 2003;89(10):1216.
75. Kaushik ML, Sharma M, Kashyap R. 'Himalayan' P Wave. JAPI. 2007;55:856.
76. Bhutto ZR, Barron JT, Liebson PR, et al. Electrocardiographic abnormalities in mitral valve prolapse. Am J Cardiol. 1992;70:265-6.
77. Peighambari MM, Alizadehasl A, Totonchi Z. Early repolarization in ECG presented as a notch in descending arm of QRS and/or ST segment or J-point elevation is more frequent in patients with MVP syndrome. J Cardiovasc Thorac Res. 2014;6(1):21-23.
78. Alizadeh-Asl A. Reverse delta -wave as a possible sign in electrocardiography to diagnose mitral valve prolapse. BMC Res Notes. 2011;25(4):16.

Chapter 24

Pacemaker Electrocardiogram Interpretation

INTRODUCTION

A pacemaker is indicated when electrical impulse conduction or formation is significantly disturbed. Pacemakers consist of pulse generator and the lead(s). The leads may be single or multiple and unipolar or bipolar. In order to interpret electrocardiograms (ECGs) with paced rhythms, it is important to understand the basic functions of pacemakers and how these functions manifest on the surface ECG. After the basic functions are understood, pacemaker malfunctions and other subtle functions can be interpreted on the ECG. The pacemaker rhythm can be recognized on the ECG. It shows pacemaker spikes—vertical signals that represent the electrical activity of the pacemaker (Fig. 24.1). Usually, these spikes are more visible in unipolar than in bipolar pacing. Duration of pacemaker spikes is usually less than 2 ms.

INDICATIONS FOR PERMANENT PACING[1-5]

- Complete atrioventricular (AV) block (acquired or congenital)
- Persisting symptomatic bradycardia
- Sick sinus syndrome

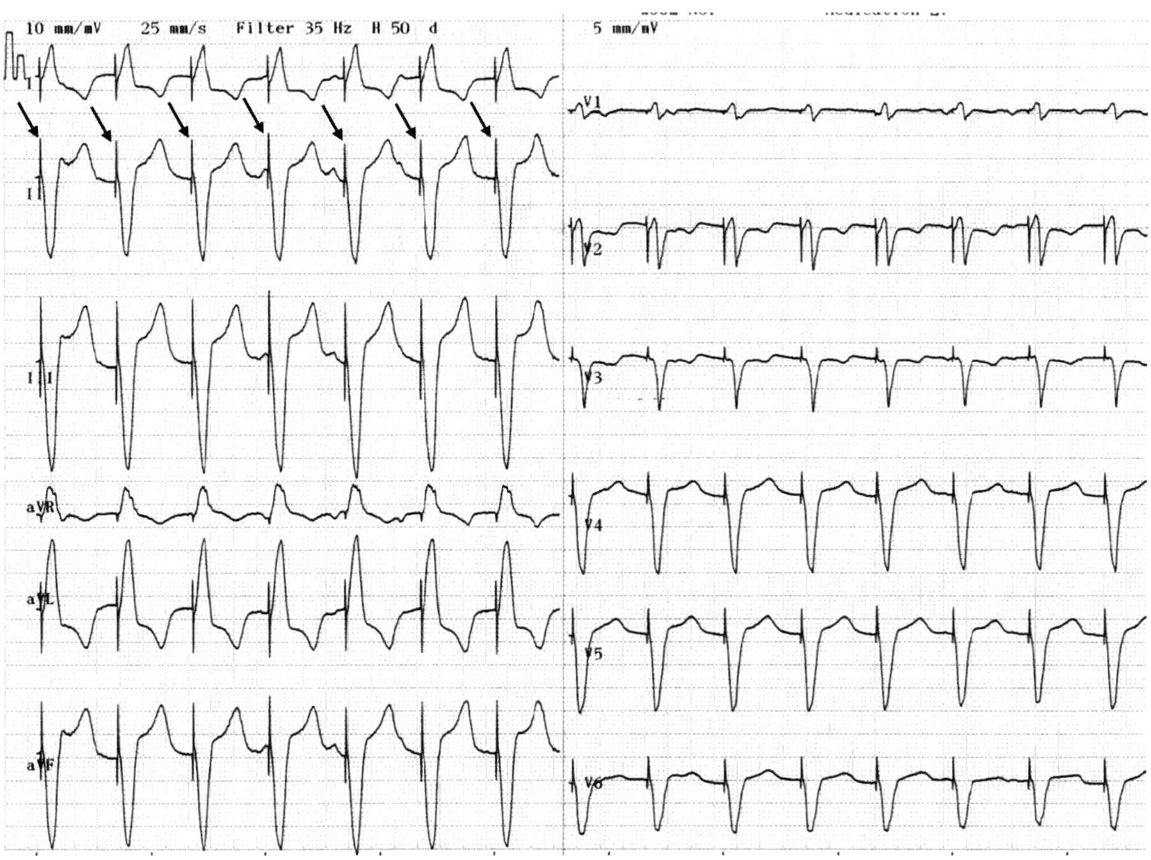

Fig. 24.1: Electrocardiogram shows prominent pacemaker spikes (*arrows*) preceding all the QRS complexes in both limb and chest leads.

- Persistent high-grade AV block, postmyocardial infarction
- Mobitz type II AV block
- Pacemakers may have a role in the suppression of resistant tachyarrhythmias
- Pacemakers have a role in the management of some patients with dilated cardiomyopathy (DCM) and hypertrophic obstructive cardiomyopathy (HOCM).

ATRIAL PACING

Atrial pacing appears on the ECG as a single pacemaker stimulus followed by a P-wave (Fig. 24.2). The morphology of the P-wave depends upon the location of the atrial lead. It may be normal, diminutive, biphasic, or negative. If the site of stimulation is near the sinoatrial (SA) node in the right atrium (RA), then the morphology of the P-waves resemble that of sinus beats. If the site of stimulation is in the coronary sinus, then the morphology of the P-waves is inverted in LII, LIII, and aVF.

The PR interval and configuration of the QRS complex are similar to those seen in sinus rhythm. They are independent of the atrial pacemaker; thus, the duration and configuration are determined by the intrinsic characteristics of the patient's conduction system. There is 100% capture if the rhythm is entirely paced. However, there may be intermittent capture when the atrial pacemaker is in a demand mode and is activated only when the intrinsic atrial rate falls below a preset level. For example, if the pacemaker is set at 60 beats/min, the pacemaker will only pace if the rate falls below 60 beats/min.

VENTRICULAR PACING

Ventricular demand pacing appears on the ECG as a single pacemaker spike followed by a QRS complex that is wide, bizarre, and resembles a ventricular beat. The pacemaker lead is usually in the right ventricular apex; thus, the paced QRS complex has a left bundle branch block (LBBB) configuration since right ventricular activation occurs before activation of the left ventricle, and is negative in the inferior leads (Fig. 24.3). Sometimes, the lead may be placed higher up in the right ventricular septum or outflow tract, and while there is still an LBBB pattern, the inferior leads may have variable axis. There may or may not be atrial activity noted, depending upon the nature of the patient's underlying rhythm. If intrinsic or native atrial activity is present with a single chamber ventricular-only pacemaker, it occurs at a rate that differs from the ventricular rate since it is dissociated from the QRS complex.

There may be episodic pacing in patients who have a ventricular demand pacemaker (Figs. 24.4A and B). The pacemaker is activated and delivers a stimulus only when the intrinsic ventricular rate falls below a predetermined lower limit; pacemaker activity is suppressed when the intrinsic heart rate is faster (ventricular inhibited). Similar to atrial pacing, if the pacemaker is set at 60 beats/min, the pacemaker will only pace the ventricle if the rate falls below 60 beats/min. If the native rate is slow, there will be 100%ventricular pacing. The ECG may have evidence of fusion or pseudofusion beats if the pacemaker rate and intrinsic heart rate are nearly identical, and the native and paced QRS complex occur simultaneously.

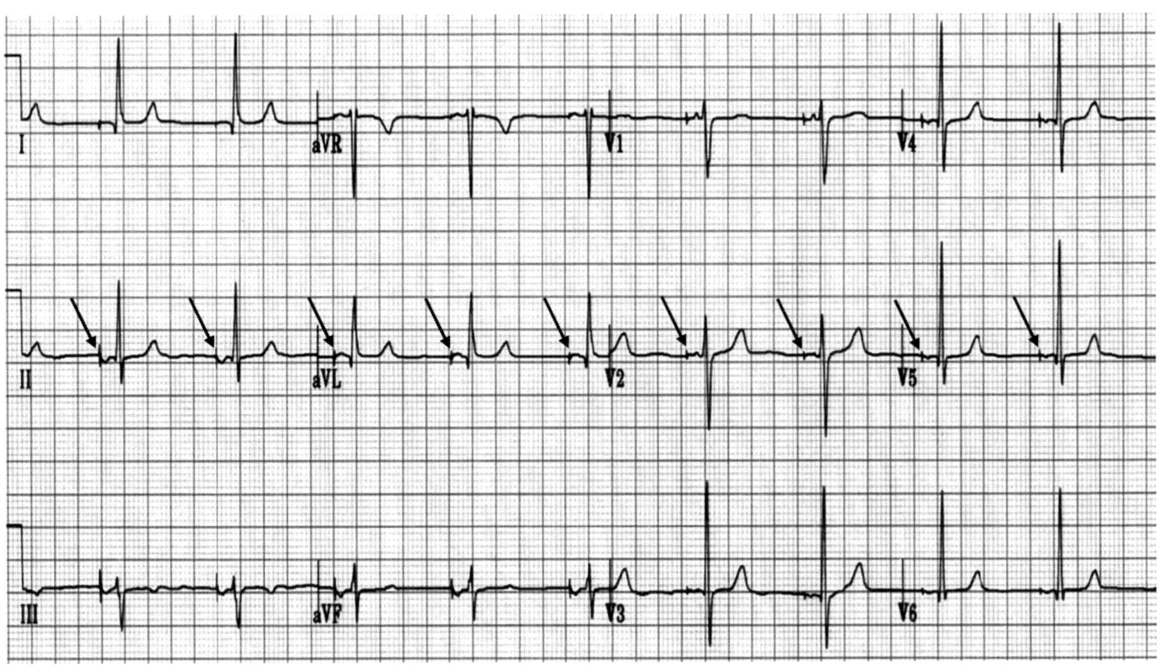

Fig. 24.2: Electrocardiogram shows atrial pacing. Note pacing spikes precede all the P waves (*arrows*) and QRS complexes are of normal configuration.

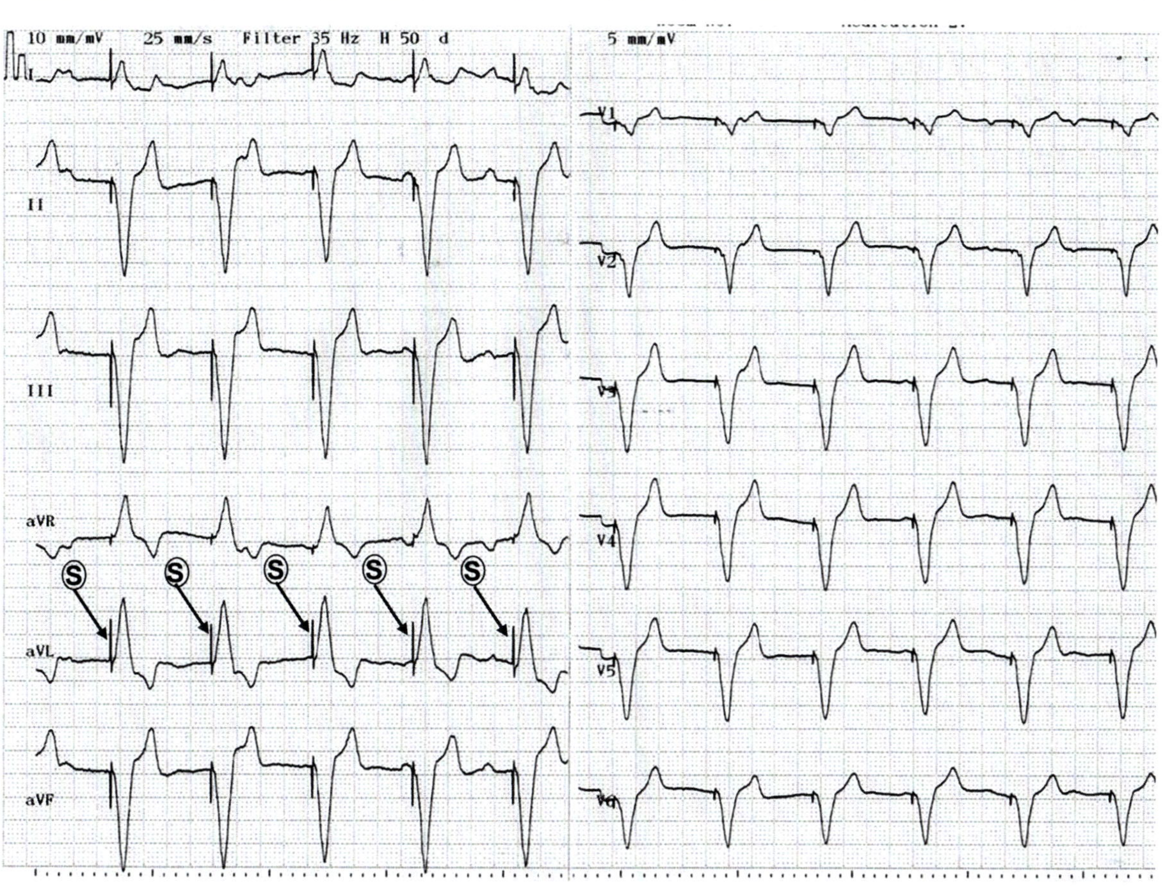

Fig. 24.3: Electrocardiogram (ECG) shows ventricular pacing. Ventricular demand pacing appears on the ECG as a single pacemaker spike preceding all QRS complexes (*arrows*). The pacemaker lead is in the right ventricular apex; thus, the paced QRS complexes resemble left bundle branch block (LBBB) configuration since right ventricular activation occurs before activation of the left ventricle, and is negative in the inferior leads. Note ST segments and T waves are discordant with the QRS complexes, i.e. the major terminal portion of the QRS complex is located on the opposite side of the baseline from the ST segment and T-wave.

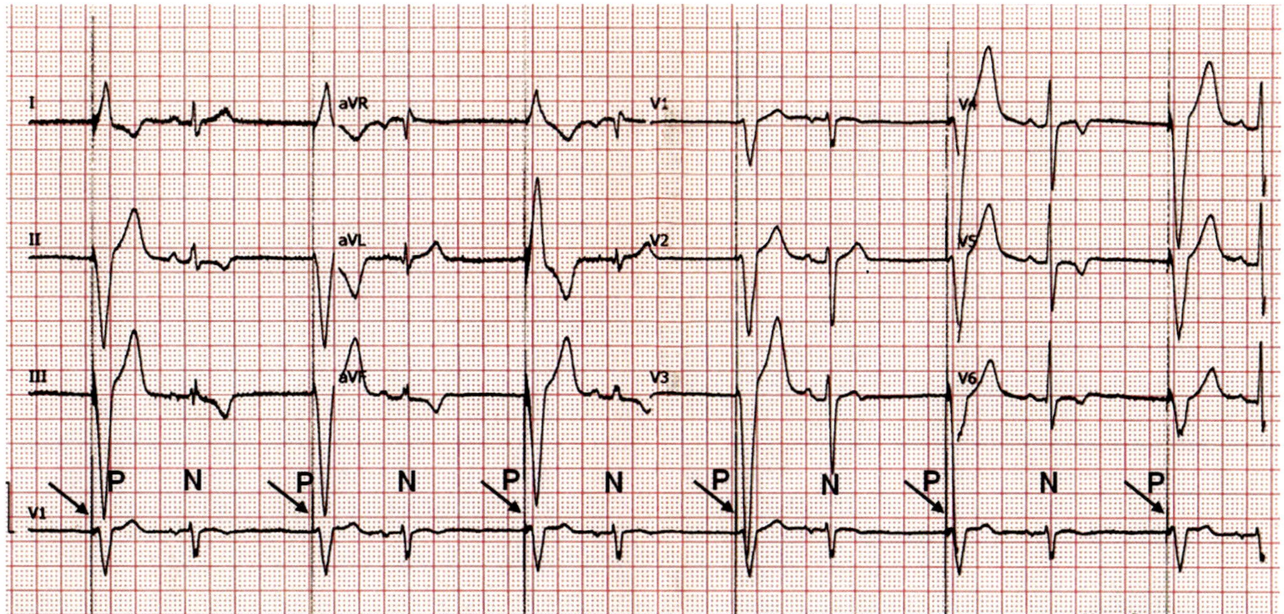

Fig. 24.4A: Electrocardiogram (ECG) displays episodic ventricular pacing. Note alternate pacing (P) and sinus conducted normal beats (N). Note all the paced QRS complexes are preceded by a pacemaker spike (*arrows*).

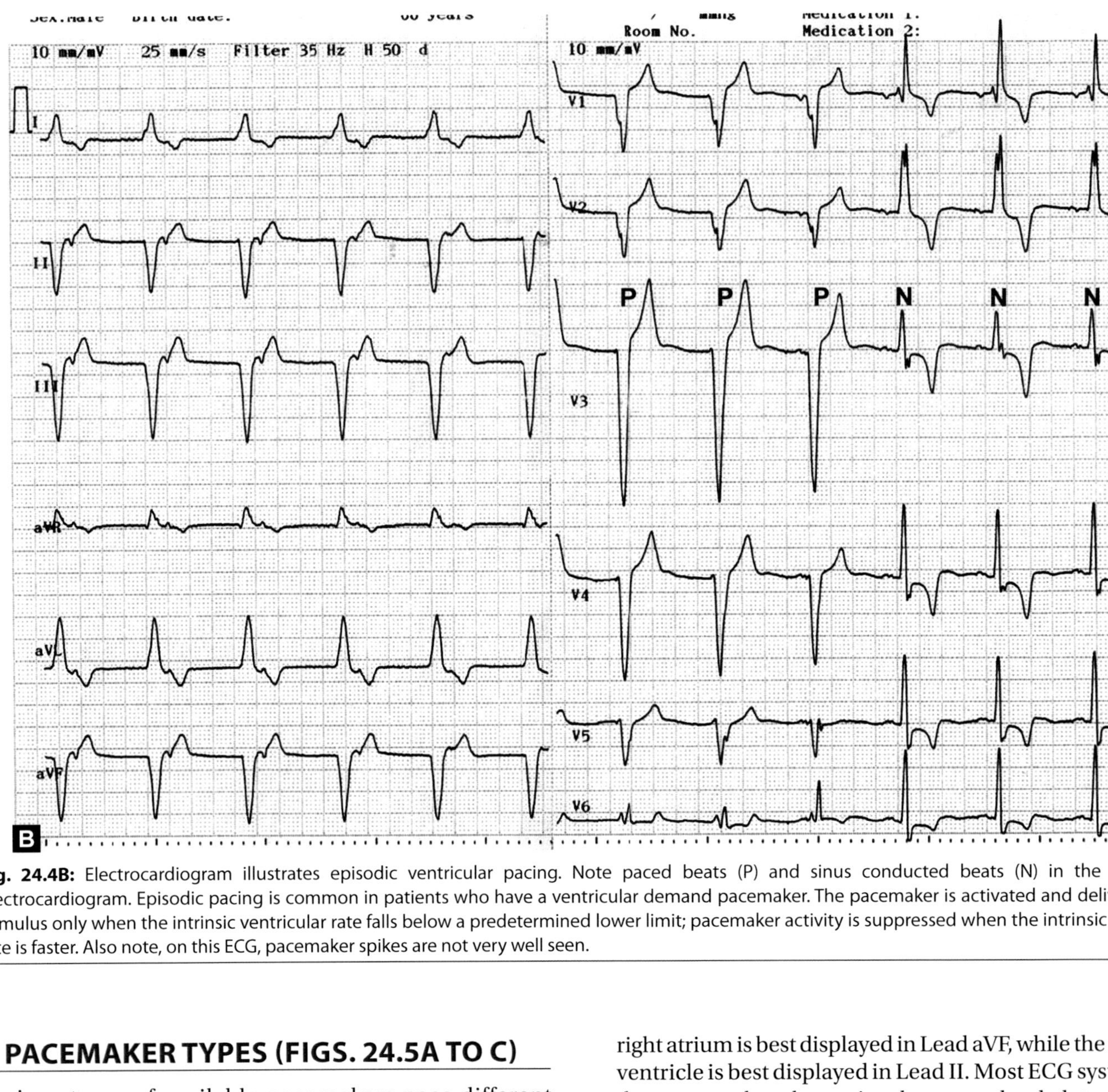

Fig. 24.4B: Electrocardiogram illustrates episodic ventricular pacing. Note paced beats (P) and sinus conducted beats (N) in the same electrocardiogram. Episodic pacing is common in patients who have a ventricular demand pacemaker. The pacemaker is activated and delivers a stimulus only when the intrinsic ventricular rate falls below a predetermined lower limit; pacemaker activity is suppressed when the intrinsic heart rate is faster. Also note, on this ECG, pacemaker spikes are not very well seen.

PACEMAKER TYPES (FIGS. 24.5A TO C)

Various types of available pacemakers pace different chambers:

- *Single-chamber pacing*: Delivers pacing therapy to only one chamber of the heart; it can be either unipolar or bipolar. Single-chamber pacing is applied to the right atrium (Fig. 24.2) or the right ventricle (Fig. 24.6) .
- *Dual-chamber pacing*: Delivers pacing therapy to both the right atrium and the right ventricle (Figs. 24.7 and 8A and B).
- *Biventricular pacing*: Delivers pacing therapy to both the right ventricle and the left ventricle. In addition, the heart is usually paced in the right atrium. This mode of pacing can be very difficult to display properly for two main reasons: first, the two ventricle paces may occur at the same time, appearing as a single pulse at the skin surface. Second, the left ventricle lead placement is generally not on the same vector as the right ventricle lead and may actually be orthogonal to it. Usually, the right atrium is best displayed in Lead aVF, while the right ventricle is best displayed in Lead II. Most ECG systems do not employ three simultaneous lead-detection circuits or algorithms, making the left ventricle the toughest lead to pick up.[4]

PACEMAKER CODES

Pacemakers have 1–3 leads which provide pacing and sensing activity. They are classified using three, four, and sometimes even five letters which describe the function of the pacemaker. These functions include which chambers are sensed, which chambers are potentially paced, which chambers cause inhibition of the pacemaker, and whether the pacemaker has the ability to be responsive to activity or not.

1. The first letter identifies what chamber is paced. The letter can be A (atrial only), V (ventricular only) or D (dual or both chambers). It is not difficult to identify what chamber is being paced when the spikes are

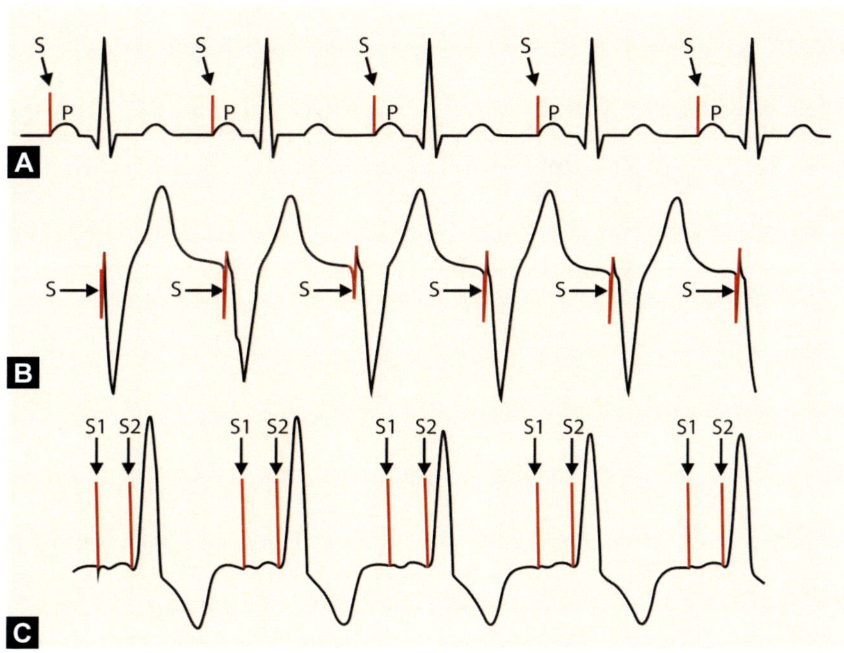

Figs. 24.5A to C: Schematic ECG representation of various types of available pacemakers pace different chambers. (A) *Atrial pacing:* Pacing spikes precede all the P waves (*S*) and morphology of the QRS complexes are of normal configuration. (B) *Ventricular pacing:* Pacing spikes (*S*) precede all the QRS complexes. Note ventricular pacing appears on the electrocardiogram (ECG) as a single pacemaker spike followed by a QRS complex that is wide, bizarre, and resembles a ventricular beat. Usually pacing leads are placed at right ventricular apex and right ventricular pacing lead placement results in a QRS morphology similar to left bundle branch block (LBBB) and left epicardial pacing lead placement results in a QRS morphology similar to right bundle branch block (RBBB). (C) *Dual chamber pacing:* Pacing spikes precede both P-waves (*S1*) and QRS complexes (*S2*). But dual chamber pacing may exhibit features of atrial pacing, ventricular pacing or both, so pacing spikes may precede only P-wave, only QRS complex, or both.

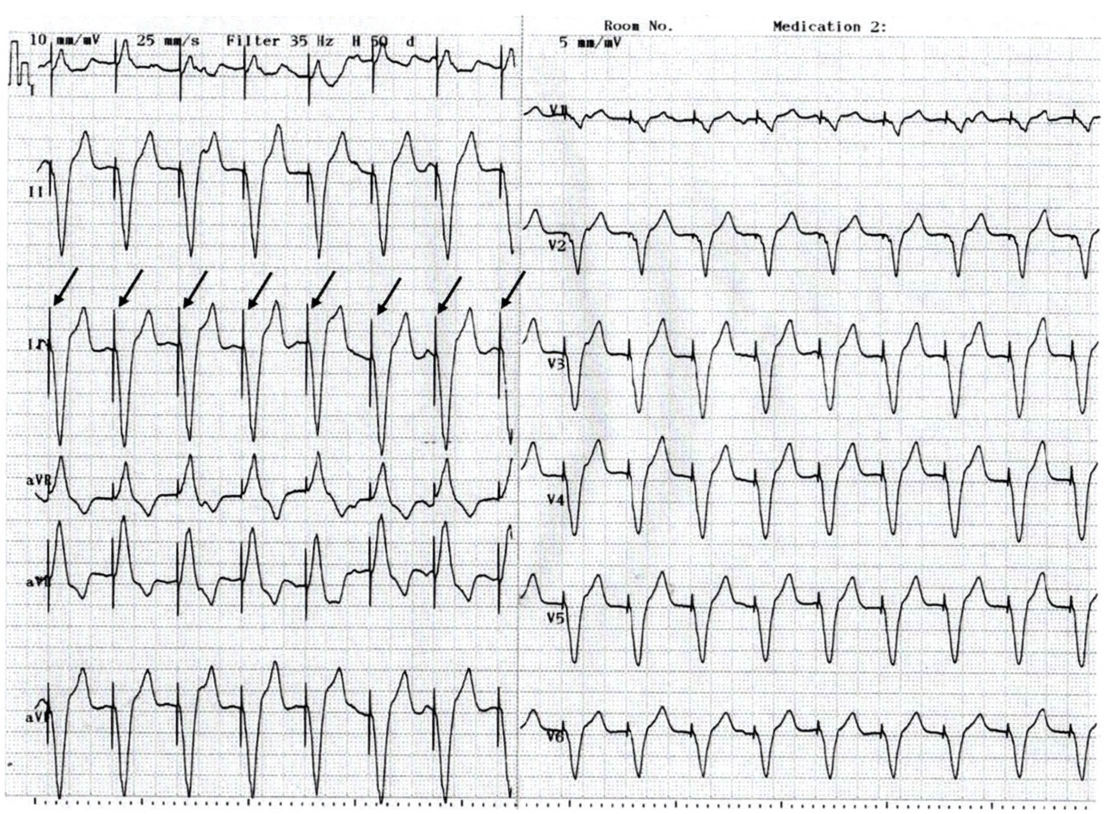

Fig. 24.6: Electrocardiogram shows ventricular pacing with magnet (rate 100 bpm). Ventricular demand pacing appears on the ECG as a single pacemaker spike preceding all QRS complexes (*arrows*). The pacemaker lead is in the right ventricular apex; thus, the paced QRS complexes resemble left bundle branch block (LBBB) pattern. Note magnet can change the pacemaker firing rate and can indirectly indicate the end-of-life (EOL) of pacemaker battery.

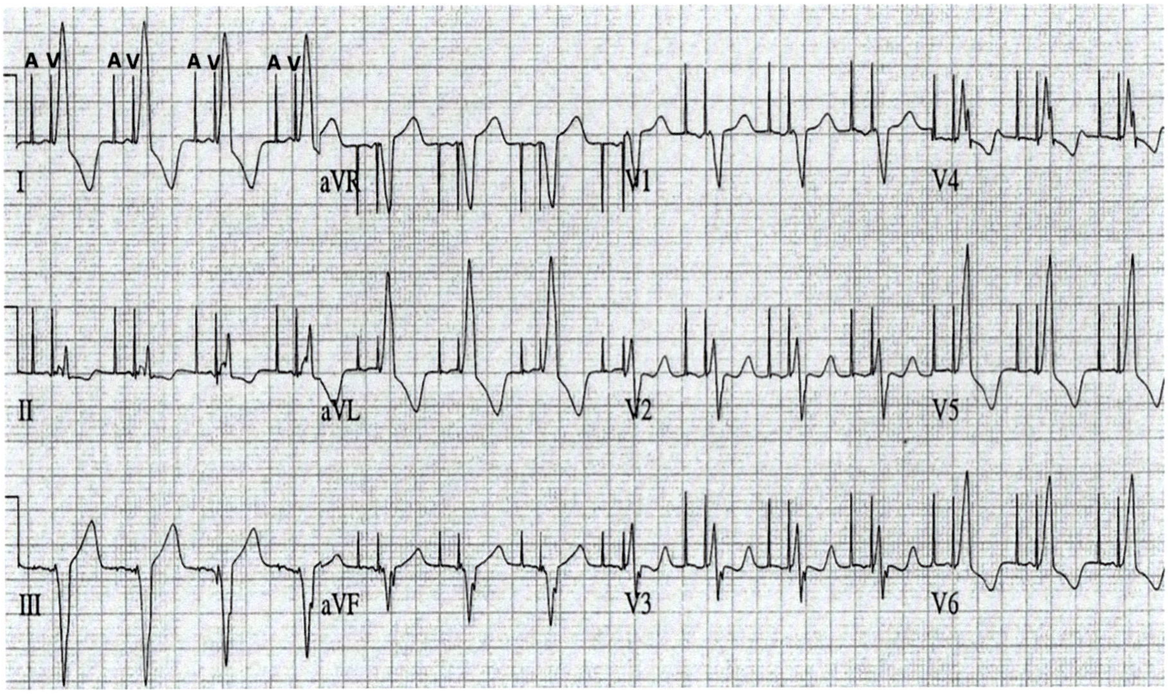

Fig. 24.7: Electrocardiogram illustrates the typical features of dual chamber pacing. This ECG of A–V sequential pacing shows atrial spikes (A) before all the P-waves and ventricular pacing spikes (V) before each QRS complex. There is 100% atrial capture; P-waves are seen following each atrial pacing spike. There is also 100% ventricular capture, a QRS complex follows each ventricular pacing spike. QRS complexes are broad with LBBB morphology, indicating the presence of a ventricular pacing electrode in the right ventricle.

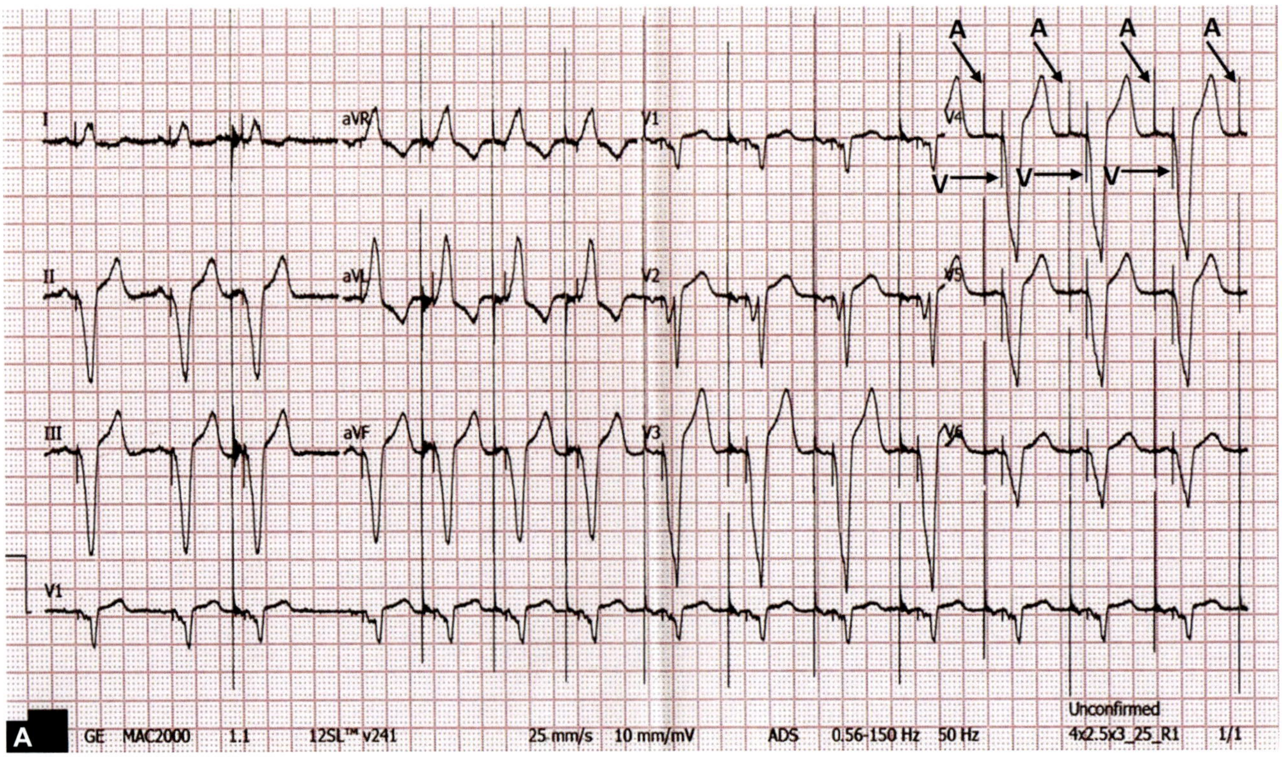

Fig. 24.8A: Electrocardiogram illustrates the typical features of dual chamber pacing. ECG displays atrial spikes (A) before the P-waves and ventricular pacing spikes (V) before QRS complexes (*arrows*). Note atrial spikes are not visible before all the P-waves. Always remember dual chamber pacing may exhibit features of atrial pacing, ventricular pacing or both, so pacing spikes may precede only P-wave, only QRS complex, or both. Pacing spikes may not be well seen in all the leads.

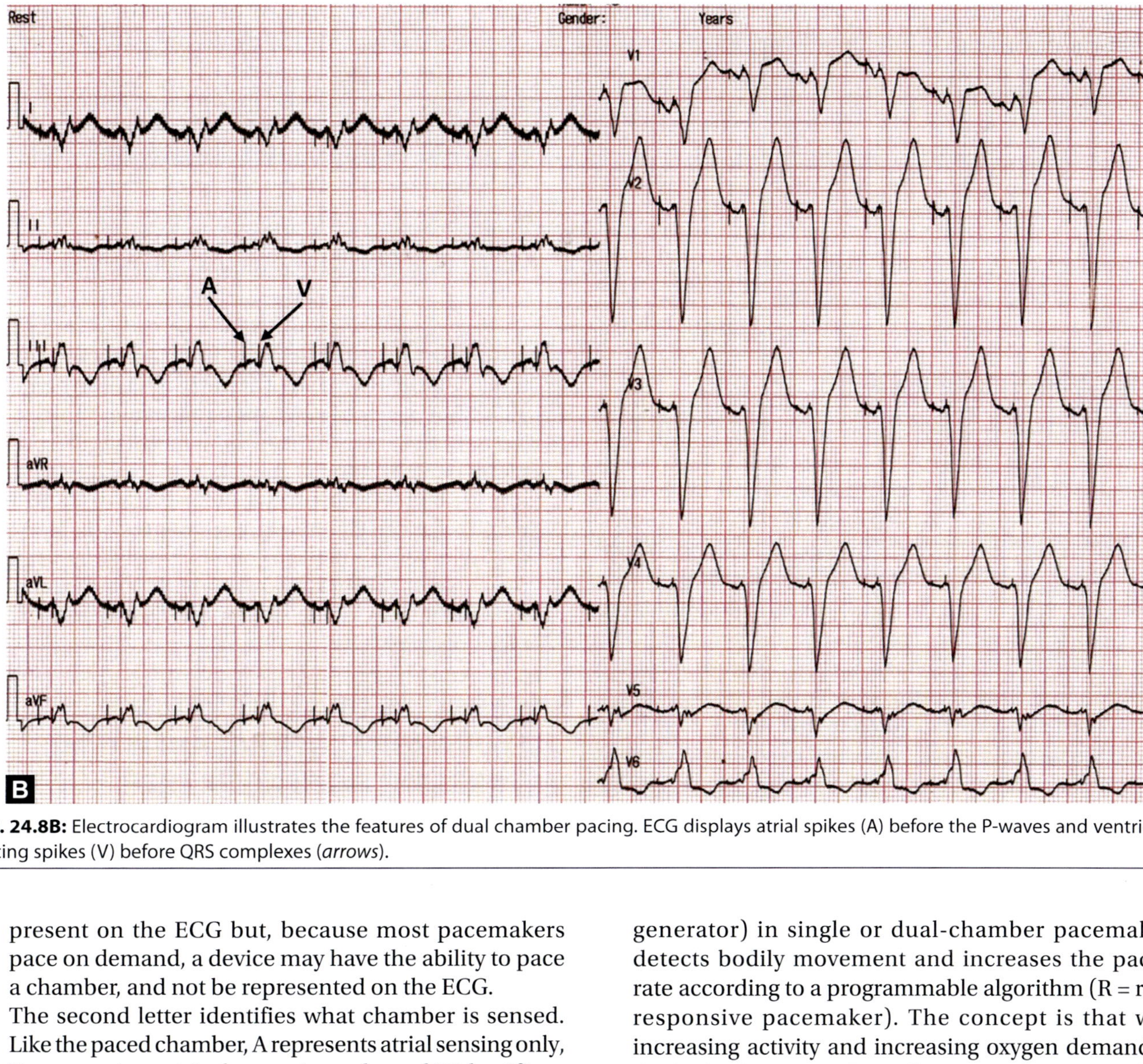

Fig. 24.8B: Electrocardiogram illustrates the features of dual chamber pacing. ECG displays atrial spikes (A) before the P-waves and ventricular pacing spikes (V) before QRS complexes (*arrows*).

present on the ECG but, because most pacemakers pace on demand, a device may have the ability to pace a chamber, and not be represented on the ECG.

2. The second letter identifies what chamber is sensed. Like the paced chamber, A represents atrial sensing only, V represents ventricular sensing only, and D identifies a pacemaker that has the ability to sense both chambers.
3. The third letter represents activity in the specific chambers that will inhibit the pacemaker. Inhibition of a pacemaker is a simple concept and identifies inhibition of pacing activity. Pacemakers are preprogrammed to pace at a certain rate. Once the time period elapses, this would allow the heart rate to fall below the set rate, the pacemaker will pace. If a natural beat occurs prior to the preprogrammed time, the pacemaker allows the heart to use its intrinsic rhythm rather than pacing. This provides two major benefits. First, the natural activation of the heart provides better hemodynamic function. The second benefit is that by decreasing the amount of pacing, there is longer battery life for the pacemaker allowing for fewer battery changes. The same letters (A, V, and D) and I (inhibited) are used for the third position.
4. The fourth letter indicates rate-responsive features; an activity sensor (e.g. an accelerometer in the pulse generator) in single or dual-chamber pacemakers detects bodily movement and increases the pacing rate according to a programmable algorithm (R = rate-responsive pacemaker). The concept is that with increasing activity and increasing oxygen demand by the body, the pacemaker will increase the rate at which it fires. This function is identified in the fourth slot as an R (rate responsive).
5. The fifth letter represents anti-tachycardia facilities.

A pacemaker in VVI mode denotes that it paces and senses the ventricle and is inhibited by a sensed ventricular event. The DDD mode denotes that both chambers are capable of being sensed and paced.

PACEMAKER TERMINOLOGY

Firing: Refers to the pacemaker's generation of electrical stimuli. This is seen as a pacemaker spike on the ECG.

Capture: Refers to the presence of a P or QRS or both after a pacemaker spike. This indicates that the tissue in the chamber being paced has been depolarized. The term is that the pacemaker has "captured" the chamber being paced. Paced QRS are wide, bizarre, and resemble PVCs.

Sensing: Refers to the pacemaker's ability to recognize the patient's own intrinsic rhythm in order to determine if it needs to fire. Most pacemakers function in the demand mode and fire when needed.

Interpretation of Pacemaker ECG

Three questions to ask when analyzing an ECG strip with pacemaker:

1. Where are the pacemaker spikes?
2. Is the chamber being paced capturing?
3. Is the pacemaker sensing the patient's inherent rhythm?

EFFECTS OF PACEMAKER ON ECG

A paced rhythm is not difficult to recognize. When a pacemaker fires, a small spike is seen on the ECG. An atrial pacemaker will generate a spike followed by a P wave and a normal QRS complex. Atrial pacemaker is usually placed to address the problem in the sinoatrial (SA) node. Once the electrical cycle starts in the pacemaker, it proceeds through the AV node, and continues distally as normal, and generates QRS of normal morphology.

With a ventricular pacemaker, a spike is seen before the QRS complex. A normal P-wave is followed by a pacemaker spike in front of a wide QRS complex. In this type of patient, the electrical cycle starts normally in the SA node but is usually blocked at the AV node. In case of ventricular pacemaker the electrode is placed in the right ventricle, which is depolarized first, followed by the left ventricle. This placement generates a wide QRS complex similar to that seen in left bundle branch block.

A sequential pacemaker stimulates the atrium first and then the ventricle. With a sequential pacemaker, two spikes are seen, one before the P-wave and the other before the QRS complex.

PACEMAKER MALFUNCTIONS/ COMPLICATIONS

- *Failure to fire*: When a pacemaker fails to send an impulse when it should, it is called failure to fire, which indicates pacemaker malfunction. Usually this means a dead battery or that the connecting wires are at fault. At times the artifacts can fool the pacemaker and it will not fire. This is displayed as no pacer spike where there should be one.
- *Loss of capture*: When loss of capture exists there is no P or QRS after the pacer has fired; just a spike (Figs. 24.9A to C). In this situation the pacer needs to be adjusted. It is possible the pacing wire has lost contact with the chamber wall which can occur when the heart is too damaged to respond.
- *Under-sensing*: This occurs when the pacemaker fires too soon after an intrinsic beat and there are pacer spikes where there should not be. These can appear in the T-wave, on the QRS or anywhere on the heart rhythm's tracing. This requires adjustment with the wires or battery replacement.
- *Failure to sense and pace*: Failure of sensing, pacing or both can result from a number of problems (Fig. 24.10). In the case of permanent pacemakers, these include development of scar at the site of electrode contact with the myocardium, insufficient programmed pacing output, etc. In the case of temporary pacing, poor lead contact due to lead displacement, local infarction or perforation, are the common causes.
- *Ventricular perforation*: An RV apical endocardial lead usually produces a QRS pattern of left bundle branch block (LBBB) and LAD (left axis deviation) and the spike. But perforation or migration of the lead through the pericardial space may produce right bundle branch block (RBBB) pattern morphology (Fig. 24.10). But it must be mentioned that the pattern of RBBB may be also caused by the displacement of the lead into the right ventricular outflow tract. It is important to recognize that the diagnosis of perforation cannot be made by the ECG alone; perforation has to be confirmed radiologically.

DIAGNOSIS OF ST-ELEVATION MYOCARDIAL INFARCTION (STEMI) IN PRESENCE OF PACEMAKER

Electrocardiogram diagnosis of several fatal conditions, e.g. STEMI, hyperkalemia may be masked by the presence of permanent pacemaker, and critical analysis of ECGs is mandatory to exclude these otherwise fatal conditions.

Pacing-induced repolarization changes may mask acute myocardial injury. Various ECG criteria have been proposed for the diagnosis of acute STEMI in presence of permanent pacemaker. The QRS complex during transvenous right ventricular apical pacing resembles that of spontaneously occurring left bundle-branch block, and the ST-T-segment changes are usually discordant from the QRS complex. From the GUSTO-1 trial experience of 131 patients with acute myocardial infarction in the presence of left bundle-branch block, three ECG criteria were found to have independent value in the diagnosis of STEMI—(1) ST-segment elevation of greater than or equal to 1 mm in the presence of a positive QRS complex; (2) ST-segment depression of greater than or equal to 1 mm in lead V1, V2, or V3, and (3) ST-segment elevation of greater than or equal to 5 mm in the presence of a negative QRS complex.[6-11] The ECG criterion with the highest sensitivity for the diagnosis of an acute myocardial infarction was ST segment elevation greater than or equal to 5 mm in leads with a negative QRS complex and even this criterion has a sensitivity of only around 50%. Sgarbossa's criteria can be used to diagnose STEMI, in the setting of both paced rhythms and LBBB.[12-17]

Another classical sign described is the Cabrera's sign.[6,16] Like other signs, this has also been adapted from

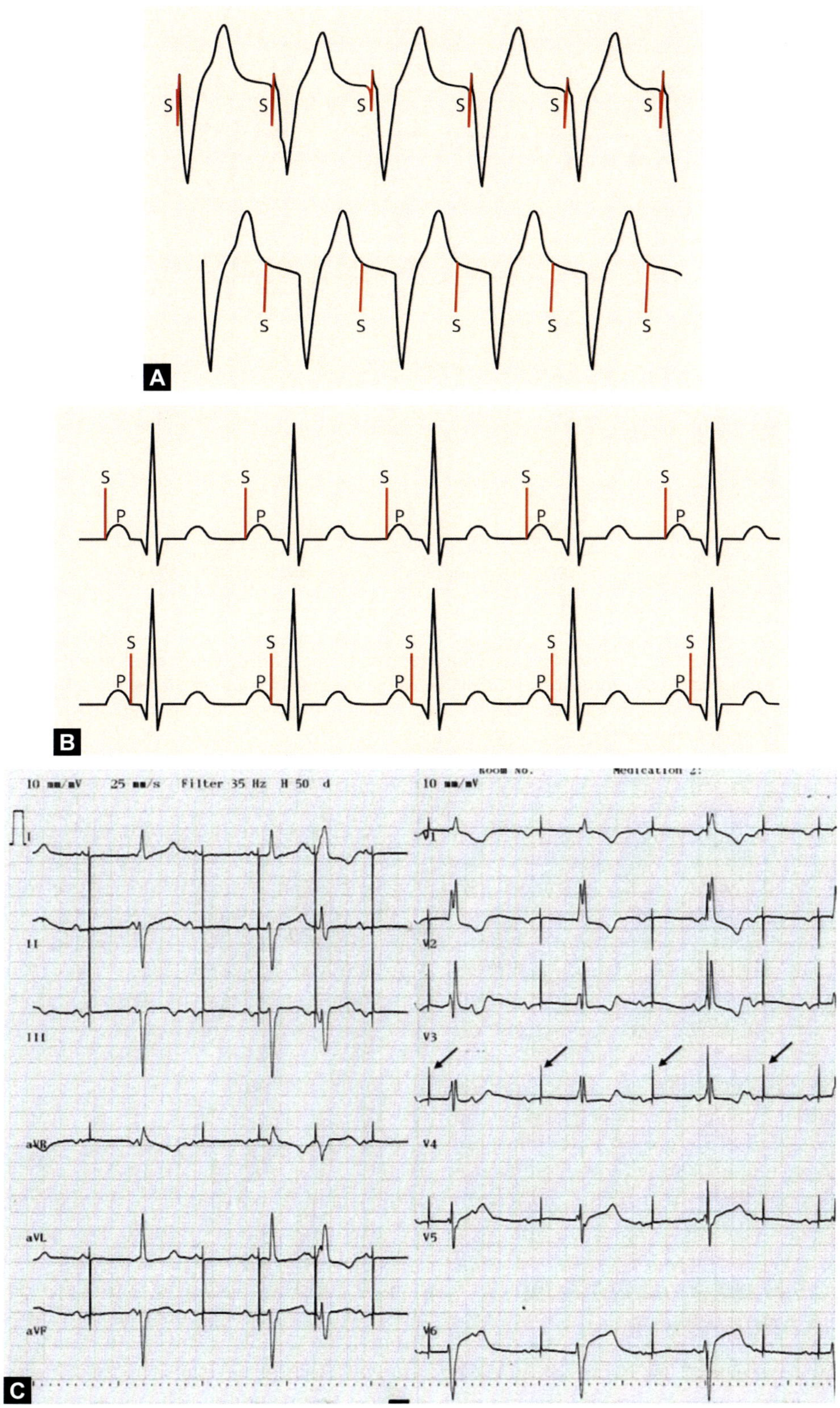

Figs. 24.9A to C: (A) Schematic representation of failure of the ventricular capture by pacemaker. Note in the tracing A (upper panel), all the QRS complexes are preceded by the appropriately placed pacemaker spikes (S) but in the lower panel of the tracing A , QRS complexes are not immediately preceded by pacemaker spikes (S) and the pacemaker fails to capture the ventricle; (B) Schematic representation of failure of the atrial capture by pacemaker. Note in the tracing of upper panel, all the P-waves are preceded by the appropriately placed pacemaker spikes (S) but in the tracing of lower panel, P-waves are not immediately preceded by pacemaker spikes (S) and atrial spikes are present right after spontaneous atrial activity (atrial malsensing); (C) This tracing demonstrates failure of a pacemaker to capture the ventricle. All the pacing spikes fail to capture the ventricle (arrows), pacing spikes are not immediately followed by a QRS. (*Courtesy:* Dr. Mokaddas Hossain Sadi, Labaid Cardiac Hospital).

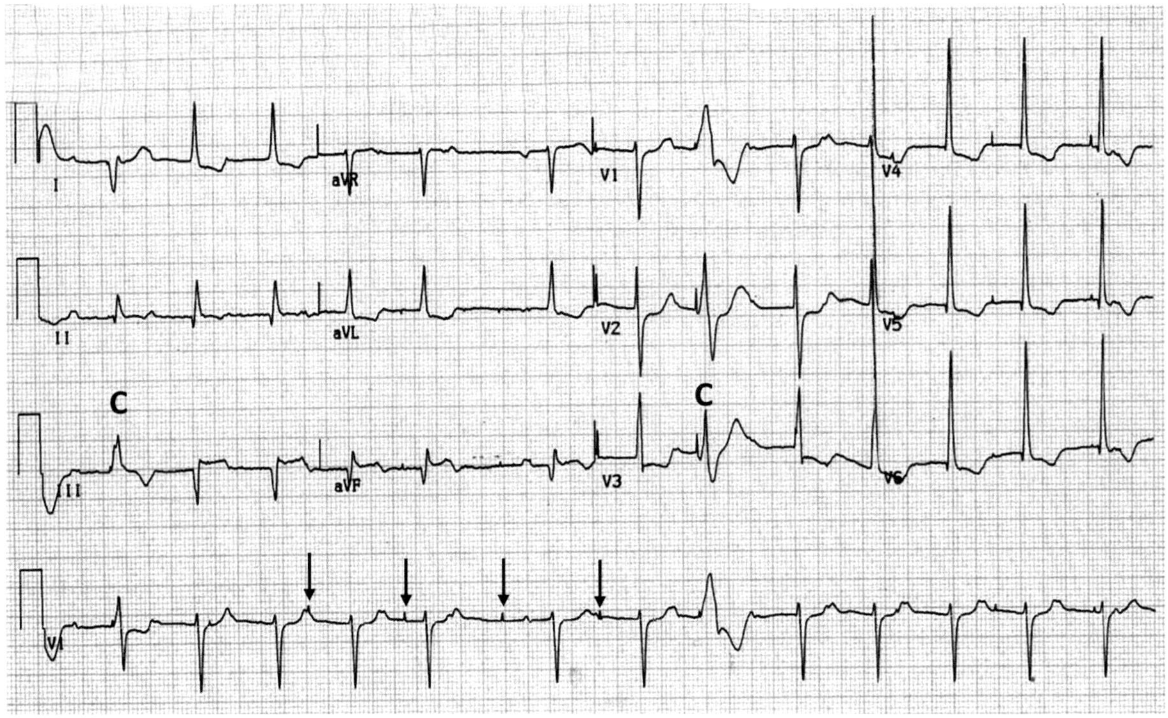

Fig. 24.10: This tracing demonstrates failure of a pacemaker to sense and to pace. Ventricular pacing spikes march through the tracing without any sensing (*arrows*). With the exception of two capture beats (C), all the pacing spikes fail to capture the ventricle. These two capture beats show RBBB morphology with rightward frontal plane axis. These findings suggest possibility of ventricular perforation or migration of the lead through the pericardial space, to be confirmed radiologically.

the criteria of diagnosing myocardial infarction in the setting of LBBB. Cabrera's sign is described as notching of the ascending limb of the S-wave usually in leads V3 and V4, and sometimes in leads V2 and V5. The notch should be greater than or equal to 0.03 seconds and present in two leads. It has low sensitivity but is a very specific sign. The diagnostic criteria described above are for anterior wall myocardial infarctions. Infarctions at other sites are usually masked by the paced rhythm. Cabrera's sign in both leads LIII and aVF may be of some value in diagnosing inferior wall myocardial infarction. Similarly ST elevation in lead V4R may occur in acute right ventricular infarction. This sign should, however, be taken with extreme caution unless accompanied by signs of inferior myocardial infarction.[6,16]

DIAGNOSIS OF HYPERKALEMIA IN PRESENCE OF PACEMAKER

Electrocardiogram is a useful guide in diagnosing hyperkalemia in patients in sinus rhythm. Initial change is usually a peaked T-wave and this is followed by widening of QRS complexes, intraventricular conduction defects, prolongation of PR interval, absence of P-wave, heart blocks, and the classical sine wave. This is because severe hyperkalemia decreases the phase 0 of the action potential resulting in widening of the QRS complex. The QRS complex continues to widen and ultimately blends with the T-wave resulting in a sine wave morphology. Typical ECG changes of hyperkalemia can also be seen even during paced rhythm. These changes include QRS widening and reduction in amplitude of the QRS complex. The QRS widening can be quite marked in some cases. These changes are especially well appreciated if an old ECG is available for comparison. Typical sine waves may also be seen on a paced ECG rhythm. These changes revert back to the baseline with correction of hyperkalemia.[18-19]

MAGNET EFFECTS ON PACEMAKERS

All pacemakers respond to a magnet by switching to an asynchronous pacing mode at a programmed AV delay and a fixed magnet rate depending on the manufacturer, device model, and the status of the battery. Usually magnet increases the pacemaker firing rate and heart rate increases. If magnet application on a pacemaker site does not produce any response on the surface ECG pacing rate or mode, the magnet may be repositioned. If no change is still observed, the following reasons may apply: (i) a depleted pacemaker battery; (ii) the pacemaker is programmed to ignore the magnet; (iii) the magnetic field does not reach the device, as in the case of those with deeper (abdominal or submuscular) implants or in very obese patients; (iv) end-of-life (EOL) or lower battery life.

ELECTROCARDIOGRAM INTERPRETATION AFTER CARDIAC RESYNCHRONIZATION THERAPY

Biventricular (BiV) pacing for cardiac resynchronization therapy (CRT) is intended to improve left ventricular function by coordinating systolic activity of the septum and free walls in patients with advanced heart failure.[20-23] CRT is indicated for patients who have left ventricular ejection fraction (LVEF) less than or equal to 35%, sinus rhythm, left bundle-branch block (LBBB) with a QRS duration greater than or equal to 150 ms, and New York Heart Association (NYHA) class II, III, or ambulatory IV, and those patients who are symptomatic in spite of taking maximum doses of guideline-directed medical therapy (GDMT).[21,22]

Cardiac resynchronization therapy has added a new dimension to the electrocardiographic evaluation of pacemaker function. During left ventricular (LV) pacing from the posterior or posterolateral coronary vein, a correctly positioned lead V1 registers a tall R-wave, and there is right axis deviation in the frontal plane with few exceptions. During simultaneous biventricular stimulation from the RV apex and LV site in the coronary venous system, the QRS complex is often positive (dominant) in lead V1 and the frontal plane QRS axis usually points to the right superior quadrant, and occasionally the left superior quadrant. The reported incidence of a dominant R-wave in lead V1 during simultaneous biventricular pacing varies from 50% to almost 100% for reasons that are not clear. A negative paced QRS complex in lead V1 during simultaneous biventricular pacing with the RV lead at the apex can be caused by incorrect placement of the lead V1 electrode (too high on the chest), lack of LV capture, LV lead displacement, ventricular fusion with the intrinsic QRS complex, coronary venous LV pacing via the middle or anterior cardiac vein, unintended placement of two leads in the RV, and severe conduction abnormalities within the LV myocardium.[20] Most of these situations can cause a QS complex in lead V1 which should be interpreted (excluding fusion) as reflecting RV preponderance in the depolarization process. Barring the above causes, a negative complex in lead V1 is unusual.[20] Optimal resynchronization should be manifested by 12-lead electrocardiogram patterns consistent with resynchronized activation, a tall (≥4 mm) R-wave in V1, and predominant negative deflection in lead I (RV1SI) (Fig. 24.11).[23] The 12-lead ECG post-implantation also predicts the clinical outcomes of biventricular pacing. Narrowing of QRS duration after CRT implantation has been taken as a reasonable marker for ventricular resynchronization. Ventricular remodeling and improvement in echocardiographic parameters are likely to be accompanied by reversal of electrical dyssynchrony in the ECG as well. This is measured by recording and comparing the QRS duration of preimplantation ECG with the postimplantation ECG.[24,25]

SUMMARY

Interpreting paced rhythms can range from very simple to very complex. The pacemaker rhythm can be recognized on the ECG by identifying the pacemaker spikes. But the modern pacemakers provide low voltage spikes on the ECG that can easily go unnoticed. Unfortunately, there is no single lead that will consistently demonstrate the pacemaker spikes. When any wide complex rhythm is present it is always a good idea to take a quick look at all leads to look for occult pacemaker spikes.

Once pacemaker activity is identified, the next step is to determine if the activity is a normal function or a malfunction. Most pacemakers are set to pace between 50 beats/min and 70 beats/min. The two most common types of pacemakers implanted are the VVI (ventricle paced, ventricle sensed; pacing inhibited if beat sensed) and DDD (dual chamber pacing and sensing, both triggered and inhibited mode) pacemakers.

Interpretation of Pacemaker Rhythm

ECG interpretation of pacemaker rhythm starts with the identification of pacemaker spikes. Pacemaker spikes are vertical signals that represent the electrical activity the pacemaker (Box 24.1). Usually these spikes are more visible in unipolar than in bipolar pacing.

Atrial Pacing

- If the site of stimulation is near the SA node in the RA, then the morphology of the P waves resemble that of sinus beats.
- If the site of stimulation is in the coronary sinus, then the morphology of the P waves are inverted in LII, LIII, and aVF.

Ventricular Pacing

- If the transvenous site of stimulation is in the RV, then a LBBB pattern appears. The sequence of activation is from the right to the left and from the apex to the

Box 24.1: Pacing spikes documentation on ECG.

- The pacemaker rhythm is recognized on ECG by documenting pacemaker spikes.
- These are vertical spikes of short duration, usually 2 ms.
- May not be visible in all the leads.
- Amplitude depends on position and type of lead. Bipolar leads result in a much smaller pacing spike than unipolar leads.
- Epicardially placed leads result in smaller pacing spikes than endocardially placed leads.

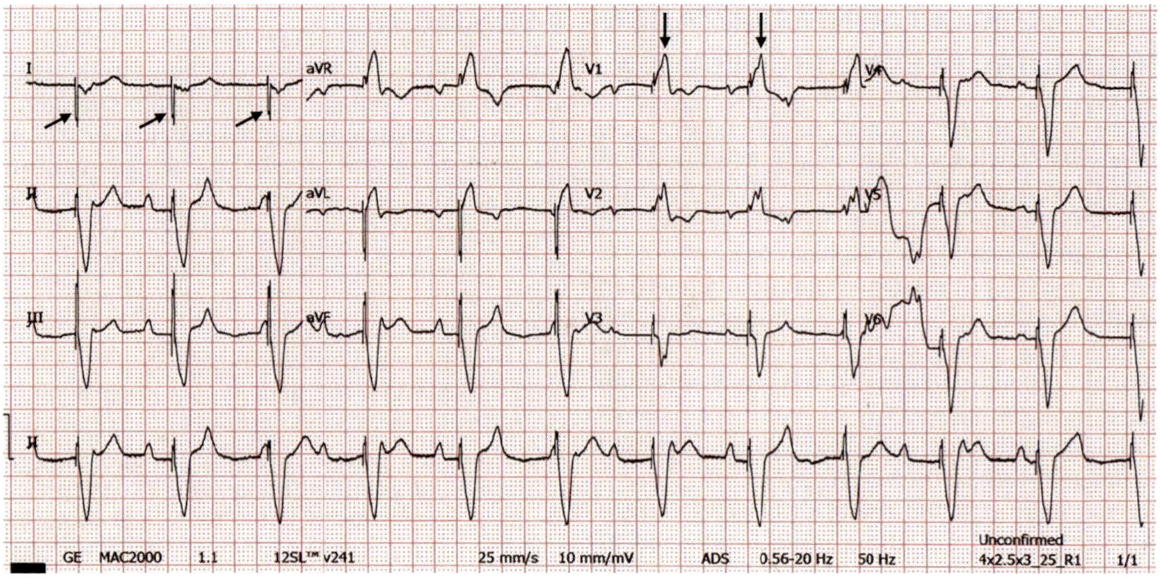

Fig. 24.11: Electrocardiogram displays optimal resynchronization features. (1) A tall (>4 mm) R-wave in V1, and (2) Predominant negative deflection in lead I (*arrows*). A negative complex in lead V1 is unusual after optimal CRT. (ECG: electrocardiogram; CRT: cardiac resynchronization therapy)

base. Unlike the usual LBBB, V6 may be predominantly negative.

- If there is left ventricular epicardial-myocardial pacing there is RBBB pattern.

Pacing-induced T Wave Changes

- Inverted broad T waves associated with QT prolongation. They are seen most commonly in the inferior leads and in the left precordial leads.
- May resemble ischemic T waves.

Types of Common Pacemakers

AAI: Atrial pacing and sensing. Also, termed as atrial demand mode. If the native atrial activity is sensed then pacing is inhibited. Used in sinus node dysfunction with intact AV conduction.

VVI: Ventricle pacing and sensing. It is similar to AAI mode, but involving ventricles instead of the atrium.

DDD: This is the most common pacing mode capable of pacing and sensing both atrium and ventricles.

Biventricular pacemakers: Pacemaker leads are placed in the right atrium, right ventricle, and indirectly to left ventricle through the coronary sinus. Useful in the management of patients with heart failure who have evidence of abnormal intraventricular conduction (most often evident as LBBB on ECG) which causes deranged ventricular contraction or dyssynchrony.

Features of the Paced ECG (Box 24.2)

Features of the paced ECG are:

- *Pacing spikes*: The pacemaker rhythm is recognized on the ECG by the pacemaker spikes. These vertical signals represent the electrical activity of the pacemaker. These spikes of short duration may be difficult to document in all leads.
- *Atrial pacing*: Pacing spike precedes the P wave. Morphology of P wave depends on the site of lead placement but may appear normal.
- *Ventricular pacing*: Pacing spike precedes the QRS complex. ST segments and T waves should be discordant with the QRS complex, i.e. the major terminal portion of the QRS complex is located on the opposite side of the baseline from the ST segment and T wave.

Box 24.2: Identification of pacemaker electrocardiogram.

Atrial pacing
- Pacing spike precedes the P-wave.
- Morphology of P-waves dependent of lead placement but may appear normal.
- QRS morphology is usually of normal configuration.

Ventricular pacing
- Pacing spike precedes the QRS complex.
- Right ventricle pacing lead placement results in a QRS morphology similar to LBBB pattern.
- ST segments and T-waves should be discordant with the QRS complex, i.e. the major terminal portion of the QRS complex is located on the opposite side of the baseline from the ST segment and T-wave.

Dual chamber pacing
- May exhibit features of atrial pacing, ventricular pacing or both.
- Pacing spikes may precede only P-wave, only QRS complex, or both.

(LBBB: left bundle branch block)

- *Dual chamber pacing*: May exhibit features of atrial pacing, ventricular pacing or both, so the pacing spikes may precede only P wave, only QRS complex, or both.

The absence of paced complexes do not always mean pacemaker failure as it may reflect satisfactory native conduction.

Diagnosis of ST-elevation Myocardial Infarction (STEMI) in Presence of Pacemaker

Paced rhythms cause ST-segment and T wave changes that can make the identification of acute STEMI difficult. Sgarbossa's criteria can be used to diagnose STEMI in the setting of paced rhythms.

- Discordant ST elevation (ST-segment deviations in the opposite direction to the QRS complex) greater than or equal to 5 mm in any lead
- Concordant ST depression greater than or equal to 1 mm in either V1, V2, or V3
- Concordant ST elevation (ST-segment deviations in same direction to the QRS complex) greater than or equal to 1 mm in any single lead.

Diagnosis of Hyperkalemia in Presence of Pacemaker

Paced rhythms can mask some of the ECG changes of hyperkalemia. Typical ECG changes of hyperkalemia including widening of QRS complex and sine waves are seen even during paced rhythm and these changes revert back with correction of hyperkalemia.

Electrocardiogram interpretation after Cardiac Resynchronization Therapy

Cardiac resynchronization therapy (CRT) is an established treatment modality in heart failure. Biventricular (BiV) pacing for CRT is intended to improve left ventricular function by coordinating systolic activity of the septum and free walls in patients with advanced heart failure. The 12-lead ECG postimplantation can predict clinical outcomes of CRT.

Cardiac resynchronization therapy is indicated for patients who have:

- Left ventricular ejection fraction ≤ 35%
- Sinus rhythm
- Left bundle branch block (LBBB)
- QRS duration ≥ 150 ms
- New York Heart Association class II, III, or ambulatory class IV symptoms
- Symptomatic in spite of taking guideline-directed medical therapy (GDMT)

Optimal resynchronization should be manifested by 12-lead ECG patterns consistent with resynchronized activation:

- A tall (≥4 mm) R-wave in V1
- Predominant negative deflection in LI
- Narrowing of QRS duration after CRT implantation has been taken as a reasonable marker for ventricular resynchronization.

REFERENCES

1. Trohman RG, Kim MH, Pinski SL. Cardiac pacing: The state of the art. Lancet. 2004;364(9446):1701-19.
2. Gregoratos G, Abrams J, Epstein AE, et al. ACC/AHA/NASPE 2002 guideline update for implantation of cardiac pacemakers and antiarrhythmia devices: Summary article. A report of the American college of cardiology/American heart association task force on practice guidelines (ACC/AHA/NASPE committee to update the 1998 pacemaker guidelines). Circulation. 2002;106(16):2145-61
3. Stockburger M, Bartels R, Gerhardt L, et al. Dual-site right atrial pacing increases left atrial appendage flow in patients with sick sinus syndrome and paroxysmal atrial fibrillation. Pacing Clin Electrophysiol. 2007;30(1):20-7.
4. Chow AW, Lane RE, Cowie MR. New pacing technologies for heart failure. BMJ. 2003;326(7398):1073-7.
5. Brignole M, Auricchio A, Baron-Esquivias G, et al. 2013 ESC Guide lines on cardiac pacing and cardiac resynchronization therapy. The task Force on cardiac pacing and resynchronization therapy of the European Society of Cardiology (ESC). Developed in collaboration with the European Heart Rhythm Association (EHRA). Eur Heart J. 2013;34:2281-329.
6. Barold SS, Falkoff MD, Ong LS, et al. Electrocardiographic diagnosis of myocardial infarction during ventricular pacing. Cardiol Clin. 1987;5(3):403-17.
7. Sgarbossa EB, Pinski SL, Barbagelata A, et al. GUSTO-1 investigators. Electrocardiographic diagnosis of evolving acute myocardial infarction in the presence of left bundle-branch block. N Engl J Med. 1996;334(8):481-7.
8. Brandt RR, Hammill SC, Higano ST, et al. Electrocardiographic Diagnosis of Acute Myocardial Infarction During Ventricular Pacing. Circulation. 1998;97:2274-5.
9. Klimczak A, Wranicz JK, Cygankiewicz I, et al. Electrocardiographic diagnosis of acute coronary syndromes in patients with left bundle branch block or paced rhythm. Cardiology J. 2007;14(2):207-13
10. Koghiadakis GE, Kaleboubas MD, Igoumenidis NE, et al. Electrocardiographic diagnosis of acute myocardial infarction in the presence of ventricular pacedrhythm. PACE. 2001;24(2):1289-90.
11. Kolb James C. Cardiac memory: Persistent T wave changes after ventricular pacing. J Emerg Med. 2002;23(2):191-7.
12. Sgarbossa EB. Recent advances in the electrocardiographic diagnosis of myocardial infarction: Left bundle branch block and pacing. Pacing Clin Electrophysiol. 1996;19(9):1370-9.
13. Sgarbossa EB, Pinski SL, Gates KB, et al. Early electrocardiographic diagnosis of acute myocardial infarction in the presence of ventricular paced rhythm. GUSTO-I investigators. Am J Cardiol. 1996;77(5):423-4.
14. Maloy KR, Bhat R, Davis J, et al. Sgarbossa criteria are highly specific for acute myocardial infarction with pacemakers. West J Emerg Med. 2010;11(4):354-7.
15. Schaaf SG, Tabas JA, Smith SW. A patient with a paced rhythm presenting with chest pain and hypotension. JAMA Intern Med. 2013;173(22):2082-5.

16. Barold SS, Herweg B, Curtis AB. Electrocardiographic diagnosis of myocardial infarction and ischemia during cardiac pacing. Cardiol Clin. 2006;24(3):387-99.
17. Kilic H, Atalar E, Ozer N, et al. Early electrocardiographic diagnosis of acute coronary ischemia on the paced electrocardiogram. Int J Cardiol. 2008;130(1):14-8.
18. Bahl A, Swamy A, Jeevan H, et al. ECG changes of hyperkalemia during paced rhythm. Indian Heart J. 2009;61(1):93-4.
19. Howard JA, Kosowsky BD. Electrocardiographic diagnosis of hyperkalemia in the presence of ventricular pacing and atrial fibrillation. Chest. 1980;78:491-2.
20. Barold SS, Herweg B. Usefulness of the 12-lead electrocardiogram in the follow-up of patients with cardiac resynchronization devices. Part I. Cardiol J. 2011;18(5):476-86.
21. Epstein AE, DiMarco JP, Ellenbogen KA, et al. 2012 ACCF/AHA/HRS focused update incorporated into the ACCF/AHA/HRS 2008 guidelines for device-based therapy of cardiac rhythm abnormalities. A report of the American college of cardiology foundation/American heart association task force on practice guidelines and the heart rhythm society. J Am Coll Cardiol. 2013;61(3):e6-75.
22. Tracy CM, Epstein AE, Darbar D, et al. 2012 ACCF/AHA/HRS focused update of the 2008 guidelines for device-based therapy of cardiac rhythm abnormalities: a report of the American College of Cardiology Foundation/American Heart Association Task Force on Practice Guidelines and the Heart Rhythm Society. [corrected] Circulation. 2012;126:1784-800.
23. Coverstone E, Sheehy J, Kleiger RE, et al. The post-implantation electrocardiogram predicts clinical response to cardiac resynchronization therapy. Pacing Clin Electrophysiol. 2015;38(5):572-80.
24. Chaturvedi V. Current research on the relevance of electrocardiography in cardiac resynchronization therapy. Indian Pacing Electrophysiol J. 2015;15(2):145-7.
25. Yang XW, Hua W, Wang J. Native QRS narrowing reflects electrical reversal and associates with anatomical reversal in cardiac resynchronization therapy. J Interv Card Electrophysiol. 2014;41:161-8.

Chapter

25

Pediatric Electrocardiogram Interpretation

INTRODUCTION

Interpretation of pediatric electrocardiograms (ECG) can be challenging for the physician. Part of this difficulty arises from the fact that the normal ECG findings, including rate, rhythm, axis, intervals, and morphology, change from the neonatal period through infancy, childhood, and adolescence. These changes occur as a result of the maturation of the myocardium and cardiovascular system with age. The basic principles of interpretation of the ECG in children are identical to those in adults, but the progressive changes in anatomy and physiology which take place between birth and adolescence result in some features which differ significantly from the normal adult pattern and vary according to the age of the child. To obtain a satisfactory recording in young children requires patience, and the parents may be helpful in providing a source of distraction. Limb electrodes may be placed in a more proximal position to reduce movement artifacts. Standard adult electrode positions are used but with the addition of either lead V3R or lead V4R to detect right ventricular or atrial hypertrophy. Standard paper speed (25 mm/sec) and deflection (10 mm/mV) are used, although occasionally large QRS complexes may require the gain to be halved.[1]

HEART RATE

Heart rate is usually faster in the children compared to adult. In children, cardiac output is determined primarily by heart rate as opposed to stroke volume. With age, the heart rate decreases as the ventricles mature and stroke volume plays a larger role in cardiac output. Age and activity-appropriate heart rates thus must be recognized. Average resting heart rate varies with age; newborns can range from 90 to 160 beats per minute (bpm) (Fig. 25.1) and adolescents from 50 to120 bpm. The average heart rate peaks about the second month of life and thereafter gradually decreases until adolescence.[2-4]

AGE-RELATED CHANGES IN VENTRICLES AND QRS AXIS

At birth the right ventricle is larger than the left. Changes in systemic vascular resistance result in the left ventricle increasing in size until it is larger than the right ventricle by age 1 month. By the age of 6 months, the ratio of the right ventricle to the left ventricle is similar to that of an adult. Right axis deviation, large precordial R-waves, and upright T-waves are, therefore, normal in the neonate. The T-wave in lead V1 inverts by 7 days and typically remains inverted until at least age 7 years (may be up to 12–16 years). Upright T-waves in the right precordial leads (V1–V3) between ages 7 days and 7 years are a potentially important abnormality and usually indicate right ventricular hypertrophy. The QRS complex also reflects some changes. At birth, the mean QRS axis lies between +60° and +160°, R waves are prominent in the right precordial leads (Fig. 25.2), and S-waves are prominent in the left precordial leads. By the age of 1 year, the axis changes gradually to lie between +10° and +100°.[1]

P-Wave

The P-wave amplitude does not change significantly during childhood and at any age amplitudes in excess of 2.5 mm should be regarded as exceeding the upper limit of normal. But P-waves appear slightly peaked in neonates. Normal P-wave duration is usually <0.09 seconds in children and <0.07 seconds in infants. A combination of tall and wide P-waves occur in combined atrial hypertrophy.[5,6]

PR Interval

The PR interval on resting 12-lead ECGs in children varies mainly in relation to heart rate and is, therefore, usually shorter in younger children. PR interval usually varies with age, gradually increasing with cardiac maturity and increased muscle mass. In neonates, it ranges from 0.08

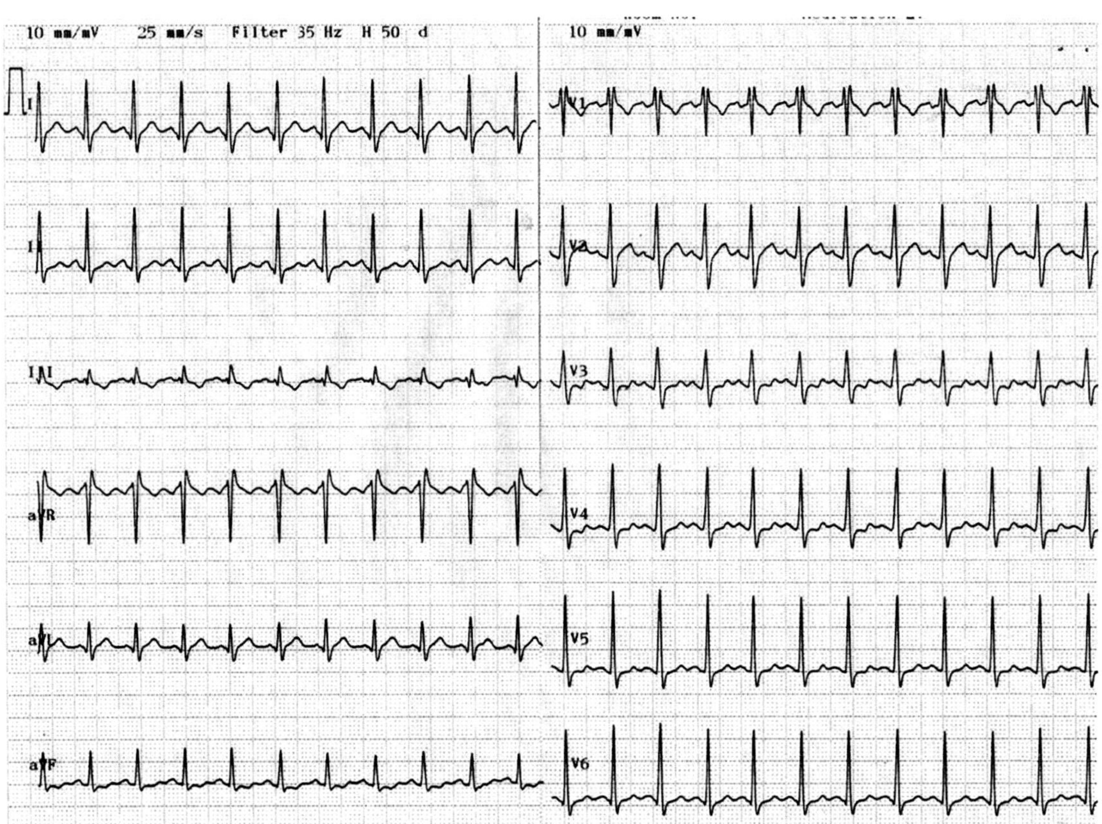

Fig. 25.1: Electrocardiogram of a healthy neonate displaying typical features of the pediatric electrocardiogram: Heart rate of 140 bpm (normal for age) and RSR' pattern (partial RBBB morphology) in V1.

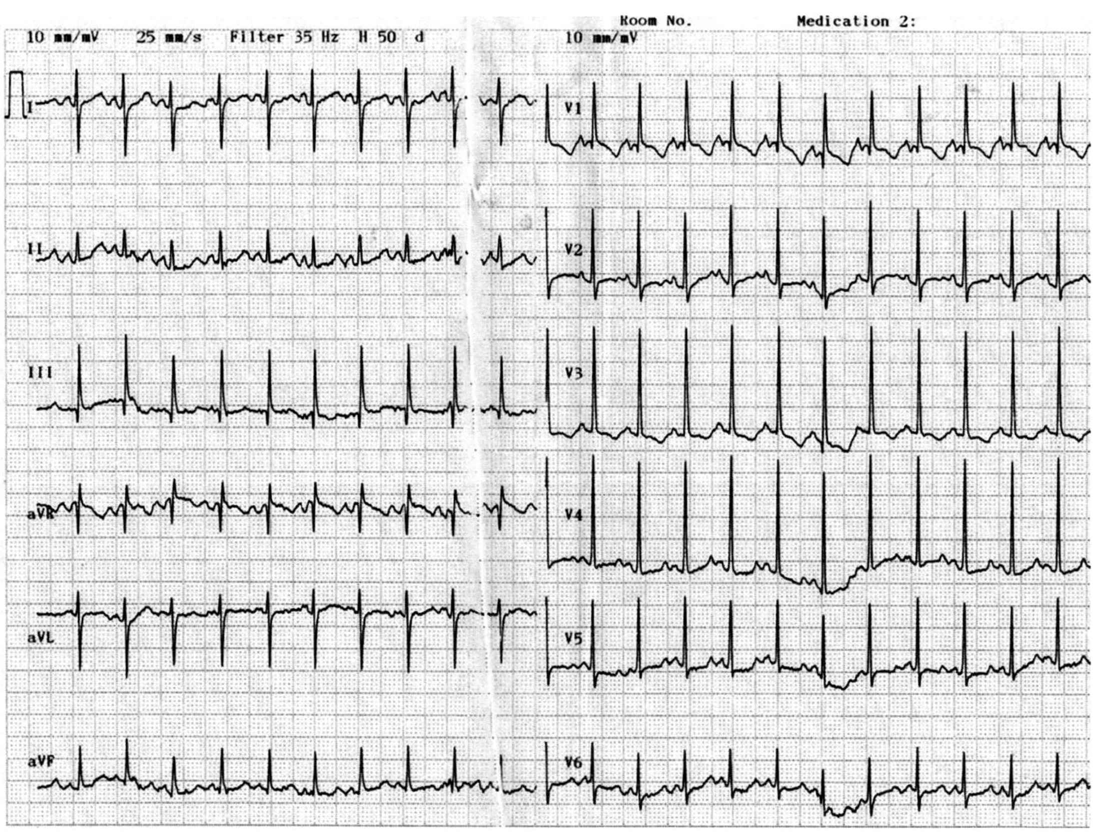

Fig. 25.2: Electrocardiogram of a neonate showing features of the pediatric electrocardiogram with marked sinus tachycardia (Heart rate-142 bpm) with right axis deviation with tall R wave in lead V1.

seconds to 0.15 seconds (80–150 ms) and in adolescents from 0.12 seconds to 0.20 seconds (120–200 ms).[2] The normal shorter PR interval in children must be taken into account when considering the diagnosis of conduction and atrioventricular (AV) block. In infants with heart rates in the range 100–150 beats/min, one would expect the PR interval to be within the range 80–110 ms extending in occasional individuals to 150 ms. In teenagers with slower heart rates, the upper limit of normal would be around 180 ms. Ambulatory ECG monitoring shows that at all ages some individuals with a normal resting PR interval will from time to time have periods when the PR interval becomes prolonged to more than 200 ms. Episodes of first degree heart block are more common during sleep and occasionally individuals may have first degree heart block as their normal resting heart rhythm (Fig. 25.3).[5,6]

Q-Wave

In most leads where a significant Q-wave appears (II, III, aVF, V5, and V6), there is a trend for the amplitude to double over the first few months of life, reaching a maximum at about 3–5 years of age, and declining thereafter back towards the initial value of the newborn period. Q-waves of up to 0.6–0.8 mV would fall within the normal range for children in the 6 month to 3 year age range.[3,4] Q-waves are normally present in leads II, III, aVF, V5, and V6. Q waves in other leads are rare and associated with disease—for example, an anomalous left coronary artery, or myocardial infarction secondary to Kawasaki syndrome.[1]

QRS Complex

The QRS complex duration varies with age. In children, the QRS complex duration is shorter, possibly because of decreased muscle mass, and gradually increases with age. In neonates it measures 0.03–0.08 seconds (30–80 ms) and in adolescents 0.05–0.10 seconds (50–100 ms). A QRS complex duration exceeding 0.08 seconds (80 ms) in young children (younger than 8 years of age) or exceeding 0.10 seconds (100 ms) in older children may be pathologic. As a result, slight prolongation of what may appear as a normal QRS complex can indicate a conduction abnormality or bundle branch block in children.[2]

Tall R-wave in V1 with sinus tachycardia with T-wave inversions in right precordial leads V1–V3 (V4) are typical features of pediatric ECG (Fig. 25.4). The amplitude of R waves in the right precordial leads of normal children decreases with age while the amplitude increases in the left precordial leads. Similar but inverse changes occur in respect of the S-wave amplitude. There is substantial individual variation in the rate at which these changes occur. On average the R/S ratio in V1 remains >1 up to about 3 years of age but will remain >1 in some normal individuals even into the 8–12 year age group.[5]

QT Interval

Detecting prolongation of the QT interval is important in the identification of individuals at risk of life threatening arrhythmia. Because of the relation between QT interval

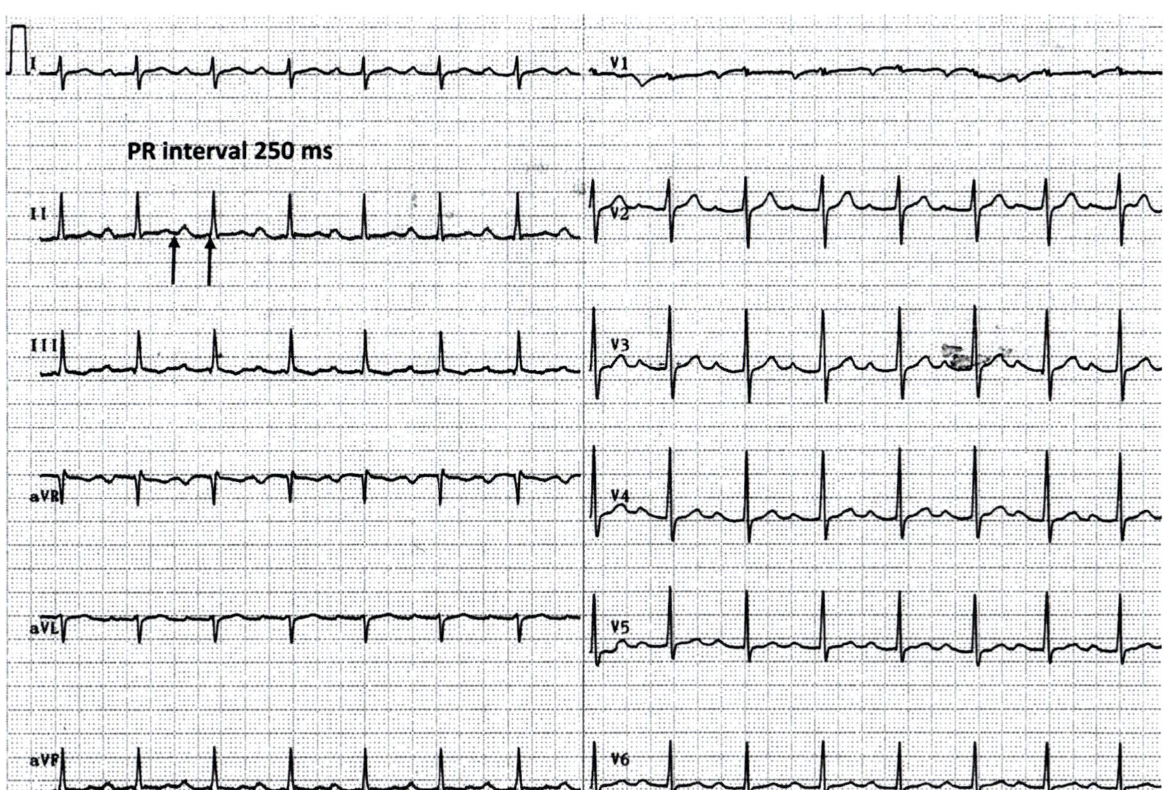

Fig. 25.3: Electrocardiogram of a 4-year-old healthy boy showing evidence of first degree AV block with PR interval 250 ms (arrows).

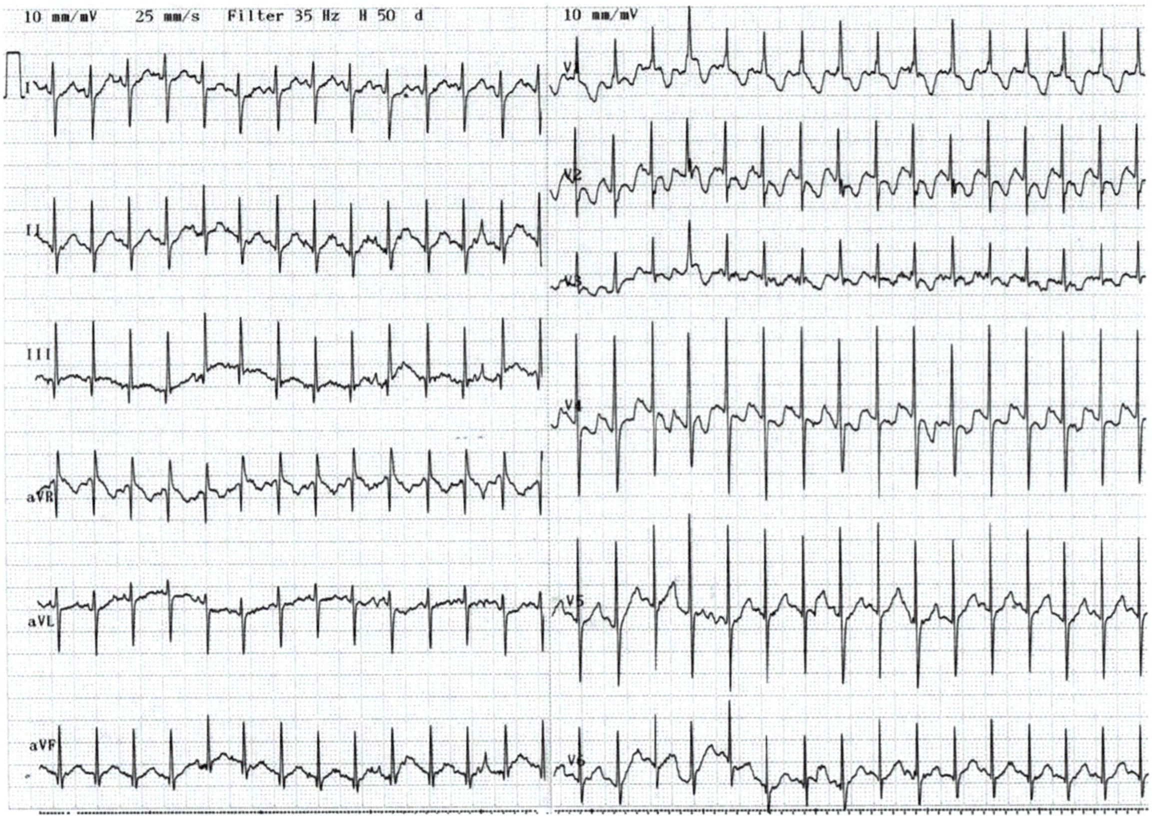

Fig. 25.4: Typical pediatric electrocardiogram showing sinus tachycardia (heart rate 179 bpm) with dominant R wave in V1 with T wave inversions with ST segment depression in right precordial leads V1–V4.

and heart rate and the considerable variability of heart rate in the pediatric age group it is difficult to judge whether a measured QT interval is normal or not. Because the QT interval varies greatly with heart rate, so corrected QT interval (QT_c) should be determined. QT_c is most commonly calculated by using Bazett's formula.[6-10]

Corrected QT (QT_c) = QT Interval/√(RR interval)

During the first half of infancy, the normal QT_c is longer than in older children and adults. In the first 6 months of life, the QT_c is considered normal at less than 0.49 seconds (490 ms). After infancy, this cutoff is generally 0.44 seconds (440 ms).[2-5]

ST Segment

ST-segment elevation may be a normal finding in teenagers as a result of early repolarization. It may also be seen in myocardial infarction, myocarditis, or pericarditis. Early repolarization is commonly seen in adolescence with an elevated J point, most obvious in the mid precordial leads (Fig. 25.5). This is a completely normal finding and must be distinguished from pathological elevation of the ST segments.[11]

T-Wave

Throughout childhood the T-wave pattern, particularly in precordial leads, is very different to that of adults and there is a progressive change in T-wave axis from birth to early adult life. The rate at which this change occurs varies considerably from one individual to another but some generalizations can be made. In the first 2–3 days of life upright T-waves in the right precordial leads (V1 and V3R) are normal. It is usual for the T-wave in these leads to invert in the majority of infants during the first week of life. Persistence of a positive T-wave in V1 or V3R beyond the first week of life should therefore raise the suspicion of abnormality. The T-wave remains inverted in these leads in the majority of children into the 12–16 year age group. In the intermediate leads, V2 and V3 the T-wave is often inverted in early childhood (Fig. 25.6) and there is a progression to the T-wave becoming upright in the sequence V3, V2, and V1. The T-wave in V5 and V6 should be upright at all ages, but in a very small number of newborn babies the T-wave in these leads may be flat or inverted for 1–3 days.

VARIATIONS FROM SINUS RHYTHM

Ambulatory electrocardiographic monitoring on normal healthy infants and children of all ages has confirmed that regular uninterrupted sinus rhythm may be punctuated from time to time by a variety of rhythm changes which could potentially be regarded as abnormal. The frequency with which these changes occur emphasizes the importance of understanding the range of normal variation of heart rhythm in children and of correlating symptoms

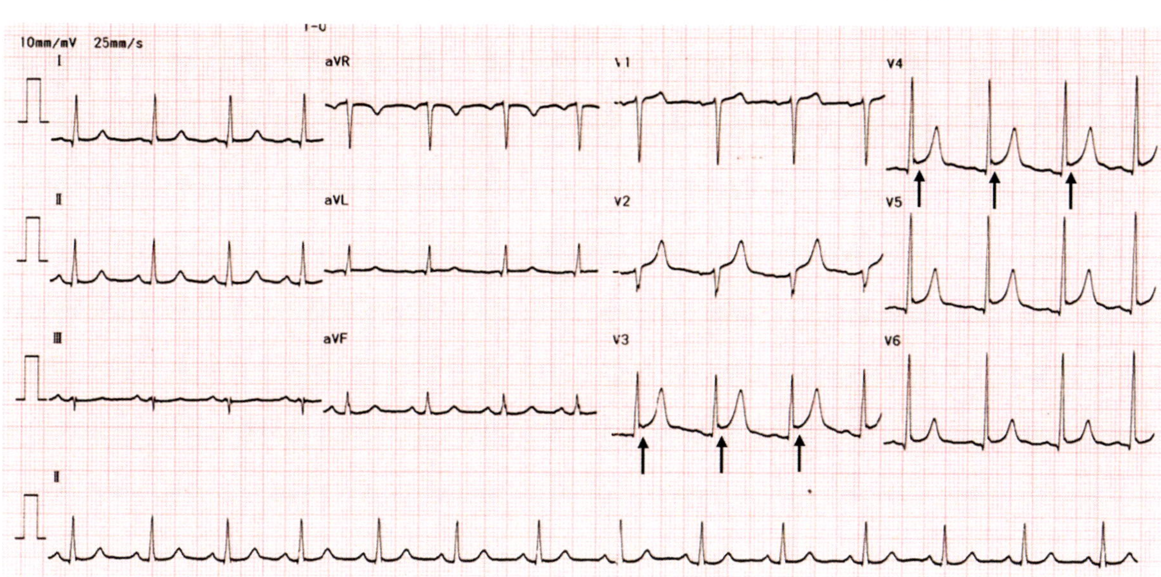

Fig. 25.5: Electrocardiogram of a 10-year-old boy showing early repolarization pattern with J point elevation (arrows) in all the chest leads, most obvious in mid precordial leads V3–V4.

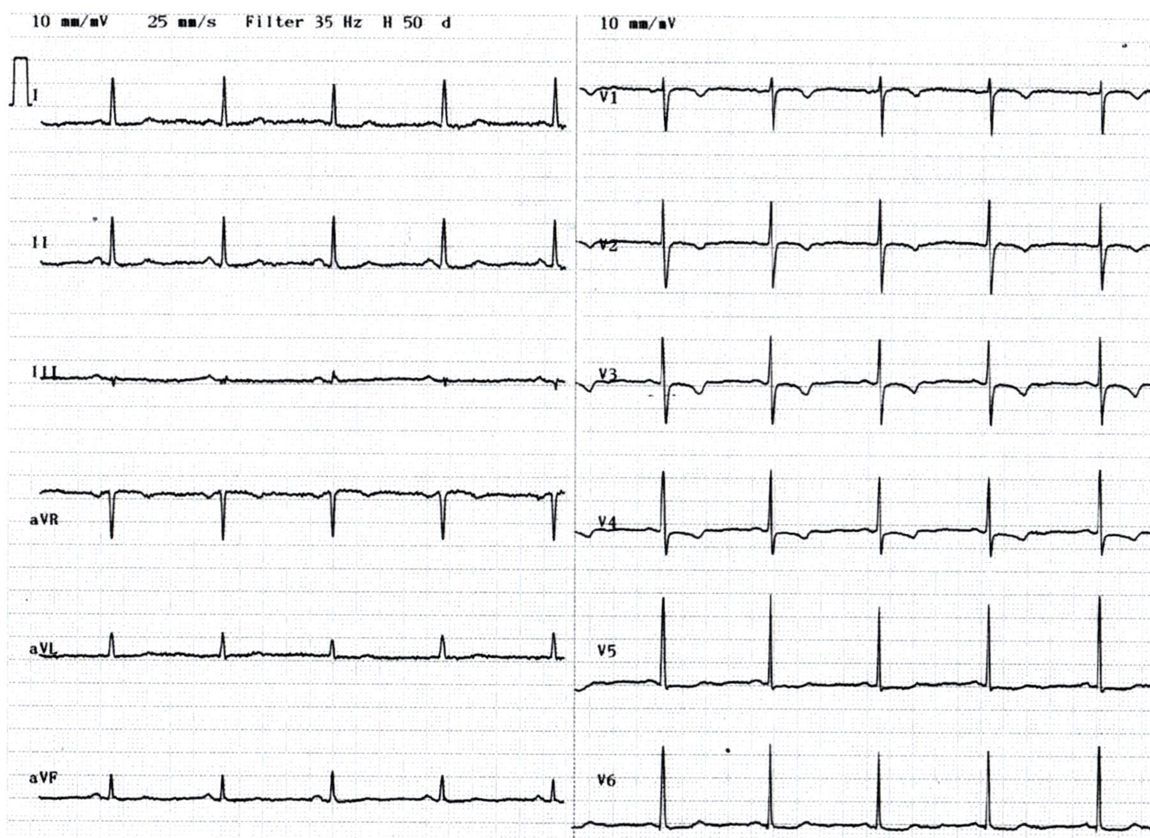

Fig. 25.6: Electrocardiogram of a 6-year-old girl showing T-wave inversion in V1–V4 (Juvenile T-wave pattern). These patterns of T-wave inversions in right precordial leads are considered normal for age. Juvenile T-wave inversions are usually present in leads V1–V3 but sometimes T wave inversions may extend up to leads V4 (V5). Also note these inverted T waves are not symmetric nor deep (<3 mm).

with rhythm change when investigating unusual events. Many of these rhythm changes are relatively common, occurring in many individuals, though not necessarily very frequently. The majority of these rhythm changes are therefore very likely to be entirely benign.[5] Phasic changes in the P–P interval are almost universal in children and can be very obvious, leading to unnecessary concerns about the irregular heart rate. The diagnosis of sinus arrhythmia is easily confirmed in most cases by observing the relation of the change to respiration (slowing in expiration and accelerating in inspiration). Pronounced sinus arrhythmia is a common feature in pediatric ECG (Fig. 25.7). Occasional

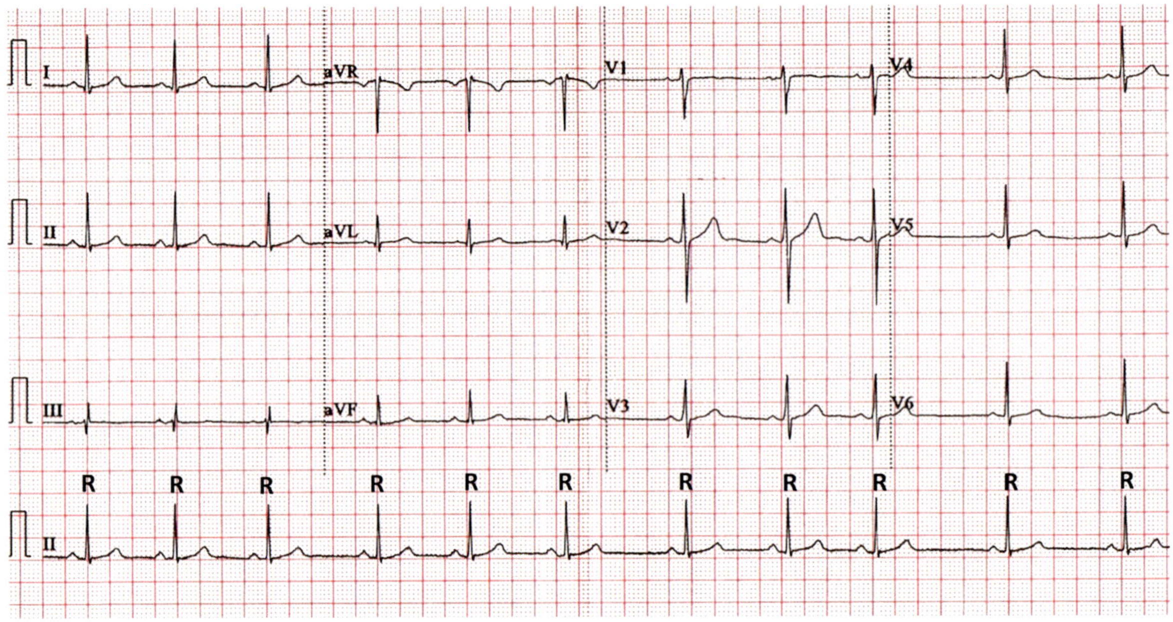

Fig. 25.7: Pediatric electrocardiogram showing marked degree of sinus arrhythmia. Note pronounced phasic variation of R–R and P-P intervals, but the rhythm is sinus.

episodes characterized by sudden prolongation of the P–P interval are also relatively common and are found in 50% of the newborn infants and in older children the frequency of such episodes appears to fall, occurring in only 16% of teenage boys. Although these sinus pauses are seen in many individuals, they are infrequent, almost invariably occurring in isolated cardiac cycles and with no more than two or three in a 24-hour period. In both neonates and older children the longest pauses recorded are no more than 1.8 seconds in duration. As sinus arrhythmia makes it difficult to measure the resting sinus cycle length in many children, the precise mechanism responsible for these pauses is uncertain in most cases. Whatever the precise mechanism it is clear that such pauses are common at all ages. Although sinus node disease does occur in young children and can result in syncope, in the vast majority of children sinus pauses are benign (Fig. 25.8).[5,12-15]

High Grade AV Block in Children

Around 10% of normal children will have episodes of Mobitz type 1 second degree AV block or Wenckebach phenomenon (Fig. 25.9). Some, but not all, of these individuals will have episodes of first degree AV block.[5] Episodes may vary in number from single isolated event to many hundreds in a 24-hour period. In some individuals the AV block will persist as 2:1 block for a few seconds after the initial Wenckebach sequence. There are very occasional reports of progression of Mobitz type 1 AV block to complete AV block but such progression must be very unusual given the relatively frequent occurrence of Mobitz type 1 block in healthy asymptomatic children.[5,16-18]

Extrasystoles

Premature supraventricular or ventricular beats are frequently seen in children of all age groups and are in most instances a benign condition. Intermittent and infrequent premature beats usually are not an indication for a cardiologic work-up. If ventricular or supraventricular premature beats are frequent and persist over a period of weeks or months, then only a cardiological evaluation is recommended.[19] Isolated ventricular premature beats may be identified on a routine resting ECG in 0.2–2.2% of normal children.[20-25] On ambulatory monitoring these extrasystoles are common, occurring in 20–30% of younger children and up to 40% of teenage boys. Typically the extrasystoles are isolated, of uniform morphology, and are associated with periods of slower heart rates. Multifocal extrasystoles are seen and in a small number of individuals couplets of ectopic activity occasionally occur. The frequency of extrasystoles is usually no more than 1–5 per hour, but occasional individuals will be seen with much more frequent ectopic activity or long periods of ventricular bigeminy. Extrasystoles which conform to this pattern and suppress on exercise are almost certainly benign.[5] Isolated supraventricular premature beats are fairly common at all ages. In older children supraventricular premature beats have been reported in between 15% and 40% of individuals studied. The usual pattern is for isolated ectopics to occur at a frequency of less than one per hour.[12]

Chamber Size

An assessment of chamber size is important when analyzing the pediatric ECG for underlying clues to congenital heart abnormalities. The right ventricle is larger than the

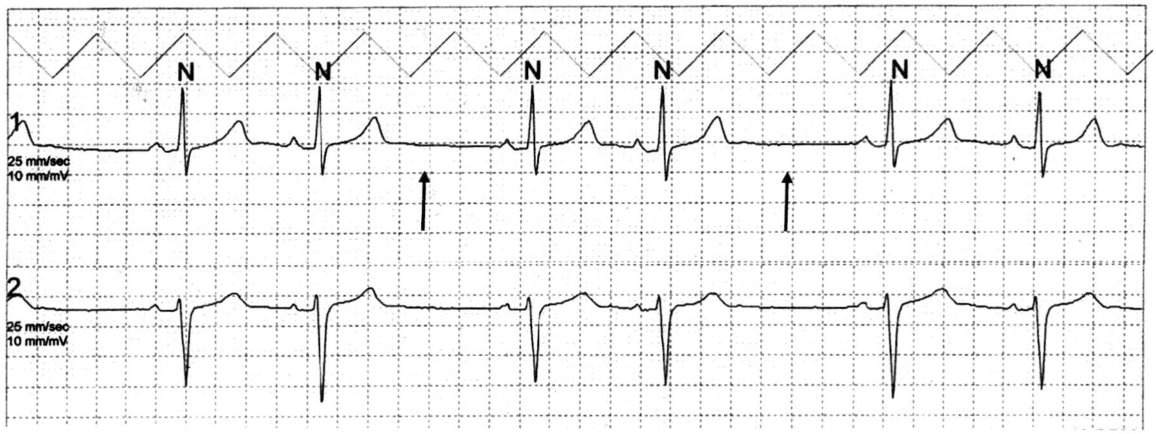

Fig. 25.8: This Holter monitoring electrocardiogram tracing of a 7-year-old boy shows two sinus pauses (arrows). Note the duration of the pauses are around 1.6 seconds (<1.8 seconds) and are usually considered benign.

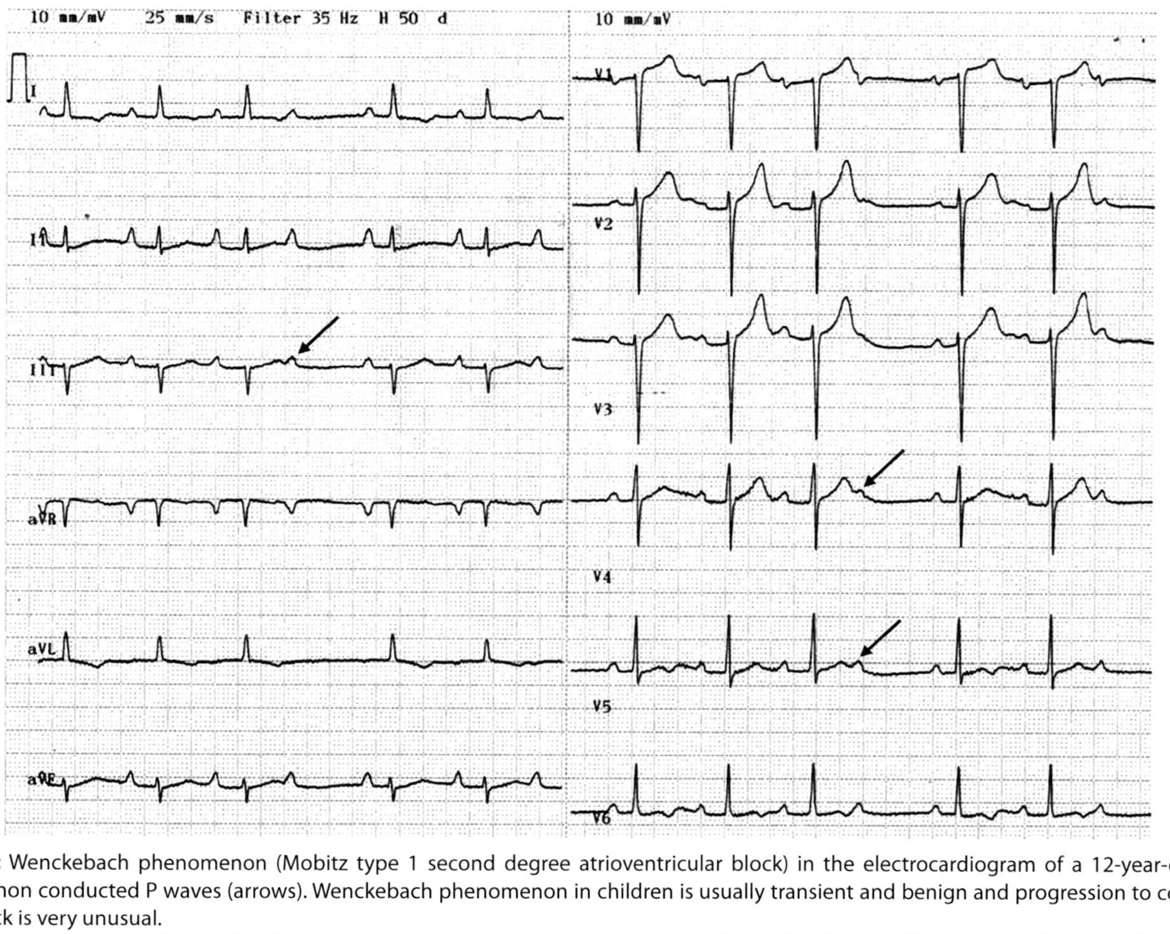

Fig. 25.9: Wenckebach phenomenon (Mobitz type 1 second degree atrioventricular block) in the electrocardiogram of a 12-year-old boy. Note the non conducted P waves (arrows). Wenckebach phenomenon in children is usually transient and benign and progression to complete heart block is very unusual.

left ventricle in the newborn infant, and the ECG will show right ventricular dominance and right axis deviation. Across the precordium, the R-wave amplitude will be increased in leads V1 and V2, and decreased in leads V5 and V6. With the cardiac changes occurring in the first 1–3 years of life, the left ventricle increases in size and the QRS axis will shift from rightward to a more leftward axis. Across the precordium, the R-wave amplitude decreases in leads V1 and V2, and increases in leads V5 and V6.[21] Diagnosis of ventricular hypertrophy by "voltage criteria" will depend on age adjusted values for R-wave and S-wave amplitudes. However, several electrocardiographic features may be useful in making a diagnosis. A qR complex or an Rsr pattern in lead V1, upright Twaves in the right precordial leads between ages 7 days and 7 years, marked right axis deviation (particularly associated with right atrial enlargement), and complete reversal of the adult precordial pattern of R- and S-waves will all suggest right ventricular hypertrophy. Left ventricular hypertrophy may be indicated by deep Q-waves in the left precordial leads or the typical adult changes of lateral ST depression and T-wave inversion.[1]

Influence of Sex

The influence of sex on some electrocardiographic variables has been noted in a small number of reports. Some differences in Q, R, and S wave amplitude measurements between boys and girls are apparent at all ages.[22,23] These differences are greatest in adolescents when the amplitudes of Q, R, and S waves are fairly consistently higher in males in most precordial leads. In the 12 to 16 year age group many of these differences are significant.[5] In childhood, sex does not have a major influence on electrocardiographic interval measurements although some small differences can be seen. The QRS duration is consistently longer in boys in all age groups. However, in absolute terms the differences are small—of the order of a 2 to 5 ms difference in median QRS duration—and probably not therefore important in day to day practice.[4] In prepubertal children sex does not appear to be of significance in determining the QT interval. Even in the adolescent group the differences are small but probably significant.[5]

COMPLETE HEART BLOCK IN PEDIATRIC ECG

Complete heart block (CHB) can be found in a number of different situations in pediatric patients. Some patients who undergo open heart surgery may develop complete heart block as a result of the surgery. The AV node may be damaged directly by the surgery, or in other instances inflammation or swelling of the cardiac tissue may damage the AV node. Less commonly, complete heart block may present in someone who has never had heart surgery as a result of a more diffuse electrical conduction system disease. Finally, complete heart block may be the result of transmission of antibodies in the womb from the mother to the fetus. This usually happens in women who have underlying connective tissue disorders such as systemic lupus erythematosus (SLE). In this situation, antibodies from the mother cross into the fetus and attack the AV node. With an incidence of 1 in 20,000 live born infants, congenital complete AV block (CCAVB) is a rare disease (Fig. 25.10). There may be evidence of a very slow heart rate in the fetus with development of complete heart block. In some instances of congenital complete heart block the problem may not be detected until the child is several years old. There is no causal therapy for CCAVB. Permanent pacing is the only possible therapy. The aim of permanent pacing therapy is to prevent sudden cardiac death and to restore an adequate heart rate to avoid any secondary effects of longstanding bradycardia.[26-30]

SUMMARY

The basic principles of interpretation of the ECG in children are identical to those in adults, but the progressive changes in anatomy and physiology which take place between birth and adolescence result in some features which differ significantly from the normal adult pattern and vary according to the age of the child (Box 25.1).

Typical indications for pediatric ECG include diagnosis and management of congenital heart diseases, syncope, exertional symptoms, tachyarrhythmias, and bradyarrhythmias (Box 25.2). Chest pain in children is rarely cardiac in origin and is often associated with tenderness in the chest wall. ECG is not usually helpful in making a diagnosis, although a normal ECG can be very reassuring to the family.

Average resting heart rate varies with age; newborns can range from 90 bpm to160 bpm and adolescents from 50 bpm to120 bpm. The average heart rate peaks about the second month of life and thereafter gradually decreases until adolescence.

The P wave amplitude does not change significantly during childhood and at any age amplitudes in excess of 2.5 mm should be regarded as exceeding the upper limit of normal.

It is important to remember that the normal PR interval in infants is shorter and lengthens as cardiac tissue matures

Box 25.1: Basic differences between pediatric and adult ECG.

1. Heart rate is much faster in neonates and infants compared to adults. Heart rate gradually decreases as the child grows older.
2. Tall R wave in lead V1 in normal pediatric ECG mimics right ventricular hypertrophy in the adult. At birth, the right ventricle is larger and thicker than the left ventricle, reflecting the greater physiological stresses placed upon it and produces dominant R in lead V1.
3. Marked right axis deviation, dominant R wave in V1 and T-wave inversions in V1–V3 (sometimes up to V4) are considered normal in pediatric ECG.
4. Conduction intervals (PR interval, QRS duration) are shorter than adults due to the smaller cardiac size.

Box 25.2: Common indications for pediatric ECG.

1. Diagnosis and management of congenital heart diseases
2. Diagnosis and management of arrhythmias
3. Diagnosis and management of rheumatic fever, Kawasaki disease, pericarditis, and myocarditis
4. Family history of sudden cardiac death
5. Electrolyte abnormalities
6. Chest pain or other symptoms related to exertion
7. Syncope and seizures
8. Cyanotic episodes

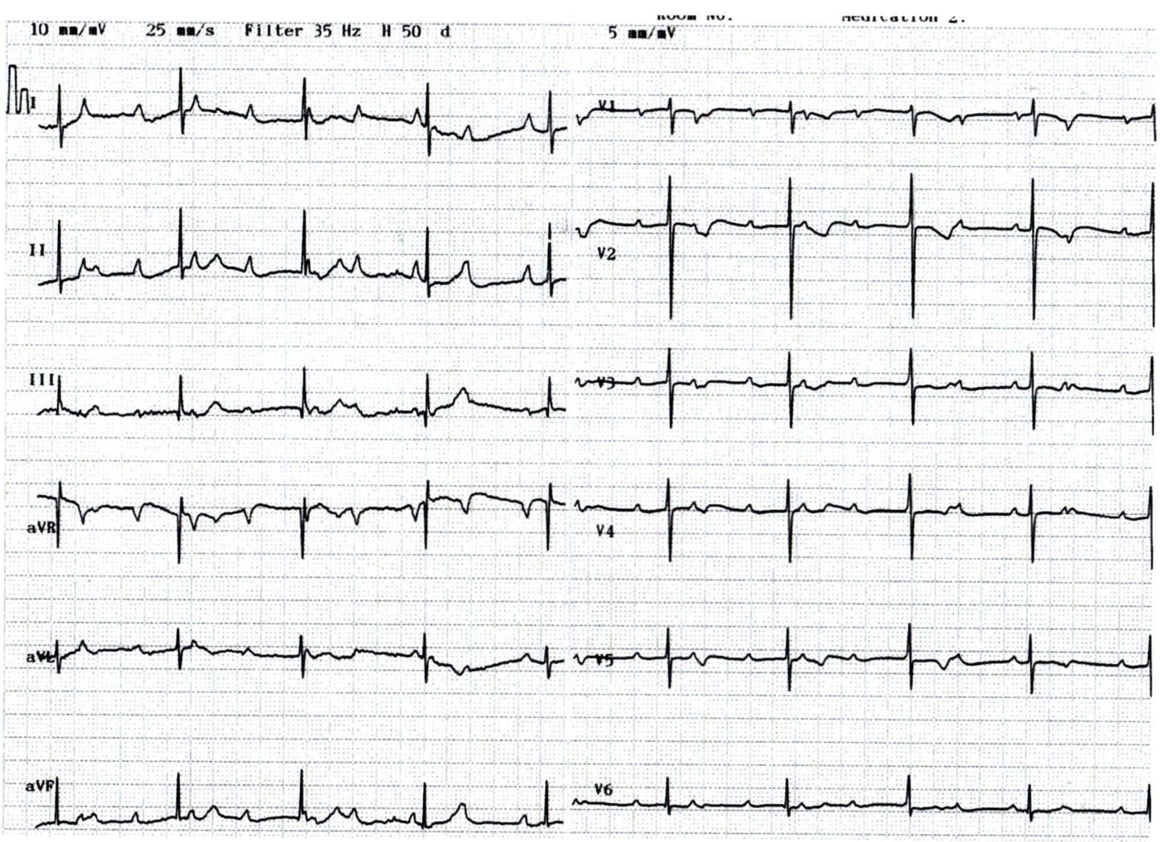

Fig. 25.10: This electrocardiogram shows complete heart block in a neonate with heart rate 57 bpm. (*Source*: Dr Nurunnahar Fatema, Labaid Cardiac Hospital.)

with age. The PR interval on resting 12-lead ECGs in children varies mainly in relation to heart rate and is therefore usually shorter in younger children. A normal appearing PR interval of 0.20 seconds (200 ms) may thus in fact represent a pathologic first-degree AV block in an infant or young child with fast heart rate.

Q waves are normally present in leads II, III, aVF, V5, and V6. Q waves in other leads are rare and associated with disease.

Detecting prolongation of the QT interval is important in the identification of individuals at risk of life threatening arrhythmia. For practical purposes Bazett's formula (measured QT interval divided by the square root of the R–R interval) remains the most commonly used method for determining the rate corrected QT interval (QT_c). In the first 6 months of life, the QT_c is considered normal at less than 0.49 seconds (490 ms). After infancy, this cutoff is generally 0.44 seconds (440 ms).

ST-segment elevation may be a normal finding in teenagers as a result of early repolarization.

Inverted T-waves in the right precordial leads (V1–3) are a normal finding in children, representing the dominance of right ventricle at these ages. T-wave inversions in the right precordial leads may persist into adulthood which is called 'Persistent Juvenile Pattern' and are most commonly seen in young Afro-Caribbean women. Persistent juvenile T-waves are asymmetric, shallow (<3 mm), and usually limited to leads V1–3. Normal ECG features in children have been summarized in Box 25.3.

Box 25.3: Normal ECG features in children.

1. Heart rate >100 beats/min
2. Marked sinus arrhythmia
3. Tall R-wave in V1
4. Right axis deviation (axis >+90°)
5. T-wave inversions in V1-3 (juvenile T-wave pattern)
6. Slurred QRS or RSR' pattern in V1
7. Short PR interval (<120 ms)
8. Short QRS duration (<80 ms)
9. Q-waves in the inferior and left precordial leads.
10. Slightly peaked P waves in neonates
11. Slightly long QTc (≤490 ms in infants)

Persistent Juvenile T-wave Pattern: A Normal Variant

1. Found in healthy children and young adults
2. More common in women than men
3. Asymmetric T-wave inversions or biphasic T-waves in leads V1–V3 (up to V4–V6 in some cases)
4. T waves are not symmetric nor deep (usually <3 mm)

Phasic changes in the P-P interval are almost universal in children and can be very obvious, leading to unnecessary concerns about the irregular heart rate. The diagnosis of sinus arrhythmia is easily confirmed in most cases by observing the relation of the change to respiration (slowing in expiration, accelerating in inspiration).

Premature supraventricular or ventricular beats are frequently seen in children of all age groups and are in most instances a benign condition. Intermittent and infrequent premature beats usually are not an indication for a cardiologic work-up.

In childhood, sex does not have a major influence on electrocardiographic interval measurements although some small differences can be seen. The QRS duration is consistently longer in boys in all age groups. However, in absolute terms the differences are small and probably not important in day-to-day clinical practice. Common variations in ECG rhythm have been summarized in Box 25.4.

Box 25.4: Common variations in rhythm which may be considered as normal in pediatric ECG.

1. Marked sinus arrhythmia
2. Short sinus pauses <1.8 sec
3. First degree AV block
4. Wenckebach phenomenon (Mobitz type 1 second degree AV block)
5. Intermittent junctional rhythm
6. Ventricular or supraventricular extrasystole

First Degree AV Block and Wenckebach Phenomenon

Around 10% of normal children will have episodes of Mobitz type 1 second degree AV block or Wenckebach phenomenon. Some, but not all, of these individuals will have episodes of first-degree AV block. These are usually transient and benign and do not progress to complete heart block (CHB).

Complete Heart Block in Pediatric ECG

Congenital complete heart block (CHB) is rare in pediatric group of patients with an incidence of 1 in 20,000 live born infants. CHB may develop in neonates and children due to:

1. Postsurgical (after cardiac surgery)
2. Maternal connective tissue disorders such as SLE
3. Diffuse electrical conduction system disease
4. Idiopathic.

REFERENCES

1. Goodacre S, McLeod K. Paediatric electrocardiography. BMJ. 2002;324(7350):1382-5.
2. Sharieff GQ, Rao SO. The Pediatric ECG. Emerg Med Clin N Am. 2006;24(1):195-208.
3. Davignon A, Rautaharju P, Boisselle E, et al. Normal ECG standards for infants and children. Pediatr Cardiol. 1979;1(2):123-31.
4. Rijnbeek PR, Witsenburg M, Schrama E, et al. New normal limits for the paediatric electrocardiogram. Eur Heart J. 2001;22(8):702-11.
5. Dickinson DF. The normal ECG in childhood and adolescence. Heart. 2005;91(12):1626-30.
6. Evans WN, Acherman RJ, Mayman GA, et al. Simplified pediatric electrocardiogram interpretation. Clin Pediatr. 2010;49(4):363-72.
7. Bazett HC. An analysis of the time-relations of electrocardiograms. Heart. 1920;(7):353-70.
8. Panicker GK, Karnad DR, Joshi R, et al. Z-score for benchmarking reader competence in a central ECG laboratory. Ann Noninvasive Electrocardiol. 2009;14(1):19-25.
9. Salvi V, Karnad DR, Panicker GK, et al. Comparison of 5 methods of QT interval measurements on electrocardiograms from a thorough QT/QTc study: Effect on assay sensitivity and categorical outliers. J Electrocardiol. 2011;44(2):96-104.
10. Panicker GK, Karnad DR, Natekar M, et al. Intra- and interreader variability in QT interval measurement by tangent and threshold methods in a central electrocardiogram laboratory. J Electrocardiol. 2009;42(4):348-52.
11. Tipple M. Interpretation of electrocardiograms in infants and children. Images Paediatr Cardiol. 1999;1(1):3-13.
12. Scott O, Williams GJ, Fiddler GI. Results of 24 hour ambulatory monitoring of electrocardiogram in 131 healthy boys aged 10 to 13 years. Br Heart J. 1980;44(3):304-8.
13. Southall DP, Johnston F, Shinebourne EA, et al. 24-hour electrocardiographic study of heart rate and rhythm in population of healthy children. Br Heart J. 1981;45(3):281-91.
14. Dickinson DF, Scott O. Ambulatory electrocardiographic monitoring in 100 healthy teenage boys. Br Heart J. 1984;51:179-83.
15. Viitasalo MT, Kala R, Eisalo A. Ambulatory electrocardiographic findings in young athletes between 14 and 16 years of age. Eur Heart J. 1984;5(1):2-6.
16. Young D, Fish B, Fisher JD. Wenckebach atrioventricular block (Mobitz type I) in children and adolescents. Am J Cardiol. 1977;40(3):393-9.
17. von Bernuth G, Toussaint R, Mund C, et al. Heart rate and heart rhythm in healthy infants and children. Klin Padiatr. 1989;201(2):98-103.
18. Massin MM, Bourguignont A, Gerard P. Study of cardiac rate and rhythm patterns in ambulatory and hospitalized children. Cardiology. 2005;103(4):174-9.
19. Pfammatter JP. Practical management of common arrhythmias in children. Praxis. 2005;94(45):1765-8.
20. Jacobson J, Gillette Garson A. Premature ventricular contractions in normal children. Pediatrics. 1978;92:36-8.
21. Chan TC, Sharieff GQ, Brady WJ, et al. Electrocardiographic Manifestations: Pediatric ECG. Emerg Med. 2008;35(4): 421-30.
22. Ayabakan C, Ozer S, Celiker A, et al. Analysis of 2017 Holter records in pediatric patients. Turk J Pediatr. 2000;42:286-93.

23. Macfarlane PW, McLaughlin SC, Devine B, et al. Effects of age, sex and race on ECG interval measurements. J Electrocardiol. 1994;27(Suppl):14-9.
24. Tsuji A, Nagashima M, Hasegawa S. Long-term follow-up of idiopathic ventricular arrhythmias in otherwise normal children. JPN Circ J. 1995;59(10):654-62.
25. O'Connor M, McDaniel N, Brady WJ. The pediatric electrocardiogram. Part I: Age-related interpretation. Am J Emerg Med. 2008;26(2):221-8.
26. Fischbach PS, Frias PA, Strieper MJ, et al. Natural history and current therapy for complete heart block in children and patients with congenital heart disease. Congenit Heart Dis. 2007;2(4):224-34.
27. Jayaprasad N, Johnson F, Venugopal K. Congenital complete heart block and maternal connective tissue disease. Int J Cardiol. 2006;112(2):153-8.
28. Villain E. Indications for pacing in patients with congenital heart disease. Pacing Clin Electrophysiol. 2008;31(Suppl 1):S17-20.
29. Kim JJ, Friedman RA, Eidem BW, et al. Ventricular function and long-term pacing in children with congenital complete atrioventricular block. J Cardiovasc Electrophysiol. 2007;18(4):373-7.
30. Balmer C, Bauersfeld U. Do All Children with Congenital Complete Atrioventricular Block Require Permanent Pacing? Indian Pacing Electrophysiol J. 2003;3(3):178-83.

Chapter 26

Exercise Tolerance Test

INTRODUCTION

Exercise tolerance test (ETT) also known as treadmill stress test (TMT) or exercise stress testing is the most widely used method for detecting myocardial ischemia, but the test is also applied in numerous other settings. The method requires close attention to technical details and application of appropriate test protocols. Attention to absolute and relative contraindications (Box 26.1) and criteria for test termination is mandatory (Box 26.2). In addition to the electrocardiogram (ECG), work capacity, heart rate, and blood pressure responses are also important diagnostic and prognostic markers. Exercise ECG testing is most valuable as a diagnostic tool for myocardial ischemia when pretest disease probability is high.[1-4]

Exercise tolerance test is usually indicated for assessment of chest pain in patients with probability for coronary artery disease (CAD), arrhythmia provocation, and assessment of symptoms (for example, presyncope) occurring during or after exercise. Prognostic indications for ETT include risk stratification after myocardial infarction, risk stratification in patients with hypertrophic cardiomyopathy, evaluation of revascularization or drug treatment, evaluation of exercise tolerance and cardiac function, and assessment of treatment for arrhythmia (Box 26.3).[5]

Exercise tolerance test has a sensitivity of 78% and a specificity of 70% for detecting CAD. It cannot, therefore, be used to rule in or rule out ischemic heart disease unless the probability of CAD is taken into account. For example, in a low-risk population, such as men aged under 30 years, and women aged under 40 years, a positive test result is more likely to be a false-positive than true, and negative results add little new information. In a high-risk population, such as those aged over 50 years with typical anginal symptoms, a negative result cannot rule out ischemic heart disease, though the results may be of some prognostic value. ETT is, therefore, of greatest diagnostic value in patients with an intermediate risk of coronary artery disease.[5] Bayes' theorem of diagnostic probability states that the predictive value of an abnormal exercise test will vary according to the probability of CAD in the population under study. Exercise testing is, therefore, usually performed in patients with a moderate probability of CAD, rather than in those with a very low or high probability.[5]

The Bruce protocol is the most widely adopted protocol and has been extensively validated. The Bruce protocol

Box 26.1: Contraindications for standard exercise testing.

- Acute myocardial infarction (within 4–6 days)
- Unstable angina (rest pain in previous 48 hours)
- Uncontrolled heart failure
- Acute myocarditis or pericarditis
- Uncontrolled hypertension (systolic blood pressure >220 mm Hg, diastolic >120 mm Hg)
- Acute systemic infection
- Severe aortic stenosis
- Severe hypertrophic obstructive cardiomyopathy
- Untreated life-threatening arrhythmia
- Dissecting aneurysm

Box 26.2: Reasons for stopping a test.

Electrocardiographic criteria

- Severe ST-segment depression (>3 mm)
- ST-segment elevation >1 mm in non-Q wave lead
- Frequent ventricular extrasystoles (unless the test is to assess ventricular arrhythmia)
- Onset of ventricular tachycardia
- New atrial fibrillation or supraventricular tachycardia
- Development of new bundle branch block [if the test is primarily to detect underlying coronary artery disease (CAD)]
- New second- or third-degree heart block
- Cardiac arrest

Symptoms and signs

- Patient requests stopping because of severe fatigue
- Severe chest pain, dyspnea, or dizziness
- Fall in systolic blood pressure (>20 mm Hg)
- Hypertensive response (SBP > 260 mm Hg; DBP > 130 mm Hg)
- Ataxia.

Box 26.3: Indications of exercise tolerance test.

Diagnostic indications of ETT
- Assessment of chest pain in patients with suspected CAD
- Arrhythmia provocation
- Assessment of symptoms (for example, presyncope) occurring during or after exercise
- Assessment of patients with atypical chest pain (to rule out the possibility of CAD)

Prognostic indications for ETT
- Risk stratification after myocardial infarction
- Assessment of treatment for arrhythmia
- Evaluation of revascularization or drug treatment
- Evaluation of exercise tolerance and cardiac function
- Assessment of cardiopulmonary function in patients with heart failure.

(ETT: exercise tolerance test; CAD: coronary artery disease)

is a diagnostic test used in the evaluation of cardiac function, developed by Robert Arthur Bruce (1916–2004), an American cardiologist, and a professor at the University of Washington. He is known as the "father of exercise cardiology" for his research and development of the Bruce protocol.

The protocol has seven stages, each lasting 3 minutes, resulting in 21 minutes' exercise for a complete test. In stage 1 the patient walks at 1.7 miles (2.7 km) per hour (mph) up a 10% incline. The speed and incline increase with each stage. Assessment of workload is measured by metabolic equivalents (METs) and workload is a reflection of oxygen consumption and hence energy use.

A modified Bruce protocol is used for exercise testing in case of elderly patients and also within 1 week of myocardial infarction. The modified Bruce protocol starts at a lower workload than the standard test. The first two stages of the modified Bruce test are performed at a 1.7 mph and 0% grade, and 1.7 mph and 5% grade, and the third stage corresponds to the first stage of the standard Bruce test protocol as listed in Table 26.1.

The patient is first connected to the ETT machine. Resting electrocardiograms, both sitting and standing, are recorded as electrocardiographic changes, particularly T-wave inversion, may occur as the patient stands up to start walking on the treadmill. A short period of electrocardiographic recording during hyperventilation

Table 26.1: Standard Bruce protocol.

Stage	*Minutes*	*% Grade*	*MPH*	*METS*
1	3	10	1.7	4
2	3	12	2.5	7
3	3	14	3.4	10
4	3	16	4.2	13
5	3	18	5.0	15
6	3	20	5.5	18
7	3	22	6.0	21

(MPH: miles per hour; METs: metabolic equivalents)

is also valuable for identifying changes resulting from hyperventilation rather than from coronary ischemia.

Beta blockers should be discontinued the day before the test, and digoxin (which may cause false-positive results, with ST-segment abnormalities) should be stopped 1 week before testing. By convention, the maximum predicted heart rate is calculated as 220 (210 for women) minus the patient's age. A satisfactory heart rate response is achieved on reaching 85% of the maximum predicted heart rate.[5] During the test, the electrocardiogram machine provides a continuous record of the heart rate and the 12-lead electrocardiogram is recorded intermittently. Blood pressure must be measured before the exercise begins and at the end of each exercise stage. Blood pressure may fall or remain static during the initial stage of exercise. This is the result of an anxious patient relaxing. As the test progresses, however, systolic blood pressure should rise as exercise increases. A level of up to 220 mm Hg is normal in adults, although athletes can have higher levels. Diastolic blood pressure tends to fall slightly. The aim of the exercise is for the patient to achieve their maximum predicted heart rate.[5] In absence of significant CAD, the exercise ECG do not reveal any significant ST-segment depression at peak exercise and at recovery (Figs. 26.1A and B).

SAFETY

Stress testing is a relatively safe procedure. Before 1980, an overall mortality rate of 1 in 20,000 tests was observed. In the contemporary era, however, this frequency has been found to be even lower, generally less than 1 in 50,000. Nonfatal complications, such as myocardial infarction, occur at the rate of less than 4 per 10,000 tests. In subjects with history of ventricular tachycardia or fibrillation, serious but nonfatal arrhythmias occurred during 2.3% of the tests. In the absence of such a history, the incidence of such complications is approximately 0.05%.[6]

Normal Electrocardiographic Changes During Exercise

- P wave increases in height
- R wave decreases in height
- J point becomes depressed
- ST segment becomes sharply upsloping
- Q–T interval shortens
- T wave decreases in height

CRITERIA FOR A POSITIVE EXERCISE TEST

ST-Segment Depression

The criterion of >1 mm horizontal (Figs. 26.2A and B) or downsloping (Figs. 26.3A and B) ST depression is the most generally accepted. But junctional (J point) depression with slowly upsloping ST segments also is generally considered

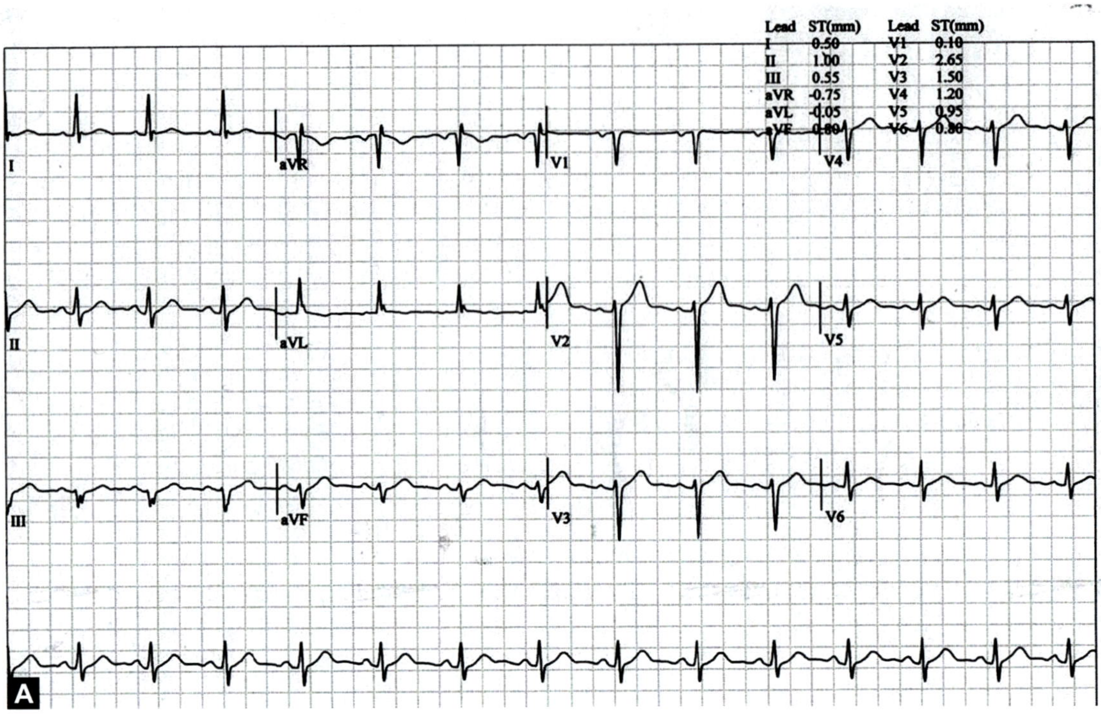

Fig. 26.1A: Pretest electrocardiogram, taken immediately before starting exercise test. This is a normal tracing without any significant ST segment change.

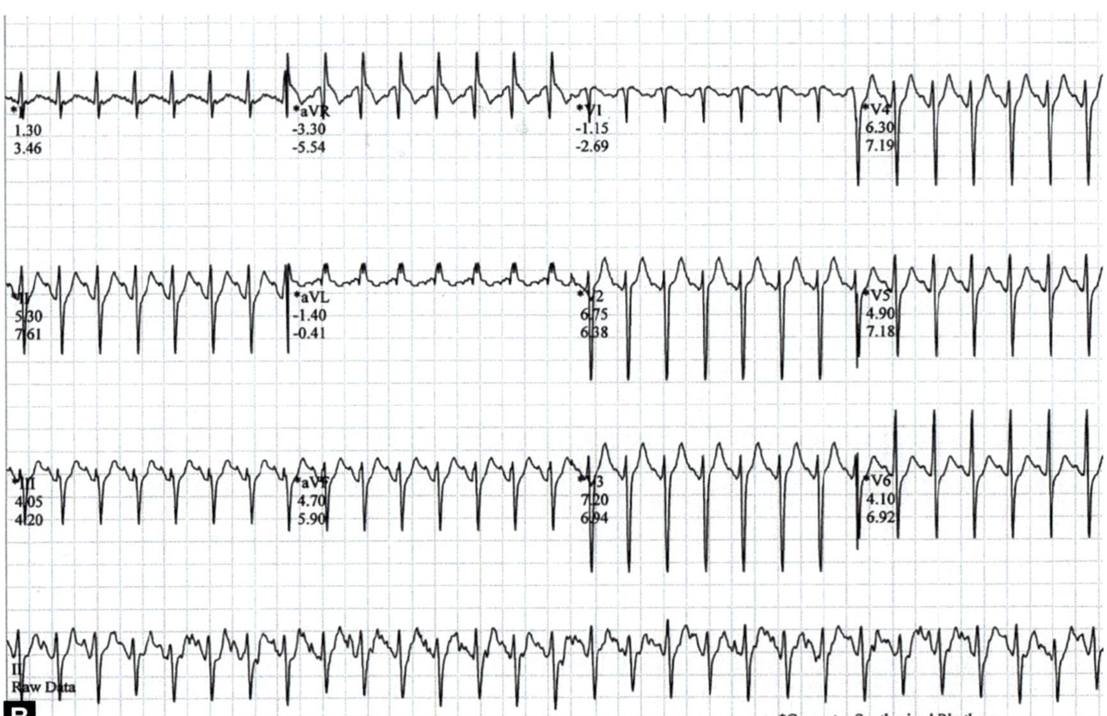

Fig. 26.1B: Electrocardiogram recorded at peak exercise of the patient (A). Patient achieved 96% of predicted heart rate at Bruce stage-4 without any ST segment depression and exercise tolerance test (ETT) is considered negative for provocable ischemia (Normal stress test).

to be an abnormal response, although the definition of slowly upsloping varies. Various investigators have reported that including upsloping ST responses that remain 1–2 mm below the baseline at 60–80 ms after the J point significantly increases test sensitivity without degrading specificity. It is usually suggested that, in the case of upsloping ST segments, 1.5-mm depression at 80 ms after the J point is a reasonable criterion for a positive response (Box 26.4).[7-12]

ST-Segment Elevation

Although horizontal or downsloping ST segment depression is the typical ischemic response in stress testing, some

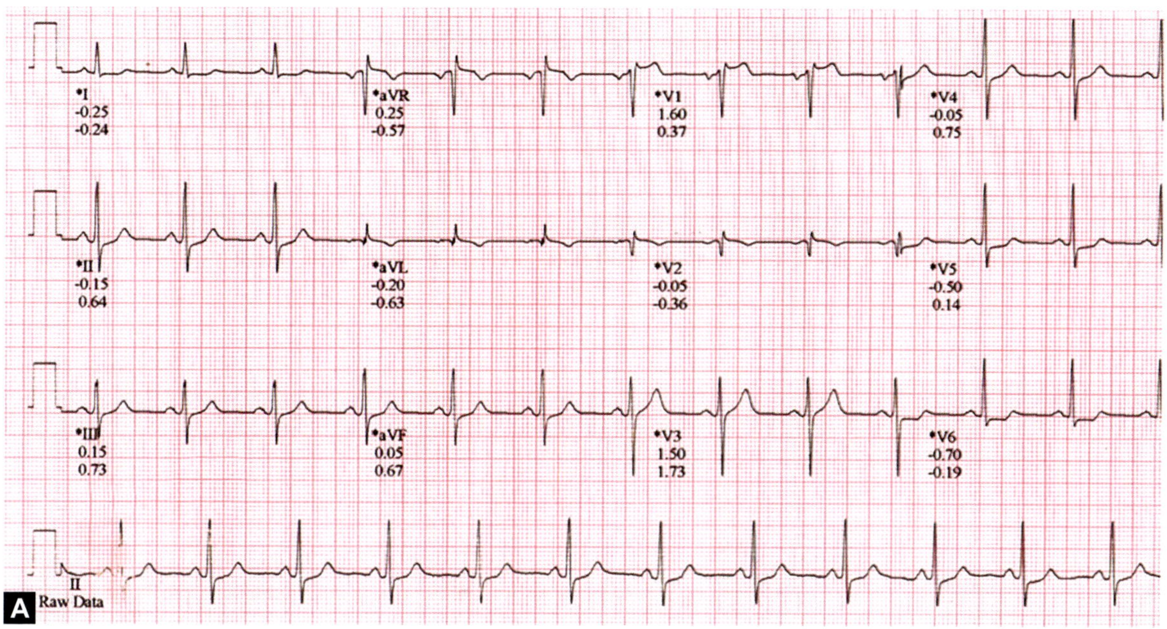

Fig. 26.2A: Pretest electrocardiogram of a patient presenting with complaints of exertional chest discomfort. Electrocardiogram taken immediately before starting exercise test and ECG findings are unremarkable.

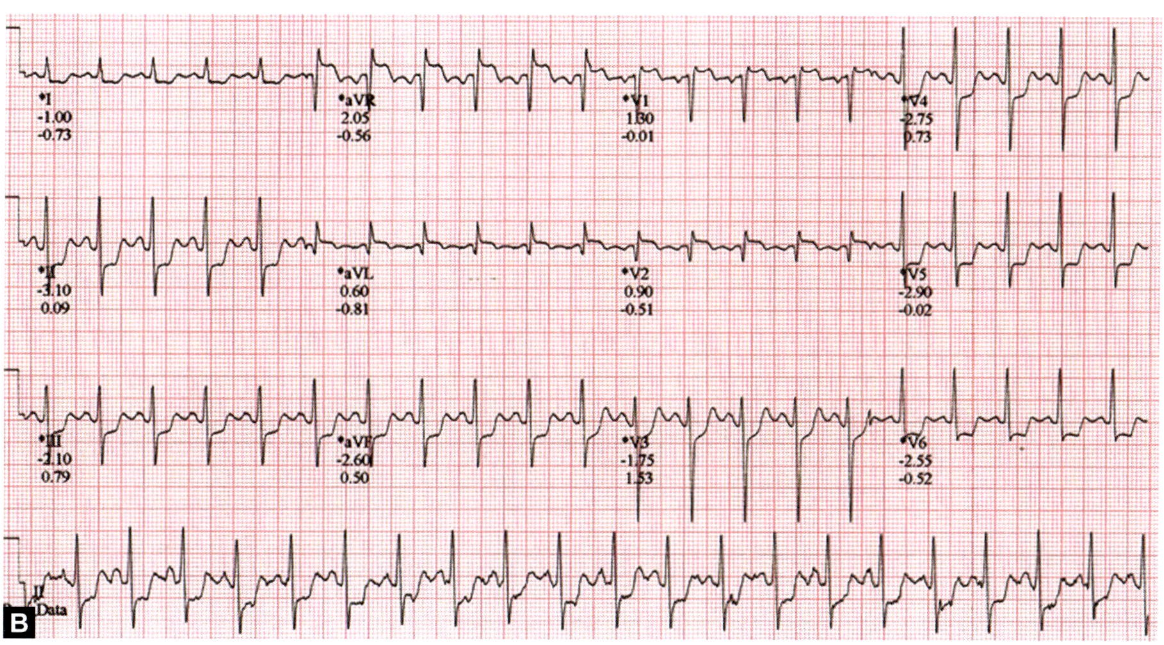

Fig. 26.2B: ECG recorded at peak exercise of the patient (A). Note marked horizontal ST segment depression (>2mm) in most of the limb and chest leads in Bruce stage-2, suggesting abnormal ETT and the test is considered positive for provocable ischemia.

patients exhibit ST-segment elevation of greater than or equal to 1 mm. Generally, in the absence of prior infarction, this finding is uncommon but implies severe transmural ischemia exceeding that associated with isolated ST depression (Figs. 26.4 A to C). High-grade proximal coronary stenosis is usually found, and this combination is associated with an ominous prognosis. The correlation between the site of the ST-segment elevation and the artery involved is generally quite good.[13-18] ST elevation in anterior leads suggest myocardial ischemia in anterior wall, which is the left anterior descending (LAD) coronary artery region. ST elevation in inferior leads suggest ischemia in the inferior or posterior myocardium, which may be the right coronary artery (RCA) or circumflex artery (Cx) region. By contrast, observation of ST segment depression during treadmill exercise test is not related to any specific myocardial territory.

Exercise-induced ST-segment elevation is seen most commonly in patients who have had previous myocardial infarctions. Most studies demonstrated an incidence of 14–27%. Patients with anterior myocardial infarction are more likely to have exercise-induced ST-segment elevation than are those with inferior myocardial infarction. The

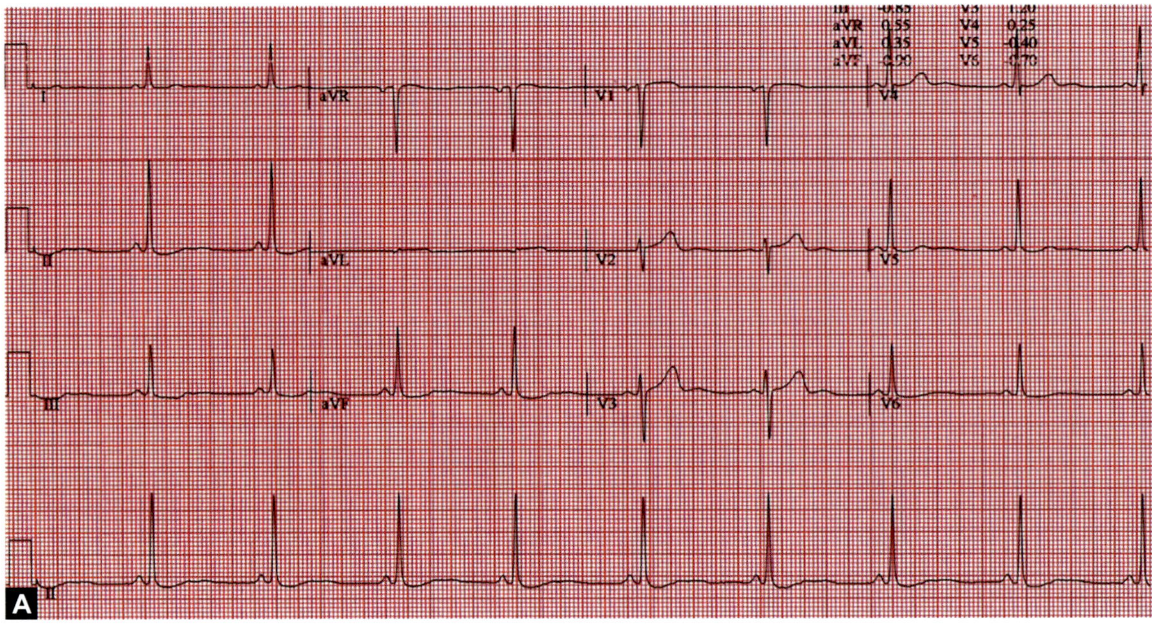

Fig. 26.3A: Pretest electrocardiogram of a patient presenting with Canadian Cardiovascular Society (CCS) class II angina. This electrocardiogram (ECG) reveals only mild nonspecific ST and T wave changes and considered unremarkable.

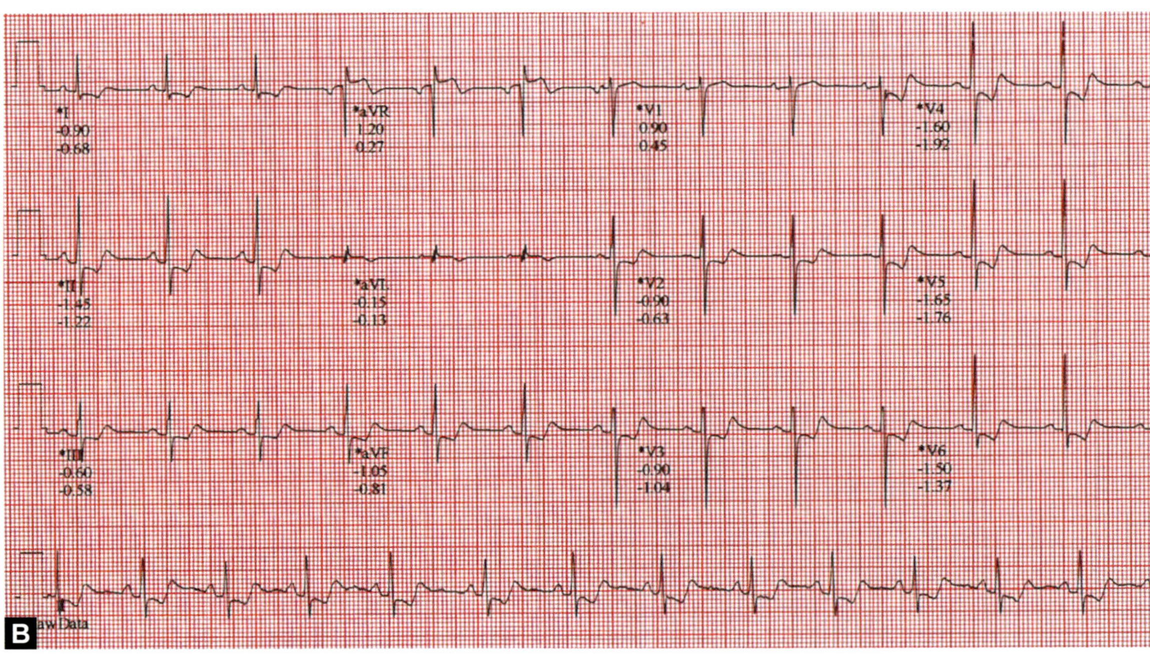

Fig. 26.3B: ECG recorded at peak exercise of the patient (A). Note downsloping ST-segment depression (>1 mm) in most of the limb and chest leads in Bruce stage-1 (at 2 mins), suggesting abnormal ETT and the test is considered positive for provocable ischemia.

ST-segment elevation almost always occurs in the leads with abnormal Q waves. It is also associated with a left ventricular wall motion abnormality, either dyskinetic or akinetic, in the corresponding site in greater than 90% of cases.[19-23] 10–30% of patients with variant angina also may have ST-segment elevation with exercise. The leads those show ST-segment elevation during exercise are usually the same leads those record elevation during angina at rest.[19]

SIGNIFICANCE OF ST-SEGMENT DEPRESSION LIMITED TO THE RECOVERY PHASE OF EXERCISE STRESS TEST

Exercise-induced ST-segment depression is considered as a reliable ECG finding for the diagnosis of obstructive coronary atherosclerosis. It has also been associated with

Box 26.4: Electrocardiogram criteria for positive exercise tolerance test.

The standard criterion for a positive ETT is horizontal or down-sloping ST segment depression of >1 mm in multiple leads.

Other recognized criteria for positive ETT response:

- ST-segment depression occurring only in recovery phase of ETT has a diagnostic value largely comparable with that of ST segment depression induced during exercise phase of ETT and should be considered as positive stress test.
- ST-segment elevation of >1 mm, particularly in the absence of Q waves.
- In the case of upsloping ST-segment depression, 1.5-mm depression at 80 ms after the J point is considered as a reasonable criterion for a positive response.

(ETT: exercise tolerance test)

a worse prognosis for patients with documented CAD. However, while the diagnostic and prognostic value of ST-segment depression occurring during the active phase of exercise test is well recognized, only a few studies have investigated the clinical significance of ST-segment depression appearing only during the recovery phase of exercise testing. In patients with a suspected or documented history of CAD, ST-segment depression limited to the recovery phase of an exercise stress test has a diagnostic and prognostic clinical meaning largely comparable with that of ST-segment depression induced during the active phase of exercise testing.[24-27]

J-Point Depression during Exercise Tolerance Test

The J point (the point of inflection at the junction of the S wave and ST segment) becomes depressed during exercise, with maximum depression at peak exercise. The normal ST segment during exercise therefore slopes sharply upwards. By convention, ST segment depression is measured relative to the isoelectric baseline (between the T and P waves) at a point 60–80 ms after the J point.[5] Upsloping ST segment depression, greater than or equal to 1.5 mm at 80 ms after the J point is a reasonable criterion for a positive stress test.

Blood Pressure Response During Exercise Tolerance Test

In response to the increased stroke volume and systolic contractile force, the systolic BP normally rises progressively with increasing workloads, reaching approximately 160–220 mm Hg with maximum effort. Because exercise lowers overall peripheral vascular resistance, the diastolic pressure exhibits little or no change (less than 10 mm Hg).

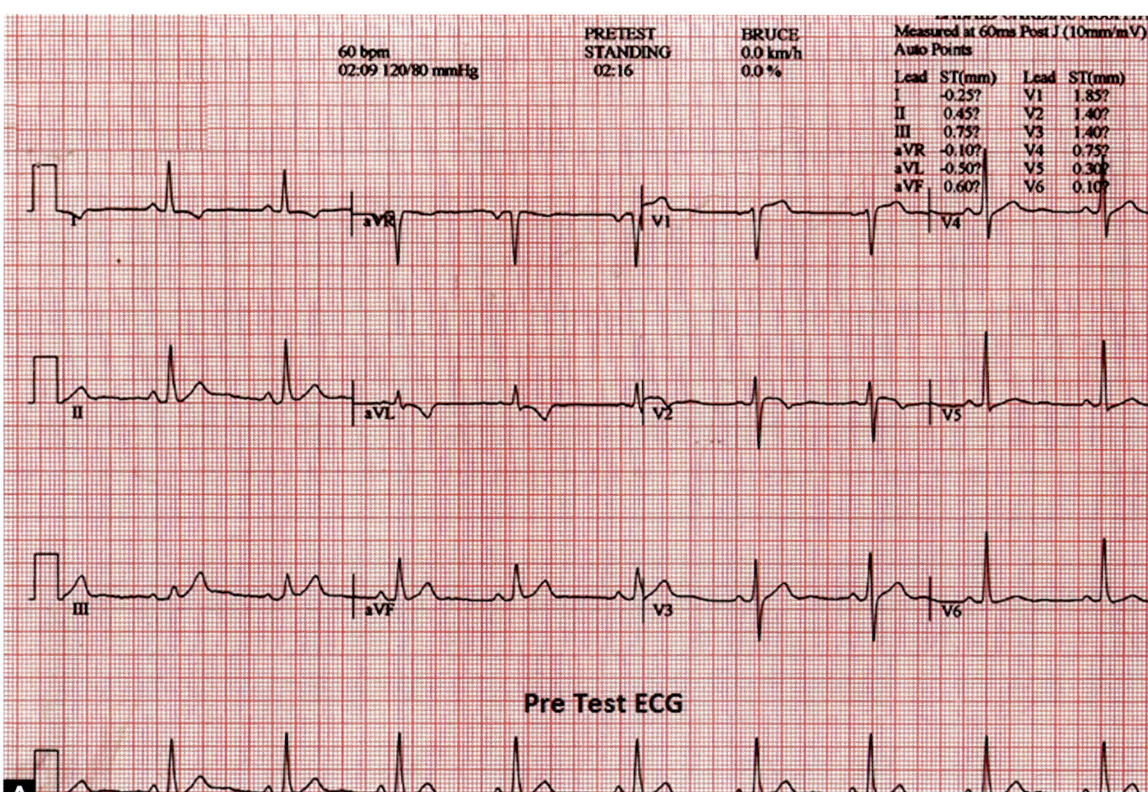

Fig. 26.4A: Pre test electrocardiogram of a patient who presented with history of chest pain on exertion of recent onset. This ECG reveals biphasic T waves in lead I and aVL and otherwise unremarkable.

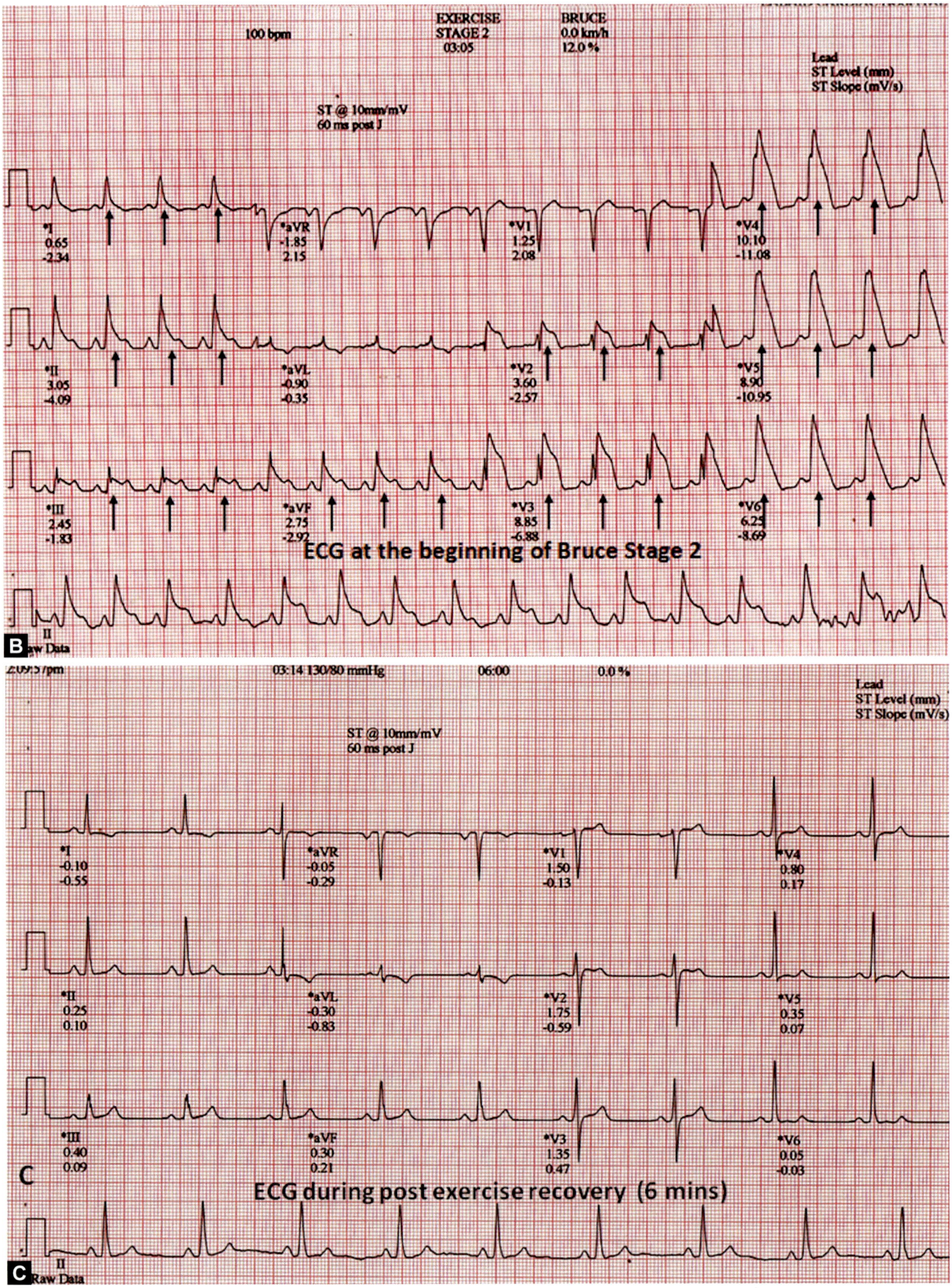

Figs. 26.4B and C: (B). At the beginning of the Bruce stage 2 (03 minutes 05 seconds), the patient (Fig.26.4A) developed severe central chest pain and ECG shows >5 mm ST segment elevation in both limb and chest leads (arrows). (C). ECG of the same patient (Fig.26.4A) 6 minutes at post-exercise recovery, showing almost normalization of ST segment elevation. Coronary angiogram of this patient revealed critical stenosis of the proximal left anterior descending (LAD) artery and subsequently percutaneous coronary intervention (PCI) was done.

If the systolic pressure fails to rise to greater than or equal to 130 mm Hg or falls by greater than or equal to 10 mm Hg in response to exercise, this frequently indicates left ventricular dysfunction and often signals the presence of severe CAD associated with extensive myocardial ischemia. Normally, the systolic pressure falls rapidly after cessation of exercise.[28-30]

False-Positive Test

A wide variety of miscellaneous situations has also been associated with falsely positive ST responses to exercise (Box 26.5). These include digitalis administration, mitral valve prolapse, hypokalemia, pectus excavatum, and intraventricular conduction defects including left bundle branch block (LBBB) and Wolff–Parkinson–White (WPW) syndrome. There is undoubtedly no common mechanism for ST shifts in these diverse situations.[31-37]

False-positive ETT may also be due to mechanical lesions and increased left ventricular mass. Presence of left ventricular hypertrophy (LVH) is a common cause of false-positive ETT. Relative coronary insufficiency is probably the cause of false-positive ETT in patients with LVH.[38,39] Mechanical lesions that place a greater burden on left ventricular dynamics and oxygen requirements may produce false-positive test and include mitral or aortic valvular lesions, pulmonary hypertension, pericardial constriction, hypertrophic cardiomyopathy, etc.[40-43]

In the case of right bundle branch block (RBBB), the resting anterior ST–T changes secondary to this conduction abnormality interfere with interpretation of the exercise response. Thus, changes in leads V1 through V3 often falsely suggest ischemia. The test is still reliable if the ST segment depression is recorded in leads V4 through V6.[44]

ST-segment elevation may be seen in the resting ECGs of healthy subjects because of early repolarization abnormality. In such cases, the ST segment returns to the isoelectric baseline with exercise, whereas those with significant CAD may have horizontal ST-segment depression. Therefore, even in the presence of ST elevation in the baseline ECG, the usual criteria for the interpretation of the exercise test are probably still applicable.[6]

Box 26.5: Causes of false positive exercise tolerance test.

- Digoxin
- Left ventricular hypertrophy
- Hypertrophic cardiomyopathy
- Wolff-Parkinson-White (WPW) syndrome
- Mitral valve prolapse
- Significant aortic or mitral valve insufficiency
- Significant aortic valve stenosis
- Anemia
- Hypokalemia
- Uncontrolled hypertension

False-Negative Test

Drugs which limit the heart rate response to exercise (beta blockers, diltiazem, and verapamil) reduce the heart rate and maximum systolic arterial BP during exercise, thus decreasing the left ventricular work and myocardial oxygen requirements, and reducing or eliminating the ST-segment depression.[45] In the process of increasing exercise capacity, nitrates may also prevent or minimize changes in exercise ECG.[46] In general, if one wishes to maximize test sensitivity, treatment with any of the drugs noted above should be withdrawn for a sufficient period to allow removal of the drug from the body before testing.

Exercise-induced Arrhythmias

Premature ventricular beats are often induced by exercise and develops in approximately 3% of subjects. The long-term prognosis of asymptomatic subjects manifesting exercise-induced ventricular arrhythmias, including nonsustained ventricular tachycardia, appears to be benign (Fig. 26.5).[47,48] In patients with CAD, the reported incidence of exercise-induced ventricular arrhythmias ranges from 38% to 65%. Significant multivessel disease is likely to be present in patients with angina and exercise-induced ventricular tachycardia (Fig. 26.6), especially if ST-segment changes consistent with myocardial ischemia also are present.[49-52]

Rarely patient may develop atrial fibrillation with fast ventricular response and supraventricular tachycardia (Fig. 26.7) during exercise. These supraventricular arrhythmias are not very diagnostic of CAD and ETT becomes equivocal.

Inversion of U Waves During Exercise

Transient inversion of U waves even in the absence of an abnormal ST-segment response has been suggested as a marker of extensive ischemia in the anterior myocardium or elsewhere.[53,54] Exercise-induced increased magnitude of the U wave in the precordial leads (greater than or equal to 0.05 mV) is suggestive of ischemia in the distribution of the left circumflex or right coronary arteries.[55,56]

Pseudonormalization of T Waves

T wave is the most labile component of ECG and may even show changes with hyperventilation. If a T wave which is negative before test becomes positive during the test (pseudonormalization), it is not generally accepted as a sign of ischemia.[57,58]

LIMITATIONS

The specificity of ST-segment depression as the main indicator of myocardial ischemia is limited. ST-segment

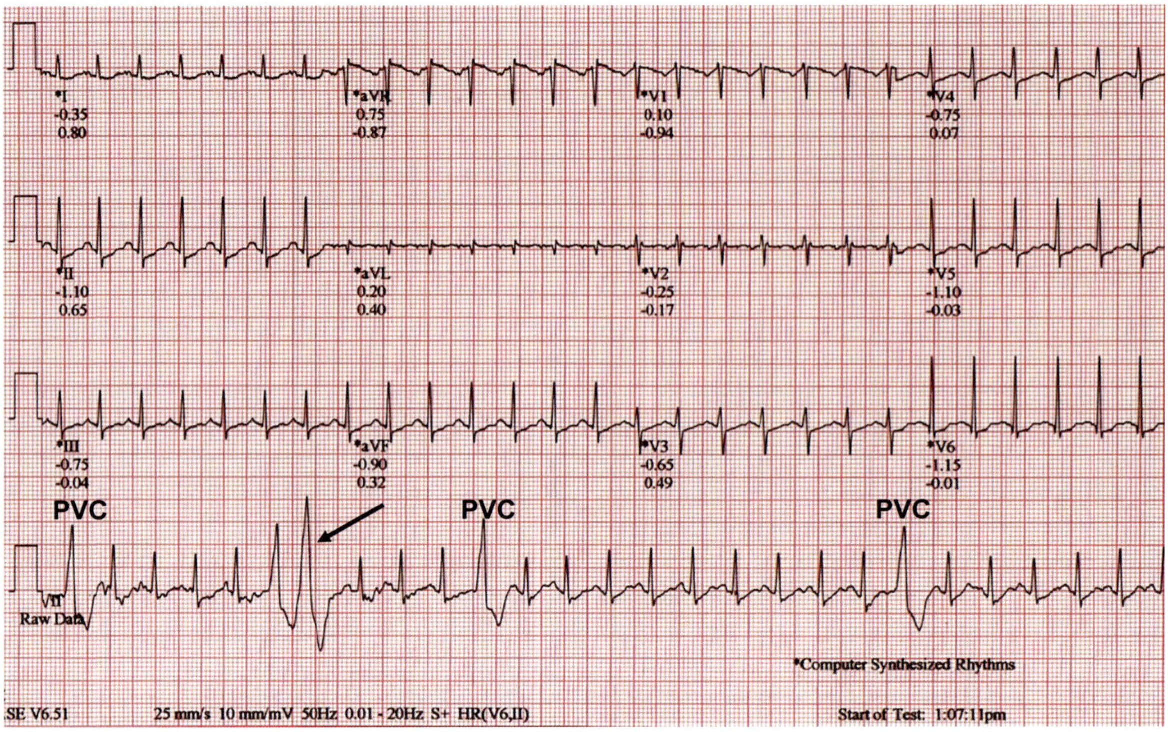

Fig. 26.5: Electrocardiogram recorded at peak exercise (Stage 3, 8 mins 50 secs). This ECG strip shows few premature ventricular complexes (PVCs) and a couplet (*arrow*) at peak exercise. Note there is no significant ST-depression at peak exercise and patient attained 97% of maximum predicted heart rate at Bruce stage 3 and stress test is considered negative for provocable ischemia. Appearance of few PVCs or couplets during exercise is considered benign.

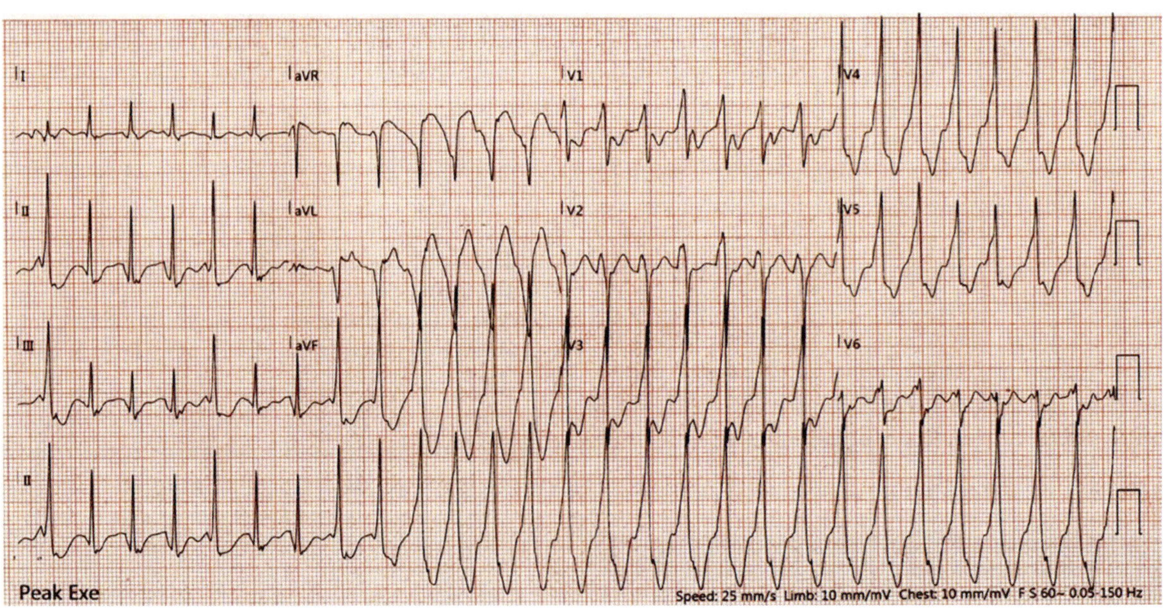

Fig. 26.6: Exercise tolerance test tracing of a patient who developed broad complex tachycardia suggestive of ventricular tachycardia (VT) at peak exercise. Note left side of the ECG shows sinus tachycardia and right side shows VT. (*Source*: Dr AK Miah, Labaid Cardiac Hospital)

depression has been estimated to occur in up to 20% of normal individuals on ambulatory electrocardiographic monitoring. There are many causes of ST segment changes apart from CAD, which confound the result of exercise testing. If the resting electrocardiogram is abnormal, the usefulness of an exercise test is reduced or may even be precluded. Repolarization and conduction abnormalities—for example, left ventricular hypertrophy, left bundle branch block, pre-excitation, and effects of digoxin—preclude accurate interpretation of the electrocardiogram during

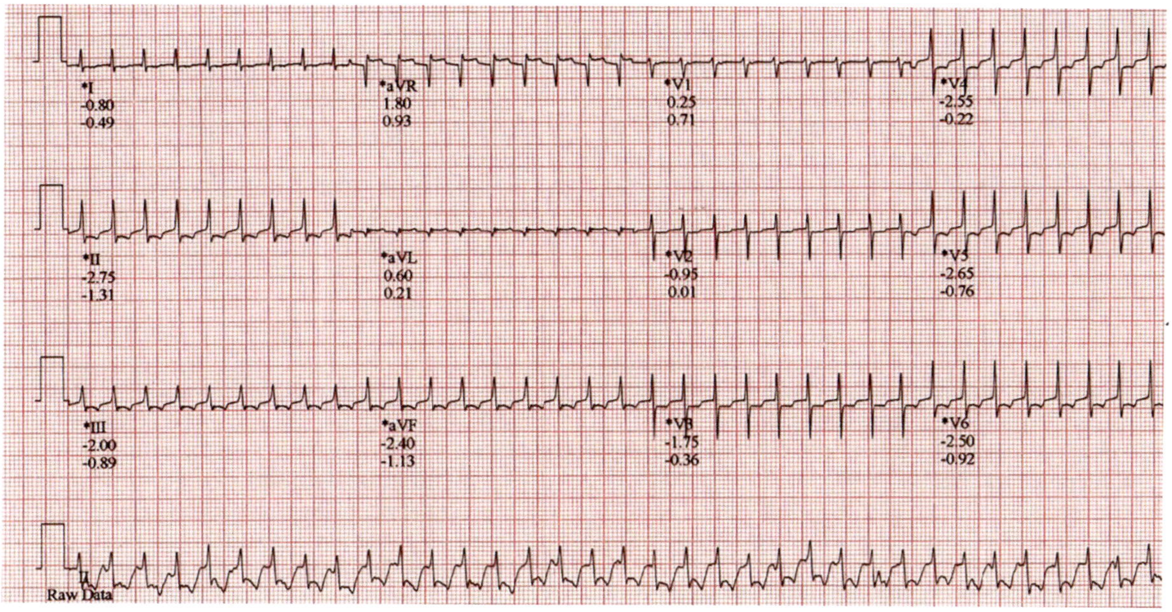

Fig. 26.7: Exercise tolerance test (ETT) tracing of a patient who developed narrow complex tachycardia suggestive of supraventricular tachycardia (SVT) at Bruce stage-2. Supraventricular arrhythmias are not diagnostic of coronary artery disease (CAD) and ETT becomes equivocal. (*Source*: Dr Fahmida Zaman, Labaid Cardiac Hospital)

exercise, and as a result, other forms of exercise test for example, adenosine or dobutamine scintigraphy, stress echocardiography, single photon emission computed tomography (SPECT) or CT coronary angiogram or conventional coronary angiography are required to evaluate this group of patients.

SUMMARY

Exercise tolerance test is the most commonly used noninvasive method to evaluate for CAD in men and women.

The Bruce protocol is the most widely adopted protocol but a modified Bruce protocol is used for exercise testing in case of elderly patients and also after recent myocardial infarction. The protocol has seven stages, each lasting 3 minutes, resulting in 21 minutes' exercise for a complete test. In stage 1, the patient walks at 1.7 miles (2.7 km) per hour (mph) up a 10% incline. The speed and incline increase with each stage (Table 26.1).

ST-segment depression (horizontal or downsloping) is the most reliable indicator of exercise-induced ischemia. ST depression observed during ETT should be at least 1 mm or more, observed in at least three consecutive beats, and observed in at least two contiguous leads. Upsloping ST-segment depression is usually not accepted as a standard sign of ischemia. ST-segment depression suggesting ischemia must be either horizontal or downsloping.

For ST-segment changes to be significant, they need not to be solely observed during exercise. The occurrence of ST-segment depression during the recovery period only, does not represent a "false-positive" response. The inclusion of findings from this period increases the diagnostic yield of the exercise test. The diagnostic and prognostic value of recovery-limited ST depression is similar to ST-segment depression during the active phase of exercise ECG stress testing and should, therefore, be interpreted as a positive test.

ST-segment elevation observed during ETT is less frequent than ST-segment depression but these changes are significant. ST elevation during ETT generally denotes to ischemia in the related segments of the myocardium, e.g. ST elevation in anterior leads suggest myocardial ischemia in anterior wall and ST elevation in inferior leads suggest ischemia in the inferior or posterior myocardium. By contrast, observation of ST segment depression during ETT is not related to any specific myocardial territory.

Left ventricular hypertrophy, LBBB, and WPW syndrome, digoxin administration, mitral valve prolapse, hypokalemia, pectus excavatum, mitral or aortic valvular lesions, pulmonary hypertension, pericardial constriction, hypertrophic cardiomyopathy, etc., can lead to false-positive ETT.

Beta-blockers, diltiazem, verapamil, and nitrate group of drugs may produce false-negative ETT.

The appearance of ventricular arrhythmias in response to exercise in asymptomatic subjects has no diagnostic or prognostic value. When they are found in association with known CAD or with other markers of ischemia, such as ST depression or anginal-type chest discomfort, they generally predict high incidence of subsequent cardiac events.

REFERENCES

1. Sharma K, Kohli P, Gulati M. An update on exercise stress testing. Curr Probl Cardiol. 2012;37(5):177-202.
2. Rahimi K, Thomas A, Adam M, et al. Implications of exercise test modality on modern prognostic markers in patients with known or suspected coronary artery disease: Treadmill versus bicycle. Eur J Cardiovasc Prev Rehabil. 2006;13(1):45-50.
3. Lauer MS. Exercise electrocardiogram testing and prognosis. Novel markers andpredictive instruments. Cardiol Clin. 2001;19(3):401-14.
4. Jalisi F. Evaluation of pretest and exercise test scores to assess all-cause mortality in unselected patients presenting for exercise testing with symptoms of suspected coronary artery disease. J Am Coll Cardiol. 2003;42(5):842-50.
5. Hill J, Timmis A. ABC of clinical electrocardiography. Exercise tolerance testing. BMJ. 2002;324(7345):1084-7.
6. Tavel ME. Stress Testing in Cardiac Evaluation: Current concepts with mphasis on the ECG. Chest. 2001;119(3): 907-25.
7. Rijneke AD, Ascoop CA, Talmon JL. Clinical significance of upsloping ST segments in exercise electrocardiography. Circulation. 1980;61(4):671-8.
8. McHenry PL, Fisch C. Clinical applications of the treadmill exercise test. Mod Concepts Cardiovasc Dis. 1977;46(5): 21-5.
9. Stuart RJ, Ellestad MH. Upsloping ST segments in exercise testing. Am J Cardiol. 1976;37(1):19-22.
10. Greenberg PS, Friscia DA, Ellestad MH. Predictive accuracy of Q-X/Q-T ratio, Q-Tc interval, S-T depression and R wave amplitude during stress testing. Am J Cardiol. 1979;44(1): 18-23.
11. Sansoy V, Watson DD, Beller GA. Significance of slow upsloping ST-segment depression on exercise stress testing. Am J Cardiol. 1997;79(6):709-12.
12. Sheffield LT. Upsloping ST segments: Easy to measure, hard to agree upon. Circulation. 1991;84(1):426-8.
13. Longhurst JC, Kraus WL. Exercise-induced ST elevation in patients without myocardial infarction. Circulation. 1979;60(3):616-29.
14. Galik DM, Mahmarian JJ, Verani MS. Therapeutic significance of exercise-induced ST-segment elevation in patients without previous myocardial infarction. Am J Cardiol. 1993;72(1):1-7.
15. Lahiri A, Balasubramanian V, Millar CMW, et al. Exercise-induced ST segment elevation: Electrocardiographic, angiographic, and scintigraphic evaluation. Br Heart J. 1980;43(5):582-8.
16. Waters DD, Chaitman BR, Bourassa MG, et al. Clinical and angiographic correlates of exercise-induced ST-segment elevation: Increased detection with multiple ECG leads. Circulation. 1980;61(2):286-96.
17. Stiles GL, Rosati RA, Wallace AG. Clinical relevance of exercise-induced S-T segment elevation. Am J Cardiol. 1980;46(6):931-6.
18. Halon DA, Mevorach D, Rodeanu M, et al. Improved criteria for localization of coronary artery disease from the exercise electrocardiogram. Noninvasive Cardiol. 1994;84(4-5):331-8.
19. Chaitman BR, Waters DD, Theroux P, et al. ST segment elevation and coronary spasm in response to exercise. Am J Cardiol. 1981;47(6):1350-8.
20. Ho JL, Lin LC, Yen RF, et al. Significance of dobutamine-induced ST-segment elevation and T-wave pseudonormalization in patients with Q-wave myocardial infarction: Simultaneous evaluation by dobutamine stress echocardiography and thallium-201 SPECT. Am J Cardiol. 1999;84:125-9.
21. Margonato A, Ballarotto C, Bonetti F, et al. Assessment of residual tissue viability by exercise testing in recent myocardial infarction: Comparison of the electrocardiogram and myocardial perfusion scintigraphy. J Am Coll Cardiol. 1992;19:948-52.
22. Ricci R, Bigi R, Galati A, et al. Dobutamine-induced ST-segment elevation in patients with acute myocardial infarction and the role of myocardial ischemia, viability, and ventricular dyssynergy. Am J Cardiol. 1997;79(6):733-73.
23. Dunn RF, Bailey IK, Uren R, et al. Exercise-induced ST-segment elevation: Correlation of thallium-201 myocardial perfusion scanning and coronary arteriography. Circulation 1980;61(5):989-95.
24. Lachterman B, Lehmann KG, Abrahamson D, et al. 'Recovery only' ST-segment depression and the predictive accuracy of the exercise test. Ann Intern Med. 1990;112(1):11-6.
25. Weizman AV, Chow CM. Does recovery-limited ST segment depression during exercise ECG stress testing confer the same prognosis as that occurring during exercise? A case and a review of the literature. J Insur Med. 2009;41(1):72-6.
26. Lanza GA, Mustilli M, Sestito A, et al. Diagnostic and prognostic value of ST segment depression limited to the recovery phase of exercise stress test. Heart 2004;90(12): 1417-21.
27. Rashid MA, Mallick NH, Alam SN, et al. Usefulness of ST segment depression limited to the recovery phase of exercise stress test. J Coll Physicians Surg Pak. 2009;19(1):3-6.
28. Weiner DA, McCabe CH, Cutler SS, et al. Decrease in systolic blood pressure during exercise testing: Reproducibility, response to coronary bypass surgery and prognostic significance. Am J Cardiol. 1982;49(7):1627-31.
29. Sanmarco ME, Pontius S, Selvester RH. Abnormal blood pressure response and marked ischemic ST-segment depression as predictors of severe coronary artery disease. Circulation. 1980;61(3):572-8.
30. Lele SS, Scalia G, Thomson H, et al. Mechanism of exercise hypotension in patients with ischemic heart disease. Circulation. 1994;90(6):2701-9
31. Feil H, Brofman BL. The effect of exercise on the electrocardiogram of bundle branch block. Am Heart J. 1953;45(5):665-9.
32. Gazes PC. False-positive exercise test in the presence of the Wolff-Parkinson-White syndrome. Am Heart J. 1969;78(1):13-5.
33. Strasberg B, Ashley WW, Wyndham CR, et al. Treadmill exercise testing in the Wolff-Parkinson-White syndrome. Am J Cardiol. 1980;45(4):742-8.
34. Sketch MH, Mooss AN, Butler ML, et al. Digoxin-induced positive exercise tests: Their clinical and prognostic significance. Am J Cardiol. 1981;48(4):655-9.
35. Soloff LA, Fewell JW. Abnormal electrocardiographic responses in exercise in subjects with hypokalemia. Am J Med Sci. 1961;242(12):724-8.
36. Gardin JM, Isner JM, Ronan JA, Jr, et al. Pseudoischemic 'false positive' S-T segment changes induced by hyperventilation

in patients with mitral valve prolapse. Am J Cardiol. 1980;45:952-8.
37. Kattus AA. Exercise electrocardiography: Recognition of the ischemic response, false positive and negative patterns. Am J Cardiol. 1974;33(6):721-31.
38. Harris CN, Aronow WS, Parker DP, et al. Treadmill stress test in left ventricular hypertrophy. Chest. 1973;63(3):353-7.
39. Smith RH, LePetri B, Moisa RB, et al. Association of increased left ventricular mass in the absence of electrocardiographic left ventricular hypertrophy with ST depression during exercise. Am J Cardiol. 1995;76(12):973-4.
40. Hellerstein HK, Prozan GB, Leibow IM, et al. The two-step exercise test as a test of cardiac function in chronic rheumatic heart disease and in arteriosclerotic heart disease with old myocardial infarction. Am J Cardiol. 1961;7(2):234-52.
41. Mattingly TW. The postexercise electrocardiogram: Its value in the diagnosis and prognosis of coronary arterial disease. Am J Cardiol. 1962;9(3):395-409.
42. Roitman D, Jones WB, Sheffield LT. Comparison of submaximal exercise ECG test with coronary cine angiocardiogram. Ann Intern Med. 1970;72(5):641-7.
43. Hogg D, Metcalfe M. The accuracy of non-invasive methods for the detection of obstructive coronary artery disease in the presence of left ventricular hypertrophy. J Hum Hypertens. 2000;14(5):295-8.
44. Tanaka T, Friedman MJ, Okada RD, et al. Diagnostic value of exercise-induced ST segment depression in patients with right bundle branch block. Am J Cardiol. 1978;41(4):670-3.
45. Gianelli RD, Treister BL, Harrison DC. The effect of propranolol on exercise induced ischemic S-T depression. Am J Cardiol. 1969;24(2):161-5.
46. Goldstein RF, Rosing DR, Redwood DR, et al. Clinical and circulatory effects of isosorbide dinitrate: Comparison with nitroglycerin. Circulation. 1971;43(5):629-40.
47. Froelicher VF, Thomas MM, Pillow C, et al. Epidemiologic study of asymptomatic men screened by maximal treadmill testing for latent coronary artery disease. Am J Cardiol. 1974;34(7):770-6.
48. Busby MJ, Shefrin EA, Fleg JL. Prevalence and long-term significance of exercise-induced frequent or repetitive ventricular ectopic beats in apparently healthy volunteers. J Am Coll Cardiol. 1989;14(7):1659-65.
49. Jelinek MV, Lown B. Exercise stress testing for exposure of cardiac arrhythmia. Prog Cardiovasc Dis. 1974;16(5): 497-522.
50. McHenry PL, Morris SN, Kavalier M, et al. Comparative study of exercise-induced ventricular arrhythmias in normal subjects and patients with documented coronary artery disease. Am J Cardiol. 1976;37(4):609-16.
51. Goldschlager N, Cake D, Cohn K. Exercise-induced ventricular arrhythmias in patients with coronary artery disease: Their relationship to angiographic findings. Am J Cardiol. 1973;31(4):434-40.
52. Udall JA, Ellestad MH. Predictive implications of ventricular premature contractions associated with treadmill stress testing. Circulation. 1977;56(6):985-9.
53. Gerson MC, Phillips JF, Morris SN, et al. Exercise-induced U-wave inversion as a marker of stenosis of the left anterior descending coronary artery. Circulation. 1979;60(5):1014-20.
54. Jain A, Jenkins MG, Gettes LS. Lack of specificity of negative U wave for anterior myocardial ischemia as evidenced by intracoronary electrogram during balloon angioplasty. J Am Coll Cardiol. 1990;15(5):1007-11.
55. Chikamori T, Yamada M, Takata J, et al. Exercise-induced prominent U waves as a marker of significant narrowing of the left circumflex or right coronary artery. Am J Cardiol. 1994;74(5):495-9.
56. Chikamori T, Takata J, Furuno, T et al. Usefulness of U-wave analysis in detecting significant narrowing limited to a single coronary artery. Am J Cardiol. 1995;75(3):508-11
57. Rhee MY, Choi RK, Kim IS, et al. Diagnostic significance of pseudonormalization during treadmill exercise test in ischemic heart disease. Korean Circ J. 1995;25(1):5-10.
58. Lavie CJ, Oh JK, Mankin HT, et al. Significance of T-wave pseudonormalization during exercise-A radionuclide angiographic study. Chest. 1988;94(3):512-6.

Chapter 27

Ambulatory Electrocardiogram Monitoring (Holter Monitoring)

INTRODUCTION

Ambulatory electrocardiogram (ECG) recording was developed to allow home ECG monitoring of patients with suspected cardiac arrhythmias. Norman J Holter (1914–1983) was an American biophysicist who invented the Holter monitor, a portable device for continuously monitoring the electrical activity of the heart for 24 hours or more. Norman J Holter introduced this method of monitoring in the 1940s. The original Holter monitor was a 75-lb backpack with a reel-to-reel frequency modulation (FM) tape recorder, analog patient interface electronics, and large batteries.[1-3]

ARRHYTHMIA AND AMBULATORY ELECTROCARDIOGRAM MONITORING

Traditionally, ambulatory monitoring has been used to determine the cause of palpitations and syncope and, to a lesser degree, to identify ventricular ectopy or ventricular tachycardia in patients at potential risk for sudden cardiac death (Figs. 27.1A and B).[4] Atrial fibrillation (AF) has become an increasingly important indication for ambulatory monitoring, predominantly as a tool to monitor the efficacy and safety of pharmacological and nonpharmacological therapies (Box 27.1).[5,6] It is also used to identify asymptomatic AF as a potential source of cryptogenic stroke (Fig. 27.2).[7,8]

CONTINUOUS MONITORS (HOLTER TECHNOLOGY)

The current state of Holter technology uses smaller recorders with flashcard technology to record and store data from 2 to 3 ECG leads attached to the patient's chest and collected continuously over 24–48 hours. Once the monitor is returned, the data are analyzed in digital format. To increase the correlation between detected heart rhythm abnormalities and symptoms, patients are asked to keep a diary of their symptoms. The recorders use patient-activated event markers (annotations) specified for the time of day.

Box 27.1: Indications of Holter monitoring.

The main indications for Holter monitoring include detection and characterization of arrhythmias to:

- Attempt to correlate a possible arrhythmia with symptoms: palpitations; syncope, near syncope or episodic dizziness; and/or other cardiac symptoms (e.g. shortness of breath, chest pain, episodic fatigue, or diaphoresis).
- Determine the risk of the arrhythmia in the individual clinical setting.
- Detect, assess, and manage atrial fibrillation.
- Monitor the efficacy of antiarrhythmic drug therapy.

Special Populations

Patients with conditions that may require documentation of an arrhythmia include:

- Structural heart diseases, e.g. postmyocardial infarction (MI), dilated or hypertrophic cardiomyopathy, valvular heart disease.
- Primary electrical heart diseases [e.g. sick sinus syndrome, high-grade atrioventricular (AV) block, Wolff–Parkinson–White (WPW) syndrome].
- Family history of sudden death or arrhythmia.

The major advantages of Holter monitoring are the ability to continuously record ECG data and the lack of need for patient participation in the transmission of data. The short duration of monitoring can be inadequate if symptoms are infrequent. Newer Holter monitors are now available with up to 2 weeks of recording capability. Limitations of Holter monitoring include frequent noncompliance with keeping a log of symptoms and using event markers, which significantly limits the diagnostic value of these devices.[9]

In the vast majority of circumstances, ambulatory monitors are used to identify a direct correlation between symptoms and the presence or absence of an arrhythmia (Box 27.2). The optimal duration of monitoring largely depends on symptom frequency. In the evaluation of palpitations, patients who experience daily symptoms can be evaluated with a Holter monitor. More often, palpitations are sporadic and

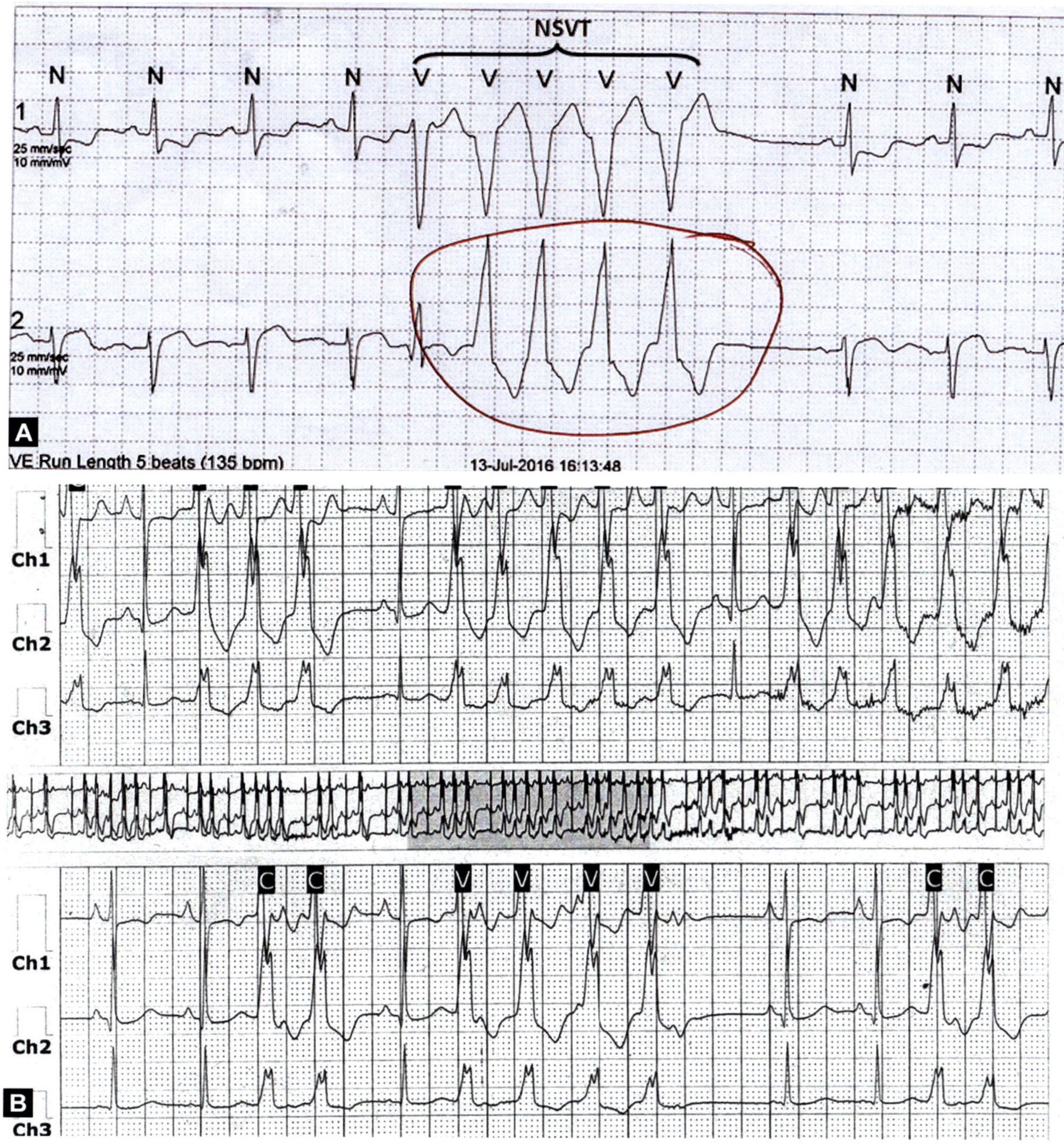

Figs. 27.1A and B: (A) Holter monitor electrocardiogram (ECG) strip shows nonsustained ventricular tachycardia (NSVT) 5 beats. (B) A 17-year old girl presented with recurrent episodes of loss of consciousness. Holter monitoring showed multiple episodes of nonsustained ventricular tachycardia (VT). This patient underwent VT ablation.

Box 27.2: Diagnostic value of Holter monitoring.

- The key to the diagnostic value of ambulatory electrocardiogram (ECG) monitoring is the correlation between symptoms and the timing of the arrhythmia.
- If no symptoms are present but an arrhythmia documented, there is likely an asymptomatic arrhythmia.
- If symptoms are present but no arrhythmia documented, an arrhythmia can likely be excluded as the mechanism.
- If no symptoms are present during the monitoring period and no arrhythmia documented, the test is considered nondiagnostic to the symptoms.

longer monitoring is required for proper diagnosis. Syncope typically requires a significantly longer monitoring period and the diagnostic yield of ambulatory monitors of any sort is extremely limited.[10] Diagnosis of the cause of palpitation and the syncope are the two most common indications of Holter monitoring. Ambulatory ECG monitoring is also frequently used to exclude the diagnosis of atrioventricular (AV) block (Fig. 27.3) and sick sinus syndrome (Fig. 27.4).

The identification of AF is also one of the most common indications for monitoring in which the documentation of asymptomatic rhythms is desired. Clinicians routinely monitor patients on antiarrhythmic drugs or after catheter

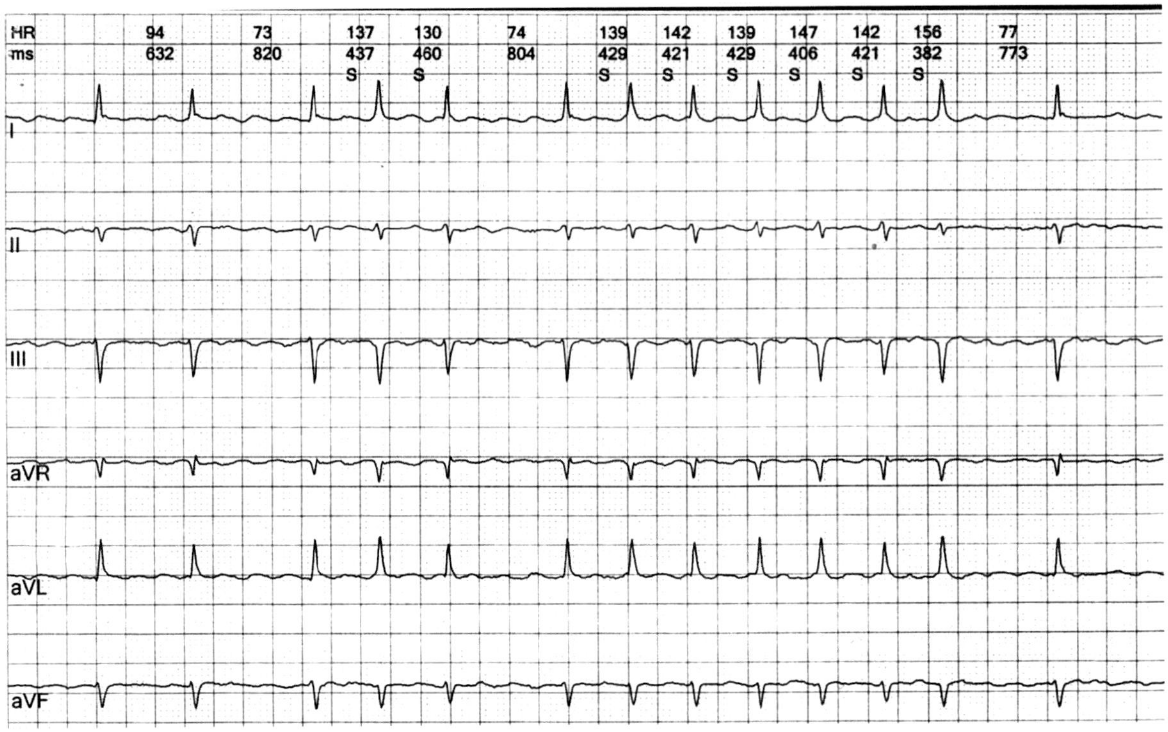

Fig. 27.2: A 60-year-old man was admitted in a hospital with stroke. His bedside ECG was unremarkable and the rhythm was sinus. Holter monitoring revealed recurrent episodes of AF.

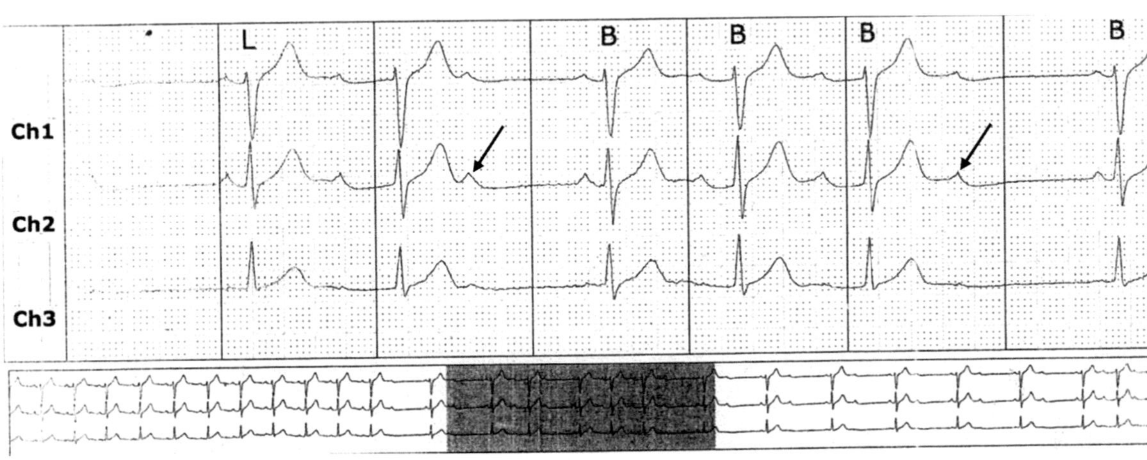

Fig. 27.3: A 70-year-old man presented with recurrent episodes of syncope. His bedside ECG was unremarkable except sinus bradycardia. His Holter monitoring showed recurrent episodes of second degree heart block. This ECG strip shows typical features of Wenckebach phenomenon with gradual prolongation of PR interval with intermittent nonconducted P waves (*arrows*). The patient underwent permanent pacemaker implantation following electrophysiological study.

or surgical AF procedures for arrhythmia recurrence. These recurrences are often asymptomatic, even in previously symptomatic patients, and may not be detected unless an aggressive monitoring strategy is undertaken. In addition, patients with cryptogenic stroke often undergo rhythm monitoring to identify asymptomatic AF as a potential cause (Fig. 27.5).[11,12]

Holter monitoring may be used to assess the potential risk of developing an arrhythmia—for example, patients prior to discharge from hospital after a myocardial infarction (Figs. 27.6A and B), patients with congestive heart failure (Figs. 27.7A and B), and patients with hypertrophic cardiomyopathy (Figs. 27.8A and B). Holter monitoring may be used to assess a patient's response to antiarrhythmic treatment—e.g. the rate of AF, or proarrhythmic responses to drugs. This monitoring may also be used to assess the function of a pacemaker device or implantable cardioversion device. Holter

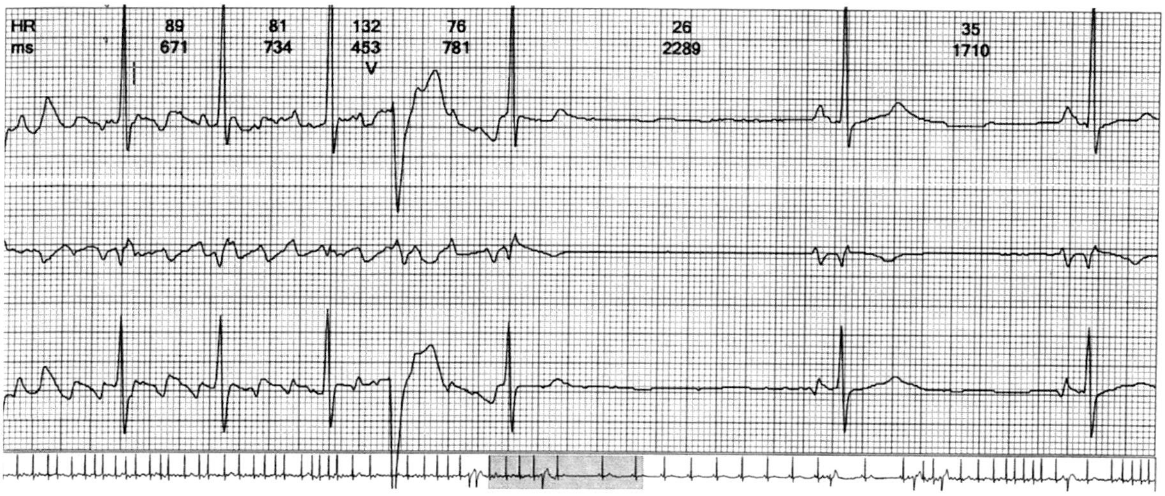

Fig. 27.4: A 79-year-old man presented with complaints of recurrent episodes of loss of consciousness. His bedside ECG showed marked sinus bradycardia. His Holter monitoring showed recurrent episodes of paroxysmal AF with prolonged pauses, suggestive of sick sinus syndrome. This patient underwent permanent pacemaker implantation and became asymptomatic.

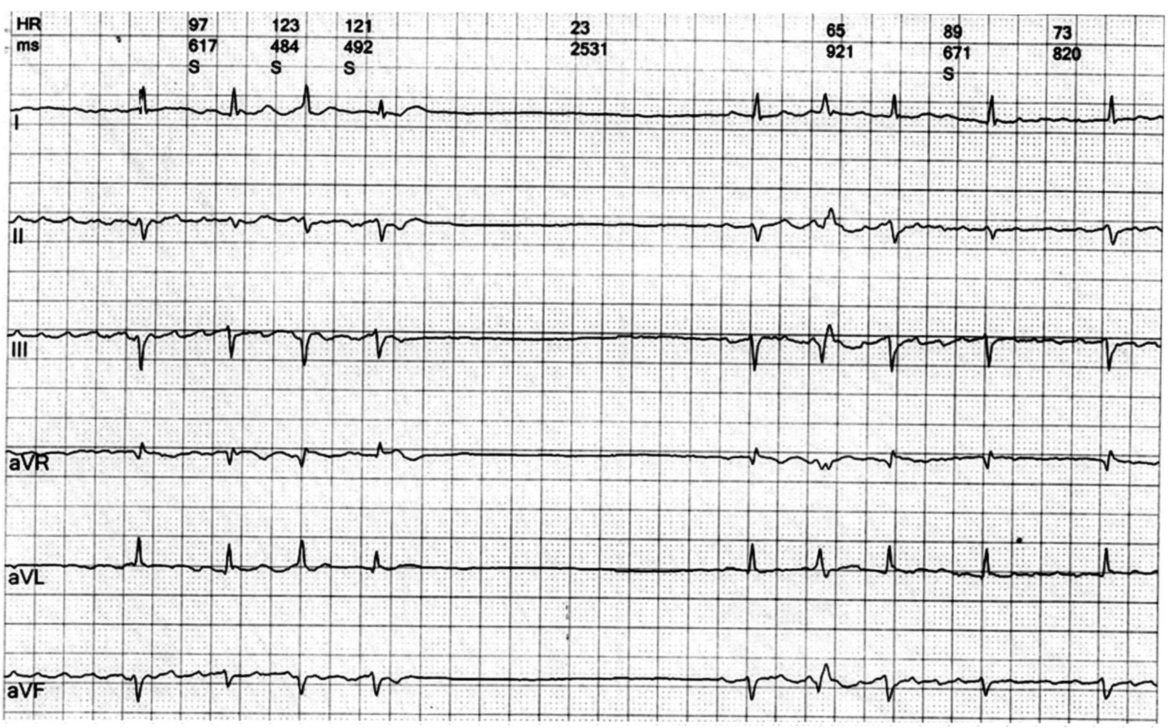

Fig. 27.5: A 80-year-old man was admitted in hospital with stroke. His bedside ECG findings were unremarkable. His Holter monitoring showed paroxysmal AF with prolonged pauses.

monitoring may also be used as a tool for the detection of myocardial ischemia, by measurement of ST segment shifts particularly in patients with suspected variant angina.[13,14]

In some circumstances, the duration of a Holter monitoring can be extended. However, the diagnostic yield of an extended time or repeat test is low. Holter monitoring is only suitable for patients with symptoms occurring within the monitoring period. If prolonged monitoring is required then event recorders, external loop recorders, and implantable loop recorders may be used.[15-20]

SUMMARY

Ambulatory ECG monitoring (Holter monitoring) is used to detect, characterize, and document cardiac arrhythmias in clinical practice. As some arrhythmias are infrequent or may occur only during certain activities (e.g. sleep or

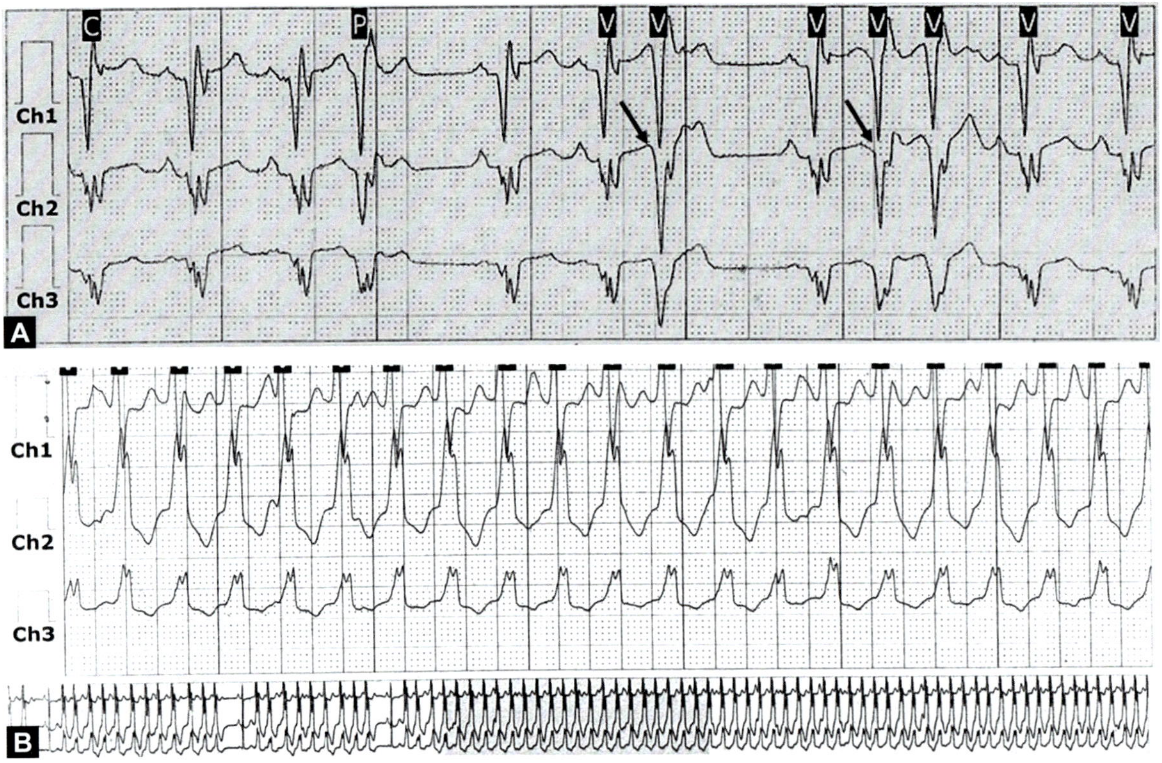

Figs. 27.6A and B: (A) Holter monitoring strip shows R on T phenomenon (*arrow*) in a patient with history of recent STEMI. (B) Holter monitoring strip illustrates an episode of nonsustained VT in a patient with history of recent STEMI. This patient subsequently underwent implantable cardioverter-defibrillator (ICD) implantation for the prevention of sudden cardiac death (SCD).

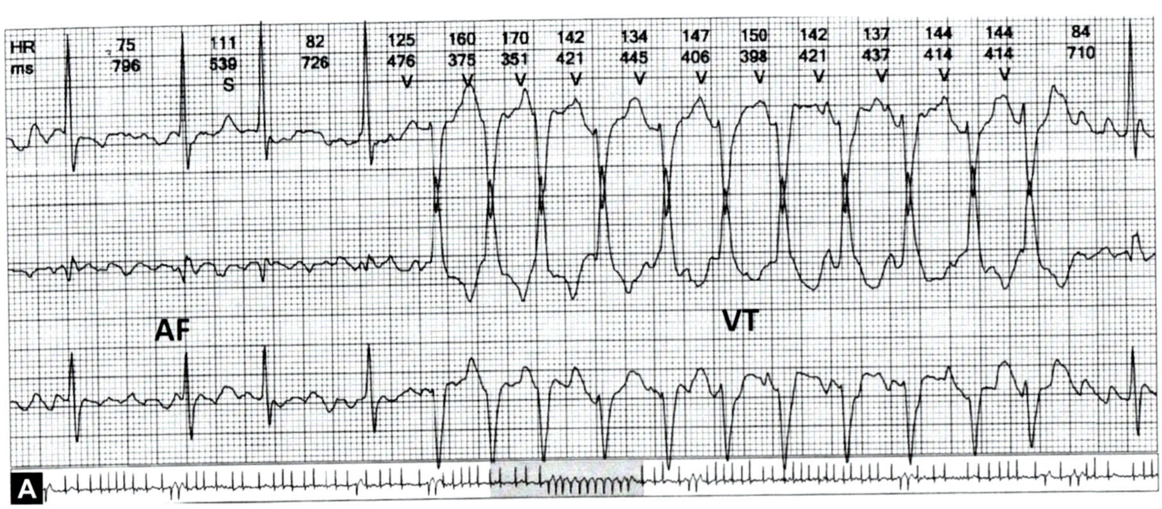

Fig. 27.7A: Holter monitoring strip illustrates episodes of paroxysmal AF (left side) and nonsustained VT (right side) in a patient with congestive heart failure. This patient underwent implantable cardioverter-defibrillator (ICD) implantation for the prevention of sudden cardiac death (SCD).

exercise), it is usual to record the electrical activity of the heart over a period of time, usually 24 hours or 48 hours.

The choice of a monitoring modality depends on the presenting symptom, symptom frequency, and degree of suspicion of a life-threatening arrhythmia. A number of considerations are useful to guide the selection of these devices.

Indications for Holter Monitoring

Holter monitoring is indicated for proper diagnosis of patients with syncope, near syncope or dizziness, patients with palpitations and patients who have had a cerebrovascular accident in whom paroxysmal AF or atrial flutter is suspected.

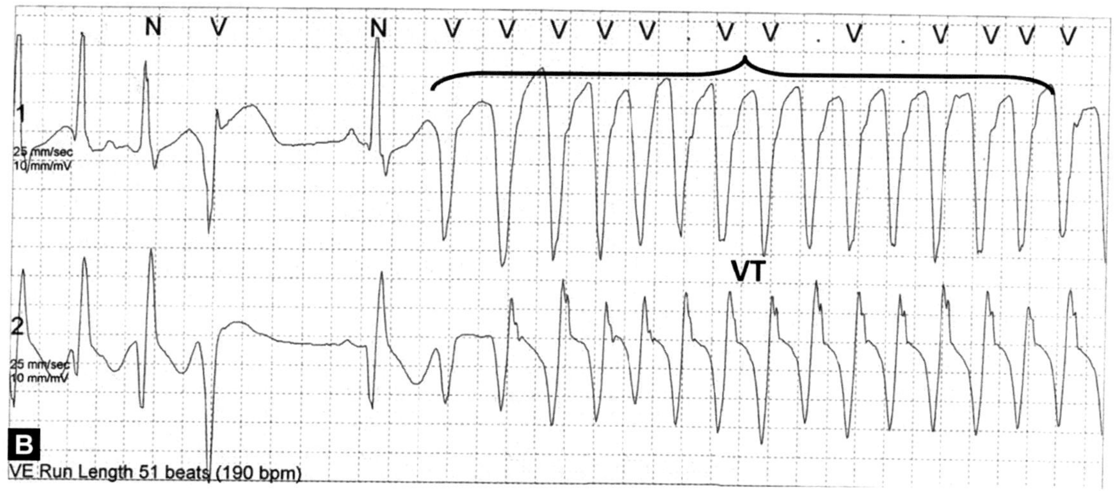

Fig. 27.7B: (B) Holter monitoring strip illustrates an episode of nonsustained VT (right side) in a patient with congestive heart failure. This patient underwent implantable cardioverter-defibrillator (ICD) implantation for the prevention of sudden cardiac death (SCD).

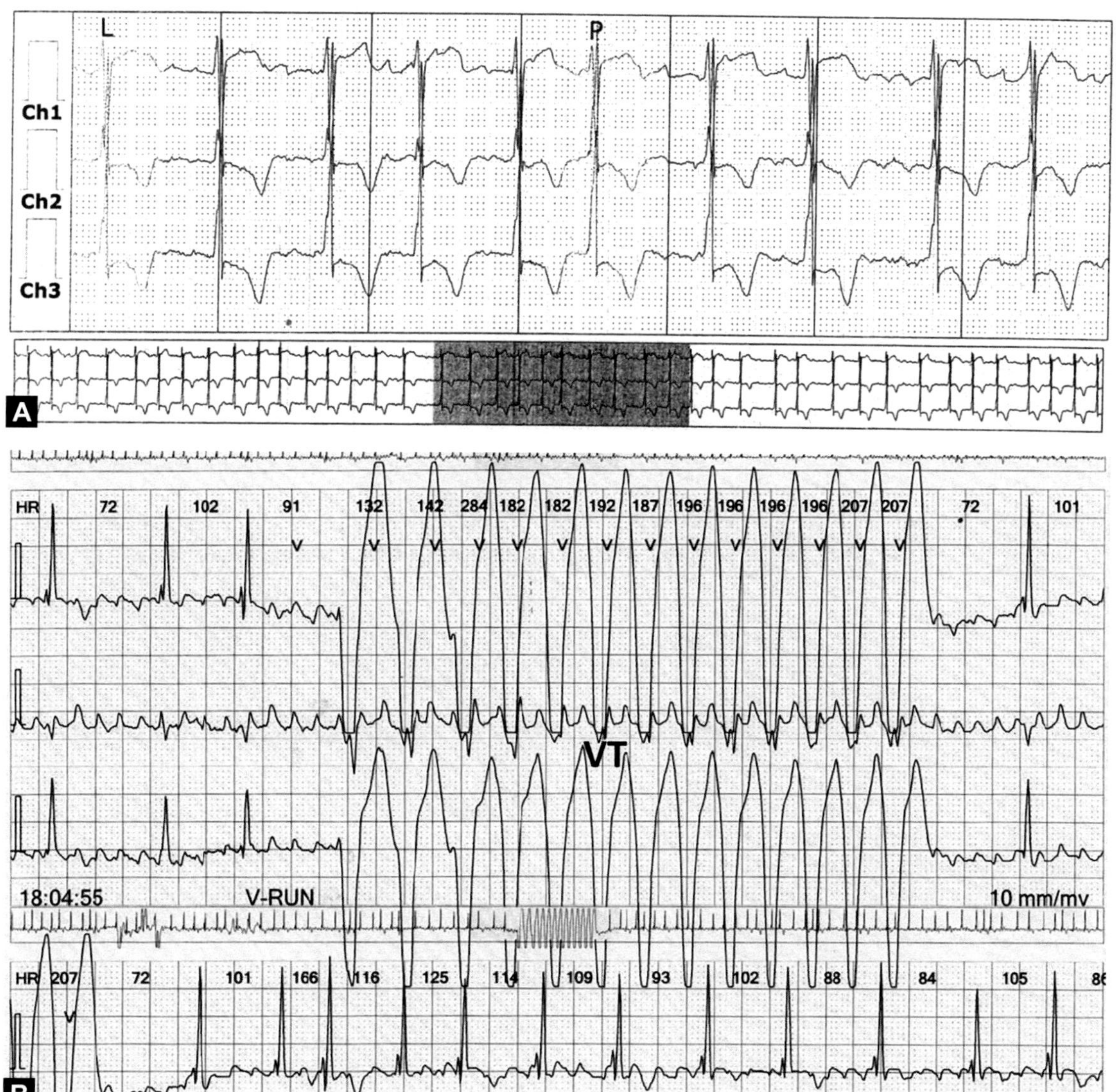

Figs. 27.8A and B: (A) A patient known to have hypertrophic cardiomyopathy (HCM) presented with complaints of recurrent episodes of palpitation. His bedside ECG showed features of HCM but rhythm was sinus. His Holter monitoring confirmed the diagnosis of paroxysmal AF. (B) A known case of apical cardiomyopathy with permanent AF presented with complaints of recurrent episodes of syncope. His bedside ECG showed features of HCM with AF. His Holter monitoring confirmed the diagnosis of recurrent nonsustained VT on the background of AF.

Ambulatory ECG monitoring is also frequently used to exclude the diagnosis of high-grade AV block and sick sinus syndrome.

Holter monitoring is useful to detect silent paroxysmal AF in patients without previously documented arrhythmic episodes, such as those with cryptogenic stroke.

REFERENCES

1. Holter NJ. New method for heart studies: continuous electrocardiography of active subjects over long periods is now practical. Science. 1961;134(3486):1214-20.
2. Buckles D, Aguel F, Brockman R, et al. Advances in ambulatory monitoring: regulatory considerations. J Electrocardiol. 2004;37(Suppl.):65-7.
3. Gawlowska J, Wranicz JK, Norman J. "Jeff" Holter (1914–1983). Cardiol J. 2009;16:386-7.
4. Zimetbaum P, Josephson ME. The evolving role of ambulatory arrhythmia monitoring in general clinical practice. Ann Intern Med. 1999;130:848-56.
5. Vasamreddy CR, Dalal D, Dong J, et al. Symptomatic and asymptomatic atrial fibrillation in patients undergoing radiofrequency catheter ablation. J Cardiovasc Electrophysiol. 2006;17:134-9.
6. Hauser TH, Pinto DS, Josephson ME, et al. Safety and feasibility of a clinical pathway for the outpatient initiation of antiarrhythmic medications in patients with atrial fibrillation or atrial flutter. Am J Cardiol. 2003;91:1437-41.
7. Douen A, Pageau N, Medic S. Usefulness of cardiovascular investigation in stroke management: Clinical relevance and economic implications. Stroke. 2007;38:1956-8.
8. Liao J, Khalid Z, Scallan C, et al. Noninvasive cardiac monitoring for detecting paroxysmal atrial fibrillation or flutter after acute ischemic stroke: a systematic review. Stroke. 2007;38:2935-40.
9. Zimetbaum P, Goldman A. Ambulatory arrhythmia monitoring: Choosing the right device. Circulation. 2010;122:1629-36.
10. DiMarco JP, Philbrick JT. Use of ambulatory electrocardiographic (Holter) monitoring. Ann Intern Med. 1990;113:53-68.
11. Hanke T, Charitros E, Stierle U, et al. Twenty-four hour Holter monitor follow-up does not provide accurate heart rhythm status after surgical atrial fibrillation therapy: up to 12 months experience with a novel permanently implantable heart rhythm monitor device. Circulation. 2009;120(Suppl.):S177-84.
12. Pontoppidan J, Nielsen JC, Poulsen SH, et al. Symptomatic and asymptomatic atrial fibrillation after pulmonary vein ablation and the impact on quality of life. Pacing Clin Electrophysiol. 2009;32:717-26.
13. Crawford MH, Bernstein SJ, Deedwania PC, et al. ACC/AHA Guidelines for ambulatory electrocardiography. A report of the American College of Cardiology/American Heart Association Task Force on Practice Guidelines (Committee to revise the guidelines for ambulatory electrocardiography). Developed in collaboration with the North American Society for Pacing and Electrophysiology. J Am Coll Cardiol. 1999;34(3):912-48.
14. Camm AJ, Corbucci G, Padeletti L. Usefulness of continuous electrocardiographic monitoring for atrial fibrillation. Am J Cardiol. 2012;110(2):270-6.
15. Arya A, Haghjoo M, Khosrawi A, et al. Predictors of arrhythmic events during second day monitoring in patients with normal first day Holter recordings. Indian Heart J. 2005;57(3):241-4.
16. Hoefman E, Bindels PJE, van Weert HCPM. Efficacy of diagnostic tools for detecting cardiac arrhythmias: systematic literature search. Neth Heart J. 2010;18(11):543-51.
17. Raviele A, Giadda F, Bergfeldt L, et al. Management of patients with palpitations: A position paper from the European Heart Rhythm Association. Europace. 2011;13:920-34.
18. Angaran P, Klein GJ, Yee R, et al. Syncope. Neurol Clin. 2011;29:903-25.
19. Edvardsson N, Frykman V, van Mechelen R, et al. Use of an implantable loop recorder to increase the diagnostic yield in unexplained syncope: Results from the picture registry. Europace. 2011;13:262-9.
20. Moya A, Sutton R, Ammirati F, et al. Guidelines for the diagnosis and management of syncope of the European Society of Cardiology (ESC). Eur Heart J. 2009;30:2631-71.

Index

Page numbers followed by *b* refer to box, *f* refer to figure, *fc* refer to flow chart, and *t* refer to table.

A

Abdominal process, acute 108
Accessory pathway
- concealed 328
- localization of 332
- location of 326*b*
- manifest 328
- types of 327*b*

Acetylcholine 317
Acidosis 31, 108, 317
Action potential shortens 398
Addison's disease 392
Adenovirus 375, 384
Ajmaline 309, 320
Alcohol 174, 181
- consumption, excessive 199

Aldosterone deficiency 392
Alkalosis 108
Ambulatory electrocardiogram 496
- monitoring 496

Ambulatory rhythm monitoring 453
American College of Cardiology 58
American Heart Association 5
Amiloride 392
Aminophylline 181
Amiodarone 30, 223, 286, 301, 304, 317, 321, 432, 433
Amitriptyline 31, 181, 313, 317, 321, 430
Amphetamines 181
Amyloidosis 304, 365
Andersen-Tawil syndrome 313, 321
Anemia 35, 78, 92, 98, 108, 491
Aneurysm, dissecting 484
Angina
- unstable 98, 99, 113, 484
- variant 111, 114

Anginal pain 98
Angioplasty, primary 98
Anomalous pulmonary venous connection 435
Antiarrhythmic drugs 223, 271, 312*f*, 432, 433
Antiarrhythmic medications 425
Antibacterials 223
Antibiotics 313, 321, 385
Antidepressant 313, 317, 321
- overdose 320

Antidromic atrioventricular reentrant tachycardia 335*f*
Antidromic supraventricular tachycardia 342
Antifungal drugs 313, 321
Antihistamines 313, 317, 321
Antihypertensive agents 271
Anti-inflammatory drugs, nonsteroidal 392
Antipsychotics 313, 317, 321
Anxiety 35
- and stress 174

Aorta, coarctation of 435, 450, 452*f*, 455
Aortic aneurysm, dissecting 320
Aortic coarctation 450
Aortic regurgitation 90
- chronic 78

Aortic stenosis 259, 267
- severe 484

Aortic valve
- annulus calcification 285
- insufficiency 491
- stenosis 435, 491

Aortic valvular
- disease 268
- lesions 493

Apical ballooning syndrome 368
Apical cardiomyopathy 351, 360*f*
Apical endocardial lead 466
Apical hypertrophic cardiomyopathy 351, 370
Arrhythmia 55, 98, 150, 168, 174, 183, 211, 322, 328, 342, 392, 394, 409, 426, 475, 496, 498
- complexity of 318
- development of malignant 59
- exercise-induced supraventricular 318
- frequency 170
- hallmark of 200*f*
- patterns of 322
- provocation 484
- related symptoms 312
- supraventricular 149, 150, 415, 418
- temporal pattern of 199
- treatment for 484

Arrhythmogenic right ventricular
- cardiomyopathy 92, 220, 309, 345, 365, 367*f*, 370
- dysplasia 238, 365, 367*f*, 370

Arterial occlusions, proximal 125
Arteriovenous shunts, peripheral 78, 92
Artery
- infarct-related 145, 161
- region, circumflex 487

Artifacts
- reduce movement 473
- shivering 420

Ashman aberrancy, typical 201
Ashman beats 204*f*
Ashman phenomenon 201, 204*f*
Astemizole 313, 317, 321
Atheroma 112
Athletes 286
Athletic training 301
Atrial abnormalities 84, 93
- left 73, 84, 93
- right 85, 93, 454

Atrial activity 14
- loss of 430
- recipient 416

Atrial arrhythmias 411
Atrial bigeminy 175*f*
Atrial complex
- characteristics of premature 192
- premature 172-174, 192, 192*b*, 193*t*, 193
- single premature 173*f*

Atrial component, right 88*f*-90*f*
Atrial depolarization wave 14
Atrial ectopic activity 409
Atrial enlargement 453
- left 72, 84, 85*f*, 88*f*, 93, 94, 349
- right 84, 85, 88*f*, 93, 94, 417, 479

Atrial extrasystoles 406
Atrial fibrillation 33, 174, 195, 197, 197, 203*f*, 213, 271, 281, 322, 325, 335, 337*f*, 360*f*, 387, 397, 411, 420, 435, 496
- causes of 197, 213*b*
  - cardiac 197
  - noncardiac 199

classification of 199, 213, 213*b*
fast 412*f*
lone 201, 213
mechanisms of 197
nonvalvular 213
slow 279*f*
typical 198*f*
Atrial flutter 195, 202, 207*f*, 213, 397, 406, 420, 435
atypical 202, 205*f*
classical 202
typical 202
waves 202
Atrial hypertrophy 84, 473
combined 473
Atrial impulse 282
Atrial infarct, diagnostic criteria for 157
Atrial infarction 149, 149*b*
clinical 149
depression in 149*f*
Atrial myocardium 425
Atrial overload 84
Atrial pacemaker 466
wandering 66
Atrial pacing 460, 460*f*, 469, 470
Atrial premature
beat 173, 415
complex 173, 418
Atrial pressure 196
Atrial rhythm, low 55
Atrial rupture 149
Atrial septal defect 80, 94, 267, 285, 435, 440*b*, 454
crochetage sign in 454
diagnosis of 435
ostium primum 454
ostium secundum 454
sinus venosus 454
types of 435, 437
Atrial spikes, electrocardiogram displays 464*f*, 465*f*
Atrial strain 84
Atrial tachyarrhythmias 453
Atrial tachycardia 206, 208, 211, 212*f*, 215, 397, 433
multifocal 66, 195, 196, 197*f*, 213, 406
Atrioventricular block 150, 282, 286, 292*t*, 293, 304, 313, 387, 475
diagnosis of 497
first degree 282, 482
in athletes 293
in children, high grade 478
Mobitz I 286
second-degree 285, 303
Mobitz II 286
second-degree 286, 304
second-degree 282, 285, 286
third-degree 282, 294, 304
types of 303*b*
Atrioventricular conduction, variable 207*f*
Atrioventricular dissociation 230
Atrioventricular junction 217
Atrioventricular nodal re-entrant tachycardia 195, 207, 208, 209*f*, 210, 214, 214*b*, 214*t*, 331, 342
types of 208
Atrioventricular node 2*f*, 3, 14, 195, 242, 282, 325
part of 338
Atrioventricular reentrant tachycardia 195, 206, 209, 210, 211*f*, 212*f*, 214, 214*t*, 328, 332*f*, 333*f*, 334*f*, 342
antidromic 214
orthodromic 214
Atrium
left 453
right 2, 279, 460
Autism spectrum disorders 313
Autoimmune diseases 286, 304, 385
Autoimmune pericarditis 375
Autonomic dysfunction 281
Axillary line
anterior 5
posterior 8
Axis deviation 58
Azithromycin 313, 317, 321, 432, 433

B

Bacterial infection 382
Bacterial pericarditis, cause of 375
Bayesian algorithm 237
Bayesian approach 236
Bazett's formula 28, 32*f*, 36, 315
Beta-adrenergic
antagonists 430
blockers 271
Beta-agonists 174
Beta-blocker 281, 286, 301, 304, 317, 318, 425, 430, 433
therapy 317
Biatrial abnormality 85
Biatrial enlargement 85, 94
Bicuspid aortic valve 450
Bifascicular block 243, 259, 260*f*, 261*f*, 262*f*, 268
causes of 268
Binge drinking 199
Bipolar lead 2
Bipolar limb leads, intersection of standard 2*f*
Blood pressure response 489
Body temperature, low 410*f*
Bradyarrhythmia 150, 433
severe 278*f*
Bradycardia 161, 223, 293*f*, 402, 453
causing 409
effects of longstanding 480
severe 413*f*
Breathing 188
Breathlessness 195
Bretylium 223
Broken heart syndrome 368, 371
Bronchospasm, acute 407
Bruce protocol 484
Brucella 384, 389
Brugada's algorithm 235, 235*fc*, 237
Brugada's criterion, ultra simple 237
Brugada's electrocardiogram
type 2 309*f*, 310*f*
types of 311*f*
Brugada's pattern 320, 430
electrocardiograms, types of 308
Brugada's population 309
Brugada's syndrome 138, 140, 153, 156, 227, 307, 308, 308*f*, 310, 312, 319, 320*b*, 321*b*, 420
arrhythmias in 320
diagnosis of 308, 312*b*
electrocardiogram 308*f*
diagnosis of 320*b*
type 1 307*f*, 308*f*, 309*f*
types of 311*f*
Brugada's sign 240, 307*f*, 312*f*
Bundle of His 4
Bundle of Kent 327
Bundle-branch block 98, 134, 217, 242, 387
basic principles 242
depolarization in 243*f*
diagnostic criteria of 267*b*
pattern 55, 101*f*
presence of 134
types of 243
Bundle-branch Purkinje system 295
Bundle-branch reentry 220
Bypass tract 325*f*

C

Cabrera's sign 137*f*, 466, 468
Cabrera's system 40
Caffeine 181
excess 174
Calcium
effect of 398
homeostasis 307
Calcium-channel blockers 271, 281, 286, 301, 304, 425
Camel hump 24
T waves 27*f*
Canadian Cardiovascular Society 488*f*
Capture beats 231
Cardiac abnormality 415
Cardiac activation, sequences of 4*fc*
Cardiac apex 126
Cardiac arrest 318, 322, 401
Cardiac arrhythmias 406, 496, 499
diagnosing 18
Cardiac axis 39
calculation of 40*f*
Cardiac causes 37, 181
Cardiac chamber
enlargement 68
hypertrophy 68
interaction 382

Cardiac channelopathy 307
diagnosis of 307
Cardiac conduction 432
system 294
Cardiac cycle 6
Cardiac diseases 307
Cardiac dysfunction 345
Cardiac electrical axis 39, 39*f*
Cardiac impulse 2
Cardiac inflammatory conditions 375, 390*b*
Cardiac ion channelopathy 312
Cardiac magnetic resonance imaging 85
Cardiac pacemaker cells 409
Cardiac resynchronization therapy 469, 471
Cardiac rhythm, respiratory variation of 56*f*
Cardiac skeleton, left side of 285
Cardiac surgery 176
after 286, 482
Cardiac tamponade 383, 384*f*, 390
Cardiac timing intervals 11
Cardiac trauma 113
Cardiomyopathy 37, 113, 181, 238, 267, 268, 280, 345, 369
diagnosis of 345
dilated 363*f*
dilated 44, 197, 238, 267, 345, 361, 370, 382, 460
hypertensive 345
ischemic 345
dilated 364*f*
normal and hypertrophic 346*f*
stress-induced 368
Cardiopulmonary
disease 196
resuscitation 415
Cardiotoxins 113
Cardiovascular complications, risks of 76
Cardiovascular disease 43, 213
Cardiovascular entities 345
Cardiovascular system 409, 420, 473
Cardioverter-defibrillator, implantable 355, 501*f*
Catastrophic bradycardias 431
Catecholamine 317
effect of 31
Catecholaminergic polymorphic ventricular tachycardia, diagnosis of 318, 322
Central nervous system 24, 409, 421
Cephalosporins 385
Cerebellar ataxia 415
Cerebellum 415
Cerebral T waves 313
Cerebrovascular accidents 108
acute 412
Cervical sympathetic denervation 318
Chagas disease 282, 386
Chamber enlargement 68
Chamber size 478
Chapman's sign 137, 137*f*
Chemotherapeutic agents 113
Chest
compressions 415
lead placement positions 6*f*
pain 113, 117, 188, 195, 387, 480
acute 98
attack of 111
recurrent 112*f*
severe central 490*f*
posterior 9*f*
Chloroquine 223, 317
Chlorpromazine 31
Ciprofloxacin 432
Cisapride 223, 317
Clarithromycin 31, 313, 317, 321, 432, 433
Clockwise rotation, causes of 44, 50
Clomipramine 317
Clozapine 317, 385
Cocaine 113, 181
Collagen vascular diseases 285
Compensatory pause
complete 174*f*
incomplete 175*f*
Concave morphology 120
Conduction abnormality 402
Conduction block 426
Conduction system
degenerative disease of 267, 285
normal 325
of heart, anatomy of 2*f*
Congenital abnormality 280
Congenital defect 455
Congenital syndrome 223
Congestive heart failure 197, 213, 382, 498, 500*f*
Connective tissue diseases 417
Consciousness, loss of 499*f*
Convex morphology 120
Cor pulmonale 42, 92, 244, 267
Cornell criteria, modified 87
Coronary angiogram 115
Coronary artery 377
disease 98, 115, 174, 197, 208, 213, 223, 268, 280, 282, 286, 368, 484, 485
absence of obstructive 368
diagnosis of 331
left anterior descending 104
left main 114
nonobstructive 112, 113*b*, 114
occlusion
left main 140
right 143
right 127, 145, 149, 487
spasm 139, 153
Coronary disease 268
Coronary syndrome, acute 20, 35, 68, 98, 113, 247, 404
Coronary vasospasm 115, 138, 139, 156
Coronary vein, posterolateral 469
Coronary venous system 469
Corynebacterium diphtheriae 384, 389
Counter-clockwise rotation, causes of 50
Coxsackievirus 375, 382, 387, 389
Crescendo angina 98
Crochetage sign 437, 438f-440*f*, 454, 454*b*
Cryptogenic stroke 498, 502
Culprit artery, identification of 156
Cushing reflex 413
Cyanotic episodes 480
Cytomegalovirus 375

D

de Winter's T and Wellens' syndrome, significance of 157*b*
Deep vein thrombosis 406
Degenerative disease, primary 259, 267
Delta wave 326
Dengue fever 386
Descending artery
left anterior 149
occlusion, left anterior 141
Desipramine 31
Developmental disorders 313
Dextrocardia 42, 435, 446, 455
mirror-image 449, 449*f*
technical 450, 451*f*, 455
Dextroposition 449
Diarrhea 394, 401
Diastole, electrocardiogram representation of 3
Digitalis 425, 433
administration 491
toxicity 426
Digoxin 108, 181, 271, 281, 286, 301, 304, 425, 429, 433, 491
administration 493
effect 25, 99, 425, 426
sign of 425*f*
toxicity 174, 425, 429*f*, 430
Diphtheria 282, 301, 386
Discordance, appropriate 135
Disopyramide 30, 223, 309, 317, 432, 433
Distal conduction system 247
Diuretic drugs 394
Dizziness 188
Dofetilide 30, 432
Dothiepin 317
Doxepin 317
Dressler's syndrome 375, 382, 387
Drinking iced water 37
Droperidol 317
Drug 29
challenge 309
toxicities 237
Dual-chamber pacing 462, 465*f*, 470, 471
Duchenne's muscular dystrophy 320, 415, 421
Dysplasia 320
triangle of 365
Dyspnea, exertional 384
Dysrhythmia 426, 429

E

Early repolarization 156
  benign 138, 139
  pattern 58, 61, 66, 156, 377, 380, 382, 389, 420
  syndrome 320
Ebstein's anomaly 94, 206, 435, 446, 447*f*, 448*f*, 453, 455
Echocardiography, two-dimensional 346*f*
Echovirus 375, 387
Ectopic beat 172, 174, 192-194, 194*t*
Ectopic ventricular beats 398
Einthoven's law 6
Einthoven's triangle 1*f*, 10
Eisenmenger syndrome 450, 452, 453*f*, 456
Electrical activity, posterior 131
Electrical conduction within heart, abnormal 11
Electrical system, parts of 3
Electricity conducting cells 2
Electrocardiogram 1, 5, 9, 35*f*, 39, 52*f*, 55, 98, 149, 195, 196*f*, 197*f*, 229, 247*f*, 272*f*, 301*f*, 315, 339*f*, 342, 376*f*, 380, 382, 389, 392, 404, 408*f*, 415
  abnormal axis on 41
  abnormalities 308
  adult 480*b*
  basic 379*f*
  causes of
    low voltage 382*b*
    motion artifacts in 421*b*
  changes 421
  classical 375*f*
  common 421
  criteria, diagnostic 114
  determination of 40*f*
  drugs on 425
  findings, possible 421
  in children, normal 481*b*
  interpret 459
  machine, standard calibration of 10*f*
  normal 1*f*
    axis on 41
    variant 55
  pacing spikes documentation on 469*b*
  paper, calculation of voltage on 10*f*
  pretest 486*f*, 487*f*
  standard 13
  strip 278*f*
  tracing 4
  typical 256*f*
    pediatric 476*f*
  waves and segments of normal 3*f*
  waves of 3
Electrocardiographic
  changes during exercise, normal 485
  criteria 87
  diagnosis 309
Electrocardiography 98
Electrode placement 6, 7
Electrolyte
  abnormalities 108, 181, 392, 480
  disturbances 181, 223, 285
  imbalance 199, 237, 286
    multiple 401
Electrophysiological phenomena 201
Elevated atrial pressure 208
Emphysema 42, 382
Endocarditis 389, 390
  diagnosis of 387
  infective 282
Endocardium 375
Endocrine abnormalities 108
Epicardial infarct artery 161
Epicardial vessel 161
Episodic pacing 462*f*
Episodic ventricular pacing, displays 461*f*
Epstein-Barr virus 375
Erythromycin 31, 223, 313, 317, 321, 432, 433
Escape beat 172, 190, 193, 194, 194*t*
Escape rhythm 271, 281
Excitation-contraction coupling 318
Exercise stress test, phase of 488
Exercise test 491
  positive 485
Exercise tolerance test 484, 485, 489, 492*f*, 493, 493*f*
  diagnostic indications of 485
  indications of 485*b*
  limitations 491
  positive 489*b*
  prognostic indications for 485
  safety 485
Extracardiac disorders 113
Extrasystoles 478
Extrinsic causes 281

F

Fabry disease 365
Faintness 195
False positive exercise tolerance test, causes of 491*b*
False-negative test 491
False-positive test 491
Familial screening 309
Fascicle bifurcates, posterior 242
Fascicular block
  left anterior 77, 252, 268
  left posterior 255, 268
Fascicular tachycardia
  left anterior 227*f*
  left posterior 226*f*
Fascicular ventricular tachycardia 225, 226*f*, 227*f*
Fasciculoventricular fiber 338
Fatal conditions, diagnosis of 466
Fatal ventricular arrhythmia, development of 315
Fatigue 188
Fever 35, 108, 384
Fibrinolytic therapy 98, 161
Fibrotic conduction system 247
Flecainide 309, 432
Flip test 11
Fluconazole 313, 317, 321
Fluoroquinolones 223, 432, 433
Fluoxetine 181
Fluphenazine 313, 317, 321
Flutter waves
  positive 205*f*
  regular 202
Focal activation 197
Food and drug administration 313
Framingham electrocardiographic score 75
Framingham formula 28
Fridericias formula 28
Friedreich's ataxia 320, 415, 416, 421
Fungal infection 389
Fusion beats, presence of 231

G

Gait ataxia 421
Gastrointestinal tract losses 394
Gatifloxacin 31
Gemifloxacin 432
Genetic disorder, rare 313
Giant P-waves 453
Glycogen storage disease 365
Goldberger's triad 363*f*
Gonococcus 375, 384, 389
Great arteries 456
  complete 456
  transposition of 435, 453
Griffith algorithm 236, 237

H

Haemophilus 375
Hemorrhage
  intraparenchymal 421
  subarachnoid 24, 138, 140, 156, 313, 414*f*, 420, 421
Haloperidol 31, 223, 313, 317, 321
Halothane 317
Hay phenomenon 286, 304
Head injury, severe 420
Heart 2, 11, 375, 449
  abnormal rotations of 51*f*
  anomalies, congenital 450
  beats 319
  clockwise rotation of 43, 49
  conductive system of 3*f*, 242*f*
  counterclockwise rotation of 43, 49
  defects, congenital 313
  depolarization wave 39
  electrical axis 41*f*
  inflammation of 375
  muscle 389
  rotation of 39, 43

Heart block 301
complete 191f, 202f, 223, 294, 297f, 298f, 300f, 303, 304, 390, 393, 414f, 430f, 453, 480, 482
congenital complete 303f
drug-induced first-degree 282
electrocardiogram criteria of first-degree 285
first degree 128f, 285, 301, 303, 388f
high grade 150
in neonate, complete 481f
infra-His complete 298f
postprocedure first-degree 285
second-degree 303, 390, 393
supra-His complete 297f
third-degree 286, 296, 301, 303
Heart disease
carcinoid 365
chronic 208
ischemic 247, 259, 267
congenital 94, 237, 244, 267, 326, 435
detectable 197
electrocardiogram features of congenital 435
hypertensive 197, 213
ischemic 29f, 267
structural 227
Heart failure 35, 37
uncontrolled 484
Heart rate 16, 196f, 197f, 473, 481, 484
calculation of 13, 32, 33f, 34f
from electrocardiogram 37
irregular 477
normal 64
standard formulas for calculating 34b
Heart strain
acute right 407
right 80
Heart transplantation 417f
electrocardiogram after 416, 421
types of 416
Hemiblock 268
causes of 268
concept 252
impulse conduction in left posterior 257f
left anterior 42, 243, 252, 255, 255f-257f, 268
left posterior 42, 243, 255, 258f, 259f, 268
typical left posterior 257f
Hemidiaphragmatic paralysis, left 449
Hemochromatosis 281, 304, 365
Hemorrhagic stroke 421
Hepatitis B virus 375
Heterotaxy syndrome 449
Heterotopic transplantation 416
Hexaxial reference system 40, 41f
His bundle 3, 295
tissue 338
His-Purkinje system 2, 3, 326, 402
Hodges formula 28
Holiday heart syndrome 199
Holter monitor electrocardiogram 497f
Holter monitoring 196, 496, 497f, 498, 498f, 499, 500f, 502
diagnostic value of 497b
electrocardiogram 221f
tracing 479f
indications for 496b, 500
strip 501f
left side of 278f
Holter strip 273f
Holter technology 496
Human cardiac sodium 307
Human herpes virus 375
Human immunodeficiency virus 375, 387
infection 386, 417
Hyperacute T wave 24f, 117
Hypercalcemia 31, 181, 317, 320, 398, 401, 402, 420
severe 401f, 403
Hyperkalemia 24, 24f, 31, 36, 37, 138, 139, 153, 217, 267, 281, 286, 304, 317, 320, 392, 393, 402, 466
degree of 393
diagnosis of 468, 471
mild 393f
levels of 393
moderate 392f, 393, 394
degree 394f
phases of 392f, 393t
severe 393
stage of 26f, 393
Hypermagnesemia 401, 403
Hypertension 78, 259, 267, 268
absence of 370
uncontrolled 484, 491
Hyperthermia 31, 317
Hyperthyroidism 35
Hypertrophic cardiomyopathy 25, 50, 197, 238, 326, 345, 346f-348f, 355, 357f, 369, 491, 493, 501f
diagnosis of 351, 355f, 370b
patterns of 369b
Hypertrophic obstructive cardiomyopathy 345, 350f, 460
severe 484
Hypertrophied right ventricular 80
Hypertrophy 82
biventricular 82, 93, 94
Hyperventilation 21
Hypocalcemia 29, 401, 403
causes of 401
degree of 401
symptoms of 401
Hypokalemia 21, 24, 29, 99, 174, 181, 199, 223, 285, 394, 396, 397, 397f, 402, 491, 493
causes of 394
degree of 397
electrocardiogram features of 402b
mild 394, 398f
degree of 399f
moderate 399f
phases of 397t, 398f
severe 397, 400f
Hypomagnesemia 29, 174, 181, 199, 223, 285, 401-403
Hypoparathyroidism 401
Hypotension 37, 401, 430
with shock 35
Hypothermia 21, 29, 37, 281, 320, 409, 410f, 415, 420, 420b
stages of 409
Hypothyroidism 37, 281, 382, 411, 420
Hypoxia 35, 196, 450

I

Ibuprofen 392
Ibutilide 30, 432
Idiopathic fibrosis 304
Idiopathic ventricular fibrillation 317
Idioventricular rhythm 161
accelerated 150, 168, 217, 227, 228f
Imipramine 31, 313, 317, 321, 430
Immune response, reduced 313
Individual waves, duration of 13
Infarcted myocardium 181
Infarction 244, 320
anteroseptal 134
current 23
diagnosis of acute 134
inferior wall 145
localization of site of 125
posterior 131, 155
Infarct-related artery, exact site of 140
Infectious diseases 282, 386b
Infiltrative diseases 281
Inflammatory disorders 382
Influenza 375
Infranodal block, presence of 286
Instantaneous vectors 39
Intact ventricular septum 340
Intermittent junctional escape rhythm 178f
Internodal pathway, anterior 2
Internodal tract
middle 2
posterior 2
Interpolated beat 182
Interstitial lung disease 417
Interventricular septum
origin 181
thickness 346f
Intestines 401
Intra-atrial
pathways 2
reentrant tachycardia 456
Intracerebral tumors 413
Intracranial pressure
electrocardiogram features of increased 412, 421
raised 29

Intraventricular conduction
defects 491
delay 349, 352*f*
disturbance, nonspecific 265
Intrinsicoid deflection 80
delayed 70
Ischemia 89, 89*t*
absence of 425
reversible 304

J

James fibers 327
Jervell and Lange-Nielsen syndrome 313, 321
Joint replacements 406
Josephson's sign 233, 236*f*
J-point 19
depression 489
elevation 153
Junctional bradycardia 395*f*
Junctional complex 177*f*
premature 172, 176, 192, 192*b*
Junctional escape
beats 191*f*
rhythm 179*f*
Junctional rhythm 176*f*
accelerated 150, 179*f*
electrocardiogram of 177*f*
Junctional tachycardia 180*f*, 433

K

Kartagener's syndrome 449
Katz-Wachtel phenomenon 83*f*, 84*f*, 94, 444, 444*f*
Katz-Wachtel sign 83, 83*f*, 93, 94, 444
Kawasaki syndrome 475
Ketoconazole 313, 317, 321
Kidney 401
disease, chronic 401, 429*f*

L

Lange-Nielsen syndrome 223
Laplace's law 78
Laxative abuse 394
Left atrial enlargement, diagnosis of 87*f*
Left axis deviation 39, 48, 70
causes of 48
pathological 45*f*
Left bundle branch 3, 4, 242, 252
Left bundle branch block 42, 55, 68, 89, 99, 103*f*, 123, 134, 138, 139, 156, 188, 243, 247, 249, 250, 251*f*, 254*f*, 260, 267, 292*f*, 320, 338, 466, 469-471
causes of 267
complete 249, 249*f*, 253*f*
diagnostic criteria
of complete 267
of incomplete 267
incomplete 252*f*
morphology 239
pattern 220*f*
presence of 77, 122
Left circumflex
artery 146*f*, 149
coronary artery 145
Left heart syndrome, hypoplastic 435
Left main stenosis, electrocardiogram evidence of 114
Left ventricular
aneurysm 140*f*, 155*f*
ejection fraction 469, 471
endocardium 2
hypertrophic cardiomyopathy 30*f*
mass 79
noncompaction 367
origin 181
strain pattern 76
systolic function 425
Left ventricular hypertrophy 6, 42, 68, 70, 72*f*, 76-78, 85, 87, 88*b*, 89, 90, 93, 94, 98, 99, 138, 139, 153, 156, 247, 320, 345, 370, 450, 491
absence of 123
cardiomyopathy 30*f*
detect 75
diagnosis of 68, 77
diastolic overload pattern 79*f*
pressure 93*t*
causes of 90
strain 72*f*, 73*f*, 88, 89*t*
pattern 76*f*
systolic overload pattern 78*f*, 452*f*
volume 68, 92
overload, causes of 90
with ischemia 76
with strain 76
Left-axis deviation 349
Lenegre-Lev syndrome 285
Leptospirosis 386
Lev's and Lenegre's disease 259, 267, 268
Lev's disease 285
Levofloxacin 432
Life-threatening arrhythmia 313, 500
untreated 484
Limb lead 7
augmented 5, 8, 8*t*, 10
inferior 437
placement of 7*t*
positions
alternate 8*f*
bipolar 5*f*
Limb, upsloping 28*f*
Lithium 223
Liu's diagnostic criteria 149*b*
Loop diuretics 394
Lower limb fractures 406, 418
Lown grading system 189, 190*t*
Lown-Ganong-Levine syndrome 326, 338, 339*f*, 342
Lung
cancer 199
disease, chronic 81, 92, 94
disorders, acute 407
resistivity of 74
Lyme disease 282, 304, 386

M

Macrolide antibiotics 432, 433
Macruz index 85
Mahaim fibers 327
preexcitation 338
Mahaim tachycardia, characteristics of 339
Mahaim-type preexcitation 326, 338, 342
McGinn-White sign 407
Medical therapy, guideline-directed 469, 471
Medications, use of 425
Mefloquine 317
Meningococcus 375
Mesocardia 449
Metabolic equivalents 485
Methamphetamines 113
Metronidazole 317
Microvascular dysfunction 115
Mitral regurgitation 92, 417
Mitral stenosis 92, 197, 213, 417
Mitral valve 325, 453
annulus calcification 285
insufficiency 491
prolapse 21, 25, 181, 238, 453, 456, 491, 493
repair 286
Mitral valvular lesions 493
Morphology, saddle-shaped 120
Morris index 85, 93
Mortality, long-term 59
Motion artefact, reduce 6
Moxifloxacin 317, 432
Mumps 375
Myalgias 384
Myocardial cell 2
membrane 431
Myocardial degeneration 44
Myocardial diseases, infiltrative 304
Myocardial fibrosis 416
Myocardial infarction 24, 112, 114, 149, 151, 157, 181, 327, 376, 382
acute 61, 61*t*, 113, 114, 117, 134, 141, 156, 181, 331, 484
acute anterior 119*f*, 124*f*, 126, 134*f*, 138*f*, 301*f*, 368
wall 120*f*
acute anteroseptal 126*f*
acute inferior 20*f*, 107*f*, 125*f*, 127, 127f-130*f*, 145, 147*f*, 148*f*, 284*f*, 286, 288*f*
anterior 122*f*, 126*f*, 127*f*, 154*f*, 259*f*, 314*f*

anterolateral 149
anteroseptal 149
diagnosis of 113*b*
acute 247
extensive anterior 149
high lateral 149
inferior 42, 132*f*, 149, 265*f*, 289*f*, 301, 331, 487
inferolateral 149
lateral wall 42
management of acute 117
posterior 8, 9*f*, 50, 132*f*, 149, 155*b*
Myocardial infiltration, diffuse 365
Myocardial ischemia 22, 24, 29, 98, 99, 244, 484
acute 313, 320
detecting 484
diagnosis of 109*f*
Myocardial necrosis, extensive 150
Myocardial perfusion 166
Myocardial reperfusion 161
Myocardial tissues 271
Myocarditis 24, 37, 113, 153, 181, 238, 244, 267, 286, 301, 304, 383, 384, 385, 385*f*, 389, 390
acute 320, 484
diagnosis of 384
electrocardiogram of 386*f*
Myocardium 375, 383, 389, 473
Myxedema 375, 382

N

Nelfinavir 317
Neoplastic pericarditis 375
Nephropathy, salt-losing 394
Nephrotic syndrome 382
Neuromuscular disorders 421
electrocardiogram changes in 415
Nodal blocking drugs 301
Nodal rhythm 176*f*
Node dysfunction 453
Nodo-Hisian junction 286
Nodoventricular fiber 338
Noncardiac causes 181
Noncoronary causes 113, 115
Non-ST elevation myocardial infarction 99, 113
Nortriptyline 430
Numerous human 117

O

Obesity 382
Obstructive coronary atherosclerosis, diagnosis of 488
Obstructive pulmonary disease, chronic 42, 197, 404, 405, 418
Occlusion, left anterior descending 142
Ofloxacin 432
Olanzapine 31
Orthodromic supraventricular tachycardia 342
Orthodromic tachycardia 340
Orthotopic heart transplantation 416, 417*f*
Osborn wave 409*f*, 410*f*, 420*b*
causes of 420
classic 420
Osmotic diuretics 394
Ostium primum type 454
Ostium secundum 435

P

P pulmonale 404, 409
P wave 14, 35
abnormal 93, 415
characteristics of normal 16
inverted 55, 65
normal 84
Pacemaker 460, 467*f*
activity 2
biventricular 470
cells 2, 193
codes 462
complications 466
electrocardiogram
identification of 470*b*
interpretation of 459, 466
functions of 459
magnet effects on 468
malfunctions 459, 466
on electrocardiogram, effects of 466
permanent 305
presence of 466, 468, 471
rhythm 42
interpretation of 469
spikes 459
temporary 302*f*
terminology 465
to sense and to pace, failure of 468*f*
types 462
of common 470
Pacing spikes 470
Palpitations, cause of 496
Parasympathomimetic action 425
Parasystole 183
Parkinson's disease 415, 416*f*, 417*f*, 421
Paroxysmal atrial
fibrillation, silent 502
flutter 271
Paroxysmal hypoglycemia 313
Paroxysmal supraventricular tachycardia 206, 420
Paroxysmal tachycardia 338
Parvovirus B_{19} 375
Patent ductus arteriosus 82, 435, 450, 455
P-congenitale 84
Pectus excavatum 491, 493
Pediatric electrocardiogram 473, 474*f*, 478*f*, 480, 480*b*, 482
indications for 480*b*
interpretation 473
Pediatric population 208
Penicillins 385
Pentamidine 31
Percutaneous coronary intervention 72, 117
primary 117, 131, 161, 164, 227, 228*f*, 300*f*, 302*f*, 394
Pericardial constriction 493
Pericardial effusion 382, 389, 390
cause of 382
electrocardiogram changes in 382
Pericardial fluid, aspiration of 384*f*
Pericardial friction rub 387
Pericardial syndromes 387
Pericarditis 37, 138, 139, 156, 197, 320, 375, 378, 383, 484
acute 139, 153, 375, 377, 378, 378*f*, 379*f*, 380, 380*t*, 382, 382*t*, 389, 389*t*, 390
diagnosis of acute 375
electrocardiogram
criteria of acute 388
diagnosis of 375
of acute 376
signs of acute 375*f*
old 24
setting of 17
subacute 24
Pericardium 375, 387
Peri-infarction
arrhythmias, classification of 150
block 265, 265*f*
Permanent pacing, indications for 459
Persistent juvenile
pattern 64, 64*f*
T-wave pattern 481
Pertussis 386
Perugia score 75
Pharmacologic agents, use of 271
Phenothiazines 223
Pheochromocytoma 35
Pimozide 30, 317
P-mitrale 84
Pneumococcus 375
Pneumomediastinum 449
Pneumonectomy, right 50
Pneumonia 199
Pneumopericardium 382
Pneumothorax 382, 407
Polymorphic ventricular tachycardia, catecholaminergic 307, 317, 319*f*, 322
Populations, special 496
Postcardiac arrest 29
Postcardiac surgery 197, 238
Postcardiac surgical state 108
Postirradiation therapy 365
Postmyocardial infarct angina 98
Postmyocardial infarction

pericarditis 382
syndrome 375, 387
Postpericardiotomy pericarditis 387
Post-tachycardia syndrome 414
P-pulmonale 84
PQRST complex 3
PR interval 16, 473
causes of prolonged 17
normal 36
short 65, 338
variation 55
PR segment 17, 36
Precordial electrode
normal 7
placement of 7
Precordial leads 8, 39
right 23, 82, 422
Preexcitation 98
alternans 335
Preexcitation syndromes 325, 338, 339, 342*t*
patterns of 340
types of 326
Pregnancy 35
Premature junctional complex, electrocardiogram characteristics of 192
Premature ventricular complex 113, 168, 172, 176, 186, 188, 190*t*, 192, 192*b*, 193, 193*t*, 204*f*, 426
electrocardiogram characteristics of 192
interpolated 188*f*, 193
typical 180*f*, 188*f*
Premature ventricular contractions 181
bigeminy 181
couplet 181
multifocal 181
multiformed 181
quadrigeminy 181
salvos 182
trigeminy 181
triplet 181
unifocal 181
Prinzmetal's angina 111, 111*f*, 114, 138, 139, 156
during chest pain 111*f*
sign of 114
Probucol 317
Procainamide 223, 309, 317, 321, 432
Prominent T-waves 119
Pronounced sinus arrhythmia 477
Propafenone 309, 432
Provocable ischemia, positive for 487*f*
Pseudo Q waves 331, 342
Pseudoephedrine 181
Pseudo-infarction pattern 351*f*
Pseudo-P pulmonale 85
Psychotropic agents 320
Pulmonary artery 453
Pulmonary atresia 340
Pulmonary disease, chronic 35
Pulmonary embolism 35, 42, 92, 113, 153, 244, 406, 407, 407*f*, 408, 418
acute 406
Pulmonary embolus 267
Pulmonary hypertension 82, 92, 417, 422, 493
development of 406
primary 81, 92, 94, 417, 418*f*, 419*f*, 422
Pulmonary stenosis 92, 94, 450, 452*f*, 455
Pulmonary thromboemboli, acute 320
Pulmonary valve stenosis 435
Purkinje fibers 2-4, 393
Purkinje system 415
P-wave 3, 473
morphologies, distinct 64

Q

Q wave 14, 36
absence of 122
abnormal 368
deep pathological 152*f*
pathological 133*f*, 151*f*, 346
presence of 233
septal 65
QRS amplitude, increased 68
QRS axis, interpretation of 45
QRS complex 3, 14, 18, 18*f*, 19, 21, 23, 33, 40, 43*f*, 44*f*, 51*f*, 79, 83, 134, 153*f*, 177*f*, 178, 182, 190*f*, 192, 233*f*, 276*f*, 286, 294, 304, 305, 315, 367*f*, 405, 431, 449*f*, 460, 468, 469, 475
appearance of 239
duration 311
equiphasic 40
fragmentation of 153*b*, 154*f*
morphology 249*f*
normal 36, 173
positive 136*f*
start of 313*f*
width of 239
QRS concordance 239
QRS configuration, axis determination from 41
QRS duration 55, 231, 252*f*, 267
QRS morphology 250*f*, 339*f*
axis determination from 45
multiple 223*f*
QRS prolongation 411
QRS slurring 380
QRS vector 39, 79
QRS voltage
factors influencing 74
increased 76
low 383
QRS/T angle, widened 70
QT interval 27, 36, 313*f*, 314, 315, 475
calculating 32*f*
corrected 28, 431
measurement 31*f*
normal 31*f*, 36
short 317
QT prolongation
absence of 315
drugs causing 30
QT syndrome
acquired long 313
arrhythmias in long 315
congenital long 29
diagnosis of long 315*b*
long 307, 312, 313, 315, 320, 321, 321*t*
short 307, 317, 318*f*, 321, 322
varieties of inherited long 313
QTc criteria 321*t*
QTc interval 314
causes of long 321, 321*b*
QTc prolongation 317*t*
drugs with 315
Quinidine 30, 223, 317, 321, 432, 433
Q-wave 131, 475
abnormality 58
appearance of pathological 117, 121
develop 122
duration 6
infarction 123
persistent 153
significant 475

R

Rabbit ear sign 233, 234*f*, 239
Refractory period, effective 209*f*
Regional contractile dysfunction 152
Renal failure 401
end-stage 113
Renal losses 394
Renal tubular acidosis 394
Reperfusion arrhythmias 168, 168*b*
Reperfusion therapy 166
failure of 161
use of 117
Repolarization 2
changes 402
patterns, types of 308
Respiratory depression 401
Respiratory distress syndrome, adult 113
Restlessness 415
Restrictive cardiomyopathy 345, 365, 365*f*, 366*f*, 370
Reverse tick sign 425, 426f-428*f*
Rheumatic carditis 35, 388*f*, 390
electrocardiogram changes in 387
Rheumatic fever 282, 286, 301, 304, 387, 390
Rheumatic heart disease 197, 267
Rheumatic valvular heart disease 238
Rheumatoid arthritis 285, 375
Rhythm abnormalities 453
Rhythm sinus 432*f*
Rhythm, irregular 197*f*
Right atrial enlargement, signs of 455

Right axis deviation 39, 48, 93, 417, 420, 481
causes of 42, 48
Right bundle branch 3, 4
Right bundle branch block 18, 42, 90, 97, 99, 102*f*, 138, 138*f*, 140, 188, 201, 219*f*, 243, 243*f*, 244, 245, 260, 267, 310, 311, 320, 360*f*, 406, 435, 454, 466, 491
causes of 267
complete 142, 203*f*, 244, 245, 245*f*, 246*f*
diagnostic criteria
of complete 267
of incomplete 267
incomplete 245, 246*f*, 248*f*, 312*f*, 436*f*, 442*f*
morphology 239
partial 474*f*
new 407
partial 437*f*, 439*f*
pattern 226*f*, 352*f*, 405*f*
partial 55
presence of 122
Right coronary artery, proximal 166*f*
Right ventricular
branch 145
cardiomyopathy, particularly arrhythmogenic 320
damage 129
dilatation, acute 407
diseases, primary 320
endocardium 2
ischemia 320
load 42
myocardial infarction 156
origin 181
outflow tract 226, 228*f*, 466
strain 407, 444
Right ventricular hypertrophy 18, 25, 42, 50, 66*f*, 79, 80*f*, 81*f*, 92, 94, 99, 267, 404, 417, 419*f*, 450, 452, 452*f*, 453*f*, 473
causes of 92
diagnosis of 92
strain 81*f*
systolic overload pattern 82*f*
Right ventricular infarction 129, 149
acute inferior and 147*f*
Risperidone 31, 313, 317, 321
Romano-Ward
patients 313
syndrome 223, 313, 321
Romhilt-Estes
criteria 87, 88*b*
point score system 87
score 75
Roxithromycin 317
Rubella 375, 386
virus 384
R-wave 14, 18
progression, poor 151

S

S wave 14
Sarcoidosis 199, 281, 304, 365, 417
Sawtooth 202
Schamroth's sign 406*f*
Schwartz criteria 315*b*
Scleroderma 285, 417
Secundum atrial septal defect 436*f*
Sepsis 35, 113
Septal fascicle 268
Septal fascicular block, left 255
Septal hemiblock, left 255, 268
Septal right atrium, low 271
Sertraline 31
Serum
K 402
potassium 393, 402
concentration 392
high 393
mild elevations of 392
Sex, influence of 480
Sgarbossa score 136
Sgarbossa's criteria 471
Sgarbossa's scoring system 136, 136*f*, 156*b*
Shock 37
Short PR interval, causes of 17
Sick sinus syndrome 271, 272*f*, 273*f*, 276f-278*f*, 280, 281, 497
Simultaneous hypokalemia 402
Sine-wave appearance 402
Single photon emission computed tomography 493
Single-chamber pacing 462
Sinoatrial block 281
first-degree 279, 281
second-degree 279, 281
third-degree 280
type II 280
Sinoatrial exit block 279, 281
third-degree 281
type II 280*f*
Sinoatrial node 2-4, 64, 173, 189*f*, 190, 271, 326, 460, 466
electrical impulses from 282
Sinus 435
arrest 271, 274*f*, 281
arrhythmia 55, 56*f*, 64, 478
degree of 478*f*
diagnosis of 482
marked 481
beat 177*f*
N-normal 185*f*
bradycardia 34, 34*f*, 55, 60*f*, 150, 271, 272*f*, 276*f*, 281, 410*f*, 411*f*, 413*f*, 420, 426, 428*f*, 431*f*, 499*f*
cause 37
severe 432*f*
node 196
dysfunction 271, 280, 453
reentrant tachycardia 195, 196, 213
pause 271
rhythm 184*f*, 185*f*, 208*f*, 233, 469, 471
basic 182
normal 190, 191*f*, 214
variations from 476
tachycardia 35, 37, 55, 105*f*, 195, 196*f*, 213, 258*f*, 370, 384*f*, 386, 386*f*, 387, 387*f*, 388*f*, 389, 406, 407, 408*f*, 415, 420, 421, 476*f*
Situs ambiguus 449
Situs inversus 446
Situs solitus 446
Sjögren syndrome 375
Sleep apnea syndrome, obstructive 417
Small vessel disease 345
Sodium channel blockers 311
Sokolow-Lyon
criteria 74, 87
voltage 74
Sotalol 30, 223, 317, 321, 432, 433
Sparfloxacin 31
Spinal cord injury 406, 418
Spironolactone 392
Spodick's sign 376, 377, 379*f*, 389
ST depression
causes of 99
primary 113
secondary 113
primary 100
and secondary 100
reciprocal 103, 114
secondary 102
Stable angina 98
electrocardiogram criteria of 113
Standard bruce protoco 485*t*
Standard calibration 9
Standard exercise testing, contraindications for 484*b*
ST-elevation
cause of saddle-shaped 121
concomitant inferior and anterior 157
initial 120
normal variant 138, 139
with concavity upward, causes of 121
with convexity upward, cause of 121
ST-elevation myocardial infarction 8, 18, 98, 117, 134, 138, 149, 153, 155, 161, 168, 267, 371, 380, 389, 389*t*
acute 377, 378, 380, 380*t*
anterior 142
diagnosis of 117, 123, 155*b*, 156*b*, 466, 471
high lateral 131
posterior 131*b*
stages of 24
evolution of 118*f*
treatment of 161
Storage disorders 365
Strain 68
Strenuous exercise 113
Stress testing 485
Stroke 113

ST-segment 3, 14, 19, 21, 476
abnormal 68
change, calculation of 170
deviation resolution, degree of 169
normal 36
normalization of 117, 122
ST-segment depression 98-100, 131*b*, 346, 357*f*, 485
causes of 21
common causes of 20
degree of 101*f*
diffuse 108, 109*f*
downsloping 106*f*
patterns of 99
reciprocal 103
resolution of 169
secondary 102*f*
significance of 488
types of 103
widespread 100*f*
ST-segment elevation 98, 111, 117, 119, 131, 135, 140, 164, 349, 371, 486
causes of 20, 36, 156, 138
common causes of 19
differential diagnosis of 138, 156
morphology of 120
resolution 166
ST-segment elevation myocardial infarction
acute anterior 354*f*
anterior 368*f*
true posterior 104
ST-segment resolution 164, 164*b*, 170, 227
single-lead 164
sum 164, 170
ST-T abnormalities 21, 76
secondary 70
Sudden cardiac death 223, 307, 345, 355, 453, 496
Sudden death 338
Sulfonamides 385
Supraventricular tachycardia 99, 195, 237, 318, 333*f*, 387, 411, 412*f*
with aberrancy 229, 233, 235*fc*, 239
with aberrant conduction 229, 239
with accessory pathway 229
Sympathetic nervous system 411, 413
Sympathomimetics 174
Syncopal spells 318
Syncope
and seizures 480
management of 259
Systemic disorders 417
Systemic hypertension 450
Systemic infection, acute 484
Systemic lupus erythematosus 285, 375, 480
Systemic sclerosis 375
Systemic vasculitides 375
Systole and diastole, electrocardiogram of 3*f*
Systolic blood pressure 484
Systolic pressure, levels of 78

T

T wave 14, 22, 26
abnormalities, secondary 79
changes, pacing-induced 470
inversion
causes of 24
pathological 37
ischemic 24, 25*f*
normal 36
patterns of different 23
pseudonormalization of 104, 491
Tachyarrhythmias 113, 433
supraventricular 150
Tachycardia 37, 195, 217, 223, 226, 230, 234, 272, 325, 338, 340, 430
bradycardia syndrome 272, 277*f*, 278*f*, 281
broad complex 217, 218f-220*f*, 227, 229, 231*f*, 235*f*, 237, 237*f*, 238*b*, 239, 239*b*
causes of
broad complex 217, 237
supraventricular 217
ventricular 217, 238
complex regular 334*f*
diagnosis, complex 237
morphology 234
narrow complex 195, 208, 218*f*
notching, broad complex 233*f*
several 272
types of ventricular 238*b*
wide complex 212*f*
Takotsubo cardiomyopathy 113, 345, 368, 368*f*, 371
features of 371
mimics 368
Tamponade 389
Tangent method 315
Terfenadine 223, 313, 317, 321
Tetanus 386
Tetralogy of Fallot 92, 94, 435, 444, 445*f*, 455
Thiamine deficiency 320
Thiazides 394
Thioridazine 30, 223, 317
Threshold method 315
Thrombolysis 162*f*
Thrombolytic therapy 161
Thrombophilic states 115
Thrombus, formation of 98
Thyrotoxic patients 411
Thyrotoxicosis 78, 92, 199, 213, 409, 411*f*, 412*f*, 420
Timothy syndrome 313, 321
Tobacco 174
Tombstone ST elevation 134
Torsades de pointes 238, 312, 315, 316*f*, 411, 420, 431
causes of 223
Trauma 375
Treadmill stress test 484
Tricuspid atresia 435, 453, 456
Tricuspid regurgitation 79
Tricuspid stenosis 94
Tricyclic antidepressants 181, 217, 223, 425, 430, 431*f*, 433
Trifascicular block 243, 259, 260, 263*f*, 264*f*, 269, 393
Trimethoprim 223
Truncus arteriosus 435
Tuberculosis 382
T-wave 131, 476
abnormalities 21
changes 104
inversion 66, 98, 100, 114, 117, 122, 346
anterior 407
appearance of early 166
nonspecific 66
morphology 315
Typhoid 386
myocarditis 386

U

U wave 32
causes of prominent 32
during exercise, inversion of 491
normal 37
Unifocal premature ventricular complexes 182*f*
Unifocal ventricular ectopic beats 183
Uremia 375

V

Vagally-mediated atrioventricular block 293
Valvular heart disease 181, 269, 417, 422
multiple 197, 417
Varicella 375
Vasculitis 417
Vector foot, augmented 14, 196
Vector left, augmented 5
Vector right, augmented 5
Venlafaxine 31
Venous thromboembolism, presentation of 406
Ventricle
age-related changes in 473
right 2
Ventricular activation time 70
increase 70
Ventricular aneurysm 138, 139, 156
Ventricular arrhythmia 113, 170, 318, 411
documented 312
malignant 331
Ventricular bigeminy 184*f*
Ventricular complex
consecutive premature 185*f*

diagnosis of premature 178
morphology of premature 181*b*
multifocal premature 183*f*
multiformed premature 183*f*
patterns of premature 193*b*
Ventricular contraction, causes of premature 181
Ventricular demand pacemaker 460, 462*f*
Ventricular depolarization 282
Ventricular diastole 4
Ventricular ectopic 433
beats 193
focus discharges 189*f*
rhythms 42, 150
Ventricular escape rhythm 191*f*
Ventricular extrasystole 176, 406, 420
Ventricular fibrillation 150, 224, 240, 307, 322, 328
electrocardiogram 225*f*
criteria of 225
start of 182
Ventricular flutter 223
electrocardiogram criteria of 223
Ventricular hypertrophy, diagnosis of 479
Ventricular paced
beats 113
rhythm 99
Ventricular pacing 460, 461*f*, 469, 470
Ventricular parasystole 189*f*, 193
Ventricular perforation 466
Ventricular preexcitation 209
Ventricular premature beat 176, 415
Ventricular rate and rhythm, analysis of 195
Ventricular reperfusion arrhythmia 169
Ventricular repolarization 413
period of 117
Ventricular rhythms 238
Ventricular septal defect 82, 435, 444, 450, 455
Ventricular systole 4
Ventricular tachyarrhythmia 312, 317, 420, 431
Ventricular tachycardia 150, 161, 217, 218*f*, 228*f*, 229, 232*f*, 233, 233*f*, 235*fc*, 237, 237*f*, 238, 238*b*, 239, 239*b*, 294, 309, 322, 387, 397, 406, 411, 430, 449, 496
bidirectional 227, 228*f*
electrocardiogram criteria of 217
mechanism of 238
mimicking 386*f*
monomorphic 220, 233*f*, 238
morphological criteria for 238
nonsustained 238, 497*f*
patterns of 238
pauses of 233*f*
polymorphic 223*f*, 420
sustained 238
with atrioventricular dissociation 230*f*
Ventricular trigeminy 184*f*
Verapamil 431, 433
Vereckei's algorithm 236*f*
Viral pericarditis 375
Vitamin D deficiency 401
Voltage and timing intervals, standardization of 9, 11
Voltage criteria 68, 345, 479
Vomiting 394

W

Wandering pacemaker 64, 65*f*, 66
diagnosis of 66
heart rate 66
Wavelet formation, multiple 197
Wellens' syndrome 104, 108*f*, 114, 145*f*, 157
Wenckebach block 279
Wenckebach phenomenon 285, 286, 290*f*, 303, 304, 479*f*, 482
Wenckebach sequence 478
Wolff-Parkinson-White syndrome 44, 50, 217, 229, 325, 326, 327, 328, 328*f*, 331, 335, 338, 339, 342, 448*f*, 455, 491, 493
presence of 331, 342
type B 330*f*
World Health Organization 345
Wrist 13

Z

Ziprasidone 30, 317